OKU 5

Orthopaedic Knowledge Update

Trauma

OKU 5

Orthopaedic Knowledge Update

Trauma

EDITORS
William M. Ricci, MD
Professor and Vice Chair
Chief, Orthopaedic Trauma Service
Department of Orthopaedic Surgery
Washington University School of Medicine
St. Louis, Missouri

Robert F. Ostrum, MD
Professor of Orthopaedics
Department of Orthopaedics
University of North Carolina at Chapel Hill School of Medicine
Chapel Hill, North Carolina

Developed by the Orthopaedic Trauma Association

ORTHOPAEDIC —TRAUMA— ASSOCIATION

AAOS
AMERICAN ACADEMY OF ORTHOPAEDIC SURGEONS

Staff

Ellen C. Moore, *Chief Education Officer*

Hans Koelsch, PhD, *Director, Department of Publications*

Lisa Claxton Moore, *Senior Manager, Book Program*

Steven Kellert, *Senior Editor*

Courtney Dunker, *Editorial Production Manager*

Abram Fassler, *Publishing Systems Manager*

Suzanne O'Reilly, *Graphic Designer*

Susan Morritz Baim, *Production Coordinator*

Karen Danca, *Permissions Coordinator*

Rachel Winokur, *Editorial Coordinator*

Charlie Baldwin, *Digital and Print Production Specialist*

Hollie Muir, *Digital and Print Production Specialist*

Emily Nickel, *Page Production Assistant*

Sylvia Orellana, *Publications Assistant*

Published 2016 by the
American Academy of Orthopaedic Surgeons
9400 West Higgins Road
Rosemont, IL 60018

Library of Congress Control Number: 2016936304
ISBN 978-1-62552-433-1
Printed in the USA

Acknowledgments

Contributors

Timothy S. Achor, MD
Assistant Professor
Department of Orthopaedic Surgery
University of Texas at Houston Health Science Center
Houston, Texas

John D. Adams, MD
Orthopaedic Trauma Fellow
Department of Orthopaedic Surgery
University of Missouri
Columbia, Missouri

Vinay Kumar Aggarwal, MD
Physician
Department of Orthopaedic Surgery
NYU Langone Medical Center, Hospital for Joint Diseases
New York, New York

Omar Fawaz Alnori, MD
Orthopedic Spine Fellow
Department of Orthopedics
Boston Medical Center
Boston, Massachusetts

Michael T. Archdeacon, MD, MSE
Professor and Chairman
Department of Orthopaedic Surgery
University of Cincinnati, College of Medicine
Cincinnati, Ohio

Frank R. Avilucea, MD
Orthopaedic Trauma Fellow
Division of Trauma
Vanderbilt University
Nashville, Tennessee

Mark E. Baratz, MD
Clinical Professor and Vice Chairman
Orthopaedic Specialists
University of Pittsburgh Medical Center
Pittsburgh, Pennsylvania

Michael Bosse, MD
Director, Orthopaedic Trauma
Department of Orthopaedic Surgery
Carolinas Medical Center
Charlotte, North Carolina

Jeffrey Brewer, MD
Fellow
Department of Orthopaedic Trauma
University of Texas Hermann Memorial Medical Center
Houston, Texas

Mark R. Brinker, MD
Clinical Professor
Fondren Orthopedic Group L.L.P.
Texas Orthopedic Hospital
Houston, Texas

Jennifer L. Bruggers, MD
Orthopaedic Trauma Surgeon
Resurgens Orthopaedics
Atlanta, Georgia

Brian W. Buck, DO
Assistant Professor of Orthopaedic Surgery
Department of Orthopaedic Surgery
University of Missouri
Columbia, Missouri

Cory A. Collinge, MD
Professor of Orthopedic Surgery
Department of Orthopedic Surgery
Vanderbilt University
Nashville, Tennessee

Alexander B. Dagum, MD, FRCS(C), FACS
Professor
Stony Brook Surgical Associates
Stony Brook University
Stony Brook, New York

Christopher DeFalco, MD
Resident Physician
Department of Orthopaedic Surgery
Indiana University School of Medicine
Indianapolis, Indiana

Christopher Doro, MD
Assistant Professor
Department of Orthopedics
University of Wisconsin
Madison, Wisconsin

Jonathan G. Eastman, MD
Assistant Professor
Department of Orthopaedic Surgery
University of California, Davis Medical Center
Sacramento, California

Reza Firoozabadi, MD, MA
Assistant Professor
Department of Orthopaedic Surgery
Harborview Medical Center/University of Washington
Seattle, Washington

Anthony V. Florschutz, MD, PhD
Orthopaedic Trauma Fellow
Department of Orthopaedic Surgery
Orlando Regional Medical Center
Orlando, Florida

Matthew Furey, MD, MSc, FRCS(C)
Fellow
St. Michael's Hospital
University of Toronto
Toronto, Ontario, Canada

Joshua L. Gary, MD
Assistant Professor
Department of Orthopaedic Surgery
University of Texas Health Science Center at Houston
Houston, Texas

Greg E. Gaski, MD
Clinical Assistant Professor
Department of Orthopaedic Surgery
Indiana University Health-Methodist Hospital
Indiana University School of Medicine
Indianapolis, Indiana

Mark Gelfand, MD
Assistant Professor
Stony Brook Surgical Associates
Stony Brook University
Stony Brook, New York

Mitchel B. Harris, MD, FACS
Chief, Orthopedic Trauma
Department of Orthopedic Surgery
Brigham and Women's Hospital
Boston, Massachusetts

Langdon A. Hartsock, MD, FACS
Professor and Director of Orthopedic Trauma
Department of Orthopedics
Medical University of South Carolina
Charleston, South Carolina

Michael R. Hausman, MD
Lippmann Professor, Orthopedic Surgery
Chief, Hand and Elbow Surgery
Department of Orthopedic Surgery
Mount Sinai Medical Center
New York, New York

Roman A. Hayda, MD
Associate Professor, Orthopedic Surgery
Brown University
Co-director, Orthopaedic Trauma
Department of Orthopaedic Surgery
Rhode Island Hospital
Providence, Rhode Island

Daniel J. Hedequist, MD
Associate Professor of Orthopedic Surgery
Department of Orthopedic Surgery
Boston Children's Hospital
Harvard Medical School
Boston, Massachusetts

Jake P. Heiney, MD, MS
Department of Orthopaedics
University of Toledo Medical Center
Toledo, Ohio

Amir Herman, MD, PhD
Fellow, Orthopaedic Trauma
Department of Surgery
University of Alabama at Birmingham
Birmingham, Alabama

Thomas Jones, MD
Orthopedic Traumatologist
Premier Orthopedic Specialists
Palmetto Health—Richland
Columbia, South Carolina

Mani Kahn, MD
Trauma Fellow
Department of Orthopaedic Trauma
Duke University
Durham, North Carolina

Madhav A. Karunakar, MD
Orthopaedic Traumatologist
Department of Orthopaedic Surgery
Carolinas Medical Center
Charlotte, North Carolina

Conor Kleweno, MD
Assistant Professor
Department of Orthopaedic Surgery
Harborview Medical Center/University of Washington
Seattle, Washington

Sanjit R. Konda, MD
Assistant Professor
Department of Orthopaedic Surgery
NYU Langone Medical Center – Hospital for Joint Diseases
New York, New York

Kenneth J. Koval, MD
Professor
Department of Orthopaedic Surgery
Orlando Health
Orlando, Florida

William D. Lack, MD
Assistant Professor
Department of Orthopaedic Surgery
Loyola University Medical Center
Maywood, Illinois

Joshua R. Langford, MD
Program Director
Orlando Health Orthopedic Residency Program
Orlando Health
Orlando, Florida

Kevin H. Latz, MD
Chief, Section of Sports Medicine
Division of Orthopaedics
Children's Mercy Hospital
Kansas City, Missouri

Mark A. Lee, MD
Professor of Orthopaedic Surgery
Department of Orthopaedic Surgery
University of California, Davis Medical Center
Sacramento, California

Philipp Leucht, MD
Assistant Professor
Department of Orthopaedic Surgery
NYU Langone Hospital for Joint Diseases
New York, New York

Frank A. Liporace, MD
Associate Professor, Director, Orthopaedic Trauma Research
Division of Orthopaedic Trauma, Department of Orthopaedic Surgery
NYU Langone Hospital for Joint Diseases
New York, New York

Jason A. Lowe, MD
Chief, Orthopaedic Trauma
Department of Surgery
University of Alabama at Birmingham
Birmingham, Alabama

Zachary O. Mallon, MD
Orthopaedic Trauma Surgeon
Department of Orthopaedic Surgery
Kaiser Permanente Vacaville Medical Center
Vacaville, California

Theodore T. Manson, MD
Associate Professor
Department of Orthopaedic Surgery
University of Maryland
Baltimore, Maryland

Philip McClure, MD
Trauma Fellow
Rhode Island Hospital, Brown University
Providence, Rhode Island

Michael D. McKee, MD, FRCS(C)
Professor
St. Michael's Hospital
University of Toronto
Toronto, Ontario, Canada

Todd O. McKinley, MD
Professor
Department of Orthopaedic Surgery
Indiana University Health - Methodist Hospital
Indiana University School of Medicine
Indianapolis, Indiana

Toni M. McLaurin, MD
Associate Director of Orthopaedics
Chief of Orthopaedic Service
Bellevue Hospital Center
Department of Orthopaedics
NYU Langone Hospital for Joint Diseases
New York, New York

Anna N. Miller, MD, FACS
Assistant Professor
Department of Orthopaedic Surgery
Wake Forest University School of Medicine
Winston-Salem, North Carolina

Bryan W. Ming, MD
Associate Professor
Department of Orthopaedic Surgery
John Peter South Hospital
Fort Worth, Texas

Hassan R. Mir, MD, MBA, FACS
Associate Professor
Department of Orthopaedic Surgery
University of South Florida
Tampa, Florida

Saam Morshed, MD, PhD, MPH
Assistant Professor
Department of Orthopaedic Surgery
University of California
San Francisco, California

Ahmed Yousry Moussa, MD
Lecturer of Neurosurgery
Department of Neurosurgery
Ain Shams University
Cairo, Egypt

Brian Mullis, MD
Chief, Orthopaedic Trauma Service
Department of Orthopaedic Surgery
Eskenazi Health
Indiana University School of Medicine
Indianapolis, Indiana

John W. Munz, MD
Assistant Professor
Department of Orthopedic Surgery
University of Texas Health Science Center at Houston
Houston, Texas

Yvonne M. Murtha, MD
Clinical Assistant Professor
Department of Orthopaedic Surgery
University of Missouri
Springfield, Missouri

Rafael Neiman, MD
Co-Director, Acute Care Orthopedic Service
Trauma Services
Sutter Roseville Medical Center
Roseville, California

Daniel P. O'Connor, PhD
Associate Professor
Department of Health and Human Performance
University of Houston
Houston, Texas

Patrick M. Osborn, MD, Lt Col, USAF, MC
Chief, Orthopaedic Trauma Service
Department of Orthopedics and Rehabilitation
San Antonio Military Medical Center
Fort Sam Houston
San Antonio, Texas

Raymond A. Pensy, MD
Assistant Professor
Department of Orthopaedic Surgery
University of Maryland School of Medicine
Baltimore, Maryland

Benjamin K. Potter, MD, FACS
Chief Orthopaedic Surgeon, Amputee Patient Care Program
Department of Orthopaedics
Walter Reed National Military Medical Center
Bethesda, Maryland

Anthony I. Riccio, MD
Staff Orthopaedist
Department of Orthopedics
Texas Scottish Rite Hospital for Children
Dallas, Texas

Jeffrey A. Rihn, MD
Associate Professor
The Rothman Institute
Thomas Jefferson University
Philadelphia, Pennsylvania

Melvin P. Rosenwasser, MD
Robert E. Carroll Professor of Hand Surgery
Department of Orthopedic Surgery
Columbia University Medical Center
New York, New York

Milton L. (Chip) Routt, Jr, MD
Professor and Dr. Andrew R. Burgess Endowed Chair
Department of Orthopedics
University of Texas McGovern Medical School at Houston
Houston, Texas

Emil H. Schemitsch, MD, FRCS(C)
Professor of Surgery
Department of Surgery
St. Michael's Hospital
Toronto, Ontario, Canada

Patrick C. Schottel, MD
Assistant Professor
Department of Orthopaedics and Rehabilitation
University of Vermont Medical Center
South Burlington, Vermont

Gregory D. Schroeder, MD
Spine Fellow
The Rothman Institute
Thomas Jefferson University
Philadelphia, Pennsylvania

William H. Seitz Jr, MD
Department of Orthopaedic Surgery
Hand and Upper Extremity
Cleveland Clinic
Cleveland, Ohio

Yaron Sela, MD
Clinical Instructor, Fellow at University of Pittsburgh Medical Center
Department of Orthopaedic Specialists
University of Pittsburgh Medical Center
Pittsburgh, Pennsylvania

David Shearer, MD, MPH
Assistant Professor
Department of Orthopaedic Surgery
University of California, San Francisco
San Francisco, California

Jodi Siegel, MD
Assistant Professor University of Massachusetts Medical School
Department of Orthopaedics
UMass Memorial Medical Center
Worcester, Massachusetts

Xavier Simcock, MD
Surgeon
Department of Orthopedics
Cleveland Clinic Foundation
Cleveland, Ohio

Charisse Y. Sparks, MD
Medical Director
TraumaOne, PLLC
Longview, Texas

James P. Stannard, MD
Professor and Chairman
Department of Orthopaedic Surgery
University of Missouri
Columbia, Missouri

Shaun Fay Steeby, MD
Orthopaedic Trauma Fellow
Department of Orthopaedics
University of Missouri – Columbia
Columbia, Missouri

Eli Swanson, MD
Assistant Clinical Professor, University of Arizona College of Medicine
Department of Orthopaedic Trauma Surgery
Maricopa Integrated Health System
Phoenix, Arizona

Peter Tang, MD, MPH
Associate Professor – Drexel University College of Medicine
Director – Allegheny General Hospital Hand, Upper Extremity, and Microvascular Fellowship
Department of Orthopaedic Surgery
Allegheny General Hospital
Pittsburgh, Pennsylvania

Chadi Tannoury, MD
Assistant Professor
Department of Orthopaedic Surgery
Boston University Medical Center
Boston, Massachusetts

Tony Tannoury, MD
Department of Orthopaedic Surgery
Boston University
Boston, Massachusetts

Nirmal C. Tejwani, MD
Professor
Department of Orthopaedics
NYU Langone, Hospital for Joint Diseases
New York, New York

Michael C. Tucker, MD
Director, Orthopaedic Trauma Service
Premier Orthopaedic Specialists
Palmetto Health – Richland
Columbia, South Carolina

Heather A. Vallier, MD
Professor of Orthopaedic Surgery
Department of Orthopaedic Surgery
Case Western Reserve University
The MetroHealth System
Cleveland, Ohio

Thomas F. Varecka, MD
Assistant Chairman of Orthopaedic Surgery
Hennepin County Medical Center
Assistant Professor of Orthopaedic Surgery
Department of Orthopaedic Surgery
University of Minnesota
Minneapolis, Minnesota

David A. Volgas, MD
Associate Professor
Department of Orthopaedic Surgery
University of Missouri – Columbia
Columbia, Missouri

David Walmsley, MD, FRCSC
Clinical Fellow
Department of Orthopaedic Surgery
St. Michael's Hospital
Toronto, Ontario, Canada

Peter H. White, MD
Department of Orthopaedics
Medical University of South Carolina
Charleston, South Carolina

Robert L. Wimberly, MD
Staff Orthopaedist
Department of Orthopedic Surgery
Texas Scottish Rite Hospital for Children
Dallas, Texas

Richard S. Yoon, MD
Department of Orthopaedic Surgery, Division of Orthopaedic Trauma
NYU Langone Hospital for Joint Diseases
New York, New York

Jay M. Zampini, MD
Instructor of Orthopaedic Surgery, Harvard Medical School
Division of Spine Surgery
Brigham and Women's Hospital
Boston, Massachusetts

David W. Zeltser, MD
Orthopedic Hand Surgeon
Department of Orthopedic Surgery
Kaiser Permanente South San Francisco Medical Center
San Francisco, California

Robert D. Zura, MD
Associate Professor, Section Head
Department of Orthopaedic Trauma
Duke University
Durham, North Carolina

Preface

Orthopaedic Knowledge Update: Trauma 5 is the latest edition of the *Orthopaedic Knowledge Update* series, and this text builds on the previous editions. *OKU Trauma 5* is comprehensive and current in its content and includes new chapters on biomechanics, osteoporosis and pathologic bone, deep vein thrombosis (DVT) prophylaxis in fracture patients, acute compartment syndrome, and biologic adjuvants for fracture healing. This publication is detailed in the latest evidence regarding diagnosis, treatment options, surgical techniques, and outcomes for the management of orthopaedic trauma and fracture patients. It is the hope of all that were involved in this endeavor that surgeons can use this book as a reference for maintaining and updating clinical competence and improving patient care. The editors would like to express their gratitude to all of the chapter authors who spent many hours reading the current literature and writing and revising their manuscripts to produce these excellent chapters. The section editors (Robert O'Toole, Mark Brinker, Mel Rosenwasser, Kyle Jeray, Brett Crist, John Flynn, Paul Tornetta III, and Ken Egol) were very conscientious and worked tirelessly while reading and editing these chapters and were persistent in making sure that the final product was outstanding.

The General Topics section includes chapters dedicated to new technologies in orthopaedic trauma, minimally invasive fracture treatment, outcomes of musculoskeletal trauma, osteoporotic fractures and DVT prophylaxis for fracture patients. The Nonunions, Malunions, and Infections section deals with surgical options, adjuvants for fracture healing, and new innovations in the treatment of these difficult cases. The Soft-Tissue Injury and the Polytrauma Patient section consists of chapters discussing the evaluation and management of the mangled extremity, traumatic amputations, disaster and mass casualty preparedness, and the critical issue of damage control orthopaedics in the polytraumatized patient. Chapters in the Upper Extremity section are inclusive from the clavicle to the hand for fracture management and the assessment and management of traumatic nerve injuries. The acute evaluation of pelvis and acetabulum fractures as well as imaging, initial and definitive treatment, and functional outcomes are discussed in the Axial Skeleton: Pelvis, Acetabulum, and Spine section. The content in the Lower Extremity section is all-inclusive, from femoral head fractures to foot fractures and dislocations. The Geriatrics section not only includes chapters on hip fractures but also osteoporosis, pathologic fractures, and periprosthetic fractures. The chapters in the Pediatrics section provide a comprehensive and detailed assessment of fractures of the upper and lower extremity and the pediatric spine.

The treatment of fractures and trauma patients is an always-evolving field with innovations, tricks, and techniques improving constantly. The surgeon must stay current with the latest management options to understand the risks and benefits associated with these procedures. Some of these "advancements" need to be looked at with a critical eye and newer may not always be better. The contributors to this book face this dilemma daily and understand the significance of their role in distilling these newer technologies to those that actually are improvements in patient care.

This publication would not have been possible without the capable stewardship of members of the AAOS staff, including Hans Koelsch, Lisa Claxton Moore, Brian Moore, Sylvia Orellana, Courtney Dunker, and Rachel Winokur, who through numerous conference calls and poking and prodding kept this publication on track.

Robert F. Ostrum, MD
William M. Ricci, MD
Editors

Emergency Medical Services and Trauma

One of the most important factors affecting orthopaedic trauma care over the past half century has been the development of prehospital emergency care. Quite simply, the ability of orthopaedic traumatologists to effectively treat patients with complex limb injuries is contingent on these patients arriving to the hospital alive. The American Academy of Orthopaedic Surgeons (AAOS) was among the first organizations to recognize the need for emergency care in the field and rapid transport of the injured to appropriately equipped facilities. AAOS initially conducted courses in the 1960s for ambulance drivers to improve prehospital care for trauma patients. The course materials became the framework for the first edition of *Emergency Care and Transportation of the Sick and Injured* (the "Orange Book"), which was published in 1971. The text was also the basis for the first National Standard Curriculum for Emergency Medical Technicians developed by the US Department of Transportation. The Orange Book—so called for its trademark orange cover—is now considered by many emergency medical services (EMS) professionals as the gold standard in EMS training.

Since 1997, AAOS has partnered with Jones & Bartlett Learning (JBL) to develop and publish outstanding educational resources for EMS providers at all levels, including emergency medical responder, emergency medical technician, advanced emergency medical technician, paramedic, and critical care transport paramedic. This partnership has resulted in a series of market-leading products that provide initial education, continuing education, and professional resources to support EMS students, educators, and providers throughout every step of their education and career. The recent release of the 11th edition of the Orange Book marks 45 years that AAOS and JBL have been a leading publisher of EMS products. This newest text is only one of more than 500 core and derivative products, print and digital, delivered throughout the world to help educate EMS providers.

Dr. Andrew Pollak serves as the medical editor of the series and works directly with AAOS staff to ensure the medical accuracy, quality, and overall integrity of each EMS product that bears the AAOS name. The goals of these products are to ensure quality patient care in the prehospital setting, to avoid preventable death from trauma, and to influence successful healthcare outcomes. There is no question that quality prehospital care limits the ongoing injury associated with severe musculoskeletal trauma, and that well-prepared prehospital care personnel can save lives and ensure that injured patients arrive quickly and safely to the most capable treatment facilities.

Andrew N. Pollak, MD, FAAOS, is Chief of Orthopaedics, University of Maryland School of Medicine; Director, Shock Trauma Go Team, R Adams Cowley Shock Trauma Center; Medical Director, Baltimore County Fire Department; and Special Deputy US Marshal.

Table of Contents

Section 4: Upper Extremity

Section 5: Axial Skeleton: Pelvis, Acetabulum, and Spine

Section 8: Pediatrics

Section Editor:
John M. Flynn, MD

Section 1

General Topics

Section Editor

Brett D. Crist, MD

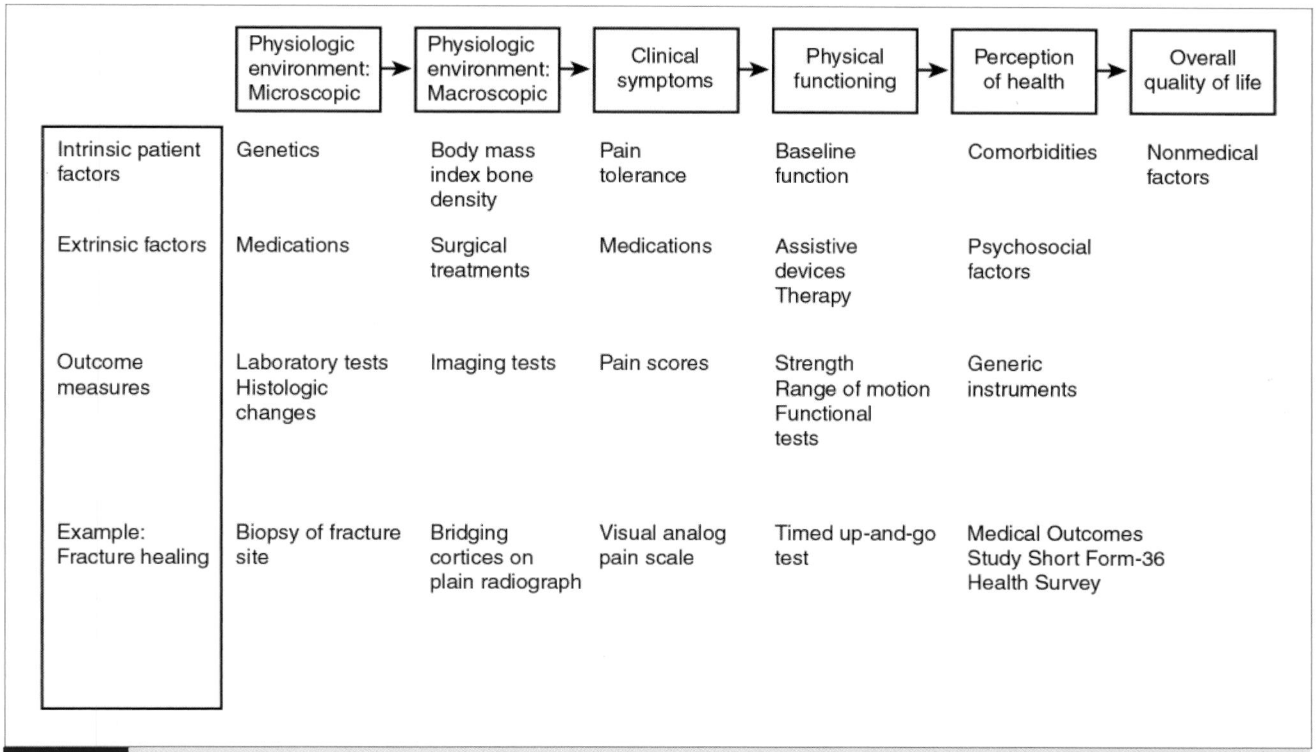

Physiologic environment: Microscopic
Physiologic environment: Macroscopic
Clinical symptoms
Physical functioning
Perception of health
Overall quality of life
Intrinsic patient factors
Genetics
Body mass index bone density
Pain tolerance
Baseline function
Comorbidities
Nonmedical factors
Extrinsic factors
Medications
Surgical treatments
Medications
Assistive devices Therapy
Psychosocial factors
Outcome measures
Laboratory tests Histologic changes
Imaging tests
Pain scores
Strength Range of motion Functional tests
Generic instruments
Example: Fracture healing
Biopsy of fracture site
Bridging cortices on plain radiograph
Visual analog pain scale
Timed up-and-go test
Medical Outcomes Study Short Form-36 Health Survey

Figure 1 A conceptual pathway for relationships among the components of health-related quality of life is shown, from the underlying causes of disease to clinical symptoms to overall quality of life. At each step on the pathway, intrinsic and extrinsic factors can influence the subsequent step, and opportunities exist for outcome measurement. Outcomes toward the left that measure the root cause of clinical symptoms, such as plain radiographs, may be highly sensitive to intervention, but not necessarily have a measurable effect on patient quality of life. Quality-of-life instruments, in contrast, may be less sensitive to change due to an intervention, but these instruments to measuring the ultimate goal of any treatment: improving quality of life.

life (HRQOL)[13] (**Figure 1**). Opportunities for measurement exist at each step along the pathway. For example, at one end of the spectrum is plain radiography, which commonly is used in trauma studies to assess bony healing and alignment even though radiographic measures of alignment may not be correlated with the patient's subjective experience of pain or functional ability. Moving toward the other end of the spectrum, outcome measures such as a pain scale, strength, or range-of-motion testing may not be correlated with the patient's overall HRQOL. Clinician- or surgeon-centered outcomes tend to differ from patient-reported outcomes, and there is an increasing emphasis on the use of patient-reported outcomes in clinical research. It is important to note that instruments that measure HRQOL can be affected by an unrelated medical or nonmedical factor (such as comorbidities or psychosocial support, respectively). In addition, these instruments often do not explain identified differences in HRQOL. For example, an intervention for a fracture may demonstrate an improvement in HRQOL, but the question remains as to whether the improvement is attributable to the patient's healing rate, limb alignment, or self-efficacy. Only by measuring outcomes across the spectrum can this question be answered. For that reason, investigators should consider a HRQOL instrument in conjunction with other secondary outcome measures across the outcomes spectrum.

Orthopaedic Trauma Outcomes

Clinical End Points

Bony union is one of the primary goals of fracture management. Because fracture union is a process that occurs across a continuum rather than as a discrete event, it can be as problematic as the primary end point of a research study.[14,15] Union has been defined as an event ranging from painless weight bearing to bridging of three of four cortices on orthogonal plain radiographs.[15] Studies assessing the reliability of radiographic assessment are limited, although some research supportsthe use of plain radiographs for assessment oflong bone fractures treated with intramedullary nailing.[16]

Bone healing remains the most direct representation of the success of treatments to promote fracture repair, but the ability to measure bone healing in clinical practice remains crude. Investigators found that any cortical bridging 4 months after treatment of a tibia fracture with intramedullary nailing predicts eventual bridging of the remaining cortices without a need for additional intervention.[17] The Radiographic Union Score for Tibial Fractures (RUST) is a relatively new measurement based on assessment of cortical bridging.[18] Each cortex (medial, lateral, anterior, and posterior) is assessed and assigned a point value (1 = fracture line, no callus; 2 = fracture line, visible callus; 3 = no fracture line, bridging callus). The total score of the four cortices, ranging from 4 to 12, may represent the continuous nature of fracture healing, and the reliability of the RUST score was found to be higher than bridging of three of four cortices or orthopaedic surgeons' subjective impression of union.[19] In addition, the Radiographic Union Scale for the Hip (RUSH) is undergoing development and validation to quantify the healing of intertrochanteric hip fractures.[20]

Reoperation is another clinical end point that is relevant to patients.[21] Mortality may not be significantly affected by orthopaedic treatment, and reoperation offers an alternative objective end point that is more likely to differentiate between fracture interventions. The common criticism of reoperation as an outcome is that it relies on the subjective assessment of the treating surgeon. This objection can be overcome by strictly defining the criteria for reoperation. Large studies often use an independent adjudication committee to assess whether the criteria for reoperation have been met for each affected patient.[22]

Functional Outcomes

Most orthopaedic interventions are intended to improve function. A variety of outcome instruments directly measure physical functioning and performance. Among the most well-known of these is the timed up-and-go test, which measures number of seconds required for a subject to stand from sitting, walk 10 ft, and return to a seated position.[23] This test is particularly useful for assessing the functional capacity of older adults, and the results of the test as administered soon after hemiarthroplasty for femoral neck fracture were found to be correlated with the long-term outcome.[24]

Wearable devices that record physical activity provide a means of measuring function that is increasingly available because of technologic improvements. Pedometers, which record each step, have been in existence for centuries, but recently more advanced devices (such as the Fitbit) have gained popularity with consumers and researchers alike.[25] Accelerometers are similar in principle but have the ability to differentiate low- and high-intensity activities. Modern accelerometers can detect movements in three-dimensional space. The use of these devices in fracture studies has been limited, but as the technology is incorporated into smartphones and other wearable devices, a plethora of data increasingly can be harnessed to measure outcomes.

Questionnaires

Outcome questionnaires can be broadly categorized as generic or disease specific.[21] Generic instruments attempt to capture the overall quality of life in a metric that is comparable across a variety of different diseases. Because these instruments must capture many different aspects of HRQOL, they may lack the granularity and responsiveness desired by researchers studying a specific condition. For that reason, a large number of disease-specific and body region–specific instruments have been developed and validated (**Table 1**).

The process of selecting the appropriate instrument for a study is driven by factors including validity, reliability, and practicality of administration. Validity is related to the content of the questionnaire and the ability of the survey to appropriately reflect changes in the study participants. Studies ideally use instruments previously found to be valid in the study population. Reliability refers to the precision and reproducibility of an instrument. Practicality includes factors such as length of time required to complete the questionnaire. The properties of several of generic instruments are outlined in **Table 2**.

Medical Outcomes Study Short Form-36 Health Survey

The Short Form-36 Health Survey (SF-36) was developed for the Medical Outcomes Study, a cohort study that in the 1980s compared clinical outcomes in different health care delivery systems.[26] The SF-36 subsequently became the most widely used generic survey in medicine.[27] The 36 questions in eight domains yield a physical component score and a mental component score. The SF-36 uses a proprietary system in which scores range from 0 to 100 with a mean of 50 and a standard deviation of 10; a higher score reflects better health. To reduce the burden on study subjects and improve the ease of administration, the SF-12 was developed using a 12-item subset of the SF-36. The SF-6D, another subset of the SF-36, uses 11 items from six domains of the full questionnaire. Unlike the SF-36 and SF-12, scores on the SF-6D have been correlated with utility, a concept from economic theory that attempts to quantify an individual's preference for a given health state from 0 to 1 (1 is perfect health, and 0 is equivalent to death). These results are useful for direct input in economic analysis.

Table 1

Injury-Specific Outcome Instruments Commonly Used in Orthopaedic Trauma Studies

Injury	Instrument(s)
Upper Extremity	Disabilities of the Arm, Shoulder and Hand
Shoulder	American Shoulder and Elbow Surgeons Shoulder Scale
	Constant-Murley Shoulder Score
Elbow	Mayo Elbow Score
	American Shoulder and Elbow Surgeons Elbow Scale
Wrist and Hand	Patient-Rated Wrist Evaluation
	Michigan Hand Questionnaire
Pelvis	Merle d'Aubigné Score (Acetabulum)
	Majeed Score (Pelvic ring)
Hip	Western Ontario and McMaster Universities Osteoarthritis Index
	Harris Hip Score
	Oxford Hip Score
Knee	Knee Injury and Osteoarthritis Outcome Score
	Lysholm Knee Scale
Foot and Ankle	American Orthopaedic Foot and Ankle Society Score

EQ-5D

The multinational EuroQol Group developed the EQ-5D instrument in the 1980s as a short, practical questionnaire that can accurately estimate an individual's quality of life.[28] The EQ-5D is significantly shorter than many other generic surveys; it has only five questions on mobility, self-care, usual activities, pain or discomfort, and anxiety or depression. Unlike the output of the SF-36 but like that of the SF-6D, the output of the EQ-5D has been correlated with utility. The EQ-5D is a useful instrument to consider if economic analysis is planned and a shorter survey is preferred, but it lacks the granularity to differentiate among many high-functioning patients, particularly those with an injury involving the upper extremity.

Musculoskeletal Function Assessment

The Musculoskeletal Function Assessment (MFA) commonly is used in orthopaedic studies as a generic instrument for evaluating musculoskeletal conditions. The full MFA has 110 items, and the Short Musculoskeletal Function Assessment (SMFA) has 46 items.[29] The ease of administering the SMFA compared with the MFA has led to its becoming the more commonly selected measure in fracture studies.[30] However, in the Study to Prospectively Evaluate Reamed Intramedullary Nails in Patients with Tibial Fractures (SPRINT) evaluation of reamed and unreamed nails for tibial shaft fractures, the SMFA was not believed to add any information beyond that provided by the SF-36 instrument, and the researchers concluded that using the generic instrument was preferred to allow broad comparisons across disease states, at least in patients with a tibial shaft fracture.[31]

Sickness Impact Profile

The Sickness Impact Profile (SIP) is a generic instrument developed in the 1970s to quantify an individual's quality of life by assessing the ability to perform daily activities.[32] The survey consists of 136 questions in a yes-or-no format; the final score is derived from the percentage of affirmative answers. The 12 domains of the SIP are ambulation, mobility, body care and movement, social interaction, alertness behavior, emotional behavior, communication, sleep and rest, eating, work, home management, and recreation and pastimes. The Lower Extremity Assessment Project (LEAP) used the SIP as the primary outcome measure and found no significant between-group differences in the scores of patients with severe lower extremity injury who were treated with amputation or limb salvage[5] (**Table 3**). However, analysis of the subset of patients with foot and ankle trauma revealed that those who required a free tissue transfer or ankle fusion had worse SIP scores than those with below-knee amputation.[33]

Table 2

Characteristics of Several Generic Outcome Instruments

	Medical Outcomes Study Short-Form 36[a]	Sickness Impact Profile[b]	EQ-5D[c]	Short Musculoskeletal Function Assessment[d]
Scoring				
Lowest score	0	0	-0.59	100
Highest score	100	100	1.0	0.0
Total range	100	100	1.59	100
Mean score	50	-	–	12.7
Minimal clinically important difference	Domain, 3–5	3–5	0.074	–
	Physical component score, 2			
Reliability				
Internal consistency	0.74–0.93	0.6–0.9	—	0.92–0.96
Test-retest reliability	0.60–0.81	0.5–0.95	0.63–0.8	0.88–0.93
Practical Aspects				
Completion time (in minutes)	5–12.5	19–30	3	10
Available languages	120	21	22	4
Cost	Not publicly available	€500–800+	Free	Free

[a] Data from Hays RD, Morales LS: The RAND-36 measure of health-related quality of life. *Ann Med* 2001;33(5):350-357; Angst F, Aeschlimann A, Stucki G: Smallest detectable and minimal clinically important differences of rehabilitation intervention with their implications for required sample sizes using WOMAC and SF-36 quality of life measurement instruments in patients with osteoarthritis of the lower extremities. *Arthritis Rheum* 2001;45(4):384-391; Brazier JE, Harper R, Jones NM, et al: Validating the SF-36 health survey questionnaire: New outcome measure for primary care. *BMJ* 1992;305(6846):160-164; Andresen EM, Rothenberg BM, Kaplan RM: Performance of a self-administered mailed version of the Quality of Well-Being (QWB-SA) questionnaire among older adults. *Med Care* 1998;36(9):1349-1360; Edelman D, Williams GR, Rothman M, Samsa GP: A comparison of three health status measures in primary care outpatients. *J Gen Intern Med* 1999;14(12):759-762.

[b] Data from Deyo RA, Patrick DL: The significance of treatment effects: The clinical perspective. *Med Care* 1995;33(4, Suppl):AS286-AS291; de Bruin AF, de Witte LP, Stevens F, Diederiks JP: Sickness Impact Profile: The state of the art of a generic functional status measure. *Soc Sci Med* 1992;35(8):1003-1014; Andresen EM, Rothenberg BM, Kaplan RM: Performance of a self-administered mailed version of the Quality of Well-Being (QWB-SA) questionnaire among older adults. *Med Care* 1998;36(9):1349-1360; Edelman D, Williams GR, Rothman M, Samsa GP: A comparison of three health status measures in primary care outpatients. *J Gen Intern Med* 1999;14(12):759-762; Coons SJ, Rao S, Keininger DL, Hays RD: A comparative review of generic quality-of-life instruments. *Pharmacoeconomics* 2000;17(1):13-35.

[c] Data from Walters SJ, Brazier JE: Comparison of the minimally important difference for two health state utility measures: EQ-5D and SF-6D. *Qual Life Res* 2005;14(6):1523-1532; Brazier JE, Harper R, Jones NM, et al: Validating the SF-36 health survey questionnaire: New outcome measure for primary care. *BMJ* 1992;305(6846):160-164; Edelman D, Williams GR, Rothman M, Samsa GP: A comparison of three health status measures in primary care outpatients. *J Gen Intern Med* 1999;14(12):759-762.

[d] Data from Swiontkowski MF, Engelberg R, Martin DP, Agel J: Short Musculoskeletal Function Assessment questionnaire: Validity, reliability, and responsiveness. *J Bone Joint Surg Am* 1999;81(9):1245-1260; Barei DP, Agel J, Swiontkowski MF: Current utilization, interpretation, and recommendations: The musculoskeletal function assessments (MFA/SMFA). *J Orthop Trauma* 2007;21(10):738-742.

PROMIS

In response to the growing demand for patient-reported outcomes, the US National Institutes of Health funded the Patient-Reported Outcomes Measurement Information System (PROMIS), a multicenter cooperative that developed an improved outcome instrument using technology and psychometric theory.[34,35] PROMIS is unique in that it allows items to be selected from several broad domains that encapsulate quality of life. As a result, PROMIS is highly flexible and can be tailored to the application. Item response theory and computer adaptive testing are two key features that affect the administration of PROMIS. In item response theory the response to a question determines the next question to be administered. This feature increases the efficiency and accuracy of the final score; by using computer adaptive testing, PROMIS can achieve the same validity and reliability as conventional techniques through fewer questions. In patients with orthopaedic trauma, the testing time for the PROMIS physical function domain was 44 seconds compared with

Table 3

Important Studies in Orthopaedic Trauma

Study	Publication Year	Study Design	PICO Framework	Major Findings
Published Studies				
Bhandari et al[6] (Study to Prospectively Evaluate Reamed Intramedullary Nails in Patients With Tibial Fractures [SPRINT])	2012	Multicenter randomized controlled study	Population: 1,319 adults with tibial shaft fracture Intervention: Reamed nailing Comparator: Unreamed nailing Outcomes: –Reoperation within 1 year –SF-36, SMFA, HUI scores –Tibial knee pain	–No overall difference in reoperation rate –Lower rate of reoperation for closed fractures treated with reamed nailing –Trend toward lower rate of reoperation for open fractures with unreamed nailing
Bosse et al[5] (Lower Extremity Assessment Project [LEAP])	2002	Multicenter prospective cohort study	Population: 569 adults with severe open lower extremity injury Intervention: Limb salvage Comparator: Amputation Outcomes: –SIP score –Limb status –Rehospitalization	–No overall difference in SIP scores at 2 years –Lower SIP scores for foot and ankle injuries with flap or ankle fusion –High level of long-term disability –Self-efficacy a strong predictor of ultimate outcome
Canadian Orthopaedic Trauma Society[7]	2007	Multicenter randomized controlled study	Population: 132 patients with displaced midshaft clavicle fracture Intervention: Open reduction and internal fixation Comparator: Nonsurgical treatment with sling Outcomes: –DASH and Constant scores –Nonunion	–Better DASH and Constant scores with surgery –Lower nonunion rate with surgery –Higher rate of symptomatic malunion without surgery
Ongoing and Future Studies			**PICO Framework**	
FAITH Investigators[8] (Fixation Using Alternative Implants for the Treatment of Hip Fractures)	2014	Multicenter randomized controlled study	Population: Adults older than 50 years with low-energy femoral neck fracture Intervention: Sliding hip screw Comparator: Multiple cancellous screws Outcomes: –Reoperation within 2 years –SF-12, EQ-5D, WOMAC scores –Fracture healing –Adverse events	

1: General Topics

Table 3 *(continued)*

Important Studies in Orthopaedic Trauma

Study	Publication Year	Study Design	PICO Framework	Major Findings
Bhandari et al[9] (Hip Fracture Evaluation with Alternatives of Total Hip Arthroplasty Versus Hemiarthroplasty [HEALTH])	2015	Expertise-based multicenter randomized controlled study	Population: Adults older than 50 years with low-energy femoral neck fracture Intervention: Total hip arthroplasty Comparator: Hemiarthroplasty Outcomes: –Reoperation within 2 years –SF-12, EQ-5D, WOMAC scores –Timed up-and-go test	
Research Consortiums			**Study Example**	
Castillo et al[10] (Major Extremity Trauma Research Consortium [METRC])	2012	Multiple ongoing multicenter studies	Outcomes of severe ankle, distal tibia, and foot injuries	
Orthopaedic Trauma Research Consortium		Multiple ongoing multicenter studies	Nails versus plates for proximal tibial fractures	

599 seconds for the SMFA.[34] Furthermore, there were no ceiling effects for PROMIS compared with a 14% ceiling effect for the SMFA. (Ceiling and floor effects occur when an instrument cannot differentiate individuals at the high [ceiling] or low [floor] end of the scale.) Because PROMIS uses item response theory to choose each question based on the response to the preceding question, it can focus on demanding activities for high-functioning subjects and thereby reduce the ceiling effect. The ceiling effect has been particularly problematic in generic instruments applied to patients with an upper extremity injury.[28] PROMIS was found superior to the Disabilities of the Arm, Shoulder and Hand score, which was designed for patients with upper extremity injury.[35]

Economic Analysis

In conjunction with the expanding emphasis on improving quality in health care by measuring patient-reported outcomes, there is pressure to reduce costs. In the future, surgeons will increasingly need to become familiar with the nomenclature of economic analysis and the quantitative research methods used to estimate the value of medical interventions across the spectrum of health care. Analysis is an increasingly important part of comparative effectiveness research and accompanies many large prospective studies in orthopaedic trauma care as well as other areas of medical practice.

Cost-Minimization Analysis

A simple comparison of the total cost of two interventions is called a cost-minimization or cost analysis. This type of study is appropriate if the clinical benefits of each treatment strategy are not significantly different. In this uncommon situation, the cost-minimization study design is straightforward and may inform a subsequent, more complex economic analysis.

Cost-Effectiveness Analysis

Cost-effectiveness analysis (CEA) attempts to estimate the cost of a given health care intervention to produce a unit of health benefit.[36] Usually the results of a CEA are quantitatively expressed as the ratio of the cost of the intervention to some term that quantifies the benefit. The numerator always contains cost, whereas the denominator can be any outcome of interest. For example, a CEA could report the cost per life saved or the cost per complication averted. The disadvantage of this method is that the more specific the outcome chosen for the denominator, the more difficult it is to make comparisons across studies.

Cost-Utility Analysis

Under the umbrella of CEA is cost-utility analysis, which is a more specific type of economic analysis. Rather than a clinical outcome, the denominator of the ratio is utility, which expresses the societal preference for a health state ranging from 1 (equating to perfect health) to 0 (equating to death).[36] For example, a patient with severe osteoarthritis might have a utility of 0.7, and a patient with a spinal cord injury might have a utility of 0.3. By multiplying the utility of the health state with the number of years spent in the health state, quality-adjusted life years (QALYs) can be calculated. This method makes it possible to compare in a single metric interventions that prolong life with those that have more effect on quality of life. QALYs are the recommended and most commonly used value for the denominator of a cost-utility analysis.[37]

The primary outcome in a cost-utility analysis is the incremental cost-effectiveness ratio (ICER). The ICER is a ratio of the incremental cost of the intervention to the comparator and the incremental utility of the intervention relative to the comparator[37]:

$$ICER = \frac{Cost_{intervention} - Cost_{comparator}}{Utility_{intervention} - Utility_{comparator}}$$

It is crucial that studies include a baseline comparison to report an accurate ICER, rather than assuming that the baseline cost and utility are 0. Even a do-nothing approach has a cost and health effect on the population and therefore should be estimated as the comparator. In fracture healing studies, the comparator typically is nonsurgical treatment, which often is associated with the cost of clinic visits for casting and radiographs and may have a reasonable outcome that is equivalent to a nonzero value for utility.

Cost-Benefit Analysis

Unlike a CEA or cost-utility analysis, in which the cost and benefit are kept separate by using a ratio, a cost-benefit analysis converts both cost and benefit into monetary units. The result is expressed as the net monetary benefit (NMB). An NMB higher than 0 indicates that the strategy will save money, and an NMB lower than 0 indicates that the strategy will lose money. The challenge of this approach in a health care context is that ethical issues arise when a monetary value is assigned. Therefore, NMB is infrequently used in health care. The principal advantage of this approach at a governmental level is that it can be used to compare programs in sectors such as education, transportation, or energy relative to health care programs.

Summary

The PICO framework can be a helpful tool for designing and interpreting high-quality clinical outcome studies. The first step in designing a study is to specify the target population. The treatment strategies in a comparative study can be assigned at random or in an observational manner. The risk of confounding bias is more likely in an observational study because the treatment groups may be unequal and therefore have a different prognosis for the measured outcome. Outcome measurements can be surgeon or patient reported; patient-reported outcomes increasingly are emphasized in health care research. Dynamic instruments implementing item response theory and using computer adaptive testing were developed during the past decade. Research into the cost of treatments as related to other outcomes and health utility metrics allows the monetary value of treatments and services to be estimated and will increasingly drive medical decision making in a resource-constrained environment.

Key Study Points

- The population-intervention-comparison-outcome (PICO) framework is a useful tool for constructing and interpreting research studies.
- The process of randomization, used to create two equivalent groups of patients for a study, minimizes the impact of confounding bias. Several methods are available to reduce bias in observational studies, but none of them can eliminate the influence of unmeasured confounding variables.
- Generic outcome questionnaires measure overall health-related quality of life. Disease-specific outcome questionnaires may be more responsive but cannot be used for comparison across disease states.
- The PROMIS instruments use computer adaptive testing to reduce administration time and improve accuracy compared with traditional questionnaires. The use of PROMIS in orthopaedic surgery remains limited.
- The results of a cost-effectiveness analysis often are reported as the incremental cost-effectiveness ratio, which can be used to estimate the cost per incremental improvement in health care related to one intervention compared with another. This result commonly is reported as cost per quality-adjusted life year.

Annotated References

1. Slobogean GP, Dielwart C, Johal HS, Shantz JA, Mulpuri K: Levels of evidence at the Orthopaedic Trauma Association annual meetings. *J Orthop Trauma* 2013;27(9):e208-e212.

The quality of podium presentations at OTA meetings improved after the introduction of guidelines for levels of evidence, but most studies remained at level IV.

2. Cunningham BP, Harmsen S, Kweon C, et al: Have levels of evidence improved the quality of orthopaedic research? *Clin Orthop Relat Res* 2013;471(11):3679-3686.

   From 2000 to 2009 the number of level I and II studies in major orthopaedic journals increased, but level IV studies continued be the most prevalent.

3. Andrawis JP, Chenok KE, Bozic KJ: Health policy implications of outcomes measurement in orthopaedics. *Clin Orthop Relat Res* 2013;471(11):3475-3481.

   The state of cost and value assessment in orthopaedics was reviewed, and orthopaedic surgeons were encouraged to actively engage in outcomes registries and the development of value-based payment strategies.

4. Katz G, Ong C, Hutzler L, Zuckerman JD, Bosco JA III: Applying quality principles to orthopaedic surgery. *Instr Course Lect* 2014;63:465-472.

   The transition of Medicare payments from fee-for-service models to value-based purchasing and outlines methods was described to maximize quality in orthopaedic practice.

5. Bosse MJ, MacKenzie EJ, Kellam JF, et al: An analysis of outcomes of reconstruction or amputation after leg-threatening injuries. *N Engl J Med* 2002;347(24):1924-1931.

6. Bhandari M, Guyatt G, Tornetta P III, et al; Study to Prospectively Evaluate Reamed Intramedullary Nails in Patients with Tibial Fractures Investigators: Randomized trial of reamed and unreamed intramedullary nailing of tibial shaft fractures. *J Bone Joint Surg Am* 2008;90(12):2567-2578.

7. Canadian Orthopaedic Trauma Society: Nonoperative treatment compared with plate fixation of displaced midshaft clavicular fractures: A multicenter, randomized clinical trial. *J Bone Joint Surg Am* 2007;89(1):1-10.

8. FAITH Investigators: Fixation using alternative implants for the treatment of hip fractures (FAITH): Design and rationale for a multi-centre randomized trial comparing sliding hip screws and cancellous screws on revision surgery rates and quality of life in the treatment of femoral neck fractures. *BMC Musculoskelet Disord* 2014;15:219.

   The design of a multicenter randomized controlled study was described. The study compared the use of sliding hip and cancellous screws to treat femoral neck fracture in patients older than 50 years with a low-energy injury.

9. Bhandari M, Devereaux PJ, Einhorn TA, et al: Hip fracture evaluation with alternatives of total hip arthroplasty versus hemiarthroplasty (HEALTH): Protocol for a multicentre randomised trial. *BMJ Open* 2015;5(2):e006263.

   The design of an expertise-based multicenter randomized controlled study was described for comparing hemiarthroplasty and total hip arthroplasty for treating femoral neck fracture in patients older than 50 years with a low-energy injury.

10. Castillo RC, Mackenzie EJ, Bosse MJ; METRC Investigators: Measurement of functional outcomes in the major extremity trauma research consortium (METRC). *J Am Acad Orthop Surg* 2012;20(Suppl 1):S59-S63.

    The history and goals of the Major Extremity Trauma Research Consortium were described with the outcome instruments used in its studies.

11. Marsh JL, Slongo TF, Agel J, et al: Fracture and dislocation classification compendium: 2007. Orthopaedic Trauma Association Classification, Database and Outcomes Committee. *J Orthop Trauma* 2007;21(10, Suppl):S1-S133.

12. Benichou J: A review of adjusted estimators of attributable risk. *Stat Methods Med Res* 2001;10(3):195-216.

13. Wilson IB, Cleary PD: Linking clinical variables with health-related quality of life: A conceptual model of patient outcomes. *JAMA* 1995;273(1):59-65.

14. Corrales LA, Morshed S, Bhandari M, Miclau T III: Variability in the assessment of fracture-healing in orthopaedic trauma studies. *J Bone Joint Surg Am* 2008;90(9):1862-1868.

15. Morshed S, Corrales L, Genant H, Miclau T III: Outcome assessment in clinical trials of fracture-healing. *J Bone Joint Surg Am* 2008;90(Suppl 1):62-67.

16. Whelan DB, Bhandari M, McKee MD, et al: Interobserver and intraobserver variation in the assessment of the healing of tibial fractures after intramedullary fixation. *J Bone Joint Surg Br* 2002;84(1):15-18.

17. Lack WD, Starman JS, Seymour R, et al: Any cortical bridging predicts healing of tibial shaft fractures. *J Bone Joint Surg Am* 2014;96(13):1066-1072.

    Patients with tibial shaft fracture were followed after intramedullary nailing to record the development of callus. Bridging of a single cortex by four-month follow-up was the best predictor of subsequent healing. No patient who met this criterion had a later nonunion or required an additional intervention.

18. Whelan DB, Bhandari M, Stephen D, et al: Development of the Radiographic Union Score for Tibial Fractures for the assessment of tibial fracture healing after intramedullary fixation. *J Trauma* 2010;68(3):629-632.

    The RUST score had better reliability for assessing fracture healing than earlier methods.

19. Kooistra BW, Dijkman BG, Busse JW, Sprague S, Schemitsch EH, Bhandari M: The Radiographic Union Scale in Tibial Fractures: Reliability and validity. *J Orthop Trauma* 2010;24(Suppl 1):S81-S86.

The validity and reliability of the RUST score were described. Although the score was found to be reliable, validation studies were limited.

20. Bhandari M, Chiavaras MM, Parasu N, et al: Radiographic Union Score for Hip substantially improves agreement between surgeons and radiologists. *BMC Musculoskelet Disord* 2013;14:70.

    The RUSH score for assessing the healing of intertrochanteric hip fractures showed better agreement between surgeons and radiologists compared with a general impression of healing.

21. Kooistra BW, Sprague S, Bhandari M, Schemitsch EH: Outcomes assessment in fracture healing trials: A primer. *J Orthop Trauma* 2010;24(Suppl 1):S71-S75.

    Concepts important to outcome studies such as validity and reliability were reviewed with variety of potential outcome instruments.

22. Vannabouathong C, Saccone M, Sprague S, Schemitsch EH, Bhandari M: Adjudicating outcomes: Fundamentals. *J Bone Joint Surg Am* 2012;94(Suppl 1):70-74.

    Methods were described for using an independent committee to adjudicate outcomes in large clinical studies to reduce bias.

23. Podsiadlo D, Richardson S: The timed "Up & Go": A test of basic functional mobility for frail elderly persons. *J Am Geriatr Soc* 1991;39(2):142-148.

24. Laflamme GY, Rouleau DM, Leduc S, Roy L, Beaumont E: The Timed Up and Go test is an early predictor of functional outcome after hemiarthroplasty for femoral neck fracture. *J Bone Joint Surg Am* 2012;94(13):1175-1179.

    The timed up-and-go test administered four days and three weeks after treatment of femoral neck fracture with hemiarthroplasty was strongly correlated with the likelihood of independent ambulation at two years.

25. Ainsworth B, Cahalin L, Buman M, Ross R: The current state of physical activity assessment tools. *Prog Cardiovasc Dis* 2015;57(4):387-395.

    Current outcome instruments to assess physical activity, such as pedometers and accelerometers, were reviewed.

26. Tarlov AR, Ware JE Jr, Greenfield S, Nelson EC, Perrin E, Zubkoff M: The Medical Outcomes Study: An application of methods for monitoring the results of medical care. *JAMA* 1989;262(7):925-930.

27. Hays RD, Morales LS: The RAND-36 measure of health-related quality of life. *Ann Med* 2001;33(5):350-357.

28. Slobogean GP, Noonan VK, O'Brien PJ: The reliability and validity of the Disabilities of Arm, Shoulder and Hand, EuroQol-5D, Health Utilities Index, and Short Form-6D outcome instruments in patients with proximal humeral fractures. *J Shoulder Elbow Surg* 2010;19(3):342-348.

    Multiple generic instruments were tested for construct validity and test-retest reliability among patients with proximal humerus fracture. All instruments performed reasonably well, although the EQ-5D had a substantial ceiling effect compared with other instruments.

29. Swiontkowski MF, Engelberg R, Martin DP, Agel J: Short Musculoskeletal Function Assessment questionnaire: Validity, reliability, and responsiveness. *J Bone Joint Surg Am* 1999;81(9):1245-1260.

30. Barei DP, Agel J, Swiontkowski MF: Current utilization, interpretation, and recommendations: The musculoskeletal function assessments (MFA/SMFA). *J Orthop Trauma* 2007;21(10):738-742.

31. Busse JW, Bhandari M, Guyatt GH, et al; SPRINT Investigators: Use of both Short Musculoskeletal Function Assessment questionnaire and Short Form-36 among tibial-fracture patients was redundant. *J Clin Epidemiol* 2009;62(11):1210-1217.

32. de Bruin AF, de Witte LP, Stevens F, Diederiks JP: Sickness Impact Profile: The state of the art of a generic functional status measure. *Soc Sci Med* 1992;35(8):1003-1014.

33. Ellington JK, Bosse MJ, Castillo RC, MacKenzie EJ; LEAP Study Group: The mangled foot and ankle: Results from a 2-year prospective study. *J Orthop Trauma* 2013;27(1):43-48.

    In patients with severe foot and ankle injuries, those who underwent limb salvage requiring a flap or ankle fusion had lower SIP scores than those initially treated with below-knee amputation.

34. Hung M, Stuart AR, Higgins TF, Saltzman CL, Kubiak EN: Computerized adaptive testing using the PROMIS physical function item bank reduces test burden with less ceiling effects compared with the Short Musculoskeletal Function Assessment in orthopaedic trauma patients. *J Orthop Trauma* 2014;28(8):439-443.

    The PROMIS physical function computerized adaptive test and the SMFA were administered to patients with orthopaedic trauma. The PROMIS test required dramatically less time to administer and had less ceiling effect.

35. Tyser AR, Beckmann J, Franklin JD, et al: Evaluation of the PROMIS physical function computer adaptive test in the upper extremity. *J Hand Surg Am* 2014;39(10):2047-2051.e4.

    The PROMIS physical function computerized adaptive test and Disabilities of the Arm, Shoulder and Hand instrument were administered to patients at an upper extremity clinic. The PROMIS instrument had a much shorter administration time, less floor or ceiling effect, and a high level of precision.

36. Muennig P: Cost-Effectiveness Analyses in Health: A Practical Approach, *ed 2*. San Francisco, CA, Jossey-Bass, 2007.

37. Weinstein MC, Siegel JE, Gold MR, Kamlet MS, Russell LB: Recommendations of the Panel on Cost-effectiveness in Health and Medicine. *JAMA* 1996;276(15):1253-1258.

Chapter 2

Delivery of Orthopaedic Trauma Care

Rafael Neiman, MD   Zachary O. Mallon, MD

Abstract

The number of orthopaedics-related emergency department visits is increasing at the same time as multiple legislative events reduced access to specialty orthopaedic care in the United States. The number of trauma centers continues to increase, additionally straining the orthopaedists providing coverage at these institutions. Novel models for orthopaedic emergency coverage have been developed to provide care, with varying results.

Keywords: orthopaedic call coverage; access to orthopaedic trauma care; acute care orthopaedics

Introduction

More than 50% of all hospitalized trauma patients in the United States have musculoskeletal injuries that could be limb-threatening or life-threatening or could result in substantial functional impairment. More than 200,000 adolescents and adults younger than 65 years are hospitalized annually in the United States because of lower extremity fractures.[1]

With this large number of acute orthopaedic injuries comes a need for access to an appropriate level of orthopaedic care. Patients flow through a rapidly evolving medical system following a complex geopolitical pathway to their ultimate destination, which may be a small community setting, a level I trauma hospital in an academic setting, or one of the many options in between.

Patient Access to Emergency Care

The number of patient visits to emergency departments across the country continues to increase at a concerning rate. According to the Centers for Disease Control and Prevention, 119 million emergency department visits were made in 2006, and 136.3 million visits were made in 2011, representing a 14.5% increase over 5 years.[2] The number of visits has increased 51% over the past 15 years. The strain on the medical system and on orthopaedic surgeons in particular becomes more tangible, and some call arrangements that worked in the past may no longer be sufficient to provide orthopaedic coverage. Emergency departments report a varying availability of on-call orthopaedic coverage, with only about one-half of those surveyed reporting adequate coverage on weekends and at night. The reasons cited for lack of coverage include the interruption of family life and lifestyle, inadequate compensation, and the disruption of the elective orthopaedic practice.[3] In many regions, traditional call panels have been supplanted by coverage solutions that match the current trends and needs to provide acute orthopaedic surgical care across the United States. At the same time as changes in health care access in this country are evolving, the availability of orthopaedic specialists is in decline.

The Patient Protection and Affordable Care Act

Access to orthopaedic specialty care in the outpatient setting varies by region depending on many factors, including the density of providers, the geographical location, and patient health insurance status. The Patient Protection and Affordable Care Act, commonly called the Affordable Care Act (ACA), was signed into law in 2010.[4] The primary goal of the ACA is to reduce the

Dr. Neiman or an immediate family member is a member of a speakers' bureau or has made paid presentations on behalf of Medtronic, serves as an unpaid consultant to the Orthopaedic Implant Company, and has stock or stock options held in the Orthopaedic Implant Company. Neither Dr. Mallon nor any immediate family member has received anything of value from or has stock or stock options held in a commercial company or institution related directly or indirectly to the subject of this chapter.

financial barriers to health care for all citizens. Unlike elective surgery with its requisite preauthorization process, trauma surgery does not have a protocol for insurance approval before intervention. Theoretically, if a higher percentage of the population is insured, trauma centers should benefit.

Massachusetts was the first state whose health care system instituted health care reform and served as a model for the ACA. After the introduction of health care reform in Massachusetts, the three level I trauma centers in Boston saw a 40% reduction in the risk of treating uninsured individuals. Additionally, uncompensated care decreased from 17% to 11.5%. Moreover, mortality in the state has declined since the implementation of health care reform. These reductions were most evident in the poorest counties.[5]

To contain health care costs, the ACA aims to shift to value-based reimbursement. The goal is to deliver the highest quality of care at the lowest possible cost. The model developed to achieve this goal is the Accountable Care Organization (ACO), which is a network of physicians and hospitals created to share the burden of delivering care for a group of patients. Another provision of the ACA is the Independent Payment Advisory Board (IPAB.) This 15-member panel has the task of slowing the increases in health care spending. The IPAB has the authority to cut Medicare spending should its targets fail to be reached. Medicare cuts could limit access to musculoskeletal care and therefore is a potential concern.

Additionally, the ACA shifts the burden of collecting and reporting quality indicators to physicians, increases the medical device tax by 2.3%, and incentivizes physicians to comply with Medicare guidelines through the "meaningful use" of electronic health records. The ACA attempts to fundamentally shift health care from a volume-centered payment system to a patient-centered, outcome-driven system. This paradigm shift could affect orthopaedic surgeons greatly, particularly those caring for traumatized patients. Trauma patients have considerable variability in injury mechanisms and patterns. Reporting quality indicators will be the responsibility of physicians. The most appropriate trauma care may not be within the geographic location of a patient's ACO, which will make outcome reporting challenging for the practitioner.[6]

The ACA has resulted in an expansion of Medicaid services in most states. With this shift has come a relative shortage of specialty providers, including orthopaedic surgeons, who have not enrolled as providers in some of the Medicaid plans. Therefore, when patients are referred to an orthopaedic specialist for an acute or subacute injury, their insurance status may still be a barrier to access.[7] This circumstance creates a cycle in which injured patients must return to the emergency department, increasing the number of visits to the emergency department and ultimately increasing costs. These patients are generally more successful in obtaining a specialty referral when referred from an emergency department, partly because of contractual obligations between hospitals and orthopaedic call groups and partly because of laws ensuring that emergency treatment does not depend on insurance status.[8]

The Emergency Medical Treatment and Active Labor Act

Emergency department visits have risen steadily over the past 15 years since patients were guaranteed medical attention under the Emergency Medical Treatment and Active Labor Act (EMTALA) in 1986. EMTALA requires emergency care physicians to evaluate and stabilize all patients regardless of their ability to pay, and hospitals must provide specialist care or arrange transfer when specialist care is unavailable. This requirement creates the potential for abuse, because hospitals that do not have continuous specialty coverage could transfer patients based on their inability to secure an orthopaedic surgeon. Even when a particular hospital has busy and active orthopaedic surgeons, the emergency department is forced to transfer a patient to a facility with guaranteed coverage if the orthopaedic surgeons are not required to take emergency call and refuse to evaluate a particular patient. In some instances, this arrangement has been shown to preferentially occur with underinsured patients.[3,9]

Alternative Solutions for Orthopaedic Call Coverage

More orthopaedic emergencies are occurring, but fewer orthopaedic surgeons are willing to take call.[3] If this trend continues, general surgeons may be enlisted for adequate orthopaedic call coverage. The American Association for the Surgery of Trauma has identified a shortage of coverage not only in orthopaedic surgery but also in general surgery, creating subspecialty fellowship training within general surgery called acute care surgery.[10] In addition to the components of general surgical acute care, which include emergency surgery, critical care surgery, and trauma surgery, criteria exist for fellowships that include elective training in basic orthopaedic procedures. Currently, 19 American Association for the Surgery of Trauma–accredited fellowships are available in the United States. The acute care surgery fellowship curriculum recommends learning techniques of emergency extremity surgery, including vascular repair, fasciotomies, débridements, joint and fracture reduction, and the application of traction pins.

Like the positions of the internal medicine hospitalist and subsequently the general surgery surgicalist, the position of the orthopaedic hospitalist has developed because hospitals have engaged physicians and groups willing to provide continuous orthopaedic coverage for all inpatient needs. The predominant subspecialty group providing this service is the orthopaedic traumatologist, because the need for transfer in community hospitals revolves around complex hip and fragility fractures, periprosthetic fractures, nonunions, and osteomyelitis, all of which are within the technical scope of a traumatologist. Although still outnumbered by traditional call panels, these hospitalist services are increasing in popularity across the country.[11]

The response to this development within the medical community is mixed, but hospitals and emergency department providers are satisfied with the continuity of coverage. The orthopaedic trauma community is less enthusiastic about this paradigm shift in treatment. Some surgeons even assert that the experienced trauma surgeon is being replaced with young inexperienced surgeons at the expense of not only the experienced surgeons but also the surrounding community. Some surgeons think that the orthopaedic surgeon has become commoditized, because hospital systems value price over experience.[12,13] As this evolution occurs, orthopaedic surgeons need to be more active in local hospital administration to help establish the quality metrics that emphasize the favorable effect of the experienced physician on the quality of patient care.

Trauma System Models

Trauma hospitals in the United States were created initially out of need, providing a network of centers spread out geographically to meet the demands of patients requiring emergency care. Over the decades, this system has evolved from a collection of independent centers into a coordinated network of hospitals offering different levels of care. A major goal of the creation of the trauma center network is to provide nationwide level I trauma care within a 60-minute transport time. Although the number of trauma centers has increased dramatically, most are concentrated in urban settings, having little effect on transport time. At the same time, some remote rural areas of the country still lack 911 emergency coverage.[14,15]

To become a trauma center, hospitals purport a need and work toward the goal within their local county medical societies. Each state assigns a designation level depending on the needs of the locale and the services the hospital is capable of providing. At least 1,100 designated trauma centers exist in the United States.[11]

The American College of Surgeons (ACS) has established high standards for trauma centers. Only after these standards are met through the ACS process does a hospital become a verified trauma center. Currently, more than 400 ACS-verified trauma centers exist. Such level I trauma centers require orthopaedic trauma care to be overseen by an Orthopaedic Trauma Association–approved and fellowship-trained orthopaedic traumatologist.[1]

As the number of trauma centers increases, so does controversy over whether the recently established centers are designated and verified in locations that most appropriately serve the needs of the patient and the trauma community. The allocation of trauma centers should be based on the needs of the population rather than on the needs of individual health care organizations or hospital groups.[16] In certain urban environments, large health care organizations have created trauma centers for a variety of questionable reasons. They may cite patient need, but may be motivated instead by issues of secondary gain, including a reduction in the number of trauma patients they would lose in transfer and an increase in the number that they repatriate back into their medical systems. These organizations receive a share of public funds allocated for trauma care. Within orthopaedic trauma, it has been shown that a dedicated trauma center brings considerable downstream revenue to the hospital through surgical care and the many ancillary services required during the course of such care.[17]

Given the large numbers of ACS level II and III trauma hospitals in urban settings, two phenomena have been observed. First, the central level I center sees fewer trauma patients, adversely affecting their training programs and reducing the number of patients available to residents and fellows. Second, emergency department throughput may be improved by the shift to other nearby centers, reducing the treatment time for injured patients in that center. In the newly established level II and III centers, similar opposing phenomena exist. Bringing a severely injured patient to a trauma center not fully prepared for complex orthopaedic or other subspecialty care necessitates transfer to a nearby level I or II hospital better equipped for these patients. The outcome for the patient can potentially be influenced for the better.[18-20] Having outlying trauma centers still accomplishes a reduction in the initial treatment time, which is beneficial for most injuries. Careful triage in the field before transport can reduce the number of second transports. Most patients are injured close to home or work, and the impact on families is reduced when the hospitalized patients are nearby. Families can offer more support to the injured patient without having to travel long distances, which could preclude their ability to provide that support. With the existence of additional level II and III hospitals, patients often can be repatriated back to the lower level trauma centers for secondary orthopaedic and other procedures as required later, when the patient is stable, thereby reducing the burden on the level I tertiary care centers.

Quality Improvement and Education

The ACS Committee on Trauma requires each trauma program to demonstrate a continuous process of monitoring, assessment, and management directed at improving care.[1] This process is called the Performance Improvement and Patient Safety (PIPS) Program. PIPS includes a written plan and an operational data system with the goal of improving the six aims of patient care: safe, effective, patient centered, timely, efficient, and equitable. The system includes regular internal peer review and regular external review and integration with the local and regional trauma system efforts. PIPS uses a model called the "Continuous Process of Performance Improvement." The steps involved begin with recognizing an area of improvement through data collection and collation, assessing the area through analysis, and then improving the area through modification and instruction. Trauma centers must be able to demonstrate a PIPS system, which requires internal and external oversight, local and regional integration, the authority to effect change, a trauma registry to collect data, and assurance that specific PIPS core measures are met within the trauma center. Quality improvement at trauma centers is bound inextricably to the quality of care that is delivered to patients, and it requires a dedicated system to make improvements effectively while minimizing bureaucratic interference.

The individual orthopaedic surgeons integrated into a hospital's trauma system must participate in these programs, because it is necessary for all subspecialties to improve care, not just for the trauma coordinators and medical directors. Continuing education for the orthopaedist is a career-long requirement for licensure and the maintenance of board certification and hospital privileges, but it must include education in trauma care to satisfy the requirements of the ACS and PIPS.

Disaster and Mass-Casualty Planning

According to the ACS, the surgical community has an obligation to be actively involved in disaster and mass-casualty planning at all levels, including those of the local, state, and federal government. As a result, trauma centers are required to have hospital disaster plans and biannual drills that integrate local hospitals and emergency services. Hospitals must exert substantial effort to develop these systems and to coordinate drills, but they are required to be aggressive about disaster and mass-casualty management, because disasters are not uncommon. The Federal Emergency Management Agency (FEMA) declared 334 disasters between 2010 and 2014. In 2010 alone, 9,913 unique mass-casualty incidents (MCIs) occurred, involving an estimated 13,677 MCI patients according to the National EMS Database of the National Emergency Medical Services Information System.[20] Although the magnitude of an individual event may not be high, designating an event as a disaster or MCI indicates that the local services are overburdened and require more resources.[20]

When an emergency occurs, the state governor declares a state of emergency that activates an emergency response at the state level. If the governor determines that the local and state resources are insufficient, FEMA will be notified. FEMA performs a preliminary assessment and reports back to the governor. The governor submits a letter asking the President to declare the event a disaster and uses the FEMA report as evidence to support the request. When the President declares a disaster, FEMA determines which federal programs are most appropriate to manage the disaster.

As with a disaster declaration, the declaration of an MCI is based on resources. An MCI declaration indicates that the number, severity, or diversity of injuries overwhelms the local medical resources. No numeric formula exists for this designation, but a lower-level trauma facility will be overwhelmed much sooner than a larger facility. The frequency with which these events occur highlights the importance of trauma centers having a thorough plan to cope with disaster and mass casualties.

A disaster plan enables hospitals and local emergency services to operate within a predictable chain of command and provides organization, checklists, accountability, and a common language to ensure that outside assistance is coordinated with internal resources. The plan should outline a protocol by which first responders triage patients, hospitals prepare for an influx of patients, and the local, state, and national governments can mobilize resources effectively. The protocols may be unfamiliar to many orthopaedic surgeons until an MCI occurs, so the job of the local medical directors and chiefs of staff is to engage the local physicians during routine drills to familiarize them with the process.[1,21]

Triaging patients involves the concept of doing the greatest good for the greatest number. Overtriage is defined as treating too many patients with minor injuries and undertriage is defined as delaying the care of critically injured patients who may benefit from immediate treatment. Triage should begin at the scene, and hospitals should begin to prepare by planning to increase their bed capacity by at least 20% during an MCI. The expected case distribution should be 20% severely injured patients, 30% moderately injured patients, and 50% patients who may be treated surgically in a delayed manner.

At the state and national levels, broader resources and requirements exist. A governor can mobilize the National Guard. An organization known as the National Disaster Medical System partners private organizations with governmental entities. FEMA is perhaps the best-known federal agency that plays a role in disaster management. A key factor in preparedness is to integrate the entire community, including public health agencies, the police, search and rescue units, the media, and the military. The Orthopaedic Trauma Association has established alignments with the American Academy of Orthopaedic Surgeons and the Society of Military Orthopaedic Surgeons to begin educating orthopaedic surgeons in disaster response.

When disasters and MCIs occur, the trauma center is an integral component of the system. Trauma centers are mandated to have a disaster plan and to ensure that the most good can be brought to the greatest number of people through communication, cost containment, and management. If the availability of acute care orthopaedic surgeons continues to decline, the already challenging task of providing proper care in this environment will be strained even further.

Summary

The delivery of orthopaedic trauma and acute care in the United States is complex. The evolution and expansion of high-quality trauma centers require surgeons to adapt and function in an evolving system to deliver excellent patient-centered care to a community. Orthopaedic trauma surgeons are charged with becoming experts in complex data-gathering processes, internal and external reviews and oversight, cost-containment strategies, and planning with local, state, and federal governmental branches. It is incumbent on all orthopaedic surgeons to do their part in serving their communities by cooperating with the trauma systems, while continuing to refine and develop their clinical skills as acute care orthopaedic surgeons. All orthopaedic surgeons must receive and maintain adequate training to remain proficient in the delivery of acute care and to develop an understanding of their role in the trauma systems in which they practice. It is the physician's responsibility to serve the needs of the community in addition to the needs of the medical practice. Patients deserve expert care irrespective of who is on call.

Key Study Points

- Patient access to emergent orthopaedic care is a dynamic entity, limited in some areas by physician call panel availability.
- The Patient Protection and Affordable Care Act of 2010 will have a varying effect on access to orthopaedic care in the United States. The costs of emergency orthopaedic care may decline, because fewer patients are expected to be uninsured, although access to nonurgent orthopaedic trauma care may remain limited unless additional orthopaedic surgeons enroll as Medicaid providers.
- The establishment of networked trauma systems has evolved, and additional designated trauma centers are being added yearly. This development may improve the coordination of disaster planning and mass-casualty treatment if orthopaedic trauma surgeons become involve in leadership at the local hospital level.

Annotated References

1. Rotondo MF, C. Cribari C, Smith SS: The Committee on Trauma, American College of Surgeons: Resources for Optimal Care of the Injured Patient 2014 (v. 1.1). Chicago: American College of Surgeons. 2014. Available at: https://www.facs.org/~/media/files/quality%20programs/trauma/vrc%20resources/resources%20for%20optimal%20care%202014%20v11.ashx. Accessed February 8, 2016.

   The ACS publishes a resource guide for trauma centers that includes guidelines required during the verification process.

2. National Hospital Ambulatory Medical Care Survey: 2011 Emergency Department Summary Tables. Tables 1, 4, 14, 24. 2011. Available at: http://www.cdc.gov/nchs/data/ahcd/nhamcs_emergency/2011_ed_web_tables.pdf. Accessed February 8, 2016.

   The Centers for Disease Control and Prevention provides data on emergency department visits and compares them with prior years' surveys.

3. Cantu RV, Bell JE, Padula WV, Nahikian KR, Pober DM: How do emergency department physicians rate their orthopaedic on-call coverage? *J Orthop Trauma* 2012;26(1):54-56.

   The authors surveyed a small group of emergency departments and found that approximately one-half of the time, departments did not have adequate orthopaedic coverage at night or on weekends.

1: General Topics

4. Patient Protection and Affordable Care Act, 42 U.S.C. § 18001 (2010). Available at: https://www.gpo.gov/fdsys/pkg/PLAW-111publ148/html/PLAW-111publ148.htm

The ACA was signed into law in 2010 to improve the quality and affordability of health insurance. It was intended to lower the uninsured rate by expanding insurance coverage and to reduce the costs of health care for individuals and the government.

5. Harris MB: Massachusetts health care reform and orthopaedic trauma: Lessons learned. *J Orthop Trauma* 2014;28(suppl 10):S20-S22.

The authors reviewed the experiences of three of the four level I trauma centers in Boston with the Massachusetts version of the ACA. They found a dramatic reduction in the proportion of uninsured orthopaedic trauma patients, as well as a reduction in the proportion of uncompensated care.

6. Issar NM, Jahangir AA: The Affordable Care Act and orthopaedic trauma. *J Orthop Trauma* 2014;28(suppl 10):S5-S7.

The authors reviewed how the ACA restructures the health care insurance market and delivery system. They reviewed the effect these changes will have on orthopaedic traumatologists.

7. Patterson BM, Draeger RW, Olsson EC, Spang JT, Lin FC, Kamath GV: A regional assessment of Medicaid access to outpatient orthopaedic care: The influence of population density and proximity to academic medical centers on patient access. *J Bone Joint Surg Am* 2014;96(18):e156.

The authors selected orthopaedic practices and made fictitious appointments for a few specific problems. Differences in wait time for an appointment were noted, based on whether the fictional patient had Medicaid or private insurance. Access to orthopaedic care was reduced substantially for patients on Medicaid.

8. Rhodes KV, Bisgaier J, Lawson CC, Soglin D, Krug S, Van Haitsma M: "Patients who can't get an appointment go to the ER": Access to specialty care for publicly insured children. *Ann Emerg Med* 2013;61(4):394-403.

In this study, children who were referred from a primary care physician to specialty care had considerable barriers to accessing specialists when they were ensured through Medicaid. The more effective means to attain referral was through the emergency department.

9. Kao DP, Martin MH, Das AK, Ruoss SJ: Consequences of federal patient transfer regulations: Effect of the 2003 EMTALA revision on a tertiary referral center and evidence of possible misuse. *Arch Intern Med* 2012;172(11):891-892.

The authors reviewed more than 25,000 diagnoses and transfers from various hospitals over an 8-year period. They found that, for certain diagnoses, transfer was more likely to occur in the underinsured patient, especially from certain hospitals.

10. Duane TM, Dente CJ, Fildes JJ, et al: Defining the acute care surgery curriculum. *J Trauma Acute Care Surg* 2015;78(2):259-263, discussion 263-264.

The authors describe the origins of the Acute Care Surgery specialty training and its evolving curriculum. Although its focus is on general surgical trauma and acute care procedures, the curriculum lists desired cases including extremity procedures such as reductions, placement of traction, fasciotomies, and amputations.

11. Agnew SG, Warren BJ: Orthopaedic trauma career and employment horizons: Identification of career destinations and opportunities. *J Orthop Trauma* 2012;26(suppl 1):S18-S20.

The authors identified multiple practice patterns currently available to the orthopaedist.

12. Hill A, Althausen PL, O'Mara TJ, Bray TJ: Why veteran orthopaedic trauma surgeons are being fired and what we can do about it? *J Orthop Trauma* 2013;27(6):355-362.

The authors addressed the problems associated with hospital-based orthopaedic trauma care and reviewed the value contributed by the surgeon to the trauma system in which they work.

13. Bray TJ: Orthopaedic Traumatology: More than a "surgicalist": Modified with permission from American Academy of Orthopaedic Surgeons. AAOS Now 2013, volume 7, number 6. *J Orthop Trauma* 2013;27(8):425-427.

The author described his position regarding the changes in the delivery of orthopaedic care, warning of the potential pitfalls associated with the surgicalist model.

14. Institute of Medicine: *Preparedness and Response to a Rural Mass Casualty Incident: Workshop Summary.* Washington, DC, The National Academies Press, 2011.

In examining specific mass-casualty incidents in the United States, the Institute of Medicine has identified geographic areas that are deficient in emergency coverage. Existing technology was reviewed and opportunities for improvement were identified and explored.

15. Branas CC, MacKenzie EJ, Williams JC, et al: Access to trauma centers in the United States. *JAMA* 2005;293(21):2626-2633.

16. American College of Surgeons, Statement on trauma center designation based upon system need, *ACS Bulletin,* Jan 1, 2015. Available at: http://bulletin.facs.org/2015/01/statement-on-trauma-center-designation-based-upon-system-need/. Accessed on February 8, 2016.

The ACS website contains periodic bulletins on relevant topics in trauma and acute care. This bulletin explains that increasing the number of trauma centers should be achieved based on patient need, not based on the need for the center to recoup patients.

17. Althausen PL, Coll D, Cvitash M, Herak A, O'Mara TJ, Bray TJ: Economic viability of a community-based level-II orthopaedic trauma system. *J Bone Joint Surg Am* 2009;91(1):227-235.

18. Demetriades D, Martin M, Salim A, Rhee P, Brown C, Chan L: The effect of trauma center designation and trauma volume on outcome in specific severe injuries. *Ann Surg* 2005;242(4):512-517, discussion 517-519.

19. Caputo LM, Salottolo KM, Slone DS, Mains CW, Bar-Or D: The relationship between patient volume and mortality in American trauma centres: A systematic review of the evidence. *Injury* 2014;45(3):478-486.

    This cohort did not observe any benefit of volume or designation for outcomes in severely injured patients. Level of evidence: I.

20. Schenk E, Wijetunge G, Mann NC, Lerner EB, Longthorne A, Dawson D: Epidemiology of mass casualty incidents in the United States. *Prehosp Emerg Care* 2014;18(3):408-416.

    This statistical report investigated the number of mass-casualty incidents in the United States during 2010. The authors used data from the National EMS Database of the National Emergency Medical Services Information System. Level of evidence: III.

21. Joint Commission Resources, Inc.: *Emergency Management in Health Care: An All-Hazards Approach* .Oak Brook, IL, Joint Commission Resources, 2012.

    This Joint Commission primer outlined the many facets of a functioning emergency response team, including managing resources and establishing leadership roles within the hospital system.

Career and Practice Management in Orthopaedic Trauma

Yvonne Murtha, MD

Abstract

Practice concerns of an orthopaedic traumatologist are unique within the field of orthopaedics. A singular relationship exists between the orthopaedic traumatologist and the facility in which he or she operates. The surgeon relies on the facility to supply the platform from which the craft of orthopaedic traumatology may be practiced, and the hospital relies on the orthopaedic traumatologist to maintain trauma certification and run a trauma program. Establishing and maintaining a career within the field of orthopaedic trauma requires the hospital and surgeon to create and sustain the relationship to accomplish the goals of both parties.

Keywords: orthopaedic trauma; contract; practice types; practice resources

Introduction

Fracture care constitutes a considerable burden of disease within the United States. It is estimated that annually nearly 47% of trauma admissions—almost 1 million patients—in the United States sustain an orthopaedic injury. When surveyed, orthopaedic traumatologists identified nearly half of all traumas accompanied by orthopaedic injuries to be complex enough to benefit from the services of a physician with specialized training and interest in the field of orthopaedic traumatology.[1] The availability of orthopaedic surgeons to cover call and assume responsibility for fracture patients has become increasingly important as hospitals organize into trauma centers and attempt to verify trauma certification. Although the need for orthopaedic trauma coverage exists at these centers, several barriers to access have developed. The increasing number of underfunded patients seeking care for musculoskeletal injuries, the rising practice overhead costs, and the declining number of orthopaedic surgeons who are comfortable taking trauma call emphasize the continued need for orthopaedic specialists with advanced training in fracture care to be supported by the hospitals and communities they serve.[2] Employment as an orthopaedic trauma surgeon continues to be a viable option for those completing fellowship training in orthopaedic traumatology.

The establishment of a trauma facility verified by the American College of Surgeons (ACS) and the addition of a fellowship-trained orthopaedic traumatologist to the facility benefits the entire community. Patient survival rates increase, length of stay declines within trauma systems,[3,4] and transfer to hospitals farther away from family support can be avoided. Hospitals benefit by more efficiently using the resources of orthopaedic traumatologists rather than those of general orthopaedic surgeons. Given similar fracture cases, traumatologists achieve shorter surgical times and lower implant charges as compared with general orthopaedic surgeons, which creates cost savings for the institution.[5] Not only do traumatologists reduce the cost of fracture care, but they also increase the facility's revenue capture. Traumatologists are less likely to transfer patients from their facilities and are more likely to treat fracture cases at the hospital rather than at an ambulatory surgery center.[6] Local orthopaedic surgeons are freed from the burden of care for fracture patients, allowing them to develop and grow practices that are substantially more rewarding financially.[7] Orthopaedic traumatologists realize benefits in these systems as well, however. Trauma centers provide a platform for fracture surgeons to practice a skill set that interests them and can provide support for the creation of a successful and sustainable trauma practice.

Dr. Murtha or an immediate family member serves as a board member, owner, officer, or committee member of the American Academy of Orthopaedic Surgeons.

Surgeon and Facility Considerations

After training is completed, choosing a practice arrangement that best fits the traumatologist's career aspirations and expectations is of primary importance. Orthopaedic trauma surgeons and trauma facilities can form symbiotic relationships through the creation and maintenance of an orthopaedic trauma service. In addition to providing a high level of patient care, meeting the needs of the surgeon and the hospital is a key goal of the professional relationship between these parties. Hospital goals typically are financially driven. They include cost containment through the delivery of efficient care and maximizing revenue potential. Hospitals also must establish and maintain trauma verification by the state or the ACS. When constructing practice arrangements, surgeons should focus on not only their financial expectations but also their long-term professional and career goals. Both parties must be willing work together. The professional relationship between the surgeon and the facility is created within a negotiated framework that is transparent and appropriately outlines the needs of all parties as well as the agreed-upon rewards for meeting defined metrics.

Longevity in orthopaedic trauma is the goal of every surgeon and should be supported by the facility and the practice partners. Burnout from the lack of general trauma surgeon and service line support and the creation of a trauma model that lacks long-term vision can create an environment that is not sustainable. A clear understanding by the surgeon and the hospital of the essential elements required to maintain a well-functioning trauma system is vital (**Table 1**). Transparent, nonadversarial negotiations facilitate the development of an agreement between the surgeon and the hospital, which is critical to the long-term success of the relationship. Strategies for achieving career sustainability within the field of trauma should be considered from the beginning of the communication process. Although short-term goals are important, a lack of vision for the future will ensure the lack of any future, or one that is less than fulfilling for all parties and increases the chances of system collapse.

Practice Selection

The orthopaedic traumatologist generally practices his or her craft within a hospital system. For this reason, the hospital's trauma-level verification and designation is an important consideration for the traumatologist. It will determine the type of practice a physician can build within that particular setting. A hospital's patient volume, injury severity, and patient mix can vary considerably between facilities. The adequacy of the trauma center's resources and the ability to manage trauma transfers and admissions are verified using the guidelines established by the Committee on Trauma of the ACS.[8] Increasing levels of system support are required to treat and manage patients with increasingly complex injuries. Trauma centers are designated level I to level IV, with level I facilities able to accept the most complex patients. Regional trauma networks are constructed, and trauma center designations are determined by governmental bodies based on the needs of the surrounding populations. The hospital's trauma-level designation indicates the support services that are available within the facility as well as the training of the orthopaedic traumatologist. The orthopaedic care of trauma patients within level 1 facilities must be "overseen by an individual who has completed a fellowship in orthopaedic traumatology as approved by the Orthopaedic Trauma Association" (OTA).[9] Other facility requirements include operating room availability, the presence of other medical services, including plastic surgery, neurosurgery, and vascular surgery, and the availability of radiology technicians, operating room staff, and therapy services. Geographical considerations can determine the volume of blunt or penetrating trauma seen as well as the payer mix.

Opportunity for practice growth and the development of a trauma niche or nontrauma focus should be considered when evaluating a practice opportunity. The needs of the trauma facility, its relationship with local orthopaedic practices, the trauma volume, projections for trauma activations, and the numbers of specific injury types seen will affect the feasibility of the development of a trauma niche or the growth of a nontrauma-related practice opportunity. The cultivation of surgical interest beyond the scope of the trauma practice can have a positive effect on the surgeon's value to the hospital by augmenting the volume of patients with health insurance the surgeon treats at the facility. If the surgeon desires the development of a niche or nontrauma practice, the regional market conditions for that type of practice must be considered. The practice environment, including the hospital and potential partners or local orthopaedic surgeons, must support the traumatologist in developing this niche. Trauma operating room coverage by other orthopaedic surgeons can be negotiated. Referrals of patients whose orthopaedic needs fit the nontrauma interests of the traumatologist should be discussed with the hospital and the local orthopaedic practices. If the local orthopaedic surgeons are not aware of the nontrauma orthopaedic interests of the traumatologist, they may view an attempt to cultivate a practice beyond the scope of trauma as an intrusion that could lead to an acrimonious relationship.

Practice opportunities generally are considered private practice or academic practice models. Both types allow

Table 1

Orthopaedic Trauma Service Needs

Hospital-based support staff
OR staff with knowledge of orthopaedic equipment and use
Radiology technicians with experience and training in the intraoperative use of the C-arm in orthopaedic cases
Physician extenders who can see and treat emergency department patients, make rounds on inpatients, and assist in surgical cases during regular hours and when the surgeon is on call
Floor nurses with orthopaedic background
Oversight of ongoing training and evaluation of hospital staff
Orthopaedic trauma room with staff available 24 hours a day, 7 days a week for urgent and emergent cases
Orthopaedic OR available for nonemergent surgical cases 3 to 5 days a week without normal release constraints
Continuing medical education support for physicians and staff
Salaried Medical Director of Orthopaedic Trauma
Participation in verification of state or ACS trauma program
Oversight of call schedule
Involvement in equipment purchases
Participation in orthopaedic implant selection and cost schedule
Morbidity and mortality review for service line
Development and oversight of protocols for transfer of definitive orthopaedic care to the orthopaedic trauma service
Hospital-based clinic for coverage of funded and underfunded patients
Adequate and regular support staff including nursing, billers/coders, administrative support, radiology technicians, and orthopaedic technicians
Appropriate facilities, time allocation, and equipment
Vacation, sick, and continuing education leave with coverage of patients and practice

ACS = American College of Surgeons; OR = operating room

hospital employment or partnership within a group. Private employment models include multispecialty groups, orthopaedic specialty groups, subspecialization of orthopaedic traumatologists, and solo practice. Remuneration within private practice typically involves a base salary with incentive pay based on a productivity metric, collections, or a hybrid of both. Academic practice often has a similar pay structure with additional expectations and financial incentives based on academic output, including attainment of tenure, publication, teaching, committee memberships, and administrative involvement. Each type of practice has its own benefits and pitfalls that must be considered carefully.

Contract Structure

When entering into contract negotiations for a professional service agreement with a hospital and/or a private practice group, physicians typically have insufficient experience and tend to have a shortsighted focus on financial remuneration and little else. Certainly, financial considerations play an important role in brokering an agreement, but other factors must be taken into consideration. The professional service agreement between the hospital or private practice and the trauma surgeon not only can reward the surgeon financially, but it also can increase the likelihood that the job evolves into a healthy, long-term relationship that is beneficial for all parties. The physician has the greatest amount of leverage to obtain demands during negotiations for the first contract. For this reason, careful consideration should be given to the maintenance of a trauma service line. Nothing is guaranteed unless it is put into writing; therefore, anything considered critical to the success of the trauma service line should be included in the contract.

Specific deadlines for satisfying requests and material consequences when promises are not kept are essential inclusions. If deadlines and consequences for failure to meet expectations are not outlined, physicians can find themselves left with empty promises and distrust. The surgeon's professional, financial, and personal costs are high if the relationship fails. Knowing what to ask for up front can increase the chances of success. When final contract negotiations are entered, obtaining legal advice from professionals familiar with medical contract negotiations is recommended.

A basic personal service agreement will set a term, or period of time, during which the contract is in effect and will include stipulations if the contract does expire or terminate prematurely. Either party can terminate a contract for "just cause." Specific reasons for just-cause termination often are related to a physician's inability to practice medicine. These grounds typically are itemized in the contract and include failure to maintain state medical or drug- prescribing licensure, Drug Enforcement Administration licensure, board certification, hospital privileges, or malpractice insurance. Conversely, either party also can terminate a contract without a reason, or "without cause." The physician should ensure that, in the case of termination without cause, the contract stipulates a reasonable notification period, appropriate severance pay, forgiveness of liabilities, and benefit extension, as well as control over language in future references. Re-employment may take several months to achieve, given the current licensure and accreditation processes. During that time, the surgeon will have no source of income. The length of time a physician may be left without pay should be considered when negotiating the specifics of any severance package.

Contracts that come to term can be renewed in one of two ways. Upon completion of the contract's term, it can be configured to automatically renew without renegotiation, unless one party objects. Other contracts will automatically expire, unless both parties agree to a renewal and the terms of renewal. If a contract is allowed to expire or is terminated, the physician may be constrained from practicing within a geographical area if a "covenant not to compete" or "noncompete" clause is a part of the contract. This provision is a time-limited restriction on the physician's ability to practice the given specialty in a geographically defined area. Enforceability of this clause can vary, depending on the state and the contract language. Alternatively, a nonsolicitation clause may be used. These clauses tend to be less restrictive because they do not prohibit practicing within a geographical area. They can limit the physician's ability to recruit previous staff, partners, or patients to their new practice location, however. If the surgeon provides trauma coverage to a community, he or she can request that these clauses not be included.

Financial Benefits

Compensation agreements include salary, call stipend, a production bonus structure, moving expenses, and signing bonuses. Depending on the structure of the employment agreement, salary and benefits can be considered a loan, with production bonuses held until the loan is repaid in full by the withholding of collections made above a guaranteed base or by forgiveness over a predetermined time period. Various entities are available to assist in determining a fair market value for an orthopaedic trauma surgeon in a particular region. The Medical Group Management Association can provide useful information regarding salaries and productivity benchmarks for specific specialties.[10] Some data must be purchased, but the information can be well worth the price. An understanding of the value of the surgeon's services on an open market can give the surgeon increased bargaining power during the negotiation process.

For traumatologists whose salaries depend on productivity metrics, achieving bonuses can hinge on factors beyond the realm of the surgeons' control. Traumatologists care for a high percentage of patients who are underfunded. The collections of a trauma practice with a high percentage of underfunded patients will be more limited than those of an elective orthopaedic practice. This fact must be taken into consideration when negotiating call stipends and productivity bonuses, not just salary. Depending on the design of the trauma service, the traumatologist also may assume the care of patients admitted or discharged from the emergency department during other nontrauma surgeons' calls. This situation can further force the trauma surgeon to see a considerably higher number of underfunded patients than surgeons in the community who have elective practices. A surgeon's hospital support should include payment for the treatment of underfunded patients.

Various resources are available that can fund indigent care. The collection of trauma activation fees are used in some centers to cover the trauma call stipend as well as physician fees billed for indigent care.[11] These activation fees are charged to cover the operational expenses incurred from trauma activations, and the amount varies by center and patient level of acuity. Most of the financial burden for these fees falls on private insurers. Even without charge variations between private and government insurers, facilities are able to maintain profitability.[12] When compared to orthopaedic traumatologists, facilities also can collect a substantially higher portion of their trauma patient billings, making financial support of the surgeon by the hospital seem logical.[13] The federal government also provides support to trauma facilities through Medicare and Medicaid Disproportionate Share Healthcare (DSH) programs, although the availability of these dollars may depend on health care legislation, as will be discussed later.

Compensation based on objective measurements of productivity and quality is an appropriate means of remuneration for a trauma surgeon. Medicare assigns work Relative Value Units (wRVUs) to various physician-patient encounters that act as a measure of productivity. Although wRVUs have some usefulness in this regard, the surgeon also must understand the shortcomings of this unit of measurement in trauma. Because of the unique nature of many injuries and the overall complexity of the severely injured trauma patient, fracture care can require substantially longer surgical times than elective procedures having similar wRVU values, thus decreasing apparent productivity. Urgent and emergent procedures also require closer surgical follow-up, necessitate longer hospital stays, and can be burdened by higher complication rates than elective procedures, thereby adding to the underweighted wRVU measurement in trauma care.[14] Multiple procedure discounts also serve to underrepresent a traumatologists' productivity. Not uncommonly, trauma patients sustain several musculoskeletal injuries requiring different procedures to address each injury. When possible, these procedures can be performed during the same surgical encounter to optimally care for the patient and improve system efficiency. When multiple procedures are performed under the same anesthetic, a discounted value is given to each subsequent procedure. This substantially reduces not only the surgeon's compensation but also the apparent productivity, despite the benefit to the patient and the system. If possible, the trauma surgeon should participate in the process of determining insurance fee schedules for fracture care and the reduction of these discounts.

In an employed physician model, aggregate benefits can amount to substantial reimbursement beyond salary. Employers can offer malpractice, life, and disability insurance, as well as retirement savings plans, paid vacation, sick leave and educational days, support for licensing and professional fees, business-related travel expenses, and coverage of practice marketing costs. Malpractice insurance that follows a claims-made model also will require the purchase of tail insurance for continued coverage if the physician should leave a practice. Tail coverage can be onerous and should be negotiated as a benefit of the personal service agreement, particularly if a contract is not renewed or is terminated prematurely by the other party.

Call and Service Structures

As expectations regarding work and life balance evolve, physicians entering the field of orthopaedic traumatology are placing lifestyle considerations at a premium. Call duties can be burdensome and can negatively affect the surgeon's life outside of work, but they do provide potential benefits. For the orthopaedic traumatologist, call provides an opportunity for revenue generation to help maintain a viable practice and allows patient access to physicians with highly specialized skills in trauma. A healthy balance that avoids burnout and equitably distributes call among those on the trauma call panel can be achieved. The number of weekday, weekend, and holiday call coverage days that are expected should be defined in the contract. To achieve a sustainable schedule and provide optimal patient care, call burden should be distributed equitably among the surgeons on the trauma call panel. An agreement can be made that allows the orthopaedic surgeons to take call, particularly during nights, weekends, and holidays, and subsequently transfer patients to the trauma service during regular hours. In this type of arrangement, patient care obligations and handoff expectations should be defined explicitly to avoid lapses in patient care.

Financial remuneration for the care of patients transferred from other orthopaedic surgeons' call coverage, particularly patients in postoperative care global periods, should be considered as part of the negotiation. Call stipends should cover operational overhead expenses incurred while taking call. Defining what referrals the call person is responsible for treating limits the preferential treatment of certain patients by physicians not taking call. The pool of referred patients can include trauma activations, emergency department visits, outside facility referrals, and inpatient consultations with musculoskeletal injuries. The scope of orthopaedic care should be defined to include or exclude pediatric, hand, and spine injuries, depending on the scope of practice of the orthopaedic traumatologist. Coverage of patient calls and inpatient care responsibilities during leave and weekends off also should be defined.

Ancillary Support

Building and maintaining an orthopaedic traumatology practice requires a team effort. Adequate staffing resources for outpatient and inpatient care are necessary. Appropriate staff support in the hospital environment includes operating room staff, radiology technicians, floor nursing, casting technicians, coders and billers, and physician extenders who are familiar with orthopaedics and fracture care. Physician extenders, in particular, have been shown to improve the delivery of patient care and reduce costs.[15,16] The hospital's cost of employing physician extenders on the orthopaedic trauma service can be neutralized by the savings they incur in reducing length of stay, complications, time to the operating room, and wait times in the emergency department. In clinics, staff should be dedicated to the trauma service. Float staff or staff designated as "prn," whose skill level, orthopaedic knowledge, and interest are variable, do not facilitate patient care. Staff should include an administrative assistant, nurses, radiology technicians, and orthopaedic technicians. To ensure the maintenance of knowledge and skills, continuing education approved by the surgeon should be available and required on an ongoing basis for all hospital-employed staff. The physician should be involved in any recruitment of new staff hired during his or her tenure. Annual reviews should be conducted with surgeon involvement. If staff vacancies occur, an appropriate time for filling the position and a plan for coverage until the position is filled should be defined.

Facility Needs

Surgeons require an operating room to treat patients, and traumatologists have special needs for utilization and availability. The OTA recommends that a trauma room and staff personnel for emergent and urgent procedures should be available 24 hours a day, 7 days a week.[17] A dedicated daytime orthopaedic trauma room that is not subject to typical release rules or shared with other surgeons is vital. The availability of the operating room and the staff during regular business hours minimizes the habitual need for operating on evenings and weekends.[18] It also allows access to the operating room when staff familiar with orthopaedic trauma equipment and practices are available. Ensuring the presence of appropriately trained staff improves efficiency and reduces case length. The use of block times can be assessed to ensure that the resource allocation is appropriate, with modifications made as agreed on by the surgeon and operating room administrators. ACS verification of a hospital's trauma abilities depends on surgical room availability for trauma and fracture procedures. This fact can drive negotiations in the surgeon's favor when determining the room's availability.

Within the surgical theater, orthopaedic traumatologists use a gamut of specialized tools for patient positioning, fracture exposure, reduction, and fixation. A thorough inventory of hospital equipment used for fracture care should be performed. A list of required equipment, including everything from operating tables to reduction clamps should be submitted during contract negotiations. Depending on the cost of items requested, some items may have to be rescheduled for future budget cycles. If this is the case, needs should be ranked and guarantees should be made, with specifics for delivery dates and compensation if expectations are not met.

Orthopaedic implants contribute considerable cost to patient care. Surgeon participation in the selection of available implants is beneficial for the surgeon and the hospital. Including the surgeon in the decision-making process and making the costs of implants transparent encourages surgeon frugality. Only a minority of surgeons know the cost of implants, and few identify that knowledge as being "very" or "extremely" important.[19] Active participation by the surgeon in the cost containment of orthopaedic implants can be accomplished in various ways, including using more expensive technologies judiciously, using generic implants, and reusing implants.[20] These surgeon practices can achieve substantial cost savings, creating an opportunity for gain sharing in a manner that is legal and beneficial to the development of a robust trauma service line.

Depending on the nature of the physician-hospital relationship, the clinic space and staff may be provided by the hospital. In any practice setting, the physician should ensure that an adequate number of rooms, sufficient clinic time, and the appropriate equipment are available to treat patients. Access to radiographs, casting, and splinting supplies as well as some durable medical equipment availability are minimum requirements. Patients with an orthopaedic fracture often have limited mobility. Special rooms with wide doors that can accommodate wheelchairs, adjustable examination beds that drop and raise, rooms that facilitate the review of radiographic imaging, and access to electronic medical records should be essential elements of the office environment.

Ongoing administrative opportunities for which the trauma surgeon can claim a leadership role include the development, maintenance, and management of policies and protocols within the hospital trauma system, peer review, establishment of fracture care protocols, the development of a center of excellence, and ACS accreditation. Although rewarding, these administrative duties can require substantial time commitments. They fall outside of the scope of practice duties, such as charting, required for direct patient care and billing. Continued improvement of the trauma service can be achieved only if the trauma surgeon is involved in decision making and takes ownership of management responsibilities. These duties are structured in the form of a paid directorship position, with time specifically allotted in the physician's schedule for overseeing the trauma service line. As a director of the orthopaedic trauma service, the physician should be responsible for call schedule creation and can develop protocols to drive improvements in patient outcomes, reduce the cost of delivery of care, and improve the morale of staff involved in patient care. Metrics that should be monitored and recorded can include patient length of stays, delays to time of treatment, trauma service line employee retention, cost containment through implant selection and the appropriate use of resources, patient and family satisfaction, and the expansion of the fracture referral network. Gain sharing in the improved profitability of the hospital can be undertaken by ethical and legal means. Reinvesting in the trauma service line by adding resources, including research support and rewards for trauma service ancillary staff, can improve morale and subsequent retention.

Coding and Billing

The skills of personnel trained in coding and billing can improve a practice's revenue generation. Coders and billers should not be used as a replacement for the surgeon's involvement in the process, however. Surgeon familiarity with documentation requirements, as well as coding and billing, will increase the charges generated, reduce insurance denials, and increase collections. Residency training imparts only a cursory understanding of these critical practice issues, and most individuals complete a residency with little understanding of documentation and coding and billing practices. Most surgeons unfamiliar with such practices can benefit from attending coding and billing courses offered through the American Academy of Orthopaedic Surgeons and the OTA and from reviewing the literature of coding and billing practices.[21,22]

The mastery of patient encounter coding and billing in and out of the surgical theater improves the bottom line of an orthopaedic trauma practice. Surgical billing codes generate higher levels of wRVU than do codes assigned to evaluation and management and nonsurgical fracture care, but the billing of services for nonfracture care in aggregate can be a substantial source of revenue generation.[23] Providers spend a considerable amount of time in the care of patients outside of the surgical theater. A few examples of these encounters include consultations, admissions, new patient visits, and the nonsurgical management of fractures. That work productivity is lost unless the surgeon possesses a thorough understanding of the appropriate billing codes and the rules for their application. Surgical procedure coding and billing is more lucrative, but substantial potential exists for the loss of credit from inappropriate documentation, the lack or inappropriate use of modifiers, and deficient knowledge of Current Procedural Terminology codes and the corresponding International Classification of Diseases, Tenth Revision codes. The accurate use of these codes reduces denials and expedites payment for services.

Documentation is key to accurate billing and, when performed in a timely fashion, it also facilitates the submission of claims to payers, increasing the likelihood of being paid. An example of how timely submission of claims can affect collections is automobile insurance. Claims submitted to automobile insurance companies are paid in full on a first-come, first-served basis until the coverage is exhausted. If a health care claim is submitted after the insurance coverage is exhausted, the bill then goes to a third-party health insurance payer, if the patient is insured. Otherwise, the claim becomes unfunded patient care.

Effects of Legislation

Practice management concerns are evolving continually because of the passage of the Patient Protection and Affordable Care Act (PPACA) in 2010 and increasing government involvement in health care. It is imperative that physicians stay abreast of pending health care legislation and its effects on their own practices as well as on the hospital systems in which they treat their patients. The American Academy of Orthopaedic Surgeons provides updates regarding the influence of legislation on the practice of orthopaedic surgery, the Academy's involvement on behalf of its members, and summaries of the 2010 law's effect on orthopaedic practice.[24] The passage of the PPACA has had a substantial effect on the delivery of patient care and payment. Various aspects of the legislation, as of this writing, continue to be challenged in the judicial system, and subsequent verdicts may affect the continued implementation of the law as well as payments to providers and hospitals.

Hospital Considerations

Trauma surgeons use the funding hospitals receive for indigent patient care through the Medicare and DSH programs as a justification for hospital support of their practices. The PPACA calls for substantial reductions in the support hospitals receive through the DSH program and possibly in the latitude hospitals have to support providers of underfunded care in their facilities. Cuts to the Medicaid and Medicare DSH programs are scheduled as part of the PPACA. The cuts in DSH support were made with the expectation that the numbers of uninsured patients would dramatically decline through Medicaid expansion and the availability of insurance through state and federal exchanges. The Supreme Court has ruled that states are not required to expand their Medicaid coverage as originally mandated by the PPACA, however. Several states have since elected to opt out of Medicaid expansion. In such states, people living below the federal poverty level who do not qualify for Medicaid will not be eligible for insurance through the exchanges. In that scenario, numerous people will still have a gap in coverage.[25] This set of circumstances may leave hospitals in the affected states at greater risk of generating substantial deficits. The loss of a funding source can greatly affect an orthopaedic traumatologist's collections but not necessarily the volume of work he or she performs, creating a situation that may not remain sustainable.[26]

Practice Considerations

The new Medicare and Medicaid Physician Value Based Payment Modifier regulations for reimbursement adjust provider payments toward a reimbursement with more focus on patient outcomes. The goal is to influence the delivery of health care by adjusting payments based on the attainment of certain metrics. The overall effect on orthopaedic trauma is yet unknown. Physician participation is lagging behind hospital participation, and questions remain regarding the appropriate application of data to physician payments. Metrics tend to be less applicable to the practice of subspecialty providers, making it difficult to determine how they will affect practices that are not defined as primary care.[27]

Summary

Orthopaedic trauma has seen an increase in interest because of changes in financial support and call arrangements that make the career choice more palatable for residents entering practice. After the completion of fellowship training, building and maintaining a career in orthopaedic trauma requires consideration beyond those parameters. Establishing a mutually satisfying relationship with a facility that progresses into a career requires the ongoing and transparent communication of needs, bilateral investment in the program, and tracking of the physician's value to the system. The surgeon's relationship with the hospital will continue to evolve, but recent legislative changes in health care, which have not yet been fully realized, will continue to affect trauma care into the next decade. Remaining educated regarding the evolving regulatory environment surrounding health care and staying active within national and state medical associations and societies unifies and strengthens the voices of physicians and surgeons affected by these changes. Surgeon involvement at all levels of health care combined with the creation and modification of a plan for the future will ensure career success and fulfillment over the long term.

Key Study Points

- Addition of orthopaedic traumatologists to the hospital staff improves patient care and can be financially rewarding for the facility and the local nontrauma orthopaedic surgeons.
- The American College of Surgeons oversees hospital trauma resource verification for trauma-level designation.
- Contract negotiation can and should include considerations beyond financial remuneration. The initial contract will affect future contracts and should include expectations regarding call, ancillary staff, and facility support.
- An understanding of documentation, coding, and billing, along with involvement in third-party payer contract negotiation, affect the physician's ability to accurately capture work performed and collect revenue.
- Ongoing federal and state involvement in health care continues to evolve and will affect the operational and financial considerations of orthopaedic trauma practice substantially.

Annotated References

1. Clement RC, Carr BG, Kallan MJ, Reilly PM, Mehta S: Who needs an orthopedic trauma surgeon? An analysis of U.S. national injury patterns. *J Trauma Acute Care Surg* 2013;75(4):687-692.

   Trauma and nontrauma surgeons identify patients who would benefit from the care of an orthopaedic traumatologist. Level of evidence: IV.

2. American Academy of Orthopaedic Surgeons Position Statement on Emergency Orthopaedic Care: http://www.aaos.org/about/papers/position/1172.asp (Accessed December 17, 2015.) The position statement discusses factors related to ensuring access to emergency orthopaedic care.

3. DiRusso S, Holly C, Kamath R, et al: Preparation and achievement of American College of Surgeons level I trauma verification raises hospital performance and improves patient outcome. *J Trauma* 2001;51(2):294-299, discussion 299-300.

4. MacKenzie EJ, Rivara FP, Jurkovich GJ, et al: A national evaluation of the effect of trauma-center care on mortality. *N Engl J Med* 2006;354(4):366-378.

5. Althausen PL, Kauk JR, Shannon S, Lu M, O'Mara TJ, Bray TJ: Operating room efficiency: Benefits of an

orthopaedic traumatologist at a level II trauma center. *J Orthop Trauma* 2014;28(5):e101-e106.

This article compares costs incurred for similar cases treated by orthopaedic traumatologists and general orthopaedic surgeons. Level of evidence: IV.

6. Ziran BH, Barrette-Grischow MK, Marucci K: Economic value of orthopaedic trauma: The (second to) bottom line. *J Orthop Trauma* 2008;22(4):227-233.

7. Althausen PL, Davis L, Boyden E, O'Mara TJ, Uppal R, Bray TJ: Financial impact of a dedicated orthopaedic traumatologist on a private group practice. *J Orthop Trauma* 2010;24(6):350-354.

   The addition of an orthopaedic traumatologist to a private practice orthopaedic group increases the profitability of nontrauma partners and simultaneously increases time off. Level of evidence: IV.

8. American College of Surgeons Resources for Optimal Care of the Injured Patient -Sixth Edition. Available at https://www.facs.org/quality%20programs/trauma/vrc/resources. Accessed December 17, 2015.

   This source describes the required institutional resources for various levels of trauma verification by the American College of Surgeons.

9. American College of Surgeons Clarification Document: *Resources for Optimal Care of the Injured Patient*. Available at: https://www.facs.org/~/media/files/quality%20programs/trauma/vrc%20resources/clarification%20document%202015%20v4_11_19_15.ashx Accessed January 10, 2016.

   This source contains the updated institutional requirements for American College of Surgeons verification.

10. MGMA Datadive Provider Compensation 2015: http://www.mgma.com/store/surveys-and-benchmarking/online/mgma-datadive-provider-compensation-2015. Accessed January 10, 2016.

    The Medical Group Management Association provides data to its members on compensation, productivity, and practice management details for various specialties and practice groups.

11. Althausen PL, Coll D, Cvitash M, Herak A, O'Mara TJ, Bray TJ: Economic viability of a community-based level-II orthopaedic trauma system. *J Bone Joint Surg Am* 2009;91(1):227-235.

12. Kleweno CP, O'Toole RV, Ballreich J, Pollack AN: Does Fracture Care Make Money for the Hospital? An analysis of Hospital Revenues and Costs for Treatment of Common Fractures. *J Orthop Trauma* 2015;29(7):e219-e224.

    Maryland's state-regulated hospital reimbursement system allows trauma referral facilities to remain profitable with fracture care in the absence of the ability to shift the funding of indigent trauma care to private insurers. Level of evidence: IV.

13. Vallier HA, Patterson BM, Meehan CJ, Lombardo T: Orthopaedic traumatology: The hospital side of the ledger, defining the financial relationship between physicians and hospitals. *J Orthop Trauma* 2008;22(4):221-226.

14. Schwartz DA, Hui X, Velopulos CG, et al: Does relative value unit-based compensation shortchange the acute care surgeon? *J Trauma Acute Care Surg* 2014;76(1):84-92, discussion 92-94.

    Emergent and elective general surgical procedures are compared to assess the differences in outcomes. Despite having equivalent RVUs, emergent procedures were found to have more complications and longer stays.

15. Althausen PL, Shannon S, Owens B, et al: Impact of hospital-employed physician assistants on a level II community-based orthopaedic trauma system. *J Orthop Trauma* 2013;27(4):e87-e91.

    Hospital-employed physician assistants used by the orthopaedic trauma service reduce costs by increasing service efficiency and improving the delivery of patient care. Revenue generation by the physician assistant is only one consideration in assessing their value to the system. Level of evidence: IV.

16. Hiza EA, Gottschalk MB, Umpierrez E, Bush P, Reisman WM: Effect of a dedicated orthopaedic advanced practice provider in a level I trauma center: Analysis of length of stay and cost. *J Orthop Trauma* 2015;29(7):e225-e230.

    The addition of a nurse practitioner to the orthopaedic trauma service significantly reduces hospital costs by reducing the length of stay. Level of evidence: IV.

17. Agnew S, Anglen J, Born C, et al: EMTALA: The Orthopaedic Traumatologist and Hospital Guidelines. http://ota.org/medical-professionals/public-and-health-policy/emtala-the-orthopaedic-traumatologist-and-hospital-guidelines/ Accessed December 17, 2015.

    The OTA defines the challenges faced in providing orthopaedic trauma call coverage and describes the resources traumatologists need from a facility to provide trauma care.

18. Wixted JJ, Reed M, Eskander MS, et al: The effect of an orthopedic trauma room on after-hours surgery at a level one trauma center. *J Orthop Trauma* 2008;22(4):234-236.

19. Okike K, O'Toole RV, Pollak AN, et al: Survey finds few orthopedic surgeons know the costs of the devices they implant. *Health Aff (Millwood)* 2014;33(1):103-109.

    This survey reports the lack of knowledge of implant cost within the orthopaedic community. Fewer than half of respondents viewed implant cost as "very" or "extremely" important. Diminished transparency in the costs of implants at a facility reduces the ability of the surgeon to make economical choices about implants.

20. Egol KA, Capriccioso CE, Konda SR, et al: Cost-effective trauma implant selection: AAOS exhibit selection. *J Bone Joint Surg Am* 2014;96(22):e189.

Various methods of implant utilization that have the potential to reduce costs are discussed in the setting of an orthopaedic fracture practice.

21. Broderick JS, Henley MB: An introduction to orthopaedic coding and billing. *J Orthop Trauma* 2014;28(suppl 9):S12-4.

    Coding and billing practices are explained. The means by which these practices can appropriately reflect the level of service provided and reduce denials are given.

22. Brennan ML, Probe RA: Common errors in billing and coding for orthopaedic trauma care. *Curr Orthop Pract* 2011;22(1):12-16.

    Tips for coding and billing practices are discussed, and tips for improving reimbursement are provided.

23. Appleton P, Chacko A, Rodriguez EK: Financial implications of nonoperative fracture care at an academic trauma center. *J Orthop Trauma* 2012;26(11):617-619.

    This article provides a breakdown of charges generated by an orthopaedic trauma service. Although surgical charges remain the largest category of charges generated, nonsurgical charges are a substantial percentage of total charges. Level of evidence: IV.

24. Issar NM, Jahangir AA: The Affordable Care Act and orthopaedic trauma. *J Orthop Trauma* 2014;28(suppl 10):S5-S7.

    A description of the PPACA's influence on the practice of orthopaedic trauma is presented. Various aspects of the act and their possible consequences for orthopaedic trauma surgery are discussed.

25. Graves JA: Medicaid expansion opt-outs and uncompensated care. *N Engl J Med* 2012;367(25):2365-2367.

    Several states have elected to opt out of the PPACA's Medicaid expansion program. The effect on hospital finances in each state is measured, given DSH reductions with and without Medicaid expansion.

26. Forsh DA, Amanatullah DF, Coleman S, Wolinsky PR: The financial impact of the loss of county indigent patient funding on a single orthopedic trauma surgery service. *J Trauma Acute Care Surg* 2014;76(2):529-533.

    County funding for underfunded patients is lost at a level 1 facility. The volume of emergent/urgent and elective procedures as well as the trauma provider's collections are reviewed in funded and unfunded periods. The frequency of emergent/urgent procedures increased, and provider collections declined during the unfunded period. Level of evidence: IV.

27. Chien AT, Rosenthal MB: Medicare's physician value-based payment modifier—will the tectonic shift create waves? *N Engl J Med* 2013;369(22):2076-2078.

    Changes to physician payments for Medicare are being made. The intent and scheduled implementation are described in this article. The effect on physician practice continues to evolve.

Chapter 4

Computer-Assisted Orthopaedic Trauma Surgery

Patrick C. Schottel, MD Joshua L. Gary, MD

Abstract

Computer-assisted surgery continues to develop as technology improves. Uses in trauma include navigation for percutaneous screw placement in pelvic and acetabular surgery. Computers can also provide assistance with starting points for intramedullary nailing, interlocking screws, and rotational reduction. Three-dimensional printing creates models of complex fractures or deformities that can aid in preoperative planning. Simulation of complex deformity corrections can be performed virtually before surgery. Simulation also is an excellent vehicle for trainee education. The exact indications have yet to be defined as the technology continues to develop.

Keywords: computer-assisted orthopaedic surgery; CAOS; navigation; radiation exposure

Introduction

Computer-assisted orthopaedic surgery (CAOS) is a developing field of orthopaedic surgery designed to improve surgeons' understanding of patient anatomy as well as aid in executing complex surgical procedures. CAOS is used by numerous orthopaedic subspecialties. Applications include spinal pedicle screw insertion, total joint arthroplasty component placement, and osseous oncologic resections. CAOS is also used in orthopaedic trauma to aid in a broad range of activities including fracture reduction, optimizing alignment and rotation of diaphyseal fractures, malunion correction, and safe insertion of percutaneous sacroiliac and periacetabular screws. CAOS also reduces intraoperative radiation exposure and enhances resident education.

Intraoperative navigation is one of the most common uses of CAOS in orthopaedic trauma. Common navigation systems require multiple components to virtually re-create the surgical field. These components typically include trackable surgical instruments and reference points, a sensor, and a computer processor.[1] Additionally, navigation systems require the input of imaging data using four possible sources: preoperative CT, intraoperative CT, two-dimensional (2D) fluoroscopy, and three-dimensional (3D) fluoroscopy.[2] The most commonly used imaging source in surgical navigation is 2D fluoroscopy.[1] Several basic applications of CAOS in orthopaedic trauma surgery are currently in use.

CAOS Trauma Applications

Sacroiliac Joint Fixation

Percutaneous sacroiliac screw fixation for posterior pelvic ring disruption has become more common since the description of the technique and report of the initial clinical outcomes in the 1990s.[3] Although conventional fluoroscopic imaging remains the current gold standard, outcomes using CAOS have been reported. One study compared surgical time, radiation exposure, and sacroiliac screw position using either conventional fluoroscopy or 3D fluoroscopic navigation. [4] Navigation resulted in no difference in surgical time, reduced radiation exposure, and fewer malpositioned screws; 31% of the 3D-navigated sacroiliac screws and 60% of the conventionally placed

Dr. Gary or an immediate family member is a member of a speakers' bureau or has made paid presentations on behalf of Smith & Nephew; has stock or stock options held in Summit Medventures; and serves as a board member, owner, officer, or committee member of the Orthopaedic Trauma Association and Wolters Kluwer Health—Lippincott Williams & Wilkins. Neither Dr. Schottel nor any immediate family member has received anything of value from or has stock or stock options held in a commercial company or institution related directly or indirectly to the subject of this chapter.

screws had cortical penetration. Another study reported the results of sacroiliac screw placement in 66 patients using CT guidance and local anesthesia.[5] No misplaced screws were reported and all patients would undergo the navigated procedure again. The mean time of screw placement was 28 minutes, and two S3 screws could be placed as a direct result of the imaging capability.

One meta-analysis compared conventional and 3D-navigated techniques for sacroiliac screw placement and the rates of screw malposition and revision surgery.[6] CT navigation had a significantly lower malposition rate than conventional fluoroscopy (0.1% versus 2.6%; $P < 0.0001$). 2D and 3D fluoroscopic navigation both had an intermediate rate of screw malposition (1.3%). The rate of revision surgery was not significantly different between the techniques and was similar to the rate of screw malposition (0.8% for CT; 1.3% for 2D and 3D fluoroscopy; and 2.7% for conventional fluoroscopy). Although these results demonstrate a lower rate of screw malposition and revision surgery with navigation, its effect on the patient's postoperative neurologic function or overall clinical outcome is not known. Irrespective of the imaging technique used to percutaneously stabilize posterior ring disruptions, thorough anatomic knowledge is needed whether or not surgical navigation is used (**Figures 1, 2,** and **3**).

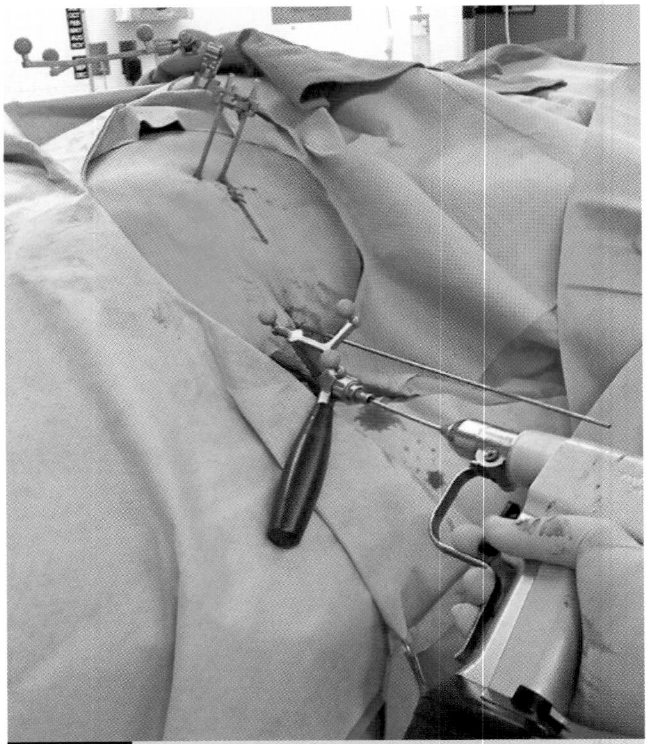

Figure 1 Demonstration of arrays placed on the iliac crest and cannulated guidewire handle. (Reproduced from Carmack DB, Kahler D, Matityahn A, Wentz BT: Computer-assisted surgery, in Schmidt AH, Teague DC, eds: *Orthopaedic Knowledge Update: Trauma*, ed 4. Rosemont, IL, American Academy of Orthopaedic Surgeons, 2010, pp 31-40.)

Acetabulum Fractures

Open reduction and internal fixation of displaced acetabular fractures is the current gold standard treatment.[7,8] Additionally, percutaneous screw fixation for particular acetabular fracture patterns has been advocated.[9,10,11] For cases amenable to percutaneous fixation, navigation technology has received increased interest as a potential technique to reduce surgical time and complications. 2D and 3D fluoroscopic navigation was studied in assisting the placement of percutaneous screws through common pelvic osseous corridors in a synthetic pelvis.[12] 2D navigation is directed after obtaining ideal images in multiple planes to demarcate the borders of the osseous corridors for screw placement. Fiduciaries are then used to guide implant placement within the corridor and alert the surgeon to deviations from an ideal trajectory. 3D navigation is obtained by electronic modeling of an osseous corridor from dozens of images obtained by isometrically rotating a fluoroscope in a continuous 190° arc about the corridor of interest.[12] 3D navigation reduced procedure time and increased screw accuracy compared with 2D navigation (**Figures 4** and **5**). Neither modality resulted in an intra-articular screw position. Similar findings were found when comparing 2D and 3D fluoroscopic imaging in synthetic and cadaver pelvises.[13]

Favorable clinical results using navigation have been reported for the management of acetabular fractures. In a study of CT navigation in 11 acetabular fractures, a substantial reduction in surgical time and fluoroscopy and increased accuracy in screw placement when compared with nonnavigated cases was reported.[14] Although some reports have demonstrated the effectiveness of navigation in treating acetabular fractures, a larger clinical study is needed to clearly define the role of navigation in acetabular fracture reduction and fixation.

Intramedullary Nailing

Another common application of CAOS is long bone intramedullary nailing. Navigation has been shown to be beneficial in the attainment of a starting point, placement of distal locking screws, and overall bony alignment and rotation. Piriformis fossa and tip of the greater trochanter starting points using either navigated 2D fluoroscopy or conventional fluoroscopy were obtained in 10 cadaver femurs.[15] For the piriformis fossa starting point, navigation

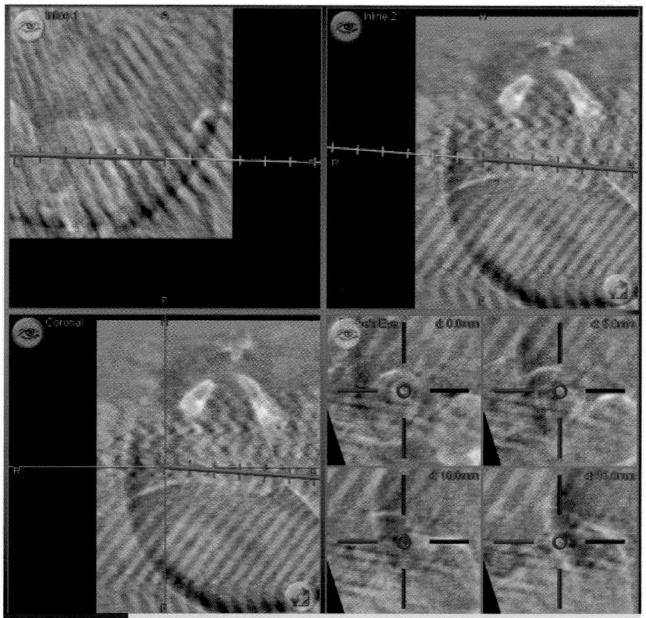

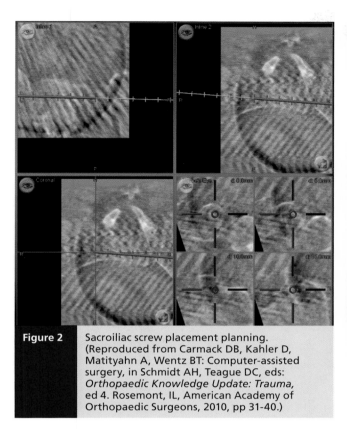

Figure 2 Sacroiliac screw placement planning. (Reproduced from Carmack DB, Kahler D, Matityahn A, Wentz BT: Computer-assisted surgery, in Schmidt AH, Teague DC, eds: *Orthopaedic Knowledge Update: Trauma,* ed 4. Rosemont, IL, American Academy of Orthopaedic Surgeons, 2010, pp 31-40.)

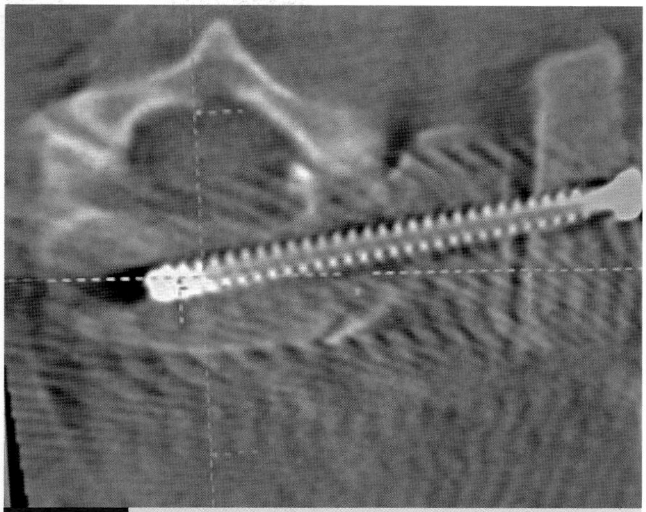

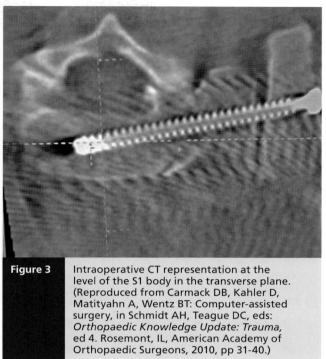

Figure 3 Intraoperative CT representation at the level of the S1 body in the transverse plane. (Reproduced from Carmack DB, Kahler D, Matityahn A, Wentz BT: Computer-assisted surgery, in Schmidt AH, Teague DC, eds: *Orthopaedic Knowledge Update: Trauma,* ed 4. Rosemont, IL, American Academy of Orthopaedic Surgeons, 2010, pp 31-40.)

resulted in higher precision and similar accuracy compared with conventional fluoroscopy. Navigation also improved the precision of obtaining a greater trochanter starting point but with less accuracy. The authors concluded that inaccuracies for navigated starting points were likely because of off-angle imaging, resulting in poor landmark identification. Improvement in intraoperative imaging and landmark registration would likely improve the accuracy and precision of navigated starting points, potentially resulting in increased use of this technology.

Navigation for the insertion of distal locking screws was prospectively studied.[16] Forty-two patients requiring intramedullary femoral nailing were divided into two groups, undergoing either conventional fluoroscopy or navigated 2D fluoroscopy. The mean time for fluoroscopy was greater in cases that used conventional fluoroscopy than in those that used navigation (108.0 versus 7.3 seconds). However, navigated procedures took longer (17.9 versus 13.7 minutes) and required approximately 40 minutes of additional time to set up the navigation system. The authors recommended fluoroscopic navigation only for selected cases in which the reduction of radiation exposure is deemed absolutely necessary.

Electromagnetic targeting is another type of navigation for the insertion of locking screws that has recently been studied.[17,18] This new technology involves inserting a probe within the intramedullary nail that is connected to a computer with calibration software. A separate targeting device generates an electromagnetic field and a representative real-time image of the nail's locking holes is created. Results of nail locking using either conventional fluoroscopy or an electromagnetic targeting system in patients with tibia and femur fractures treated using intramedullary nailing were compared.[17] Electromagnetic targeting resulted in a substantially faster mean insertion time (234 versus 343 seconds) and a lower radiation dose (0 versus 9.2 mrads). No misses occurred in either cohort. Other groups have reported similar findings.[18]

Navigation technology for improving the alignment and rotation of intramedullary has also been studied. Results from a prospective case series using 2D fluoroscopy were reported; 16 patients undergoing navigation-assisted fixation for femoral shaft fracture were postoperatively evaluated with bilateral lower extremity CT.[19] The patients had a mean rotational difference of 3.5° and mean length difference of 5.8 mm between the two extremities. In a randomized controlled study of cadaver specimens with segmental femoral defects comparing the results of intramedullary femoral nailing using 2D fluoroscopic navigation and conventional fluoroscopic imaging, the mean length difference was substantially smaller using navigation compared with conventional fluoroscopy (3.8 versus 9.8 mm).[20] However, rotational differences

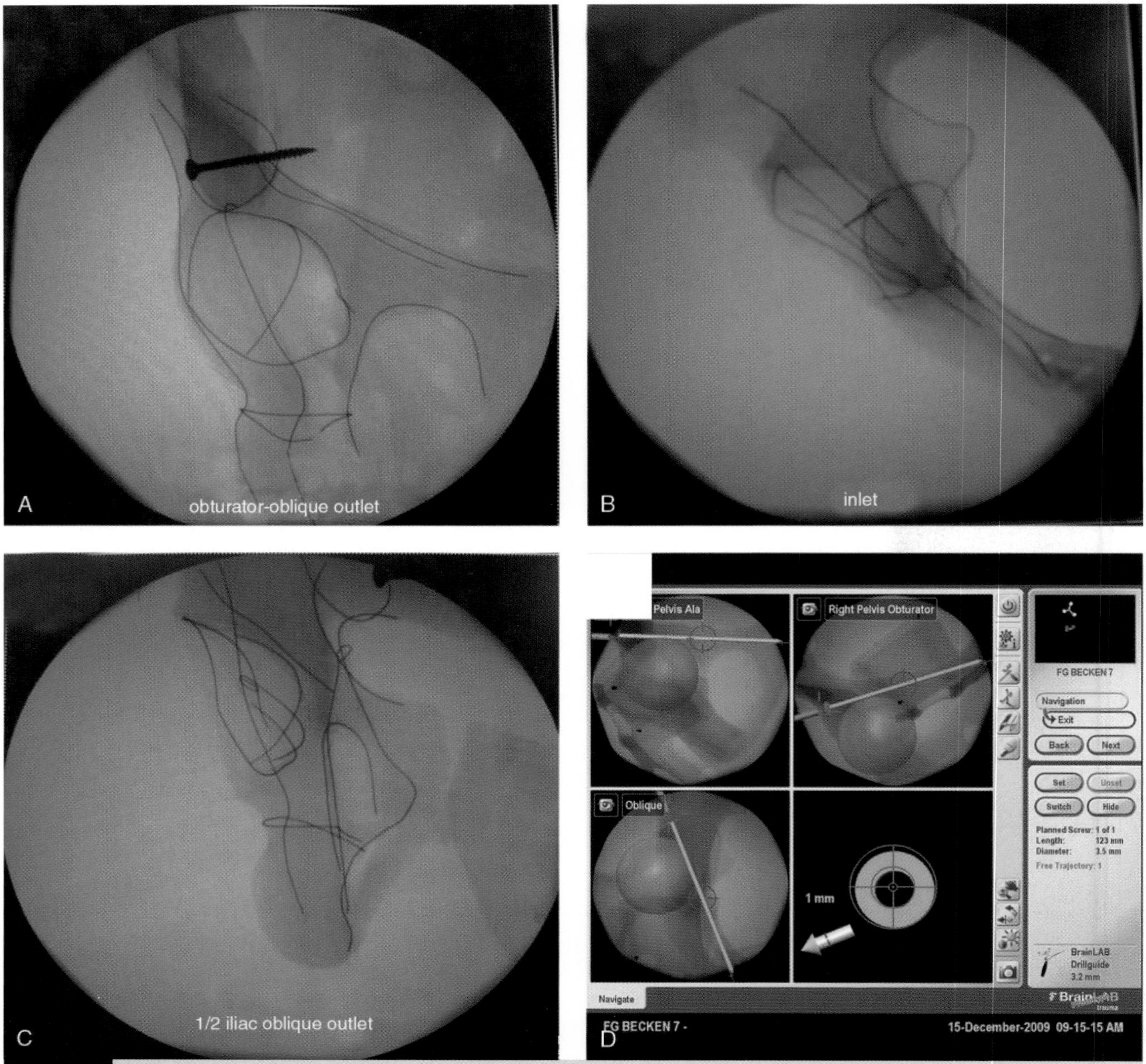

Figure 4 Intraoperative fluoroscopic views showing obturator oblique outlet (**A**), inlet (**B**), iliac oblique outlet (**C**), and navigation screenshots (**D**) of the screw pathway where two-dimensional navigation was used for placement of an anterior column screw in the acetabulum. (Reproduced with permission from Gras F, Marintschev I, Kajetan K, et al: Screw placement for acetabular fractures: Which navigation modality (2-dimensional vs. 3-dimensional) should be used? An experimental study. *J Orthop Trauma* 2012;26[8]:466-473.)

were noted to be similar (navigation, 7.7°; conventional fluoroscopy, 9.0°).

Navigation has been shown to be beneficial in some aspects of femoral intramedullary nailing. Intraoperative planning and assessment of functional reduction of length, alignment, and rotation may be more accurate with navigation (**Figure 6**). Because of the substantial reduction of radiation exposure, navigation holds promise especially for pregnant and pediatric patients. Further work is needed to improve the overall procedural time and results of navigation for this application.

Upper Extremity Fractures

Although use of navigation for acute upper extremity fractures is uncommon, some authors have highlighted its potential role in aiding the treatment of particular

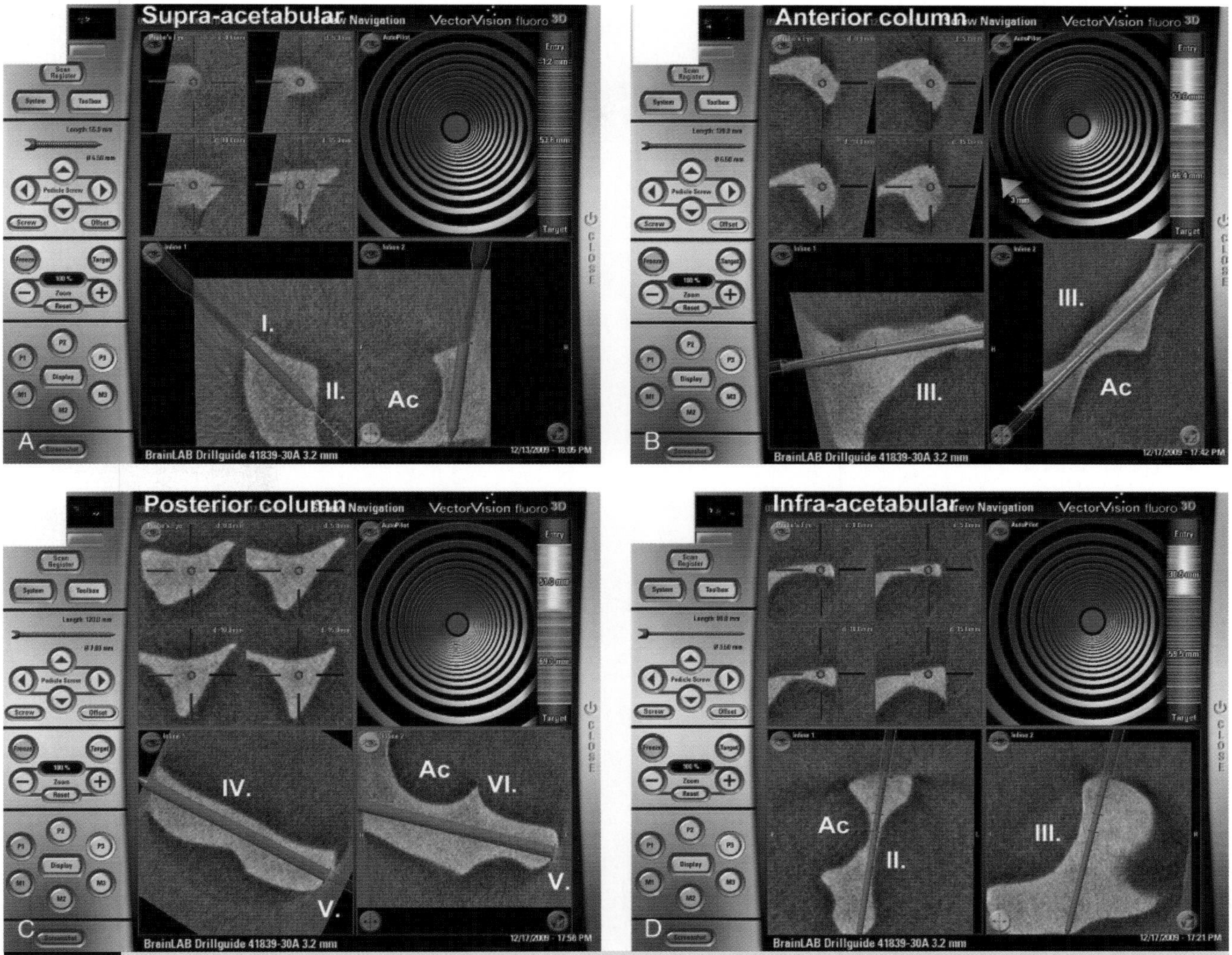

Figure 5 Optimized three-dimensional navigation images for screws placed in various osseous corridors of the pelvis. A, Supra-acetabular screw. **B**, Anterior column screw. **C**, Posterior column screw. **D**, Infra-acetabular screw. (Reproduced with permission from Gras F, Marintschev I, Kajetan K, et al: Screw placement for acetabular fractures: Which navigation modality (2-dimensional vs. 3-dimensional) should be used? An experimental study. *J Orthop Trauma* 2012;26[8]:466-473.)

fractures. In a 2013 study, technique and results using 2D fluoroscopic navigation to percutaneously stabilize nondisplaced intra-articular glenoid fracture in two patients were described.[21] Postoperative CT confirmed that the percutaneously inserted screws were extra-articular in both cases. Use of navigation with this injury cohort facilitated percutaneous in situ stabilization of the nondisplaced glenoid fractures, thereby limiting the potential for displacement and need for an open approach and associated morbidities.

Malunion Correction

CAOS techniques can also help in precisely performing an osteotomy for malunion via creation of a simulated malunion model and osteotomy templates. A technique of creating a custom-made osteotomy template using a computer-simulated model for diaphyseal forearm malunion has been described.[22] The authors reported the results of 20 patients with a preoperative angular deformity of 21° and a mean arc of forearm motion of 76°. Following corrective osteotomy using the custom templates and plate fixation, the angular deformity and mean arc of forearm motion substantially improved to 1° and 152°, respectively. No postoperative complications were reported, and 75% of patients were very satisfied. Another study reported a similar method of computer modeling and creation of a custom-made osteotomy template in patients with distal humerus malunion.[23] Three

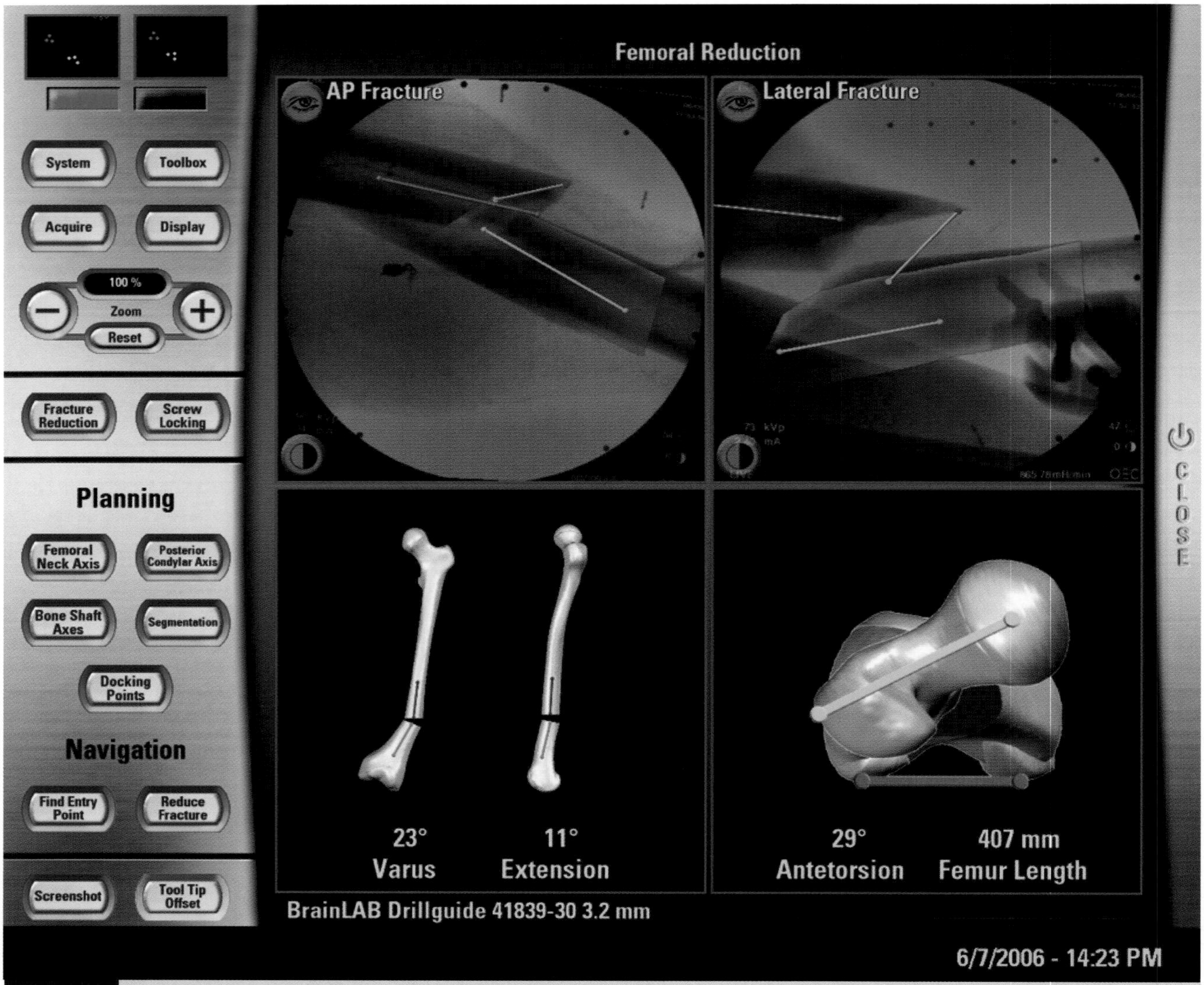

Figure 6 Stored anteroposterior and lateral images of a displaced, comminuted femoral shaft fracture. The distal fracture fragment has been manually segmented (in green) so that it can be tracked during reduction. Information on alignment, length, and antetorsion is also displayed before reduction. (BrainLAB, Feldkirchen, Germany.) (Reproduced from Carmack DB, Kahler D, Matityahn A, Wentz BT: Computer-assisted surgery, in Schmidt AH, Teague DC, eds: *Orthopaedic Knowledge Update: Trauma*, ed 4. Rosemont, IL, American Academy of Orthopaedic Surgeons, 2010, pp 31-40.)

patients underwent lateral closing wedge osteotomy for correction of their cubitus varus deformity following a malunited supracondylar distal humerus fracture. The planned correction was achieved in all cases and all patients were asymptomatic at final clinical follow-up. Use of computer-modeled osteotomy templates decreased surgical time and the need for fluoroscopy, and improved accuracy of the deformity correction. However, the cost was increased because of the need for preoperative CT, template fabrication, and computer software. Although this technique may not be appropriate for all deformity correction cases, selective use, especially in cases with multiplanar deformity and two-bone extremity segments such as the forearm, may be warranted.

Preoperative Assessment

In addition to navigation guidance during surgery, technologic advances have allowed surgeons to print 3D models of complex fractures to increase visualization of the anatomy and to precontour implants and plan the placement of clamps or other reduction devices. Results from a study on the use of rapid-prototype 3D solid models for acetabular fractures and spine deformities have been reported.[24] Forty-one acetabular fracture models were produced and used to contour plates and assess extra-articular screw trajectory. Postoperatively, all screws were noted to be extra-articular and a decrease in the amount of fluoroscopy time was reported for the cases with accompanying 3D models. The models were estimated to cost less than $100. The authors of a 2014 study reported on using sterilizable 3D pelvic models for five patients with acetabular fracture.[25] In addition to using the model preoperatively for planning purposes, the model was used intraoperatively to better assess and understand the fracture. Postoperatively, all screws were extra-articular and no surgical site infections were reported as a result of intraoperative model use. Although the reported cost of production has been low, the initial investment in a 3D printer can be much higher. Current estimates of cost for printers that can accurately reproduce a pelvic fracture model are $100,000 to $300,000. The costs and lack of reimbursement have limited the widespread adoption of this technology. This remains an area of future growth and clinical interest, as availability increases and cost decreases with more widespread use of the technology.

Radiation Exposure

Intraoperative conventional fluoroscopy exposes the patient, surgeon, and operating room staff to potentially harmful radiation. Although prior studies have shown that the surgeon would have to perform approximately 400 long bone intramedullary nailing procedures per year to exceed the maximum recommended extremity dose for the surgeon,[26] even low doses of radiation have been found to be harmful.[27] Therefore, minimizing the use of fluoroscopy should be a goal for all surgical procedures. The use of CAOS has been found to be particularly effective in reducing fluoroscopy use. The effective radiation dose of patients undergoing dorsal spinal fusion and percutaneous sacroiliac screw insertion using conventional fluoroscopy or 3D fluoroscopic navigation was compared.[28] The effective dose was determined by radiating a phantom torso using the same number of fluoroscopic images and technique as used intraoperatively. The total effective dose for sacroiliac screw insertion was found to be fivefold greater for conventional fluoroscopy than with navigation (2.5 versus 0.51 mSv) and correlated with published clinical studies.[4] However, the patient and surgeon benefit of reduced radiation exposure needs to be balanced by other factors, such as potentially increased surgical time and costs.

Resident Education

Another potential benefit of CAOS is in aiding medical student and resident education. The authors of a 2013 study evaluated 52 senior medical students and first-year residents in their ability to percutaneously insert guidewires into the femoral neck and head.[29] Groups were randomized between using conventional fluoroscopy and 2D fluoroscopic guidance for guidewire placement. Performance was judged on proximity of the guidewire to the subchondral bone, guidewire parallelism, and insertion distance from the lesser trochanter as well as number of attempts, total radiation time, and total procedure time. At a later date, the groups switched imaging modalities and the procedure was repeated. Guidewire placement was similar between groups, but those students/residents who were trained with navigation made fewer attempts and were exposed to less fluoroscopy. When the procedure was repeated using the other imaging modality, no difference was seen. Therefore, navigation was found to be an effective modality to train novice surgeons while reducing radiation exposure. These results highlight the advantage of using CAOS for surgical training by allowing novice surgeons to gain valuable experience about the proper trajectory and location of common percutaneous screw paths for treating fractures such as a valgus-impacted femoral neck or posterior pelvic ring injury.

Summary

CAOS is an exciting area, and new applications of navigation technology are being studied. Navigation has been shown to reduce radiation exposure to the patient and surgeon, aid in fracture fixation planning, and positively contribute to resident education. Widespread adaptation of CAOS is currently limited by navigation costs and setup time. However, future development of less expensive equipment and greater familiarity with navigation technology will likely result in its greater use in the future. Currently, a thorough understanding of osseous and soft-tissue anatomic principles combined with careful study of preoperative and intraoperative imaging is sufficient for safe fracture treatment.

Key Study Points

- CAOS can include, but is not limited to, the creation of osteotomy guides for malunion, intraoperative navigation technology, and fracture model creation for surgical planning and education purposes.
- Different navigation modalities are available, such as CT navigation and 2D or 3D fluoroscopic navigation. 2D fluoroscopic navigation is the type currently used most often.
- Decreasing costs and greater familiarity with CAOS technology will likely expand its role in the future.

Annotated References

1. Atesok K, Schemitsch EH: Computer-assisted trauma surgery. *J Am Acad Orthop Surg* 2010;18(5):247-258.

   The authors of this review summarize the technique of CAOS as well as its numerous applications in the field of orthopaedic trauma.

2. Hüfner T, Gebhard F, Grützner PA, Messmer P, Stöckle U, Krettek C: Which navigation when? *Injury* 2004;35(suppl 1):S-A30-4.

3. Routt ML Jr, Kregor PJ, Simonian PT, Mayo KA: Early results of percutaneous iliosacral screws placed with the patient in the supine position. *J Orthop Trauma* 1995;9(3):207-214.

4. Zwingmann J, Konrad G, Kotter E, Südkamp NP, Oberst M: Computer-navigated iliosacral screw insertion reduces malposition rate and radiation exposure. *Clin Orthop Relat Res* 2009;467(7):1833-1838.

5. Ziran BH, Smith WR, Towers J, Morgan SJ: Iliosacral screw fixation of the posterior pelvic ring using local anaesthesia and computerised tomography. *J Bone Joint Surg Br* 2003;85(3):411-418.

6. Zwingmann J, Hauschild O, Bode G, Südkamp NP, Schmal H: Malposition and revision rates of different imaging modalities for percutaneous iliosacral screw fixation following pelvic fractures: A systematic review and meta-analysis. *Arch Orthop Trauma Surg* 2013;133(9):1257-1265.

   A systematic review and meta-analysis was performed to compare conventional fluoroscopy with 2D or 3D fluoroscopic navigation and CT navigation for percutaneous sacroiliac screw insertion. The rate of screw malposition was substantially lower for CT navigation than for the other modalities. However, no substantial difference in the rate of revision surgery was noted. Level of evidence: I.

7. Letournel E: Acetabulum fractures: Classification and management. *Clin Orthop Relat Res* 1980;151:81-106.

8. Matta JM, Mehne DK, Roffi R: Fractures of the acetabulum. Early results of a prospective study. *Clin Orthop Relat Res* 1986;205:241-250.

9. Starr AJ, Reinert CM, Jones AL: Percutaneous fixation of the columns of the acetabulum: A new technique. *J Orthop Trauma* 1998;12(1):51-58.

10. Bates P, Gary J, Singh G, Reinert C, Starr A: Percutaneous treatment of pelvic and acetabular fractures in obese patients. *Orthop Clin North Am* 2011;42(1):55-67, vi.

    A case series of 23 obese (body mass index > 30 kg/m^2) patients with pelvic and acetabular fractures treated with percutaneous reduction and fixation had no postoperative infections or unplanned returns to the operating room. Two of seven patients with acetabular fractures had a loss of reduction requiring total hip arthroplasty.

11. Gary JL, VanHal M, Gibbons SD, Reinert CM, Starr AJ: Functional outcomes in elderly patients with acetabular fractures treated with minimally invasive reduction and percutaneous fixation. *J Orthop Trauma* 2012;26(5):278-283.

    Functional outcomes and rate of conversion to total hip arthroplasty of limited open reduction and percutaneous fixation of acetabular fractures in patients older than 60 years (n = 35) at injury were no different from historical controls treated with open reduction and internal fixation at a mean follow-up of 6.8 years.

12. Gras F, Marintschev I, Klos K, Mückley T, Hofmann GO, Kahler DM: Screw placement for acetabular fractures: Which navigation modality (2-dimensional vs. 3-dimensional) should be used? An experimental study. *J Orthop Trauma* 2012;26(8):466-473.

    Common osseous corridors in 40 synthetic pelvic models were drilled using either 2D or 3D fluoroscopy. The duration of procedure, total fluoroscopic time, and quality of drilling were assessed. 3D fluoroscopy resulted in reduced surgical time and increased precision, but at the cost of substantially higher cumulative fluoroscopic time.

13. Ochs BG, Gonser C, Shiozawa T, et al: Computer-assisted periacetabular screw placement: Comparison of different fluoroscopy-based navigation procedures with conventional technique. *Injury* 2010;41(12):1297-1305.

    Cadaver and synthetic pelvic specimens were used to assess accuracy, total procedural time, and total fluoroscopic time for percutaneous screw insertion within common osseous corridors using conventional fluoroscopy, 2D fluoroscopy, or 3D fluoroscopy. 3D fluoroscopy resulted in higher accuracy but longer procedural times and total fluoroscopic times.

14. Brown GA, Willis MC, Firoozbakhsh K, Barmada A, Tessman CL, Montgomery A: Computed tomography image-guided surgery in complex acetabular fractures. *Clin Orthop Relat Res* 2000;370:219-226.

15. Crookshank MC, Edwards MR, Sellan M, Whyne CM, Schemitsch EH: Can fluoroscopy-based computer

navigation improve entry point selection for intramedullary nailing of femur fractures? *Clin Orthop Relat Res* 2014;472(9):2720-2727.

Cadaver femurs had the piriformis fossa and tip of the greater trochanter antegrade intramedullary nailing starting points digitized using direct visualization. Starting points were then obtained with conventional fluoroscopy and 2D fluoroscopic navigation and compared with the digitized standard. Navigation substantially improved precision but did not substantially improve accuracy for both starting points.

16. Suhm N, Messmer P, Zuna I, Jacob LA, Regazzoni P: Fluoroscopic guidance versus surgical navigation for distal locking of intramedullary implants. A prospective, controlled clinical study. *Injury* 2004;35(6):567-574.

17. Chan DS, Burris RB, Erdogan M, Sagi HC: The insertion of intramedullary nail locking screws without fluoroscopy: A faster and safer technique. *J Orthop Trauma* 2013;27(7):363-366.

    Patients with tibia and femur fractures treated with intramedullary nailing were divided between standard freehand nailing with fluoroscopic assistance or an electromagnetic targeting system for locking screw insertion. Electromagnetic-targeted nail locking was faster and used less fluoroscopy. No difference was reported in accuracy between the two cohorts. Level of evidence: III.

18. Langfitt MK, Halvorson JJ, Scott AT, et al: Distal locking using an electromagnetic field-guided computer-based real-time system for orthopaedic trauma patients. *J Orthop Trauma* 2013;27(7):367-372.

    This prospective, randomized controlled trial compared standard freehand nail locking technique with an electromagnetic-targeting system in patients with tibia and femur fractures treated with an antegrade intramedullary nail. The electromagnetic-targeting system was faster and resulted in few misses. Level of evidence: II.

19. Weil YA, Greenberg A, Khoury A, Mosheiff R, Liebergall M: Computerized navigation for length and rotation control in femoral fractures: A preliminary clinical study. *J Orthop Trauma* 2014;28(2):e27-e33.

    Sixteen patients with femur fractures were treated with intramedullary nailing and 2D navigation. Using the uninjured contralateral side, the surgeons could determine the mean malrotation and shortening of the surgical extremity using intraoperative navigation. This result was compared with postoperative CT measurements. The measured mean malrotation of the navigation system and postoperative CT was 2.9° and 3.45°, respectively. Navigation predicted limb shortening of 7.3 mm compared with the actual 5.83 mm of shortening as measured using postoperative CT. None of the measurements were significantly different. Level of evidence: IV.

20. Keast-Butler O, Lutz MJ, Angelini M, et al: Computer navigation in the reduction and fixation of femoral shaft fractures: A randomized control study. *Injury* 2012;43(6):749-756.

    This cadaver study reviewed 20 femoral shaft fractures treated with antegrade intramedullary nailing. Nail insertion was assisted by either conventional fluoroscopy or 2D fluoroscopic navigation. Postoperative CT was used to compare the rotation and length difference between the surgical and uninjured femurs. Navigation substantially improved the mean difference in limb length but had no effect on the degree of malrotation.

21. Gras F, Marintschev I, Aurich M, Rausch S, Klos K, Hofmann GO: Percutaneous navigated screw fixation of glenoid fractures. *Arch Orthop Trauma Surg* 2013;133(5):627-633.

    In this report, two patients with a nondisplaced glenoid fracture were treated with percutaneous screws aided by 2D fluoroscopic navigation. Postoperative CT scans were obtained and the clinical outcome of the patients was reported. None of the percutaneously placed screws were intra-articular and neither patient required revision. The mean Disabilities of the Arm, Shoulder and Hand score was 40.2 points.

22. Miyake J, Murase T, Oka K, Moritomo H, Sugamoto K, Yoshikawa H: Computer-assisted corrective osteotomy for malunited diaphyseal forearm fractures. *J Bone Joint Surg Am* 2012;94(20):e150.

    Twenty patients with diaphyseal forearm malunion underwent corrective osteotomy using custom-made osteotomy templates. The mean angle of deformity in the cohort was 21°. Based on CT imaging of the contralateral uninjured side, modeling software was used to determine the location and type of osteotomy necessary to correct the malunion. Custom osteotomy guides were created using rapid prototyping with medical-grade resin. Nineteen patients (95%) achieved primary osseous union. The postoperative mean angle of deformity improved to 1° and forearm arc of motion (pronation/supination) improved from 76° preoperatively to 152° postoperatively. The estimated total cost of the osteotomy jig and preoperative CT scan was $250. Level of evidence: IV.

23. Tricot M, Duy KT, Docquier PL: 3D-corrective osteotomy using surgical guides for posttraumatic distal humeral deformity. *Acta Orthop Belg* 2012;78(4):538-542.

    Three pediatric patients with distal humeral malunion were treated with a corrective osteotomy using a fabricated osteotomy guide. A preoperative CT scan was obtained and a rapid prototype model of the humerus was then created. An osteotomy guide was made using the model and the plates were also precontoured. A correction of the preoperative deformity was reportedly obtained in all patients and all had regained full elbow range of motion at latest follow-up.

24. Brown GA, Firoozbakhsh K, DeCoster TA, Reyna JR Jr, Moneim M: Rapid prototyping: The future of trauma surgery? *J Bone Joint Surg Am* 2003;85-A(suppl 4):49-55.

25. Niikura T, Sugimoto M, Lee SY, et al: Tactile surgical navigation system for complex acetabular fracture surgery. *Orthopedics* 2014;37(4):237-242.

Five patients with acetabular fractures had a 3D pelvic model printed. The models were used for preoperative planning and surgery simulation, plate contouring, and intraoperative consultation. No instances of intra-articular screw penetration or postoperative infection were reported, and osseous union was achieved in all cases. The 3D printed models were concluded to be beneficial in treating patients with complex acetabular fractures. Level of evidence: IV.

26. Müller LP, Suffner J, Wenda K, Mohr W, Rommens PM: Radiation exposure to the hands and the thyroid of the surgeon during intramedullary nailing. *Injury* 1998;29(6):461-468.

27. Singer G: Occupational radiation exposure to the surgeon. *J Am Acad Orthop Surg* 2005;13(1):69-76.

28. Kraus MD, Krischak G, Keppler P, Gebhard FT, Schuetz UH: Can computer-assisted surgery reduce the effective dose for spinal fusion and sacroiliac screw insertion? *Clin Orthop Relat Res* 2010;468(9):2419-2429.

The effective radiation dose for percutaneous sacroiliac screw insertion was compared using conventional fluoroscopy and 3D fluoroscopic navigation. The typical use for both imaging modalities based on a patient series was performed on a model using thermoluminescence dosimeters. Conventional fluoroscopy and 3D fluoroscopy resulted in an effective dose of 2.5 mSV and 0.51 mSv, respectively. The effective radiation dose for sacroiliac screws is reduced fivefold with the use of 3D navigation.

29. Nousiainen MT, Omoto DM, Zingg PO, Weil YA, Mardam-Bey SW, Eward WC: Training femoral neck screw insertion skills to surgical trainees: Computer-assisted surgery versus conventional fluoroscopic technique. *J Orthop Trauma* 2013;27(2):87-92.

Medical students and first-year surgical residents were randomized to being taught to treat femoral neck fractures using three cannulated screws under either conventional fluoroscopy or a navigation technique. A pretest using a cadaver model was performed before either of the 30-minute tutorials. A test following the procedure was performed and multiple parameters were collected including parallelism, distance of the guidewire tip to the subchondral femoral head bone, number of attempts, and total radiation time were collected. No difference was reported between groups in parallelism or guidewire distance to the subchondral bone. However, the authors found that the navigated group required fewer attempts to perform the procedure and less total radiation time.

Chapter 5

Principles of Minimally Invasive Fracture Care

Mark A. Lee, MD   Jonathan G. Eastman, MD

Abstract

Minimally invasive surgical techniques are used throughout the body to achieve fracture reduction and stability with minimal soft-tissue disruption. The primary benefit of these approaches is minimizing the disruption of critical soft-tissue attachments in the fracture zone that are frequently disrupted or cleared using traditional open approaches. Many of these techniques require special surgical equipment, sometimes special instrumentation and hardware, and most important, unique surgical techniques. In the upper extremity, specialized implants have been developed for the proximal humerus that allow minimally invasive insertion and optimal stabilization for metaphyseal fractures. Diaphyseal fractures of the upper and lower extremity can be managed with minimally invasive techniques using nonspecialized hardware. In the lower extremity, implants that optimize stabilization of the distal femur, proximal tibia, and distal tibia continue to be optimized. The evolution of percutaneous techniques with closed reduction techniques in the pelvis continues to reduce patient surgical morbidity and improve outcomes.

Dr. Lee or an immediate family member is a member of a speakers' bureau or has made paid presentations on behalf of Synthes, Zimmer, and AONA, serves as a paid consultant to Synthes and Zimmer, has received research or institutional support from Synthes, has received nonincome support (such as equipment or services), commercially derived honoraria, or other non–research-related funding (such as paid travel) from Synthes Fellowship Support, and serves as a board member, owner, officer, or committee member of the Orthopaedic Trauma Association. Neither Dr. Eastman nor any immediate family member has received anything of value from or has stock or stock options held in a commercial company or institution related directly or indirectly to the subject of this chapter.

Keywords: minimally invasive; percutaneous; MIO

Introduction

The ability to achieve and maintain reduction of displaced fractures using small incisions is technically demanding but yields myriad patient benefits. Although the smaller incisions are cosmetically favorable, the real benefit of a minimized surgical footprint is maintenance of the soft-tissue attachments to the fractured fragments in the injury zone and less tenuous extensile exposures. There are several minimally invasive surgical techniques that achieve reduction and stability with minimal soft-tissue disruption.

Although minimally invasive techniques can be used with multiple fracture types (typically via indirect reduction), they are particularly challenging in settings for which absolute stability is preferred. Simple patterns can be successfully managed with minimally invasive osteosynthesis (MIO) techniques (for example, transverse diaphyseal humeral and femoral shaft fractures treated with intramedullary rods). Most applications of MIO techniques outside the pelvis are used to bridge complicated fractures. Although the spectrum of stability is broad among bridging implant options, these approaches typically result in predictable healing responses involving secondary fracture.

The greatest use of minimally invasive techniques likely relates to periarticular fractures with metaphyseal or diaphyseal extension. For these fractures, the reduction and bridging can be performed with minimal additional insult to the injury zone. These periarticular fractures frequently have some degree of intra-articular fracture extension, and although the metaphyseal bridging can be done via small incision technique, the displaced articular component still requires open reduction via an adequate arthrotomy that facilitates articular visualization and reduction. Any compromise on the precision of the articular reduction should be avoided.

Precontoured/anatomically contoured and locking plates have assisted in the development and use of the MIO technique. With locking plates, hybrid fixation techniques (the use of nonlocking screws to create translation and plate-bone apposition and the use of locking screws to neutralize and maintain reductions and plate positions) has resulted in the ability to affect fracture reduction indirectly with an implant that does not require complete bone/plate apposition. For many approaches, the complex, multiplane contours simplify indirect reduction by allowing the surgeon to focus on length, gross frontal and lateral plane reduction, and using a combination of locking and nonlocking screws to make fine adjustments to the reduction.

Proximal Humeral Fractures

Some of the most important advances in minimally invasive approaches for reduction and fixation have occurred in the treatment of proximal humeral fractures. The increasingly used extended anterolateral surgical approach via the raphe between the anterior and middle deltoid muscle heads is an ideal, biologically optimal surgical approach. With gentle soft-tissue handling, the anterior and medial soft-tissue attachments can remain intact during reduction and instrumentation. The lateral reduction provides easy access to the surface of the proximal humerus just lateral to the bicipital groove. This position provides unimpeded access to the subacromial space for placement of sutures in the rotator cuff, access to posteriorly displaced greater tuberosity fragments, and easy positioning for most plate designs. The fracture site is easily manipulated from this lateral position, and the endosteal space is accessible for placement of intramedullary implants that can help in reduction and/or fixation. Provisional fixation with 1.6-mm or 2.0-mm Kirschner wires can be performed from within the exposure or percutaneously. Shaft reduction to the head segment can also be performed from within the exposure. If a plate is selected for fixation, the shortest plate needs to be used to simplify passage beneath the axillary nerve without harmful traction. Provisional plate positioning and eventual screw placement in the shaft can be performed percutaneously.[1] Intramedullary stabilization is also feasible using newer rod designs with interlocking screws and proximally directed screw paths with improved stability characteristics. The starting location for these newer implants is more on-axis and medial (near the articular margin), with proximal insertion paths that traverse the more muscular portions of the rotator cuff muscles (instead of the tendinous areas). Early experience with these rods is favorable and comparable with plating experience[2] (**Figure 1**). Irrespective of implant choice, reduction (particularly calcar reduction) remains critical for maintenance of stability and uneventful healing.

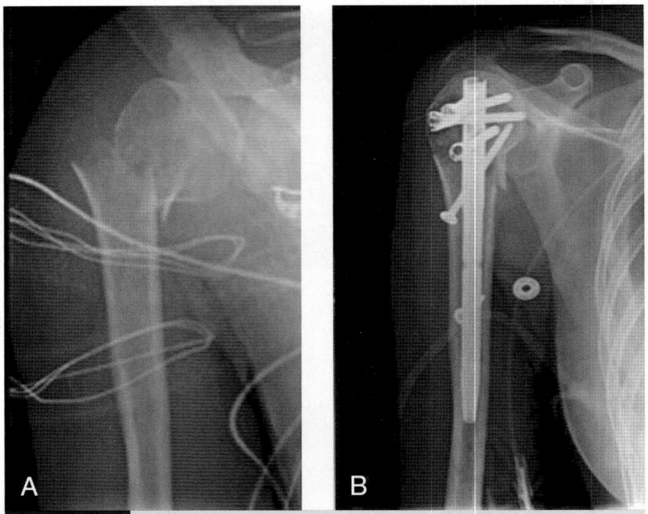

Figure 1 AP shoulder radiographs demonstrate a displaced two-part proximal humerus fracture. **A**, Preoperative view. **B**, Postoperative view demonstrates on-axis nail with multiplanar proximal interlocks that interface with the nail.

Humeral Diaphyseal Fractures

Intramedullary nailing approaches provide a truly minimally invasive alternative to traditional plate fixation. Intramedullary nailing is particularly helpful for highly comminuted and segmental humeral shaft fractures. The benefits of locked intramedullary nailing in multiply injured patients is a long-recognized benefit of immediate weight bearing for crutch use and transfer, but substantial concerns remain about insertional morbidity, especially at the shoulder. Newer nail designs use a more medial start site that traverses the more vascular, muscular part of the rotator cuff instead of the more avascular tendinous or insertional part of the cuff. According to a 2013 retrospective study, retrograde nailing techniques also have evolved to a more aggressive preparation of the distal start site, with a low rate of iatrogenic supracondylar fracture.[3] Ultimately, both retrograde and antegrade techniques yield essentially equivalent results.[4]

The use of minimally invasive plating of the humeral shaft has increased internationally as a reasonable alternative to intramedullary nailing, and anatomic studies have demonstrated safe portals using an anterior MIO technique.[1,4] The indications for this technique are essentially the same as for intramedullary nailing, especially highly comminuted diaphyseal fractures with intact proximal and distal segments.[5]

The surgical technique is straightforward with knowledge of the nerve positions in the upper arm. The proximal portal is in the distal part of the deltopectoral interval, and the distal incision is at the lateral margin of the biceps. Radial nerve visualization is not required unless entrapment-related palsy is suspected or an open technique is being used at the fracture site to compress the bone ends. Using mainly indirect reduction techniques and relatively stable fixation, a bridge plate concept can be selected. Simple fractures and absolute stability can also be used with a small anterolateral incision at the fracture site. This same lateral incision can be extended slightly and used to dissect and visualize the radial nerve if desired. Locking plates are beneficial in this setting to avoid the need for precise contour of the plate (**Figure 2**). Recent clinical studies demonstrate excellent performance of the minimal invasive submuscular technique.[5,6]

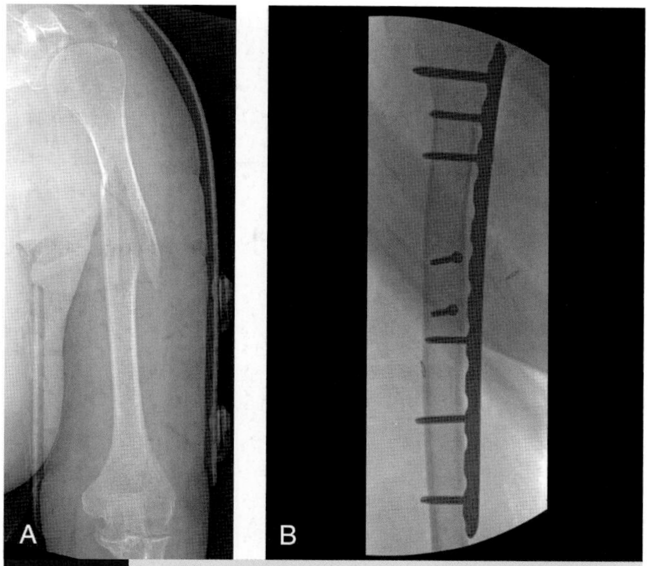

Figure 2 **A**, AP radiograph demonstrates a displaced proximal humeral shaft fracture for which bracing failed after 2 weeks. **B**, Intraoperative AP fluoroscopic view obtained following minimally invasive anterior approach. A small incision was made at the midshaft and lag screws were placed across the fracture. Proximal and distal incisions were made for plate passage and fracture neutralization.

Pelvic Ring Injuries

With improvement in intraoperative imaging quality, increased anatomic understanding, and technologic advances, closed reduction and percutaneous fixation is being used more often for the successful stabilization of pelvic ring injuries.[7] Although recent series show a decreased complication rate, the use of open approaches to the posterior pelvic ring has historically been linked with increased complication rates.[8,9] Surgical incisions and extensive dissection in traumatized and potentially compromised tissues increase the likelihood of perioperative complications.[8,9] Percutaneous techniques allow fracture reduction and stabilization without a formal open or extensile surgical approach, which decreases the likelihood of postoperative wound complications. Similarly, surgical times and associated blood loss are reduced. Limiting the surgical exposure also does not decompress the intrapelvic hematoma and therefore decreases the risk of additional hemorrhage.[7] Thorough knowledge of pelvic osseous anatomy is mandatory. Great anatomic variability exists in the posterior pelvic ring and the presence of sacral dysmorphism must be appreciated. Failure to do so can result in catastrophic iatrogenic injuries to the surrounding neurovascular anatomy.[10] Percutaneous reduction, instrumentation, and fixation both rely on a complete comprehension of the complex osseous morphology of the pelvis. Understanding the location, size, and orientation of the possible osseous fixation pathways within the pelvis allows surgeons to successfully place instruments and implants to manipulate and internally stabilize pelvic ring injuries.[11] Complete understanding of the osseous anatomy available for percutaneous fixation, accurate translation of the preoperative plan into the operating room, and correct interpretation of high-quality intraoperative fluoroscopic imaging are essential.[12,13]

Safe, stable fixation is performed only after accurate reduction has been achieved. Otherwise, the intraosseous safe zone for iliosacral screw placement is decreased.[7,14] Manipulation of the pelvis to obtain an anatomic reduction should begin with closed techniques and progress to percutaneous options. Formal open reduction should only be performed if needed to obtain appropriate reduction. Closed reduction techniques range from positioning to manual manipulation of the pelvis and lower extremities. In addition to the benefits of keeping patients with polytrauma supine, placing them on a midline lumbosacral bump induces lordosis and can help correct kyphotic deformities commonly seen with U-, H-, or Y-shaped sacral fracture patterns.[15-17] With anteroposterior compression pelvic ring patterns, placement of a circumferential pelvic sheet can aid in reduction[18] as well as be used intraoperatively by cutting working portals through the sheet.[19] For some injuries, a circumferential pelvic sheet does not provide a complete reduction; for others, it cannot be performed. Internal rotation and taping of the lower extremities can be an incredibly effective alternative or supplemental treatment.[20] As reported in a 2013 study, manual manipulation of the pelvis using force through the iliac crest is commonly used simultaneously.[21]

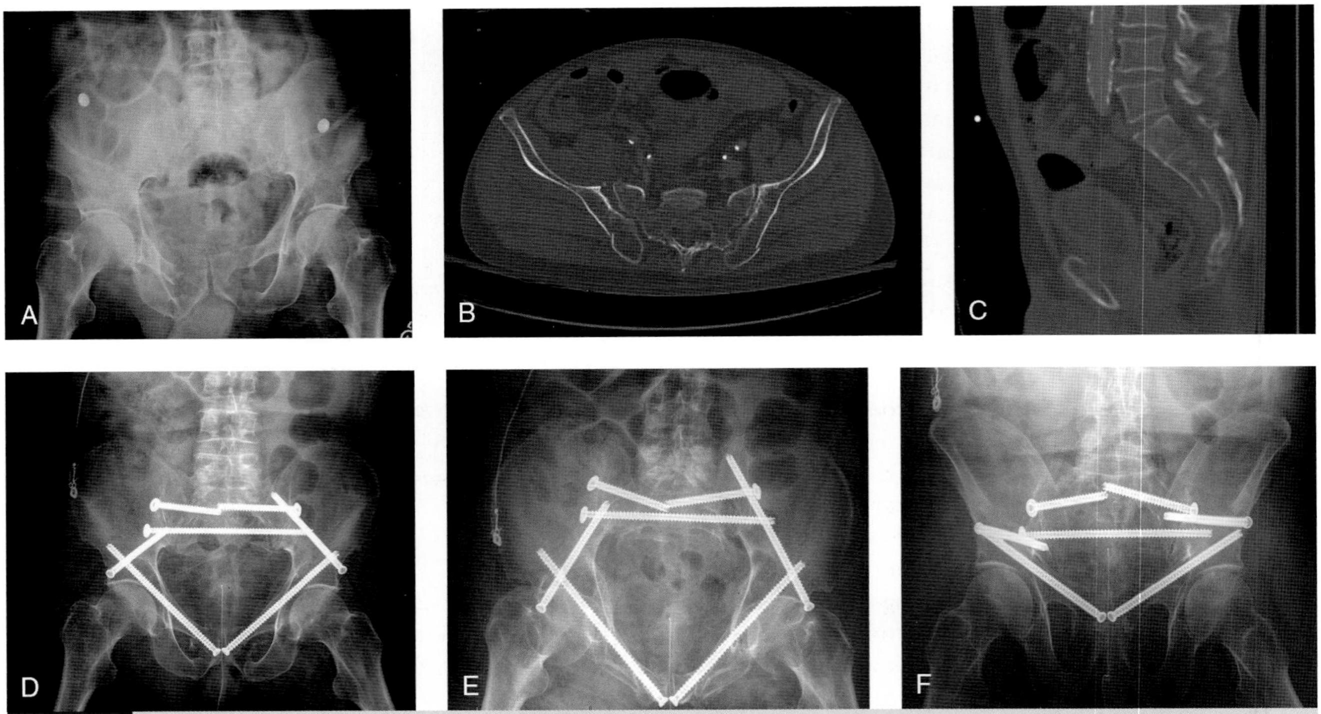

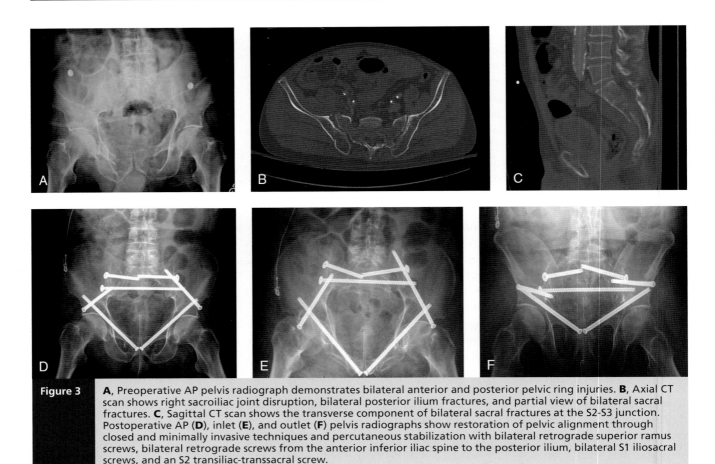

Figure 3 **A**, Preoperative AP pelvis radiograph demonstrates bilateral anterior and posterior pelvic ring injuries. **B**, Axial CT scan shows right sacroiliac joint disruption, bilateral posterior ilium fractures, and partial view of bilateral sacral fractures. **C**, Sagittal CT scan shows the transverse component of bilateral sacral fractures at the S2-S3 junction. Postoperative AP (**D**), inlet (**E**), and outlet (**F**) pelvis radiographs show restoration of pelvic alignment through closed and minimally invasive techniques and percutaneous stabilization with bilateral retrograde superior ramus screws, bilateral retrograde screws from the anterior inferior iliac spine to the posterior ilium, bilateral S1 iliosacral screws, and an S2 transiliac-transsacral screw.

If the previously mentioned techniques do not accurately reduce the pelvic injury, percutaneous techniques are commonly used. Skeletal traction through the limb itself or through the use of a traction table can correct cranial displacement of the hemipelvis.[22] Schanz pins placed in appropriate osseous fixation pathways can be used to manipulate the hemipelvis in many directions, and can be accomplished by simply using a T-handle chuck, an obliquely oriented external fixator or universal distractor,[23] or table-skeletal fixation and commercially available skeletal reduction frames.[24,25] The C-clamp can be challenging to use but it has been successfully described in the management of both anterior and posterior pelvic ring injuries.[26,27] Some anterior ring injuries are managed definitively with external fixation. An anterior internal fixator has been successfully used, but recent studies have shown substantial potential complications.[28,29] Percutaneously placed screws can be used to achieve both accurate reduction and stable fixation. In certain clinical scenarios, a properly placed iliosacral screw can reduce and stabilize a displaced sacroiliac joint and assist in the acute resuscitation of a critically injured patient. Similarly, acute intraoperative correction of misdirected cannulated screws or malaligned fractures can be performed percutaneously.[30]

Ultimately, myriad techniques for percutaneous manipulation, reduction, and fixation are available. A thorough knowledge of pelvic osseous anatomy, injury patterns with accompanying deformity, correctly correlating intraoperative findings, and appropriate application of the previously mentioned techniques are mandatory for safe, effective percutaneous pelvic fixation (**Figure 3**).

Diaphyseal Femur Fractures

The optimization of minimally invasive approaches to femoral diaphyseal fractures is primarily related to development of techniques and instrumentation for percutaneous antegrade intramedullary nailing. Specialized long insertion handles have been designed to allow both on-axis and off-axis insertion vectors from proximal start sites. These start sites are feasible even in large patients and can minimize the tendency for problematic medial-to-lateral insertion vectors, which can result in frontal plane malreduction (usually varus). Multiple insertion portals for antegrade nailing, including piriformis and trochanteric sites, are available.[31,32] Although the percutaneous insertion instrumentation and techniques have simplified instrumentation and also creation of accurate insertion vectors, damage to the external rotators and/or the gluteus medius tendon still occurs on insertion, as well as a theoretical risk of injury to the femoral head blood supply. Newly designed helical-shaped nails use a lateral entry site (10 mm lateral to the trochanteric tip on the AP view) and the middle third of the trochanter (on the lateral view).[33] The lateral entry site preserves the soft-tissue attachments to the tip of the greater trochanter. According to a 2014 study, experiences with a helical-shaped nail and lateral entry insertion technique in Europe have been favorable and comparable with traditional nailing techinques.[34] Outcomes analysis in greater detail is required to determine the benefit of this versus other techniques. Experience with lateral entry nailing is also increasing in skeletally immature patients to minimize the risk of damage to the blood supply of the femoral head.[35]

Minimally invasive plate osteosynthesis for pediatric femoral shaft fractures is well described, especially in patients from walking age through young teenagers. This technique is essentially identical to that performed in adults, with more limited indications. Curved, large fragment plates facilitate percutaneous application. Indirect reduction is first performed with a mechanical distraction device. The plate is introduced via proximal and distal access incisions of approximately 6 cm. The tip of the plate is pressed against the bone to maintain its position in the submuscular space (**Figure 4**). Although used less commonly in adults, percutaneous applications have had recent success.[36] Most commonly, these techniques are used in the setting of ipsilateral neck fractures, and increasingly for interprosthetic femoral shaft fractures.

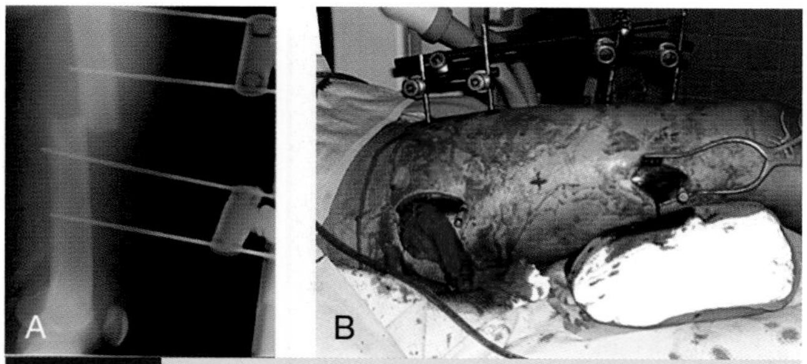

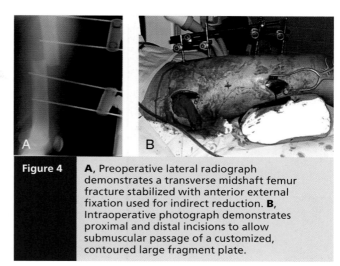

Figure 4 **A**, Preoperative lateral radiograph demonstrates a transverse midshaft femur fracture stabilized with anterior external fixation used for indirect reduction. **B**, Intraoperative photograph demonstrates proximal and distal incisions to allow submuscular passage of a customized, contoured large fragment plate.

Distal Femur Fractures

Some early experiences with MIO technique were developed to treat metaphyseal fractures around the knee joint. Minimally invasive plate fixation of distal femoral fractures developed as a standard approach to treat most C-type (complete articular) fractures of the distal femur. Medial submuscular plate application is one new concept in minimally invasive fixation for distal femur fractures and periprosthetic fractures. This technique has application in situations with medial bone loss and poor bone quality in which two-column fixation is preferable, as well as other situations. Further indications need more extensive clinical experience. The safe zones for plate application have been described on the medial side of the distal femur, demonstrating safe application using this method.[37] Varus failure, which is common, could be lessened using this approach.

Interest has increased in retrograde distal femur nailing for distal acute fractures as well as periprosthetic fractures just proximal to total knee arthroplasty (TKA) implants. This trend seems to be indicated most often in patients with poor bone quality for whom questions of lower healing rates with lateral locking plate applications remain.[38] Retrograde nailing of distal femur fractures has traditionally been limited by the ability to achieve adequate fixation in more distal fracture variants; however, more recent nail designs have included very distally directed, multiplanar, and fixed-angle interlocking screw positions, which have allowed more distal fixation options (**Figure 5**). In addition, most contemporary TKA designs have an intercondylar aperture that allows passage of a retrograde nail. In the setting of nail placement through a TKA, the start site should be established after an open arthrotomy to protect the TKA components (in contrast to nonperiprosthetic fractures, which can be repaired with a limited opening incision). Also, the start site for the retrograde nail through a TKA is much more posterior, and this may require a nail with special design characteristics (lower radius of curvature, beveled tip) as well as augments (such as blocking screws) to maintain reduction (**Figure 6**).

Diaphyseal Tibia Fractures

Intramedullary Nailing

Intramedullary nailing is the gold standard for treating diaphyseal tibia fractures.[39] Although most tibia fractures can be stabilized in this manner, certain clinical scenarios benefit from plate fixation. Patients with altered or

5: General Topics

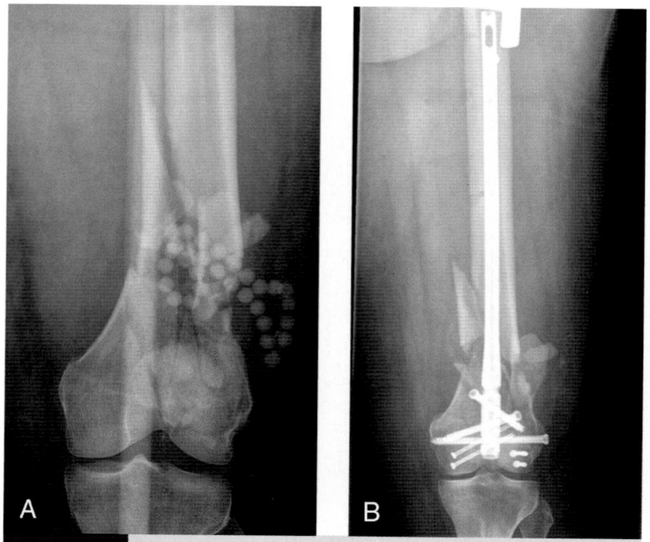

Figure 5 **A**, Preoperative AP knee radiograph demonstrates a C-type (intra-articular) distal femur fracture with proximal extension. **B**, AP knee radiograph following open reduction and internal fixation of a distal articular injury with subsequent passage of retrograde intramedullary nail.

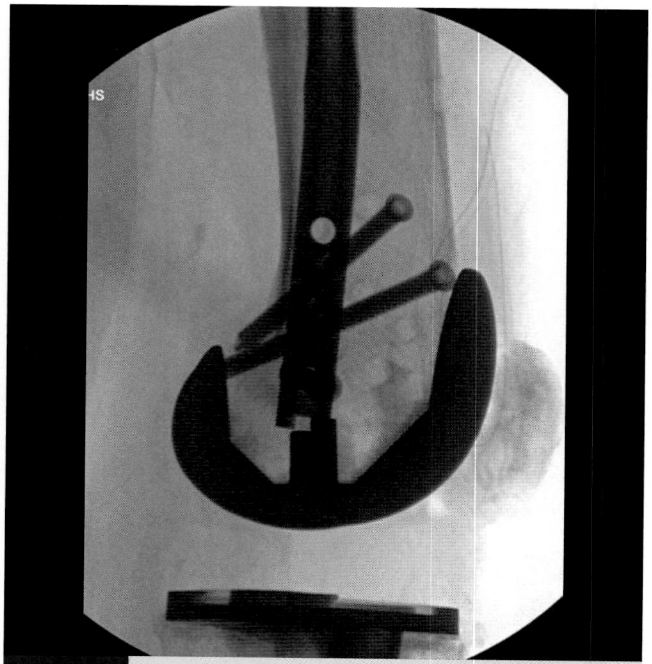

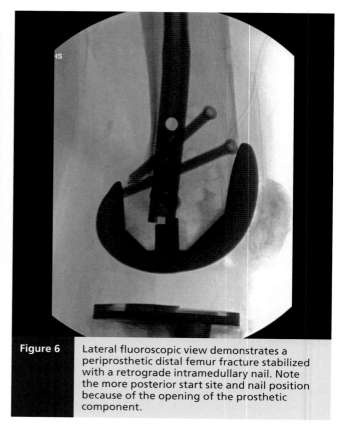

Figure 6 Lateral fluoroscopic view demonstrates a periprosthetic distal femur fracture stabilized with a retrograde intramedullary nail. Note the more posterior start site and nail position because of the opening of the prosthetic component.

sclerotic intramedullary canals as a result of prior injury, patients of small stature who cannot accommodate an intramedullary implant, the presence of malunion or nonunion, previous cruciate ligament reconstruction, and the presence of a TKA prosthesis are all indications for plate osteosynthesis. In addition, plating is indicated in patients with burns or soft-tissue compromise at the nail insertion site and pediatric patients with open physes. In patients who are elite athletes, plating should be considered to minimize the likelihood of anterior knee pain.[39,40] Technologic advances in surgical technique and implant design allow minimally invasive plate osteosynthesis with both conventional and locking constructs. Minimally invasive techniques can be used to treat acute fractures as well as some cases of malunion and nonunion[41,42] (**Figure 7**). Although not commonly performed, more recent reports have been published on intramedullary nailing around a TKA prosthesis with both antegrade and retrograde approaches. Biomechanics and limited clinical studies show promise for this unique technique.[43-45]

Fractures of the Proximal Quartile

As with the deforming forces seen in subtrochanteric femur fractures, the deformities encountered with tibia fractures of the proximal quartile can be problematic. If these deformities are not treated appropriately, valgus and apex anterior malreductions will occur.[46,47] In addition to percutaneous reduction instruments and techniques, alternative surgical approaches can also be used. The suprapatellar/retropatellar or semiextended approaches allow the leg to be placed in a more extended position, which minimizes apex anterior and valgus deformity commonly seen. Although concerns are valid for damage to intra-articular structures with these approaches, anatomic and clinical series have shown similar risks as well as early favorable results.[39]

Distal Tibial Fractures

Although intramedullary nailing with extremely distal interlocking designs is now feasible for distal tibia fractures and is an optimal minimally invasive solution in the setting of a damaged soft-tissue envelope, questions still exist about the stability of interlocking screws in distal metaphyseal locations. New interlocking designs with the capability to achieve an interference fit with the intramedullary nail have improved angular stability.[48]

Submuscular plating for the distal tibia can be performed on the anterolateral or medial distal surfaces, depending on the fracture pattern.[49] Plate fixation can be achieved via two indirect reduction approaches. The

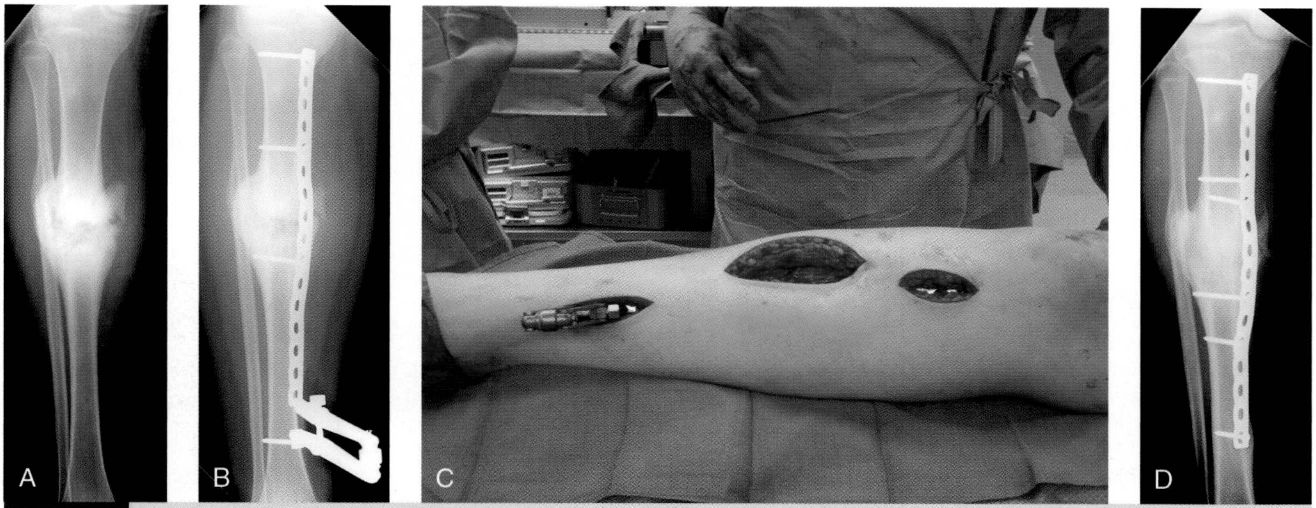

Figure 7 Images of hypertrophic nonunion in a right tibia. **A**, AP radiograph demonstrates callus formation. **B**, Intraoperative fluoroscopic AP view demonstrates minimally invasive compression plating. The plate was contoured and secured proximally, followed by application of the articulated device distally and stabilization after appropriate tensioning. **C**, Intraoperative photograph demonstrates limited exposure of tibial nonunion via three medial incisions. **D**, Postoperative AP radiograph demonstrates healing of nonunion and maintenance of coronal alignment.

reduction can first be almost completed using mechanical distraction with some type of ankle-spanning external fixation device. The plate is applied to an almost completely reduced fracture and minor reduction adjustments are made with strategic clamp or screw placement. Alternatively, the plate can be fixed distally first, and using the push/pull technique proximally can be effective; the plate is passed epiperiosteally, and perfectly aligned and fixed to the distal fragment. Optimally, an anatomically contoured plate is used that incorporates the 20° internal rotation and 20° radius of curvature to assist in the frontal and rotational reduction. Following distal fixation, a screw is placed just above the plate, and a lamina spreader or bone-holding clamp is used to push or pull the distal fragment and plate to the anatomic length. Multiplanar imaging is performed to ensure sagittal plane fracture reduction and perfect plate alignment on the proximal fragment before placing screws percutaneously into the proximal fragment.

Summary

MIO techniques are used throughout the body to achieve fracture reduction and stability. These contemporary approaches minimize the insult to soft-tissue attachments in the fracture zone that are frequently disrupted using traditional open approaches. Many of these techniques require special surgical equipment, specific instrumentation, and unique surgical techniques. Specialized implants have been developed for the proximal humerus, which allow minimally invasive reduction and stabilization of metaphyseal fractures. Diaphyseal fractures of the upper and lower extremity can be managed with minimally invasive techniques using nonspecialized hardware. Continued implant evolution allows distal femur, proximal tibia, and distal tibia fractures to be stabilized using minimally invasive techniques. Closed reduction and percutaneous stabilization techniques for pelvic ring injuries reduce patient surgical morbidity and improve outcomes.

Key Study Points

- Minimally invasive surgical techniques minimize the soft-tissue disruption associated with open approaches to reduction and instrumentation.
- Indirect reduction techniques are frequently required prior to instrumentation.
- Detailed knowledge of anatomy is critical for safe insertion of instrumentation.
- Traditional implants can be used successfully for many fracture types.
- Evolution in implant design has simplified minimally invasive surgical insertion.

Annotated References

1. Laflamme GY, Rouleau DM, Berry GK, Beaumont PH, Reindl R, Harvey EJ: Percutaneous humeral plating of fractures of the proximal humerus: Results of a prospective multicenter clinical trial. *J Orthop Trauma* 2008;22(3):153-158.

2. Hessmann MH, Nijs S, Mittlmeier T, et al: Internal fixation of fractures of the proximal humerus with the MultiLoc nail. *Oper Orthop Traumatol* 2012;24(4-5):418-431.

   In this study, an anterior acromial approach was used to treat 160 patients with various simple and complex proximal humeral fractures; these patients were followed for 6 months. All fractures healed with a favorable shoulder functional outcome score and a low complication rate; loss of reduction was rare.

3. Biber R, Zirngibl B, Bail HJ, Stedtfeld HW: An innovative technique of rear entry creation for retrograde humeral nailing: How to avoid iatrogenic comminution. *Injury* 2013;44(4):514-517.

   This retrospective study described a custom device used for precise placement of the insertion site for retrograde humeral nailing; 41 patients underwent accurate placement and no iatrogenic fractures were reported. Surgical times were shorter than those reported for the antegrade technique. A custom tool for the insertion site could optimize the safety of the retrograde nailing technique.

4. Bhandari M, Devereaux PJ, McKee MD, Schemitsch EH: Compression plating versus intramedullary nailing of humeral shaft fractures—a meta-analysis. *Acta Orthop* 2006;77(2):279-284.

5. Zhiquan A, Bingfang Z, Yeming W, Chi Z, Peiyan H: Minimally invasive plating osteosynthesis (MIPO) of middle and distal third humeral shaft fractures. *J Orthop Trauma* 2007;21(9):628-633.

6. Kim JW, Oh CW, Byun YS, Kim JJ, Park KC: A prospective randomized study of operative treatment for noncomminuted humeral shaft fractures: Conventional open plating versus minimal invasive plate osteosynthesis. *J Orthop Trauma* 2015;29(4):189-194.

   In this study, 68 fractures were randomized to open or minimally invasive plate osteosynthesis plating: 31 fractures (97%) in the open group healed within 16 weeks and 36 fractures (100%) in the minimally invasive plate osteosynthesis group healed by 15 weeks. No differences were reported in the surgical time or complication rates. All fractures healed with excellent function.

7. Routt ML Jr, Nork SE, Mills WJ: Percutaneous fixation of pelvic ring disruptions. *Clin Orthop Relat Res* 2000;375:15-29.

8. Stover MD, Sims S, Matta J: What is the infection rate of the posterior approach to type C pelvic injuries? *Clin Orthop Relat Res* 2012;470(8):2142-2147.

   This multicenter retrospective review investigated surgical site infection associated with open posterior approaches in a diverse group of complete posterior pelvic ring injuries in 236 patients and reported an infection rate of 3.4%. These patients required surgical débridement, closure, and antibiotics with no additional soft-tissue reconstruction needed or catastrophic complications reported. Patient selection and the surgical technique described were key for minimizing wound complications.

9. Fowler TT, Bishop JA, Bellino MJ: The posterior approach to pelvic ring injuries: A technique for minimizing soft tissue complications. *Injury* 2013;44(12):1780-1786.

   In this retrospective review of 31 patients who underwent 34 modified posterior approaches to the posterior pelvic ring, a surgical site infection rate of 2.94% was reported. Minimizing subcutaneous dissection and creating a full-thickness fasciocutaneous flap were emphasized. No complications related to the repair of the gluteus maximus tendinous origin on the iliac crest were reported. Level of evidence: IV.

10. Miller AN, Routt ML Jr: Variations in sacral morphology and implications for iliosacral screw fixation. *J Am Acad Orthop Surg* 2012;20(1):8-16.

    This review article describes the key radiographic characteristics of sacral dysmorphism, which allows full understanding and correlation on CT review. Applying this knowledge allows the surgeon to safely place iliosacral screws in possible osseous corridors. Level of evidence: V.

11. Bishop JA, Routt ML Jr: Osseous fixation pathways in pelvic and acetabular fracture surgery: Osteology, radiology, and clinical applications. *J Trauma Acute Care Surg* 2012;72(6):1502-1509.

    Because of the unique osseous morphology of the pelvis, the term osseous fixation pathway is introduced to describe the geometrically complex "bone tubes" located throughout the pelvis. Each corticated bony cylinder is described and the corresponding fluoroscopic views used to best appreciate each pathway are defined. The size and dimension of each pathway vary among patients, and the ability to safely place an intraosseous implant depends on recognizing the fluoroscopic anatomy. Level of evidence: V.

12. Eastman JG, Routt ML Jr: Correlating preoperative imaging with intraoperative fluoroscopy in iliosacral screw placement. *J Orthop Traumatol* 2015;16(4):309-316.

    This retrospective review of 24 patients demonstrated the translation of preoperative planning of iliosacral screws to the operating room. The anticipated inlet and outlet view angles measured on preoperative sagittal reconstruction CT scans were compared with the intraoperative fluoroscopic angles used. The reported differences were 4.4° for the inlet and 0.45° for the outlet. Level of evidence: IV.

13. McAndrew CM, Merriman DJ, Gardner MJ, Ricci WM: Standardized posterior pelvic imaging: Use of CT inlet and CT outlet for evaluation and management of pelvic ring injuries. *J Orthop Trauma* 2014;28(12):665-673.

This retrospective review of 68 patients demonstrated the variability of safe zone measurements for iliosacral screws when using routing axial imaging in comparison with specific CT sequences oriented perpendicular and parallel to the sacrum. When compared with CT inlet specific views, the safe zones for S1 and S2 screws are underestimated using routine axial CT images. Appreciating the variability of the posterior pelvic ring preoperatively is mandatory and intraoperative application allows safe iliosacral screw placement. Level of evidence: IV.

14. Reilly MC, Bono CM, Litkouhi B, Sirkin M, Behrens FF: The effect of sacral fracture malreduction on the safe placement of iliosacral screws. *J Orthop Trauma* 2006;20(1suppl):S37-S43.

15. Nork SE, Jones CB, Harding SP, Mirza SK, Routt ML Jr: Percutaneous stabilization of U-shaped sacral fractures using iliosacral screws: Technique and early results. *J Orthop Trauma* 2001;15(4):238-246.

16. Ruatti S, Kerschbaumer G, Gay E, Milaire M, Merloz P, Tonetti J: Technique for reduction and percutaneous fixation of U- and H-shaped sacral fractures. *Orthop Traumatol Surg Res* 2013;99(5):625-629.

    This retrospective review and discussion demonstrated the benefit of supine positioning in treatment of U- and H-shaped sacral fractures. Placing a lumbosacral bump under patients and using bilateral distal femoral skeletal traction helps induce a lordotic vector, which minimizes the kyphotic deformity commonly seen in these fracture patterns. Level of evidence: IV.

17. Routt ML Jr, Simonian PT, Mills WJ: Iliosacral screw fixation: Early complications of the percutaneous technique. *J Orthop Trauma* 1997;11(8):584-589.

18. Routt ML Jr, Falicov A, Woodhouse E, Schildhauer TA: Circumferential pelvic antishock sheeting: A temporary resuscitation aid. *J Orthop Trauma* 2002;16(1):45-48.

19. Gardner MJ, Osgood G, Molnar R, Chip Routt ML Jr: Percutaneous pelvic fixation using working portals in a circumferential pelvic antishock sheet. *J Orthop Trauma* 2009;23(9):668-674.

20. Gardner MJ, Parada S, Chip Routt ML Jr: Internal rotation and taping of the lower extremities for closed pelvic reduction. *J Orthop Trauma* 2009;23(5):361-364.

21. Tonetti J, van Overschelde J, Sadok B, Vouaillat H, Eid A: Percutaneous ilio-sacral screw insertion. Fluoroscopic techniques. *Orthop Traumatol Surg Res* 2013;99(8):965-972.

    This retrospective review and technical discussion of percutaneous fixation of pelvic ring injuries reported on several closed reduction methods as well as the authors' method of iliosacral screw placement with corresponding intraoperative fluoroscopic views. Level of evidence: IV.

22. Evans AR, Routt ML Jr, Nork SE, Krieg JC: Oblique distraction external pelvic fixation. *J Orthop Trauma* 2012;26(5):322-326.

    This retrospective series demonstrated the use of oblique anterior pelvic external fixation to correct hemipelvic deformity and instability. The extension and external rotation vectors generated through the construct facilitates the reduction of flexion and internal rotation deformities commonly seen with lateral compression–type pelvic ring injuries. Level of evidence: IV.

23. Matta JM, Yerasimides JG: Table-skeletal fixation as an adjunct to pelvic ring reduction. *J Orthop Trauma* 2007;21(9):647-656.

24. Lefaivre KA, Starr AJ, Reinert CM: Reduction of displaced pelvic ring disruptions using a pelvic reduction frame. *J Orthop Trauma* 2009;23(4):299-308.

25. Wright RD, Glueck DA, Selby JB, Rosenblum WJ: Intraoperative use of the pelvic c-clamp as an aid in reduction for posterior sacroiliac fixation. *J Orthop Trauma* 2006;20(8):576-579.

26. Richard MJ, Tornetta P III: Emergent management of APC-2 pelvic ring injuries with an anteriorly placed C-clamp. *J Orthop Trauma* 2009;23(5):322-326.

27. Gardner MJ, Mehta S, Mirza A, Ricci WM: Anterior pelvic reduction and fixation using a subcutaneous internal fixator. *J Orthop Trauma* 2012;26(5):314-321.

    In this multicenter retrospective study, 24 patients with various pelvic fractures underwent treatment with a subcutaneous internal fixator. Indications included anterior ring injuries that would benefit from anterior external fixation for definitive treatment. Benefits include no open wounds at pin sites and increased biomechanical strength for reduction and fixation with larger pins and bars closer to pin construct. Complications included grade 1 heterotopic ossification in six patients and lateral femoral cutaneous nerve neurapraxia in two, which fully resolved. Level of evidence: IV.

28. Hesse D, Kandmir U, Solberg B, et al: Femoral nerve palsy after pelvic fracture treated with INFIX: A case series. *J Orthop Trauma* 2015;29(3):138-143.

    In this retrospective series, six patients with eight femoral nerve palsies underwent treatment with an anterior subcutaneous internal fixator. After implant removal, persistent femoral nerve dysfunction was reported in several patients; two cases of complete recovery were reported. Surgeons should be aware of potential neurovascular complications with the technique. Level of evidence: IV.

29. Gardner MJ, Chip Routt ML Jr: The antishock iliosacral screw. *J Orthop Trauma* 2010;24(10):e86-e89.

    In this case report, iliosacral screw reduction of complete sacroiliac joint disruption was performed in a hemodynamically unstable patient. Percutaneous manipulation occurs with Schanz pins in the medius pillar and/or anterior inferior iliac spine and limited manipulation is performed based on the patient's hemodynamic status. This technique is useful with substantial distraction component injury patterns, but it can be used with any posterior pelvic ring injury. Level of evidence: V.

30. Scolaro JA, Routt ML: Intraosseous correction of misdirected cannulated screws and fracture malalignment using a bent tip 2.0 mm guidewire: Technique and indications. *Arch Orthop Trauma Surg* 2013;133(7):883-887.

In this study, surgical technique was reported using a manually bent tip 2.0-mm guidewire to alter the path of misdirected cannulated screws in the posterior and anterior pelvis. Screw paths can be changed and fracture reductions can be achieved in some circumstances, which can facilitate screw trajectory corrections in the middle of the placement sequence. This technique should not be used as a substitute for a poor starting point or insufficient knowledge of the osseous pelvic anatomy. Level of evidence: V.

31. Rhorer AS: Percutaneous/minimally invasive techniques in treatment of femoral shaft fractures with an intramedullary nail. *J Orthop Trauma* 2009;23(5suppl):S2-S5.

32. Bellabarba C, Herscovici D Jr, Ricci WM: Percutaneous treatment of peritrochanteric fractures using the gamma nail. 2000. *J Orthop Trauma* 2003;17(8suppl):S38-S50.

33. Ostrum RF, Marcantonio A, Marburger R: A critical analysis of the eccentric starting point for trochanteric intramedullary femoral nailing. *J Orthop Trauma* 2005;19(10):681-686.

34. Rether JR, Höntzsch D: Femoral nailing using a helical nail shape (LFN®). *Oper Orthop Traumatol* 2014;26(5):487-496.

In this prospective multicenter study, 227 helical femoral nails were used for antegrade femoral nailing. Follow-up after 12 months was available in 74%. The surgeons rated ease of identifying the entry site as excellent or good in 89%. Functional and radiologic results after 12 months do not prove substantial benefits over conventional antegrade femoral nails.

35. Keeler KA, Dart B, Luhmann SJ, et al: Antegrade intramedullary nailing of pediatric femoral fractures using an interlocking pediatric femoral nail and a lateral trochanteric entry point. *J Pediatr Orthop* 2009;29(4):345-351.

36. Angelini AJ, Livani B, Flierl MA, Morgan SJ, Belangero WD: Less invasive percutaneous wave plating of simple femur shaft fractures: A prospective series. *Injury* 2010;41(6):624-628.

Of 57 patients treated with percutaneous wave plate fixation for simple femoral shaft fractures, 54 healed by an average of 13 weeks. Two patients presented with implant failure; one patient displayed signs of delayed union. Eleven patients had postoperative deformities, including valgus deformities that developed in six patients and external rotation malalignment that developed in five. Overall, the technique was safe and effective.

37. Kim JJ, Oh HK, Bae JY, Kim JW: Radiological assessment of the safe zone for medial minimally invasive plate osteosynthesis in the distal femur with computed tomography angiography. *Injury* 2014;45(12):1964-1969.

In this retrospective review, 30 patients underwent CT angiography for free tissue transfer. The femur was divided into six levels between the lower margin of the lesser trochanter to the adductor tubercle, and the total length of this region was measured. The shortest distance from the outer border of the femur to the femoral artery was evaluated at each level. The average distance from the bone to the femoral artery and the anteromedial aspect of the distal half of the femur is the safe zone, and a long plate can be positioned safely in this zone at the anterior aspect up to the level of 8 cm inferior to the lesser trochanter.

38. Henderson CE, Kuhl LL, Fitzpatrick DC, Marsh JL: Locking plates for distal femur fractures: Is there a problem with fracture healing? *J Orthop Trauma* 2011;25(suppl 1):S8-S14.

This paper reviewed 18 publications of distal femur fractures repaired with lateral locking plates to evaluate successful healing with these implants. Problems with healing were noted in 0% to 32% in these studies. Many of the noted implant failures occurred late; one-half at 6 months. Healing problems, including nonunion, delayed union, and implant failure, are not infrequent and represent ongoing problems with distal femur fracture treatment.

39. Tejwani N, Polonet D, Wolinsky PR: Controversies in the intramedullary nailing of proximal and distal tibia fractures. *J Am Acad Orthop Surg* 2014;22(10):665-673.

This review article discusses treatment of metadiaphyseal tibia fractures. Reduction and fixation adjuncts are presented, including plating versus nailing. Alternative surgical procedures are covered, including suprapatellar nailing. Level of evidence: V.

40. Schmidt AH, Finkemeier CG, Tornetta P III: Treatment of closed tibial fractures. *Instr Course Lect* 2003;52:607-622.

41. Hasenboehler E, Rikli D, Babst R: Locking compression plate with minimally invasive plate osteosynthesis in diaphyseal and distal tibial fracture: A retrospective study of 32 patients. *Injury* 2007;38(3):365-370.

42. Gardner MJ, Toro-Arbelaez JB, Hansen M, Boraiah S, Lorich DG, Helfet DL: Surgical treatment and outcomes of extraarticular proximal tibial nonunions. *Arch Orthop Trauma Surg* 2008;128(8):833-839.

43. Zafra-Jiménez JA, Pretell-Mazzini J, Resines-Erasun C: Distal tibial fracture below a total knee arthroplasty: retrograde intramedullary nailing as an alternative method of treatment: a case report. *J Orthop Trauma* 2011;25(7):e74-e76.

In this case report, an 85-year-old woman with type I diabetes mellitus, hypertension, and chronic venous insufficiency with lower extremity venous stasis ulcers sustained a distal-third tibia fracture below a TKA prosthesis. The patient underwent retrograde hindfoot fusion with a nail. Although the implant crosses the subtalar and tibiotalar joints, the fracture healed and the patient returned to her previous level of function with no reported deficits. Concerns with crossing distal joints as well as having stress

5: General Topics

riser between the nail and TKA prosthesis were discussed. Level of evidence: V.

44. Kuhn S, Appelmann P, Pairon P, Mehler D, Rommens PM: The Retrograde Tibial Nail: Presentation and biomechanical evaluation of a new concept in the treatment of distal tibia fractures. *Injury* 2014;45(suppl 1):S81-S86.

    In this biomechanical comparison of a prototype retrograde tibial intramedullary implant and a commonly used antegrade nail using a 10-mm defect, axial and torsional testing were performed. Comparable stability in axial load and statistically increased rotational stability were reported. Biomechanical comparability of the new implant was reported; however, further studies are needed. Level of evidence: V.

45. Doulens KM, Joshi AB, Wagner RA: Tibial fracture after total knee arthroplasty treated with retrograde intramedullary fixation. *Am J Orthop (Belle Mead NJ)* 2007;36(7):E111-E113.

46. Freedman EL, Johnson EE: Radiographic analysis of tibial fracture malalignment following intramedullary nailing. *Clin Orthop Relat Res* 1995;315:25-33.

47. Lang GJ, Cohen BE, Bosse MJ, Kellam JF: Proximal third tibial shaft fractures. Should they be nailed? *Clin Orthop Relat Res* 1995;315:64-74.

48. Wähnert D, Stolarczyk Y, Hoffmeier KL, Raschke MJ, Hofmann GO, Mückley T: Long-term stability of angle-stable versus conventional locked intramedullary nails in distal tibia fractures. *BMC Musculoskelet Disord* 2013;14:66.

    In this cadaver biomechanical loading study, torsional and axial loading of angle-stable screws and conventional locking screws were reported. The angle-stable screws showed a substantially higher torsional stiffness compared with conventional screws at all times. The angle-stable screws with the biodegradable sleeve provide substantially increased long-term stability with differences under torsional loading that could be clinically relevant.

49. Helfet DL, Suk M: Minimally invasive percutaneous plate osteosynthesis of fractures of the distal tibia. *Instr Course Lect* 2004;53:471-475.

Chapter 6

New Technologies in Orthopaedic Trauma

Jake P. Heiney, MD, MS

Abstract

Several new technologies are being used in orthopaedic trauma care. These technologies include balloon osteoplasty, suprapatellar tibial intramedullary nailing in the semiextended position, alternatives for placing intramedullary nails to reduce radiation exposure, carbon fiber implants, biologic active implants, amniotic cells to promote wound healing, disposable negative-pressure wound therapy devices, rib plating for flail chest, limb lengthening, and Google Glass in orthopaedic surgery. It is important for the orthopaedic surgeon to be knowledgeable about conditions resulting from orthopaedic trauma, and theory can be applied to develop new technology to solve those problems.

Keywords: new technology; trauma

Introduction

In many respects, medical care in the United States is considered the best in the world. One reason is the constant innovation and advancement of new technologies. Orthopaedic trauma surgeons must embrace new technologies to improve and pioneer the best treatments for patients and help constrain increasing medical costs.[1]

Dr. Heiney or an immediate family member is a member of a speakers' bureau or has made paid presentations on behalf of Medtronic, Smith & Nephew, and Osteomed, serves as a paid consultant to Invuity and Medtronic, serves as an unpaid consultant to Invuity, has received research or institutional support from Medtronic, and serves as a board member, owner, officer, or committee member of the Orthopaedic Trauma Association.

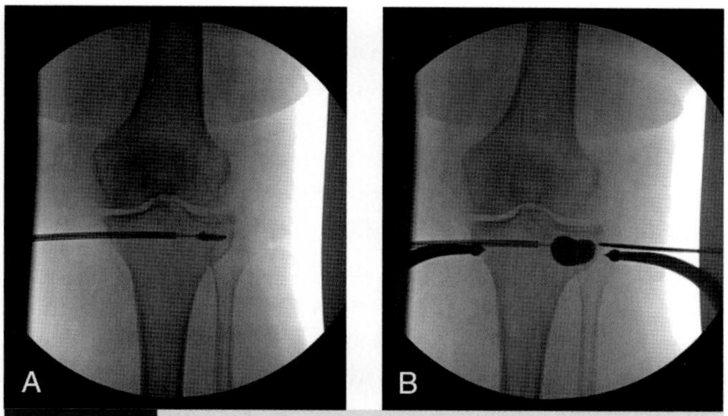

Figure 1 Intraoperative fluoroscopic AP images of tibial plateau fracture reduction using balloon osteoplasty. **A**, The inflatable bone tamp is partially inflated. **B**, The inflatable bone tamp is fully inflated to aid in reduction of a tibial plateau fracture.

Balloon Osteoplasty

The use of inflatable balloons as bone tamps for fracture reduction had its first commercial use in the area of spine surgery. In recent years, these balloons have been used as inflatable bone tamps to reduce articular surfaces in procedures termed balloon osteoplasties. A 2010 clinical case series provided a detailed description of a successful technique that achieved percutaneous balloon reduction of articular surfaces and then backfilled the voids with fast-setting calcium phosphate.[2] The fast-setting calcium phosphate provides immediate articular support in an isothermic manner because of the proximity of the articular surface. Since the initial description of the technique, other studies have reported on the clinical success of balloon osteoplasty,[3] including its ability to obtain and maintain fracture reduction and its use with standard implants until radiographic union of periarticular fractures is obtained. Success has been reported with fractures of the distal radius, tibial plateau (**Figure 1**), tibial pilon, and calcaneus.[4]

The clinical findings concerning balloon osteoplasty have been supported biomechanically. A balloon tamp and fast-setting, drillable calcium phosphate was found to be biomechanically superior to traditional metal tamps, cortical cancellous chips, and fast-setting drillable calcium phosphate when reduction was performed percutaneously using only intraoperative fluoroscopy.[5] Substantially less malreduction and overreduction also was reported when the inflatable bone tamp was used compared with traditional methods. The better performance of the inflatable bone tamp was predicted because of the clinical problem of articular violation when using a traditional bone tamp for the reduction of tibial plateau fractures. Independent reviewers also judged the visual reduction of the articular surface to be subjectively superior when reduction was achieved with an inflatable bone tamp compared with reduction achieved with a traditional bone tamp.

These clinical and laboratory results have led to the adoption of balloon osteoplasty for reduction in several types of articular fractures, including tibial plateau, tibial pilon, calcaneus, distal radius, acetabulum, and proximal humerus fractures.[2,4,6,7] In many instances, the inflatable bone tamp provides a more biomechanically sound construction and can potentially be introduced in a less disruptive manner than a traditional bone tamp. With proper technique, this tool has the potential to decrease the risk of wound complications through the use of potentially smaller incisions with less soft-tissue disruption compared with traditional metal bone tamps.

Suprapatellar Tibial Intramedullary Nailing in the Semiextended Position

Suprapatellar or retropatellar intramedullary (IM) nailing techniques have been developed to possibly avoid malunion complications and knee pain associated with traditional IM nailing techniques for tibial fractures. Traditional approaches to IM nailing are performed via the medial or lateral parapatellar and involve patellar tendon splitting.[8,9] The most common complications after this procedure is anterior knee pain.[8-10]

The suprapatellar approach to tibial IM nailing was originally described as an open medial parapatellar arthrotomy, with lateral subluxation of the patella during the procedure. This technique was later revised to a more minimally invasive approach.[8,11] Other suprapatellar portal options (including retropatellar approaches) in which the nail is advanced from proximal and posterior to the patella and onto the tibial plateau have been described.[8,9] During nail placement, the knee is positioned in 10° to 15° of flexion to relax the quadriceps.[8,9] This technique helps prevent the procurvatum deformity that typically occurs with proximal one-third tibial shaft fractures treated with traditional approaches.

A recent study indicates that most patients treated with suprapatellar nailing recovered with almost full knee range of motion and no reports of knee pain.[9] Some patients were observed for arthroscopic changes of the knee immediately after the insertion of the nail. No important findings were reported, except for two patients who had grade II chondromalacia of the trochlea immediately after the procedure. At 1-year follow-up, normal MRI findings were reported for both patients. However, a cadaver study found similar risks and damage to the menisci, articular surface, anterior cruciate ligament insertion, fat pad, and intermeniscal ligament with suprapatellar nailing compared with other nailing techniques.[10] Therefore, like many new technologies, proper training for the correct use of the technique is likely crucial for excellent outcomes and the avoidance of increased complication rates.

Alternatives for Placing IM Nails to Reduce Radiation Exposure

The freehand technique for placing interlocking bolts in IM nails remains a challenging procedure for surgeons and can lead to substantial radiation exposure for the patient, the surgeon, and the operating room personnel. Radiation-induced cancer is increasing among orthopaedic surgeons, who have a relative risk for any type of cancer that is 5.37 times greater than that of the general population.[12] Malignancies in personnel exposed to radiation range from cancers of solid organs (ie, thyroid and pancreas) to skin and hematopoietic cancers. In female orthopaedic surgeons, the standardized prevalence ratio for all cancers is 1.9, and 2.88 specifically for breast cancer when compared with the general population.[12] A number of studies have demonstrated substantial exposure to fluoroscopy during freehand placement of locking bolts.[13]

As a result, a number of techniques and systems (implants, devices, and external guides) have been developed to help minimize radiation exposure. Attempts have been made using proximally based outriggers; however, because of nail deformation inside the medullary canal, they are not always accurate. A computer-navigated electromagnetic system without fluoroscopic radiation was developed and has been shown in clinical practice to guide the freehand placement of interlocking bolts with accuracy similar to that achieved with conventional fluoroscopically guided bolt insertion. Equal or shorter procedure times were also reported.[14,15]

Another technique that has demonstrated a reduction in radiation exposure uses a computer in concert with C-arm landmarks. This technique uses a targeting jig

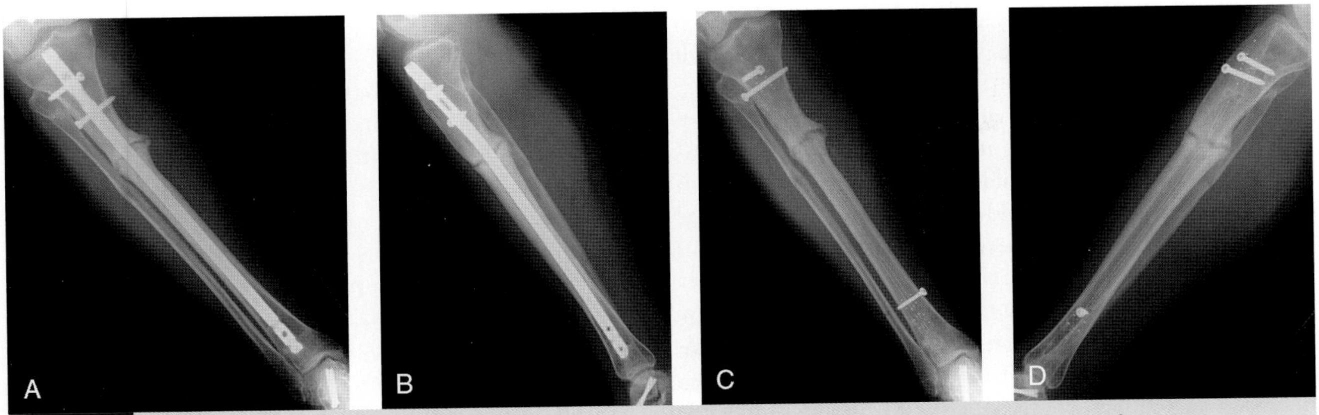

Figure 2 AP (**A**) and lateral (**B**) radiographs of a 4-year-old tibial fracture show a symptomatic nonunion after attempt at dynamization. Postoperative AP (**C**) and lateral (**D**) radiographs after carbon fiber nailing of the tibia shaft nonunion and bone grafting.

that sends positional information back to the computer, which then generates an image of the drill relative to the hole on the C-arm image and allows directional guidance of the drill. This technique is similar to that used in electromagnetic systems, except that this system can be connected to a fluoroscope that is already in place.[16]

A combined magnetic-manual system has been developed. This system uses a low-frequency magnetic field to find the position of the first hole, and the other holes are then located using a mechanical template. In a 2013 study, residents and attending orthopaedic surgeons were able to place locking bolts successfully in 239 of 240 attempts without exposure to radiation.[17]

Along with the risk of radiation exposure, locking bolt placement also is associated with neurovascular injury in 2% to 30% of patients.[18] The Fixion IM nail (Disc-O-Tech) is an expandable nailing system designed to address both radiation and complication issues. The nail is inserted and then expanded. Stability is obtained with an interference fit between the bone and the implant without interlocks. Because the Fixion IM nail does not use locking bolts or radiation, no associated complications or revisions have been reported in the literature. However, the average revision rate was 10.2%, with shortening reported in 3% of patients and fracture propagation in 2%.[18]

Carbon Fiber Implants

For many years, stainless steel has been the predominant metal used in orthopaedic implants for trauma-related surgeries. Stainless steel is easy to manufacture, is relatively low in cost, resists corrosion, is strong, and can be contoured intraoperatively. In some instances, titanium is used as an alternative implant material because of the benefits associated with its modulus of elasticity, which more closely matches that of bone, and its ability to be used in patients who are allergic to nickel.

Recently, carbon-fiber-reinforced (CFR) polyetheretherketone (PEEK) implants, which have multiple carbon fiber sheets layered in different directions and embedded in PEEK, have been introduced. These implants have the potential advantages of high fatigue strength, a low modulus of elasticity, and the allowance of improved intraoperative and postoperative imaging.[19] CFR-PEEK implants may be made with imbedded metal lines to allow for fluoroscopic and radiographic identification of the outline of the implant and locking bolt holes. However, the carbon composite does not obscure visualization with fluoroscopy, radiography, CT, or MRI. However, the typical amount of scatter with advanced imaging modalities is seen at the locations of screws and bolts, which are made of titanium. The use of CFR-PEEK implants has been reported to provide better visualization of fracture reduction and healing in clinical practice,[20,21] which can be critically important in patients with fracture nonunion or oncologic diseases (**Figure 2**).

The PEEK polymer has been shown to have excellent biocompatibility by eliciting minimal cellular response both in vitro and in vivo. This may be advantageous compared with metals such as nickel, which are known to cause allergic reactions.[20] In direct biomechanical comparisons with currently used metal implants, the PEEK polymer was found to have similar mechanical properties, with the added benefit of less wear debris.[22]

Although both titanium and carbon fiber implants have a modulus of elasticity closer to that of bone, carbon fiber does not have the cold-welding issue of titanium. Also, a low modulus of elasticity means that there is less stress shielding with high strain and strength in bending.

In clinical practice, ample callous formation leading to fracture union was found in patients treated with carbon fiber implants.[20,21]

Potential disadvantages of carbon fiber implants are the difficulty in visualization of implant failure and inability to contour the implants intraoperatively. With only a fine metal line imbedded in the implant, it may be difficult to visualize a failure, especially if the implant breaks but does not displace. In addition, the carbon fiber implants must be heated to their melting point to allow remolding; this is impractical for intraoperative contouring.[20] Although decreased stiffness can be advantageous, it is also recognized that too little stiffness can lead to complications such as nonunion.[19]

Biologic Active Implants

Device-associated infections are an increasing problem in the field of orthopaedics. Infection is a complication that results in substantial patient morbidity, potential mortality, and costs to the health system in billions of dollars.[23] When an infection occurs, the formation of a bacterial biofilm may necessitate a high dosage of antibiotics that could result in an overdose and possible associated complications such as renal failure, hepatotoxicity, or *Clostridium difficile* colitis.[24]

A solution is to deliver the antibiotic directly to the infection. In a common treatment pathway, the implant associated with the infection is removed if it is not stabilizing the fracture, the fracture is débrided, and antibiotic-loaded polymethyl methacrylate beads or spacers are placed. After the infection has been successfully treated, a new implant is placed. If the infection treatment is not successful, the process can be repeated until the infection is eradicated. This regimen has a high cost and is burdensome to the patient. Therefore, an antimicrobial coating on the surface of newly placed implants in setting of prior infection may suppress or prevent infection from re-forming and may possibly be an effective prophylactic in primary implants.[24,25] Antimicrobial coating has been used in other applications, such as urinary tract catheters, with great success;[24] however, it is still at an experimental stage for orthopaedic applications.

Infected local bone reabsorption takes place when an infection develops around an implant. Active and passive implant coatings have been developed to prevent bone loss and implant loosening.[24,25] These osteoconductive coatings "guide" bone formation on the coated surface to improve implant fixation and possibly prevent infection (passive coating). Other (active) osteoinductive coatings stimulate the undifferentiated cells to promote bone formation on the coating, most notably arginyl-glycyl-aspartic acid and bone morphogenetic protein coatings.[24,25]

The adherence of bacteria to implant surfaces and subsequent biofilm formation (glycocalyx) are challenging to manage, and treatment with systemically administered antibiotics is often unsuccessful. Therapeutic coatings applied to the implant surfaces are capable of inhibiting bacterial adhesion and are a potential strategy to treat and prevent implant-related infections. Crystalline arc-deposited titanium dioxide and biomimetic hydroxyapatite coatings have been evaluated for their potential use as antibacterial surface modifications for bone-anchored implants. These coatings have been shown to provide a bactericidal effect against *Staphylococcus epidermidis* and *Staphylococcus aureus* for clinically relevant times and doses, even when exposed to biomechanical forces during insertion. The treatment of implant surfaces with bioactive and biocompatible coatings holds promise in effecting clinical success in applications related to bone-anchored implants. These coatings provide an immediate response to bacterial implant contamination, may contribute to the minimization of postoperative infections, and may improve the bone-implant interface.[25]

Amniotic Cells to Promote Wound Healing

Orthopaedic trauma often leads to complex wounds. Normal wound healing is a complex biologic process that includes inflammation, proliferation, and remodeling. This process requires a complex interplay among numerous types of cells regulated by extracellular matrix, cytokine expression, stromal deposition, and epithelialization. Patients with traumatic orthopaedic injuries often have risk factors such as advanced age, nicotine use, hypertension, steroid use, diabetes, obesity, and renal failure that can compromise wound healing. The application of amniotic membrane cells may tip the biologic environment in favor of wound healing (**Figure 3**).

Amniotic membranes share the same cell origin as the fetus; hence, these cells work to protect the fetus from maternal immunologic insults. As a result, these tissues inherently contain a number of molecular modulators that combat inflammation.[26] Because amniotic tissue has shown clinical success as a potent anti-inflammatory and anti-scarring agent in other medical areas, it is now being used in orthopaedic applications for improved wound healing, tendon reinforcement, and nerve protection.[26] In clinical practice, the application of amniotic tissue products has aided in traumatic wound healing and protected tendon and nerve repairs.[27,28] Widespread successful

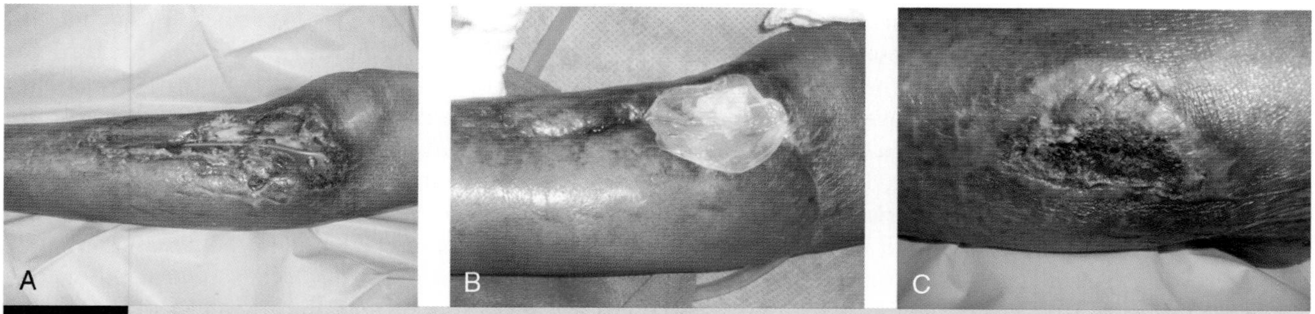

Figure 3 **A,** Clinical photograph of the lower limb of a patient taken after open reduction and internal fixation of a proximal tibia fracture. The limb was affected by compartment syndrome. **B,** Clinical photograph of the limb after 3 weeks of wound care that included the application of amniotic tissue. **C,** Clinical photograph of the healed wound after 8 weeks of wound care and amniotic cell treatment.

clinical use of these products and continuing research are beginning to clarify the mechanisms of action of amniotic tissue products.

It appears that one part of the mechanism of action occurs through retained amounts of high-molecular-weight, heavy chain hyaluronic acid (HC-HA), which are important in healing.[26] One signaling pathway uses HC-HA/pentraxin 3 (PTX3), which is a unique matrix component responsible for the therapeutic actions of these amniotic membranes. Soluble HC-HA/PTX3 suppresses the proliferation and promotes the apoptosis of lipopolysaccharide-induced macrophages. In addition, the immobilization of this component leads to upregulation of interleukin-10 and downregulation of interleukin-12 upon stimulation of interferon-alpha and lipopolysaccharides to polarize macrophages toward an activated macrophage, which plays an integral role in promoting a healing response.[29]

In addition, dehydrated human amnion chorion membrane (dHACM) has a number of growth factors and cytokines, including platelet-derived growth factor AA, transforming growth factor β-1, vascular endothelial growth factor, and fibroblast growth factor-2, along with inflammatory mediators such as interleukins and metalloproteinases. dHACM has demonstrated amplification of angiogenic cues, including inducing endothelial cell proliferation and upregulating the production of endogenous angiogenic growth factors. Also, dHACM has been shown to effectively recruit circulating progenitor cells, likely through the mechanism of stromal-derived factor expression.[26] Although the exact mechanisms of action continue to be elucidated, promising clinical results have been reported, including the healing of difficult wounds, the reduction of inflammation and wound-site pain, and the acceleration of healing time.[30,31]

Disposable Negative-Pressure Wound Therapy Devices

The benefits of negative-pressure wound therapy (NPWT) have been well reported in the literature, with more than 1,000 peer-reviewed publications describing its clinical efficacy and safety in various type of wounds over the past decade.[32] Wound healing benefits as a result of macrocellular and microcellular changes include decreasing the bioburden (eg, bacterial colonization) and swelling (interstitial edema), managing fluid, promoting a more rapid increase in granulation tissue and wound contraction, and inducing positive blood flow effects. In orthopaedics, specific applications have included aiding in wound closure, dressings for split-thickness skin grafts, and decreasing swelling in traumatic injuries. Negative-pressure wound dressings also are used as an incisional dressing for at-risk incisions or those with large amounts of exudate.[33]

Recently, easy-to-apply disposable devices have been developed for use in negative-pressure therapy. Negative pressure is generated from a disposable battery or by using spring power. These devices have shown clinical benefits equal to those of traditional negative-pressure devices in noninfected, nonischemic, nonplantar diabetic and venous wounds in the lower limbs.[34] Compared with traditional negative-pressure devices, the disposable units are smaller and allow more mobility for patients. Hospital discharge planning is also easier because the device is maintained for up to 1 week after discharge without need for a rental unit or a dressing change.

Disposable NPWT has played a major role in the healing success of high-risk, clean surgical incisions. Potential complications of surgical incisions include surgical dehiscence, hematomas, seromas, delayed healing, and infection (accounting for 17% to 22% of healthcare-associated infections).[35] The cost-effectiveness of traditional

NPWT has been demonstrated and, despite the increased upfront costs, it is likely that disposable NPWT may have equal if not greater financial benefits.[36] The use of disposable NPWT systems has improved wound healing and decreased overall costs for surgical and traumatic wounds.[37] When used over skin grafts, disposable NPWT systems provide a more efficient transition after hospital discharge, improved ease of use, and increased patient mobility compared with traditional negative-pressure devices.[38] Decreased infection rates also have been reported with the use of disposable NPWT systems over sternotomy incisions when the dressing remained in place for 6 to 7 days postoperatively compared with traditional sterile tape dressings; a similar result was found in wound care after vascular bypass surgery.[39,40]

Rib Plating for Flail Chest

For many years, rib plating has been successfully used to stabilize the chest wall of patients with flail chest, but it has been underutilized secondary to its complexity, time requirements, and limited knowledge about the technique.[41,42] Stabilization of a flail chest reduces ventilator time, pneumonia, mortality, and overall medical costs.[41,42]

Initially, rib plates were made of stainless steel that needed to be contoured to the curves of the ribs prior to placement. These types of implants were known to be uncomfortable and stiff, resulting in screw pullout caused by stress.[41] Kirschner wire also has been used to stabilize the chest wall; however, it can cause implant migration, which leads to other complications (including mortality).[41]

Recently, anatomic plates and IM rib splints have been designed to make the procedure less time consuming, decrease complexity, and reduce complications. The new anatomic plates are made of flexible titanium, which allows ribs flexion.[41] This theoretically limits hardware failure caused by stress. IM rib splints are also made of flexible titanium, allowing the same benefits as the anatomic plates.[41] Rib splints are more often used for simple fracture patterns, especially posterior fractures that otherwise would require elevation of the latissimus dorsi for plating.

The newer generation of implants also uses locking screws that help prevent implant migration.[41] The new designs of anatomic plates and rib splints simplify surgical procedures with more reliable stabilization and will likely see increased use in properly selected patients.

Limb Lengthening

Limb lengthening is a complicated procedure. Internal devices for limb lengthening include the Fitbone (Wittenstein), the Albizzia nail or newer Guichet nail (Guichet Clinic), and the Intramedullary Skeletal Kinetic Distractor (Orthofix); however, these devices are known to cause pain during lengthening; often require anesthesia for manipulation; and prevent monitoring of the lengthening rate, which can lead to high complication rates.[43,44] Patients are often noncompliant because of the complexity of their role in the lengthening process, and may not perform tasks as instructed or they perform tasks too frequently, which can lead to failed surgery.

For limb-length correction, external fixation devices have been used in the past and are still used, but they are associated with the risks of pin tract infection, skin pain, soft-tissue tethering, joint stiffness, and severe discomfort. Also, use of external devices often requires long periods of time in an awkward and sometimes uncomfortable device. Psychosocial complications are associated with the extended use of external fixation devices.[43]

Recent advances in limb lengthening have addressed some of the complex problems of older implants. A magnet-operated limb-lengthening nail (PRECICE; Ellipse Technologies) recently has been approved by the Food and Drug Administration. This IM nail is used for lengthening the femur and the tibia and uses the PRECICE External Remote Controller (ERC; Ellipse Technologies) to noninvasively lengthen the implant. The technology uses magnetic interaction between the implant and the ERC, which is a portable, handheld unit that controls the lengthening rate of the nail. The clinical efficacy of the PRECICE system is not fully understood at this time because of the limited available data. However, early studies showed high rates of distraction accuracy, maintenance of joint motion and bone alignment, and few complications compared with older lengthening devices.[43-45] Growth rates were easily controlled by the ERC, and patients were able to understand proper use of the system, which made the distraction rate very predictable.[43-45] Anecdotal reports from patients noted less pain compared with traditional lengthening procedures during the distraction process, with recovery of nearly full range of knee, ankle, and hip motion after physical therapy.[45] Reported complications included deep infection and delayed bone healing, which were treated with secondary procedures.[45] These early studies have limitations, including nonrandomized patient selection, a limited number of patients, and the short length of the follow-up periods. However, a magnet-operated limb-lengthening nail remains a promising tool in the armamentarium of treatment for limb-length problems.

Google Glass

As part of the information age, the introduction of Google Glass (Google Inc.) has demonstrated a number of potential benefits. Google Glass is a recently developed wearable computer that includes an optical display, camera, microphone, speaker, touchpad, gyroscope, and accelerometer. The computer can record photographs and videos using hands-free technology, which makes Google Glass a potentially important technology for surgical practice, including documentation and teaching.

Google Glass is worn above the line of sight and does not obscure vision. When the device is activated, the default command menu can be selected verbally, by finger touch, or by blinking an eye. With the default menu, the wearer can search Google, make a phone call, send a message, and take a picture or video that also can be transmitted to others. The system can also perform any activity that can be performed by the user's cell phone because it acts as an extension of the cell phone (a wireless Internet connection is required). Information that appears on the screen can be read by the user or heard as a voice reads the information.

The increasing complexity of orthopaedic trauma surgery coupled with restricted working hours for residents has created fewer opportunities for residents to acquire necessary surgical skills.[46,47] Research has identified the need for orthopaedic surgical skills laboratories and simulation technologies as required components of orthopaedic residency training programs. Thus far, only 50% of training programs offer access to such learning tools.[48]

Google Glass offers the novel ability to teach residents and attending physicians and allows experts in complex orthopaedic procedures to train other practicing surgeons. Remote video streaming enables an individual or an audience anywhere in the world to see what the operating surgeon is seeing. Initiatives of centers of excellence in the United States have attempted to establish surgical procedures to treat difficult cases to maximize patient outcomes; however, logistics, patient objections, and costs have made this goal difficult to achieve. The adoption of real-time augmented reality systems and wearable computing devices can allow a local surgeon to interact with an expert surgeon at a remote location while both view the local surgical field.[49]

Google Glass has been used successfully in clinical orthopaedic surgical practice.[49] Potential clinical applications including the ability to provide documents for other surgeons or patients; interaction with electronic medical records; review of imaging tests such as MRIs or CT scans; performance of telemedicine; completion of checklists; and, possibly, the ability to connect the operating room fluoroscopic monitor to the device to simplify monitor placement. Google Glass has been used to teach anatomy to students by integrating training in ultrasound and palpation techniques.[50]

Potential disadvantages of this type of technology include the legal concerns about adhering to the provisions of the Health Insurance Portability and Accountability Act and overcoming resistance to cultural change. Resolution of problems will require time, commitment, and innovative leadership.

Summary

Technologic advancements can affect the lives of patients in countless ways, and it is human nature to determine possible applications of new inventions and procedures. When applications of new technologies are explored, it is important to be mindful of the many advantages and as well as the disadvantages of those technologies. There are a number of inherent risks that come with a new technology that have applications in clinical practice, and many of these risks may only become apparent after widespread use. Also, because of the current emphasis on fiscal prudence, the usual increased upfront costs of new technologies must be recognized. However, it must also be acknowledged that new technologies may help constrain costs while improving both efficiency and the quality of patient care.

Key Study Points

- Advantages and disadvantages associated with some of the new technologies available to orthopaedic trauma surgeons should be explored for optimal patient care.
- Theory can be used to develop new technologies to address conditions resulting from orthopaedic trauma.

Annotated References

1. Koopmann MC, Kudsk KA, Szotkowski MJ, Rees SM: A team-based protocol and electromagnetic technology eliminate feeding tube placement complications. *Ann Surg* 2011;253(2):287-302.

   One to two million feeding tubes with stylets are placed annually in the United States. Feeding tube placement that used a team-based protocol with electromagnetic tracking decreased the morbidity and mortality of this common hospital procedure.

1: General Topics

2. Heiney J, O'Connor J: Balloon Reduction and Minimally Invasive Fixation (BRAMIF) for extremity fractures with the application of fast-setting calcium phosphate. *J Orthop* 2010;7(2):e8. Available at: https://www.researchgate.net/publication/45945597_Balloon_Reduction_And_Minimally_Invasive_Fixation_BRAMIF_for_Extremity_Fractures_with_the_Application_of_Fast-Setting_Calcium_Phosphate. Accessed January 15, 2016.

A novel technique using balloon reduction is described in detail. Successful outcomes were reported in fracture fixation of the calcaneus, tibial pilon, tibial plateau, and distal radius using an inflatable bone tamp and fast-setting calcium phosphate.

3. Hahnhaussen J, Hak DJ, Weckbach S, Heiney JP, Stahel PF: Percutaneous inflation osteoplasty for indirect reduction of depressed tibial plateau fractures. *Orthopedics* 2012;35(9):768-772.

The authors describe the technique of percutaneous balloon-guided inflation osteoplasty for the fixation of depressed lateral tibial plateau fractures.

4. Heiney JP, Redfern RE, Wanjiku S: Subjective and novel objective radiographic evaluation of inflatable bone tamp treatment of articular calcaneus, tibial plateau, tibial pilon and distal radius fractures. *Injury* 2013;44(8):1127-1134.

The authors use radiographs and statistics to show that an inflatable bone tamp and fast-setting calcium phosphate can be used for reduction of articular fractures, and that reduction can be maintained until union at 12 weeks. The analysis of independent evaluators incorporated a number of specific radiographic measurements. The objective and subjective analyses correlated with statistical analyses. The Fisher exact test demonstrated the technique was reproducible and resulted in acceptable, maintained reductions in 17 distal radius, 7 tibial pilon, 9 tibial plateau, and 8 calcaneus fractures.

5. Heiney JP, Kursa K, Schmidt AH, Stannard JP: Reduction and stabilization of depressed articular tibial plateau fractures: Comparison of inflatable and conventional bone tamps: Study of a cadaver model. *J Bone Joint Surg Am* 2014;96(15):1273-1279.

Cadaver tibial plateau fractures treated with an inflatable bone tamp had qualitatively and quantitatively better reductions than contralateral control fractures treated with a conventional bone tamp. Treatment with the inflatable bone tamp typically resulted in a smoother articular surface with less residual defect volume. Inflatable bone tamp reduced fractures exhibited less subsidence during cyclic loading and greater stiffness under static loading compared with fractures treated with a conventional bone tamp.

6. Sandmann GH, Ahrens P, Schaeffeler C, et al: Balloon osteoplasty: A new technique for minimally invasive reduction and stabilisation of Hill-Sachs lesions of the humeral head. A cadaver study. *Int Orthop* 2012;36(11):2287-2291.

This preliminary cadaver study demonstrated that using a balloon kyphoplasty system was a successful alternative treatment option for Hill-Sachs lesions and also reduced soft-tissue damage.

7. König B, Schaser K, Schäffler A, Stöckle U, Haas N: Percutaneous reduction and stabilization of a dislocated acetabular fracture: Case report [German]. *Unfallchirurg* 2006;109(4):328-331.

8. Morandi M, Banka T, Gaiarsa GP, et al: Intramedullary nailing of tibial fractures: Review of surgical techniques and description of a percutaneous lateral suprapatellar approach. *Orthopedics* 2010;33(3):172-179.

The authors describe a technique of proximal lateral suprapatellar nailing of tibial shaft fractures.

9. Sanders RW, DiPasquale TG, Jordan CJ, Arrington JA, Sagi HC: Semiextended intramedullary nailing of the tibia using a suprapatellar approach: Radiographic results and clinical outcomes at a minimum of 12 months follow-up. *J Orthop Trauma* 2014;28(5):245-255.

The authors describe results from a series of patients treated with intramedullary nailing of a tibia fracture using a semiextended approach through a suprapatellar portal. At 1 year follow-up, the patients reported an absence of anterior knee pain and had clinically acceptable tibial alignment, union, and knee range of motion. Level of evidence: IV.

10. Beltran MJ, Collinge CA, Patzkowski JC, Masini BD, Blease RE, Hsu JR; Skeletal Trauma Research Consortium (STReC): Intra-articular risks of suprapatellar nailing. *Am J Orthop (Belle Mead NJ)* 2012;41(12):546-550.

Suprapatellar nailing was done in 15 cadaver specimens. Injury was noted after nail passage, in one menisci, two medial articular surfaces, and three intermeniscal ligaments. No damage to anterior cruciate ligaments was reported.

11. Tornetta PIII, Collins E: Semiextended position of intramedullary nailing of the proximal tibia. *Clin Orthop Relat Res* 1996;328:185-189.

12. Singer G: Occupational radiation exposure to the surgeon. *J Am Acad Orthop Surg* 2005;13(1):69-76.

13. Soni RK, Mehta SM, Awasthi B, et al: Radiation-free insertion of distal interlocking screw in tibial and femur nailing: A simple technique. *J Surg Tech Case Rep* 2012;4(1):15-18.

A method of radiation-free distal interlocking screw insertion is described in which a same-length nail is placed over the skin. This method could potentially be used without an image intensifier.

14. Chan DS, Burris RB, Erdogan M, Sagi HC: The insertion of intramedullary nail locking screws without fluoroscopy: A faster and safer technique. *J Orthop Trauma* 2013;27(7):363-366.

The use of electromagnetic navigation for the insertion of intramedullary nail locking screws demonstrated accuracy

1: General Topics

equivalent to conventional fluoroscopic-guided insertion. Electromagnetic-guided locking screw insertion resulted in substantially shorter total procedural times and completely eliminated radiation exposure. Level of evidence: III.

15. Maqungo S, Horn A, Bernstein B, Keel M, Roche S: Distal interlocking screw placement in the femur: Free-hand versus electromagnetic assisted technique (SureShot). *J Orthop Trauma* 2014;28(12):e281-e283.

    The freehand technique of placing distal interlocking screws was compared with an electromagnetic targeting system with respect to time, radiation, and accuracy. The electromagnetic targeting device substantially reduced radiation exposure during the placement of distal interlocking screws without sacrificing surgical time, and it was equivalent in accuracy compared with the freehand technique. Level of evidence: II.

16. Windolf M, Schroeder J, Fliri L, Dicht B, Liebergall M, Richards RG: Reinforcing the role of the conventional C-arm: A novel method for simplified distal interlocking. *BMC Musculoskelet Disord* 2012;13:8.

    A new technique is introduced that uses information from conventional radiographic images to help accurately guide the placement of an interlocking bolt into an interlocking hole. Surgery time and radiation exposure using the newly developed technique were compared with a conventional freehand technique on the lower legs of human cadavers. The new technique resulted in a reduction in radiation exposure compared with the conventional freehand technique.

17. Negrin LL, Vécsei V: Is a magnetic-manual targeting device an appealing alternative for distal locking of tibial intramedullary nails? *Arch Trauma Res* 2013;2(1):16-20.

    A combined magnetic-manual system for the placement of locking bolts was developed. A low-frequency magnetic field is used to find the position of the first hole, and the other holes are located with a mechanical template. Residents and attending orthopaedic surgeons were able to place locking bolts successfully in 239 of 240 attempts without radiation exposure.

18. Beazley J, Mauffrey C, Seligson D: Treatment of acute tibial shaft fractures with an expandable nailing system: A systematic review of the literature. *Injury* 2011;42(suppl 4):S11-S16.

    The complications of an expandable nailing system were systematically reviewed in the literature. The system eliminated complications and revision surgeries associated with the use of locking screws, but there was a high revision rate associated with other complications.

19. Hak DJ, Mauffrey C, Seligson D, Lindeque B: Use of carbon-fiber-reinforced composite implants in orthopedic surgery. *Orthopedics* 2014;37(12):825-830.

    The authors use clinical examples to demonstrate that CRF-PEEK implants lead to successful fracture healing. The potential benefits over traditional metal implants are discussed and include the radiolucent property permitting improved, artifact-free radiographic imaging; a lower modulus of elasticity that is closer to that of bone; and greater fatigue strength.

20. Hillock R, Howard S: Utility of carbon fiber implants in orthopedic surgery: Literature review. *Reconstructive Review* 2014;4(1):23-32.

    The authors review and discuss clinical applications for the successful use of carbon fiber implants in orthopaedics, including visualization. Limitations of carbon fiber implants also are presented.

21. Caforio M, Perugia D, Colombo M, Calori GM, Maniscalco P: Preliminary experience with Piccolo Composite™, a radiolucent distal fibula plate, in ankle fractures. *Injury* 2014;45(suppl 6):S36-S38.

    Surgeons discuss their successful clinical experience with radiolucent plates for the treatment of complex ankle fractures, particularly trimalleolar fractures.

22. Steinberg EL, Rath E, Shlaifer A, Chechik O, Maman E, Salai M: Carbon fiber reinforced PEEK Optima: A composite material biomechanical properties and wear/debris characteristics of CF-PEEK composites for orthopedic trauma implants. *J Mech Behav Biomed Mater* 2013;17:221-228.

    The carbon fiber PEEK tibial nail, dynamic compression plate, proximal humeral plate, and distal radius volar plate were compared biomechanically and for wear debris with commercially available devices. The carbon nail was found to have similar mechanical properties, with less wear debris.

23. Anderson DJ, Kaye KS, Classen D, et al: Strategies to prevent surgical site infections in acute care hospitals. *Infect Control Hosp Epidemiol* 2008;29(suppl 1):S51-S61.

24. Odekerken JC, Welting T, Arts J, Walenkamp G, Emans PJ: Modern orthopaedic implant coatings: Their pro's, con's and evaluation methods, in Aliofkhazraei M, ed: *Modern Surface Engineering Treatments*. 2013. Available at: http://www.intechopen.com/books/modern-surface-engineering-treatments/modern-orthopaedic-implant-coatings-their-pro-s-con-s-and-evaluation-methods. Accessed January 16, 2016.

    The authors review the pros and cons of osteoconductive, osteoinductive, and antimicrobial coatings for orthopaedic implants. These include apatite, hydroxyapatite, silver, antibiotics, arginyl-glycyl-aspartic acid, and bone morphogenetic coatings.

25. Lilja M: *Bioactive Surgical Implant Coatings With Optional Antibacterial Function: Digital Comprehensive Summaries of Uppsala Dissertations from the Faculty of Science and Technology 1091* .Uppsala, Sweden, Acta Universitatis Upsaliensis, 2013, p. 60.

    Photocatalysis of titanium dioxide and antibiotic release from various hydroxyapatite coating structures were investigated. Demonstrated promising results were reported for these coatings as strategies to achieve antibacterial surface modifications for surgical implants.

26. Tan EK, Cooke M, Mandrycky C, et al: Structural and biological comparison of cryopreserved and fresh amniotic membrane tissues. *J Biomater Tissue Eng* 2014;4(5):379-388.

Cryopreserved amniotic membrane and umbilical cord tissues were compared with dehydrated amniotic membrane/chorion tissue using biochemical and functional assays. The results showed that cryopreservation better preserved the structural and biologic signaling molecules of fetal tissue.

27. Demirkan F, Colakoglu N, Herek O, Erkula G: The use of amniotic membrane in flexor tendon repair: An experimental model. *Arch Orthop Trauma Surg* 2002;122(7):396-399.

28. Singh R, Chouhan US, Purohit S, et al: Radiation processed amniotic membranes in the treatment of non-healing ulcers of different etiologies. *Cell Tissue Bank* 2004;5(2):129-134.

29. He H, Zhang S, Tighe S, Son J, Tseng SC: Immobilized heavy chain-hyaluronic acid polarizes lipopolysaccharide-activated macrophages toward M2 phenotype. *J Biol Chem* 2013;288(36):25792-25803.

Despite the known anti-inflammatory effect of amniotic membrane, its action mechanism remains largely unknown. In this bench study, heavy chain-hyaluronic acid complex purified from human amniotic membrane (consisting of high-molecular-weight hyaluronic acid covalently linked to the heavy chain 1 of inter-a-trypsin inhibitor) were used to demonstrate that immobilization of lipopolysaccharides leads macrophages to the M2 phenotypes.

30. Maan ZN, Rennert RC, Koob TJ, Januszyk M, Li WW, Gurtner GC: Cell recruitment by amnion chorion grafts promotes neovascularization. *J Surg Res* 2015;193(2):953-962.

In this study, dHACM was tested for its ability to recruit hematopoietic progenitor cells to a surgically implanted graft in a murine model of cutaneous ischemia. This study showed that dHACM effectively recruits circulating progenitor cells. The recruited cells express markers and localize to sites of neovascularization, providing a potential mechanism for the clinical efficacy of dHACM in the treatment of chronic wounds.

31. Sheikh ES, Sheikh ES, Fetterolf DE: Use of dehydrated human amniotic membrane allografts to promote healing in patients with refractory non healing wounds. *Int Wound J* 2014;11(6):711-717.

The use of a novel dehydrated amniotic membrane allograft for the treatment of chronic nonhealing wounds resulted in healing in a variety of wounds with one to three applications of dehydrated amniotic membrane material. Healed wounds had not recurred at the 1-year follow-ups.

32. Birke-Sorensen H, Malmsjo M, Rome P, et al; International Expert Panel on Negative Pressure Wound Therapy [NPWT-EP]: Evidence-based recommendations for negative pressure wound therapy: Treatment variables (pressure levels, wound filler and contact layer)—steps towards an international consensus. *J Plast Reconstr Aesthet Surg* 2011;64(suppl):S1-S16.

Evidence-based recommendations for NPWT, obtained by a systematic review of the literature, included pressure settings, use when infection is present, and choices of wound fillers and contact layers.

33. Becker D, D'Oro L, Farrer MD, et al: Expert recommendations for the use of mechanically powered negative pressure wound therapy. Available at: http://www.o-wm.com/files/owm/Spiracur-Mechanically-Powered-NPWT-Supplement.pdf. Accessed January 14, 2016.

Recommendations from a panel of medical clinicians on treatment guidelines for the use of mechanically powered NPWT are presented.

34. Armstrong DG, Marston WA, Reyzelman AM, Kirsner RS: Comparative effectiveness of mechanically and electrically powered negative pressure wound therapy devices: A multicenter randomized controlled trial. *Wound Repair Regen* 2012;20(3):332-341.

This multicenter, randomized controlled trial supported statistically equivalent wound healing via Kaplan-Meier analysis in a comparison of an ultraportable mechanically powered negative pressure wound care system with an electrically powered vacuum-assisted closure system. Noninfected, nonischemic, nonplantar lower extremity diabetic and venous wounds were treated with the NPWT systems. Results supported the concept that NPWT aids in wound healing regardless of the delivery mechanism.

35. Scalise A, Tartaglione C, Bolletta E, et al: The enhanced healing of a high-risk, clean, sutured surgical incision by prophylactic negative pressure wound therapy as delivered by Prevena™ Customizable™: Cosmetic and therapeutic results. *Int Wound J* 2015;12(2):218-223.

The authors examined therapy technology as delivered by a disposable NPWT system as a prophylactic measure. The immediate application of NPWT was used to prevent complications in high-risk, clean, closed surgical incisions. Preventive NPWT may have a critical role in the management of healing of these type of incisions.

36. Ousey KJ, Milne J: Exploring portable negative pressure wound therapy devices in the community. *Br J Community Nurs* 2014;19(suppl):S14, S16-S20.

The use of NPWT within community environments is increasing as the length of hospital stays decrease. The authors used a portable NPWT system to provide a cost-effective alternative to traditional wound therapy systems. Faster healing times and a reduction in overall treatment costs were reported.

37. Payne C, Edwards D: Application of the single use negative pressure wound therapy device (PICO) on a heterogeneous group of surgical and traumatic wounds. *Eplasty* 2014;14:e20.

A single-use, NPWT dressing (PICO; Smith & Nephew) was applied to a variety of posttraumatic acute, chronic, and high output wounds in 21 patients. The patients were treated on an outpatient basis after the dressing was applied. The authors concluded that a disposable NPWT device may benefit patients by promoting wound healing and managing costs.

38. Gabriel A, Thimmappa B, Rubano C, Storm-Dickerson T: Evaluation of an ultra-lightweight, single-patient-use negative pressure wound therapy system over dermal regeneration template and skin grafts. *Int Wound J* 2013;10(4):418-424.

    The authors used a new, disposable NPWT system over a dermal regeneration template and/or skin grafts in 33 patients (41 graft procedures). Preliminary data suggest that the NPWT system provides a quicker, seamless transition to home care and results in a shorter hospital stay and potential cost savings.

39. Grauhan O, Navasardyan A, Tutkun B, et al: Effect of surgical incision management on wound infections in a poststernotomy patient population. *Int Wound J* 2014;11(suppl 1):6-9.

    After median sternotomy, the postoperative dressing of a clean, closed incision for 6 to 7 days substantially reduced the incidence of wound infection compared with traditional treatment.

40. Weir G: The use of a surgical incision management system on vascular surgery incisions: A pilot study. *Int Wound J* 2014;11(suppl 1):10-12.

    This prospective case-controlled study assessed wound complications in patients undergoing vascular bypass procedures in which both femoral areas were incised to gain access to the femoral arteries. A NPWT surgical incision management system was placed on one femoral area, and a standard postoperative wound dressing was placed on the contralateral femoral area. No significant complications occurred in wounds treated with NPWT system; three significant complications were reported in the control wounds.

41. Bottlang M, Walleser S, Noll M, et al: Biomechanical rationale and evaluation of an implant system for rib fracture fixation. *Eur J Trauma Emerg Surg* 2010;36(5):417-426.

    Biomechanical research directed at developing customized implant solutions for rib fracture fixation is essential to reduce the complexity and increase the reliability of rib osteosynthesis. The anatomic plate set can simplify rib fracture fixation by minimizing the need for plate contouring. Intramedullary fixation with rib splints provides a less-invasive fixation alternative for a posterior rib fracture when access for plating is limited.

42. Bottlang M, Helzel I, Long WB, Madey S: Anatomically contoured plates for fixation of rib fractures. *J Trauma* 2010;68(3):611-615.

    Contouring plates intraoperatively for rib fractures can be time consuming and difficult. After examining 109 cadaver ribs, the authors found that a simple set of six plates to incorporate the average rib twists at various length plates could potentially minimize the need for intraoperative contouring of plates.

43. Kirane YM, Fragomen AT, Rozbruch SR: Precision of the PRECICE internal bone lengthening nail. *Clin Orthop Relat Res* 2014;472(12):3869-3878.

    The accuracy and precision of distraction, effects on bone alignment, effects on adjacent-joint range of motion, and frequency of implant-related and non–implant-related complications were evaluated for a new IM nail. The authors concluded that the PRECICE nail is a valid option to achieve accurate and precise limb lengthening to treat a variety of conditions with limb shortening or length discrepancy. Level of evidence: IV.

44. Paley D, Harris M, Debiparshad K, Prince D: Limb lengthening by implantable limb lengthening devices. *Tech Orthop* 2014;29(2):72-85.

    A new nailing system with external magnetic actuation was described for the successful treatment of limb-length discrepancies.

45. Rozbruch SR, Birch JG, Dahl MT, Herzenberg JE: Motorized intramedullary nail for management of limb-length discrepancy and deformity. *J Am Acad Orthop Surg* 2014;22(7):403-409.

    Motorized IM nails allow accurate, well-controlled distraction. Successful early clinical results have been reported.

46. Armstrong DG, Rankin TM, Giovinco NA, Mills JL, Matsuoka Y: A heads-up display for diabetic limb salvage surgery: A view through the Google looking glass. *J Diabetes Sci Technol* 2014;8(5):951-956.

    The Google Glass device facilitated hands-free, rapid communication, documentation, and consultation. An eyeglass-mounted screen has the potential to improve communication, safety, and efficiency of intraoperative and clinical care. In the future, a union of medical devices with consumer technology is possible.

47. Hodgins JL, Veillette C: Arthroscopic proficiency: Methods in evaluating competency. *BMC Med Educ* 2013;13:61.

    The current paradigm of arthroscopic training lacks objective evaluation of technical ability and its adequacy is concerning given the accelerating complexity of the field. Abstracts were independently evaluated to find a method to evaluate competency.

48. Karam MD, Pedowitz RA, Natividad H, Murray J, Marsh JL: Current and future use of surgical skills training laboratories in orthopaedic resident education: A national survey. *J Bone Joint Surg Am* 2013;95(1):e4-1.

    Two online versions of the Surgical Skills Simulation surveys were created. The purpose of this study was to provide baseline information on the current use of surgical skills training laboratories in orthopaedic resident education programs and determine interest in expansion of these facilities and training techniques. There was strong

1: General Topics

agreement among both program directors and residents that surgical skills laboratories and simulation technology should be required components of orthopaedic resident training programs.

49. Ponce BA, Menendez ME, Oladeji LO, Fryberger CT, Dantuluri PK: Emerging technology in surgical education: Combining real-time augmented reality and wearable computing devices. *Orthopedics* 2014;37(11):751-757.

The first surgical case adopting the combination of real-time augmented reality and wearable computing devices such as Google Glass was described. Throughout the surgical procedure, the use of Google Glass allowed a remote surgeon to successfully interact with a local surgeon.

50. Benninger B: Google Glass, ultrasound and palpation: The anatomy teacher of the future? *Clin Anat* 2015;28(2):152-155.

Google Glass was used in the teaching of anatomy to medical students, a method that demonstrated combining traditional medical teaching with cutting edge technology.

Chapter 7

Biomechanics of Fracture Healing

Jason A. Lowe, MD   Amir Herman, MD, PhD

Abstract

Fracture healing after osteosynthesis requires a combination of anatomic restoration of length alignment and rotation and a fracture-fixation construct crafted to promote primary or secondary bone healing. The mode of fracture healing is determined by selection and application of implants. Technologic advances in fracture fixation enable surgeons to modulate construct stability in favor of more flexibility or rigidity as dictated by the fracture pattern. Locking-screw technology increases construct stability in bone of poor quality that is subjected to repetitive stress and has been implicated in increasing rigidity sufficiently to delay secondary bone healing in bridge-plating constructs. To address this unintended consequence, a concept that has been called "far cortical locking" or "dynamic locking" has been suggested. Secondary bone healing can also be achieved by intramedullary nail fixation. Technologic advancements have resulted in screws that lock in a threaded bolt in the nail. This construct offers higher rotational and bending stability while allowing axial compression, which is necessary for healing. This represents a trend toward more rigid fixation constructs in intramedullary nails. The surgeon's knowledge of new technologies and advancements is paramount in optimizing fracture-fixation stability and promoting uneventful fracture healing.

Keywords: biomechanics; stress; strain; nonunion; fracture fixation

Dr. Lowe or an immediate family member is a member of a speakers' bureau or has made paid presentations on behalf of DePuy Synthes, serves as a paid consultant to Acumed, and has received research or institutional support from Stryker and DePuy Synthes. Neither Dr. Herman nor any immediate family member has received anything of value from or has stock or stock options held in a commercial company or institution related directly or indirectly to the subject of this chapter.

Introduction

The principles of fracture fixation focus on restoring length alignment and rotation with an optimal fixation construct for the given fracture. Fracture stabilization is achieved with a variety of implants, ranging from plates and nails to external fixators. Within each implant category, there are additional ways that surgeons can determine primary and secondary fracture healing on the basis of implant material, size, shape, and screw. One factor that remains constant is that implant selection and mode of application determine how the bone will heal.

Basic Concepts of Fracture Healing

In the process of fracture healing, combined material and structural properties of the bone and implant affect the biologic pathway through which the body ultimately heals. For example, bridging constructs are applied with a degree of flexibility, allowing for micromotion under physiologic load (relative stability), and subsequently promote secondary bone healing. Absolute stability constructs are applied with anatomic reduction and compression to afford primary bone healing.[1] If implants are applied without regard for these basic tenets, the act of surgical stabilization may contribute to nonunion and subsequent hardware failure.

When stress is plotted over strain, the resulting curve is one of the basic tools used to describe biomechanical material properties and provides additional information such as the yield point (transition from elastic to plastic deformation) and failure point (ultimate strength) of the material.[1] Alternatively, stiffness is an example of a structural property and depends on the size and shape of each object as well as the direction the object is being loaded (bending, torsion, axial load). For example, the bending stiffness of a plate is directly proportional to its width and the third order of its thickness; for a cannulated intramedullary nail, the bending stiffness is proportional to the fourth power of the outer diameter minus the fourth power of its inner diameter.

Combining basic mechanical principles with the biology of fracture healing is critical to understanding how mechanical conditions support bony consolidation. Strain across a fracture gap is defined as the allowed motion divided by the fracture gap. The fracture healing pathway, intramembranous or enchondral, is determined by the amount of strain or motion across the fracture. During fracture fixation surgery, surgeons strive to reduce strain by controlling the stiffness or flexibility of the fixation construct. For example, stiff fixation constructs that allow less than 2% strain induce intramembranous or primary bone healing, and constructs that allow 2% to 10% strain induce endochondral ossification or secondary bone healing. Decreasing stiffness such that strain is greater than 30% supports proliferation of fibrous tissue and results in a greater possibility of nonunion.[1-4] These concepts are difficult to transfer to complex bony anatomy and unique fixation constructs, including plating, nailing, cortical screws versus locking screws, plate length, working length, and screw density. Each can be manipulated to affect the stiffness of, the strength of, and ultimately the strain on a fixation construct.

Comminuted Periarticular Fracture Fixation

Comminuted periarticular fractures are challenging to treat because they typically require absolute stability across the articular segment for primary bone healing and flexible fixation across areas of metadiaphyseal comminution for secondary bone healing. Absolute stability at the articular surface and relative stability across the metadiaphysis is a common fixation schema, producing intramembranous and enchondral ossifications, respectively.[5,6] Promoting different healing modalities in the same bone necessitates that the fixation constructs provide different mechanical properties.

One of the most common fractures that requires a combination of healing modalities is the distal femur fracture. When locking-plate technology was initially used for distal femur fractures, it was thought that the screws would provide increased stability and could improve the chances for surgical success compared with nonlocked constructs. The authors of a 2011 study investigated both clinical and biomechanical data to elucidate results in distal femur fractures treated with locking plates.[7] They found up to a 19% rate of nonunion, a 15% rate of delayed union, and a 20% incidence of hardware failure. Secondary surgery for locking plate osteosynthesis was required in up to 32% of fractures. An increasing body of literature supports the idea that these failures are a result of insufficient and asymmetric motion provided by excessively stiff plating constructs. The authors of a 2010 study demonstrated asymmetric callus in distal femur fractures in which the medial or far cortex was observed to produce more healing bone than did the lateral cortex.[8] The authors postulated that small motion at the lateral cortex results from the proximity of a stiff plate. Subsequent studies have supported the idea that locked-plate fixation increases the fracture construct rigidity to the point that interfragmentary motion and subsequent secondary bone healing are limited.[9-11]

Means to reduce construct stiffness and increase interfragmentary motion include increasing working length (the length between the first screw and the fracture) and using a less stiff material (such as titanium versus stainless steel), as well as using new locking-screw technology. The authors of a 2013 study reviewed the axial and torsional stiffness of commercially available plates and observed variability in the stiffness between implants depending on manufacturer and plate material.[12] Another study showed that distal femur fractures stabilized with titanium plates had a statistically greater volume of callus (49%) at 24 weeks after fixation than did stainless steel plates (26%).[8] The findings of these studies support that titanium plates are less stiff and induce greater callus than do stainless steel plates, but there are no conclusive data indicating that titanium plates result in higher union rates. Increasing the fracture working length also increases fracture construct flexibility and can be accomplished by omitting one or two screws adjacent to the fracture. Increasing the plate's working length has been shown to decrease construct stiffness,[13] preserve micromotion, and increase callus formation.[8] Differences in fracture callus, however, have only been observed during the first 6 weeks of healing, and the true clinical importance of the finding is unknown.[8] Additionally, in poor-quality diaphyseal bone, hybrid fixation (use of locking and nonlocking screws) as opposed to the use of only nonlocking screws, can increase construct strength.[14-16] Placing a locking screw in the last diaphyseal screw hole may lead to a stress riser and contribute to a periprosthetic fracture.[16] It has been recommended that the last diaphyseal screw be a cortical screw unless it overlaps an intramedullary implant, in which case a unicortical locking screw may be required.

Intramedullary constructs are another method of promoting lower construct stiffness and may be applied in extra-articular and some intra-articular fractures (**Figure 1**). Fractures fixed with intramedullary nails (IMNs) have been observed to have greater fracture callus than do fractures fixed with plates[7] (**Figure 2**). Selection of intramedullary implants, however, must be balanced with the ability to maintain rigid stability of any associated articular fracture component.

Each of the aforementioned techniques is a means to modulate construct stiffness using existing technology. These techniques have developed secondary to the

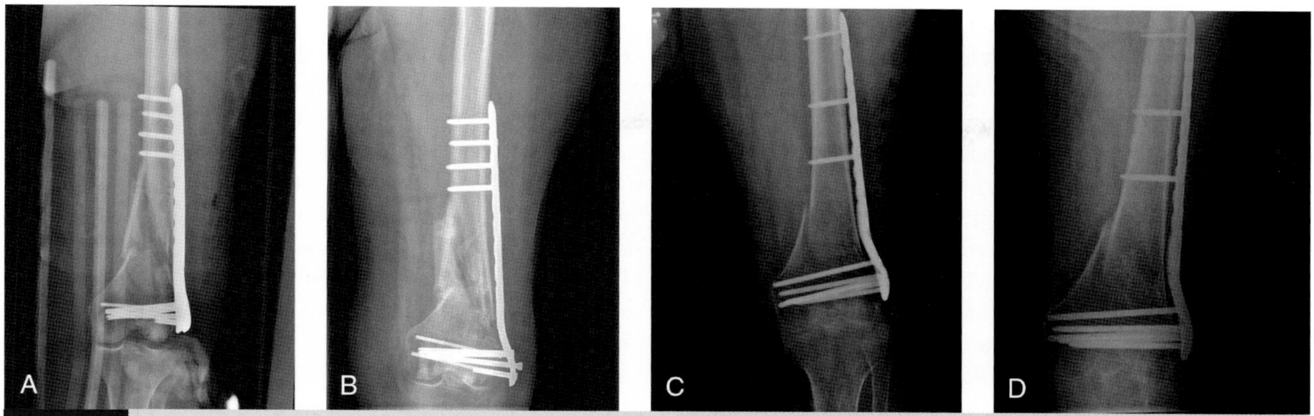

Figure 1 Two cases of distal femur fracture treated with a locking plate. **A**, Postoperative radiograph demonstrates four locking screws used to completely fill the plate. **B**, Radiograph of the same patient obtained 4.5 months postoperatively, with one distal screw backing and the fracture varus displaced. **C**, Postoperative radiograph demonstrates the use of hybrid locking and highly dispersed cortical screws; the most proximal screw is a cortical nonlocking screw. **D**, Radiograph of the same patient at 5-month follow-up. Note the callus formation and bone healing.

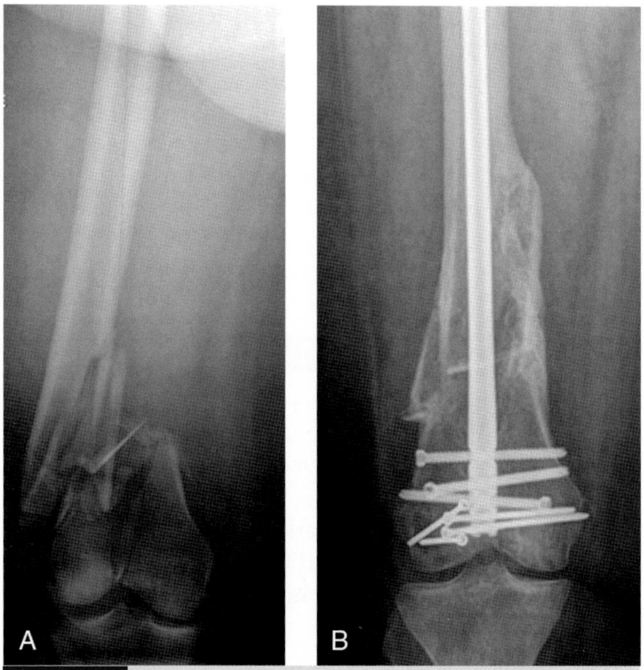

Figure 2 AP radiographs of a distal femur periarticular fracture treated with an intramedullary nail. **A**, Preoperative view. **B**, Six months after fixation, callus formation and fracture healing can be observed.

observed asymmetric callus, high incidence of nonunion (near cortex), and subsequent hardware failure in locked plating, particularly in the distal femur.[8,17] One newer method of decreasing construct stiffness and increasing symmetric fracture micromotion as well as callus formation is the use of far cortical locking screws. These implants thread into the far cortex as well as into the plate, are allowed to toggle within the near cortex (by a variety of proprietary methods or by simply overdrilling the near cortex), and may be coupled with a gap between the plate and bone interface that allows for controlled parallel interfragmentary motion. Compared with a construct involving all-locking screws, these constructs have shown lower compressive strength but higher bending and torsional strength for both osteoporotic and nonosteoporotic bone.[9,10] Another study demonstrated a simultaneous decrease in stiffness of 80% to 88% in the tibia or femoral diaphysis as well as the femoral metaphysis.[17] An ovine model has shown up to a 36% increase in overall fracture callus as well as higher rates of symmetric callus.[9] This technology offers an alternative solution to the overly stiff locking plate; however, it is in its infancy. To date, there are no prospective studies comparing far cortical locking screws with other methods of decreasing construct stiffness. As this and other new technologies are explored, the benefits of improved implants will need to be balanced with their cost and safety profile. Careful clinical evaluation of new technology is necessary given that complications not observed during mechanical testing can be observed in clinical practice and lead to implant recall.[18]

Diaphyseal Fracture Fixation

Tibia and femoral diaphyseal fracture are most commonly fixed with locked intramedullary nail fixation. These implants, by design, are load sharing and provide relative stability with the goal of secondary bone healing. One limitation of these fixation devices is a high incidence of delayed union and fracture malalignment, particularly for fractures in the metadiaphyseal region.[19,20] Biomechanical and radiographic studies have shown that increasing stability in intramedullary nail fixation promotes faster union and stronger callus compared with standard nails.[21,22] Increasing stability of these fractures has been pursued by increasing nail size (reaming), which is a well-established practice, as well as with new technology aimed at controlling torsion and axial motion.

One technique to improve stability is to enhance the interference fit between the interlocking bolts and the nail. One study used a sheep tibiae osteotomy model to compare an unreamed standard nail construct with an angle-stable tibial nail (ASTN).[21] This technology uses a nail in which the drilled locking bolt holes in the nail are threaded. In vivo comparisons included measurements of ground reaction forces and interfragmentary movements during gait. During the healing process, the ASTN group showed higher ground reaction forces and lower axial torsion and shearing while walking. Postmortem biomechanical studies confirmed higher stiffness in most planes studied. Radiologic studies also demonstrated a greater number of healing cortices in the ASTN group. Interestingly, histopathologic results showed that the total amount of connective tissue was greater in the standard nail group, but the total area of mineralized bone was higher in the ASTN group. This finding supports that the ASTN is more rigid in vivo, which leads to the formation of bony callus.

A standard unreamed nail, the ASTN, and four configurations of external fixation were compared.[22] Biomechanical properties of the fixation methods of the four constructs were compared and were further related to callus formation and healing callus properties. It was determined that the direction of external fixation relative to the limb (anteromedial or medially mounted fixation) influenced the direction in maximum resistance to shear stress achieved. The ASTN was the most rigid construct for anteroposterior shear and axial compression. The standard unreamed nail was the least rigid construct. When torsional moment and torsional stiffness were compared at 9 weeks postosteotomy, the ASTN-treated bones had biomechanical properties similar to the externally fixed bones, whereas the bones treated with the standard unreamed nail showed the lowest biomechanical properties.

The authors of a 2013 study reviewed the torsional and axial stiffness of angle-stable versus a conventional locking tibia nail.[23] The same nail, when used with angle-stable screws, had 60% higher torsional stiffness and 10% higher axial stiffness. The concern that the high axial stiffness might increase the rate of nonunion, combined with the realization that increased torsional stiffness might contribute to union, led to the development of a nail with high torsional stiffness and low axial stiffness.[24,25] The Flexible Axial Stimulation intramedullary nail (OrthoXel) is constructed with an internal sleeve with circular holes within the locking oval nail holes.[25] This construct provides interfragmentary axial motion of 1 mm, which is associated with a 22% reduction in axial stiffness and a 14% increase in torsional stiffness, compared with fixation via regular intramedullary nails. It is postulated that these properties would lead to expedited union and decreased nonunion rates; however, to date there are no clinical data to support this claim.

Pelvic Fixation

Vertically unstable pelvic fractures have a high rate of hardware failure and pose a challenge for the trauma surgeon. The need to provide fixation to the spinopelvic junction demands a highly stable fixation method. Transsacral screw fixation has offered an alternative to triangular osteosynthesis. It has been shown that two transsacral screws provided greater stiffness (248.7 N/mm) than did triangular fixation with tension band and lumbopelvic fixation (125 N/mm).[26] This study assumes a safe corridor for sacral and transsacral screw fixation.

Summary

Both plating and nailing technology are used in the context of secondary bone healing. Plates are a more rigid construct that focus on less rigid fixation for secondary bone healing. Nails are a less rigid construct by nature and focus on more rigid fixation, allowing for motion in the axial plane. A similar optimal stiffness could be suggested for secondary bone healing in both plating and nailing technologies.

Additional studies are needed to validate whether the use of these concepts increases the rate of fracture union. Other studies are also needed to apply plating and nailing technologies in bones other than the tibia and the distal femur. The results of emerging studies in vertically unstable pelvic fixation support improved biomechanical properties of transsacral fixation versus lumbopelvic fixation and indicate that transsacral fixation should be considered for these challenging fractures.

Key Study Points

- Combining basic mechanical principles with the biology of fracture healing is critical to understanding how mechanical conditions support bony consolidation.
- A balance in optimal stiffness for both nailing and plating constructs continues to be explored by focusing on reducing the rigidity of plating constructs and increasing stiffness of nailing constructs.
- Transsacral screw fixation offers a biomechanically stronger alternative to lumbopelvic fixation of vertically unstable pelvic ring injuries; however, additional clinical trials are required.

Annotated References

1. Tencer A, Johnson KD: *Biomechanics in Orthopaedic Trauma, Bone Fracture and Fixation,* ed 1. London, England, Martin Dunitz, 1994.

2. Claes LE, Heigele CA, Neidlinger-Wilke C, et al: Effects of mechanical factors on the fracture healing process. *Clin Orthop Relat Res* 1998; (355 suppl):S132-S147.

3. Carter DR, Beaupré GS, Giori NJ, Helms JA: Mechanobiology of skeletal regeneration. *Clin Orthop Relat Res* 1998;(355 suppl):S41-S55.

4. Egol KA, Kubiak EN, Fulkerson E, Kummer FJ, Koval KJ: Biomechanics of locked plates and screws. *J Orthop Trauma* 2004;18(8):488-493.

5. Miller DL, Goswami T: A review of locking compression plate biomechanics and their advantages as internal fixators in fracture healing. *Clin Biomech (Bristol, Avon)* 2007;22(10):1049-1062.

6. Collinge CA, Gardner MJ, Crist BD: Pitfalls in the application of distal femur plates for fractures. *J Orthop Trauma* 2011;25(11):695-706.

   The authors present case examples of failure in fixation of distal femur fractures and offer technical tips for improving outcome. They then discuss anatomic characteristics of the distal femur. Level of evidence: III.

7. Henderson CE, Kuhl LL, Fitzpatrick DC, Marsh JL: Locking plates for distal femur fractures: Is there a problem with fracture healing? *J Orthop Trauma* 2011;25(suppl 1):S8-S14.

   The authors conducted a literature review for complications after distal femur plate fixation. They report on 18 publications involving complication rates of zero to 32%. Level of evidence: IV.

8. Lujan TJ, Henderson CE, Madey SM, Fitzpatrick DC, Marsh JL, Bottlang M: Locked plating of distal femur fractures leads to inconsistent and asymmetric callus formation. *J Orthop Trauma* 2010;24(3):156-162.

   The authors report on callus sizes after distal femur fixation achieved with locking plates. The medial cortex had on average 64% more callus than did the anterior or posterior cortex. Level of evidence: III.

9. Bottlang M, Lesser M, Koerber J, et al: Far cortical locking can improve healing of fractures stabilized with locking plates. *J Bone Joint Surg Am* 2010;92(7):1652-1660.

   The authors report on a new screw technology: the far cortical locking screw. They reported on an ovine tibial osteotomy model with a 3-millimeter gap. At week 9, the group that received the far cortical locking construct had 36% higher callus volume and 44% higher bone mineral content than did the group that received locked plating.

10. Bottlang M, Doornink J, Fitzpatrick DC, Madey SM: Far cortical locking can reduce stiffness of locked plating constructs while retaining construct strength. *J Bone Joint Surg Am* 2009;91(8):1985-1994.

11. Doornink J, Fitzpatrick DC, Madey SM, Bottlang M: Far cortical locking enables flexible fixation with periarticular locking plates. *J Orthop Trauma* 2011;25(suppl 1):S29-S34.

    The authors conducted a biomechanical cadaver study to compare far cortical locking screws versus standard locking screws for fixation of distal femur fractures. The study showed 81% lower stiffness in the far cortical screws construct and similar strength of the constructs.

12. Schmidt U, Penzkofer R, Bachmaier S, Augat P: Implant material and design alter construct stiffness in distal femur locking plate fixation: A pilot study. *Clin Orthop Relat Res* 2013;471(9):2808-2814.

    The authors performed a biomechanical comparison of the stiffness of new-generation distal femur locking plates. The AxSOS (stainless steel Stryker) and PolyAx (titanium, Depuy) showed highest and lowest stiffness, respectively.

13. Stoffel K, Dieter U, Stachowiak G, Gächter A, Kuster MS: Biomechanical testing of the LCP—how can stability in locked internal fixators be controlled? *Injury* 2003;34(suppl 2):B11-B19.

14. Sommers MB, Fitzpatrick DC, Madey SM, Bottlang M: Combined use of locked and non-locked screws for plating of fractures in osteoporotic bone. *J Biomech* 2006;39(suppl 1):S136.

15. Doornink J, Fitzpatrick DC, Boldhaus S, Madey SM, Bottlang M: Effects of hybrid plating with locked and nonlocked screws on the strength of locked plating constructs in the osteoporotic diaphysis. *J Trauma* 2010;69(2):411-417.

    The authors compared locking screws and a hybrid combination of locking and nonlocking screw constructs. The hybrid construct was 7% stronger in bending and 42% stronger in torsion.

16. Bottlang M, Doornink J, Byrd GD, Fitzpatrick DC, Madey SM: A nonlocking end screw can decrease fracture risk caused by locked plating in the osteoporotic diaphysis. *J Bone Joint Surg Am* 2009;91(3):620-627.

17. Bottlang M, Doornink J, Lujan TJ, et al: Effects of construct stiffness on healing of fractures stabilized with locking plates. *J Bone Joint Surg Am* 2010;92(suppl 2):12-22.

    The authors review the current evidence of far cortical technology. They report on the biomechanical properties, the in vivo animal models, and available clinical evidence. Far cortical locking screws reduce the stiffness of a plate fixation construct and as such propagates fracture healing. Level of evidence: IV.

18. U.S. Food and Drug Administration. Enforcement report—week of December 4, 2013. Available at: http://www.accessdata.fda.gov/scripts/enforcement/enforce_rpt-Product-Tabs.cfm?action=select&recall_number=Z-0390-2014&w=12042013&lang=eng. Accessed Jan. 31, 2016.

19. Henderson CE , Lujan T, Bottlang M, Fitzpatrick DC, Madey SM, Marsh JL: Stabilization of distal femur fractures with intramedullary nails and locking plates: Differences in callus formation. *Iowa Ortho J* 2010;30:61-68.

    The authors present retrospective case-matched comparisons of 12 patients treated with intramedullary nail fixation and 12 patients treated with locking compression plate fixation for distal femur fracture. The fractures treated with intramedullary nail fixation had 2.4 times more callus formation. Level of evidence: II.

20. Vallier HA, Cureton BA, Patterson BM: Randomized, prospective comparison of plate versus intramedullary nail fixation for distal tibia shaft fractures. *J Orthop Trauma* 2011;25(12):736-741.

    The authors present prospective randomized trial of 104 patients with distal tibia fractures treated either with intramedullary nail or large fragment plate. Fractures that were fixed with intramedullary nails showed higher rates of larger than 5° of malalignment. Level of evidence: I.

21. Kaspar K, Schell H, Seebeck P, et al: Angle stable locking reduces interfragmentary movements and promotes healing after unreamed nailing. Study of a displaced osteotomy model in sheep tibiae. *J Bone Joint Surg Am* 2005;87(9):2028-2037.

22. Epari DR, Kassi JP, Schell H, Duda GN: Timely fracture-healing requires optimization of axial fixation stability. *J Bone Joint Surg Am* 2007;89(7):1575-1585.

23. Wähnert D, Stolarczyk Y, Hoffmeier KL, Raschke MJ, Hofmann GO, Mückley T: Long-term stability of angle-stable versus conventional locked intramedullary nails in distal tibia fractures. *BMC Musculoskelet Disord* 2013;14:66.

    The authors used a porcine cadaver model to study the biomechanical properties of intramedullary nail fixation with either conventional locking screws or angle-stable locking screws. They observed 60% higher torsional stiffness in the tibiae with the angle-stable screws.

24. Dailey HL, Daly CJ, Galbraith JG, Cronin M, Harty JA: A novel intramedullary nail for micromotion stimulation of tibial fractures. *Clin Biomech (Bristol, Avon)* 2012;27(2):182-188.

    A cadaver tibia model showed that using an intramedullary nail with an insert of a micromotion locking-bolt nail provided 50% less stiffness for axial compression loads than do conventional locking bolts.

25. Dailey HL, Daly CJ, Galbraith JG, Cronin M, Harty JA: The Flexible Axial Stimulation (FAST) intramedullary nail provides interfragmentary micromotion and enhanced torsional stability. *Clin Biomech (Bristol, Avon)* 2013;28(5):579-585.

    A cadaver tibia model showed 14% higher torsional stiffness and 22% lower axial load stiffness when flexible axial stimulation nails were used.

26. Min KS, Zamorano DP, Wahba GM, Garcia I, Bhatia N, Lee TQ: Comparison of two-transsacral-screw fixation versus triangular osteosynthesis for transforaminal sacral fractures. *Orthopedics* 2014;37(9):e754-e760.

    The authors used a cadaver model to compare the biomechanical properties of transsacral screws fixation versus triangular fixation. The study showed that two transsacral screws had stiffness two times higher than that among specimens using the triangular fixation model.

Chapter 8

Osteoporosis and Pathologic Bone

Philipp Leucht, MD

Abstract

Osteoporosis is a common bone disorder, and its incidence is increasing. Early recognition, medical management, and fracture prevention are the main pillars of treatment. Several diagnostic modalities are available for the current and future medical management of bone loss in the aged male and female patient. It is important to be aware of common disease states that lead to pathologic fracture and the medical treatment options available.

Keywords: osteoporosis; osteopenia; bisphosphonates; teriparatide; bone metastasis; pathologic fracture; adjuvant therapy

Introduction

Osteoporosis is defined as a bone disorder characterized by compromised bone strength, predisposing patients to an increased risk of fracture. In 2014, approximately 54 million adults in the United States aged 50 years or older were affected by osteoporosis and low bone mass (osteopenia).[1] Osteoporosis is diagnosed with dual-energy x-ray absorptiometry, which should be performed in all women older than 65 years and in patients with increased fracture risk to determine bone mineral density.[2] According to the World Health Organization the following characteristics define osteoporosis: having a T-score less than or equal to -2.5 standard deviation at the femoral neck or the lumbar spine or the presence of a fragility fracture. Low bone mass is characterized by a T-score between -1 and -2.5 standard deviation at either site.[3] Currently, 10.2 million adults in the United States have osteoporosis, and 43.3 million have low bone mass, putting them at a substantial risk for fracture.[4] With almost one-half of the adult U.S. population at risk for fracture because of low bone mass, preventive measures may offer the only option of avoiding future fracture and disability for these individuals.

The continuous loss of bone mass most commonly affects postmenopausal women, but men also are affected.[5,6] Although most individuals with osteoporosis or low bone mass are non-Hispanic white women, a substantial number of men and women from other ethnic or racial groups are affected. Low bone mass accounts for approximately 2 million fractures each year in the United States. Of these fractures, 80% occur in Medicare recipients, making osteoporosis the 10th ranked major illness among Medicare beneficiaries.[7] Typical fragility fractures include hip fractures, vertebral compression fractures, distal radius fractures, pelvic ring injuries, proximal humerus fractures, and tibial plateau fractures. By definition, fragility fractures result from a low-energy mechanism of injury—most commonly a fall from a standing height.

Osteoporosis is a chronic degenerative disease based on a dysregulation of bone-forming and bone-resorbing mechanisms. In the young and healthy patient, osteoblastic bone formation and osteoclastic bone resorption are tightly regulated and are calibrated to maintain bone mass. This homeostasis is able to adapt to changes in lifestyle, such as increased exercise that leads to increased bone mass in an attempt to strengthen the mechanically stressed skeleton. In the elderly, however, this balance is shifted toward increased resorption with inadequate bone deposition, likely as a result of decreased bone-forming ability from osteoblasts. Basic science research has identified multiple signaling pathways involved in this intricate balance of bone homeostasis, and a plethora of potential treatment approaches has arisen from these discoveries. Some of the more promising approaches target the Wnt signaling pathway, the RANK (receptor activator of nuclear factor kappa-B)/RANKL (receptor activator of nuclear factor-kappa B ligand) interaction, and the parathyroid hormone axis.[8]

Dr. Leucht or an immediate family member serves as a board member, owner, officer, or committee member of the American Academy of Orthopaedic Surgeons Biological Implants Committee.

Medical Treatment of Osteoporosis

Diphosphonates

Diphosphonates are the most widely used antiresorptive medications for the treatment of osteoporosis and other conditions characterized by increased bone resorption caused by osteoclastic activity.[9] Intensive research over the past decade has proven the efficacy of diphosphonates in fracture prevention,[10] and they now represent first-line treatment for patients with osteoporosis, because they are cost effective and safe to use.

Ten years after the introduction of diphosphonates, the first reports of atypical femur fractures (AFFs) appeared in the literature.[11] What previously seemed to be a rare occurrence now is recognized as a long-term side effect of diphosphonate use.[12] Although the mechanism is not fully understood, evidence points toward a negative effect of diphosphonates on bone remodeling, resulting in increased microdamage without repair, leading to a stress reaction and eventual fracture. Multiple studies attempted to correlate the anatomy of the proximal femur to the risk of an AFF, but to date, a causative effect of bone geometry on fracture risk has not been determined.[13] However, the benefit of diphosphonates outweighs the risk of the relatively rare AFF during early treatment period; after 5 years of use, however, this risk-benefit profile changes, which led to the introduction of "diphosphonate holidays" for 2 to 3 years to allow bone remodeling to occur.[14] In particular, caution should be exercised in patients without a vertebral fracture and a T-score greater than -2.5, in whom the benefit of diphosphonate treatment is not yet clear.

Parathyroid Hormone

Parathyroid hormone 1-84 and teriparatide1-34 are anabolic recombinant proteins that stimulate osteogenesis and therefore result in a net bone mass increase.[15,16] Animal studies and randomized controlled trials in humans have shown that daily injection of teriparatide results in restoration of bone mass and strength.[17] The current indication for teriparatide use includes postmenopausal women with osteoporosis and increased fracture risk. Conflicting results in patients treated with a combination of antiresorptive and anabolic agents has resulted in a recommendation for monotherapy.[16]

Denosumab

Denosumab is a human monoclonal antibody that acts against RANKL and therefore inhibits osteoclast function and survival. Denosumab is indicated for postmenopausal women with osteoporosis, men with osteoporosis, men at high risk for fracture who receive androgen-deprivation therapy for nonmetastatic prostate cancer, and women with increased fracture risk who receive adjuvant aromatase inhibitor therapy for breast cancer. The Fracture Reduction Evaluation of Denosumab in Osteoporosis Every 6 Months, or FREEDOM trial, showed a significant reduction in vertebral fractures, nonvertebral fractures, and hip fractures compared with placebo.[18] Head-to-head trials showed that denosumab is as effective as the diphosphonate zoledronate.[19] Denosumab is injected subcutaneously biannually. It has a shorter skeletal retention time than bisphosphonates and is not associated with gastrointestinal symptoms. These features translate into improved patient tolerance, thus resulting in a greater therapeutic effect.

Surgical Treatment of Osteoporosis

Most fragility fractures occur in the elderly with osteoporosis, and these patients often present with a multitude of associated medical conditions. Orthopaedic surgeons treating such injuries need to be aware of these conditions and should tailor their surgical and medical treatment plans to account for the decreased physiologic reserve of these patients.

In recent years, a fracture liaison service (FLS) was established to offer patients a multidisciplinary treatment approach. A multicenter study comparing hospital admissions to a center with and without an FLS demonstrated a mortality reduction of 35% for patients receiving the multidisciplinary approach.[20] In addition, a statistically significant reduction in nonvertebral fractures in the FLS group occurred over the following 2 years. The American Academy of Orthopaedic Surgeons recently published a clinical practice guideline on the management of hip fractures in the elderly.[21]

Recommendations support surgical treatment in a timely fashion.[20,22] Additionally, after medical optimization has been obtained and delirium has been minimized, moderate to strong recommendations for the prevention of future fragility fractures through osteoporosis screening, calcium and vitamin D substitution, and an interdisciplinary care program also were made.

Pathologic Bone

Pathologic fractures occur as a result of an underlying process that weakens the mechanical strength of bone. Benign lesions, such as nonossifying fibromas (NOFs), fibrous dysplasia, solitary bone cysts, aneurysmal bone cysts (ABCs), and giant cell tumors can present with a pathologic fracture. In nonaggressive lesions such as NOFs and bone cysts, fracture healing can be expected

Table 1

The Mirels Criteria for Predicting Fracture Risk

Score[a]	Site	Pain	Radiographic Appearance	Size[b]
1	Upper extremity	Mild	Blastic	<1/3
2	Lower extremity	Moderate	Mixed	1/3 to 2/3
3	Peritrochanteric region	Functional	Lytic	>2/3

[a] A score of 9 or higher indicates recommended prophylactic fixation.
[b] Fraction of cortical thickness.

in a manner similar to that of a primary, nonpathologic fracture. Aggressive lesions, including giant cell tumors and ABCs, heal primarily after stabilization; however, local control should be established with adjuvant treatment, including curettage and burring, liquid nitrogen, or an argon beam.[22,23] Because of the often encountered larger bone defects in aggressive benign tumors, bone void fillers are recommended for enhanced stability. For such defects, tricalcium phosphate, polymethyl methacrylate (PMMA) cement, and allograft or autograft bone can be used and have been shown to result in good functional outcome.[24]

Primary malignant bone tumors are rare, and most pathologic fractures encountered in daily orthopaedic practice are a direct result of a metastatic bone lesion in adults. The management of metastatic bone fractures requires identification of the lesion, determination of the primary tumor, and stable fracture fixation to allow early weight bearing, with the goal of restoring limb function and minimizing pain. Fracture fixation in pathologic bone differs substantially from fixation in healthy bone. Although disease-free bone regenerates in response to injury and stabilization, pathologic bone usually requires a more stable and durable construct, because the underlying disease usually progresses, resulting in further weakening of the bone or prolonged fracture healing.

Diagnostic Work-up for Bone Lesions

Evaluation of the patient with a pathologic fracture should focus on identifying the primary tumor. A thorough history, physical examination, laboratory tests, and imaging studies will successfully identify the primary tumor in more than 90% of cases.[25] If the primary tumor cannot be identified, then a well-planned surgical biopsy is indicated, in which the principles of an open biopsy should be followed.[26] The diagnostic accuracy of a biopsy is correlated directly to the surgeon's biopsy experience; therefore, transfer of patients to a treatment facility with orthopaedic oncology service may be indicated in select cases.[27]

Management of Metastatic Bone Lesions and Fractures

The decision to surgically treat a pathologic fracture is often straightforward. When a patient presents with a lytic lesion without fracture, however, the treatment decision becomes much more difficult. The Mirels scoring system can be a helpful guide when treating these patients.[28] The Mirels method predicts the fracture risk based on the degree of pain, the lesion size, the lytic versus the blastic nature of the lesion, and the anatomic location[28] (**Table 1**). Prophylactic fixation is recommended for patients with a score equal to or greater than 9. Although this scoring system is very helpful, the most reliable predictor for an impending fracture is mechanical pain, which indicates that the involved bone cannot withstand the physiologic load it is subjected to and therefore is at high risk for fatigue failure.

Although the clinical presentation of patients with metastatic bone disease varies, the effect of skeletal metastases on the quality of life is often considerable. Pathologic fracture, loss of limb function, and bone pain are associated with a poor quality of life. Treatment options, including radiation and chemotherapy, diphosphonate treatment, and surgical stabilization are limited and often palliative. Recent evidence, however, suggests that treatment with diphosphonates or the monoclonal antibody denosumab in patients with breast or prostate cancer may not only restrain the invasive nature of the metastasis, but also prevent the implantation of metastatic cells into the skeleton, thus reducing the overall number of skeletal related events.[29,30] Until larger studies have confirmed the effectiveness, safety, and cost effectiveness of diphosphonate and denosumab for the prevention of bone metastasis, however, these treatments should be reserved for patients with advanced metastatic bone disease.

As in primary bone lesions, a normal healing response in pathologic fractures cannot be expected because of the underlying invasive osteolytic process. Therefore, the surgical fixation of these fractures requires unique fixation strategies to allow early weight bearing and promote prolonged fracture stability. These strategies often involve augmentation with polymethyl methacrylate cement, intramedullary fixation when possible, locking plate fixation, adjuvant chemotherapy, or radiation.[31,32] The ultimate goals of any surgical strategy for metastatic bone disease are pain relief and early weight bearing to maintain function. Multiple studies have evaluated the immediate and short-term pain and functional outcomes in this patient cohort.[33,34] These studies suggest that the surgical management of pathologic lesions or fractures provides benefits for pain relief and maintains range of motion, ambulatory status, and possibly independence. Because of the patient's underlying oncologic comorbidities and general medical conditions, however, the surgeon must consider the substantially elevated risk of perioperative morbidity (~17%) and mortality (~4%).[34,35] For long-term success, local tumor control is necessary and can be achieved by postoperative irradiation, which has been shown to contribute to postoperative pain control and the suppression of metastatic growth. Radiation results in depletion of the osteoprogenitor pool at the fracture site, thus resulting in a delay in fracture healing that increases the risks of implant fatigue failure.[35]

Summary

Osteoporosis is a common disorder that mainly affects postmenopausal women, although men also can be affected and often are underdiagnosed. Unbalanced osteoclastic bone resorption is the leading cause of osteoporosis, and current treatment approaches such as diphosphonates and denosumab focus on inhibition of the osteoclast. Future treatment algorithms likely will include anabolic agents in addition to osteoclast inhibitors. Recent advances in surgical implant development and design have made fracture fixation for fragility fractures more reliable and will continue to improve postoperative recovery and function.

Fracture treatment in pathologic bone requires a multidisciplinary approach involving oncologists, internists, radiologists, and orthopaedic surgeons. The surgical fixation of pathologic lesions and fractures has been shown to greatly improve the quality of life, and if the projected life expectancy allows, adjuvant treatment such as irradiation can improve the surgical outcome. Similar to fracture fixation in osteoporotic bone, pathologic bone fixation requires a unique approach centered on improved stability, which can be achieved with load-sharing devices and bone augmentation.

Key Study Points

- Current treatment algorithms for the medical management of osteoporosis in men and postmenopausal women rely on antiresorptive therapy. Future treatments will focus on anabolic agents, such as parathyroid hormone and analogs.
- Patient-centered care of the osteoporotic fracture patient that involves a multidisciplinary team of surgeons, internists, and endocrinologists (the fracture liaison service) results in reduced morbidity and mortality.
- Fractures within pathologic bone segments represent a unique challenge to the treating surgeon and often require medical management in addition to surgical fixation to restore the regenerative potential to the injured bone.

Annotated References

1. Wright NC, Looker AC, Saag KG, et al: The recent prevalence of osteoporosis and low bone mass in the United States based on bone mineral density at the femoral neck or lumbar spine. *J Bone Miner Res* 2014;29(11):2520-2526.

   The authors applied prevalence estimates for osteoporosis and low bone mass based on bone mineral density of the femoral neck or lumbar spine and found that 53.6 million adults older than 50 years were affected by these conditions.

2. Lewiecki EM: Bone density measurement and assessment of fracture risk. *Clin Obstet Gynecol* 2013;56(4):667-676.

   FRAX is a computer-based algorithm developed by the World Health Organization to determine fracture risk based on CRF and BMD. The combination of BMD and CRF predicts fractures better than BMD or CRFs alone.

3. World Health Organization: *WHO scientific group on the assessment of osteoporosis at primary health care level.* Available at: http://www.who.int/chp/topics/Osteoporosis.pdf. Accessed March 10, 2016.

4. National Osteoporosis Foundation: 54 Million Americans Affected by Osteoporosis and Low Bone Mass. 2014, Available at http://nof.org/news/2948. Accessed February 11, 2016.

   The National Osteoporosis Foundation released updated data on the prevalence of osteoporosis in the United States

5. Langdahl BL, Teglbjærg CS, Ho PR, et al: A 24-month study evaluating the efficacy and safety of denosumab for the treatment of men with low bone mineral density: Results from the ADAMO trial. *J Clin Endocrinol Metab* 2015;100(4):1335-1342.

In the United States, 1 in 4 men older than 50 years will have an osteoporosis-related fracture. The purpose of this study was to evaluate denosumab therapy in men with low bone mineral density. In such men, denosumab treatment increased bone mineral density and was well tolerated. The effects were similar to those previously seen in postmenopausal women with osteoporosis and in men with prostate cancer receiving androgen deprivation therapy. Level of evidence: I.

6. Watts NB, Adler RA, Bilezikian JP, et al; Endocrine Society: Osteoporosis in men: An Endocrine Society clinical practice guideline. *J Clin Endocrinol Metab* 2012;97(6):1802-1822.

   The Endocrine Society recommends testing higher-risk men older than 70 years and men aged 50 to 69 years who have risk factors such as low body weight, prior fracture as an adult, and history of tobacco use, using central dual-energy x-ray absorptiometry. Laboratory testing should be done to detect contributing causes. Obtaining adequate calcium and vitamin D and weight-bearing exercise should be encouraged; smoking and excessive alcohol consumption should be discouraged. Pharmacologic treatment is recommended for men aged 50 years or older who have had spine or hip fractures, those with T-scores of -2.5 or below, and men at high risk of fracture based on low bone mineral density and/or clinical risk factors. Treatment should be monitored with serial dual-energy x-ray absorptiometry testing.

7. Centers for Medicare and Medicaid Services: Research, Statistics, Data & Systems: https://www.cms.gov/Research-Statistics-Data-and-Systems/Research-Statistics-Data-and-Systems.html. Accessed March 10, 2016.

8. Lane NE: Osteoporosis: Yesterday, today and tomorrow. *Rheumatology (Oxford)* 2011;50(7):1181-1183.

   This review article summarizes the past and current accomplishments in osteoporosis research and treatment. It is predicted that new medications such as denosumab will have a positive effect on treatment.

9. Morris CD, Einhorn TA: Bisphosphonates in orthopaedic surgery. *J Bone Joint Surg Am* 2005;87(7):1609-1618.

10. Schmidt GA, Horner KE, McDanel DL, Ross MB, Moores KG: Risks and benefits of long-term bisphosphonate therapy. *Am J Health Syst Pharm* 2010;67(12):994-1001.

    The benefits of long-term diphosphonate therapy in patients at high risk of fracture likely outweigh the risks. In lower-risk patients such as those with a bone mineral density in the osteopenic or normal range after 2 to 5 years of treatment and no history of fracture, consideration could be given to the cessation of therapy for 2 to 5 years.

11. Lenart BA, Lorich DG, Lane JM: Atypical fractures of the femoral diaphysis in postmenopausal women taking alendronate. *N Engl J Med* 2008;358(12):1304-1306.

12. Gedmintas L, Solomon DH, Kim SC: Bisphosphonates and risk of subtrochanteric, femoral shaft, and atypical femur fracture: A systematic review and meta-analysis. *J Bone Miner Res* 2013;28(8):1729-1737.

    This meta-analysis suggests that an increased risk of subtrochanteric, femoral shaft, and AFFs exists among diphosphonate users. Further research examining the risk of AFF with long-term use of bisphosphonates is indicated. The public health implication of this observed increase in AFF risk is not yet clear.

13. Hagen JE, Miller AN, Ott SM, et al: Association of atypical femoral fractures with bisphosphonate use by patients with varus hip geometry. *J Bone Joint Surg Am* 2014;96(22):1905-1909.

    Patients on chronic diphosphonate therapy who presented with AFF had more varus proximal femoral geometry than those who took bisphosphonates without sustaining a fracture. Although no causative effect can be determined, a finding of varus geometry may help to better identify patients at risk for fracture after long-term diphosphonate use.

14. Adler RA, El-Hajj Fuleihan G, Bauer DC, et al: Managing osteoporosis in patients on long-term bisphosphonate treatment: Report of a Task Force of the American Society for Bone and Mineral Research. *J Bone Miner Res* 2016;31(1):16-35 .

    This American Society for Bone and Mineral Research task force report outlines the beneficial effects of bisphosphonates but warns about potential side effects, such as osteonecrosis of the jaw and AFFs. These rare events clearly are outweighed by the beneficial reduction in fracture risk, however.

15. Dobnig H, Sipos A, Jiang Y, et al: Early changes in biochemical markers of bone formation correlate with improvements in bone structure during teriparatide therapy. *J Clin Endocrinol Metab* 2005;90(7):3970-3977.

16. Song J, Jin Z, Chang F, Li L, Su Y: Single and combined use of human parathyroid hormone (PTH) (1-34) on areal bone mineral density (aBMD) in postmenopausal women with osteoporosis: Evidence based on 9 RCTs. *Med Sci Monit* 2014;20:2624-2632.

    Teriparatide alone could improve the bone mineral density of the lumbar spine, total hip, and femoral neck considerably. The BMD outcomes of the concomitant use of teriparatide and antiresorptive agents are site-dependent and vary depending on the specific antiresorptive agent used and the timing of antiresorptive therapy initiation.

17. Miyauchi A, Matsumoto T, Shigeta H, Tsujimoto M, Thiebaud D, Nakamura T: Effect of teriparatide on bone mineral density and biochemical markers in Japanese women with postmenopausal osteoporosis: A 6-month dose-response study. *J Bone Miner Metab* 2008;26(6):624-634.

18. Cummings SR, San Martin J, McClung MR, et al; FREEDOM Trial: Denosumab for prevention of fractures in postmenopausal women with osteoporosis. *N Engl J Med* 2009;361(8):756-765.

19. Ishtiaq S, Fogelman I, Hampson G: Treatment of post-menopausal osteoporosis: Beyond bisphosphonates. *J Endocrinol Invest* 2015;38(1):13-29.

This review provides an overview of the mechanisms of action of these therapeutic agents on the skeleton and assesses their efficacy in osteoporosis and fracture prevention.

20. Huntjens KM, van Geel TA, van den Bergh JP, et al: Fracture liaison service: Impact on subsequent nonvertebral fracture incidence and mortality. *J Bone Joint Surg Am* 2014;96(4):e29.

Patients seen at the fracture liaison service had a significantly lower mortality (35%) and subsequently a lower risk of nonvertebral fracture (56%) than those not seen at the fracture liaison service over 2 years of follow-up. A fracture liaison service appears to be a successful approach to reducing the number of subsequent fractures and premature mortality in this cohort of patients.

21. American Academy of Orthopaedic Surgeons: *Clinical Practice Guideline on Management of Hip Fractures in the Elderly.* Rosemont, IL, American Academy of Orthopaedic Surgeons, September 2014. http://www.aaos.org/research/guidelines/HipFXGuideline.pdf. Accessed March 10, 2016.

22. Wang EH, Marfori ML, Serrano MV, Rubio DA: Is curettage and high-speed burring sufficient treatment for aneurysmal bone cysts? *Clin Orthop Relat Res* 2014;472(11):3483-3488.

Curettage, burring, and bone grafting compare favorably in the literature with other approaches for aneurysmal bone cysts such as cryotherapy and argon-beam coagulation. The authors conclude that high-speed burring alone as an adjuvant to intralesional curettage is a reasonable approach to achieving a low recurrence rate for aneurysmal bone cysts.

23. Rapp TB, Ward JP, Alaia MJ: Aneurysmal bone cyst. *J Am Acad Orthop Surg* 2012;20(4):233-241.

This review summarizes the diagnostic approaches for identifying aneurysmal bone cysts, recommends evidence-based treatment options, and outlines prognostic criteria.

24. Damron TA, Lisle J, Craig T, Wade M, Silbert W, Cohen H: Ultraporous β-tricalcium phosphate alone or combined with bone marrow aspirate for benign cavitary lesions: Comparison in a prospective randomized clinical trial. *J Bone Joint Surg Am* 2013;95(2):158-166.

Although substantial improvements in radiographic parameters were observed in both tricalcium phosphate cement groups over 2 years of follow-up, the addition of bone marrow aspirate was not found to provide any substantial benefit.

25. Stella GM, Senetta R, Cassenti A, Ronco M, Cassoni P: Cancers of unknown primary origin: Current perspectives and future therapeutic strategies. *J Transl Med* 2012;10:12.

This review provides state-of-the-art information about the clinical and therapeutic management of this malignant syndrome. The main focus rests on the most recent improvements in the molecular biology and pathology of cancers of unknown primary origin, which can lead to successful tailored therapeutic options.

26. Scolaro JA, Lackman RD: Surgical management of metastatic long bone fractures: Principles and techniques. *J Am Acad Orthop Surg* 2014;22(2):90-100.

This review article outlines the appropriate diagnostic algorithms required to identify metastatic bone lesions, and then discusses the principles of surgical management of these lesions. Emphasis is placed on the importance of sound fixations, as these lesions will not result in fracture healing and thus purely rely on the stability of the implant.

27. Avedian RS: Principles of musculoskeletal biopsy. *Cancer Treat Res* 2014;162:1-7.

Obtaining the right diagnosis is key to tailoring the appropriate cancer treatment. This review outlines the approach for optimal biopsy procurement.

28. Mirels H: Metastatic disease in long bones. A proposed scoring system for diagnosing impending pathologic fractures. *Clin Orthop Relat Res* 1989;249:256-264.

29. Gartrell BA, Saad F: Managing bone metastases and reducing skeletal related events in prostate cancer. *Nat Rev Clin Oncol* 2014;11(6):335-345.

The medical treatment of prostate cancer metastasis is accompanied by other complications, including bone loss. This review addresses the skeletal morbidity associated with prostate cancer. The authors describe medical treatment options to combat the side effects associated with metastatic prostate cancer.

30. Craig Henderson I: Bisphosphonates: Game changers? *Oncology (Williston Park)* 2015;29(1):16-42, 42.

This article summarizes the current indications for bisphosphonate use in patients with metastatic disease. After careful review of the current evidence, the author recommends the use of diphosphonate or denosumab only in patients with advanced metastatic disease after breast cancer.

31. Zore Z, Filipović Zore I, Matejcić A, Kamal M, Arslani N, Knezović Zlatarić D: Surgical treatment of pathologic fractures in patients with metastatic tumors. *Coll Antropol* 2009;33(4):1383-1386.

32. Piccioli A, Maccauro G, Rossi B, Scaramuzzo L, Frenos F, Capanna R: Surgical treatment of pathologic fractures of humerus. *Injury* 2010;41(11):1112-1116.

This study evaluates different surgical treatment options for patients with metastatic fractures of the humerus, focusing on surgical procedures, complications, function, and survival rates. In particular, endoprosthetic replacement after resection was compared with nailing of diaphyseal fractures. Both options led to good pain relief and an acceptable complication rate.

33. Janssen SJ, Teunis T, Hornicek FJ, Bramer JA, Schwab JH: Outcome of operative treatment of metastatic fractures of the humerus: A systematic review of twenty three clinical studies. *Int Orthop* 2015;39(4):735-746.

This systematic review provides an overview of the functional outcome and complications after surgery for metastatic humerus fractures. The authors comment that functional outcome, pain, and quality of life were poorly reported and that future research is needed in this field.

34. Wood TJ, Racano A, Yeung H, Farrokhyar F, Ghert M, Deheshi BM: Surgical management of bone metastases: Quality of evidence and systematic review. *Ann Surg Oncol* 2014;21(13):4081-4089.

The authors postulate that, despite the inherent limitations of the current evidence, a benefit for the surgical management of bone metastases to the long bones and pelvis/acetabulum is evident. Substantial risk of perioperative morbidity and mortality still exists and should be considered, however.

35. Healey JH, Brown HK: Complications of bone metastases: Surgical management. *Cancer* 2000;88(12suppl):2940-2951.

1: General Topics

Chapter 9

Deep Vein Thrombosis Prophylaxis in Fracture Patients

Brian W. Buck, DO

Abstract

There are limited consensus guidelines available for direct deep vein thrombosis prophylaxis for orthopaedic surgeons managing patients with fractures. The indications regarding deep vein thrombosis/venous thromboembolism prophylaxis in patients sustaining upper and lower extremity fractures, as well as patients sustaining pelvic ring, acetabulum, and hip fractures, should be carefully reviewed.

Keywords: deep venous thrombosis; venous thromboembolism; pulmonary embolism; fracture

Introduction

Venous thromboembolism (VTE) events affect an estimated 900,000 to 1 million people annually in the United States, with between 100,000 to 300,000 mortalities reported annually secondary to complications from VTE.[1-4] In one study, the incidence of VTE was estimated at 1.35 million cases per year in the United States.[5] VTE encompasses the clinical entity of a deep vein thrombosis (DVT) and/or a pulmonary embolism (PE). Guidelines exist for prophylaxis in trauma patients who are critically injured and for patients undergoing major orthopaedic surgery, which includes total hip arthroplasty, total knee arthroplasty, and hip fracture surgery.[6]

No consensus guidelines are available to direct the clinician with regard to orthopaedic patients who sustain isolated fractures and who subsequently require treatment with surgical and nonsurgical management strategies.

Neither Dr. Buck nor any immediate family member has received anything of value from or has stock or stock options held in a commercial company or institution related directly or indirectly to the subject of this article/chapter.

It is important to review the indications regarding DVT/VTE prophylaxis in patients sustaining upper and lower extremity fractures, as well as in patients with pelvic ring, acetabulum, and hip fractures.

Prevalence of VTE and Risk Factors for Orthopaedic Trauma Patients

The clinical diagnosis of a DVT is often extremely difficult, with sudden death the presenting symptom in 25% of patients who sustain a PE related to VTE.[1] It has been documented that in patients in whom a DVT develops, the risk of it advancing to a fatal PE is 1.68%.[4] In addition, up to one-third of patients in whom VTE has been diagnosed will have a recurrence within 10 years.[1] PE is the third leading cause of death in injured patients who survive more than 24 hours after trauma, accounting for up to 10% of hospital deaths in the trauma population.[7,8] One of four patients who sustain a PE will die from related complications within 1 year. VTE is the leading cause of preventable death in hospitalized patients, as up to 70% of the entire VTE population comprises this group.[9] In one study, the 30-day mortality rate of a documented DVT was 6%, whereas that of a PE was 12%.[8] The economic effect of VTE is currently more than $1.5 billion per year.

More than 150 years ago, Virchow described the triad of venous stasis, endothelial injury, and hypercoagulability as it relates to thrombus formation. Patients undergoing major orthopaedic surgery and trauma patients often display all of these risk factors, and subsequent studies have attempted to identify risk factors for the development of VTE in these patients. The results of well-designed studies are intended to provide a framework for guidelines allowing physicians to minimize the risk of VTE and concurrently minimize complications related to mechanical and pharmacologic VTE prophylaxis.

According to one study, known risk factors for the development of VTE in trauma patients include age, need for blood transfusion, surgery, femur fracture, tibia fracture,

Table 1

Guidelines for Current Venous Thromboembolism Prophylaxis in Orthopaedic Patients

Source	Guidelines
Orthopaedic Trauma Association[a]	Major orthopaedic surgery LMWH is considered the agent of choice and should be initiated within 24 h provided there are no contraindications (Strong) Combined LMWH and calf pneumatic compressive devices over either regimen alone (Strong) Continuation of VTE prophylaxis for at least 1 mo after discharge (Limited) Recommend against routine screening protocols for DVT in asymptomatic trauma patients (Strong) Isolated lower extremity injury Do not recommend routine chemical prophylaxis in patients who do not have additional risk factors and are dependently mobile (Moderate) Recommend against routine screening protocols for DVT in asymptomatic trauma patients (Strong)
American College of Chest Physicians[b]	Major orthopaedic surgery Extend outpatient prophylaxis for up to 35 d postop (2B) Dual prophylaxis with pharmacologic agent and IPCD while inpatient (2C) Recommend against screening Doppler ultrasonography before discharge (1B) Hip fracture surgery Prophylaxis for a minimum of 10–14 d (1B) Start LMWH either 12 h or more preop or 12 h or more postop (1B) Recommend use of LMWH, fondaparinux, LDUH, adjusted-dose aspirin (1B) or IPCD (1C) LMWH is preferred to other agents (2B/2C) Isolated lower extremity injury No prophylaxis in patients who require leg immobilization (2C)
American Academy of Orthopaedic Surgeons[c]	Elective total joint arthroplasty Pharmacologic agents and/or mechanical compressive devices for VTE prevention for those who are not at elevated risk (Moderate) No specific agent recommended (Inconclusive) Patients and physicians discuss duration of treatment (Consensus) Recommend against routine duplex ultrasonography screening postoperatively (Strong)
Eastern Association for the Surgery of Trauma[d]	LDH has little proven efficacy in prevention of VTE as sole agent in high-risk trauma patients (level II) IPCD may have some benefit in isolated Studies (level III) LMWH can be used in trauma patients with pelvic fractures, complex lower extremity fractures, and spinal cord injury when bleeding risk is acceptable (level II) IVCF should be considered in very high-risk trauma patients who cannot receive pharmacologic prophylaxis or have an injury pattern that would leave them immobilized for long period of time (level III) Duplex ultrasonography may be used to diagnose symptomatic patients with suspected DVT without venography (level I)

and spinal cord injury.[3] In another study analyzing patients from the National Trauma Data Bank, risk factors for the development of VTE were identified as age older than 40 years, lower extremity fracture with Abbreviated Injury Score higher than 3, more than 3 ventilatory days, head injury with Abbreviated Injury Score higher than 3, venous injury, and any major surgical procedure.[10] Eastern Association for the Surgery of Trauma (EAST) guidelines identified spinal fractures and spinal cord injuries as the most significant risk factors for the development of VTE.[11] Older age, increased Injury Severity Score, and the need for blood transfusion appeared to increase the risk of VTE; however, the association remained unclear.[11] Other risk factors in trauma patients include femoral catheter

Table 1 *(continued)*

Guidelines for Current Venous Thromboembolism Prophylaxis in Orthopaedic Patients

Source	Guidelines
Cochrane Review	No evidence that prophylaxis reduces mortality or secondary outcome of pulmonary embolus Pharmacologic prophylaxis is more effective than mechanical prophylaxis LMWH is more effective than UH Insufficient studies for comparison between pharmacologic agents vs placebo or pharmacologic prophylaxis vs mechanical prophylaxis

DVT = deep vein thrombosis, IPCD = intermittent pneumatic compression devices, IVCF = inferior vena cava filter, LDH = low dose heparin, LDUH = low-dose unfractionated heparin, LMWH = low molecular-weight heparin, UH = unfractionated heparin, VTE = venous thromboembolism.

[a] OTA recommendation strengths; Strong = greater than two high-quality (level I) studies to support the recommendation; Moderate: one high-quality (level I) or two moderate-quality (level II or III) studies to support the recommendation; Limited = one moderate-quality (level II or III) or two low–quality (level IV) studies to support the recommendation; Inconclusive = one low-quality (level IV) study or lack of evidence to support the recommendation; Consensus = expert work-group opinion (no studies)

[b] American College of Chest Physicians recommendation strengths: 1B = strong recommendation, moderate-quality evidence, benefits clearly outweigh risk and burdens or vice versa; 1C = strong recommendation, low-quality or very low-quality evidence, benefits clearly outweigh risks and burdens or vice versa; 2B = weak recommendation, moderate-quality evidence, benefits closely balanced with risks and burdens; 2C = weak

Reproduced from Scolaro JA, Taylor RM, Wigner NA: Venous thromboembolism in orthopaedic trauma. *J Am Acad Orthop Surg* 2015;23[1]:1-6.

placement, obesity, known history of VTE, history of malignancy, oral contraceptive use, hormone replacement therapy, heart failure, recent myocardial infarction, and prolonged immobility.[5,12]

Without thromboprophylaxis, the incidence of VTE is up to 40% to 50% among general surgery trauma patients and up to 60% in patients undergoing major orthopaedic surgery.[7,9] The risk of fatal PE is 2% in patients with multisystem trauma or major trauma without thromboprophylaxis.[8] **Table 1** outlines levels of thromboembolic risk and **Table 2** presents recommended strategies of prophylaxis of venous thromboembolism. In another study, general trauma surgery patients without VTE prophylaxis demonstrated a 30% incidence of VTE, with an associated fatality risk of 1%.[3] In one study, the authors recognized a 65% incidence of DVT and a 16% incidence of PE in trauma patients at the time of autopsy.[13] The rate of documented VTE varies depending on the mode of detection as well as the form of VTE prophylaxis administered.

According to a 2013 study, there is a 60% incidence of DVT in high-risk trauma patients without VTE prophylaxis.[4] Despite treatment, VTE has been documented to occur in up to 15% in the trauma population. According to a 2014 study, the incidence of VTE after major trauma has been reported as high as 60% despite appropriate prophylaxis.[14]

In patients undergoing major orthopaedic surgery, the reported incidence of VTE in patients treated without thromboprophylaxis is 60% to 80%, with a reported rate of PE up to 10%.[9,15,16] Despite standardized guidelines and prophylaxis measures, symptomatic VTE continues to be reported in approximately 10% to 30% of patients, with reported rates of fatal PE as high as 1% to 13% in patients following major orthopaedic surgery.[9,17-19]

Current Guidelines on VTE Prophylaxis

Despite the abundance of available data on VTE, there are few published guidelines available for the prevention of VTE in patients with fractures. Chest guidelines provide optimal strategies for thromboprophylaxis after major orthopaedic surgical procedures[6] and are based on the highest level of evidence and stratified between levels I–V. The level of evidence is given an alphanumeric strength of recommendation based on the quality of the studies available. In addition to American College of Chest Physicians (ACCP) guidelines, several guidelines are available to instruct orthopaedic surgeons regarding thromboprophylaxis regimens (**Table 1**). Surgical Care Improvement Program guidelines from the Centers for Medicare and Medicaid Services have been instituted in an attempt to mitigate VTE events and include a pay-for-performance measure available to clinicians to measure the quality of care.[20] Current guidelines focus on individual assessment for patients and recommend against protocols that increase pharmacologic prophylaxis without regard to VTE risk.[16] Risk-benefit analysis is indicated to minimize the risk of VTE while considering the development of major and minor bleeding events and other complications associated with the use of pharmacologic prophylaxis.

VTE prevention is currently achieved in the form of either mechanical or pharmacologic prophylaxis, used in combination when indicated. The use of inferior vena

Table 2

Levels of Thromboembolic Risk and Recommended Strategies of Prophylaxis of Venous Thromboembolism

Level of Risk	DVT Risk (%) in the Absence of Prophylaxis	Suggested Pharmacologic Options
Low Risk • Minor surgery in mobile patients • Medical patients who are fully mobile	<10	No specific prophylaxis Early and aggressive ambulation
Moderate Risk • General, open, gynecologic, or urologic surgery • Medical patients, bed rest or sick • Moderate VTE risk + high bleeding risk	10–40	LMWH, LDUH bid or tid, fondaparinux
High Risk • Hip/knee arthroplasty, HFS • Major trauma	40–80	LMWH, fondaparinux, VKAs (INR: 2-3)

bid = twice a day, DVT = deep vein thrombosis, HFS = hop fracture surgery, INR = international normalized ratio, LMWH = low molecular weight heparin, LDUH = low-dose unfractionated heparin, tid = three times a day, VTE = venous thromboembolism, VKAs = vitamin K antagonists. Reproduced from Tufano A, Coppola A, Cerbone AM, Ruosi C, Franchini M: Preventing postsurgical venous thromboembolism: Pharmacological approaches. *Semin Thromb Hemost* 2011;37(3):252-266.

cava (IVC) filters has also been recommended when pharmacologic therapy is contraindicated. However, controversy exists as to the appropriateness of filter placement secondary to complications. The most common form of mechanical prophylaxis is with an intermittent pneumatic compression device (IPCD); however, graded compression stockings and foot pumps are also used. External compression devices function by reducing vein diameter, resulting in an increased vein flow velocity. Although some studies have shown a reduced rate of DVT in trauma patients, mechanical VTE prophylaxis is recommended only in combination with pharmacologic prophylaxis or when pharmacologic prophylaxis is contraindicated.[3,6]

Pharmacologic agents include low-molecular-weight heparin (LMWH), low-dose unfractionated heparin (LDUH), vitamin K antagonists (VKAs), pentasaccharide factor Xa inhibitor (fondaparinux), and aspirin. Other agents with potential for the prevention of VTE in orthopaedic patient populations include rivaroxaban, apixaban, and dabigatran. Rivaroxaban is an oral pharmacologic agent that acts as a direct Xa inhibitor. A recent study evaluated the rate of VTE in a group of patients sustaining pelvic trauma treated with daily dosing of rivaroxaban followed by evaluation up to 4 months postoperatively with ultrasonography and ventilation/perfusion scan as indicated.[21] In this study, the rate of proximal DVT was 2.4%, with a rate of fatal PE of 1.2%.[21] Apixaban, another oral agent designed to directly inhibit factor Xa, may show some benefit for the use of VTE prevention in this high-risk group of orthopaedic patients. Dabigatran, an oral pharmacologic agent that acts as a direct thrombin inhibitor, may prove beneficial in VTE prevention. Currently, dabigatran has only been examined with respect to orthopaedic patients undergoing total joint arthroplasty.

Currently, pharmacologic prophylaxis with LMWH is recommended over other pharmacologic agents during major orthopaedic surgery procedures. Recommendations include concurrent usage of IPCD, with thromboprophylaxis extended for up to 35 days postoperatively. When thromboprophylaxis is contraindicated, IPCDs are recommended or no thromboprophylaxis is indicated. Based on the quality of the data available in the literature, IVC filters are not recommended in patients in whom pharmacologic and mechanical prophylaxis are contraindicated.[6]

Upper Extremity Fractures and Venous Thromboembolic Disease

There is little published literature on the rate of VTE following upper extremity fractures. Available literature suggests that upper extremity DVTs account for 5% to 10% of all DVTs.[22,23] Upper extremity DVTs (UEDVT) are defined as proximal and distal, with proximal UEDVTs involving the axillary and more proximal deep veins. Distal UEDVT involve thrombosis of the brachial and more distal deep arm veins. The axillary and subclavian veins are the most common sites of UEDVT.[22]

UEDVT can be primary or secondary in nature, with

the primary form less common than secondary UEDVT. Paget-Schroetter syndrome is the most common primary form of UEDVT, and is defined as an effort-related thrombosis secondary to overuse with an underlying diagnosis of venous thoracic outlet syndrome. Repetitive microtrauma causes fibrosis of the subclavian vein, whereas concomitant activation of the coagulation cascade leads to the development of thrombosis.[23]

Risk factors associated with the secondary form of UEDVT are catheter placement with central venous lines or ports, cancer, history of VTE, thrombophilia, trauma to the extremity, surgery or immobilization of the extremity, pregnancy, oral contraceptive use, and ovarian hyperstimulation syndrome.[23] In one study, up to 25% of patients in whom UEDVT was diagnosed received a subsequent diagnosis of cancer.[23] The reported rate of UEDVT after central venous catheter placement has been documented as high as 28%.[23] Catheter-related risk factors include subclavian venipuncture, difficult catheter placement, left-sided catheter placement, location of the catheter tip not at the atriocaval junction, prior central catheter placement, and large lumen catheter placement.[23]

The complications of UEDVT are generally regarded as less morbid in comparison with those of lower extremity DVT. The risk of symptomatic PE is documented between 2% to 9% in one study and up to 36% in another study evaluating VTE in upper extremity orthopaedic surgery.[2,23] The risk of fatal PE following a documented UEDVT is estimated at 1%.[24] The risk of DVT recurrence is increased within the first 6 months compared to lower extremity DVT, in which late recurrence is more common. Cancer, female sex, and obesity all are risk factors for recurrent UEDVT. Postthrombotic syndrome has been reported in up to 50% of patients who sustain an UEDVT. The 3-month mortality rate is at least as high in patients with UEDVT compared to lower extremity VTE, which is attributed to the high prevalence of malignancy in this group of patients.

Patients in whom a UEDVT develops may present with chest discomfort, labored breathing, chest heaviness, paresthesias, and marked swelling of the affected limb. Physical examination may demonstrate edema, redness or cyanosis of the extremity, and development of collateral veins over the upper extremity. In severe cases associated with superior vena cava syndrome, facial swelling, cough, hoarseness, dysphagia, stridor, and life-threatening airway obstruction have been reported.

Upper extremity ultrasonography has largely replaced venography as the gold standard in diagnosing UEDVT, with a sensitivity of 97% and a specificity of 96%.[23] Contrast CT and MRI are also useful in diagnosing UEDVT and concomitant pathology.

When UEDVT is diagnosed, anticoagulation therapy is recommended with bridging LMWH therapy while starting VKA therapy for 3 months. Unlike lower extremity VTE, extended treatment is not recommended beyond 3 months after an initial documented UEDVT. The authors of a 2011 study treated 67 patients with documented UEDVT with VKA or dalteparin for 3 months to examine the safety and efficacy of pharmacologic therapy in patients with UEDVT. At 3-month follow-up, no patient displayed evidence of VTE. The authors concluded that patients in whom UEDVT was diagnosed may be safely and appropriately treated with VKA or dalteparin therapy for 3 months.[25] In patients with UEDVT associated with malignancy, extended LMWH therapy is recommended over the use of VKA. LMWH therapy is recommended as long as the cancer remains active. If the UEDVT is related to catheter use, LMWH therapy may be discontinued at 3 months if the catheter has been removed. Therapy should continue if the catheter remains[23] (**Figure 1**).

Multiple case reports discuss fractures of the upper extremity with the development of symptomatic VTE and fatal PEs.[24,26-29] In a retrospective review, the documented rate of VTE in patients with upper extremity fractures was approximately 5%, which was similar to the rate of VTE in all trauma patients.[22] Furthermore, the rate of VTE was no higher in patients treated with upper extremity trauma compared to patients undergoing elective surgery. Based on these findings, it was concluded that upper extremity trauma was not an independent risk factor for the development of VTE. However, risk stratification and appropriate VTE thromboprophylaxis is recommended in patients with risk factors including history of VTE, thrombophilia, associated injuries in high-risk trauma patients, and a catheter-associated UEDVT.[22]

The British Elbow and Shoulder Society have published VTE guidelines and general recommendations for the use of thromboprophylaxis associated with upper extremity surgery.[30] Patients are stratified as very low, low, moderate, high, and extreme risk. Patients with high and extreme risk are recommended to undergo pharmacologic VTE prophylaxis.

VTE risks for major open surgery of the shoulder and elbow include anesthetic and surgical time longer than 90 minutes, prolonged immobility longer than 3 days, acute trauma, age older than 60 years, active malignancy, history of VTE, thrombophilia, obesity, major illness, pregnancy, and critical care patients undergoing surgical intervention. Surgical fixation of upper extremity fractures is classified as moderate risk for the development of VTE, and the duration of risk for most patients undergoing surgical fixation lasts for 1 month. Although the guidelines offered by the British Elbow and Shoulder

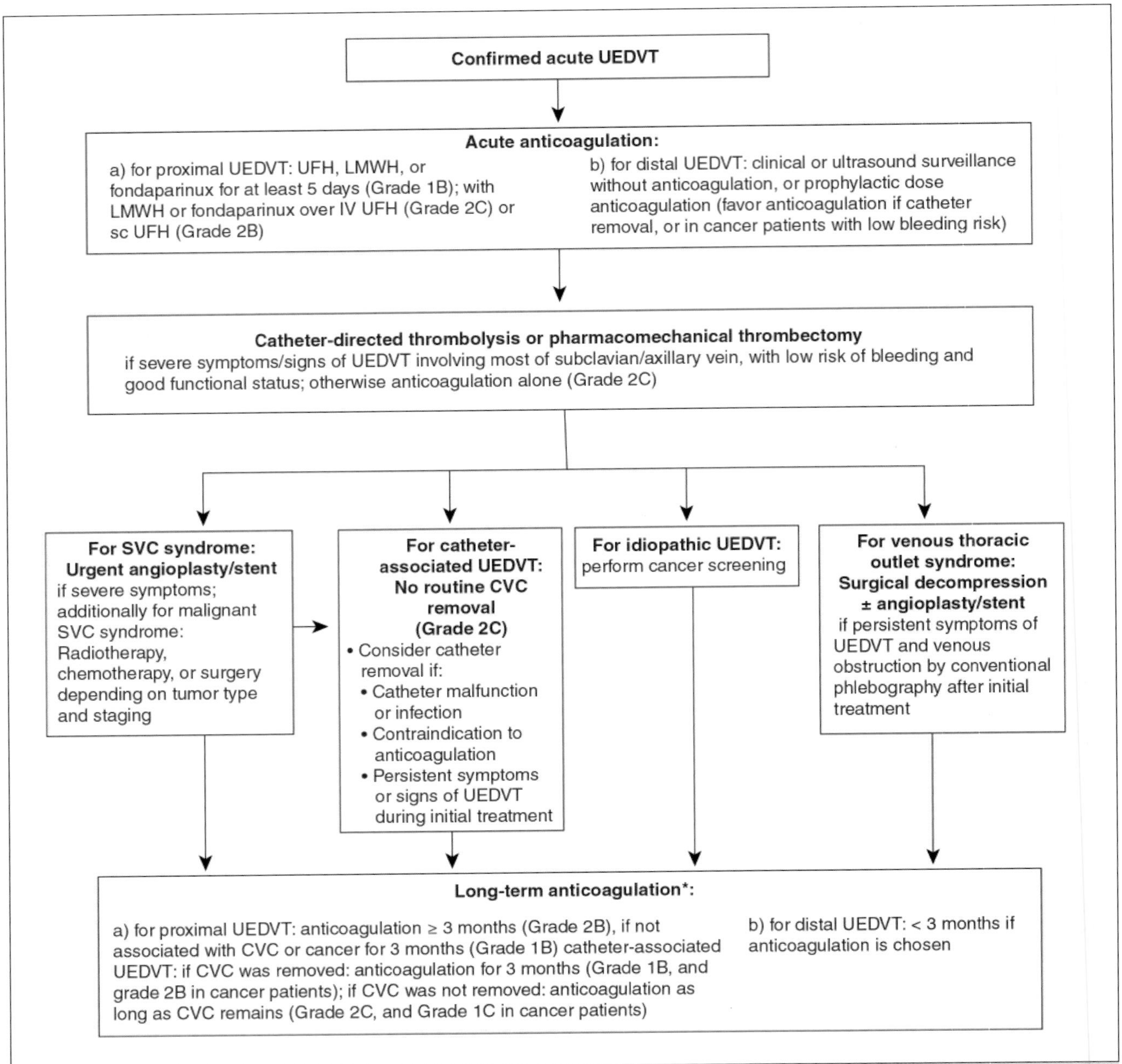
Confirmed acute UEDVT
Acute anticoagulation:
a) for proximal UEDVT: UFH, LMWH, or fondaparinux for at least 5 days (Grade 1B); with LMWH or fondaparinux over IV UFH (Grade 2C) or sc UFH (Grade 2B)
b) for distal UEDVT: clinical or ultrasound surveillance without anticoagulation, or prophylactic dose anticoagulation (favor anticoagulation if catheter removal, or in cancer patients with low bleeding risk)
Catheter-directed thrombolysis or pharmacomechanical thrombectomy
if severe symptoms/signs of UEDVT involving most of subclavian/axillary vein, with low risk of bleeding and good functional status; otherwise anticoagulation alone (Grade 2C)
For SVC syndrome: Urgent angioplasty/stent
if severe symptoms; additionally for malignant SVC syndrome: Radiotherapy, chemotherapy, or surgery depending on tumor type and staging
For catheter-associated UEDVT: No routine CVC removal (Grade 2C)
• Consider catheter removal if:
• Catheter malfunction or infection
• Contraindication to anticoagulation
• Persistent symptoms or signs of UEDVT during initial treatment
For idiopathic UEDVT: perform cancer screening
For venous thoracic outlet syndrome: Surgical decompression ± angioplasty/stent
if persistent symptoms of UEDVT and venous obstruction by conventional phlebography after initial treatment
Long-term anticoagulation*:
a) for proximal UEDVT: anticoagulation ≥ 3 months (Grade 2B), if not associated with CVC or cancer for 3 months (Grade 1B) catheter-associated UEDVT: if CVC was removed: anticoagulation for 3 months (Grade 1B, and grade 2B in cancer patients); if CVC was not removed: anticoagulation as long as CVC remains (Grade 2C, and Grade 1C in cancer patients)
b) for distal UEDVT: < 3 months if anticoagulation is chosen

Figure 1 Algorithm for management of acute upper extremity deep vein thrombosis. CVC = central venous catheter; IV = intravenous; LMWH = low-molecular weight heparin, SC = subcutaneous, SVC = superior vena cava; UEDVT = upper extremity deep vein thrombosis, UFH = unfractioned heparin. (Reproduced with permission from Engelberger RP, Kucher N: Management of deep vein thrombosis of the upper extremity. *Circulation* 2012:126:768-773.)

Society are not rigorously stratified by level of evidence and quality of study, they provide guidance for the appropriateness of VTE thromboprophylaxis in patients with risk factors and upper extremity fractures.

The authors of a 2014 study assessed 3,400 consecutive upper extremity orthopaedic surgical procedures to estimate the incidence of postoperative VTE associated with upper extremity orthopaedic surgery. Included were 20% of the patients classified as "fixation of fracture/dislocation."[31] The reported incidence of postoperative VTE was 0.0018%, with two documented DVTs and four PEs. Based on these findings, routine VTE prophylaxis was not recommended in patients undergoing upper extremity orthopaedic procedures unless there is a personal or family history of VTE.

Two review articles provide opposite recommendations.

The authors of a 2013 study reported that upper extremity surgery was not an independent risk factor for the development of VTE and recommended against routine VTE prophylaxis despite an increased risk after surgery for up to 3 months.[2] In another 2013 study,[32] the authors reviewed 4,800 shoulder procedures for surgical fixation of proximal humerus fractures for VTE and the incidence was 0.64%. Risk factors for the development of VTE in this group included patients with diabetes mellitus, rheumatoid arthritis, and ischemic heart disease. Despite the limitations of the available studies, a multimodal approach was recommended in patients with substantial risk factors.

Published guidelines do not recommend routine use of pharmacologic thromboprophylaxis in patients undergoing upper extremity surgery, including patients undergoing fixation of upper extremity fractures. However, no strong body of evidence exists to provide recommendations regarding mechanical and chemical prophylaxis following upper extremity fracture surgery. Consequently, until national guidelines are developed addressing VTE in orthopaedic upper extremity fracture surgery, clinical judgment is recommended. Patient-specific risk factors should be taken into account, and weighed against the risks and benefits of mechanical and pharmacologic prophylaxis. After careful consideration, VTE prophylaxis should be considered in high-risk patients undergoing surgical fixation of upper extremity fractures. Patients in whom UEDVT develops following upper extremity fractures or following fracture fixation should be treated appropriately with LMWH for 3 to 6 months.

Pelvic Ring and Acetabulum Fractures

DVT occurs in up to 60% of patients who sustain pelvic ring and acetabulum fractures without prophylaxis.[33] The documented rate of proximal DVT exceeds 35%, with a risk of symptomatic PE up to 12% and fatal PE up to 2%.[21,33] A 12.5% incidence of VTE was documented in patients who sustained high-energy pelvic ring skeletal trauma despite thromboprophylaxis.[34] Patients with pelvic and acetabulum trauma are considered at high risk of VTE complications and consideration is recommended for early pharmacologic and mechanical thromboprophylaxis.

Because current prophylaxis guidelines are lacking, a systematic review was performed to evaluate the effectiveness of thromboprophylaxis regimens to reduce the rate of VTE in patients who sustain pelvic ring and acetabulum fractures. The results indicated a trend toward lower rates of DVT with the use of mechanical prophylaxis versus no thromboprophylaxis in a group of patients with pelvic ring and acetabulum fractures.[35] However, there was no statistical difference in the incidence of VTE between the two groups. The use of IVC filters was also evaluated, and no difference in symptomatic pulmonary emboli was noted among patients with or without filter placement. The results of these findings suggested that no meaningful thromboprophylaxis guidelines could be made specifically for patients sustaining pelvic ring or acetabulum fractures.[35]

Other studies have shown that timing of initiating therapy is important. A prospective study was performed on patients undergoing surgical fixation of pelvic ring and acetabulum fractures. Patients were treated with LMWH within 24 hours of injury or after hemodynamic stability was achieved. Subsequent screening for proximal DVT was performed to detect the incidence of DVT, and PE was documented following CT of the chest. The incidence of DVT was 10%, whereas the incidence of PE was 5%.[36] Patients who received pharmacologic prophylaxis within 24 hours of injury had a 3% incidence of proximal DVT, whereas the incidence in those administered prophylaxis beyond 24 hours was 22%.[36] The results of this study suggest that LMWHs can be administered early in the management of trauma patients who sustain pelvic ring and acetabulum fractures for VTE prophylaxis. A consecutive group of patients with pelvic trauma treated with a standardized thromboprophylaxis protocol with rivaroxaban were studied. Rivaroxaban was given within 24 hours of injury or once hemodynamically stable. Ultrasonography was performed preoperatively and postoperatively and ventilation-perfusion scans were performed when indicated to confirm a PE. The incidence of proximal DVT was 2.4% and the incidence of PE was 1.2% within the study period.[34] A substantially higher incidence of a symptomatic DVT was demonstrated with ultrasonography in those patients in whom treatment was started more than 24 hours after admission. The authors concluded that the use of rivaroxaban decreased the incidence of symptomatic and asymptomatic VTE in patients treated with pelvic ring trauma.

Evidence-based recommendations are lacking with respect to prevention of VTE events in patients with pelvic ring and acetabulum trauma. Clinical strategies for prevention include mechanical and pharmacologic therapy, which appear to be most effective when instituted early. The timing of therapy ultimately depends on the thrombotic risk present, and the mode of prophylaxis is based on the balance between development of VTE and risk of bleeding. IVC filters have been used in an effort to decrease the chance of the development of life-threatening effects of PE. IVC filters have been recommended when there is a contraindication to pharmacologic anticoagulation or when a proximal DVT has developed. Unfortunately, despite the reported benefits, IVC filters are associated with complications that may temper enthusiasm for their usage. For example, EAST guidelines provide a level III recommendation for prophylactic IVC filter placement in very high-risk trauma patients in whom pharmacologic therapy is contraindicated. In contradistinction, ACCP guidelines recommend against the use of filter placement and recommend no therapy in patients in whom mechanical and pharmacologic therapy are contraindicated, with a grade 2C recommendation. As a result, controversy continues with regard to optimal therapy recommendations.

Hip Fractures

Hip fracture surgery is considered major orthopaedic surgery, and consensus guidelines have been well established regarding the use of thromboprophylaxis in this patient population. Prospective randomized controlled trials have demonstrated that the risk of DVT in patients treated without prophylaxis is as high as 60% to 75%.[17-19,37] The development of PE associated with a hip fracture and hip fracture surgery ranges from 4% to 24%, with an incidence of fatal PE up to 13%.[19]

PE is the fourth most common cause of death after a hip fracture, and patients are at an increased risk of a VTE event developing up to 3 months following injury.[37] One study found that VTE was diagnosed in more than 70% of patients after acute inpatient discharge, with a median time to presentation for DVT of 24 days and 17 days for the presentation of PE.[37]

The most current ACCP Chest guidelines,[6] released in 2012, recommend LMWH, fondaparinux, LDUH, VKA, or aspirin as pharmacologic antithrombotic prophylaxis for a minimum of 10 to 14 days in patients undergoing hip fracture surgery, with a grade 1B recommendation. Furthermore, LMWH is suggested in these patients over other agents, with a grade 2C recommendation. Thromboprophylaxis is suggested to continue for up to 35 days postoperatively, which has a grade 2B recommendation. In addition to pharmacologic agents, dual prophylaxis with an IPCD during hospital admission is suggested in patients undergoing major orthopaedic surgery, based on a grade 2C recommendation.[6]

If patients have an increased risk of bleeding that outweighs the benefit of pharmacologic antithrombotic prophylaxis in the setting of hip fracture surgery, IPCD or no prophylaxis is indicated, with a grade 2C recommendation.[6]

In patients who are noncompliant with injections or IPCD, apixaban or dabigatran are preferred over alternative agents of prophylaxis, with a grade 1B recommendation. Alternatively, rivaroxaban or VKA are recommended if unavailability exists.

IVC filters are not recommended for primary prevention over no prophylaxis in patients with an increased bleeding risk in whom both mechanical and pharmacologic thromboprophylaxis are contraindicated, with a grade 2C recommendation.[6]

It is important to begin thromboprophylaxis upon admission after a hip fracture, as patients are at an increased risk of VTE as they wait for surgery. One study demonstrated a 55% incidence of DVT in patients who did not present to the hospital for more than 48 hours after injury.[17] In a similar group of patients admitted within 48 hours, the rate of DVT was 6%.[17] The incidence of preoperative DVT was as high as 62% in patients who waited 48 hours to undergo surgery when not treated with thromboprophylaxis. This study suggests that the risk of VTE starts at the time of initial injury as opposed to the surgical intervention. It also underscores the importance of initiating thromboprophylaxis at the time of admission as opposed to waiting until the day following surgery to minimize the risk of surgical bleeding.

Missed doses of anticoagulation may also increase the risk of the development of VTE events. Patients who missed at least one dose of LMWH therapy had a 24% incidence of DVT versus 5% in patients with uninterrupted therapy.[18] In the hip fracture population, missed doses may be a frequent finding due to multiple medical comorbidities, the surgical intervention, the difficult postoperative recovery, and frequent therapy sessions throughout the hospital admission. Strategies should be implemented to decrease the chances of missing doses of anticoagulation to effectively minimize the likelihood of the development of a VTE event.

Lower Extremity Fractures

Consensus guidelines are lacking with regard to the treatment and prevention of VTE events in the population of patients who sustain lower extremity fractures. However, the topic has been reviewed in multiple studies and recommendations made. One study found that the incidence of lower extremity DVT was 58% in trauma patients, and up to 69% in patients with associated lower extremity injuries.[38] In this study, the rate of documented thrombi was 80% in patients with femur fractures, 75% with tibia fractures, 75% with ankle fractures, and over 60% with pelvic ring injuries.[38] The results indicate that all patients with trauma should be considered at high risk for VTE complications. Current guidelines recommend that all trauma patients with at least one risk factor for VTE

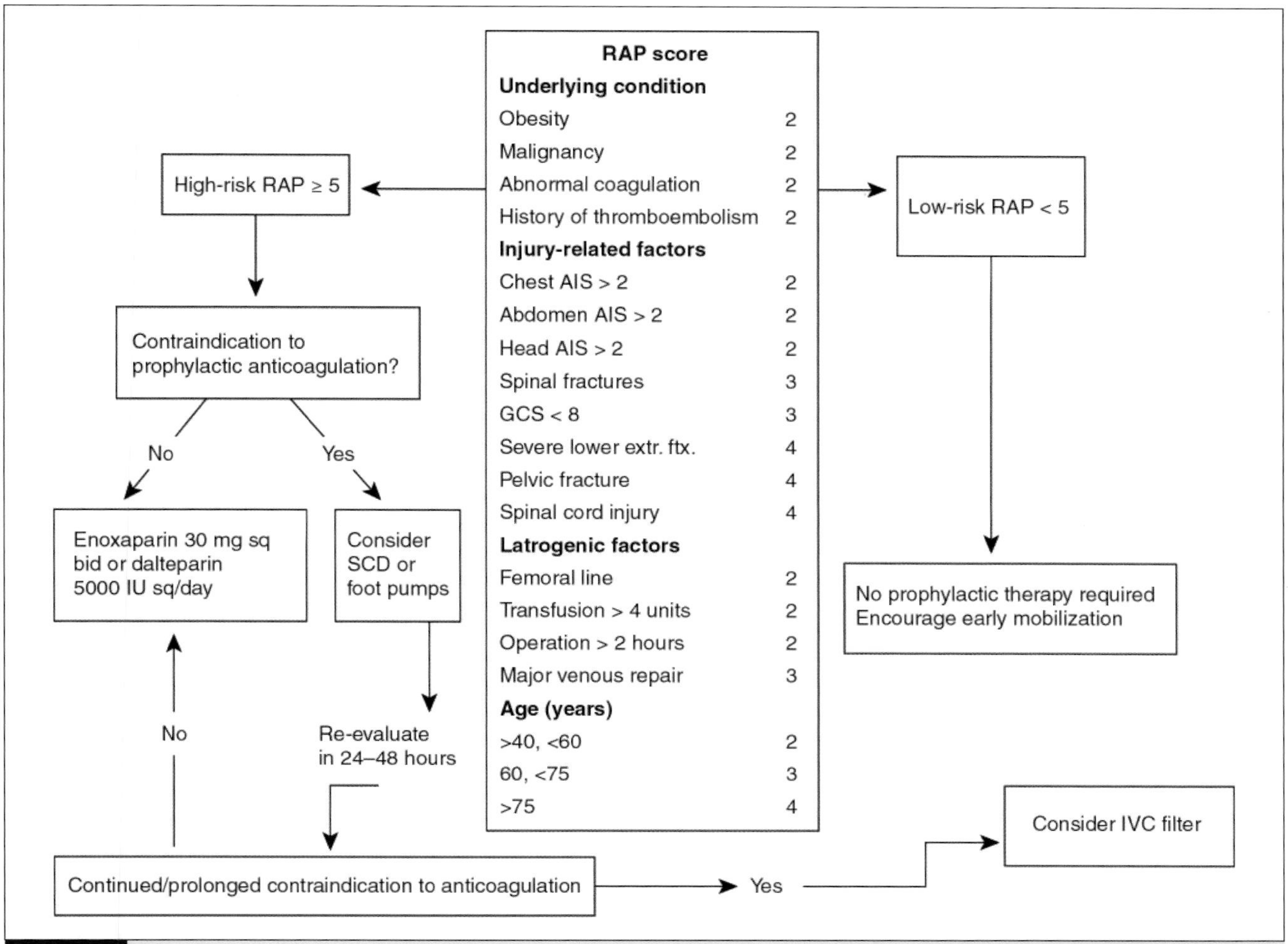

Figure 2 Algorithm for venous thromboembolism prophylaxis. AIS = Abbreviated Injury Scale; bid = twice a day; GCS = Glasgow Coma Scale; IVC = inferior vena cava; RAP = Risk Assessment Profile; SCD = sequential compression device: sq = subcutaneously. (Reproduced with permission from Toker S, Hak DJ, Morgan SJ: Deep vein thrombosis prophylaxis in trauma patients. *Thrombosis* 2011;(2011):Article ID 505373:11.)

receive some form of thromboprophylaxis, with the use of LMWH or LDUH (grade 2C recommendation) (**Figure 2**).

A study was performed to examine the incidence of DVT in patients with fractures of the lower extremity distal to the hip.[15] The overall incidence of DVT in this patient population was 28%: 40% for femoral shaft, 43% for tibial plateau, 22% for tibial shaft, and 12.5% for tibial plafond fractures. However, only 4 of the documented 33 positive venograms demonstrated thrombi proximal to the popliteal fossa, and all of the DVTs were classified as occult or asymptomatic. Using multiple logistic regression analysis, age older than 60 years, operating room time longer than 105 minutes, and time from injury to surgery were found to be associated risk factors to predict the development of DVT. The authors concluded that this patient population should receive anticoagulation for the prevention of VTE.

Even when patients undergo prophylaxis, VTE can occur. One study found an 11.5% incidence of VTE in patients with high-energy skeletal trauma despite prophylaxis measures, including 10% in those with nonpelvic trauma.[34] In comparison, another study examined 1,700 patients with isolated low-energy fractures to determine the incidence of symptomatic VTE events in patients treated with standard VTE prophylaxis.[39] The incidence of VTE was 0.012%, with female sex and increased body mass index significant risk factors for VTE.[39]

The concept of damage control orthopaedics is commonly applied in trauma patients. In a study reporting on the incidence of DVT after temporary joint spanning external fixation for lower extremity injuries treated with early mobilization and LMWH administration,[40] the incidence of DVT was 2.1%, but zero in patients with an isolated lower extremity injury. The authors recommend the routine use of pharmacologic thromboprophylaxis in patients with high-energy lower extremity injuries treated with early stabilization and mobilization protocols.

Using the National Trauma Data Bank, musculoskeletal injury risk factors for the development of pulmonary embolism were identified in patients with pelvic ring injuries and lower extremity fractures.[14] PEs occurred at a rate of 0.46% over the course of hospitalization and patients with pelvic fractures had a higher rate of PE compared to patients with isolated lower extremity fractures. Patients with PE had a 12.7% mortality rate compared to 5.7% in patients without PE. Univariate analysis revealed a higher rate of PE with increasing age, pelvic fracture, obesity, history of VKA use, bilateral femur fractures, and polytrauma with multiple fractures. Likewise, regression analysis demonstrated that multiple fractures, VKA therapy, obesity, admission to a university hospital, and direct admission to the intensive care unit or operating room were a predictor of PE. The results of the study confirmed the need for appropriate VTE prophylaxis to protect against the development of PE in these high-risk patient populations.

In a similar study, high-risk patients were evaluated for the development of early and late PE following trauma.[41] More than 279,000 patients were included and there was a -0.36% incidence of PE. In this cohort study, early lower extremity fracture fixation was the only independent risk factor for the development of early PE and had a threefold higher risk of early PE compared to those patients who did not undergo early surgical intervention. The results highlight the need for pharmacologic and mechanical thromboprophylaxis in patients undergoing early surgical fixation of lower extremity and pelvic ring fractures.

Unfortunately, despite highlighting the rates and risk factors related to VTE in lower extremity trauma patients, these studies are lacking detailed information regarding the mode of thromboprophylaxis provided. The efficacy and safety of rivaroxaban versus LMWH therapy was examined in patients with lower extremity fractures.[42] The incidence of all VTE in the rivaroxaban and LMWH groups was 4.9% and 8.6%, respectively. Rivaroxaban reduced the incidence of VTE by 45% compared to patients treated with LMWH therapy with no increase in the risk of bleeding events. Although the incidence of proximal DVT in the two groups was not statistically significant (0.9% versus 2.9%), the incidence of single distal DVT was significantly lower in the rivaroxaban group. The findings suggest that rivaroxaban reduces the incidence of DVT mainly by reducing the development of distal VTE.[42] Therefore, the decreased incidence of VTE in the rivaroxaban group may be due to a decreased rate of distal VTE events where the need for treatment remains controversial.[42] The results suggest that rivaroxaban may be used safely as an alternative to LMWH therapy in patients undergoing surgical fixation of lower extremity fractures to reduce the rate of VTE.

Despite the incidence of VTE in patients who sustain lower extremity fractures below the knee, there is no clear indication for the use of mechanical and pharmacologic therapy in this population. A prospective randomized controlled study was performed to determine the incidence of DVT and the need for thromboprophylaxis following surgical fixation of fractures below the knee.[12] Patients were randomized following surgical fixation of a lower extremity fracture to treatment with LMWH therapy versus placebo. Patients were evaluated venographically for the development of DVT. There was no statistically significant difference in the incidence of DVT between the groups, with the overall incidence of DVT 11%: 8.7% in the LMWH group and 12.6% in the placebo group. Patient age and type of fracture, specifically tibial plateau fracture, were identified as risk factors for DVT. All documented DVTs were asymptomatic, without proximal migration, and did not require therapy. The findings suggest that pharmacologic therapy in patients undergoing surgical fixation of lower extremity fractures below the knee may not be justified.

The incidence of symptomatic DVT after lower extremity foot and ankle surgery is 0.5%, with an incidence of PE of approximately 0.2% to 0.3%.[43] In a position statement from the American Orthopaedic Foot and Ankle Society, current data are insufficient to recommend for or against routine VTE prophylaxis for patients undergoing foot and ankle surgery.[44] Consistent with most current guidelines, assessment of risk factors associated with the development of VTE are indicated and when present, warrant mechanical or pharmacologic therapy. However, the stratification of risk factors and mode of treatment remain ill defined.

Multiple studies have been conducted to evaluate the incidence and treatment of VTE in patients sustaining ankle fractures.[5,43] Based on the quality and results of the literature available, authors recommend that physicians should not administer routine VTE prophylaxis. With regard to ankle and foot fractures, there is no evidence to support routine VTE thromboprophylaxis in patients with isolated injuries. ACCP guidelines currently advocate for no thromboprophylaxis in patients with isolated lower extremity injuries with a grade 2B recommendation.[6]

Summary

Limited consensus VTE prophylaxis guidelines exist for physicians managing trauma patients with fractures. Currently, there are no guidelines addressing a need for thromboprophylaxis in patients undergoing surgical fixation of upper extremity fractures. However, in patients with significant risk factors, mechanical and chemical prophylaxis should be considered despite current recommendations against prophylaxis.

Future studies are recommended with well-powered prospective randomized controlled trials in an effort to elucidate the true incidence of VTE, including DVT and PE, in patients sustaining fractures. In addition, high-level studies are necessary to examine the appropriate need for VTE prophylaxis as well as the optimal prophylactic regimen in this particular patient population. Until that time, thoughtful consideration for VTE prophylaxis should be based on patient risk assessment.

Key Study Points

- VTE events affect between 900,000 to 1 million people yearly in the United States, with up to 300,000 mortalities reported annually secondary to complications from VTE.
- ACCP guidelines provide treatment strategies for VTE prophylaxis in patients undergoing major orthopaedic surgical procedures. However, there are limited guidelines for patients sustaining isolated fractures.
- Guidelines do not recommend for the routine use of pharmacologic VTE prophylaxis in patients treated with upper extremity fractures. Despite this, clinical judgment and consideration for VTE prophylaxis are warranted in high-risk patient populations.
- Early administration of mechanical and pharmacologic thromboprophylaxis measures have been shown to decrease the incidence of VTE events in patients sustaining pelvic ring injuries and acetabulum fractures.
- Despite the incidence of VTE, there is no indication for VTE prophylaxis in patients who sustain lower extremity fractures below the knee.

Annotated References

1. Beckman MG, Hooper WC, Critchley SE, Ortel TL: Venous thromboembolism: A public health concern. *Am J Prev Med* 2010;38(4suppl):S495-S501.

   This review article provides US data and statistics from the Centers for Disease Control and Prevention on venous thromboembolism disease. Discussion of postthrombotic syndrome and long-term complications of deep vein thrombosis are reviewed.

2. Anakwe R, Middleton S, Beresford-Cleary N, et al: Preventing venous thromboembolism in elective upper limb surgery. *J Shoulder Elbow Surg* 2013;22(3):432-438.

   Various worldwide guidelines for VTE prevention are reviewed and the highest level of evidence recommendations for appropriate prophylaxis in patients undergoing upper extremity orthopaedic surgery are provided.

3. Toker S, Hak DJ, Morgan SJ: Deep vein thrombosis prophylaxis in trauma patients. *Thrombosis* 2011;2011:505373.

   In this review article, mechanical and pharmacologic regimens are discussed as well as the use of IVC filters in high-risk patient populations. EAST and ACCP Chest guidelines are presented, with a discussion of the controversy regarding the optimal prophylactic regimen.

4. DeMuro JP, Hanna AF: Prophylaxis of deep vein thrombosis in trauma patients: A review. *J Blood Disord Transfus* 2013;4:151.

   Pharmacologic thromboprophylaxis regimens are presented in difficult trauma subpopulations in this review article. Populations include patients with renal failure, nonsurgical solid organ injury, intracranial hemorrhage, spinal cord injury, and bariatric trauma. Recommendations are provided based on available evidence-based literature.

5. Martin SL, Hardy MA: Venous Thromboembolism Prophylaxis in Foot and Ankle Surgery: A Literature Review. *The Foot and Ankle Journal* 2008;1(5):4.

6. Falck-Ytter Y, Francis CW, Johanson N, et al: American College of Chest Physicians: Prevention of VTE in orthopaedic surgery patients: Antithrombotic Therapy and Prevention of Thrombosis, 9th edition: American College of Chest Physicians Evidence-Based Clinical Practice Guidelines. *Chest* 2012;141(2 suppl):e278S-e325S.

   The 9th edition *Chest* guidelines, provided by the American College of Chest Physicians, provide venous thromboembolism prophylaxis recommendations based on the highest level of evidence for orthopaedic surgery patients. Recommendations are provided based on a grading system based on qualitative level of evidence.

7. Datta I, Ball C, Rudmik L, et al: Complications related to deep venous thrombosis prophylaxis in trauma: A systematic review of the literature. *J Trauma Manag Outcomes* 2010;4:1.

   Mechanical compression devices, chemical prophylaxis regimens, and IVC filter placement are discussed in this systematic literature review. Indications and complications are evaluated for these prophylactic venous thromboembolism options.

8. Surgical and Medical Critical Care Services at Orlando Regional Medical Center: DVT Prophylaxis in Surgical Patients 2005, updated 2014. Available at: http://www.surgicalcriticalcare.net/Guidelines/deep_venous_prophylaxis_2014.pdf. Accessed February 17, 2016.

9. Tufano A, Coppola A, Cerbone AM, Ruosi C, Franchini M: Preventing postsurgical venous thromboembolism: Pharmacological approaches. *Semin Thromb Hemost* 2011;37(3):252-266.

   Pharmacologic thromboprophylaxis agents are discussed in the prevention of postsurgical VTE events in this review article. Various general surgery and orthopaedic patient populations are addressed with respect to VTE risks and appropriate anticoagulation strategies.

10. Knudson MM, Ikossi DG, Khaw L, Morabito D, Speetzen LS: Thromboembolism after trauma: An analysis of 1602 episodes from the American College of Surgeons national trauma data bank. *Ann Surg* 2004;240(3):490-496, discussion 496-498.

11. Rogers F, Cipolle M, Vlemahos G, et al: Practice management guidelines for the prevention of venus thromboembolism in trauma patients: The EAST practice management guidelines work group. *J Trauma* 2002;53(1):142-164.

12. Goel DP, Buckley R, deVries G, Abelseth G, Ni A, Gray R: Prophylaxis of deep vein thrombosis in fractures below the knee: a prospective randomised controlled trial. *J Bone Joint Surg Br* 2009;91(3):388-394.

13. Sevitt S, Gallagher N: Venous thrombosis and pulmonary embolism. A clinico-pathological study in injured and burned patients. *Br J Surg* 1961;48:475-489.

14. Godzik J, McAndrew CM, Morshed S, Kandemir U, Kelly MP: Multiple lower-extremity and pelvic fractures increase pulmonary embolus risk. *Orthopedics* 2014;37(6):e517-e524.

   The purpose of this retrospective study was to identify patients at risk for the development of PE following musculoskeletal trauma. A PE developed in 918 of 199,952 patients (0.46%) reviewed in the National Trauma Data Bank after sustaining pelvic ring and lower extremity injuries. Multiple fractures were found to significantly increase the risk of PE events. Factors that were associated with an increased rate of PE included obesity, history of warfarin use, hospital disposition, ICU odds ratio, and hospital setting.

15. Abelseth G, Buckley RE, Pineo GE, Hull R, Rose MS: Incidence of deep-vein thrombosis in patients with fractures of the lower extremity distal to the hip. *J Orthop Trauma* 1996;10(4):230-235.

16. Holley AB: Shifts in the approach to venous thromboembolism prophylaxis for trauma patients. Available at: http://www.medscape.com/viewarticle/775654. Accessed February 17, 2016.

   This Medscape article discusses the evolution of ACCP guidelines and recommendations for thromboprophylaxis based on available best evidence literature.

17. Grant PJ, Jaffer AK: When should prophylactic anticoagulation begin after a hip fracture? *Cleve Clin J Med* 2006;73(9):785-786, 788, 790-792.

18. Phend C: Missed doses cripple postop DVT prevention. Available at: http://www.medpagetoday.com/Cardiology/VenousThrombosis/45311. Accessed February 17, 2016.

   This review article investigates the association of missed doses of chemical thromboprophylaxis and the rate of development of DVT. Patients were found to have an 8.49-fold higher risk of development of a DVT with two to four missed doses. A 10.13-fold higher risk when 5 to 8 doses were missed and 14.73-fold higher risk when 9 to 17 doses were missed was calculated based on national data. The results underscore the timely administration of pharmacologic prophylaxis and the need for compliance to decrease the incidence of VTE events.

19. Egol KA, Strauss EJ: Perioperative considerations in geriatric patients with hip fracture: What is the evidence? *J Orthop Trauma* 2009;23(6):386-394.

20. Clark CR: Coagulation, thromboembolism, and blood management in orthopaedic surgery, in Flynn JM, ed: *Orthopaedic Knowledge Update 10* .Rosemont, ILAmerican Academy of Orthopaedic Surgeons, 2011, pp 137-145.

   Venous thromboembolism mechanical and pharmacologic prevention regimens are reviewed. AAOS guidelines on the prevention of pulmonary embolism in patients undergoing total joint arthroplasty are summarized in table form. The chapter also focuses on perioperative blood management strategies in orthopaedic surgery.

21. Godoy Monzon D, Iserson KV, Cid A, Vazquez JA: Oral thromboprophylaxis in pelvic trauma: A standardized protocol. *J Emerg Med* 2012;43(4):612-617.

   A standardized protocol was evaluated in this prospective nonrandomized study to assess the efficacy of oral rivaroxaban in preventing VTE events in patients with pelvic ring and acetabulum trauma. Of the 84 patients included in the study, 6 deep vein thrombosis events (9.4%) were recorded in 64 patients receiving early chemoprophylaxis, whereas 8 events were noted in 20 patients (45%) who received late pharmacologic therapy after 24 hours or after hemodynamic stability was achieved.

22. Scolaro JA, Taylor RM, Wigner NA: Venous thromboembolism in orthopaedic trauma. *J Am Acad Orthop Surg* 2015;23(1):1-6.

   This review article details current recommendations for venous thromboembolism prophylaxis in the orthopaedic trauma patient population. Existing guidelines are reviewed providing prophylaxis strategies. Recommendations for orthopaedic trauma patients are reviewed based on surgical and nonsurgical injuries, and literature is reviewed with respect to upper and lower extremity injuries. Recommendations are based on recent level I–III studies.

23. Engelberger RP, Kucher N: Management of deep vein thrombosis of the upper extremity. *Circulation* 2012;126(6):768-773.

This clinical update reviews the diagnosis and management of a deep vein thrombosis in the upper extremity. Superior vena cava syndrome, Paget-Schroetter syndrome, and catheter-associated thrombosis are highlighted in this review. Mechanical and pharmacologic regimens are discussed, as well as the role of catheter intervention procedures to mitigate the risks of post-thrombotic syndrome.

24. Peivandi MT, Nazemian Z: Clavicular fracture and upper extremity deep venous thrombosis. *Orthopedics* 2011;34(3):227-231.

This case report identifies a patient with a clavicle fracture in whom a UEDVT develops, treated with a figure-of-8 harness. Discussion points include 3-month treatment with enoxaparin and the hypothesis that clot formation in the upper extremity may be a result of direct trauma to the venous wall from a clavicle fracture. As a result, the authors recommend clavicle fractures be added to the list of risk factors for the development of a UEDVT.

25. Rathbun SW, Stoner JA, Whitsett TL: Treatment of upper-extremity deep vein thrombosis. *J Thromb Haemost* 2011;9(10):1924-1930.

This level I study assesses the efficacy of dalteparin sodium compared to warfarin therapy in the prevention of new venous thromboembolism events in patients with a documented upper extremity deep vein thrombosis (UEDVT). Major and minor bleeding events are compared between the two treatment regimens.

26. Jones RE, McCann PA, Clark DA, Sarangi P: Upper limb deep vein thrombosis: A potentially fatal complication of a clavicle fracture. *Ann R Coll Surg Engl* 2010;92(5):W36-8.

In this case report, a UEDVT is associated with a patient sustaining a clavicle fracture. Appropriate diagnostic interventions, including a three-dimensional CT venogram, are discussed in addition to treatment strategies including a 3-month course of anticoagulation.

27. Sobue S, Kaketa T, Noike K, et al: Fatal pulmonary embolism after surgery for a clavicle fracture: A case report. *Open J Clin Diagn* 2012;2:63-65.

A fatal PE is documented in a patient after undergoing surgical fixation of a clavicle fracture in this case report. Questions are raised regarding the appropriate mechanical and/or pharmacologic regimens necessary for patients undergoing clavicle surgery.

28. Claes T, Debeer P, Bellemans J, et al: Deep venous thrombosis of the axillary and subclavian vein after osteosynthesis of a midshaft clavicular fracture: A case report. *Am J Sports Med* 2010;38(6):1255-1258.

This is a case report of a patient in whom a UEDVT develops after undergoing surgical fixation of a midshaft clavicle fracture. Catheter-guided thrombolysis was performed in an attempt to reestablish the patency of the subclavian and axillary vein with partial success. Eventual treatment consisted of 2-month duration of low-molecular-weight heparin and bandages to ameliorate swelling. The role of pharmacologic prophylaxis in this patient population is postulated to avoid potential development of an UEDVT.

29. Chuter G, Weir D: Upper extremity deep vein thrombosis following a humeral fracture: A case report and literature review. *Injury Extra* 2005;36(7):249-252.

30. VTE Guidelines for Shoulder and Elbow Surgery. The Consensus Views of the British Elbow and Shoulder Society. Updated 2013. Available at: http://www.bess.org.uk/media/VTE_Guidelines_updated_Feb_2013.doc. *Accessed February 17, 2016.*

Venous thromboembolism guidelines from the British Elbow and Shoulder Society for shoulder and elbow surgery are summarized in this review article. Risk factors are reviewed and linked to prophylaxis recommendations for orthopaedic procedures involving the shoulder and elbow.

31. Hastie G, Pederson A, Redfern D: Venus thromboembolism incidence in upper limb orthopaedic surgery: Do these procedures increase venous thromboembolism risk? *J Shoulder Elbow Surg* 2014;23(10): 1481-1484.

This level IV case series examines the incidence of postoperative venous thromboembolism in upper extremity orthopaedic surgery. More than 3,300 events are reviewed, with a 0.0018% incidence of venous thromboembolism noted. The most common risk factor identified for the development of a venous thromboembolism event is a personal or family history of a VTE event.

32. Dattani R, Smith CD, Patel VR: The venous thromboembolic complications of shoulder and elbow surgery: A systematic review. *Bone Joint J* 2013;95-B(1):70-74.

This systematic review examined 14 level III and IV studies to determine the incidence and risk factors for venous thromboembolic events associated with surgery of the shoulder and elbow. The incidence of VTE was -0.38% from 92,440 arthroscopic shoulder procedures, -0.52% from 42,261 arthroplasty procedures, -0.64% from 4,833 procedures to treat proximal humerus fractures, and -0.26% from 2,701 elbow arthroplasty procedures. Risk factors associated with development of VTE included diabetes, rheumatoid arthritis, and ischemic heart disease.

33. Toro JB, Gardner MJ, Hierholzer C, et al: Long-term consequences of pelvic trauma patients with thromboembolic disease treated with inferior vena caval filters. *J Trauma* 2008;65(1):25-29.

34. Stannard JP, Singhania AK, Lopez-Ben RR, et al.: Deep-vein thrombosis in high-energy skeletal trauma despite thromboprophylaxis. *J Bone Joint Surg Br* 2005;87(7):965-968.

35. Slobogean GP, Lefaivre KA, Nicolaou S, O'Brien PJ: A systematic review of thromboprophylaxis for pelvic and acetabular fractures. *J Orthop Trauma* 2009;23(5):379-384.

36. Steele N, Dodenhoff R, Ward A, Morse MH: Thromboprophylaxis in pelvic and acetabular trauma surgery. The

1: General Topics

role of early treatment with low molecular weight heparin. *J Bone Joint Surg Br* 2005;87(2):209-212.

37. Marsland D, Mears SC, Kates SL: Venous thromboembolic prophylaxis for hip fractures. *Osteoporos Int* 2010;21(suppl 4):S593-604.

    This level III study reviews preventive treatment strategies for the development of venous thromboembolism events and itemizes their associated complications in patients treated with a hip fracture.

38. Geerts WH, Heit JA, Clagett GP, et al: Prevention of venous thromboembolism. *Chest* 2001;119(1suppl):132S-175S.

39. Prensky C, Urruela A, Guss MS, Karia R, Lenzo TJ, Egol KA: Symptomatic venous thrombo-embolism in low-energy isolated fractures in hospitalised patients. *Injury* 2013;44(8):1135-1139.

    This retrospective study aimed to determine the incidence and risk factors associated with VTE events in a patient population sustaining low-energy fractures. A total of 1,701 patients were evaluated, with 479 upper extremity fractures and 1,222 lower extremity fractures included in their analysis. The incidence of clinically significant venous thromboembolism events was 1.4%, with 13 DVTs and 12 PEs recorded. Seventy-four percent of the patients reviewed received chemoprophylaxis. Female sex and elevated body mass index were found to be predictors of VTE events.

40. Sems SA, Levy BA, Dajani K, Herrera DA, Templeman DC: Incidence of deep venous thrombosis after temporary joint spanning external fixation for complex lower extremity injuries. *J Trauma* 2009;66(4):1164-1166.

41. Forsythe RM, Peitzman AB, DeCato T, et al: Early lower extremity fracture fixation and the risk of early pulmonary embolus: Filter before fixation? *J Trauma* 2011;70(6):1381-1388.

    The Pennsylvania state trauma registry was used to perform a retrospective analysis to determine patients at highest risk for the development of a PE following trauma. Patients with early and delayed presentation of a PE, defined within the first 72 hours of admission or after, were compared using logistic regression analysis to determine risk factors. The only risk factor for development of an early PE was early fixation within the first 48 hours for pelvic ring and lower extremity injuries. In this group of patients, the risk was threefold higher, reinforcing the need for early admission preventive anticoagulation strategies.

42. Long A, Zhang L, Zhang Y, et al: Efficacy and safety of rivaroxaban versus low-molecular-weight heparin therapy in patients with lower limb fractures. *J Thromb Thrombolysis* 2014;38(3):299-305.

    In a retrospective cohort study, 2,050 patients were evaluated and the rates of VTE, bleeding and surgical complications, and length of hospital stay were compared in two patient populations. The study included 608 patients who received rivaroxaban compared to 717 patients who received a low-molecular-weight heparin (LMWH). The rate of symptomatic VTE events was 4.9% in the rivaroxaban group, and 8.6% in the group who received LMWH. Although not statistically significant, the incidence of major bleeding events was lower in the rivaroxaban group (0.2 versus 0.6%). The length of hospital stay was found to be shorter in the rivaroxaban group (12.2 versus 13.1 days). Results favored rivaroxaban compared to LMWHs; however, prospective randomized trials were recommended to substantiate these findings.

43. Kadous A, Abdelgawad AA, Kanlic E: Deep venous thrombosis and pulmonary embolism after surgical treatment of ankle fractures: A case report and review of literature. *J Foot Ankle Surg* 2012;51(4):457-463.

    In this case report, a 66-year-old woman who did not receive pharmacologic thromboprophylaxis presents to the emergency department 17 days after sustaining a trimalleolar ankle fracture-dislocation with a massive PE. The article reviews the literature regarding the development of DVT and PE associated with ankle fractures.

44. American Orthopaedic Foot and Ankle Society: Position Statement: The Use of VTED Prophylaxis in Foot and Ankle Surgery. Available at: http://www.aofas.org/medical-community/health-policy/Documents/VTED-Position-Statement-approv-7-9-13-FINAL.pdf. Accessed February 17, 2016.]

    The American Orthopaedic Foot and Ankle Society position statement concludes that there are insufficient data to recommend for or against VTE prophylaxis for patients after foot and ankle surgery.

Section 2

Nonunions, Malunions, and Infections

Section Editor

Mark R. Brinker, MD

Chapter 10

Nonunions

Jeffrey Brewer, MD   Daniel P. O'Connor, PhD   Mark R. Brinker, MD

Abstract

Nonunion represents a challenging orthopaedic problem because of variable etiology and a multitude of treatment options. An understanding of the basic treatment principles can optimize patient outcomes. Over the past 5 years, various treatment modalities have been described that incorporate plating, nailing, arthroplasty, Masquelet technique, and external fixation (including the Ilizarov method).

Keywords: infected nonunion; hypertrophic nonunion; oligotrophic nonunion; atrophic nonunion; surface characteristics

Introduction

Although most fractures heal, a nonunited fracture can have devastating functional, psychologic, and financial implications. The patient with a bony nonunion often endures months or years of burden related to his or her condition. The effect on health-related quality of life has been reported for tibial nonunion to show mental and physical effects worse than congestive heart failure, type II diabetes mellitus, and myocardial infarction.[1] Patients and physicians both must understand the physical and psychologic stresses associated with this condition.

Each nonunion has unique problems and treatment challenges. Nonunion can have many aspects that must be considered, including the mechanical environment, infection, metabolic abnormalities, soft-tissue compromise, patient compliance, and patient expectations. A well-coordinated treatment regimen that includes multispecialty involvement must be incorporated.

The evaluation of a case of nonunion requires a thorough understanding of the principles of acute fracture management, bone biology, and fracture healing. Before a surgeon can treat nonunion, a diagnosis must be made, which is not always straightforward because of the complex nature of bone healing.

Definition

Nonunion is not clearly defined in the literature. Although many definitions rely on a time after injury, a more pragmatic definition is when the treating surgeon determines that a fracture has no possibility of healing without further intervention.[2] Objective indications of nonunion include failure to improve clinically such as continued severe pain and inability to bear weight, and lack of radiographic evidence of progression of fracture healing such as absence of bridging bone on plain radiographs or CT scans over 2 or more consecutive months following fracture, at which time some bridging would be expected. A fracture with signs of progression toward healing that are taking longer than usual can be identified as a delayed union, which may or may not require new surgical or medical intervention. Identifying when a fracture needs further intervention is one of the most difficult aspects of nonunion treatment. The point at which the healing process has appeared to stop indicates nonunion that will require further intervention to attain healing.

Etiology

Factors associated with development of nonunion include mechanical instability, inadequate bone contact, infection, and insufficient vascularity. Any single factor or a combination can result in failure of a fracture to heal. Multiple other contributing factors can create an environment that predisposes a fracture to nonunion (**Table 1**).

Neither of the following authors nor any immediate family member has received anything of value from or has stock or stock options held in a commercial company or institution related directly or indirectly to the subject of this chapter: Dr. Brewer and Dr. Brinker. Dr. O'Connor or an immediate family member serves as a paid consultant to Nimbic Systems.

Table 1

Factors That Predispose a Fracture to Nonunion

Predisposing Factors	Possible Causes
Mechanical instability	Inadequate fixation Poor bone quality Bone loss Distraction
Insufficient vascularity	Soft-tissue stripping Vascular injury Vascular disease
Poor bone contact	Distraction Malalignment Bone loss Soft-tissue interposition
Contributing Factors	
Infection	
Nicotine	
Certain medications	
Metabolic bone disease	
Malnutrition	
Vitamin deficiencies	
Medical comorbidities	
Obesity	
Venous stasis	
Burns	
Irradiation	
Alcohol abuse	
Poor functional status	

Evaluation

History

The initial evaluation of a patient with fracture nonunion should include a thorough history. Potential causes of nonunion should be investigated by examining health and nutritional status, medical comorbidities, medications, drug and alcohol use, injury mechanism and characteristics, prior treatments, and history of infection. Associated injuries and functional limitations must be identified to educate the patient regarding functional expectations. All contributing factors should be considered.

Physical Examination

Physical examination starts with the inspection of soft tissues to evaluate the zone of injury, signs of infection, or draining sinus tracts. The location and type of any soft-tissue transfer should be noted. Motion and pain at the nonunion site should be assessed as well as adjacent joint range of motion. Compensatory fixed deformities at adjacent joints must be identified and corrected for optimal return of function. If the treatment plan includes bone grafting, the donor site is evaluated for prior surgical procedures or injury that could preclude graft procurement. Vascular examination is essential to evaluate for vascular insufficiency, which can contribute to nonunion. Neurologic assessment for motor and sensory dysfunction helps identify preoperative deficits.

Radiographic Evaluation

Radiographic evaluation begins with plain radiographs. Initial injury films are necessary to assess the severity of the injury and to account for bone fragments that may have been removed during treatment. Subsequent images show interval treatments and the progression toward the current nonunion. Hardware should be evaluated for loosening, breakage, and positioning to determine the mechanical environment of the nonunion. Additional features examined radiographically include bone quality, deformity, surface characteristics, and healing effort.

CT is a powerful tool in the assessment of nonunion because sclerotic bone and surrounding hardware often obscure the fracture site on plain radiographs. The cross-sectional area with bridging bone can be estimated to determine healing at a nonunion site. Nonunion that has healed typically demonstrates at least 25% cross-sectional area with bridging bone.

Laboratory Evaluation

Laboratory workup includes markers to identify metabolic and infectious causes of nonunion. Metabolic workup includes levels for nutrition laboratory tests (albumin, prealbumin, absolute lymphocyte count), calcium, vitamin D, parathyroid hormone, thyroid-stimulating hormone, and testosterone. Infectious workup includes white blood cell count, erythrocyte sedimentation rate, and C-reactive protein. In addition, an aspiration or biopsy specimen can be obtained from the nonunion site for cultures and histologic evaluation.

Nonunion Types

Viable

Hypertrophic Nonunion

Hypertrophic nonunion results from inadequate mechanical stability and exhibits surrounding callus formation. Progressive resorption occurs at the fracture site as interposing fibrocartilage develops with failure to mineralize. These cases of nonunion can be categorized as elephant foot type, with extensive callus formation, or horse hoof type, with a lesser degree of callus formation. The primary goal of treatment is to provide an improved mechanical environment with increased stability. Treatment of hypertrophic nonunion does not routinely require opening the fracture site or bone grafting.

Oligotrophic Nonunion

Oligotrophic nonunion develops as the result of poor bone contact in the presence of appropriate vascularity. Radiographically, little or no callus formation is demonstrated. Reapproximation of the bone ends and improved stability is needed to achieve union. Bone grafting can be used in cases with opposing bone fragment surfaces that are irregular and do not permit large surface-to-surface contact area, large missing bone fragments or segmental defects, or questionable biologic activity.

Nonviable

Atrophic Nonunion

Nonviable nonunion includes atrophic nonunion that displays no callus formation with resorption and osteopenia at the fracture site. Some cases of avascular nonunion will have substantial sclerosis of the bone ends surrounding the nonunion, which lack the vascularity and biologic activity necessary to stimulate osteogenesis. Principles of treatment include improvement of the biologic environment and improved mechanical stability.

Infected Nonunion

Infected nonunion presents the challenges of eradicating the infection and healing the nonunion. The primary goal is to achieve union followed by elimination of the infection. However, eradication or suppression of the infection may be necessary for healing to occur. Treatment of infected nonunion depends on the character of the infection. Infections can present as draining, active nondraining, or quiescent.

Synovial Pseudarthrosis

Synovial pseudarthrosis is a unique type of nonunion with a sealed medullary canal and synovial pseudocapsule. Standard treatment consists of débridement of interposing fibrous tissue and pseudocapsule and opening the medullary canal. Biologic stimulation and increased stability are then often used to achieve union.

Surface Characteristics

Understanding the surface characteristics of nonunion is important for understanding its healing potential as well as possible treatment strategies. Surface characteristics include axial stability, the surface area of bone fragments, degree of bony contact, and fracture line orientation (**Figure 1**). Cases of nonunion with larger areas of bone contact and axial stability tend to have improved healing potential. Improving the surface characteristics during surgery for nonunion is one method to increase the potential to achieve union.

Treatment

Goals

The objective of treatment is to heal the nonunited fracture and regain function of the extremity. Treatment is designed with an understanding of both physical and psychologic components of the condition. Host factors and healing potential must be considered because the patient whose fracture has not healed is at risk of a complicated or prolonged course to union. The patient must understand the duration of treatment and alternatives, which can include amputation.

A multidisciplinary approach to nonunion treatment is beneficial in many cases because the etiology is often multifactorial and treatment necessitates additional expertise. Patients often have multiple comorbidities requiring medical management to optimize healing potential. An endocrinologist can help diagnose and correct metabolic abnormalities that can impede fracture healing. In a study of 37 patients with nonunion, 31 were found to have a metabolic or endocrine abnormality:[3] 8 patients were treated nonsurgically with endocrine/metabolic correction, all of whom achieved healing. The assistance of a plastic surgeon can help manage a compromised soft-tissue envelope or closure of wounds after débridement. In the case of infected nonunion, an infectious disease specialist is essential for antibiotic management.

After diagnosis of nonunion, understanding the etiology is the first step in creating a treatment regimen. Infected, hypertrophic, oligotrophic, atrophic nonunion, and nonunion associated with segmental defects all require different specific treatment approaches. However, fortification of the mechanical environment is a treatment concept shared by all nonunion types.

Treatment Methods

External Fixation

External fixation is a powerful tool for the treatment of nonunion. However, its use must be predicated on the principles of nonunion treatment and designed to provide adequate mechanical stability. It is especially useful in cases of infected nonunion and segmental bone loss (**Figure 2**). An ideal environment is provided for eradication of infection because bony stabilization can be achieved without internal fixation hardware. In addition, a dynamic system can be incorporated to provide compression, deformity correction, and/or distraction osteogenesis for segmental bone defects. The Ilizarov external fixator has

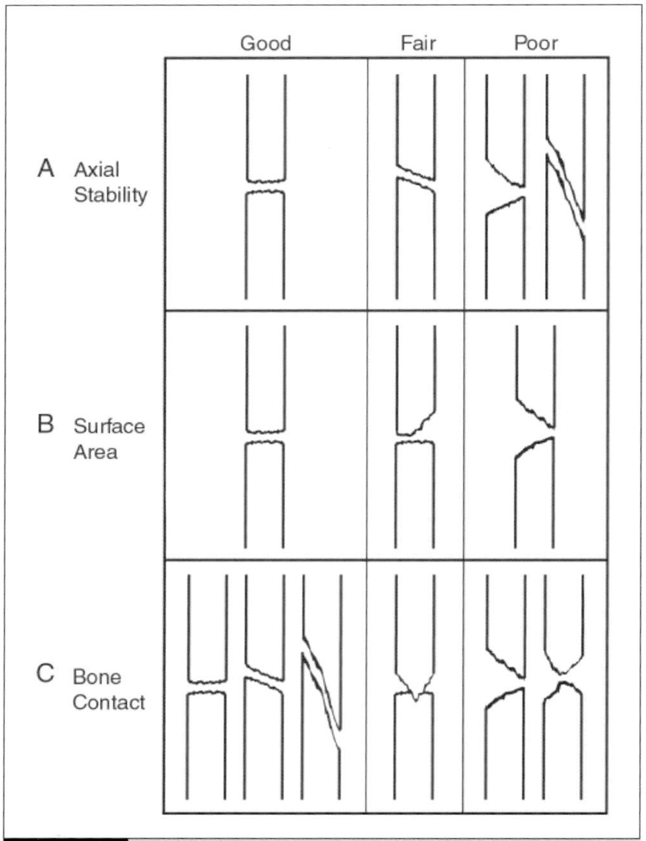

Figure 1 Illustration depicts nonunion surface characteristics. **A**, Axial stability **B**, Surface area. **C**, Bone contact.

the advantages of thin-wire fixation, increased stability, and capability of multidimensional deformity correction. The disadvantages of external fixation include pin tract infections, potential long duration of treatment, and possible difficulty ascertaining healing status because of hardware obscuring the nonunion site or artifact on radiographic images.

Monolateral External Fixation

The use of monolateral external fixators has recently been described for the treatment of infected nonunion with bone defects after débridement. In a retrospective study of 21 patients with infected nonunion of the forearm, treatment consisted of débridement and bone transport via a monolateral external fixator.[4] Draining sinus was present in 19 patients and average bone defect size was 3.1 cm (range, 1.8 to 4.6 cm). Débridement and hardware removal were performed, followed by corticotomy for bone transport remote from the infected nonunion site. Intravenous antibiotics were administered for 6 weeks postoperatively followed by oral antibiotics until the end of treatment. All patients in this group obtained union and resolution of infection despite recurrence of infection in three patients. Bone grafting was required at the docking site or regenerate site in almost 30% of cases. The most common complication was pin tract infection, which occurred in more than one-half of patients. Another report described the use of a monolateral external fixator with distraction osteogenesis for infected femoral nonunion in 13 patients.[5] A similar treatment regimen was used with débridement, remote corticotomy, and intravenous antibiotics. Bone defect size was an average 7.9 cm (range, 5.5 to 17.0 cm). Union and eradication of infection was achieved in all patients. However, five patients required additional procedures because of delayed union or soft-tissue interposition.

Ilizarov Method

The Ilizarov frame has proved useful in treatment of all types of long bone nonunion at various locations and in those with segmental defects. The versatility of thin-wire fixation facilitates short segment fixation, stability in osteoporotic bone, and soft-tissue preservation. The dynamic capability of these frames allows compression, lengthening, dynamization, and deformity correction without additional surgical procedures.

Multiple studies have reported on the use of Ilizarov external fixation for the treatment of infected nonunion with 95% to 100% union rates.[6-13] In this setting, the Ilizarov frame is useful for performing bone transport after débridement of infected bone results in a subsequent bone defect. A retrospective study evaluated 120 cases of infected tibial nonunion treated with an Ilizarov frame.[10] Corticotomy was performed in metaphyseal bone at the time of débridement. Subsequent bone loss was an average of 9.5 cm (range, 6 to 18 cm) which was restored with bone transport. All patients, except one who died as a result of pulmonary embolism, healed with only one patient experiencing a recurrent infection. Fourteen patients required bone grafting, 25 patients had pin tract infections, and 34 patients had broken wires.

The Ilizarov external fixator also has use in soft-tissue management associated with infected nonunion after débridement. In cases of infected nonunion with soft-tissue deficits, acute shortening or bone transport can be performed for skin closure and compression at the resected bone ends.[8,10] This allows soft-tissue coverage with correction of the limb-length discrepancy in a controlled manner.

Recent reports have shown successful outcomes for treatment of aseptic and infected femoral nonunions using Ilizarov external fixation. Treatment of aseptic femoral nonunion after intramedullary nailing in eight patients

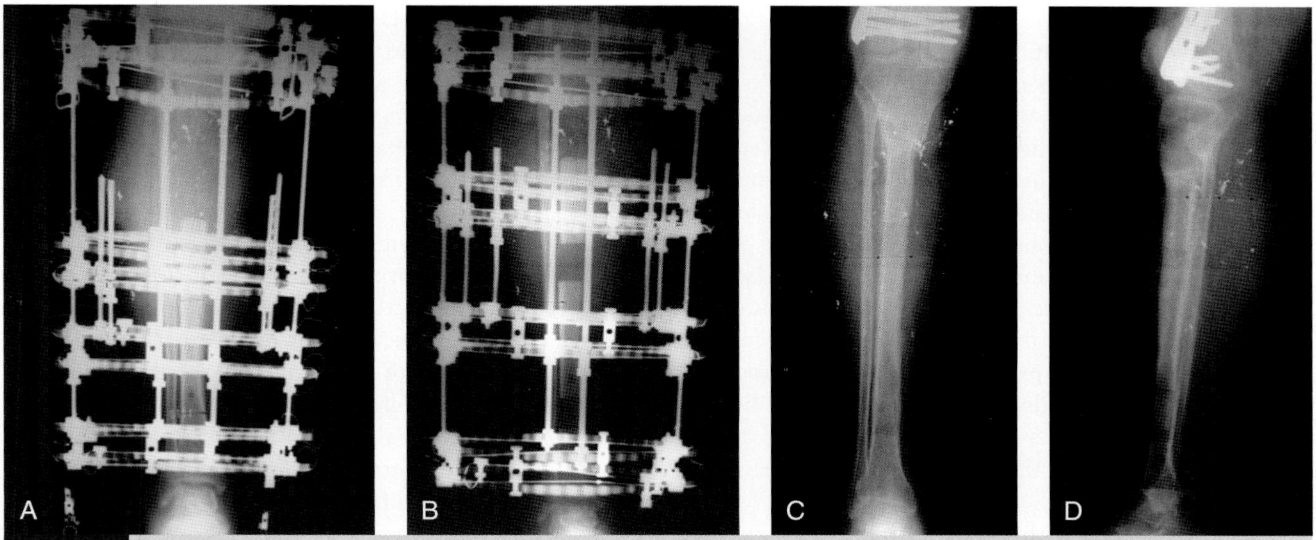

Figure 2 Radiographs demonstrate an open tibia fracture nonunion with segmental defect treated using Ilizarov external fixation and bifocal bone transport. **A**, AP view obtained prior to bone transport. **B**, AP view obtained during transport. AP (**C**) and lateral (**D**) views obtained after consolidation.

consisted of nail removal, Ilizarov external fixation, and conversion to a monolateral frame after cortical bridging was noted at the nonunion site.[14] In three patients, a metaphyseal corticotomy was performed to correct limb-length discrepancy. All eight patients experienced healing at an average of 32 weeks. In a retrospective review, Ilizarov external fixation was used in a staged fashion to treat 50 patients with infected femoral nonunion.[6] The staged protocol consisted of hardware removal, débridement of necrotic bone and tissue, and 10 days of culture-specific antibiotics during stage one. Bone defects following débridement ranged from 2.5 to 17.0 cm. The second stage was application of the Ilizarov frame with percutaneous corticotomy for bifocal bone transport. The average time in an external fixator was 24.5 months (range, 2 to 39 months), with union achieved in 49 of the 50 patients. Complications included pin tract infections in all patients, decreased knee range of motion, iatrogenic injury to the profunda femoris artery resulting in sepsis and hip disarticulation in one patient, and residual limb-length discrepancy greater than 1.1 cm in 32 patients.

The capability to alter treatment with the Ilizarov frame was shown in a prospective study that evaluated the treatment of supracondylar humerus nonunion in eight patients. Treatment included implant removal, nonunion débridement, ulnar nerve neurolysis, elbow contracture release, and Ilizarov external fixation with compression at the nonunion site. Two patients had no signs of radiographic healing identified at 6 weeks. This resulted in a change from compression to alternating compression-distraction at the nonunion site, which ultimately resulted in union. All patients achieved union at a mean of 7 months, with improvement in functional scores.[11]

Plating

Plate fixation for nonunion has been used with various techniques to improve stability at the nonunion site including compression, bridge, locking, dual, wave, and augmentative plating. Direct exposure of the nonunion site in plating procedures allows the surgeon to débride the nonunion site when necessary, as with infected nonunion, atrophic nonunion, and select oligotrophic nonunion. In addition, direct exposure allows surgical shaping of the bone ends to improve the surface characteristics for obtaining a high surface area of bone-to-bone contact (for example, flattening to produce parallel surfaces). In cases of hypertrophic nonunion, a contoured plate allows rigid fixation without requiring débridement of the highly vascular, biologically active callus. Advantages include rigid fixation and versatility regarding anatomic location. Disadvantages that can limit plate use include wide surgical dissection, limited weight bearing postoperatively, and the static nature of fixation.

Compression plating has the advantages of providing contact between bone ends and improved stability at the nonunion by means of compression. Techniques to achieve compression include lag screw fixation, eccentric screw placement for compression through the plate, and use of an articulated tensioning device. In addition, shaping the bone ends to improve the contact surface area facilitates improved compression across the nonunion site and increased bony contact.

Successful use of compression plating in upper extremity nonunion has been demonstrated in multiple studies, with union rates of 95% to 100%.[15-25] The need for bone graft is determined by the type of nonunion present and the need for biologic stimulation. In cases of nonviable nonunion with bone loss, the use of cortical iliac crest autograft can be used to maintain length by using plating techniques.[20-22] An intramedullary or extramedullary fibular strut allograft can be used to improve screw purchase for nonunion in osteoporotic bone. An alternative method is bone shortening to improve surface characteristics and provide viable bone ends. Shortening can then be corrected with subsequent procedures or the bone can be left short, depending on the patient's functional demands and preferences.

In cases of nonunion after intramedullary nail fixation, augmentative plating with the nail in situ has been shown to be an excellent treatment option.[15,18,22,26-28] Benefits of this method include the mechanical advantage provided by the nail with increased rigidity resulting from the addition of a supplementary plate. The plate can be applied to a statically locked nail for increased rigidity or the nail can be dynamized using a compression plating technique. The open plating procedure also gives the surgeon the option to débride the nonunion site and apply bone graft.

Augmentative plating for long bone nonunion is particularly advantageous in metaphyseal or metadiaphyseal locations where a mismatch exists between the nail diameter and the medullary canal diameter. This was demonstrated in a retrospective study that compared augmentative plating with exchange nailing of nonisthmic femoral nonunion.[28] Of 11 patients who underwent augmentative plating and autogenous iliac crest bone grafting with the nail in situ, all achieved union. However, of seven patients with nonisthmic femoral nonunion who underwent exchange nailing, with an increase in nail diameter of at least 1 mm, only two cases of nonunions healed.

Nailing

Treatment of long bone nonunion with intramedullary nailing is optimal in many situations because of its mechanical strength and load-sharing capabilities. This property is especially important in lower extremity nonunion. However, using an intramedullary device in the case of an infected nonunion may not be ideal because of the potential for intramedullary sepsis. An exception is made in the case of exchange nailing of an infected nonunion in which the medullary canal likely has already been seeded. In such cases, the surgeon can consider using a planned series of surgical procedures. The first stage is implanting an antibiotic-impregnated polymethyl methacrylate (PMMA) nail to provide antimicrobial therapy and temporary internal splinting. In the second stage, the antibiotic nail is replaced with a permanent interlocking nail.

Exchange nailing has been shown to be a successful technique for lower extremity long bone nonunion.[29-31] In two separate studies that evaluated exchange nailing for 50 cases of aseptic femoral nonunion[30] and 46 cases of aseptic tibial nonunion,[31] union rates of 100% and 98% were obtained, respectively. The authors of both studies stressed the importance of appropriate patient selection to achieve success with this technique. Exchange nailing was not used when defects were larger than 50% of the cross-sectional cortical contact surface area. Technical details included increased nail diameter of at least 2 mm, use of a nail from a different manufacturer for different interlocking trajectory, and medullary reaming to increase the cortical nail contact area and stimulate the biologic environment. Reamed tissue can also be sent for cultures to rule out infection. Additionally, in cases of mismatch between the nail diameter and the diameter of the medullary canal at the nonunion site, as well as metaphyseal and metadiaphyseal nonunion, a custom nail with increased interlocking options near the nonunion site and the use of blocking screws should be considered.

The location of a femoral nonunion has been identified as a potential factor related to success of exchange nailing. In a study comparing exchange nailing for cases of isthmic and nonisthmic femoral nonunion, the isthmic group (31 cases) had an 87% union rate and the nonisthmic group (10 cases) had a 50% union rate.[32] In a separate study comparing exchange nailing with augmentative plating for nonisthmic femoral nonunion, only five of seven patients in the exchange nailing group achieved union.[28] However, mismatch between nail diameter and medullary canal diameter at the nonunion site can be overcome with increasing interlocking options.

Various techniques of compression nailing have also been described for the treatment of nonunion. In a study of 12 humeral nonunions treated with compression nailing, a 100% union rate was reported.[33] The procedure was performed closed, without bone grafting. Compression was obtained by placement of the distal interlocking screws followed by backslapping the nail. Additional compression was obtained by means of a compression screw after placement of the proximal interlocking screws. Another study evaluated nailing for humeral nonunion with compression obtained by interfragmentary tension band wiring at the nonunion site:[34] 28 patients underwent anterior iliac crest autograft and 36 patients underwent cancellous allograft at the nonunion site. The overall union rate with this technique was 97%; one patient from each bone grafting group did not achieve union.

Arthroplasty

Although preservation of bone stock is ideal in most situations, bypassing the bone-to-bone healing process can be advantageous in some cases. Arthroplasty is useful in cases of short-segment periarticular nonunion with osteopenic bone, nonunion associated with posttraumatic arthritis, and older patients who cannot tolerate a prolonged reconstruction process. The results of joint arthroplasty for treatment of nonunion has good outcomes but relatively high complication rates.

Three studies have reported on the use of reverse total shoulder arthroplasty for the treatment of proximal humerus nonunions.[35-37] The average age of patients in these studies ranged from 68 to 79 years. Aseptic nonunion of the proximal humerus after both surgical and nonsurgical treatment was included. Each study reported improvement in functional outcomes after arthroplasty; however, relatively high complication rates were reported (range, 20% to 41%). These complications included axillary nerve injury, infection, and dislocation.

A megaprosthesis used with aseptic distal femoral nonunion in eight patients had good results reported.[38] Patient age ranged from 68 to 85 years and all had severe knee arthritis and disuse osteoporosis. Aspiration was performed to rule out infection. Resection proximal to the nonunion site was followed by cemented femoral and tibial intramedullary component placement. No major postoperative complications were reported except for one patient who sustained a periprosthetic fracture, which was successfully treated with open reduction and internal fixation. All patients reported improved postoperative functional scores.

Induced Membrane Technique/Masquelet Technique

The induced membrane technique to treat nonunion with associated segmental defects has demonstrated union rates of 90%.[39-41] The two-stage technique uses a foreign body reaction induced by surgically placing a PMMA spacer in the bone defect. After 4 to 8 weeks, the cement spacer is removed, revealing a chamber for bone grafting including a membrane that provides vascularity and growth factors.

A retrospective study of 84 posttraumatic bone defects in various anatomic locations including the tibia ($n = 61$), femur ($n = 13$), humerus ($n = 6$), and forearm ($n = 4$) were treated with an induced membrane technique.[40] The initial injury was an open fracture in 89%; 41 patients were infected at the beginning of treatment of the bone defect. More than one-half of defects were larger than 5 cm; the largest defect measured 23 cm in the tibia. Various forms of stabilization were used including external fixation, rigid and flexible intramedullary nail, and plate fixation. Autologous bone graft was used alone or variably combined with bone substitutes and growth factors. After an average of six procedures, union occurred in 90% of cases at a mean of 14 months following the initial procedure. Failure occurred only in tibial bone defects. In a retrospective review of 27 cases of segmental bone loss nonunion involving the tibia ($n = 19$) and femur ($n = 8$), the Masquelet technique was used with bone graft from the reamer-irrigator-aspirator (RIA).[41] Of 27 cases of nonunion, open fractures were present in 15 and infection was present in 7. After thorough débridement, an antibiotic cement spacer was placed in the bone defect, which ranged from 1 to 25 cm. The spacer was removed at 6 to 8 weeks, carefully preserving the membrane induced by the foreign body reaction to the spacer, and bone grafting from the femur with the RIA, which was supplemented with iliac crest bone graft and/or BMP in some cases. An average of three surgeries was performed before the bone grafting procedure. Definitive fixation consisted of plate, nail, or a combined plate-and-nail construct. At 1 year, 90% of segmental defect nonunions were healed.

Other Treatment Methods

Bone Marrow Aspirate

Percutaneous injection of bone marrow aspirate is a minimally invasive technique that may have use in a subset of cases of nonunion with adequate stability and bone contact. In a study of 11 cases of distal tibia aseptic nonunion, this technique resulted in an 82% union rate.[42] Bone marrow was harvested from the posterior iliac crest (range, 40 to 80 mL). Under fluoroscopic guidance the aspirate was injected using an 18-gauge needle after using the needle to create microtrauma at the nonunion site. Union occurred in nine patients at an average of 4 months after the injection procedure.

Treatment of Infected Nonunion

Many regimens exist for the treatment of infected nonunion; however, basic principles can be applied depending on the type of infection present. Draining and active nondraining infected nonunions are treated in a similar manner with serial débridements, organism-specific antibiotics, and reconstruction. Cultures should be obtained during the initial débridement after withholding antibiotics for 2 weeks. In addition, if a sinus tract is present, a biopsy must be obtained to evaluate for carcinoma. Débridement is performed with excision of all necrotic tissue, including necrotic bone, and removal of orthopaedic hardware and foreign material. Following débridement, the resulting dead space can initially be managed using antibiotic-impregnated PMMA with definitive coverage, often requiring various forms of vascularized flap coverage. Cases of nonunion with associated intramedullary sepsis can be treated with serial débridement with antibiotic cement nail exchanges before definitive treatment. Bone loss secondary to débridement is managed with limb shortening or various reconstructive options including the Masquelet technique or distraction osteogenesis. Quiescent infected nonunion presents in patients with a history of infection but without signs of infection for at least 3 months or with a positive nuclear medicine scan without history of infection. These cases of nonunion can be treated similarly to atrophic nonunion without serial débridements. Bone grafting and internal or external fixation can be performed during the initial surgical procedure.

A history of open fracture or prior surgical treatment can also raise the index of suspicion for possible quiescent infection, irrespective of prior history of diagnosed infection or current signs of infection. For patients who have these risk factors, cultures obtained from the nonunion site during surgical fixation of the nonunion can be used to identify the presence of bacteria or other microbes. In the event that cultures have positive results, culture-specific antibiotics can be administered under the direction of an infectious disease specialist.

Summary

Nonunion treatment requires a thorough understanding of the etiology of a nonunion as well as the various treatment options. Each case is unique and has its own challenges because of the variability in nonunion type, injury characteristics, prior treatments, patient comorbidities, and treatment options. Successful management requires the treating surgeon to develop a systematic approach and maintain composure to achieve the ultimate goal of functional restoration.

Key Study Points

- Stable fixation with optimization of nonunion surface characteristics, mechanical stability, and the biologic environment is key to the treatment of nonunion.
- A systematic approach to the treatment of nonunion with a multidisciplinary team is often necessary for successful outcomes in cases of complex nonunion.

Annotated References

1. Brinker MR, Hanus BD, Sen M, O'Connor DP: The devastating effects of tibial nonunion on health-related quality of life. *J Bone Joint Surg Am* 2013;95(24):2170-2176.

   In this study, 237 patients with tibial nonunion were evaluated using Short Form-12 Physical and Mental Component scores. The effect of tibial shaft nonunion was worse than many chronic medical conditions including type II diabetes mellitus, myocardial infarction, and congestive heart failure. Level of evidence: III.

2. Brinker MR, O'Connor DP: Nonunions: evaluation and treatment, in Browner BD, Jupiter JB, Levine AM, Trafton PG, eds: *Skeletal trauma: basic science, management, and reconstruction* ,ed 4. Philadelphia, W.B. Saunders, 2009, pp 615-708.

3. Brinker MR, O'Connor DP, Monla YT, Earthman TP: Metabolic and endocrine abnormalities in patients with nonunions. *J Orthop Trauma* 2007;21(8):557-570.

4. Liu T, Liu Z, Ling L, Zhang X: Infected forearm nonunion treated by bone transport after debridement. *BMC Musculoskelet Disord* 2013;14:273.

   In this retrospective review, 21 patients with infected forearm nonunion with a mean bone defect of 3.1 cm were treated with implant removal, débridement, and monolateral external fixation followed by bone transport through a remote corticotomy. All cases of nonunion healed without infection recurrence.

5. Arora S, Batra S, Gupta V, Goyal A: Distraction osteogenesis using a monolateral external fixator for infected non-union of the femur with bone loss. *J Orthop Surg (Hong Kong)* 2012;20(2):185-190.

   In this study, 13 cases of infected femoral nonunion had a mean bone defect of 7.9 cm. Treatment consisted of débridement, monolateral external fixation, and bone transport after corticotomy. Union was achieved in all patients with eradication of infection.

6. Blum AL, BongioVanni JC, Morgan SJ, Flierl MA, dos Reis FB: Complications associated with distraction osteogenesis for infected nonunion of the femoral shaft in the presence of a bone defect: A retrospective series. *J Bone Joint Surg Br* 2010;92(4):565-570.

   In this retrospective review, 50 cases of infected femoral shaft nonunion with bone defect were treated with débridement, Ilizarov external fixation, and distraction osteogenesis through a remote corticotomy. Healing occurred in 49 of 50 patients with additional bone grafting required in 15.

7. Bumbasirević M, Tomić S, Lesić A, Milosević I, Atkinson HD: War-related infected tibial nonunion with bone and soft-tissue loss treated with bone transport using the Ilizarov method. *Arch Orthop Trauma Surg* 2010;130(6):739-749.

In this retrospective review, 30 war-injured patients with infected tibial nonunion and an average bone loss of 6.9 cm were treated by using débridement, corticotomy, and Ilizarov bifocal bone transport. A union rate 97% was reported, with no refracture or recurrence of infection at 99-month follow-up.

8. Feng ZH, Yuan Z, Jun LZ, Tao Z, Fa ZY, Long MX: Ilizarov method with bone segment extension for treating large defects of the tibia caused by infected nonunion. *Saudi Med J* 2013;34(3):316-318.

   In this retrospective review, 21 cases of infected tibial nonuion were treated using Ilizarov bone transport. The average bone defect following débridement was 6.6 cm. Union was achieved in all patients at a mean of 7.8 months.

9. Megas P, Saridis A, Kouzelis A, Kallivokas A, Mylonas S, Tyllianakis M: The treatment of infected nonunion of the tibia following intramedullary nailing by the Ilizarov method. *Injury* 2010;41(3):294-299.

   In this retrospective review, nine cases of infected tibial nonunion with an average segmental bone defect of 5 cm were treated by nail removal followed by corticotomy and Ilizarov bone transport in six cases and monofocal distraction-compression in three cases. All patients achieved union without recurrence of infection.

10. Mora R, Maccabruni A, Bertani B, Tuvo G, Lucanto S, Pedrotti L: Revision of 120 tibial infected non-unions with bone and soft tissue loss treated with epidermato-fascial osteoplasty according to Umiarov. *Injury* 2014;45(2):383-387.

    In this retrospective review, 120 cases of infected tibial nonunion with bone and soft-tissue defects were treated with Ilizarov frame application followed by bone transport and gradual wound closure during transport. Union occurred in all but one patient who died before completion of treatment.

11. Safoury YA, Atteya MR: Treatment of post-infection nonunion of the supracondylar humerus with Ilizarov external fixator. *J Shoulder Elbow Surg* 2011;20(6):873-879.

    In this prospective study, eight cases of infected supracondylar humerus nonunion were treated with débridement, ulnar nerve neurolysis, contracture release, and Ilizarov external fixation with compression at the nonunion site. Union was achieved in all patients without recurrence of infection. Level of evidence: Therapeutic Study Level IV

12. Wu CC: Single-stage surgical treatment of infected nonunion of the distal tibia. *J Orthop Trauma* 2011;25(3):156-161.

    In this retrospective review, cases of infected distal tibial nonunion were treated with Ilizarov external fixation after débridement, implant removal, tibial canal reaming, and bone grafting. Union was achieved in all cases with resolution of infection

13. Xu K, Fu X, Li YM, Wang CG, Li ZJ: A treatment for large defects of the tibia caused by infected nonunion: Ilizarov method with bone segment extension. *Ir J Med Sci* 2014;183(3):423-428.

    In this report, 30 cases of infected tibial nonunion with bone defect were treated with débridement and Ilizarov bone transport. All patients achieved union at a mean of 8.8 months.

14. Lammens J, Vanlauwe J: Ilizarov treatment for aseptic delayed union or non-union after reamed intramedullary nailing of the femur. *Acta Orthop Belg* 2010;76(1):63-68.

    In this retrospective series, eight patients were treated with Ilizarov external fixation for femoral nonunion after intramedullary nailing. Three patients required bone transport. Union was achieved in all patients without recurrence of infection.

15. Ateschrang A, Albrecht D, Stöckle U, Weise K, Stuby F, Zieker D: High success rate for augmentation compression plating leaving the nail in situ for aseptic diaphyseal tibial nonunions. *J Orthop Trauma* 2013;27(3):145-149.

    In this study, 28 patients with tibial nonunion after intramedullary nailing were treated with augmented compression plating. Union was obtained in 27 patients within 5 months. Plate removal was required in almost 80% of patients because of pain. Level of evidence: IV.

16. Baker JF, Mullett H: Clavicle non-union: Autologous bone graft is not a necessary augment to internal fixation. *Acta Orthop Belg* 2010;76(6):725-729.

    In this report, 15 cases of clavicle nonunion were treated with plate fixation without bone grafting. Union was obtained in all 15 cases.

17. Bernard de Dompsure R, Peter R, Hoffmeyer P: Uninfected nonunion of the humeral diaphyses: Review of 21 patients treated with shingling, compression plate, and autologous bone graft. *Orthop Traumatol Surg Res* 2010;96(2):139-146.

    In this retrospective review, 21 patients with humeral nonunion were treated with compression plating and autologous bone graft. Union was achieved in 95% of cases at a mean of 4.5 months. Level of evidence: IV.

18. Hakeos WM, Richards JE, Obremskey WT: Plate fixation of femoral nonunions over an intramedullary nail with autogenous bone grafting. *J Orthop Trauma* 2011;25(2):84-89.

    In this study, seven patients were treated with augmentative compression plating and autogenous bone graft for femoral nonunion after intramedullary nailing. All patients achieved union within 5 months.

19. Kloen P, Wiggers JK, Buijze GA: Treatment of diaphyseal non-unions of the ulna and radius. *Arch Orthop Trauma Surg* 2010;130(12):1439-1445.

    In this retrospective study, 51 cases of forearm nonunion in 47 patients were treated with compression plating and/or autogenous bone grafting. Internal fixation was used alone in 14 cases, plate fixation plus bone graft in 30 cases, and bone graft alone in 7 cases. Union was achieved in all patients.

20. Livani B, Belangero W, Medina G, Pimenta C, Zogaib R, Mongon M: Anterior plating as a surgical alternative in the treatment of humeral shaft non-union. *Int Orthop* 2010;34(7):1025-1031.

    In this study, 15 patients were treated with anterior plating for humeral nonunion. Compression plating was used in 12 cases of viable nonunion and wave plating with tricortical bone graft was used in 3 cases of nonviable nonunion. All cases of nonunion healed at a mean of 9 weeks.

21. Prasarn ML, Achor T, Paul O, Lorich DG, Helfet DL: Management of nonunions of the proximal humeral diaphysis. *Injury* 2010;41(12):1244-1248.

    In this retrospective review, 19 patients with proximal humerus diaphyseal nonunion were treated with compression plating and various grafting substrates. Union was achieved in all patients at a mean of 15.2 weeks.

22. Said GZ, Said HG, el-Sharkawi MM: Failed intramedullary nailing of femur: Open reduction and plate augmentation with the nail in situ. *Int Orthop* 2011;35(7):1089-1092.

    In this study, 14 patients with aseptic femoral nonunion after intramedullary nailing were treated with augmentative plating. Autologous bone graft was used in nine patients. Union occurred in all patients at a mean of 4.3 months.

23. Singh AK, Arun GR, Narsaria N, Srivastava A: Treatment of non-union of humerus diaphyseal fractures: A prospective study comparing interlocking nail and locking compression plate. *Arch Orthop Trauma Surg* 2014;134(7):947-953.

    This prospective study compared intramedullary nailing and locked compression plating for treatment of humeral shaft nonunion. Twenty patients were in each group: union was achieved in 95% in the intramedullary nailing group and in 100% in the compression plating group.

24. Stufkens SA, Kloen P: Treatment of midshaft clavicular delayed and non-unions with anteroinferior locking compression plating. *Arch Orthop Trauma Surg* 2010;130(2):159-164.

    In this retrospective review, 21 cases of clavicle nonunion were treated with compression plating and autogenous bone grafting. Union was obtained in all patients at an average of 3.5 months.

25. Willis MP, Brooks JP, Badman BL, Gaines RJ, Mighell MA, Sanders RW: Treatment of atrophic diaphyseal humeral nonunions with compressive locked plating and augmented with an intramedullary strut allograft. *J Orthop Trauma* 2013;27(2):77-81.

    In this retrospective study, 20 patients with aseptic, atrophic diaphyseal humeral nonunion were treated with compression plating and intramedullary strut allograft. Union was obtained in 19 patients. Level of evidence: IV.

26. Gao KD, Huang JH, Tao J, et al: Management of femoral diaphyseal nonunion after nailing with augmentative locked plating and bone graft. *Orthop Surg* 2011;3(2):83-87.

    In this retrospective study, 13 cases of diaphyseal femoral shaft nonunion after intramedullary nailing were treated with augmentative plating and autologous bone grafting. All healed at an average of 7.5 months.

27. Lin CJ, Chiang CC, Wu PK, et al: Effectiveness of plate augmentation for femoral shaft nonunion after nailing. *J Chin Med Assoc* 2012;75(8):396-401.

    In this study, 22 cases of femoral shaft nonunion after intramedullary nailing were treated with augmentative plating and iliac crest or local bone autografting. Union was obtained in all patients at a mean of 22.1 weeks.

28. Park J, Kim SG, Yoon HK, Yang KH: The treatment of nonisthmal femoral shaft nonunions with im nail exchange versus augmentation plating. *J Orthop Trauma* 2010;24(2):89-94.

    In this retrospective review, nonisthmic femoral nonunion was treated with exchange nailing or augmentative plating. Union was achieved in all 11 patients in the augmentative plating group compared with only 2 of 7 in the exchange nailing group.

29. Naeem-ur-Razaq M, Qasim M, Sultan S: Exchange nailing for non-union of femoral shaft fractures. *J Ayub Med Coll Abbottabad* 2010;22(3):106-109.

    In this study, 43 cases of aseptic femoral nonunion were treated with exchange nailing. Union occurred in 90% of cases at a mean of 4.97 months.

30. Swanson EA, Garrard EC, Bernstein DT, O'Connor DP, Brinker MR: Results of a systematic approach to exchange nailing for the treatment of aseptic femoral nonunions. *J Orthop Trauma* 2015;29(1):21-27.

    In this retrospective study, 50 cases of aseptic femoral nonunion with cortical contact greater than 50% were treated with exchange nailing. Nails were at least 2 mm larger in diameter than the previous nail and statically locked. Union was achieved in all cases at a mean of 7 months. Level of evidence: IV.

31. Swanson EA, Garrard EC, O'Connor DP, Brinker MR: Results of a systematic approach to exchange nailing for the treatment of aseptic tibial nonunions. *J Orthop Trauma* 2015;29(1):28-35.

    In this retrospective study, 46 cases of aseptic tibial nonunion with cortical contact greater than 50% were treated with exchange nailing. Nails were at least 2 mm larger in diameter than the previous nail and statically locked. Union was achieved in 98% of cases at a mean of 4.8 months. Level of evidence: IV.

32. Yang KH, Kim JR, Park J: Nonisthmal femoral shaft nonunion as a risk factor for exchange nailing failure. *J Trauma Acute Care Surg* 2012;72(2):E60-E64.

In this retrospective review, 41 patents with aseptic femoral nonunion were treated with exchange nailing. Union was achieved in 87% of cases of isthmic nonunion compared with 50% of nonisthmic cases.

33. Fenton P, Qureshi F, Bejjanki N, Potter D: Management of non-union of humeral fractures with the Stryker T2 compression nail. *Arch Orthop Trauma Surg* 2011;131(1):79-84.

In this retrospective review, 12 patients with humeral nonunion were treated with compression nailing. All patients healed at a mean of 4.5 months.

34. Lin WP, Lin J: Allografting in locked nailing and interfragmentary wiring for humeral nonunions. *Clin Orthop Relat Res* 2010;468(3):852-860.

This prospective study evaluated the treatment of humeral nonunion with locked intramedullary nailing, interfragmentary compression wiring, and bone autograft in 28 cases versus allograft in 26 cases. Union was achieved in all patients but one from each group for an overall union rate of 96.9%. Level of evidence: III.

35. Martinez AA, Bejarano C, Carbonel I, Iglesias D, Gil-Albarova J, Herrera A: The treatment of proximal humerus nonunions in older patients with reverse shoulder arthroplasty. *Injury* 2012;43(suppl 2):S3-S6.

In this study, 18 patients (mean age, 78.8 years) with atrophic proximal humerus nonunion were treated with reverse total shoulder arthroplasty. Mean Constant score improved postoperatively but major complications were reported in five patients, including transient axillary nerve palsy, infection, and dislocation.

36. Raiss P, Edwards TB, da Silva MR, Bruckner T, Loew M, Walch G: Reverse shoulder arthroplasty for the treatment of nonunions of the surgical neck of the proximal part of the humerus (type-3 fracture sequelae). *J Bone Joint Surg Am* 2014;96(24):2070-2076.

In this multicenter study, 32 patients were treated for humerus surgical neck nonunion with reverse shoulder arthroplasty. Mean Constant scores improved, but a 41% complication rate was reported. Level of evidence: IV.

37. Zafra M, Uceda P, Flores M, Carpintero P: Reverse total shoulder replacement for nonunion of a fracture of the proximal humerus. *Bone Joint J* 2014;96-B(9):1239-1243.

In this prospective study, 35 patients (mean age, 69 years) with proximal humerus nonunion were treated with reverse total shoulder arthroplasty. A 20% complication rate was reported, including transient axillary nerve palsy, dislocation, and infection.

38. Vaishya R, Singh AP, Hasija R, Singh AP: Treatment of resistant nonunion of supracondylar fractures femur by megaprosthesis. *Knee Surg Sports Traumatol Arthrosc* 2011;19(7):1137-1140.

In this retrospective study, eight patients (age range, 68 to 85 years) with aseptic distal femoral nonunion were treated with megaprosthesis. No postoperative complications were reported and median Knee Society pain and functional scores improved. Level of evidence: IV.

39. Donegan DJ, Scolaro J, Matuszewski PE, Mehta S: Staged bone grafting following placement of an antibiotic spacer block for the management of segmental long bone defects. *Orthopedics* 2011;34(11):e730-e735.

In this retrospective review, 11 patients with segmental bone defects (range, 4 to 15 cm) of the lower extremity were treated with a staged induced membrane technique. Patients underwent cement spacer placement followed by various combinations of bone grafting at 4 to 5 weeks. Healing occurred in 10 patients.

40. Karger C, Kishi T, Schneider L, Fitoussi F, Masquelet AC; French Society of Orthopaedic Surgery and Traumatology (SoFCOT): Treatment of posttraumatic bone defects by the induced membrane technique. *Orthop Traumatol Surg Res* 2012;98(1):97-102.

In this retrospective review, 84 patients with diaphyseal long bone segmental defects (up to 23 cm) were treated with a staged induced-membrane technique. Various forms of bone graft were used in the second stage. Union was reported in 90% of cases. Level of evidence: IV.

41. Stafford PR, Norris BL: Reamer-irrigator-aspirator bone graft and bi Masquelet technique for segmental bone defect nonunions: A review of 25 cases. *Injury* 2010;41(suppl 2):S72-S77.

In this retrospective study, 27 cases segmental bone loss nonunion (range, 1 to 25 cm) of the lower extremity were treated with a staged induced-membrane technique with RIA bone grafting. Union was reported in 90% of cases at 1 year.

42. Braly HL, O'Connor DP, Brinker MR: Percutaneous autologous bone marrow injection in the treatment of distal meta-diaphyseal tibial nonunions and delayed unions. *J Orthop Trauma* 2013;27(9):527-533.

In this study, 11 cases of distal tibial aseptic nonunion were treated with percutaneous autologous bone marrow injection. Union was achieved in 9 patients at an average of 4.1 months. Level of evidence: IV.

Chapter 11

Malunions

Eli Swanson, MD

Abstract

Effective treatment of malunited fractures requires careful patient selection and detailed clinical and radiographic evaluation, as well as a thorough understanding of the available treatment options. A malunion can become symptomatic when shortening, translation, angulation, rotational malalignment, or a combined deformity impair function or cause pain. Proper treatment requires accurate characterization of the malunion regarding location, severity, and direction of deformity. Radiographic evaluation of malunions includes concepts related to limb alignment, mechanical axes, anatomic axes, joint orientation lines/angles, center of rotational angle, and correction axes. Variations in treatment options include acute or gradual correction, internal or external fixation, and type of osteotomy selected.

Keywords: malunion; tibia; femur; alignment; corticotomy; osteotomy; distraction osteogenesis; deformity correction

Introduction

A malunion results from a fracture that heals in a nonanatomic position to a degree that impairs function or becomes symptomatic. A malunion can cause symptoms of pain or disability by asymmetric loading of an adjacent joint, resulting in increased contact pressure, overloading ligaments, muscle/tendon irritation, tension strain on the bone, and impairment of normal ambulation or motion.[1-6] A malunion also can result from bony union with associated shortening, translation, angulation, rotational malalignment, or a combined deformity. Accurate characterization of the malunion regarding location, severity, and direction of deformity is required to identify the most effective treatment. The position of the distal segment relative to the proximal segment is used to describe the direction of the deformity. Lower extremity malunions tend to be more symptomatic than upper extremity malunions as length discrepancy and asymmetric joint loading are affected by body weight, thereby magnifying the effects of the malunion. Upper extremity malunions may be more clinically significant in patients with paraplegia, who may rely on the upper extremities for ambulation, or patients with specific occupational dependence on upper extremity function. Most patients with upper extremity deformity following a fracture are able to compensate because of the forgiving mobility of the shoulder joint.

Symptoms present quickly when the deformity interferes with gait mechanics and the compensatory capacity of adjacent joints is overwhelmed. An example of this is when a procurvatum deformity of the femur interferes with the ability to lock the knee during the stance phase of gait or while standing.[7] Most symptoms resulting from malunions occur more gradually as a result of asymmetric adjacent joint contact pressure and subsequent pain.[1-3,5,6]

Clinical Evaluation

Accurate evaluation of a malunion begins with a thorough medical history, including the nature and timing of the initial injury as well as all treatments between the initial treatment and the current presentation. Soft-tissue status (open or closed initial injury, whether soft-tissue coverage was required, infection or draining sinus present) along with the patient's current functional status and location of pain should be documented. The level of supportive resources as well as the patient's overall motivation/insight should also be taken into account as gradual correction requires good compliance and consistent follow-up. The patient should be queried about the location and type of symptoms related to the malunion.

During the physical examination, a neurovascular examination as well as assessment of the range of motion for

Neither Dr. Swanson nor any immediate family member has received anything of value from or has stock or stock options held in a commercial company or institution related directly or indirectly to the subject of this chapter.

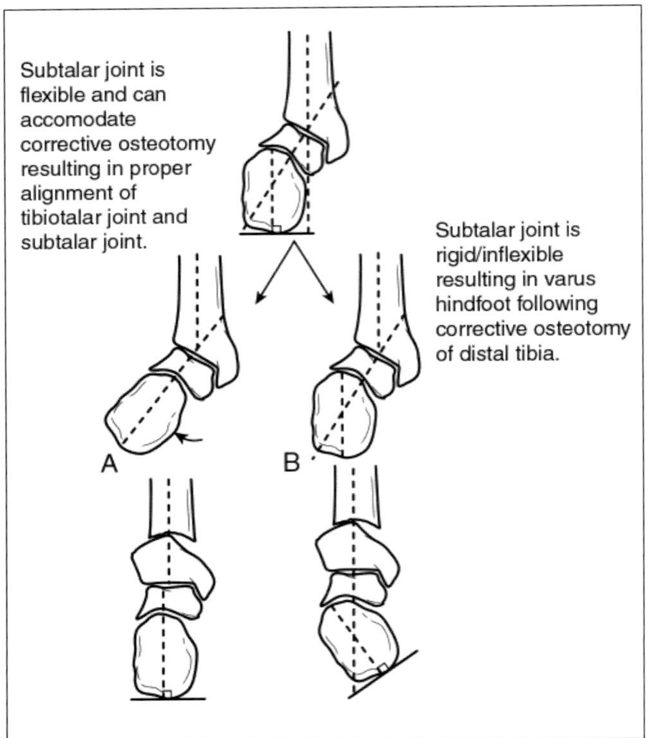

Subtalar joint is flexible and can accomodate corrective osteotomy resulting in proper alignment of tibiotalar joint and subtalar joint.
Subtalar joint is rigid/inflexible resulting in varus hindfoot following corrective osteotomy of distal tibia.
A
B

Figure 1 Drawings depict flexible and rigid subtalar joints associated with correction of a distal tibial malunion. **A**, The subtalar joint is flexible and can accommodate corrective osteotomy, resulting in overall acceptable hindfoot alignment after tibial malunion is corrected. **B**, The subtalar joint is fixed in the compensatory varus position, which does not change after osteotomy, resulting in varus malalignment of the subtalar joint and varus hindfoot following correction of tibial malunion.

joints adjacent to the malunion should be performed. The potential range of motion or lack thereof in an adjacent joint may affect treatment decisions. If an adjacent joint has a rigid compensatory deformity, then correction of the malunion will result in a secondary deformity at the level of the joint. With a distal tibial valgus malunion, for example, the subtalar joint may partially compensate for the tibial deformity.[8] The mobility of the subtalar joint should be assessed to determine whether it has the flexibility to return to a normal position after the malunion is corrected to avoid creating a varus malalignment at the level of the subtalar joint. A fixed varus position of the foot will result if the subtalar joint is not flexible (**Figure 1**). The malunion site should be stressed to assess stability of union and presence of pain. If pain is present, further imaging may be helpful to rule out a nonunion and potentially alter management. Gait abnormalities should be documented as well as rotational alignment of the femur and tibia.

Because of concerns about soft tissue in the area of the previous fracture site, the importance of patient selection cannot be underestimated. A history of open fracture, soft-tissue coverage, and infection are factors that should be considered during the preoperative assessment. Even though correction may ideally occur at the level of the deformity, compromised soft tissue at the level of the previous fracture site may require that the osteotomy be made at a location further away from the deformity than preferred. The patient must have a good understanding of the treatment plan, including duration of treatment and possibility of failure. A solidly healed malunion could potentially become an unstable or infected nonunion following osteotomy, which could ultimately result in amputation. The patient should be aware of these types of risks and be willing to proceed before treatment is initiated. In patients with medical comorbidities (diabetes, smoking history, malnourishment), optimization strategies should be implemented before treatment to increase the likelihood of successful surgery.

Radiographic Evaluation

Mechanical Axes

The femoral mechanical axis is shown by a line drawn from the center of the femoral head down to the center of the knee joint. The tibial mechanical axis is created by drawing a line from the center of the knee joint down to the center of the ankle joint. The mechanical axis of a bone is always a straight line because it always connects two points. The mechanical axis of the tibia is slightly lateral to the mid-diaphyseal line/anatomic axis (**Figure 2**).

Anatomic Axes

The anatomic axis of a bone is created by a line drawn through the center of the diaphysis along the length of the bone. Several points along the diaphysis can be created by a line drawn perpendicular to the long axis of the bone spanning from cortex to cortex. This line is then bisected and this center point is connected for two or more points along the length of the bone to create the anatomic axis of the bone. In the femur, the anatomic axis exits proximally through the piriformis fossa and distally at the lateral aspect of the medial femoral condyle on the AP view. Depending on the shape of the bone the anatomic axis may be straight, as seen on the AP view of the femur, or curved, as seen on the lateral view of the femur. The tibial anatomic axis is straight on both the frontal and sagittal planes (**Figure 2**). A summary of joint orientation angles is shown in **Figure 3**.

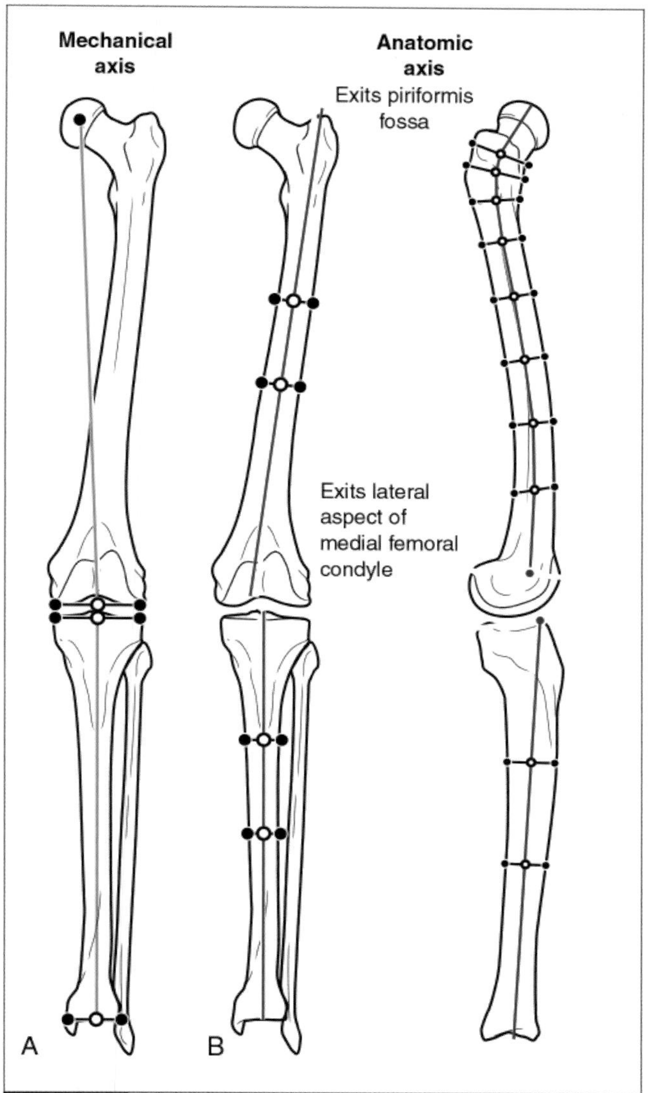

Figure 2 Drawings depict axes of the femur and tibia. **A**, The mechanical axis of the femur and tibia is determined by drawing a line from the center of the femoral head to the center of the knee joint and from the center of the knee joint to the center of the ankle joint. **B**, The anatomic axis of the femur and tibia is determined by drawing a line through the midpoint of two lines drawn perpendicular to the long axis of the bone spanning from both cortices. This resultant line connecting the midpoints represents the anatomic axis, which is collinear with the medullary canal. The tibial anatomic axis is straight on both the frontal and sagittal planes while the femoral anatomic axis is straight on the frontal plane but varies on the sagittal plane due to the femoral bow.

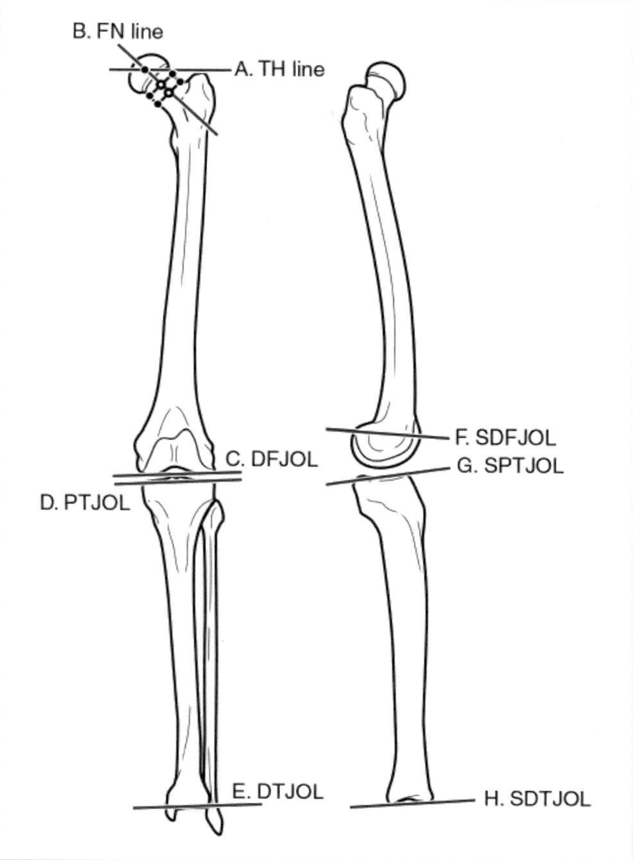

Figure 3 Drawings depict joint orientation lines. **A**, The trochanteric head line (TH) is the line connecting the tip of the greater trochanter with the center of the femoral head. **B**, The femoral neck line (FN) is the line connecting the center of the femoral head with several points bisecting the femoral neck. **C**, The distal femoral joint orientation line (DFJOL) is the line tangential to the medial and lateral femoral condyles. **D**, The proximal tibial joint orientation line (PTJOL) is the line tangential to the subchondral bone of the medial and lateral tibial plateau. **E**, The distal tibial joint orientation line (DTJOL) is the line tangential to the distal tibial articular surface. **F**, The sagittal distal femoral joint orientation line (SDFJOL) is the line drawn through the anterior and posterior condylar-metaphyseal junctions. **G**, The sagittal proximal tibial joint orientation line (SPTJOL) is the line drawn tangential to the subchondral bone of the proximal tibia on the lateral view. **H**, The sagittal distal tibial joint orientation line (SDTJOL) is the line drawn between the distalmost point on the anterior and posterior aspect of the distal tibia on the lateral view.

Joint Orientation Angles

The intersection of joint orientation lines (**Figure 3**) and either the mechanical or anatomic axis of the bone in question allows one to calculate the respective joint orientation angles (**Figure 4**). These joint orientation angles can be used to determine axis alignment of a bone if the segment is too short to use the anatomic or mechanical axis lines. In most instances, a natural template for “normal” is

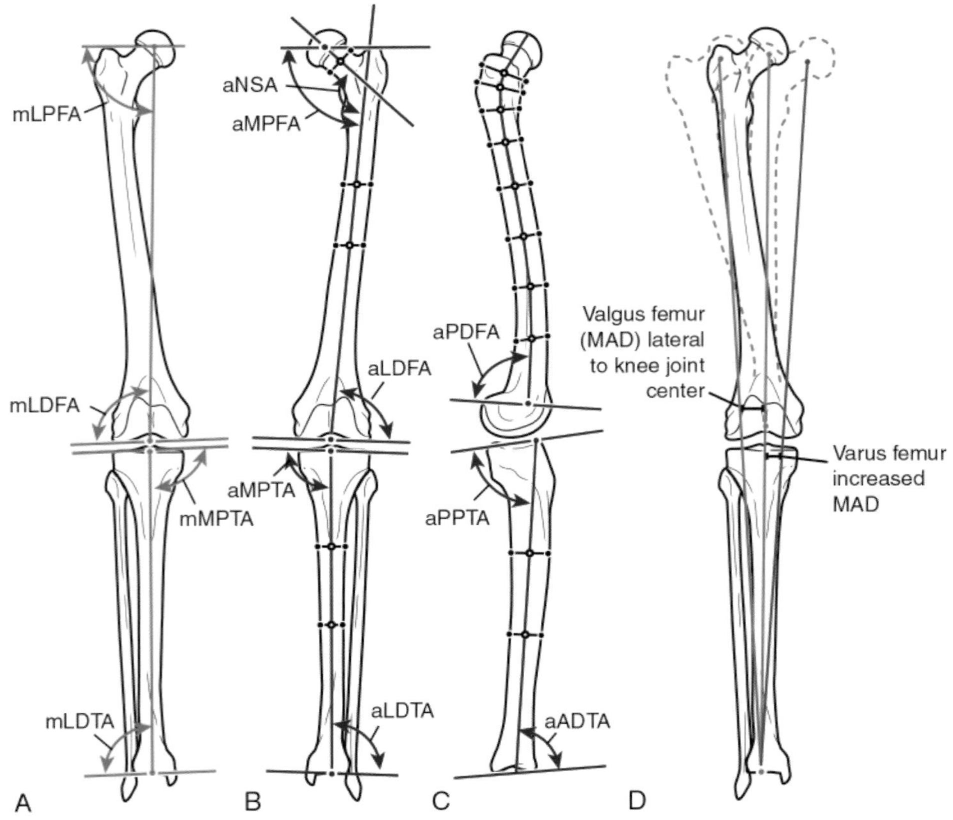

Figure 4 Drawings depict the femoral and tibial angles. **A**, The mechanical lateral proximal femoral angle (mLPFA) and mechanical lateral distal femoral angle (mLDFA) are formed between the mechanical axis of the femur and the proximal and distal femoral orientation lines, respectively. The mechanical medial proximal tibial angle (mMPTA) and mechanical lateral distal tibial angle (mLDTA) are formed between the mechanical axis of the tibia and the proximal and distal tibial joint orientation angles, respectively. **B**, The anatomic lateral proximal femoral angle and anatomic lateral distal femoral angle (aLDFA) are formed between the anatomic axis of the femur and the proximal and distal femoral orientation lines, respectively. The anatomic medial proximal tibial angle (aMPTA) and anatomic lateral distal tibial angle (aLDTA) are formed between the anatomic axis of the tibia and the proximal and distal tibial joint orientation angles, respectively. aNSA = ; aMPFA = anatomic medial proximal femoral angle. **C**, The anatomic posterior distal femoral angle (aPDFA) is the angle between the sagittal distal femoral joint orientation line and the anatomic axis of the femur on the lateral view. The anatomic proximal posterior tibial angle (aPPTA) is the angle between the sagittal proximal tibial joint orientation line and the anatomic axis of the tibia on the lateral view. The anatomic anterior distal tibial angle (aADTA) is the angle between the sagittal distal tibial joint orientation line and the anatomic axis of the tibia on the lateral view. **D**, The mechanical axis deviation (MAD) is the distance from the knee joint center (medially or laterally) to the mechanical axis of the limb on the AP view. The normal range is 1 to 15 mm medial to the knee joint center. With relative valgus mechanical axis the MAD is negative as it is lateral to the knee joint center, whereas relative varus mechanical axis is greater than 15 mm medial to the knee joint center.

already provided in the unaffected limb. If both limbs are affected, the mean value for the population sample is the next best option[9] (**Table 1**). The same convention should be used when assessing alignment: either the anatomic axis or the mechanical axis should be used, but not both, when assessing alignment of a malunited fracture.

Limb Alignment

Full-length, 51-inch bilateral AP standing radiographs taken with both feet pointed straight forward as well as full-length weight-bearing lateral views of each lower extremity showing the hip, knee, and ankle with the limb in full extension allow for assessment of limb alignment by drawing a line from the center of the femoral head to the center of the ankle joint. Mechanical axis deviation (MAD) refers to the distance from the center of the knee joint to this line drawn from the center of the femoral head to the center of the ankle on the AP view. The normal range for MAD is 1 to 15 mm medial to the knee joint center (**Figure 4, D**).

Table 1

Normal Range Values for Lower Extremity Joint Orientation Angles and Mechanical Axis Deviation Distance

Angle	Angle Formed by	Mean (degrees)	Range (degrees)
Femur: frontal			
Mechanical lateral proximal femoral angle	Mechanical axis – Trochanteric tip to head center line	90	85-95
Mechanical lateral distal femoral angle	Mechanical axis – Distal femoral joint orientation line	88	85-90
Anatomic medial proximal femoral angle	Anatomic axis – Trochanteric tip to head center line	84	80-89
Anatomic neck shaft angle	Anatomic axis – Femoral neck line	130	124-136
Anatomic lateral distal femoral angle	Anatomic axis – Distal femoral joint orientation line	81	79-83
Femur: sagittal			
Anatomic posterior distal femoral angle	Mid-diaphyseal line – Sagittal distal femoral joint orientation line	83	79-89
Tibia: frontal			
Mechanical medial proximal tibial angle	Mechanical axis – Proximal tibial joint orientation line	87	85-90
Mechanical lateral distal tibial angle	Mechanical-axis – Distal tibial joint orientation line	89	83-92
Anatomic medial proximal tibial angle	Anatomic axis – Proximal tibial joint orientation line	87	85-90
Anatomic lateral distal tibial angle	Anatomic axis – Distal tibial joint orientation line	89	88-92
Tibia: sagittal			
Anatomic posterior proximal tibial angle	Mid-diaphyseal line – Sagittal proximal tibial joint orientation line	81	77-84
Anatomic anterior distal tibial angle	Mid-diaphyseal line – Sagittal distal tibial joint orientation line	80	78-82
Knee: frontal			
Mechanical axis deviation	Distance on horizontal plane from line drawn from center of femoral head through center of ankle joint to knee joint center		Normal range: 1-15 mm medial to center of knee joint

Center of Rotation of Angulation

The center of rotational angle (CORA) is the intersection of the proximal and distal bone segment axes (**Figure 5**). In the process of deformity correction the bone may be rotated around this point to correct angular deformity. Anatomic or mechanical axes may be used to determine the CORA, but axis types should not be mixed. Anatomic axes are easier to use for diaphyseal segments; for peri-articular segments, axis lines can be created by measuring joint orientation angles from the patient's contralateral limb or by using mean values from **Table 1** to determine the mechanical or anatomic axis relative to the joint orientation line. For multi-apical deformities the anatomic axes should be used for the femur, as it is difficult to assess the mechanical axis for a central diaphyseal segment if either the proximal or distal joint segment is not attached to that diaphyseal segment. To determine the CORA, a line is drawn along the axes of the segments in question. If these lines intersect at the level of obvious deformity, then the deformity is uni-apical. If the lines intersect outside of the bone, a second CORA, or a translational component, exists (**Figure 6**). Two angles are created at the CORA.

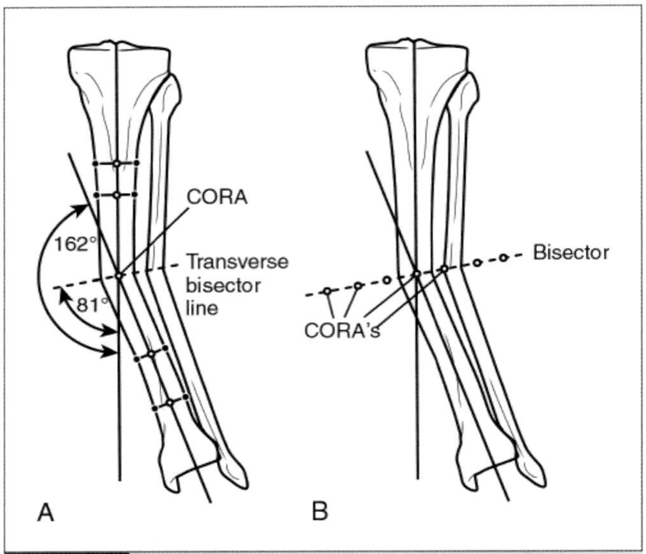

Figure 5 Drawings depict the center of rotational angle (CORA), which is the intersection of the proximal and distal bone segment axes. **A,** The bisector line is drawn passing through the CORA and dividing the medial and lateral angles, creating a transverse bisector line. **B,** Any point on this transverse bisector line is considered to be a CORA as rotation about any point on the bisector line will result in angular correction without secondary translation.

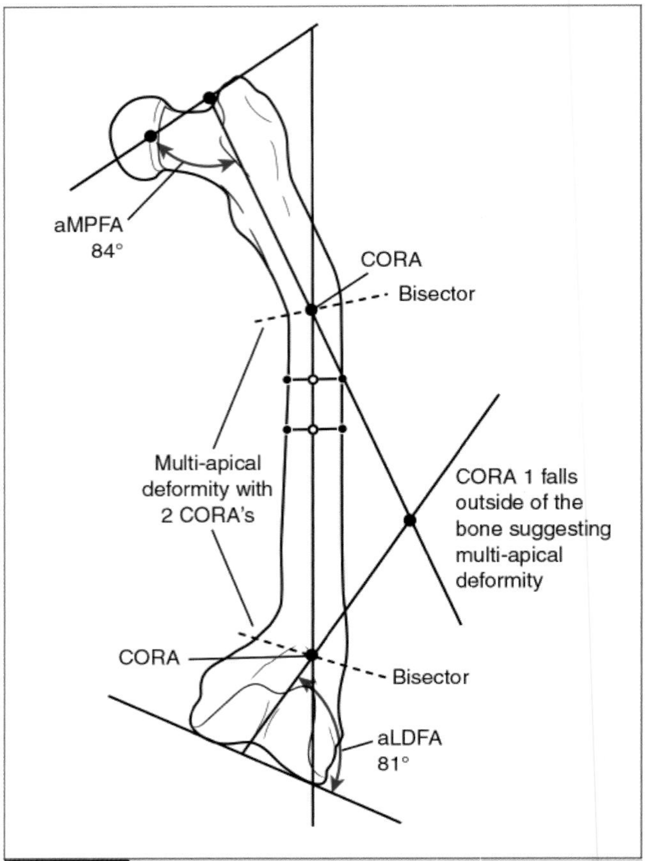

Figure 6 Drawing depicts the center of rotational angle (CORA) and its relationship to deformity. If more than one CORA exists on an AP or lateral view, then a multi-apical deformity exists. If there are distal or proximal segments, the anatomic medial proximal femoral angle (aMPFA) and the anatomic lateral distal femoral angle (aLDFA) can be used to determine the anatomic axis of the short segments, as seen in this example.

These can be labeled as proximal, distal, medial, and lateral. With the example seen in **Figure 5**, the proximal and distal angles are equal to each other and represent the magnitude of angular deformity. The medial and lateral angles are also equal to each other. The bisector line is drawn passing through the CORA and dividing these medial and lateral angles, creating a transverse bisector line. Any point on this transverse bisector line is considered to be a CORA as rotation about any point on the bisector line will result in angular correction without secondary translation. Ideally, the correction of angular deformity is done at the CORA. However, if soft tissue, poor bone healing potential, or internal fixation construct options prevent placing the osteotomy at the level of the CORA, and an angular correction must be done proximal or distal to the CORA, this will result in a translational deformity. Often this translational deformity is clinically insignificant, but this predictable result of an osteotomy not centered at the CORA should be recognized.

Correction Axis

The correction axis, which is seen when angular correction rotates or pivots to correct deformity, depends on the location and type of osteotomy performed. Deformity correction with an osteotomy results in realignment through angular correction alone if the correction axis lies on the CORA/bisector line, realignment through angular and translational correction if the correction axis lies on the CORA/bisector line but the osteotomy is away from the CORA, or angular correction with residual translational deformity if the correction axis is away from the CORA/bisector line.[8,9]

Evaluation of Deformity Types

Deformities are described in terms of direction and magnitude using the position of the distal segment relative to the proximal segment. Identification of the CORA is essential in correction of angular deformities. Angulation is characterized by type (flexion/extension/varus/valgus) and magnitude as well as whether there is any effect on the mechanical axis or MAD. If an angular deformity appears on the frontal and sagittal planes with the CORA at the same level, then an oblique deformity exists. If the CORA is at a different level on AP and lateral radiographs, then a translational deformity also exists. Determination of angular deformity can also be visualized with three-dimensional reconstructions on CT scan. If more than one CORA exists on the AP or lateral view, then a multi-apical deformity exists (**Figure 6**).

Malunions affecting length include fractures healed in a shortened position, such as in the presence of bone loss or bayonet apposition of the fracture fragments. Fractures healed in an overdistracted position result in a malunion with excessive length. Both shortened and distracted malunions will result in a relative length discrepancy. The evaluation of length deformity is made with 51-inch bilateral full-length weight-bearing x-rays or with a CT scanogram. Length deformities are described by their direction and magnitude, are measured from the joint centers, and are compared with the contralateral extremity. If malunion occurs in the lower extremity, then shortening the longer limb is an option, as is lengthening the relatively shortened limb. Care must be taken to distinguish between shortened malunion and congenital length discrepancy. A limb that has been shortened as a result of a malunited fracture has neurovascular structures that at some point were equal in length to the uninjured side, whereas congenital length discrepancies have neurovascular structures that have always been short. This may affect the plan of acute versus gradual length correction as well as the magnitude of correction for congenital length discrepancies. Shortening can be done acutely, as much as the surrounding soft tissues will tolerate. Acute lengthening of up to 2 cm has been described to be safe.[8,9] Lengthening of more than 2 cm should be done gradually to avoid increased risk of neurovascular injury. Chronic valgus malunions about the knee should also be taken into account, as correction of valgus alignment can result in neurovascular injury if done too quickly.

Rotational malunions are described in terms of the distal segment relative to the proximal segment and occur about the longitudinal axis of the bone. Magnitude (degrees) and direction (internal or external) are noted compared with the unaffected side. Rotational malunion of the femur is the most common malunion of long bones of the lower extremity usually following intramedullary nailing.[8] Assessment of rotational deformity can be done clinically[10] as well as radiographically.[8,11-13] Malrotation of the femur can be assessed clinically by having the patient lie prone with knees flexed to 90°. The femur is passively internally and externally rotated, and the degree of rotation of the tibia is noted and compared with the unaffected side. The relative difference indicates the magnitude of femoral rotational deformity. This technique assumes that both tibiae are straight. If an angular deformity of the tibia exists this must be factored into the respective degree of internal/external rotation noted. Tibial rotational deformity can also be checked with the patient in this position by measuring the axis of the second ray of the foot with the axis of the femur (**Figure 7**). Another option to clinically assess rotational deformity of the tibia requires the patient to stand with both patella facing directly anterior, and the axis of the second ray of the foot is compared in terms of its rotational relationship with the patella or tibial tubercle. Any difference represents a tibial rotational deformity. Rotational deformity can also be evaluated with CT[10,14,15] or radiographs.[8] CT can be used to measure the angle of the femoral neck in relation to the condylar axis of the distal femur to assess femoral rotational deformity. The relationship between the proximal tibia and the distal tibia can be evaluated in the same scan by comparing the axis of the proximal tibia with that of the distal tibial/fibular joint (**Figure 8**).

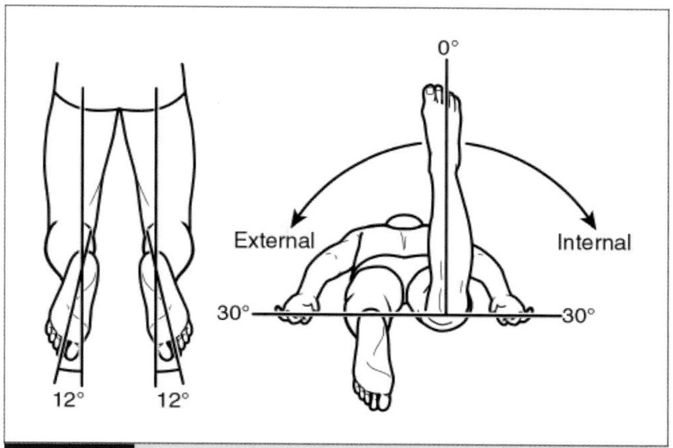

Figure 7 Drawings depict clinical assessment of malrotation of the femur, which can be assessed clinically by having the patient lie prone with knees flexed to 90°. The femur is passively internally and externally rotated, and the degree of rotation of the tibia is noted and compared with the unaffected side. The relative difference indicates the magnitude of femoral rotational deformity. Tibial rotational deformity can also be checked with the patient in this position by measuring the axis of the second ray of the foot with the axis of the femur.

Translational deformity resulting from malunion is described in terms of direction (anterior, posterior, medial, lateral) and magnitude (millimeters). Except for the femoral and humeral heads, translational deformity is described in terms of the distal segment's relationship to

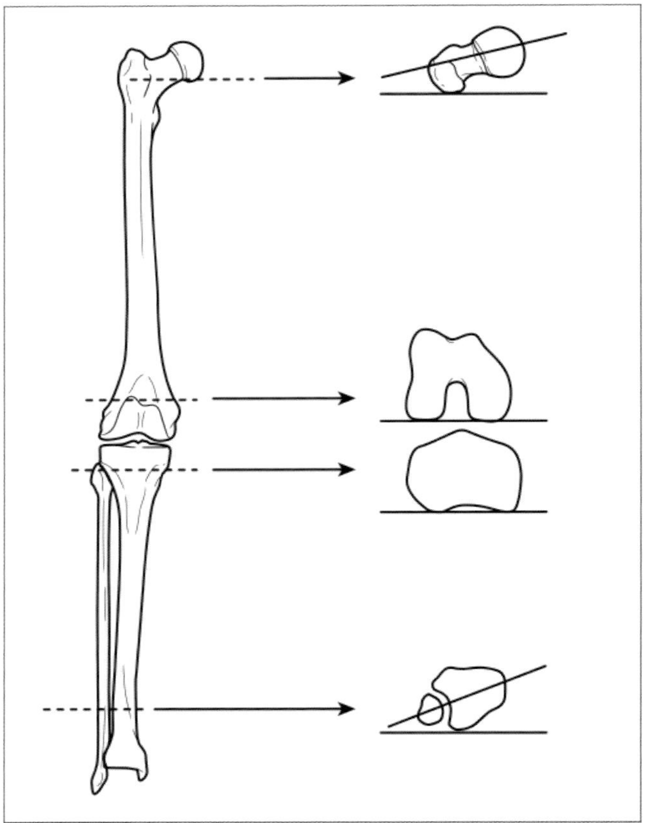

Figure 8 Drawing depicts how a CT scanogram can be used by measuring the angle of the femoral neck in relation to the condylar axis of the distal femur to assess femoral rotational deformity. The relationship between the proximal tibia and the distal tibia can be evaluated in the same scan by comparing the axis of the proximal tibia with that of the distal tibial/fibular joint.

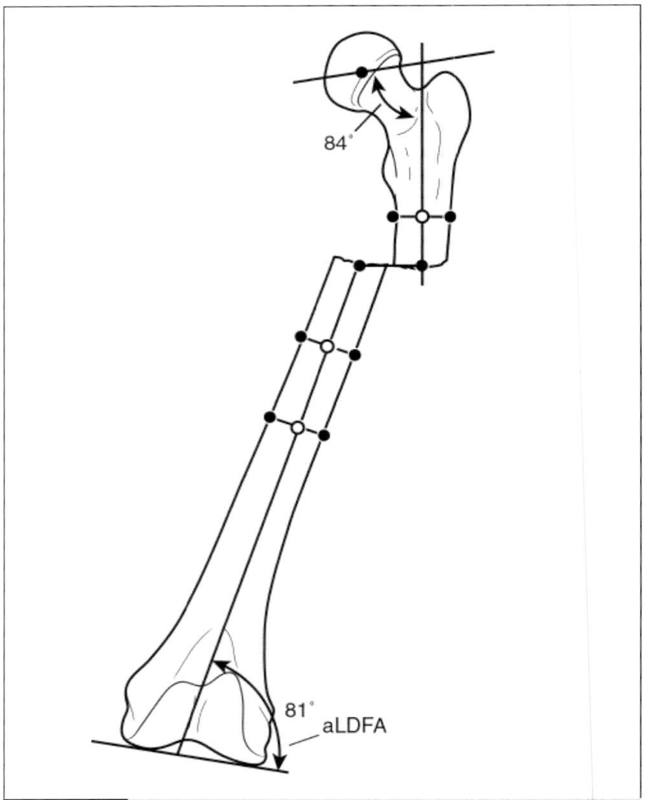

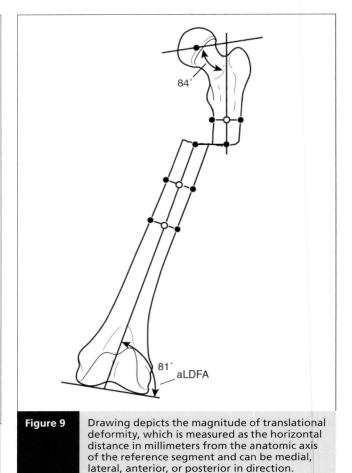

Figure 9 Drawing depicts the magnitude of translational deformity, which is measured as the horizontal distance in millimeters from the anatomic axis of the reference segment and can be medial, lateral, anterior, or posterior in direction.

the proximal segment. For the femoral and humeral heads the convention is reversed. Regardless of the plane of the translational deformity, the magnitude is measured as the horizontal distance in millimeters from the anatomic axis of the reference segment (**Figure 9**).

Treatment

Depending on the type of deformity and related factors (angulation, length, translation, rotation) and soft-tissue status, a malunion may be managed acutely or gradually. If neurovascular structures are located on the concave side of a deformity (for example, a valgus deformity about the knee), acute correction may cause neurovascular injury.

Gradual correction can be performed with a tensioned small wire ring fixator (Ilizarov/Taylor Spatial Frame [Smith & Nephew]). Malunions with shortened, angulated, or combined deformities are often best treated with gradual correction with a tensioned small wire ring fixator.

Ideally, osteotomies are made at the level of the CORA. However, osteotomy type and location can be influenced by deformity type and fixation options for the proposed method of correction, as well as biologic factors such as bone and soft-tissue quality. If these factors result in the osteotomy being made away from the CORA, then the original angular deformity remains; as the alignment is corrected, a secondary translational deformity can result (**Figure 10**). Correction of acute deformity is generally well tolerated in the femur and humerus because of a forgiving surrounding soft-tissue envelope, whereas the tibial soft-tissue envelope is less forgiving and usually better treated with gradual correction with a frame.[16,17]

Osteotomy

There are three concepts associated with osteotomy for the treatment of malunion.[8] The first is that when the osteotomy and angular correction axis pass through

2: Nonunions, Malunions, and Infections

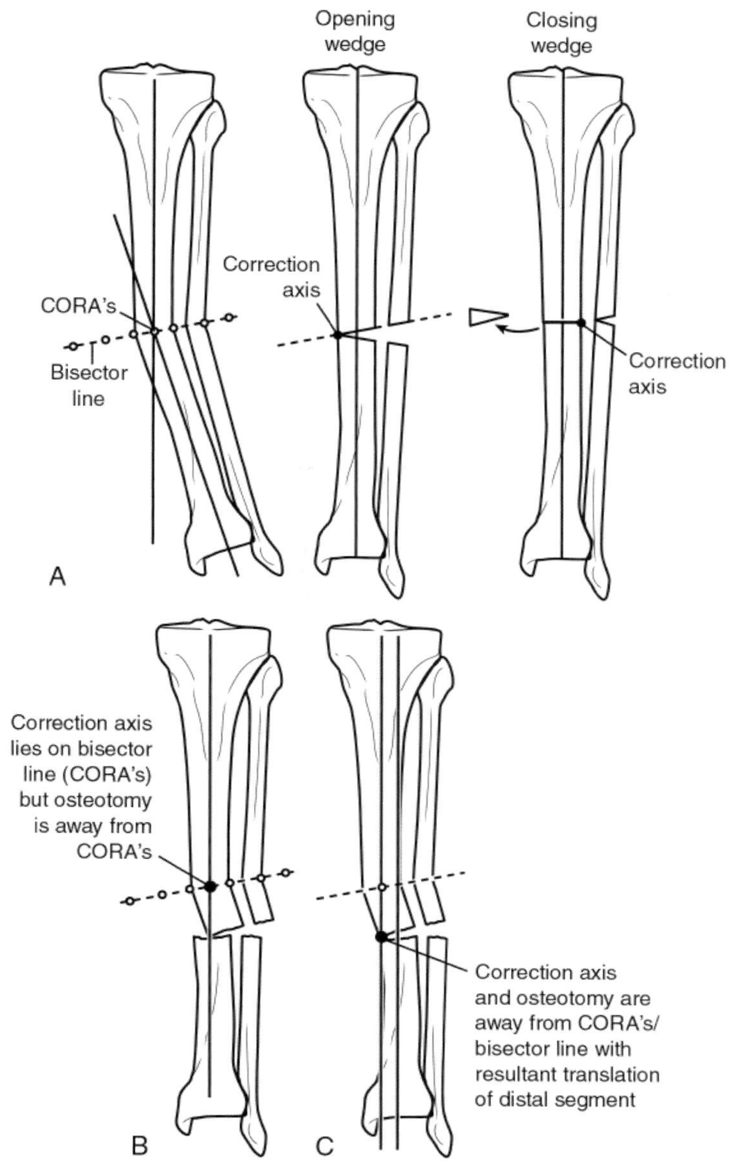

Figure 10 Drawings depict three concepts associated with osteotomy for the treatment of malunion **A**, When the osteotomy and angular correction axis pass through any of the center of rotational angles (CORAs) (any point on the CORA bisector line), then realignment occurs without translation. **B**, When the correction axis is through the CORA but the osteotomy is at a different level, the axis will realign by angulation and translation at the osteotomy site. **C**, When the osteotomy and correction axis are at a level above or below the CORA, a translational deformity will result.

any of the CORAs (any point on the CORA bisector line), then realignment occurs without translation. This can be achieved with an opening or closing wedge osteotomy (**Figure 10, A**). Second, when the correction axis is through the CORA but the osteotomy is at a different level, the axis will realign by angulation and translation at the osteotomy site (**Figure 10, B**). Third, when the osteotomy and correction axis are at a level above or below the CORA, a translational deformity will result (**Figure 10, C**).

Wedge Osteotomy

This osteotomy can be made at the CORA along the bisector line. If the correction axis is on the convex side, a wedge is resected along the entire bone diameter so that the cortices proximal and distal to the wedge resected on

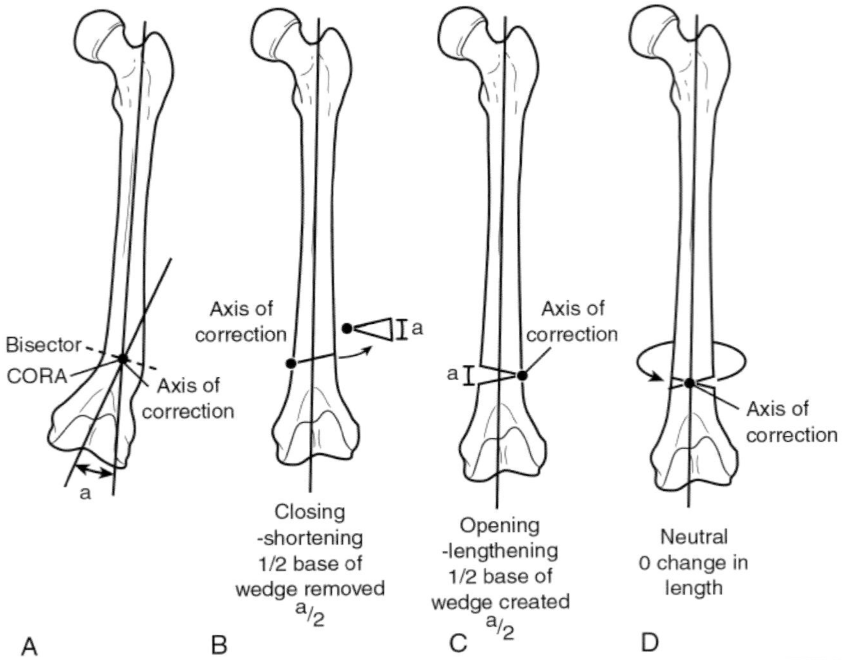

Figure 11 Drawings depict wedge osteotomy. **A**, A wedge osteotomy can be made at the center of rotational angle (CORA) along the bisector line. **B**, If the correction axis is on the convex side, a wedge is resected along the entire bone diameter so that the cortices proximal and distal to the wedge resected on the concave side of the deformity are compressed. This results in shortening that is equal to one-half the base of the resected wedge. **C**, If the axis of correction is on the convex side of the deformity, angular correction results in an opening wedge. The osteotomy traverses the entire diameter of the bone, and angular correction adds length equal to one-half the base of the opening wedge created. **D**, If the axis of correction is central, then a smaller wedge that spans one-half the diameter of the bone is resected on the convex side and placed into the opening wedge defect created on the concave side. This results in a neutral wedge osteotomy, which does not change length.

the concave side of the deformity are compressed. This results in shortening equal to one-half the base of the resected wedge (**Figure 11**). If the axis of correction is on the convex side of the deformity, angular correction results in an opening wedge. The osteotomy traverses the entire diameter of the bone, and angular correction adds length equal to one-half the base of the opening wedge created. One technique is to place parallel Kirschner wires proximal and distal to the osteotomy site. Magnitude of correction is easily measured by the angulation created between the previously parallel wires. If the axis of correction is central, then a smaller wedge that spans one-half the diameter of the bone is resected on the convex side and placed into the opening wedge defect created on the concave side. This results in a neutral wedge osteotomy, which does not change length. The wedge osteotomy can be useful for angular deformities with or without minor length deformity. As long as the axis of correction lies on the bisector line at the level of the CORA, then alignment of the anatomic axis can be restored.

Drawbacks of wedge osteotomy include a shortened bone segment if closing wedge is used (one-half the base of resected wedge), extensive surgical exposure, and the potential for functional lengthening of ligaments that cross the osteotomy site if the procedure is performed close to the joint.

Dome Osteotomy

This type of osteotomy obviates the need for a wedge resection and does not create a large bony void, which requires bone graft, as seen with an opening wedge osteotomy. The dome osteotomy allows for good bony opposition for healing. A more accurate description of the dome is half of a cylinder as opposed to hemisphere, which would be a true dome. Dome osteotomy allows angular correction around a specific axis of correction. If the axis of correction is at the CORA, then alignment without translation can be achieved. However, if the dome osteotomy goes through the CORA, then a secondary translational deformity will occur because the axis of correction cannot be at the point of the osteotomy (**Figure 12**). If the axis of correction is on the bisector line of the CORA, then angular correction can be achieved without secondary translational deformity. As seen with wedge osteotomies, when the axis of correction is on the concave side of the deformity, some shortening will occur as well as possible symptomatic overhanging bone (**Figure 13**). If the axis of correction is on the convex side of the deformity, then length is gained although the bony contact is diminished and may require bone graft. A dome osteotomy with the axis of correction centered on the CORA will result in no change in length with good bony contact and correction of angular deformity without secondary translational deformity. To avoid translation, the axis of correction should fall on the CORA/bisector line. If the osteotomy is through the CORA/bisector line, then the axis of rotation will be proximal or distal to the CORA and will reliably result in a translational deformity.

Transverse Osteotomy

Transverse osteotomies can be made to correct rotational or translational malunions. Rotational malunion osteotomies can be made with an intramedullary saw and exchange nail. Alternatively, an open osteotomy can be made with plate or external fixation after rotational correction. Application of a tensioned wire ring fixator with software correction guidance can allow for precise correction of rotational deformity in the acute setting (temporarily used intraoperatively) or in the gradual correction setting. The osteotomy is made after the frame is applied and strut adjustment can accurately correct the deformity, which some would consider more precise than the parallel Kirschner wire technique. This procedure is often performed to correct a rotational deformity following a fracture initially managed with an intramedullary nail with rotational malreduction. One of the most common complications of this type of osteotomy is nonunion.[18] Because the osteotomy is usually performed in hard diaphyseal cortical bone, it is important to avoid thermal necrosis that can occur with an oscillating saw. The use of a sharp blade with copious irrigation is recommended to reduce the risk of thermal necrosis; another method involves the use of a sharp drill bit and osteotomy completion with an osteotome.

Oblique Osteotomy

Oblique osteotomies correct translational deformities when gaining length is desired and can also be used to correct combined deformities including angular and rotational components. Combined deformity will be discussed later.

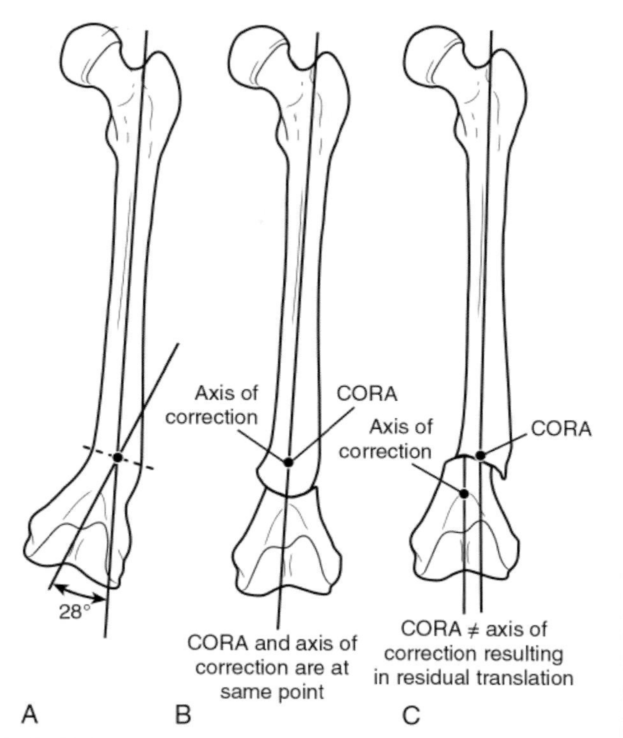

Figure 12 **A**, Distal femoral malunion is shown. **B**, If the axis of correction is at the center of rotational angle (CORA) then alignment without translation can be achieved. **C**, However, if the dome osteotomy goes through the CORA and the axis of correction is away from the CORA, then a secondary translational deformity will occur.

Treatment by Deformity Type

Angulation

Acute correction of angular deformity can be achieved with wedge or dome osteotomies. Angular deformity components of a combined deformity with angulation and rotation can be managed with an oblique osteotomy. Gradual correction can be achieved with an Ilizarov-type tensioned small wire ring fixator. Gradual correction also can be achieved with transverse osteotomy if length is being added as well or if an opening wedge correction is planned. Gradual correction of angular deformity alone with a dome osteotomy may result in early consolidation because of the large surface area of opposing segments.

Rotation

Rotational deformities can be corrected acutely with a transverse osteotomy and internal or external fixation. Gradual correction can be achieved with external fixation. Rotational malunion correction can be made at various levels.[18-21] The level of the osteotomy may be affected by

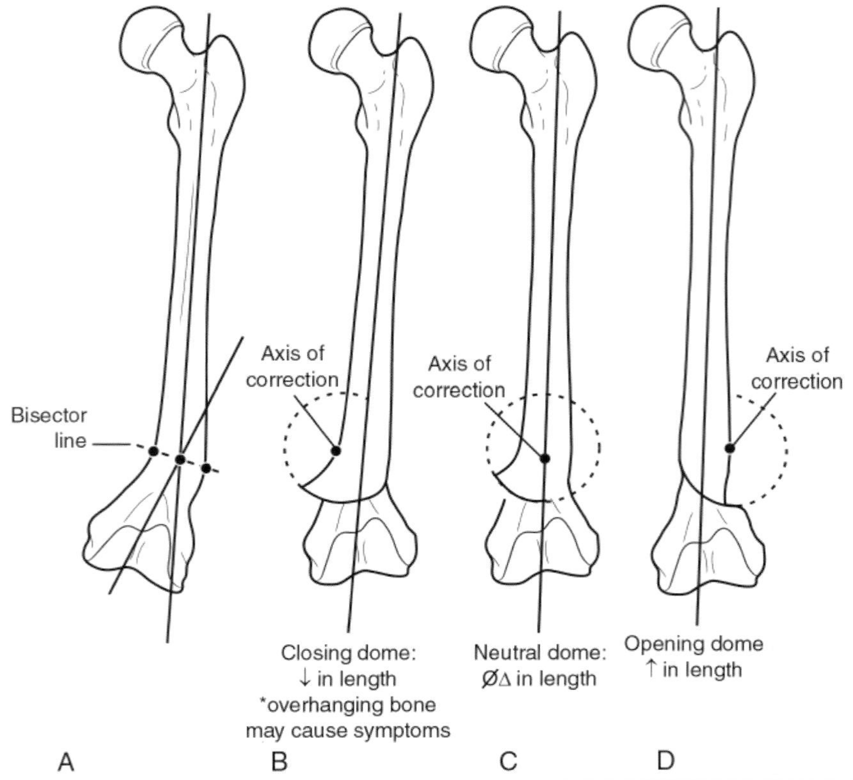

Figure 13 Drawings depict axis of correction with dome osteotomy. **A**, If the axis of correction is on the bisector line of the center of rotational angle (CORA), then angular correction can be achieved without secondary translational deformity. **B**, When the axis of correction is on the concave side of the deformity, some shortening will occur as well as possible symptomatic overhanging bone. The deformity as well as the bisector line/CORA is shown. **C**, A dome osteotomy with the axis of correction centered on the CORA will result in no change in length with good bony contact and correction of angular deformity without secondary translational deformity. **D**, If the axis of correction is on the convex side of the deformity then length is gained although the bony contact is diminished and may require bone graft.

surrounding soft tissues/neurovascular structures, bone healing potential, or muscular origins/insertions.

Length

Most patients can tolerate lower extremity length discrepancies up to 2 cm with a shoe insert. Discrepancies up to 4 cm can be managed with a shoe sole lift, although some patients have difficulty with this method of treatment.[22-26] Patients with discrepancies greater than 4 cm generally benefit from length correction.[22-26] Upper extremity length discrepancies are better tolerated up to 4 cm. Length discrepancy in the upper extremities of more than 4 cm has been reported to be successfully treated with length correction.[27,28]

Length deformities can be treated acutely depending on the magnitude and direction of deformity and the surrounding soft-tissue envelope. Acute distraction can generally be done safely up to 2 cm. Distracting the respective bone ends and filling the void with bone graft can achieve acute lengthening (**Figure 14, A**). Alternatively, a step-cut osteotomy can allow acute lengthening without creating bony discontinuity (**Figure 14, B**). Stabilization can be achieved with intramedullary fixation or a plate-and-screw construct. Usually this process can be made easier with a universal distractor to achieve length intraoperatively. Length can also be restored gradually (**Figure 14, C**). Success has also been reported for gradual lengthening with a lengthening nail.[29,30] Alternatively, acute shortening can be achieved with the same techniques if the surrounding soft-tissue envelope will allow it. Although acute lengthening is limited more by potential risk to neurovascular structures, acute shortening is primarily limited by surrounding soft tissue. More compliant soft-tissue envelopes, such as the thigh and upper arm, generally are more forgiving with acute shortening as opposed to a thinner envelope, as seen in the leg. In the forearm and the leg, osteotomy or partial excision to allow shortening and compression of the bone in question

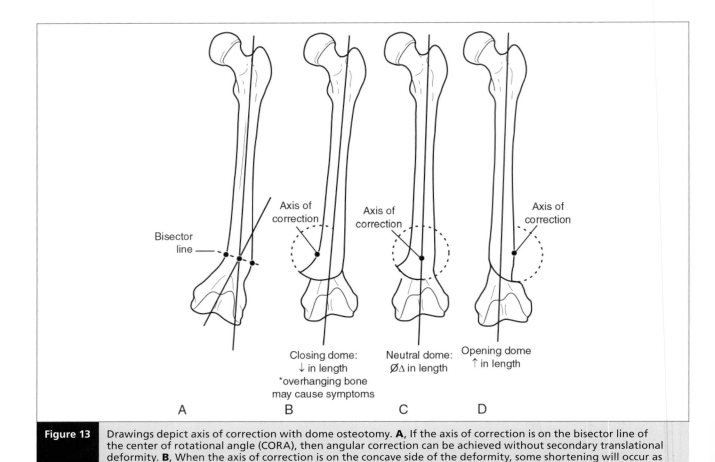

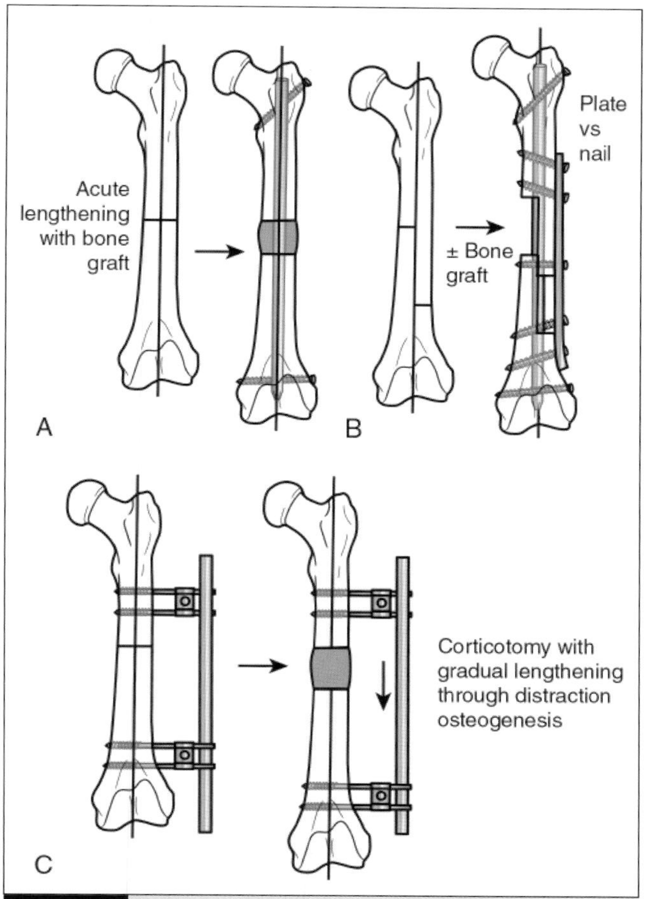

Figure 14 Drawings depict acute lengthening achieved by making a transverse osteotomy and filling the void with bone graft (**A**) or by making a step-cut osteotomy (**B**). Both osteotomy types can be stabilized with intramedullary fixation, external fixation, or a plate-and-screw construct. Gradual lengthening can be achieved with a corticotomy and lengthening through distraction osteogenesis (**C**).

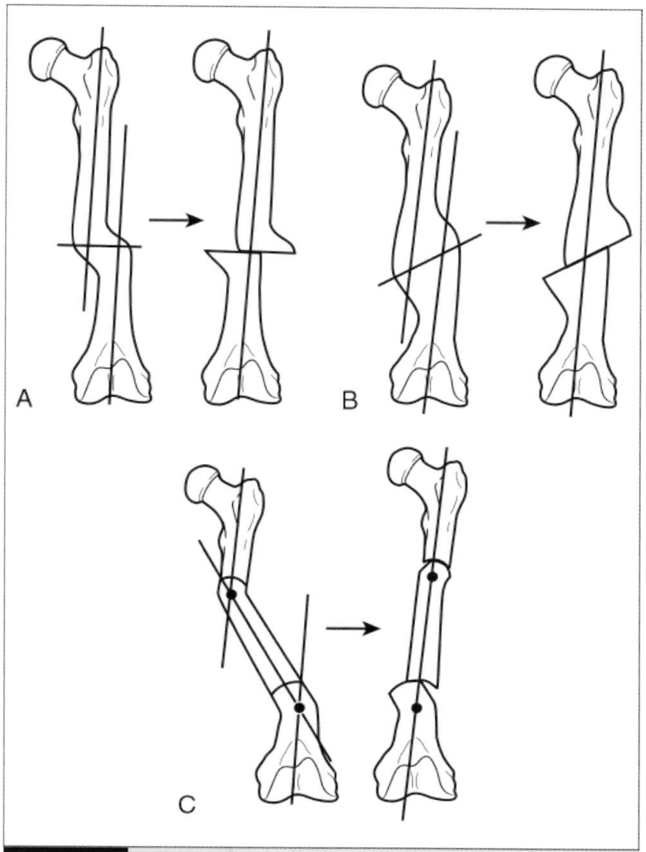

Figure 15 Drawings depict correction of translational deformities. **A**, A transverse osteotomy is shown; the overall length of the bone in question is unchanged. **B**, An oblique osteotomy, which can add length, is shown. **C**, Multiple angular deformities of equal magnitude can result in an overall translational deformity, which can be corrected by addressing both angular deformities.

will help avoid obstruction of length correction. This most commonly occurs in the tibia with a partial fibulectomy to allow acute shortening and compression of the tibia.

Translation

Translational deformities can be corrected with a transverse osteotomy, which does not change the overall length of the bone in question (**Figure 15, A**), whereas an oblique osteotomy can add length (**Figure 15, B**). Transverse osteotomies can be made at the level of the deformity or away from the deformity and still correct the overall alignment, whereas oblique osteotomies should be made at the level of the deformity. In some cases multiple angular deformities of equal magnitude can result in an overall translational deformity, which can be corrected by addressing both angular deformities (**Figure 15, C**).

Treatment of Combined Deformity

All combined deformities can be treated gradually with external fixation. Although a tensioned small wire ring fixator is capable of correcting any combination of deformities, monolateral fixators can be used to correct angular/rotational/length deformities, although the construct is not as stable and does not tolerate weight bearing as well as tensioned wire ring fixators. Combined deformities can also be treated acutely with the clamshell osteotomy[31] (**Figure 16**).

Acute Correction of Angulation and Rotation

Acute correction of angular deformity with associated rotational deformity can be achieved with an oblique osteotomy.[32-34] The procedure involves rotating the distal

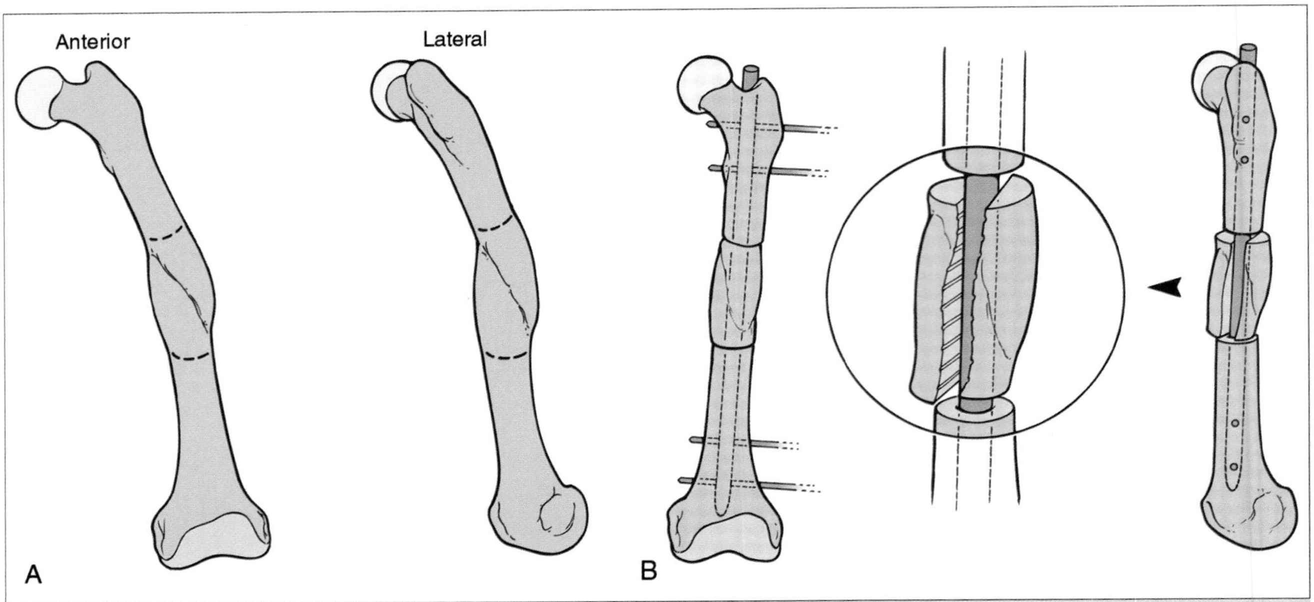

Figure 16 Drawings depict the clamshell osteotomy. (Reproduced with permission from Russell GV, Graves ML, Archdeacon MT, Barei DP, Brien GA Jr, Porter SE: The clamshell osteotomy: A new technique to correct complex diaphyseal malunions. Surgical technique. *J Bone Joint Surg Am* 2010;92[1][suppl 1, pt 2]:158-175.)

bone segment through the plane of the osteotomy with the correction axis centered on the CORA to simultaneously correct both deformities. Fluoroscopic views of the bone in question with maximal angular deformity as well as the orthogonal view without angular deformity are needed. The plane of the osteotomy is initially oriented perpendicular to the maximal angular deformity (**Figure 17, A and B**). Osteotomy angulation is calculated by arctan (angulation/rotation). The rotation to correct both deformities occurs about the axis of inclination, which is perpendicular to the osteotomy angulation. The axis of inclination can be calculated as arctan (rotation/angulation). Next, the rotational component of the deformity is accounted for by rotating the axis one-half of the magnitude of rotational deformity in the opposite direction of the rotational deformity (**Figure 17, C**). The magnitude of rotational correction about the axis of inclination can be calculated by using the graphic method with rotation on the x-axis and angulation on the y-axis. The point at which both sides intersect allows measurement of the osteotomy angle and the magnitude of rotational correction (**Figure 17, D**). After the osteotomy is made, the distal bone segment is rotated around the axis of inclination. In the example seen in **Figure 17** a combined deformity with 45° of angulation and 25° of external rotation results in the following calculated values[34]:

Axis inclination: arctan (25/45) = 29°

Osteotomy angle: arctan (45/25) = 61°

Magnitude of rotational component: (rotation/2) made in the opposite direction of the deformity (in this case external rotation). In this case an external rotation deformity of 25° translates into a 12.5° internal rotation change to the axis of the osteotomy.

Magnitude of angular correction about the axis of inclination: using the graphical method, a triangle is created with 25° (rotation) on the x-axis, 45° (angulation) on the y-axis, and a hypotenuse of 51°: ($a^2 + b^2 = c^2$). This means that the distal bone segment will be rotated 51° through the oblique osteotomy site to achieve correction of both the angular and rotational deformities.

Correction of Length and Angulation

Depending on the magnitude of length deformity, angulation and length can be managed with an opening or closing wedge osteotomy, although correction of length is limited by the amount of angular deformity as shortening/lengthening is equal to one-half the base of the wedge resected, so depending on the diameter of the bone at the level of the osteotomy, the amount of length change is proportionate with greater length changes effected in wider metaphyseal bone because the base of the wedge is larger (**Figure 18**).

Correction of Length and Translation

As previously mentioned, an oblique osteotomy can restore length as well as translation, but this is limited to the magnitude of deformity (**Figure 15, B**).

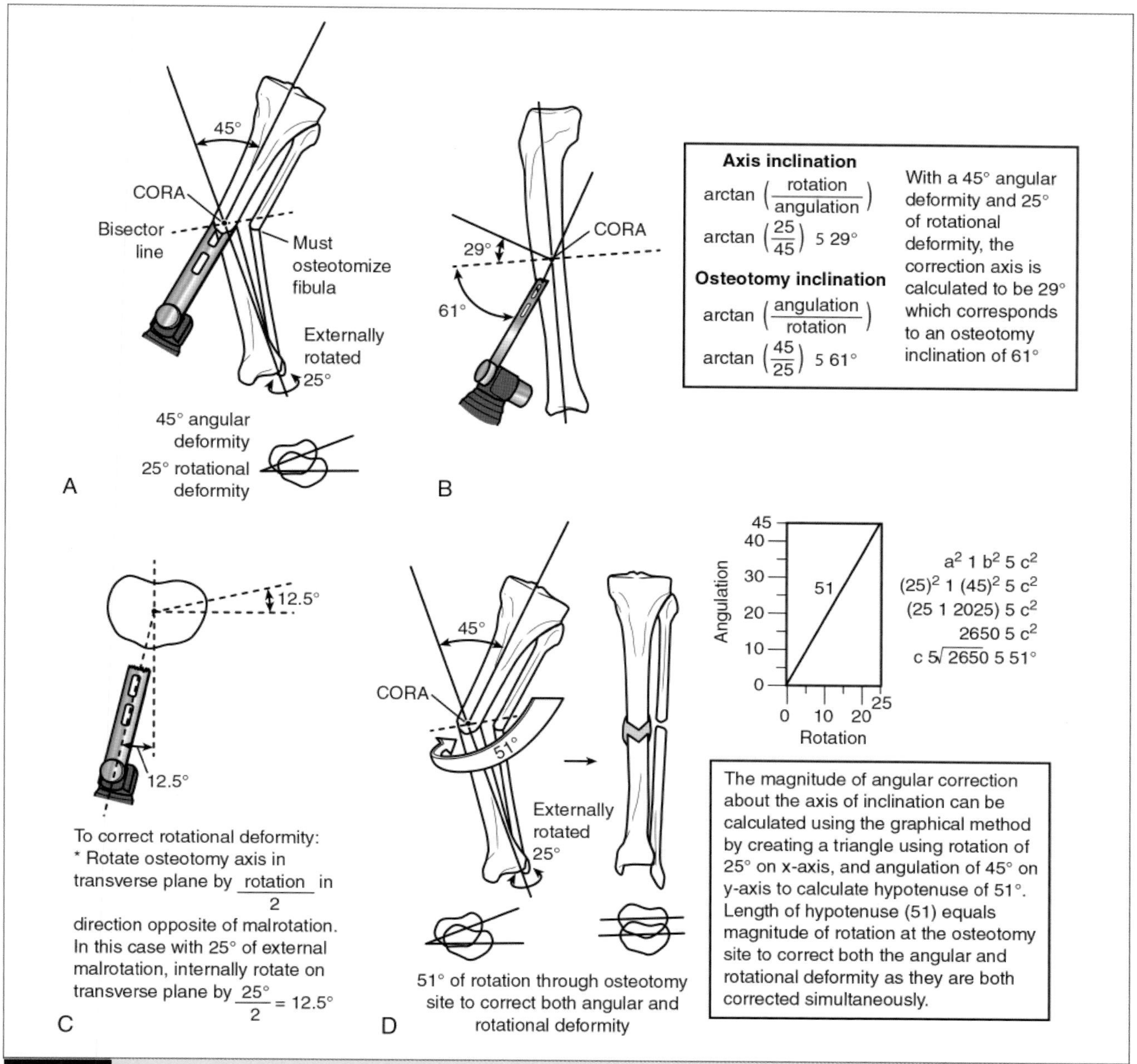

45°
CORA
Bisector line
Must osteotomize fibula
Externally rotated 25°
45° angular deformity
25° rotational deformity
A
29°
CORA
61°
B
Axis inclination
arctan (rotation/angulation)
arctan (25/45) 5 29°
Osteotomy inclination
arctan (angulation/rotation)
arctan (45/25) 5 61°
With a 45° angular deformity and 25° of rotational deformity, the correction axis is calculated to be 29° which corresponds to an osteotomy inclination of 61°
12.5°
12.5°
To correct rotational deformity:
* Rotate osteotomy axis in transverse plane by rotation/2 in direction opposite of malrotation.
In this case with 25° of external malrotation, internally rotate on transverse plane by 25°/2 = 12.5°
C
45°
CORA
51°
Externally rotated 25°
51° of rotation through osteotomy site to correct both angular and rotational deformity
D
Angulation
Rotation
51
a2 1 b2 5 c2
(25)2 1 (45)2 5 c2
(25 1 2025) 5 c2
2650 5 c2
c 5√2650 5 51°
The magnitude of angular correction about the axis of inclination can be calculated using the graphical method by creating a triangle using rotation of 25° on x-axis, and angulation of 45° on y-axis to calculate hypotenuse of 51°. Length of hypotenuse (51) equals magnitude of rotation at the osteotomy site to correct both the angular and rotational deformity as they are both corrected simultaneously.

Figure 17 Drawings depict an example of a single oblique osteotomy to correct a combined angular and rotational deformity with a 45° valgus angulation and 25° external rotational deformity. **A**, The center of rotational angle (CORA) (bisector line) is established. **B**, Fluoroscopic views of the bone in question with maximal angular deformity as well as the 90° view without angular deformity should be visualized. The plane of the osteotomy is initially oriented perpendicular to the maximal angular deformity. To calculate the inclination of the osteotomy one must calculate arctan (angulation/rotation). In this case, arctan (45/25) = 61°. Similarly, to calculate the axis of correction inclination one must calculate arctan (rotation/angulation). In this case, arctan (25/45) = 29°. **C**, After the osteotomy inclination is determined (in this case 61°), the rotational component of the osteotomy can be calculated. Because the deformity is 25° of external rotation, the plane of the corrective osteotomy should be rotated by 50% of the magnitude of rotational deformity in the opposite direction. In this case, a 25° external rotation deformity would result in internal rotation of the plane of the corrective osteotomy of 12.5°. So the saw blade would be internally rotated 12.5°, then 61° going from distal and anterior to proximal and posterior to establish the orientation of the osteotomy. **D**, After the osteotomy is made the magnitude of rotation through the osteotomy is calculated by the graphical method where the degree of angulation is on the y-axis (45°) and the magnitude of rotation is on the x-axis (25°), which allows the area above and below the line to be calculated: $a^2 + b^2 = c^2$, where $a = 25$, $b = 45$ and c is the hypotenuse. $25^2 + 45^2 = c^2$. c = square root of (2650), which equals 51°.

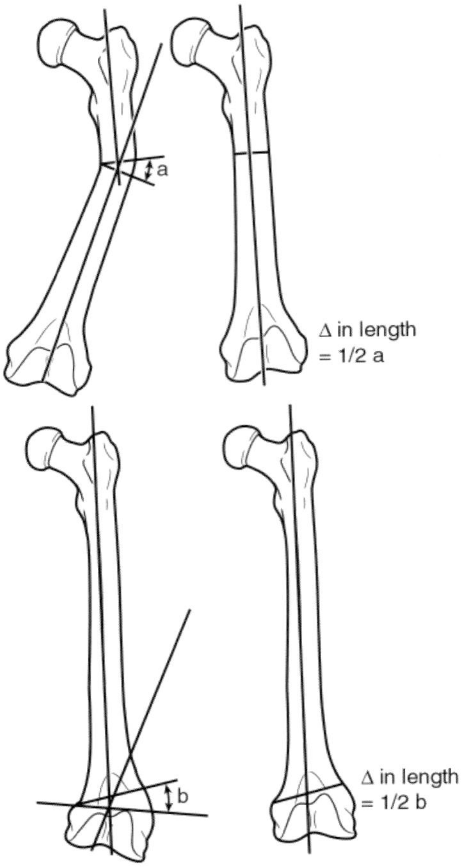

Figure 18 Drawings depict an example of angulation and minor length discrepancies addressed with an opening or closing wedge osteotomy, although correction of length is limited by the amount of angular deformity as shortening/lengthening is equal to one-half the base of the wedge resected, so depending on the diameter of the bone at the level of the osteotomy, the amount of length change is proportionate, with greater length changes effected in wider metaphyseal bone as the base of the wedge is larger.

Treatment According to Deformity Location

In general, deformity location may influence the type of osteotomy and fixation construct. Deformities in the diaphyseal region generally have relatively smaller-diameter cortical bone segments, which allow angular and translational deformities to be easily seen with radiographs. In the diaphyseal region, correction of angular deformities can reliably be achieved with wedge osteotomies through the CORA/bisector line. Intramedullary fixation can assist in the maintenance of alignment by realigning the medullary canal, which is essentially equivalent to the anatomic axis for the proximal and distal segments. The load-sharing characteristics of intramedullary fixation make it a good option for acute corrections in diaphyseal bone, although plate-and-screw or external fixation constructs can also be used.

For deformities occurring closer to the joint in the metaphyseal or epiphyseal region, correction and fixation can be difficult. Periarticular deformities often require joint orientation angles to properly identify and characterize the deformity; these angles can be calculated by imaging of the unaffected limb or from population-generated averages as seen in **Table 1**. Proximity to the joint may also limit options for osteotomy or fixation. Ligamentous attachments, tendon origins/insertions, and neurovascular anatomy may limit the ability to perform the correction at the level of the deformity, potentially requiring the osteotomy/correction axis to be at a point other than the CORA/bisector line. In addition, limited bone stock in the periarticular region may limit fixation construct options. Anatomic plate-and-screw constructs as well as blade plates can be used for periarticular fixation if an acute correction is performed, whereas a tensioned small wire ring fixator is extremity versatile in obtaining fixation in small periarticular bone segments and can be used for acute and gradual correction.

Treatment of Intra-articular Malunion

CT can help evaluate intra-articular malunions. The decision to treat an intra-articular malunion with corrective osteotomy may depend on the salvage options for each specific joint involved. An acetabular malunion can be treated with a total hip arthroplasty rather than corrective osteotomy if substantial posttraumatic arthritis has resulted from the malunion. Intra-articular malunions of the distal femur or proximal tibia may affect the overall alignment of the limb, and correction of alignment in addition to restoration of the articular congruity may be required.[8] Proximal tibial plateau malunions can affect overall alignment and can be corrected with an opening wedge osteotomy (**Figure 19**). A sagittal split in the distal femur or proximal tibia can be corrected with restoration of articular congruity as well as alignment.

Treatment of Acetabular and Pelvic Ring Malunion

Acetabular malunion can manifest as pain related to joint incongruity and can be treated early with corrective osteotomy but most often can be treated with total hip arthroplasty if the posttraumatic arthritis is advanced.[19,35,36] Pelvic ring malunions can manifest clinically with chronic pain, dyspareunia, sexual problems of mechanical origin, sitting imbalance, or gait abnormalities resulting from relative lower extremity length discrepancy.[36-38] Pelvic ring, and acetabular malunions require

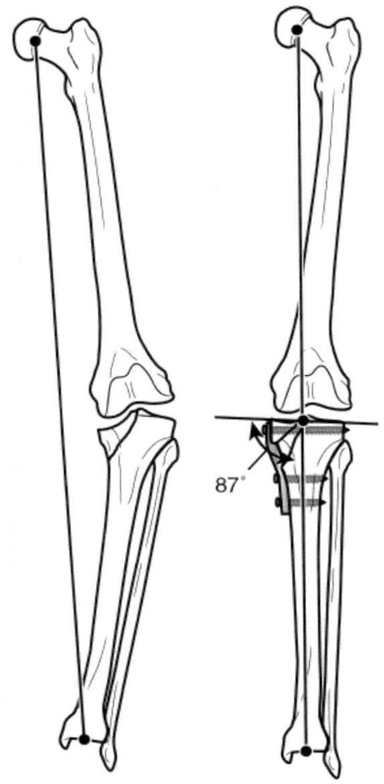

Figure 19 Drawings depict how an intra-articular proximal tibial malunion can affect overall alignment and can be corrected with an opening wedge osteotomy. This opening wedge tibial osteotomy can be used to correct articular congruity as well as alignment. In this example, the goal of the osteotomy is to restore the medial proximal tibial angle.

complex osteotomy procedures and should be treated by a specialist in pelvis/hip preservation or reconstruction.

Treatment Methods

Plate-and Screw-Construct

The plate-and-screw construct is advantageous because of its utility in periarticular locations and its ability to provide rigid fixation with the potential for interfragmentary compression. Disadvantages include the requirement for extensive soft-tissue dissection and restricted early weight bearing. A periarticular anatomically contoured locked plating is particularly useful for small bone segments close to the joint, possibly excluding intramedullary fixation as an option.

Intramedullary Nail

Intramedullary nails have optimal load-sharing characteristics and can help restore intramedullary alignment, which secondarily helps correct angular and translational deformity. These qualities make intramedullary nails ideal for acute correction of lower extremity diaphyseal or metadiaphyseal malunions, whereas use is limited in periarticular malunions.

Table 2

Advantages of the Ilizarov Technique

Minimally invasive/percutaneous bony fixation with minimal soft-tissue dissection
Capable of correcting angular, length, rotational, translational, or a combination of these deformities acutely or gradually
Obviates the need for bone graft in the setting of correction of a shortened deformity with distraction osteogenesis
Capable of bony fixation in small periarticular bone segments
External bony fixation remote from the deformity allows this technique to be used in the setting of infection
Deformity correction can be adjusted over time
Allows for immediate weight bearing as weight is distributed from the bone to the tensioned wires, then across the frame via struts or threaded rods, and back to the distal bone segment via tensioned wires; the tensioned wires also allow axial loading/unloading to be experienced at the osteotomy/corticotomy site with weight bearing
Versatile in terms of anatomic location, deformity type, and soft-tissue status where an open procedure may not be possible and limited to a lesser degree by soft tissue

Tensioned Small Wire Ring Fixator

Tensioned small wire ring fixator or Ilizarov techniques allow versatility in the treatment of angular, length, rotational, translational, or any combination of these deformities.[8,9,39-43] Advantages of the Ilizarov technique are outlined in **Table 2**. The primary disadvantage of this technique is patient inconvenience: the frame is usually in place for months and requires consistent patient compliance and regular follow-up.

Distraction Osteogenesis

In cases where restoration of length is required, distraction osteogenesis is a useful technique because the patient can bear weight throughout the process, no bone grafting is required, and substantial length corrections can be made.[39,42,44-47] Distraction causes cell proliferation, bone generation through intramembranous osteogenesis, and vascular proliferation through a tension-stress effect.

Following corticotomy (which is different from osteotomy) and lengthening, a substantial increase in blood flow has been documented.[48,49] To minimize necrosis at the corticotomy site, a low-energy osteotomy technique should be used, such as a Gigli saw or drill holes followed by osteotome without completely disrupting the intramedullary canal/intraosseous blood supply. Distraction osteogenesis ideally is performed at the metaphyseal or metadiaphyseal region because bone regenerate formation is more robust in these regions. Considering that these frames may be in place for months or years in extreme cases, it is important to consider the long-term stability of the construct and that good frame application techniques be followed. Although techniques vary among experts in this particular area of orthopaedic surgery, a latency period of 1 to 3 weeks is recommended before distraction to allow the beginning of regenerate formation. Because the formation of bone is different in every patient, the treating surgeon should monitor and progress at a rate suitable for each individual patient. The rate of distraction will be different for a healthy high school student compared with a 65-year-old individual with diabetes mellitus who has a suboptimal vascular status. Usually a rate of 1 mm per day is a good place to start and can be modified depending on the regenerate seen on follow-up radiographs. Most cases require approximately two to three times the amount of time required for the distraction phase to allow solid consolidation of the regenerate. This requires the regenerate to reestablish a cortex and regenerate hypertrophy, which occurs with weight transfer through the regenerate segment, which is allowed by the "trampoline effect" of the tensioned wire construct. Foreshortened hypertrophic nonunions can also be treated with distraction osteogenesis.[49,50]

Current systems allow for complex combined deformities to be simultaneously corrected with the use of telescopic struts. The Taylor Spatial Frame has been the most widely used version of this type of tensioned small wire ring fixator, although other systems are available. The Taylor Spatial Frame uses a software program to guide the deformity correction.[43,51-58] The deformity can be corrected by placing ring segments perpendicular to the proximal and distal bone segments that are gradually adjusted to achieve parallel rings and realigned bone segments. Any residual deformity can be accounted for during the deformity correction process. Each case must be approached with respect to its unique deformity, soft-tissue status, physiologic healing potential, and regenerate formation capacity.

Summary

To effectively treat malunited fractures, the surgeon must have a thorough understanding of the clinical and radiographic evaluation of the malunion as well as the various treatment options. Careful patient selection is crucial and includes detailed clinical and radiographic evaluation. Radiographic evaluation of malunions requires a thorough understanding of limb alignment, mechanical axes, anatomic axes, joint orientation lines/angles, CORA, and correction axes. Symptomatic malunions can result from deformities including shortening, translation, angulation, and rotational malalignment or a combined deformity when they impair function or cause pain. Proper treatment requires accurate characterization of the malunion (location, severity, and direction of deformity). Symptomatic malunions can be treated acutely versus gradually using internal versus external fixation and with various osteotomy types, including transverse, wedge, oblique, step-cut, and dome osteotomies.

Key Study Points

- An understanding of principal components regarding the clinical and radiographic evaluation of malunions, including assessment of deformity type, is important to guide treatment.
- Osteotomy type, gradual or acute correction, and internal or external fixation are important factors related to treatment strategy.

Annotated References

1. Tarr RR, Resnick CT, Wagner KS, Sarmiento A: Changes in tibiotalar joint contact areas following experimentally induced tibial angular deformities. *Clin Orthop Relat Res* 1985;199:72-80.

2. Puno RM, Vaughan JJ, Stetten ML, Johnson JR: Long-term effects of tibial angular malunion on the knee and ankle joints. *J Orthop Trauma* 1991;5(3):247-254.

3. McKellop HA, Llinás A, Sarmiento A: Effects of tibial malalignment on the knee and ankle. *Orthop Clin North Am* 1994;25(3):415-423.

4. Ting AJ, Tarr RR, Sarmiento A, Wagner K, Resnick C: The role of subtalar motion and ankle contact pressure changes from angular deformities of the tibia. *Foot Ankle* 1987;7(5):290-299.

5. Paley D, Tetsworth K: Mechanical axis deviation of the lower limbs: preoperative planning of uniapical angular

deformities of the tibia or femur. *Clin Orthop Relat Res* 1992;280:48-64.

6. Wu DD, Burr DB, Boyd RD, Radin EL: Bone and cartilage changes following experimental varus or valgus tibial angulation. *J Orthop Res* 1990;8(4):572-585.

7. Probe RA: Lower extremity angular malunion: Evaluation and surgical correction. *J Am Acad Orthop Surg* 2003;11(5):302-311.

8. Paley D: Principles of deformity correction, in Browner BD, Jupiter JB, Levine AM, Trafton PG, eds: *Skeletal Trauma* .Philadelphia, PA, WB Saunders, 2003, pp 2519-2576.

9. Brinker MR, O'Connor DP: Principles of malunions, in Court-Brown CM, Heckman JD, McQueen MM, Ricci WM, Tornetta P III, McKee MD, eds: *Rockwood and Green's Fractures in Adults* , ed 8. Philadelphia, PA, Lippincott Williams & Wilkins, 2014, vol I, pp 869-894.

10. Wissing H, Buddenbrock B: Determining rotational errors of the femur by axial computerized tomography in comparison with clinical and conventional radiologic determination [German]. *Unfallchirurgie* 1993;19(3):145-157.

11. Jaarsma RL, Pakvis DF, Verdonschot N, Biert J, van Kampen A: Rotational malalignment after intramedullary nailing of femoral fractures. *J Orthop Trauma* 2004;18(7):403-409.

12. Staheli LT, Corbett M, Wyss C, King H: Lower-extremity rotational problems in children: Normal values to guide management. *J Bone Joint Surg Am* 1985;67(1):39-47.

13. Brinker MR, Gugenheim JJ, O'Connor DP, London JC: Ilizarov correction of malrotated femoral shaft fracture initially treated with an intramedullary nail: A case report. *Am J Orthop (Belle Mead NJ)* 2004;33(10):489-493.

14. Dugdale TW, Degnan GG, Turen CH: The use of computed tomographic scan to assess femoral malrotation after intramedullary nailing: A case report. *Clin Orthop Relat Res* 1992;279:258-263.

15. Carey RP, de Campo JF, Menelaus MB: Measurement of leg length by computerised tomographic scanography: Brief report. *J Bone Joint Surg Br* 1987;69(5):846-847.

16. Ilizarov GA: Pseudoarthrosis and defects of long bones, in Ilizarov GA, ed: *Transosseous Osteosynthesis: Theoretical and Clinical Aspects of Regeneration and Growth of Tissue* .Berlin, Germany, Springer-Verlag, 1992, pp 453-494.

17. Paley D, Maar DC: Ilizarov bone transport treatment for tibial defects. *J Orthop Trauma* 2000;14(2):76-85.

18. Krengel WF III, Staheli LT: Tibial rotational osteotomy for idiopathic torsion: A comparison of the proximal and distal osteotomy levels. *Clin Orthop Relat Res* 1992;28(283):285-289.

19. Barker B, Staples K: Malunions, in Archdeacon MT, Anglen JO, Ostrum RF, Herscovici D Jr, eds: *Prevention and Management of Common Fracture Complications.* Thorofare, NJ, SLACK Incorporated, 2012, pp 53-66.

    The fundamental concepts regarding the prevention and management of common fracture complications are reviewed.

20. Inan M, Ferri-de Baros F, Chan G, Dabney K, Miller F: Correction of rotational deformity of the tibia in cerebral palsy by percutaneous supramalleolar osteotomy. *J Bone Joint Surg Br* 2005;87(10):1411-1415.

21. Pirpiris M, Trivett A, Baker R, Rodda J, Nattrass GR, Graham HK: Femoral derotation osteotomy in spastic diplegia: Proximal or distal? *J Bone Joint Surg Br* 2003;85(2):265-272.

22. Bhave A, Paley D, Herzenberg JE: Improvement in gait parameters after lengthening for the treatment of limb-length discrepancy. *J Bone Joint Surg Am* 1999;81(4):529-534.

23. Brady RJ, Dean JB, Skinner TM, Gross MT: Limb length inequality: Clinical implications for assessment and intervention. *J Orthop Sports Phys Ther* 2003;33(5):221-234.

24. Friend L, Widmann RF: Advances in management of limb length discrepancy and lower limb deformity. *Curr Opin Pediatr* 2008;20(1):46-51.

25. McCarthy JJ, MacEwen GD: Management of leg length inequality. *J South Orthop Assoc* 2001;10(2):73-85, discussion 85.

26. Vitale MA, Choe JC, Sesko AM, et al: The effect of limb length discrepancy on health-related quality of life: Is the '2 cm rule' appropriate? *J Pediatr Orthop B* 2006;15(1):1-5.

27. Damsin JP, Ghanem I: Upper limb lengthening. *Hand Clin* 2000;16(4):685-701.

28. Raimondo RA, Skaggs DL, Rosenwasser MP, Dick HM: Lengthening of pediatric forearm deformities using the Ilizarov technique: Functional and cosmetic results. *J Hand Surg Am* 1999;24(2):331-338.

29. Horn J, Grimsrud Ø, Dagsgard AH, Huhnstock S, Steen H: Femoral lengthening with a motorized intramedullary nail. *Acta Orthop* 2015;86(2):248-256.

    A matched comparison of 30 femoral lengthenings with 15 using a motorized intramedullary nail and 15 using a ring fixator was performed to determine whether there would be fewer problems in the nail group than in the external fixator group. A larger number of complications were noted in the external fixator group, which consisted of nine pin tract infections that all resolved with oral antibiotic drug therapy. One superficial infection was noted in the nail group that also resolved with oral antibiotic drug therapy. Outcomes in terms of length restoration were similar between both groups. Range of motion returned faster in the nail group as well. Although this study showed fewer complications in the nail group, there are limitations in terms of the degree of deformity correction compared with a ring fixator.

30. Kirane YM, Fragomen AT, Rozbruch SR: Precision of the PRECICE internal bone lengthening nail. *Clin Orthop Relat Res* 2014;472(12):3869-3878.

    This retrospective study reviewed the results of 17 femoral and 8 tibial lengthening procedures done with a mechanically lengthening intramedullary nail with a magnet-operated internal lengthening device consisting of a magnet connected to a gear box and screw shaft assembly. The lengthening is controlled by an external controller unit. Cases were evaluated for accuracy of distraction, effects on adjacent joints, and complications. All of the cases achieved their respective lengthening goals (mean, 35 mm). Removal of the nail is recommended once adequate consolidation occurs, and patients are recommended to avoid MRI until the nail is removed due to the possibility of magnet interaction and risk of bodily injury as a result. Additional research is needed to follow up on this relatively small series.

31. Russell GV, Graves ML, Archdeacon MT, Barei DP, Brien GA Jr, Porter SE: The clamshell osteotomy: A new technique to correct complex diaphyseal malunions. Surgical technique. *J Bone Joint Surg Am* 2010;92(1)(suppl 1, pt 2):158-175.

    The clamshell osteotomy is described as a way to effectively correct diaphyseal malunions by realigning the anatomic axis of the long bone with the use of a reamed intramedullary nail as a template. The central intercalary segment created by two osteotomies is split to create two relative barrel staves between which the intramedullary nail is sandwiched. This technique provides an alternative option in the treatment of diaphyseal malunions.

32. Rab GT: Oblique tibial osteotomy for Blount's disease (tibia vara). *J Pediatr Orthop* 1988;8(6):715-720.

33. Sangeorzan BP, Judd RP, Sangeorzan BJ: Mathematical analysis of single-cut osteotomy for complex long bone deformity. *J Biomech* 1989;22(11-12):1271-1278.

34. Sanders R, Anglen JO, Mark JB: Oblique osteotomy for the correction of tibial malunion. *J Bone Joint Surg Am* 1995;77(2):240-246.

35. Matta JM, Dickson KF, Markovich GD: Surgical treatment of pelvic nonunions and malunions. *Clin Orthop Relat Res* 1996;329:199-206.

36. Marti RK: Malunion, in Redi TP, Buckley RE, Moran CG, eds: *AO Principles of Fracture Management* .New York, NY, Thieme, 2007, vol 1, pp 482-503.

37. Cole JD, Blum DA, Ansel LJ: Outcome after fixation of unstable posterior pelvic ring injuries. *Clin Orthop Relat Res* 1996;329:160-179.

38. Kanakaris NK, Angoules AG, Nikolaou VS, Kontakis G, Giannoudis PV: Treatment and outcomes of pelvic malunions and nonunions: A systematic review. *Clin Orthop Relat Res* 2009;467(8):2112-2124.

    This articles reviews the presenting symptoms of pelvic malunions and discusses the outcomes of pelvic malunion surgery.

39. Brinker MR, Gugenheim JJ: The treatment of complex traumatic problems of the forearm using Ilizarov external fixation. *Atlas Hand Clin* 2000;5(1):103-116.

40. Green SA: The Ilizarov method, in Browner BD, Jupiter JB, Levine AM, Trafton PG, eds: *Skeletal Trauma: Fractures, Dislocations, Ligamentous Injuries* , ed 2. Philadephia, PA, WB Saunders, 1998,vol 1, pp 661-701.

41. Gugenheim JJ Jr, Brinker MR: Bone realignment with use of temporary external fixation for distal femoral valgus and varus deformities. *J Bone Joint Surg Am* 2003;85(7):1229-1237.

42. Ilizarov GA: The principles of the Ilizarov method. *Bull Hosp Jt Dis Orthop Inst* 1988;48(1):1-11.

43. Feldman DS, Shin SS, Madan S, Koval KJ: Correction of tibial malunion and nonunion with six-axis analysis deformity correction using the Taylor Spatial Frame. *J Orthop Trauma* 2003;17(8):549-554.

44. Ilizarov GA: The tension-stress effect on the genesis and growth of tissues: Part I. The influence of stability of fixation and soft-tissue preservation. *Clin Orthop Relat Res* 1989;238:249-281.

45. Ilizarov GA: The tension-stress effect on the genesis and growth of tissues: Part II. The influence of the rate and frequency of distraction. *Clin Orthop Relat Res* 1989;239:263-285.

46. Marsh DR, Shah S, Elliott J, Kurdy N: The Ilizarov method in nonunion, malunion and infection of fractures. *J Bone Joint Surg Br* 1997;79(2):273-279.

47. Paley D, Chaudray M, Pirone AM, Lentz P, Kautz D: Treatment of malunions and mal-nonunions of the femur and tibia by detailed preoperative planning and the Ilizarov techniques. *Orthop Clin North Am* 1990;21(4):667-691.

48. Aronson J: Temporal and spatial increases in blood flow during distraction osteogenesis. *Clin Orthop Relat Res* 1994;301:124-131.

49. Murray JH, Fitch RD: Distraction histiogenesis: Principles and indications. *J Am Acad Orthop Surg* 1996;4(6):317-327.

50. Rozbruch SR, Helfet DL, Blyakher A: Distraction of hypertrophic nonunion of tibia with deformity using Ilizarov/Taylor Spatial Frame: Report of two cases. *Arch Orthop Trauma Surg* 2002;122(5):295-298.

51. Tetsworth KD, Paley D: Accuracy of correction of complex lower-extremity deformities by the Ilizarov method. *Clin Orthop Relat Res* 1994;301(301):102-110.

52. Eidelman M, Bialik V, Katzman A: Correction of deformities in children using the Taylor spatial frame. *J Pediatr Orthop B* 2006;15(6):387-395.

53. Fadel M, Hosny G: The Taylor spatial frame for deformity correction in the lower limbs. *Int Orthop* 2005;29(2):125-129.

54. Feldman DS, Madan SS, Koval KJ, van Bosse HJ, Bazzi J, Lehman WB: Correction of tibia vara with six-axis deformity analysis and the Taylor Spatial Frame. *J Pediatr Orthop* 2003;23(3):387-391.

55. Nakase T, Ohzono K, Shimizu N, Yoshikawa H: Correction of severe post-traumatic deformities in the distal femur by distraction osteogenesis using Taylor Spatial Frame: A case report. *Arch Orthop Trauma Surg* 2006;126(1):66-69.

56. Rogers MJ, McFadyen I, Livingstone JA, Monsell F, Jackson M, Atkins RM: Computer hexapod assisted orthopaedic surgery (CHAOS) in the correction of long bone fracture and deformity. *J Orthop Trauma* 2007;21(5):337-342.

57. Rozbruch SR, Fragomen AT, Ilizarov S: Correction of tibial deformity with use of the Ilizarov-Taylor spatial frame. *J Bone Joint Surg Am* 2006;88(suppl 4):156-174.

58. Taylor JC: Perioperative planning for two- and three-plane deformities. *Foot Ankle Clin* 2008;13(1):69-121, vi.

Chapter 12

Biologic Adjuvants for Fracture Healing

John W. Munz, MD   Patrick C. Schottel, MD

Abstract

Biologic adjuvants improve fracture healing by providing osteoconduction, osteoinduction, or osteogenic cells. Examples of biologic adjuvants include autogenous bone graft, allograft bone, demineralized bone matrix, platelet-rich plasma, autogenous bone marrow, calcium phosphate, calcium sulfate, parathyroid hormone, and bone morphogenetic protein. These adjuvants can be delivered both locally and systemically during the course of treatment and can maximize the healing capability of bone. The treating surgeon must possess a strong understanding of the biology of fracture healing and not violate basic fracture management principles. Although a useful tool, biologic adjuvants are not a substitute for a well-thought-out preoperative plan and surgical execution, but can aid the overall treatment strategy.

Keywords: autogenous bone graft; allograft bone; demineralized bone matrix (DBM); platelet-rich plasma (PRP); autogenous bone marrow; calcium phosphate; calcium sulfate; parathyroid hormone (PTH); bone morphogenetic protein (BMP); Wnt

Introduction

Biologic adjuvants are locally or systemically administered products that help improve the healing capability of bone. These adjuvants provide one or more of the following components necessary for fracture healing: osteoconduction, osteoinduction, or osteogenic cells. Osteoconductive grafts provide a scaffold that allows ingrowth of mesenchymal stem cells (MSCs) and blood vessels that are necessary for new bone formation. Osteoinductive materials provide the needed molecular signaling to initiate the differentiation of MSCs to osteoblasts. These molecular signals are typically provided by growth factors such as bone morphogenetic protein (BMP), platelet-derived growth factor, and vascular endothelial-derived growth factor. Osteogenesis occurs when a sufficient number of bone-forming cells are present at the fracture site. Autogenous bone graft and bone marrow are valuable sources of osteogenic cells.

Examples of biologic adjuvants include autogenous bone graft, allograft bone, demineralized bone matrix (DBM), platelet-rich plasma (PRP), autogenous bone marrow, calcium phosphate, calcium sulfate, parathyroid hormone (PTH), and BMP. Various options are available to orthopaedic trauma surgeons that may improve the biologic environment in the treatment of difficult-to-heal fractures, bone defects, and nonunions.

Dr. Munz or an immediate family member is a member of a speakers' bureau or has made paid presentations on behalf of Synthes. Neither Dr. Schottel nor any immediate family member has received anything of value from or has stock or stock options held in a commercial company or institution related directly or indirectly to the subject of this chapter.

Autogenous Adjuvants

Autogenous Bone Graft

Autogenous bone is the current gold standard for treating bone defects and nonunions. Autogenous bone is osteoconductive, osteoinductive, and contains numerous osteogenic cells. In addition to its biologic properties, autogenous bone graft carries no risk of disease transmission or immunologic rejection. The primary disadvantages of autogenous bone graft are the morbidity associated with its harvest, increased surgery time, and the quantitative limit of obtainable graft. Autogenous bone can be obtained as cancellous (iliac crest or long bone intramedullary reaming), corticocancellous, or cortical graft (nonvascularized or vascularized fibula). Cancellous autogenous graft is most commonly obtained

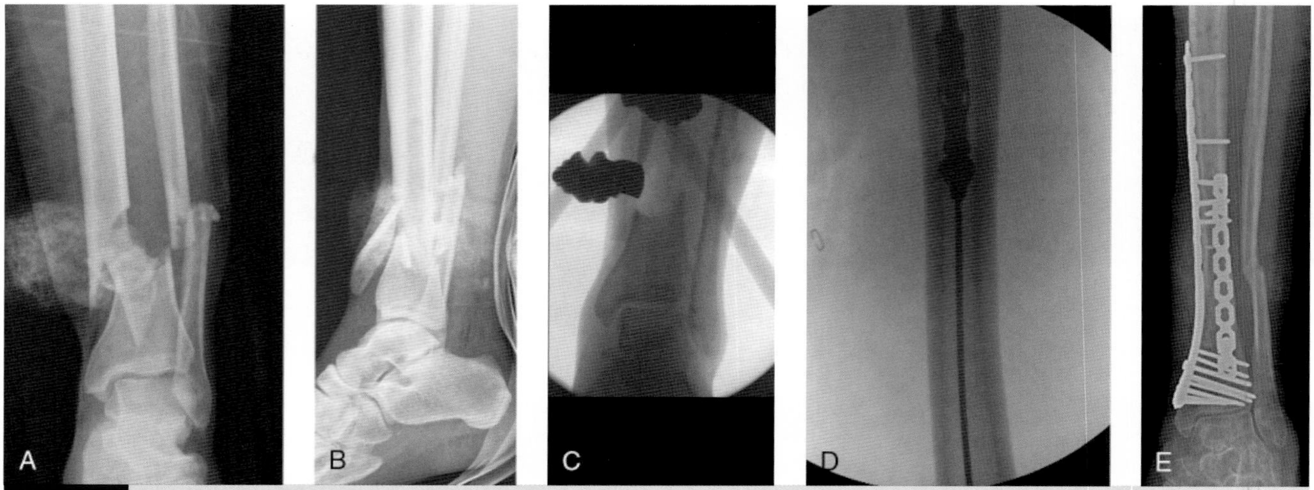

Figure 1 Images show fracture treatment with the Reamer/Irrigator/Aspirator. AP (**A**) and lateral (**B**) radiographs demonstrate an open type IIIb distal tibia fracture with gross contamination. **C,** Fluoroscopic view demonstrates placement of an ankle-spanning external fixation after initial irrigation and débridement of all nonviable bone. **D,** Fluoroscopic view shows that the Reamer/Irrigator/Aspirator autograft was later harvested from the patient's ipsilateral femur using an antegrade technique. **E,** AP radiograph obtained following delayed open reduction and internal fixation with the Reamer/Irrigator/Aspirator autograft resulted in osseous union.

from the iliac crest.[1] However, there is debate regarding the optimal iliac crest harvest location and whether cancellous autograft harvested from the medullary canal of long bones is superior to bone harvested from the iliac crest.[1]

Complications and functional outcomes of patients with long bone osteomyelitis undergoing a limb salvage procedure who had autogenous bone graft harvested from either the anterior or posterior iliac crest were compared.[2] After a minimum 2-year clinical follow-up, the overall complication rate was significantly higher in the anterior iliac crest harvest cohort than in the group with graft taken from the posterior iliac crest (23% versus 2%). Patients with anterior iliac crest bone harvest had greater postoperative pain and a longer duration of pain symptoms. However, patients in this series were not randomized between harvest sites and there was no significant difference in "major" complications between the two groups.

More recently, a new autogenous bone harvesting technique has been used to mitigate the potential complications or need for a separate prone positioning with iliac crest bone harvest. The Reamer/Irrigator/Aspirator (RIA; Synthes) is a sharp reaming device that continuously irrigates the intramedullary canal and aspirates cancellous bone that is collected in a filtration unit. The RIA is most commonly used in the femur with either an antegrade or retrograde technique. Recent studies have shown promising findings using the RIA (**Figure 1**). The histologic and transcriptional profile of bone graft obtained from the iliac crest and RIA were compared in a 2012 study.[3] Graft obtained by the RIA overexpressed genes associated with MSCs and bone growth factors (BMP-2) substantially more than graft harvested from the iliac crest. RIA autogenous bone graft was concluded to be a viable alternative to iliac crest bone graft (ICBG). A recent systematic review evaluated the overall complication rate of autogenous graft obtained from the iliac crest (anterior and posterior combined) versus RIA.[4] An overall complication rate of 19.4% in 6,449 patients undergoing iliac crest harvest and only 6% in 233 RIA patients were reported. In another study, 133 patients with nonunion or posttraumatic segmental bone defect requiring surgical intervention using either the RIA or ICBG were followed in a prospective randomized trial.[5] When compared with autograft obtained from the iliac crest, autograft harvested using the RIA achieved similar union rates with substantially less donor-site pain. In addition, RIA yielded a greater volume of graft (37.7 cm) compared with anterior ICBG (20.7 cm), whereas the volumes obtained with RIA and posterior ICBG were similar. RIA was also found to have a shorter harvest time compared with posterior ICBG, 29.4 minutes versus 40.6 minutes, respectively.

When autogenous graft is needed, the decision of location and method of graft harvest should depend on the surgeon's experience and specific clinical scenario including the patient's preference based on an informed discussion of the risks and benefits of each method.

Autogenous Bone Marrow

Bone marrow aspirate from the iliac crest is known to contain osteogenic stem cells. It can either be injected as a single agent or combined with osteoconductive materials such as DBM or allograft bone. Its advantages include low harvest-associated morbidity and percutaneous application when used alone.

A clinical study found that 17 of 20 patients (85%) with long bone nonunion were successfully treated with percutaneously injected bone marrow aspirate.[6] The patients averaged 10 months between injury and treatment and the bone marrow was harvested from the posterior iliac crest. Another clinical study published in 2013 reported an 82% union rate (9 of 11 patients) with percutaneously injected bone marrow aspirated from the posterior iliac crest.[7] In this study, 11 patients with distal metadiaphyseal tibia nonunions 8 months after the initial injury underwent treatment with 40–80 mL of unconcentrated marrow. The mean time to union was 4.1 months.

Recent research has focused on the number of progenitor cells in the bone marrow and its influence on clinical outcomes. In one study, 60 patients with atrophic tibial nonunions were treated by percutaneous injection of concentrated bone marrow aspirate from the anterior iliac crest.[8] The 53 patients who achieved osseous union had a significantly higher number of fibroblast colony-forming units than the 7 patients who had persistent nonunion. In a 2013 study, bone marrow aspirated from the posterior iliac crest had 1.6 times more MSCs than aspirate from the anterior iliac crest.[9] It was concluded that bone marrow should preferably be harvested from the posterior iliac crest. However, no clinical studies have compared the union rate of bone marrow aspirated from either the anterior or posterior iliac crest and therefore no definitive guideline has been established. The use of bone marrow aspirate in acute fracture care has not been studied and remains an area of potential future research.

Platelet-Rich Plasma

The platelet concentration of PRP typically is five times greater than that of blood.[10] The PRP component is typically isolated using a two-phase centrifugation process that separates the platelets from the larger blood cells.[11] Platelets lack nuclei but contain numerous other cellular organelles as well as granules that contain multiple growth factors and cytokines. In particular, the α-granule has been found to contain growth factors such as transforming growth factor (TGF), vascular endothelial growth factor, platelet-derived growth factor, insulin-like growth factor, and epidermal growth factor that are released upon activation. It is believed that these cytokines may aid in the process of bone, tendon, ligament, and muscle repair. However, evidence supporting the use of PRP for an acute or reconstructive trauma patient is limited.

The effect of BMP versus PRP in a clinical population of long bone nonunions was compared in a prospective randomized clinical study.[12] The authors randomized 120 atrophic nonunions to revision surgery with the addition of BMP-7 or PRP. Patients were followed clinically and radiographically for evidence of union. At an average clinical follow-up of 12.4 months, 87% of the BMP-7 cohort and 68% of the PRP group had obtained union. This difference was statistically significant. BMP-7 was found to be more effective than PRP in the treatment of atrophic long bone nonunion. Additional randomized trials are needed to evaluate the effectiveness of PRP as an adjuvant in acute fracture treatment.

Allogenous Adjuvants

Allogenous Bone Graft

Allograft bone is cadaver bone that can be used to fill cancellous voids or structural defects. It is commercially available as cancellous, corticocancellous, and structural grafts (fibular shaft or femoral or tibial cortical strut). The advantages of allograft bone include its availability in different shapes and sizes, osteoconductivity, lack of quantitative volume limits, and lack of donor-site morbidity. Along with a risk of disease transmission, immunologic rejection of allograft bone may occur if a fresh graft is implanted. Because most allograft bone is either frozen or freeze dried, the risk of disease transmission and immunologic rejection is low.

The clinical outcomes of allograft bone in orthopaedic trauma patients were examined in a randomized trial of 90 patients with comminuted distal radius fractures between an open reduction and internal fixation (ORIF) with cancellous allograft group and an autogenous ICBG group.[13] No difference between the groups was reported in final radiographic measures as well as clinical outcomes such as wrist range of motion and grip strength. However, patients treated with allograft bone had a significantly shorter surgery time than did the autogenous graft group (89 minutes versus 117 minutes). Allograft bone was found to be a viable alternative to autogenous iliac crest for comminuted distal radius fractures. Other clinical case series have reported osseous union and acceptable clinical outcomes using allograft bone in other metaphyseal fractures such as the tibial plateau and proximal humerus.[14,15] Additional work is needed to clearly define the best clinical scenarios for use of allograft bone with or without osteoinductive additives.

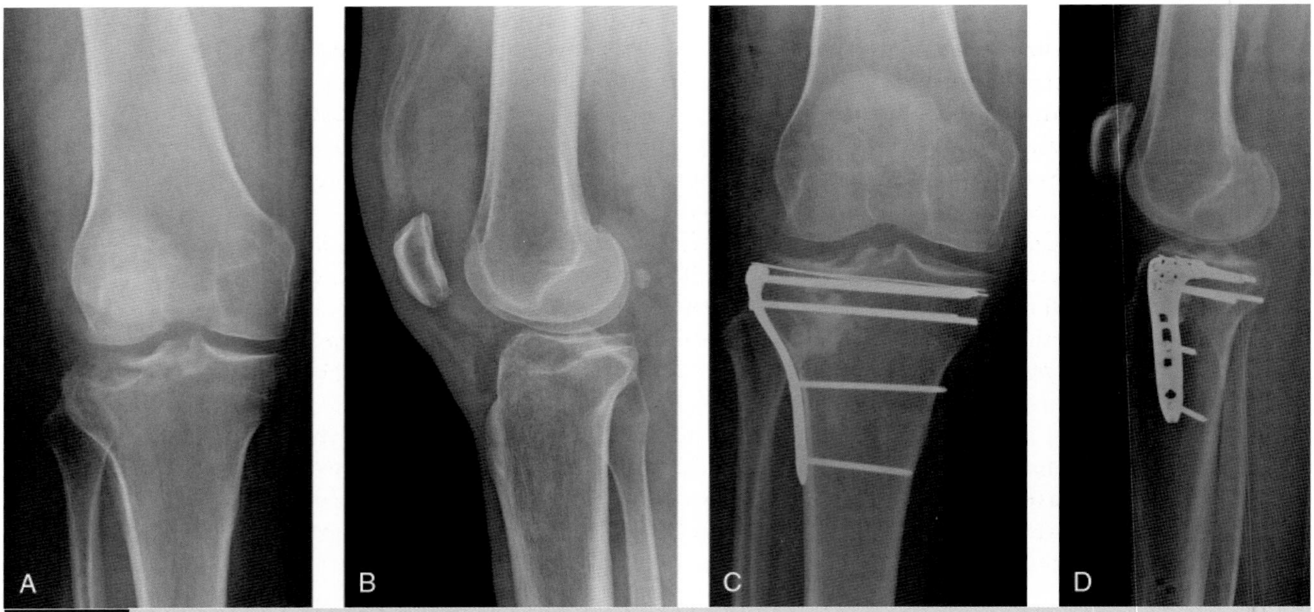

Figure 2 AP (**A**) and lateral (**B**) radiographs of a split depressed tibial plateau fracture after a motor vehicle collision. AP (**C**) and lateral (**D**) radiographs obtained after open reduction and internal fixation and implantation of calcium phosphate cement.

Demineralized Bone Matrix

DMB is allograft bone that has been chemically decalcified. The remaining tissue consists of type I collagen and noncollagenous proteins including osteoinductive growth factors such as BMPs and TGFs.[16] DBM is sold in multiple physical forms (such as putty or gel) for numerous different applications. However, DBM is associated with a theoretical risk of disease transmission because it is derived from allograft bone. In addition, the quantity of osteoinductive growth factor varies between products inherent to each donor. The clinical efficacy of DBM has not been firmly established. One of the few clinical studies of DBM compared outcomes of treating humeral shaft atrophic nonunions with ORIF plus either DBM or autogenous anterior ICBG.[17] In 100% of the autogenous bone graft cohort and 97% of the DBM group, osseous union was achieved. However, 44% of the autogenous bone graft cohort had donor-site morbidity at the anterior iliac crest harvest site. DBM and autogenous bone graft both achieved consistent osseous union, with DBM having a lower rate of complications. More clinical evidence is needed before more ubiquitous use of DBM can be recommended in the orthopaedic trauma population.

Local Adjuvants

Calcium Phosphate

Calcium phosphate functions as an osteoconductive scaffold, is reabsorbed as new bone is formed, and closely resembles the mineral component of native bone. There are three common formulations of calcium phosphate: calcium phosphate cement (CPC), tricalcium phosphate, and coralline hydroxyapatite.[18] Each formulation varies in its mechanical strength, resorption rate, and physical form. CPCs have the most clinical evidence supporting its use and is best for filling metaphyseal and subchondral defects (**Figure 2**). The primary advantages of CPCs is that they have been shown to have high compression strength, no disease transmission risk, and no donor-site morbidity.

Numerous randomized studies have evaluated the clinical effectiveness of CPCs. One study randomized tibial plateau fractures between an autogenous iliac crest bone graft group and a CPC group.[19] The authors found that the autogenous bone graft cohort had a significantly higher rate of articular subsidence compared to the CPC group (30% versus 9%) at 12-month or greater follow-up. Clinical outcome scores were not collected. Another randomized study compared the radiographic and clinical outcomes of patients with intra-articular calcaneal fractures treated with either ORIF alone or ORIF and CPC.[20] The investigators found that at 1-year follow-up the loss of the Böhler angle in the ORIF/CPC group was less than in the ORIF alone group (6.2° versus 10.4°). This difference was statistically significant. No difference in the 36-Item Short Form Health Survey (SF-36) or Lower Extremity Measure (LEM) scores was noted. It was concluded that CPC was a safe augment to ORIF in intra-articular calcaneal fractures. A meta-analysis of 14 randomized trials that used CPC found that its use was associated with less fracture site pain and a lower rate of loss of fracture reduction.[21]

Calcium Sulfate

Calcium sulfate is an osteoconductive graft that has a long history of use in orthopaedics.[22] Similar to calcium phosphate, it is readily available and presents no risk of disease transmission and no donor-site morbidity. However, unlike calcium phosphate, which is reabsorbed more slowly and thereby allowing time for new bone formation, calcium sulfate dissolves more rapidly through an independent chemical process. Although its predictable resorption rate allows it to be a reliable carrier for compounds such as antibiotics, there have been reports of seroma formation and serous drainage from surgical wounds.[23-27] Additionally, there have been a limited number of prospective studies investigating its clinical effectiveness in an orthopaedic trauma cohort.[27,28]

The results of using calcium sulfate as a bone graft substitute in patients with acetabular fractures were reported.[29] In 31 patients in whom follow-up imaging was performed, 84% of patients had either all or most of the calcium sulfate replaced by bone. The remaining 16% of patients with incomplete or no bone replacement were all found to have calcium sulfate in direct communication with the hip joint. It was concluded that calcium sulfate was an effective bone graft substitute in acetabular fractures with complete bony containment. Another study examined antibiotic-impregnated calcium sulfate for the treatment of infected long bones.[27] After appropriate surgical débridement and treatment of the osteomyelitis, calcium sulfate pellets with tobramycin were added to the subsequent bone defect. At the latest follow-up, infection had been successfully treated in 92% of patients. Additionally, of the seven patients without concomitant or staged autogenous bone graft, five patients (71%) achieved union with antibiotic-impregnated calcium sulfate alone.

The use of calcium sulfate as a bone graft substitute in acute fractures is limited by concerns of serous drainage and rapid reabsorption limiting its osteoconductive properties. However, combined with antibiotics, calcium sulfate may be an effective treatment of traumatic osteomyelitic defects and infected nonunions.

Bone Morphogenetic Protein

BMPs are osteoinductive polypeptides that belong to the TGF-β superfamily of proteins. Numerous BMP types have been described but only two, BMP-2 and BMP-7, are commercially available. BMPs induce osteogenesis by signaling pluripotent MSCs to differentiate into osteoprogenitor cells. BMPs have been approved by the US FDA in two orthopaedic trauma scenarios: open tibial shaft fracture (BMP-2) and long bone nonunion or traumatic bone defect (BMP-7).

The BESTT trial studied 450 open tibia shaft fractures.[30] The patients were randomized between intramedullary nail fixation alone or intramedullary nail fixation and BMP-2 of either 6-mg or 12-mg doses. The primary outcome measure was the need for a secondary surgery within 12 months of the initial injury. Patients treated with a 12-mg BMP dose had a substantially lower rate of secondary interventions compared to patients treated via the conventional standard of care (26% versus 46%). They also found that the 12-mg BMP cohort had fewer hardware failures, fewer infections, and faster wound healing. Of note, approximately 67% of the study cohort was treated with unreamed intramedullary nails. Subsequently, the data from the BESTT trial were combined with the results of a similarly conducted unpublished study performed at trauma centers throughout the United States.[31] The larger cohort size allowed for subgroup analysis including the outcomes of patients with Gustilo-Anderson type III (A and B) open tibial fractures as well as patients treated with reamed intramedullary nails. Patients with type III open tibial fractures treated with 12 mg of BMP-2 had a significantly lower rate of secondary autogenous bone grafting (2% versus 20%), invasive secondary procedures (9% versus 28%), and lower infection rate (21% versus 40%) when compared to controls. However, for open tibial fractures of all Gustilo-Anderson types treated with reamed intramedullary nailing, the addition of BMP-2 did not significantly reduce the number of secondary autogenous bone grafting procedures, invasive secondary procedures, or infections. These results were confirmed by a similarly designed randomized trial of open tibial shaft fractures treated with reamed intramedullary nails.[32] No difference between the BMP-2 and control cohorts in regard to the number of secondary procedures or risk of infection was found. The clinical outcomes of patients with open tibial shaft fractures treated with reamed intramedullary nailing was not significantly improved with the addition of BMP-2.

BMP-7 is also approved for use in patients with long bone nonunion. One hundred twenty-four tibial nonunions treated with intramedullary nailing were randomized between a group receiving BMP-7 and a group receiving autogenous bone grafting.[33] A successful clinical outcome was obtained equally between the two groups. The BMP-7 and autogenous bone grafting cohorts both had a low rate of secondary procedures (5% versus 10%). At 12-month follow-up, 13% of autogenous bone graft patients had persistent pain at the donor site. In addition, the autogenous bone graft cohort had a significantly longer surgery time, more blood loss during surgery, and a longer hospital stay.

Although the use of commercially available BMPs in acute open fractures has waned, strong evidence still supports its use as an alternative to autogenous bone grafting in the treatment of long bone nonunion. The cost of this adjuvant needs to be weighed against the potential morbidity of autogenous bone graft harvest.

Systemic Adjuvants

Parathyroid Hormone

PTH is a naturally occurring 84-amino-acid polypeptide that helps regulate calcium homeostasis. Typically, PTH increases serum calcium through its effect on a combination of target organs including the kidney, gastrointestinal tract, and skeleton. Its skeletal effects are mediated via osteoblast-stimulated secretion of nuclear factor κB ligand and increased osteoclast activity. Although osteoclast stimulation occurs with continuous PTH exposure, it has been found that if administered intermittently (daily), osteoblasts are more preferentially activated, leading to the opposite effect of bone formation.

The 1-34 N-terminal residues of PTH have been found to be the most biologically active and therefore the target for drug development. Teriparatide is an FDA-approved recombinant form of human PTH consisting of the 1-34 amino acids used for the treatment of osteoporosis. There has been increasing interest in teriparatide to aid fracture healing. An animal study randomized 270 Sprague-Dawley rats with closed femur fractures to different dosages of a daily subcutaneous PTH (1-34) injection versus placebo control.[34] The PTH (1-34) group had enhanced fracture healing with increased torsional strength, bone mineral content, and density.

Two human randomized clinical trials evaluating PTH and fracture healing have been published. In a 2011 study, 65 elderly women with unilateral pelvic fractures and osteoporosis were assessed.[35] Twenty-one patients were administered daily subcutaneous PTH and 44 patients served as the control group. All patients were given calcium and vitamin D supplementation. The patients were followed for CT evidence of fracture healing and reduction of pain as well as mobility as judged by the Timed Up and Go (TUG) test. At 8 weeks, the PTH patients had a substantially higher rate of fracture healing (100% versus 9.1%) and substantially lower self-reported pain. The TUG test at 12 weeks was substantially faster for patients taking PTH (22.9 seconds versus 54.3 seconds). A 2010 study investigated the effect of PTH in postmenopausal women with dorsally angulated distal radius fractures;[36] 102 patients received either 20 µg PTH, 40 µg PTH, or placebo. Patients were followed for radiographic and CT evidence of fracture healing, administered a functional questionnaire, and underwent grip strength testing. No difference in time to complete cortical bridging, functional results, or grip strength was noted between the three groups. Paired comparisons found that the 20-µg PTH group had a shorter time to healing than the placebo group but this was not seen in the 40-µg cohort.

PTH offers significant promise to aid in acute fracture healing. However, further prospective studies are needed to determine what fracture locations, drug dosage, and patient characteristics would benefit most from this therapy. Additionally, work is needed to clarify the role of PTH in treating delayed unions and nonunions.

Wnt Pathway

One developing area of systemic drug development to facilitate acute fracture healing is manipulation of the Wnt signaling pathway. The Wnt pathway stimulates the differentiation and development of osteoprogenitor cells, thereby increasing bone formation. Sclerostin is a protein that inhibits the Wnt pathway and is an attractive pharmaceutical target.[37] Antibodies against sclerostin have shown promise in initial animal studies.

Seventy rats with a 6-mm femoral defect were randomized to one of four treatments: continuous sclerostin antibody administration, early sclerostin antibody administration, late sclerostin antibody administration, and control.[38] The femurs were tested at 12 weeks for evidence of radiographic healing, histologic healing, and torsional strength. Animals receiving sclerostin antibody had a substantially higher rate of bone formation. It was concluded that sclerostin antibody enhanced bone formation and represented a possible aid for fracture healing in humans.

Additional targets in the Wnt signaling pathway are being studied.[39] However, the effect of Wnt signaling modifiers in a human fracture population is not yet known. Additional work is needed but this area represents an exciting development in future research.

Summary

Biologic adjuvants aid fracture healing during the initial and delayed management of acute fractures, nonunions, and segmental bone defects in conjunction with a well-thought-out preoperative plan and surgical execution. As future therapies continue to evolve, the use of more cell-based approaches and gene therapy by orthopaedic surgeons will likely increase. Continued research will be paramount in evaluating the efficacy and safely of these new modalities. Only after extensive study and critical review of the clinical results can orthopaedic surgeons make educated and informed decisions about future applications.

Key Study Points

- Autogenous bone graft is the current gold standard biologic adjuvant because it is osteoconductive, osteoinductive, and possesses osteogenic cells. Autograft aspirated from the intramedullary canal of long bones (RIA) has been found to provide similar quality graft with fewer complications, and is a new alternative to cancellous graft harvest from the iliac crest.
- Use of BMP in acute open fractures does not substantially improve clinical outcomes; however, strong evidence still supports its use as an alternative to autogenous bone grafting in the treatment of long bone nonunion.
- Locally or systemically administered biologic adjuvants offer surgeons a powerful tool to aid fracture healing but are not a substitute for a carefully considered preoperative plan and surgical execution.

Annotated References

1. Pape HC, Evans A, Kobbe P: Autologous bone graft: Properties and techniques. *J Orthop Trauma* 2010;24(suppl 1):S36-S40.

   This article reviews the clinical literature on the use of autologous bone graft. Level of evidence: V.

2. Ahlmann E, Patzakis M, Roidis N, Shepherd L, Holtom P: Comparison of anterior and posterior iliac crest bone grafts in terms of harvest-site morbidity and functional outcomes. *J Bone Joint Surg Am* 2002;84-A(5):716-720.

3. Sagi HC, Young ML, Gerstenfeld L, Einhorn TA, Tornetta P: Qualitative and quantitative differences between bone graft obtained from the medullary canal (with a Reamer/Irrigator/Aspirator) and the iliac crest of the same patient. *J Bone Joint Surg Am* 2012;94(23):2128-2135.

   This study performed comparative transcriptional analysis of cancellous autograft collected from both the iliac crest and intramedullary canal via the RIA in 10 patients. The authors found that the RIA autograft had a similar transcriptional profile and is a reasonable alternative to ICBG.

4. Dimitriou R, Mataliotakis GI, Angoules AG, Kanakaris NK, Giannoudis PV: Complications following autologous bone graft harvesting from the iliac crest and using the RIA: A systematic review. *Injury* 2011;42(suppl 2):S3-S15.

   This systematic review analyzed 92 articles with 6,449 patients to determine the complication differences between autogenous iliac crest bone and RIA harvest. The investigators found that RIA harvesting had a lower complication rate and represented a promising autogenous bone harvest technique. Level of evidence: I.

5. Dawson J, Kiner D, Gardner W II, Swafford R, Nowotarski PJ: The reamer-irrigator-aspirator as a device for harvesting bone graft compared with iliac crest bone graft: Union rates and complications. *J Orthop Trauma* 2014;28(10):584-590.

   This randomized controlled trial investigated 133 nonunions or segmental bone defects treated with either autogenous iliac crest or RIA bone grafting. The authors found that the overall rate and time to union were not different between the harvest sites. However, the authors found that RIA had less donor-site pain, yielded more graft than from the anterior iliac crest, and cost less than graft from the posterior iliac crest. Level of evidence: I.

6. Garg NK, Gaur S, Sharma S: Percutaneous autogenous bone marrow grafting in 20 cases of ununited fracture. *Acta Orthop Scand* 1993;64(6):671-672.

7. Braly HL, O'Connor DP, Brinker MR: Percutaneous autologous bone marrow injection in the treatment of distal meta-diaphyseal tibial nonunions and delayed unions. *J Orthop Trauma* 2013;27(9):527-533.

   This case series reported the outcomes of distal metadiaphyseal tibial nonunions treated with percutaneously injected bone marrow aspirate. All fractures were aseptic, had intact hardware, and were mechanically stable. Bone marrow was aspirated from the posterior iliac crest and 40 to 80 mL was injected at the nonunion site. The authors found that bone marrow injection was successful in 82% of cases (9 of 11 patients) after a mean of 4 months clinical follow-up. Level of evidence: IV.

8. Hernigou P, Poignard A, Beaujean F, Rouard H: Percutaneous autologous bone-marrow grafting for nonunions. Influence of the number and concentration of progenitor cells. *J Bone Joint Surg Am* 2005;87(7):1430-1437.

9. Pierini M, Di Bella C, Dozza B, et al: The posterior iliac crest outperforms the anterior iliac crest when obtaining mesenchymal stem cells from bone marrow. *J Bone Joint Surg Am* 2013;95(12):1101-1107.

In this article, bone marrow aspirate was collected from the posterior and anterior iliac crest of 22 patients and examined. The authors found that aspirate from the posterior iliac crest contained a greater number of progenitor cells than an equal volume collected from the anterior iliac crest. The authors concluded that bone marrow aspirate from the posterior iliac crest is the preferred location.

10. Alsousou J, Thompson M, Hulley P, Noble A, Willett K: The biology of platelet-rich plasma and its application in trauma and orthopaedic surgery: A review of the literature. *J Bone Joint Surg Br* 2009;91(8):987-996.

11. Hsu WK, Mishra A, Rodeo SR, et al: Platelet-rich plasma in orthopaedic applications: Evidence-based recommendations for treatment. *J Am Acad Orthop Surg* 2013;21(12):739-748.

    This review article examined the evidence for use of PRP in different orthopaedic applications including bone healing and soft tissue injuries. Level of evidence: V.

12. Calori GM, Tagliabue L, Gala L, d'Imporzano M, Peretti G, Albisetti W: Application of rhBMP-7 and platelet-rich plasma in the treatment of long bone non-unions: A prospective randomised clinical study on 120 patients. *Injury* 2008;39(12):1391-1402.

13. Rajan GP, Fornaro J, Trentz O, Zellweger R: Cancellous allograft versus autologous bone grafting for repair of comminuted distal radius fractures: A prospective, randomized trial. *J Trauma* 2006;60(6):1322-1329.

14. Euler SA, Hengg C, Wambacher M, Spiegl UJ, Kralinger F: Allogenic bone grafting for augmentation in two-part proximal humeral fracture fixation in a high-risk patient population. *Arch Orthop Trauma Surg* 2015;135(1):79-87.

    This case series reported the outcomes of varus angulated two-part proximal humerus fractures treated with ORIF with cancellous allograft. Nine of 10 patients experienced healing, with no cases of osteonecrosis and good clinical outcome scores. Level of evidence: IV.

15. Lasanianos N, Mouzopoulos G, Garnavos C: The use of freeze-dried cancelous allograft in the management of impacted tibial plateau fractures. *Injury* 2008;39(10):1106-1112.

16. Kinney RC, Ziran BH, Hirshorn K, Schlatterer D, Ganey T: Demineralized bone matrix for fracture healing: Fact or fiction? *J Orthop Trauma* 2010;24(suppl 1):S52-S55.

    This article reviewed the clinical literature on the use of DMB. Level of evidence: V.

17. Hierholzer C, Sama D, Toro JB, Peterson M, Helfet DL: Plate fixation of ununited humeral shaft fractures: Effect of type of bone graft on healing. *J Bone Joint Surg Am* 2006;88(7):1442-1447.

18. Larsson S: Calcium phosphates: What is the evidence? *J Orthop Trauma* 2010;24(suppl 1):S41-S45.

    This article reviewed the clinical literature on the use of calcium phosphates. Level of evidence: V.

19. Russell TA, Leighton RK; Alpha-BSM Tibial Plateau Fracture Study Group: Comparison of autogenous bone graft and endothermic calcium phosphate cement for defect augmentation in tibial plateau fractures. A multicenter, prospective, randomized study. *J Bone Joint Surg Am* 2008;90(10):2057-2061.

20. Johal HS, Buckley RE, Le IL, Leighton RK: A prospective randomized controlled trial of a bioresorbable calcium phosphate paste (alpha-BSM) in treatment of displaced intra-articular calcaneal fractures. *J Trauma* 2009;67(4):875-882.

21. Bajammal SS, Zlowodzki M, Lelwica A, et al: The use of calcium phosphate bone cement in fracture treatment. A meta-analysis of randomized trials. *J Bone Joint Surg Am* 2008;90(6):1186-1196.

22. Beuerlein MJ, McKee MD: Calcium sulfates: What is the evidence? *J Orthop Trauma* 2010;24(suppl 1):S46-S51.

    This article reviewed the clinical literature on the use of calcium sulfate. Level of evidence: V.

23. Ziran BH, Smith WR, Morgan SJ: Use of calcium-based demineralized bone matrix/allograft for nonunions and posttraumatic reconstruction of the appendicular skeleton: Preliminary results and complications. *J Trauma* 2007;63(6):1324-1328.

24. Borrelli J Jr, Prickett WD, Ricci WM: Treatment of nonunions and osseous defects with bone graft and calcium sulfate. *Clin Orthop Relat Res* 2003;411:245-254.

25. Yu B, Han K, Ma H, et al: Treatment of tibial plateau fractures with high strength injectable calcium sulphate. *Int Orthop* 2009;33(4):1127-1133.

26. Kelly CM, Wilkins RM, Gitelis S, Hartjen C, Watson JT, Kim PT: The use of a surgical grade calcium sulfate as a bone graft substitute: Results of a multicenter trial. *Clin Orthop Relat Res* 2001;382:42-50.

27. McKee MD, Wild LM, Schemitsch EH, Waddell JP: The use of an antibiotic-impregnated, osteoconductive, bioabsorbable bone substitute in the treatment of infected long bone defects: Early results of a prospective trial. *J Orthop Trauma* 2002;16(9):622-627.

28. McKee MD, Li-Bland EA, Wild LM, Schemitsch EH: A prospective, randomized clinical trial comparing an antibiotic-impregnated bioabsorbable bone substitute with standard antibiotic-impregnated cement beads in the treatment of chronic osteomyelitis and infected nonunion. *J Orthop Trauma* 2010;24(8):483-490.

    In this prospective clinical trial, patients with chronic osteomyelitis or infected nonunion who were undergoing surgical débridement were randomized to either antibiotic-impregnated calcium sulfate or antibiotic-impregnated polymethyl methacrylate. The authors found that 86% of patients (12 of 14) in both groups successfully eradicated their infection. Additionally, both groups had similar rates of osseous union. Although the study sample size was small, the investigators concluded that antibiotic-impregnated calcium sulfate was equivalent to standard therapy. Level of evidence: II.

29. Moed BR, Willson Carr SE, Craig JG, Watson JT: Calcium sulfate used as bone graft substitute in acetabular fracture fixation. *Clin Orthop Relat Res* 2003;410:303-309.

30. Govender S, Csimma C, Genant HK, et al; BMP-2 Evaluation in Surgery for Tibial Trauma (BESTT) Study Group: Recombinant human bone morphogenetic protein-2 for treatment of open tibial fractures: A prospective, controlled, randomized study of four hundred and fifty patients. *J Bone Joint Surg Am* 2002;84-A(12):2123-2134.

31. Swiontkowski MF, Aro HT, Donell S, et al: Recombinant human bone morphogenetic protein-2 in open tibial fractures. A subgroup analysis of data combined from two prospective randomized studies. *J Bone Joint Surg Am* 2006;88(6):1258-1265.

32. Aro HT, Govender S, Patel AD, et al: Recombinant human bone morphogenetic protein-2: A randomized trial in open tibial fractures treated with reamed nail fixation. *J Bone Joint Surg Am* 2011;93(9):801-808.

    In this study, 277 patients with open tibial fractures were treated with reamed intramedullary nails and randomized to either receiving BMP-2 or not. The authors found that BMP-2 did not significantly increase the time to healing.

33. Friedlaender GE, Perry CR, Cole JD, et al: Osteogenic protein-1 (bone morphogenetic protein-7) in the treatment of tibial nonunions. *J Bone Joint Surg Am* 2001;83-A(Pt 2suppl 1):S151-S158.

34. Alkhiary YM, Gerstenfeld LC, Krall E, et al: Enhancement of experimental fracture-healing by systemic administration of recombinant human parathyroid hormone (PTH 1-34). *J Bone Joint Surg Am* 2005;87(4):731-741.

35. Peichl P, Holzer LA, Maier R, Holzer G: Parathyroid hormone 1-84 accelerates fracture-healing in pubic bones of elderly osteoporotic women. *J Bone Joint Surg Am* 2011;93(17):1583-1587.

    In this randomized controlled trial, the authors compared osteoporotic female pelvic fractures treated with either PTH or the conventional standard of care. The authors found that patients treated with PTH had earlier mean time to fracture healing as well as improved pain and functional testing. Level of evidence: II.

36. Aspenberg P, Genant HK, Johansson T, et al: Teriparatide for acceleration of fracture repair in humans: A prospective, randomized, double-blind study of 102 postmenopausal women with distal radial fractures. *J Bone Miner Res* 2010;25(2):404-414.

    This study randomized 102 women with distal radius fractures to receiving daily injections of either a placebo or two different doses of teriparatide. The investigators found that the lower dosage (20 µg) shortened the median time to heal compared to placebo, whereas the higher dosage (40 µg) was found to have no significant effect. Level of evidence: II.

37. Compton JT, Lee FY: A review of osteocyte function and the emerging importance of sclerostin. *J Bone Joint Surg Am* 2014;96(19):1659-1668.

    This article reviews sclerostin and its role in bone metabolism. Level of evidence: V.

38. Virk MS, Alaee F, Tang H, Ominsky MS, Ke HZ, Lieberman JR: Systemic administration of sclerostin antibody enhances bone repair in a critical-sized femoral defect in a rat model. *J Bone Joint Surg Am* 2013;95(8):694-701.

    Using a critical-sized femoral defect rat model, the authors administered three different schedules of sclerostin antibody and compared new bone formation to a placebo group. The authors found that the sclerostin antibody groups had significantly increased new bone formation and a greater number of femoral defects healed.

39. Leucht P, Jiang J, Cheng D, et al: Wnt3a reestablishes osteogenic capacity to bone grafts from aged animals. *J Bone Joint Surg Am* 2013;95(14):1278-1288.

    This article used transgenic mice to investigate the influence of Wnt3a protein on gene expression in bone graft harvested from young and aged mice. The authors found that Wnt3a increased osteogenic gene expression and increased callous formation in an animal bone defect model.

Chapter 13

Diagnosis and Management of Infection Associated With Fractures and Nonunions

Timothy S. Achor, MD Joshua L. Gary, MD

Abstract

Musculoskeletal infection after fractures can have life-altering and limb-threatening complications. Wound drainage, sinus tracts, history of open fracture, and nonunion are factors that should raise suspicion for infection. Laboratory markers including elevated erythrocyte sedimentation rate and C-reactive protein level are sensitive but nonspecific for diagnosis. The trends of these values can be used to determine the effectiveness of treatment. Definitive diagnosis is made by identification of an organism by deep tissue culture. Newer technologies for diagnosis of infection including polymerase chain reaction await validation. Imaging modalities including MRI, CT, and positron emission tomography can also aid in diagnosis and planning surgical treatment. Surgical treatment mandates excision of all nonviable and infected bone if possible. Bony defects resulting from resection of infected bone remain a challenging problem and several strategies exist for treatment, including distraction osteogenesis, bone grafting, and amputation. An individualized treatment plan should be based on host factors, functional requirements, location of infection, and realistic goals of both patient and surgeon.

Keywords: infection; nonunion; diagnosis of infection, treatment; infected nonunion; bone defect

Dr. Achor or an immediate family member serves as a paid consultant to Synthes. Dr. Gary or an immediate family member is a member of a speakers' bureau or has made paid presentations on behalf of Smith & Nephew, has stock or stock options held in Summit Medventures, and serves as a board member, owner, officer, or committee member of the Orthopaedic Trauma Association.

Introduction

Despite recent medical and surgical advances, infection associated with fractures and nonunions continues to be a devastating complication of musculoskeletal trauma. Unfortunately, there is rarely a simple way to diagnose or treat this problem, and a musculoskeletal infection can be limb and life threatening. Musculoskeletal infection has a profound psychosocial and socioeconomic effect on society, and the importance of prevention cannot be overstated. Recent data have shown tibial nonunion to be a severely disabling medical condition that has a negative effect on health-related quality of life.[1] Patients with tibial nonunion report a detrimental effect on both physical and mental health. The additional burden of infection associated with nonunion would presumably only complicate the situation. The severity of musculoskeletal infection must be discussed with patients, and reasonable treatment goals and functional expectations should be an early part of clinical evaluation.

Diagnosis of the Patient With Musculoskeletal Infection

Patient History

The diagnosis of infection associated with musculoskeletal trauma can be challenging. Furthermore, an accurate diagnosis is complicated by differing opinions and definitions of infection and osteomyelitis. There are currently no universally accepted guidelines to aid in the diagnosis of musculoskeletal infection, and there is no single gold standard test. Therefore, several regional, personal, and anecdotal preferences are used to aid in the diagnosis. The authors of a 2011 study attempted to simplify the diagnosis with their proposed "Osteomyelitis Diagnosis Score," which is based on five parameters: history and risk factors; clinical examination and pertinent laboratory values; imaging studies; microbiology; and histopathology.[2] A scoring system may allow the clinician to make a diagnosis with improved confidence.

Patients can present acutely (days to weeks) or on a delayed basis (months to years) following fracture fixation. Several host factors are commonly associated with an increased risk of infection, including immunocompromised health status, diabetes mellitus, peripheral vascular disease, and advanced age.[3] Although host factors play an important role in the development of a musculoskeletal infection, many of these issues can be mitigated with meticulous preoperative and postoperative medical management. The importance of compliance should be discussed with the patient. Adherence to medical recommendations and postoperative restrictions are critical to help decrease the risk of infection. Patients should be counseled regarding their risk of the development of an infection—a well-documented informed consent is key to the treatment process. Treatment plans can occasionally be altered by well-informed, educated patients. Realistic goals and treatment strategies should be discussed early with the patient. A comprehensive treatment plan can involve multiple procedures spanning months or years and typically there is no guarantee of success. This can be a considerable time and financial sacrifice for the patient. Depending on the age of the patient, overall health status, and likelihood of success, amputation is a treatment option that can be considered (**Figure 1**).

A history of an open fracture should raise suspicion for infection. Open fractures are known to have an increased risk of infection, and multiple studies have shown that with increasing energy of injury, rates of infection increase accordingly.[4,5] Although the size of the wound does not always correlate with the mechanism of injury or the energy imparted to the body, it is an important part of the history. Gross contamination at the time of injury should also raise concern for infection, as should vascular compromise. Open fractures requiring free tissue transfer often have large areas of soft-tissue stripping and loss of periosteum. A decrease in vascularity to the region can predispose to both infection and nonunion.

Unlike host factors and injury characteristics, there are several factors under the surgeon's control. Time to antibiotic delivery[6] and time to initial débridement[7] are both considered important in helping to decrease the chance for infection. A history of a delay in surgical débridement should raise concern for infection. If a patient is too unstable for surgical débridement of an open fracture, obvious gross contamination should be removed in the emergency department, and the wound covered with moist gauze. Fracture immobilization is important via traction or splinting in an effort to decrease further soft-tissue damage. Aggressive surgical débridement is the mainstay of early surgical intervention for open fractures. Following excision of all devitalized tissue, irrigation can be performed. Any unhealthy tissue or devitalized bone left behind is a risk factor for future infection. Gentle soft-tissue handling techniques can lessen any further damage not already created by the injury. These aforementioned factors are most easily controlled by the original treating surgeon. A subsequent treating surgeon must gather information, and a complete history and review of the medical records and surgical reports is key; with the patient's permission, a conversation with the original treating surgeon can be insightful. Knowledge of the number of previous surgeries (including dates and descriptions) and retained implants (and dates of implantation) are important. A history of infection is important information. A history of antibiotic therapy is paramount; both drug and duration should be considered. A surgeon should have a team available, including an internist, an infectious disease specialist, a plastic surgeon, an endocrinologist, and others as needed, to assist in comanagement of these patients.

Clinical Evaluation

Acute infections can present in a variety of ways. A history of a violent injury with significant soft-tissue damage or open fracture should increase suspicion for infection. Patients may present with the hallmark signs of infection including erythema, heat, and swelling, and can also have persistent serous drainage, purulent drainage, nonhealing wounds, wound dehiscence, and foul odor about the wound (**Figure 2**). Any evidence of bone or hardware visible through the wound is concerning. Most patients will have acutely diminishing functional capacity and increasing pain and disability about the region. Exquisite tenderness around a previously benign wound should be considered infection until proven otherwise. Occasionally, acute infections have very little symptomatology and require diligence in evaluation.

Chronic infections can present with many of the aforementioned symptoms. A draining sinus tract in the area of a previous incision or traumatic wound is extremely concerning for infection (**Figure 3**). Nonhealing wounds can also allow for previously sterile fractures to become seeded with organisms. Plain film radiographs should be obtained, as infection can frequently lead to hardware loosening and/or failure. Patients occasionally report that while the pain from the fracture is annoying, the drainage is even more bothersome for their daily activities.

Unfortunately, not all infections referable to the musculoskeletal system present with classic findings. Chronic infections can also present with the spectrum

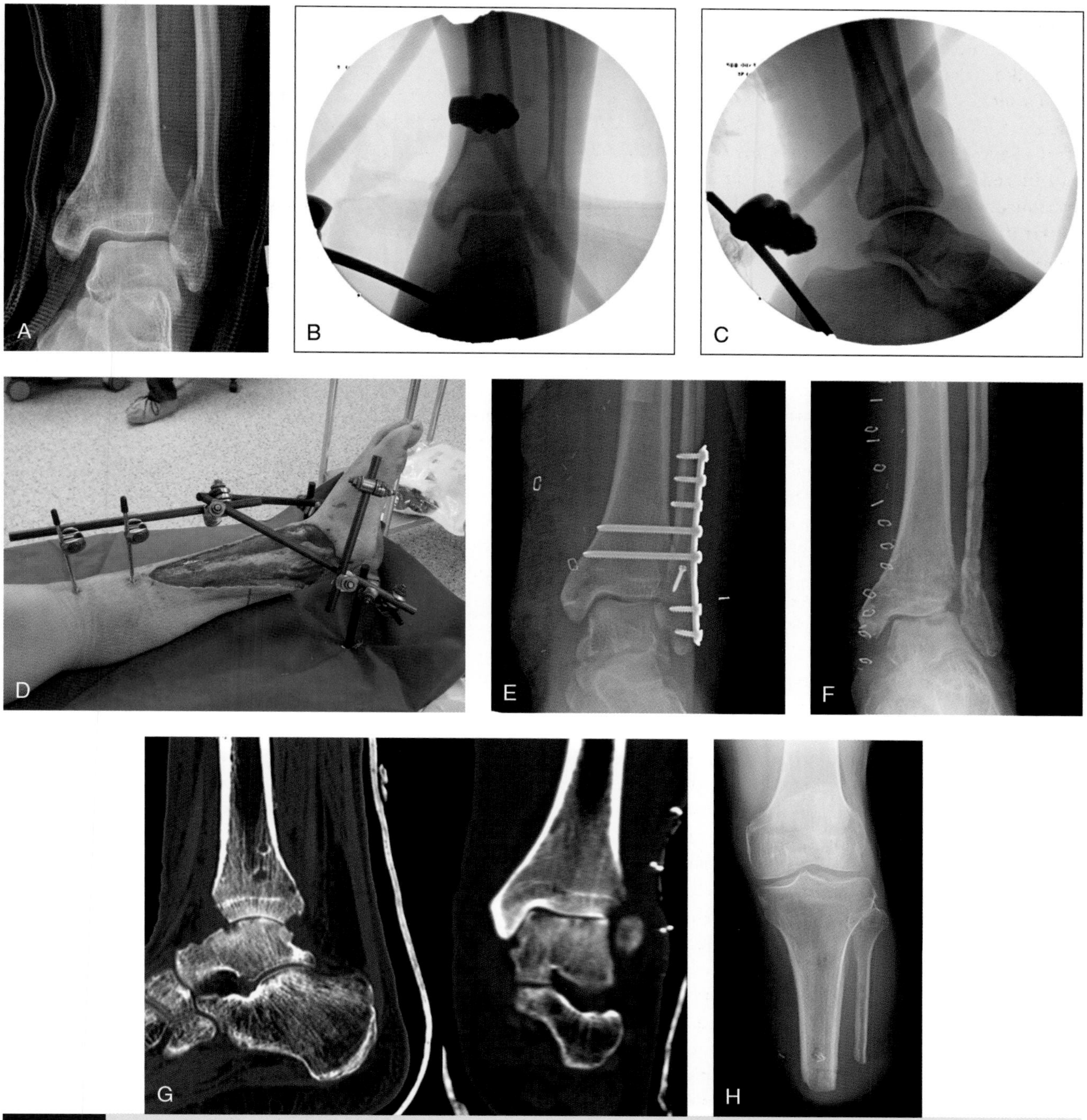

Figure 1 A 43-year-old man sustained a contaminated open ankle fracture-dislocation after a motorcycle crash. **A**, Radiograph of the injured ankle following closed reduction. **B** and **C**, Intraoperative fluoroscopic images following emergent irrigation and débridement and external fixation. **D**, Clinical photograph of the ankle; the patient underwent serial débridements and had severe soft tissue loss. **E**, Postoperative AP radiograph following open reduction and internal fixation of the ankle fracture. **F**, Radiograph of the ankle 4 months later; all implants were removed because of severe infection and purulent drainage. **G**, CT scans showing chronic, destructive postinfectious changes about the ankle. **H**, Radiograph showing below-knee amputation. Salvage options were discussed with the patient.

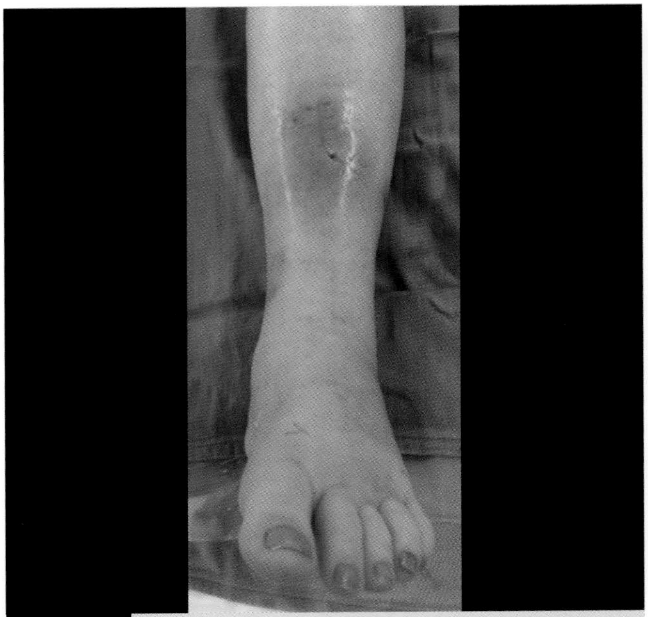

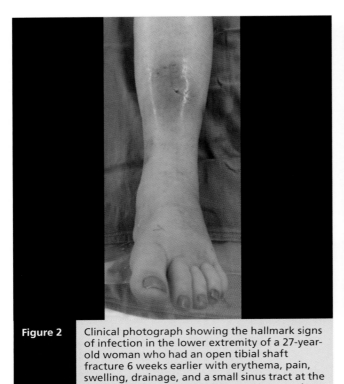

Figure 2 Clinical photograph showing the hallmark signs of infection in the lower extremity of a 27-year-old woman who had an open tibial shaft fracture 6 weeks earlier with erythema, pain, swelling, drainage, and a small sinus tract at the site of a previously healed traumatic wound.

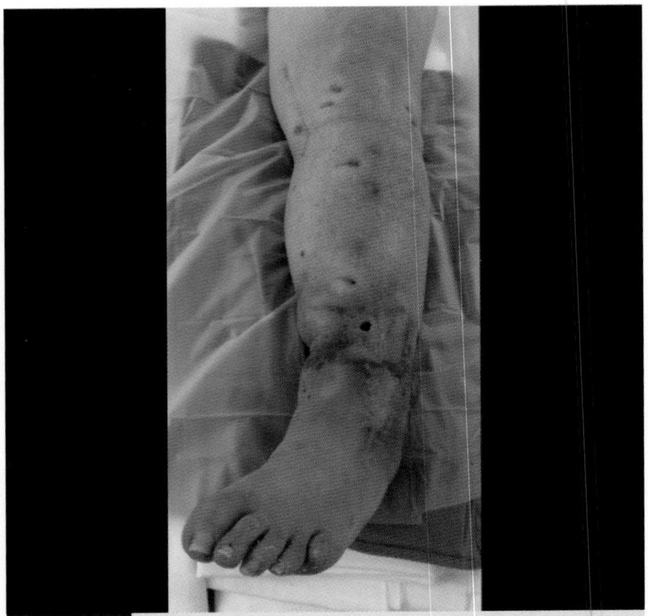

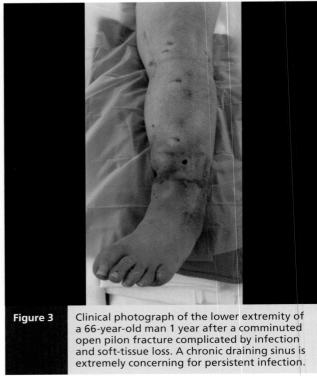

Figure 3 Clinical photograph of the lower extremity of a 66-year-old man 1 year after a comminuted open pilon fracture complicated by infection and soft-tissue loss. A chronic draining sinus is extremely concerning for persistent infection.

of pain, from severe to minimal or none. Occasionally, patients can function relatively well, even with a nonunion. Any patient presenting with a nonunion should be evaluated for the possibility of infection. In addition, chronic draining sinus tracts with underlying osteomyelitis can dedifferentiate to malignant squamous cell carcinoma. Termed a Marjolin ulcer, these wounds should be closely evaluated and biopsied. The authors of a 2015 study noted that over a 10-year period, a Marjolin ulcer was diagnosed in nine patients and despite wide resection, four eventually died from the cancer.[8]

Laboratory Evaluation

Serologic Evaluation

Standard laboratory values include complete blood count (CBC) with differential, erythrocyte sedimentation rate (ESR), and C-reactive protein (CRP) level. One study involving 265 children reported on the utility of using both ESR and CRP to aid in the diagnosis of bone and joint infection. The authors found that using both serum laboratory values can allow for a sensitivity as high as 98%.[9] Another group has reported on serum procalcitonin as a test that is both sensitive and specific for septic arthritis and acute osteomyelitis.[10] In the early postoperative period, the ESR and CRP level can be elevated; however, the CRP level should return to normal within 3 weeks after the surgery and the ESR within several months. As such, ESR and CRP level are unreliable markers of infection in the early postoperative period. However, in the setting of infection and osteomyelitis, these laboratory values can be used to monitor the success or failure of treatment.[11] A secondary elevation in CRP level following an initial downward trend is highly suggestive of infection and should be closely evaluated. The CBC can reveal an elevated white blood cell (WBC) count in either the acute or chronic setting. Interleukin-6 has recently been shown to be another serum value that can help in the diagnosis of early infection, specifically after open fractures.[12] A recent study reported on a standardized protocol in evaluation of potentially infected nonunions.[13] Ninety-five nonunions were evaluated, and 30 were ultimately deemed infected. The predicted probability of having an infected nonunion with elevation of zero, one, two, or all three of the aforementioned serum laboratory values was 20%, 19%, 56%, and 100%, respectively. The authors reported their protocol can assist surgeons in decision making as well as to counsel patients more effectively on realistic goals of treatment.[13]

Microbiology

The diagnosis of infection is established and confirmed with isolation of an organism from the nonunion site.

Swabs of a draining wound or sinus tract are generally unreliable and can be misleading.[14,15] Similarly, needle biopsy of the nonunion site can be unreliable.[16] An open biopsy with multiple tissue samples and swabs from various regions of the wound/nonunion site is a reliable way to obtain accurate information about the sterility of the milieu. At least three to six samples should be taken. Generally, antibiotics are held for 2 weeks before the biopsy and perioperative prophylactic antibiotics are held until after the samples are obtained. A Gram stain should be performed; the presence of organisms and number of white blood cells per high-power field should be noted. Cultures should be sent for aerobic, anaerobic, acid-fast bacilli, fungal, and any other routine agar culture medium available at the surgical facility. Any unusual organism suspected due to institutional or regional reasons should be noted and discussed with pathology laboratory personnel. It should be noted that cultures can routinely take days to show any bacterial growth; in some instances, acid-fast bacilli and fungus can take weeks and must be checked periodically until finalized. One study showed that the median time to positivity was 1 day and 96.6% of positive cultures were deemed positive by 7 days.[17] Typically, cultures that become positive beyond 7 days are likely to be an unusual organism or a contaminant. A 14-day incubation period is recommended when known slow-growing pathogens such as *Propionibacterium spp.*, *Corynebacterium* bacteria, coagulase-negative staphylococci, or anaerobes are suspected.[17]

Although intraoperative cultures have long been considered the gold standard in diagnosis of infection, occasionally purulent wounds that appear clearly infected do not grow any organisms in vitro. Furthermore, evaluation of cultures where only a portion of the cultures were positive or growth is delayed or noted only in broth can complicate the diagnosis or raise suspicion for contamination. In these and other situations, molecular diagnostic techniques or fluorescence in situ hybridization can be useful. In one study involving 34 nonunions, molecular diagnostics (including polymerase chain reaction and fluorescence in situ hybridization) were more sensitive for identifying bacteria than cultures.[18] It was concluded that this finding may be due to the inability of cultures to detect organisms in biofilms or bacteria with prior exposure to antibiotics.

Several studies have shown culture of bath sonication fluid from removed implants has a high sensitivity for detecting causative organisms.[19,20] It is believed that sonication of implants dislodges bacteria from biofilms and allows for more accurate microbiologic diagnosis. Culture of sonication fluid in blood culture bottles has been found to be reliable even in the setting of recent antibiotic use.[21]

The detection and identification of causative organisms is vital to eradication of infection in nonunions, and these techniques may prove invaluable in the future. It remains uncertain whether these tests will become the new standard for diagnosis of infection as cost/benefit ratio continues to be questionable for these advanced diagnostic techniques.

Imaging

All patients should be followed with serial plain radiographs or digital radiography. Radiographs are relatively inexpensive and straightforward to obtain in the outpatient setting. Although neither sensitive nor specific for infection, plain films are valuable for many reasons. Orthogonal images may reveal the extent of fracture healing, which is evaluated and documented. The presence of a radiographically united fracture is important because of the possible need for hardware removal. Radiographs can be compared from one visit to the next; any changes or new findings should raise concern. The presence of an infection can be associated with a variety of radiographic findings. Early infections may present with subtle findings such as lucency around screws, backing out and loosening of screws, soft-tissue swelling, and gas in the soft tissues (**Figure 4**). More advanced infections can present with catastrophic hardware failure including broken screws, plates, and nails. Other findings can include periosteal reaction and bony erosions (**Figure 5**). Although a change in alignment of a fracture can result for a variety of reasons, infection should be included in the differential diagnosis (**Figure 6**).

CT can be used to identify fluid collections and abscess formation, soft-tissue swelling, and the presence or absence of union. Air droplets and gas around a suspected infection should be considered an infectious etiology unless there is another explanation. Although CT is not ideal to reveal the extent of bony involvement, the ability to evaluate bony erosions, involucrum, and sequestrum is enhanced. This valuable information can assist in determining the amount of bony resection, if any, required for successful treatment. The extent of union is evaluated and can be a useful adjunct to plain films in determining the course of treatment and maintenance or removal of implants.

Prior work has established nuclear imaging as a useful adjunct in establishing the diagnosis of infection. However, Tc 99M labeled red blood cell studies are not useful in the setting of an acute fracture following surgical intervention. The study detects increased bone metabolism and remodeling, which is present during typical fracture healing for up to 1 year. In such a setting, this study will be positive and nondiagnostic. However, a lack of uptake

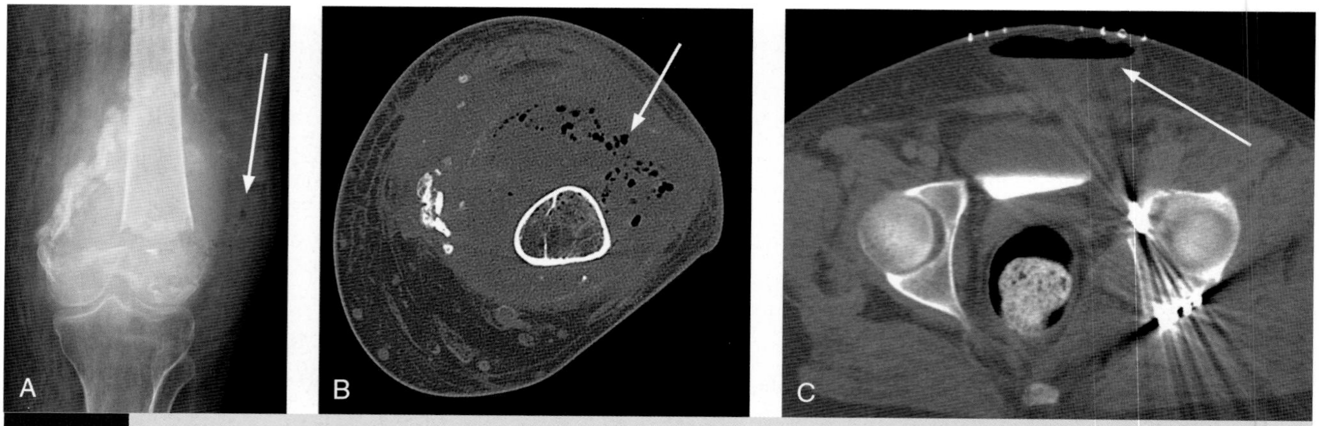

Figure 4 **A**, AP film of a distal femur fracture weeks following hardware removal due to infection. Note gas in the soft tissues (arrow), which is indicative of infection. **B**, Axial CT image of the same patient shown in **A**; large fluid collection and gas are noted (arrow). **C**, Axial CT image of a pelvis 2 weeks after acetabular fixation. The patient had fever, increasing white blood cell count, and fluctuance referable to the incision. Gas collection in the subcutaneous tissues is seen (arrow). A large abscess was subsequently evacuated.

can indicate devascularized or necrotic bone with poor healing potential. A tagged WBC bone scan can help differentiate normal healing from infection (**Figure 7**). One study found nuclear imaging scans to have a high specificity (92%) but a low sensitivity (19%).[13] It was concluded that nuclear imaging studies do not appear to be cost effective, as they were the most expensive and least valuable test in the study.[13]

Fluorodeoxyglucose (FDG) PET scintigraphy can be considered a potentially superior imaging modality to CT or MRI, as there is minimal implant-related artifact to hinder interpretation. With this technique, a radioactive substance is administered and uptake is evaluated at the nonunion site. Previous drawbacks to PET, including vague anatomic localization, have been improved with the addition of a concurrent CT scan. One study evaluated the value of PET with CT scan in 10 patients who underwent internal fixation of a tibia fracture and later presented with signs of a possible deep infection.[22] The authors reported that PET/CT confirmed their working diagnosis in 9 of 10 patients, helped treatment decisions, and distinguished between infected nonunion, aseptic nonunion, soft-tissue infection, and chronic osteomyelitis.

The fine anatomic detail of MRI allows for accurate identification of infection, in addition to evaluation of the soft tissues in much greater detail than nuclear imaging. Intravenous gadolinium can enhance imaging interpretation in scenarios of potential infection. Fluid collections, sinus tracts, and the full extent of the infection are straightforward to identify. A drawback continues to be metallic artifact in the setting of implant-related infection, as this can hinder accurate interpretation.

Treatment

Débridement and Irrigation

Several recent studies have demonstrated success with radical débridement to bleeding healthy bone followed by various techniques for reconstruction of bony defects.[23-30] Infection of large articular blocks remains a challenge as débridement can greatly limit reconstructive options.

Although there is debate regarding the method of irrigation (pulsatile lavage versus low flow with or without antibiotics or detergents), irrigation is unlikely to play much of a role in the treatment of an established musculoskeletal infection.

The Reamer-Irrigator-Aspirator (RIA; Synthes) is commonly used to débride the intramedullary canal of the femur and tibia (**Figure 8**). When combined with culture-specific antibiotics and an antibiotic cement rod, a 96% success rate (no evidence of recurrent infection) was reported.[31] The RIA has a limited role in the upper extremity long bones as the minimum reamer size is 12 mm.

Biofilm and Bacterial Adherence

Biofilms are associated with staphylococcal adhesion to implants.[32,33] Mature biofilms resist antibiotics, chemical disinfectants, surgical débridement, and host immune system defenses, and causative bacteria can disperse in their planktonic form to begin the process anew in different locations.[32] No current treatments other than implant removal (with high rate of recurrence) exist for biofilm-related infections; it is hoped that future therapies attack the porous matrix with enzymes or develop implants that are resistant to biofilm formation.[32]

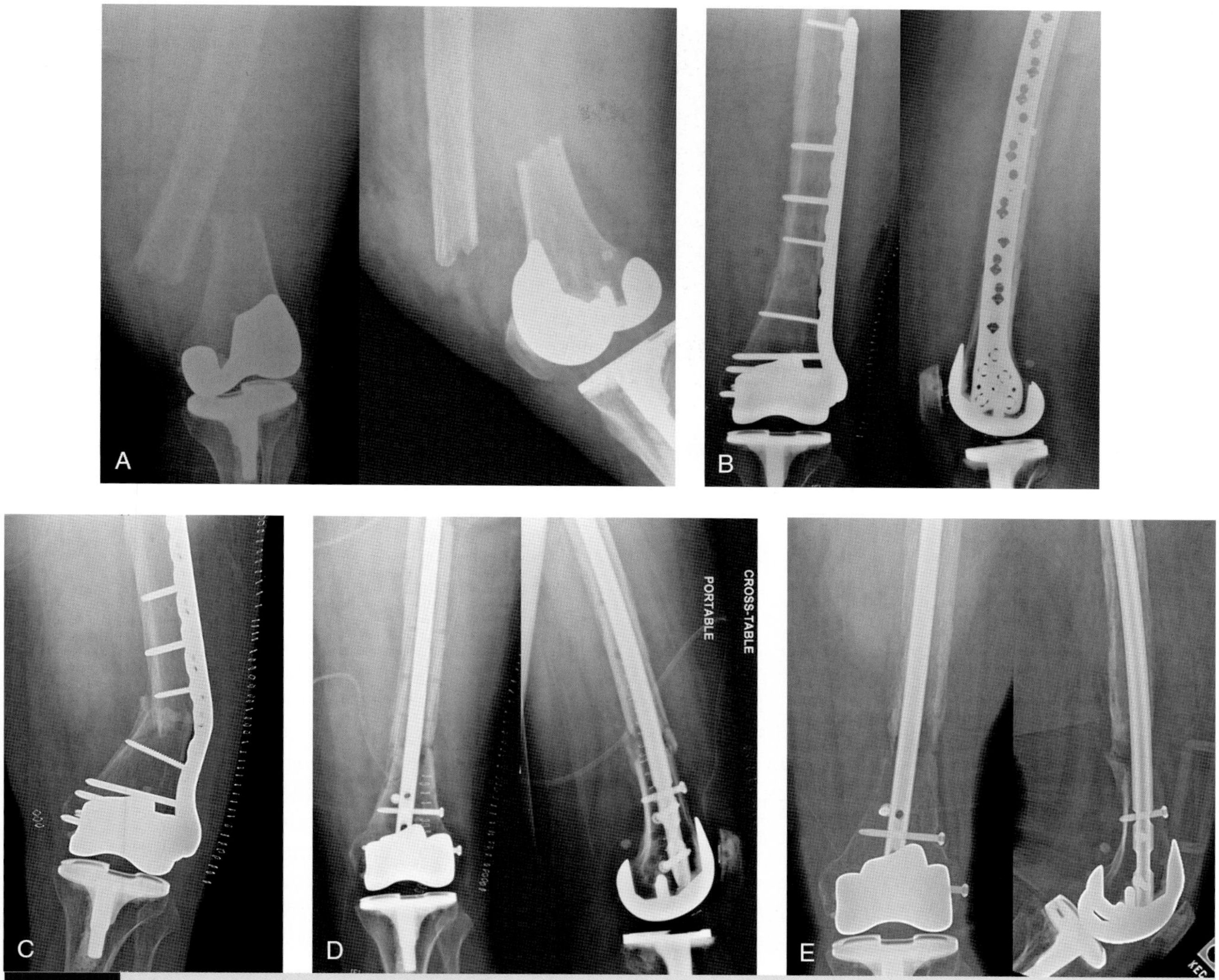

Figure 5 A 55-year-old man sustained a distal femoral shaft fracture above a total knee replacement. **A**, AP and lateral radiographs reveal the fracture. Note the radiographic appearance of the bone adjacent to the fracture, concerning for infection or malignancy. **B**, AP and lateral postoperative radiographs following open biopsy and fixation with a distal femur locking plate. The cultures and pathology were both negative. **C**, Postoperative AP radiograph 3 weeks after a fall, showing plate breakage and catastrophic failure. **D**, AP and lateral postoperative radiographs following removal of all implants, open biopsy, and antegrade nailing. Cultures at that time grew *Acinetobacter* and *Enterobacter* species. The patient was treated with antibiotics but declined additional procedures. **E**, 10-month follow-up AP and lateral radiographs showing progressive bony erosion and nonunion, consistent with chronic osteomyelitis.

Staphylococcus aureus biofilms have been shown to promote bone loss in vitro by inducing apoptosis for osteoblasts, decreased osteogenic differentiation, and up-regulating receptor activator of nuclear factor-κB ligand (RANK-L), leading to an indirect increase in osteoblastic activity and bone resorption.[32,33] Further damage to surrounding soft tissues can occur when neutrophils unable to penetrate the biofilm lyse and spill their toxic enzymes.[32]

In vitro staphylococcal adherence to high-tensile strength sutures has also been demonstrated with decreasing adherence,[34] and this should be considered when sutures are used as part of a reconstruction.

Implant Retention Versus Removal

Little scientific evidence exists regarding implant retention versus removal. Unstable, infected fixation warrants removal because it provides no mechanical benefit. When fixation provides mechanical stability, the decision to retain or remove the implant is more challenging. Arthroplasty infections within 3 weeks of initial surgery or hematogenous seeding can be treated with débridement

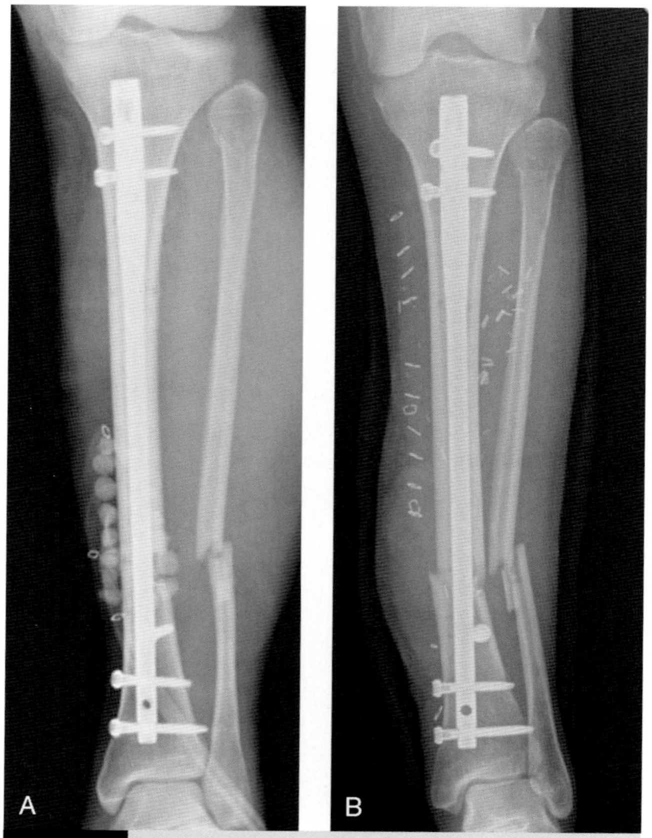

Figure 6 Radiographs of the lower extremity of a 32-year-old woman who sustained a 3B open tibial shaft fracture. **A**, AP view following intramedullary nailing and placement of an antibiotic bead pouch. **B**, Two-week follow-up view after soft-tissue coverage; the patient reported increasing pain. Loss of reduction and intraoperative findings included medullary purulence deep to the free flap necessitated removal of all implants. Change in alignment of fracture fragments should raise suspicion for infection.

and irrigation and a course of parenteral antibiotic therapy.[35] A multicenter retrospective study demonstrated a 71% union rate with débridement, hardware retention, and culture-specific antibiotics for deep wound infections within 6 weeks of fracture internal fixation; a history of open fracture (42% failure rate) or presence of a intramedullary nail (54% failure rate) substantially increased the risk for failure with implant retention.[36]

Antibiotic Depot Devices

Implants made or encased in antibiotic-loaded cement can also be used to provide local antibiotic delivery while simultaneously providing stability to unhealed fractures. Antibiotic cement nails can be used as a bridge to definitive intramedullary nailing when there is concern for high risk of infection with history of external fixator pins or to treat known medullary osteomyelitis.[31,37] Union was achieved in 14 of 16 patients with infected long-bone nonunions using this technique and systemic antibiotics; 3 patients required supplemental bone grafting.[38] An infected periprosthetic hip fracture was successfully treated to union with an antibiotic cement-coated plate.[39]

Local antibiotic therapy is used both acutely for severe open fractures and for treatment of chronic osteomyelitis. Several carriers for antibiotics can be used. Antibiotic cement (polymethyl methacrylate or PMMA) beads can be made with a variety of heat-stable antibiotics, with disadvantages being a second surgery required for removal and the possibility of bacterial colonization.[40,41] A randomized prospective trial comparing PMMA antibiotic beads to bioabsorbable antibiotic calcium sulfate cement showed no difference in infection eradication but increased reoperations in the PMMA beads group.[40] Chitosan sponges, derived from shellfish polysaccharides, have been tested in vitro as an antibiotic delivery device and been shown to decrease bacterial counts,[42] whereas a bioabsorbable phospholipid gel was shown to be superior in an animal model to PMMA beads.[41] Biodegradable polyurethane with vancomycin reduced bacterial contamination in an animal model.[43]

High local concentrations of antimicrobials can be cytotoxic and decrease osteogenic cell activity. Rifampin, minocycline, doxycycline, nafcillin, penicillin, ciprofloxacin, colistin, and gentamicin have the most deleterious effects and amikacin, tobramycin, and vancomycin are the least damaging and require very high concentrations to elicit cytotoxic effects.[44]

For acute open fracture with soft-tissue defects, concerns exist with concurrent use of antibiotic beads and negative-pressure wound therapy (NPWT). A goat open tibia model showed sixfold less bacteria when antibiotic beads with an occlusive dressing were used instead of antibiotic beads and NPWT.[45] NPWT is also more effective at reducing *Pseudomonas* contamination than *S aureus*.[46] The addition of silver-impregnated dressings to NPWT decreases *Pseudomonas* and *S aureus* bacterial loads.[47]

Surgical Treatments of Bone Defect

Treatment strategies must be individualized to the patient, location of bone defect, and surrounding soft-tissue envelope. Different considerations are made when dealing with periarticular infection compared with diaphyseal infection. Amputation may be more likely for recalcitrant infections of the foot and ankle than other sites due to the functionality of below-knee prosthetics compared with other prosthetics, especially those for the upper

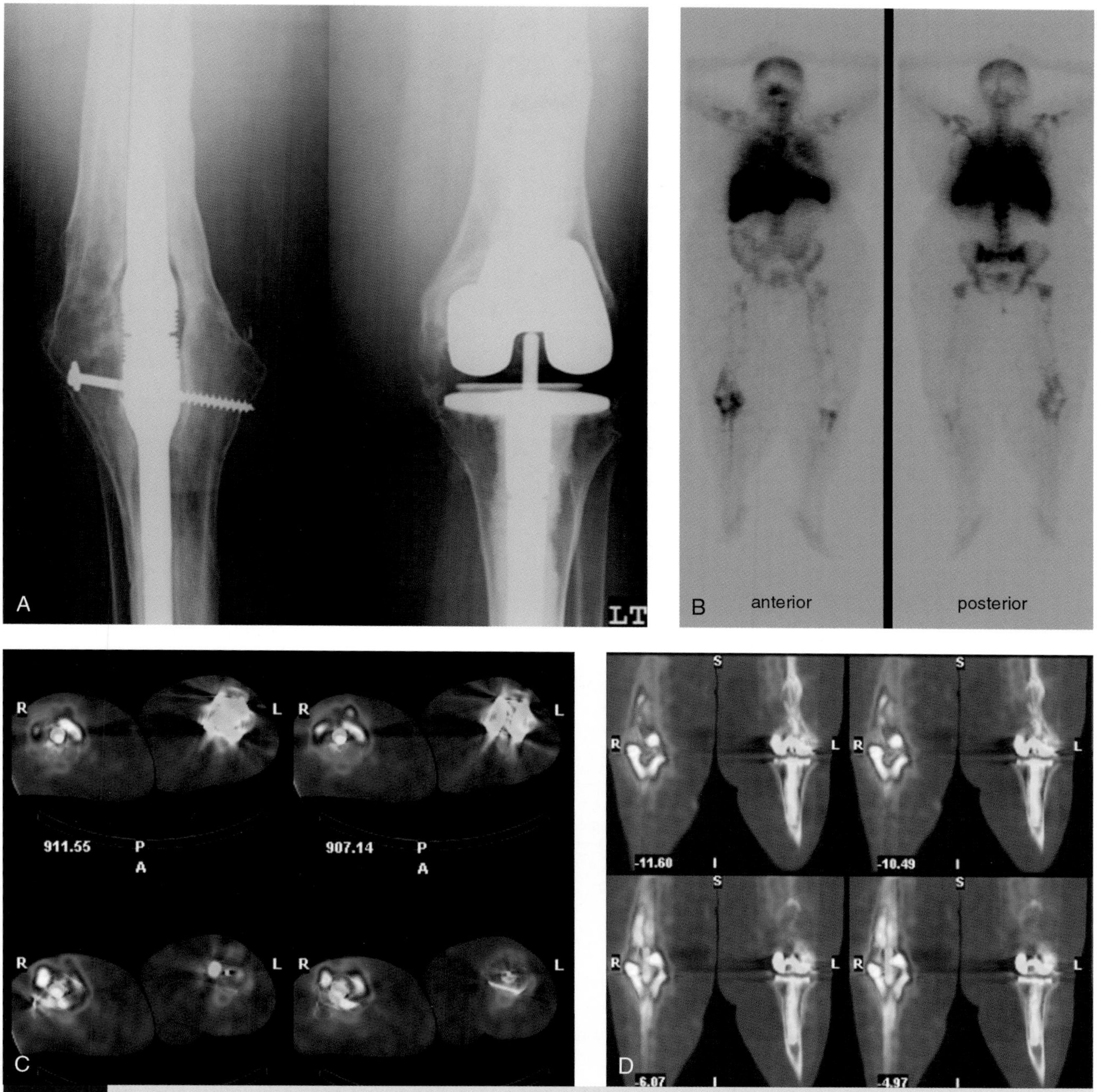

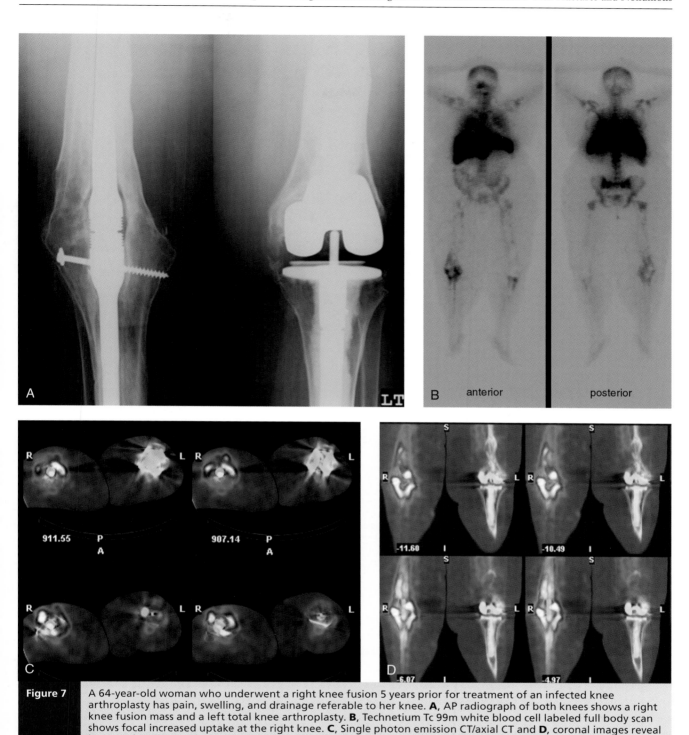

Figure 7 A 64-year-old woman who underwent a right knee fusion 5 years prior for treatment of an infected knee arthroplasty has pain, swelling, and drainage referable to her knee. **A**, AP radiograph of both knees shows a right knee fusion mass and a left total knee arthroplasty. **B**, Technetium Tc 99m white blood cell labeled full body scan shows focal increased uptake at the right knee. **C**, Single photon emission CT/axial CT and **D**, coronal images reveal increased activity at the right knee. These findings are consistent with chronic osteomyelitis.

extremity.[48] Shortening remains another option that is especially appealing for upper-extremity defects. Unequal lower extremity limb length creates problems with gait that necessitate a prosthetic device or further reconstructive solutions.

Regardless of the bony reconstruction method used, all recent literature supports radical resection to noninfected, healthy bleeding bone.[23-30]

Structural bone graft can be taken from various donor sites. Tricortical iliac crest remains a traditional donor

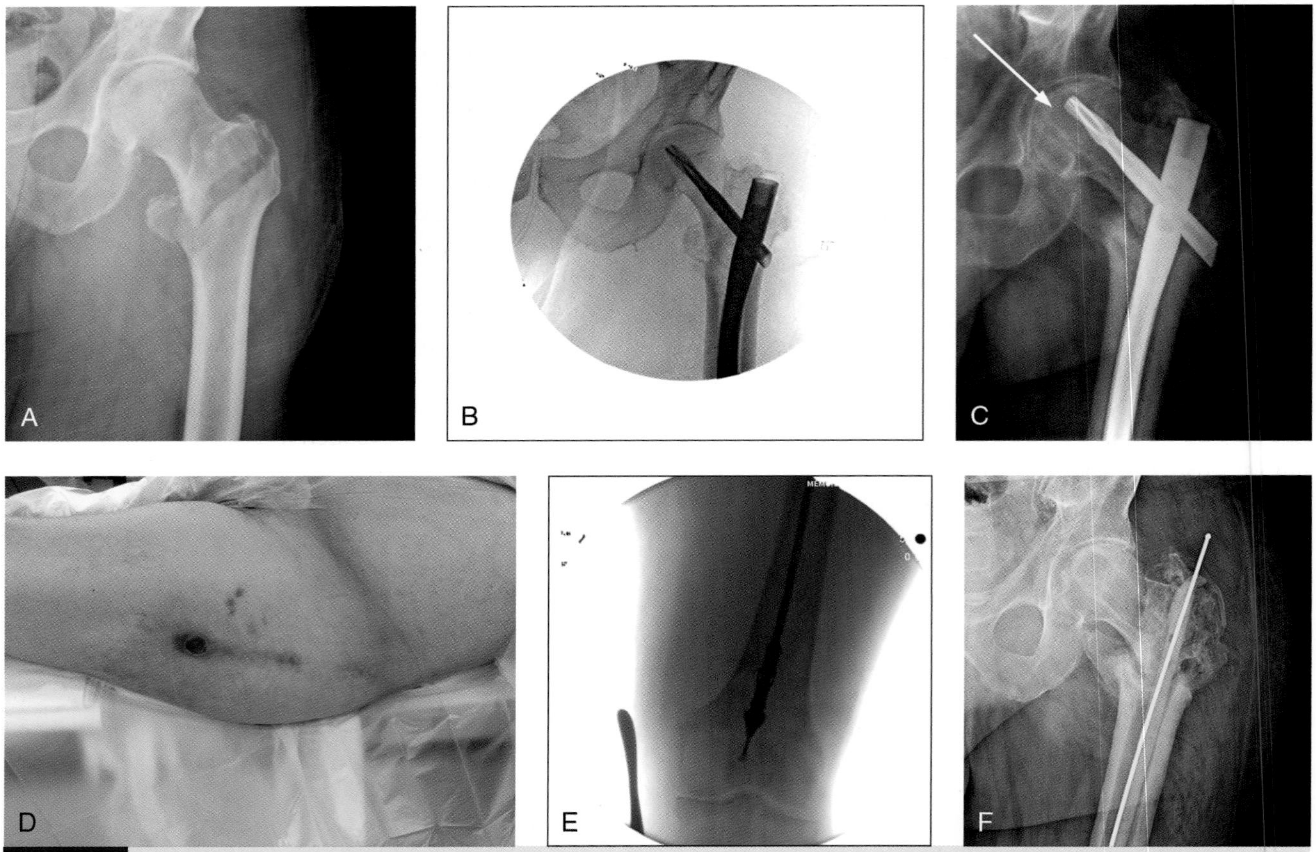

Figure 8 Imaging studies and clinical photograph of the lower extremity of a 55-year-old man with a history of hepatitis B who was involved in a motor vehicle crash. **A**, AP radiograph reveals an intertrochanteric proximal femur fracture. **B**, AP fluoroscopic image reveals intra-operative adequacy of reduction and cephalomedullary nail placement. **C**, AP radiograph taken 6 months after surgery reveals a perihardware lucency (arrow), progressive loss of reduction, and lack of bridging bone. The patient was experiencing worsening pain and new drainage, which indicated infected nonunion. **D**, Clinical photograph shows a draining sinus in line with a previously well-healed scar that is indicative of infection. **E**, Intraoperative fluoroscopic image following hardware removal shows débridement of the medullary canal using the Reamer Irrigator Aspirator. **F**, An antibiotic impregnated cement rod has been implanted.

site, but is limited by the length of graft obtainable. Diaphyseal nonunions of the forearm with bone defects ranging from 1 to 7 cm have been successfully treated in more than 90% of a single surgeon case series with tricortical iliac crest autograft.[26]

Nonvascularized fibular shaft provides an option for larger defects, but no recent literature documents its use in the extremities. Free-vascularized fibular grafting remains a structural bone graft option that requires microvascular anastomosis and harvest of a large segment of uninjured fibula. A series of 10 patients with lower extremity bony defects between 6 cm and 17 cm showed that 100% of patients were able to bear weight without assistive devices or pain without any recurrence of osteomyelitis at almost 2.5 years average follow-up.[29]

Nonstructural cancellous autograft or allografts can be used acutely or in a delayed fashion following appropriate débridement. A 2011 study reported that a single-stage treatment of 25 infected nonunions of the distal tibia had 100% success by performing débridement, removing hardware, placing a thin-wire ring external fixator, and using cancellous autograft from the proximal tibia mixed with vancomycin powder and gentamicin solution.[30] Animal data have shown some promise for a biodegradable polyurethane scaffold loaded with vancomycin and bone morphogenetic protein-2 (BMP-2), or a dual purpose bone graft, when compared with a collagen scaffold or a scaffold without loaded antibiotics.[43]

The induced membrane or Masquelet technique remains a popular two-stage technique. After radical débridement of necrotic and/or infected bone, an antibiotic-loaded cement spacer is placed into the bony defect for 4 to 8 weeks before cement spacer removal and bone grafting (**Figure 9**). The development of a vascularized membrane around the cement spacer allows delivery of growth factors to the bone graft site. The authors of a 2012 study retrospectively reported a union rate of 90% with defects ranging from 2 to 23 cm in more than half of their 84 cases; all 8 failures occurred in the tibia (n = 61) and all were previously open injuries.[24] There were no failures in the femur (n = 13), humerus (n = 6), and forearm (n = 4). The authors used a heterogeneous group of graft material ranging from cancellous bone to vascularized grafts with and without bone substitutes and growth factors. They stress that the cement spacer should extend onto the healthy bone proximal and distal to the defect site, with decortication of surrounding bone and opening of the medullary canal at bone grafting. The authors also note that when used in the tibia, the cement block should be in contact with the fibula. Another series reporting defects ranging from 1 cm to 25 cm (where femoral shaft harvested with the RIA was used as graft) showed a 70% union rate at 6 months and 90% union rate at 12 months.[28]

Bone transport using thin-wire ring external fixation remains a popular treatment of large bony defects, especially those in the tibia. Several retrospective series have been published with excellent union rates. In one study, 100% union was obtained in 12 patients with an average tibial defect of 8 cm (range, 3–12 cm) with an average time in the ring external fixation of 418 days (± 99).[27] A retrospective series also showed 100% union rate for nine patients with an average tibial defect of 5 cm (range, 2–12 cm) with a shorter external fixation time averaging 6 months.[25] None of the patients in either of these series required free tissue transfer for salvage, but some did require local rotational flap. Another study demonstrated that free tissue transfer and bone transport can provide excellent results. Free flap coverage was generally performed 6 weeks before the initiation of distraction osteogenesis. Twenty-six of 28 patients with tibial defects averaging 6 cm (range, 3–14 cm) went on to ambulate independently and return to work; amputations were performed in two patients with free flap failure before distraction.[23] A radical débridement strategy was used acutely for type IIIB open tibia fractures, leaving an average defect of 9.4 cm (range, 5–17 cm) followed by delayed distraction osteogenesis with a 95% union rate and average reconstruction time of 26.5 months (range, 12–73 months).[49] Acute shortening followed by delayed distraction osteogenesis provides another salvage option for severe open tibia fractures. In a series of 13 patients treated in this manner with average shortening ranging from 4.0 cm to 12.5 cm, every patient achieve a functional status where they could perform light work and walk with a slight limp.[50] Enthusiasm for bone transport in the femur is tempered, and high complication rates have been reported with reduced knee range of motion, persistent pain and a mean residual limb-length discrepancy of 1.9 cm after treatment.[51]

Medical Therapy

The principles of antimicrobial therapy remain unchanged. Prevention remains the first line of defense. Preoperative prophylactic antibiotics are known to decrease infection with fracture fixation.[52] After an implant-related infection has been diagnosed, identification of the causative organism(s) and antibiotic susceptibilities is paramount.

Traditional recommendations for treatment of osteomyelitis or implant-associated infection are 4 to 6 weeks on intravenous antibiotics; however, there is limited science to support this duration versus shorter or longer time periods.[53]

Virulence varies by pathogen. *Staphylococcus* species cause approximately two-thirds of orthopaedic implant-related infections.[54] A retrospective comparative study of 163 *Staphylococcus* species infections (combined arthroplasty and fracture fixation) treated with 6 to 12 weeks of intravenous antibiotic therapy showed that cure rates 1 year after treatment were greatest for coagulase-negative staphylococci at 82%. Methicillin-sensitive *S aureus* (MSSA) infections had cure rates of 72%, whereas methicillin-resistant *S aureus* (MRSA) only had a cure rate of 57% with more long-term sequelae when compared with MSSA and coagulase-negative staphylococci infections.[54] Treatment of fracture fixation related infections had a substantially higher cure rate than arthroplasty-related infections.[54]

An initial course of parenteral pharmacotherapy is thought to decrease bacterial burden, and subsequently, the risk of emergence of drug-resistant bacteria before conversion to oral antimicrobial agents.[55] The timing of conversion from intravenous to oral antibiotics is controversial and there is a recent trend toward an earlier switch to oral agents.

Although no specific guidelines exist for implant infections related to fracture fixation, the Infectious Diseases Society of America published guidelines in 2013 for the treatment of arthroplasty-related implant infections and generally recommend 4 to 6 weeks of intravenous therapy.[35]

A recent study demonstrated that 2 to 3 months of oral antimicrobial therapy commenced after only 10 to 14 days of intravenous therapy was effective in the treatment of prosthetic hip infections.[56] Bactericidal antibiotic combination therapy is recommended when compared with monotherapy. For implant-associated MRSA infection, fluoroquinolone/rifampicin as the first-line therapy with

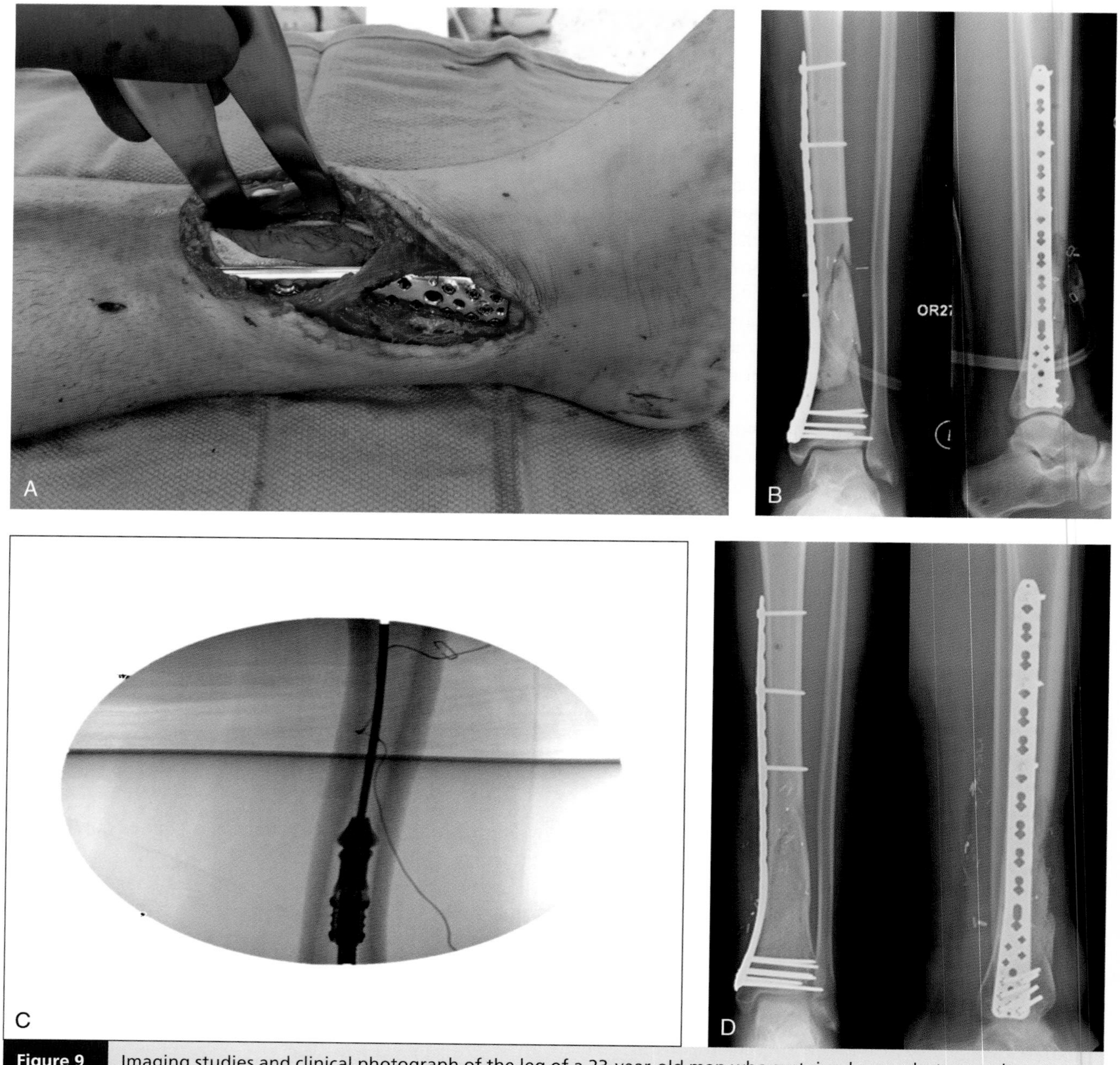

Figure 9 Imaging studies and clinical photograph of the leg of a 23-year-old man who sustained a gunshot wound to the leg and underwent radical débridement of nonviable bone, leaving a significant bony defect. **A**, Clinical photograph shows how an antibiotic cement spacer or Masquelet technique was used to increase local concentration of antibiotic, fill the dead space, and induce membrane formation. **B**, AP and lateral radiographs of the tibia following plate fixation with antibiotic cement spacer. **C**, Intraoperative fluoroscopic image shows use of the Reamer Irrigator Aspirator for bone graft harvest, 8 weeks after débridement. An ipsilateral retrograde femoral approach was selected. **D**, AP and lateral radiographs of the tibia following re-elevation of the free flap, removal of the spacer, and bone grafting of the defect.

fusidic acid/rifampicin as the backup for fluoroquinolone resistance or allergy has been recommended.[57] Other MRSA combination treatments include rifampicin in combination with clindamycin, trimethoprim/sulfamethoxazole, a tetracycline, or linezolid. Rifampicin allergy or resistance should be treated with fluoroquinolone combination therapies. Oral antibiotic monotherapy is a treatment of last resort and MSSA infection may be treated with first-generation cephalosporins or antistaphylococcal penicillins.[55]

Intravenous infusion of antibiotics necessitates specialized care when compared with oral antibiotic therapy. Although no studies have analyzed the cost of intravenous versus oral antibiotic therapy for postfracture fixation infections, data have demonstrated that management of an infected total hip arthroplasty is 3.6 times more costly than a primary total hip arthroplasty because of costs related to laboratory tests, intravenous antibiotics, healthcare personnel, and an orthopaedic rehabilitation hospital.[58] It is intuitive that these results likely translate to postfracture infection care. There are published guidelines by the Infectious Diseases Society of America for monitoring outpatient parenteral antibiotics; these guidelines have not been updated in more than decade.[59]

Summary

Several challenges remain in the treatment and diagnosis of infection after fracture. Clinicians should maintain a high index of suspicion when infection is a consideration. Diagnosis is imperfect with current technologies; however, intraoperative cultures with antibiotic sensitivities provide the best guidance for antimicrobial management. Cultures should be held for at least 2 weeks to allow for growth of slow-growing organisms. Although serologic markers such as ESR and CRP are elevated with infection, they are nonspecific and are better as trends to monitor for success or failure of treatment. Imaging modalities such as CT and MRI are imperfect as metal artifact often limits utility when fractures or nonunions are evaluated. Treatment of infections associated with fractures or nonunions includes débridement, antimicrobial therapy, and elimination of the biofilm, which usually necessitates removal of implants. Bone defects may be addressed with amputation, bone grafting procedures, or distraction osteogenesis, and the choice of strategy is often dictated by anatomic location and patient factors. Treatment requires a team approach with the combined knowledge and skills of orthopaedic surgeons, plastic surgeons, and infectious disease specialists.

Key Study Points

- Surgical débridement of all infected and nonviable tissue, including bone, should be performed regardless of the planned method of bony reconstruction.
- Identification of causative organisms with site-specific cultures and antibiotic sensitivities guides medical therapy in consultation with an infectious disease specialist.
- Biofilms are associated with staphylococcal adhesion to implants and resist antibiotics, chemical disinfectants, and mechanical débridement; they evade immune system defenses and are only eradicated with implant removal.
- Bone defects may be managed with amputation, structural graft, cancellous graft via the induced membrane (or Masquelet) technique, or distraction osteogenesis; the strategy chosen is individualized based on anatomic location and patient factors.

Annotated References

1. Brinker MR, Hanus BD, Sen M, O'Connor DP: The devastating effects of tibial nonunion on health-related quality of life. *J Bone Joint Surg Am* 2013;95(24):2170-2176.

   This study evaluated 243 tibial shaft nonunions treated by a single surgeon. Using the Medical Outcomes Study Short Form (SF)-12 Physical Component Summary and Mental Component Summary, the authors reported patient scores below the mean United States population, indicating self-perceived physical and mental disability. The outcomes reveal tibial nonunion to be more devastating than many other medical conditions, and most orthopaedic conditions. Level of evidence: III.

2. Schmidt HG, Tiemann AH, Braunschweig R, et al; Arbeitsgemeinschaft septische Chirugie der DGOUC10: Definition of the Diagnosis Osteomyelitis-Osteomyelitis Diagnosis Score (ODS). *Z Orthop Unfall* 2011;149(4):449-460.

   The authors present a scoring system to aid in the reliable diagnosis of osteomyelitis using five separate parameters: history and risk factors, clinical examination and pertinent laboratory values, imaging studies, microbiology, and histopathology.

3. Bishop JA, Palanca AA, Bellino MJ, Lowenberg DW: Assessment of compromised fracture healing. *J Am Acad Orthop Surg* 2012;20(5):273-282.

   The authors present a review of the evaluation and classification of nonunions. They include a discussion of risk factors and clinical/radiographic/laboratory evaluation findings to aid in the proper diagnosis to determine the most appropriate treatment.

4. Bosse MJ, MacKenzie EJ, Kellam JF, et al: An analysis of outcomes of reconstruction or amputation after leg-threatening injuries. *N Engl J Med* 2002;347(24):1924-1931.

5. Gustilo RB, Anderson JT: Prevention of infection in the treatment of one thousand and twenty-five open fractures of long bones: Retrospective and prospective analyses. *J Bone Joint Surg Am* 1976;58(4):453-458.

6. Patzakis MJ, Wilkins J: Factors influencing infection rate in open fracture wounds. *Clin Orthop Relat Res* 1989;243:36-40.

7. Kindsfater K, Jonassen EA: Osteomyelitis in grade II and III open tibia fractures with late debridement. *J Orthop Trauma* 1995;9(2):121-127.

8. Khundkar R, Williams G, Fennell N, Ramsden A, Mcnally M: Squamous cell carcinoma complicating chronic osteomyelitis: clinical features and outcome of a case series. *Bone Joint J* 2015;97-B(suppl 15):75.

   Over a 10-year period, a Marjolin ulcer was diagnosed in nine patients and despite wide resection, four eventually died from the cancer.

9. Pääkkönen M, Kallio MJ, Kallio PE, Peltola H: Sensitivity of erythrocyte sedimentation rate and C-reactive protein in childhood bone and joint infections. *Clin Orthop Relat Res* 2010;468(3):861-866.

   The authors present a study involving 265 children with culture-positive bone and joint infections, and determined that CRP was more sensitive than ESR for detecting infection, but elevations of both improved sensitivity to 98%. Also, CRP normalized faster after successful treatment, and as such was more useful in monitoring recovery. Level of evidence: II.

10. Maharajan K, Patro DK, Menon J, et al: Serum procalcitonin is a sensitive and specific marker in the diagnosis of septic arthritis and acute osteomyelitis. *J Orthop Surg Res* 2013;8(19):19.

    The authors report on a group of 82 patients with suspected acute osteomyelitis and septic arthritis. They found that serum procalcitonin at a cut-off of 0.4 ng/mL is a sensitive and specific marker for infection and may be used as a new diagnostic test to allow initiation of treatment.

11. Michail M, Jude E, Liaskos C, et al: The performance of serum inflammatory markers for the diagnosis and follow-up of patients with osteomyelitis. *Int J Low Extrem Wounds* 2013;12(2):94-99.

    The authors followed 61 patients with foot infections for three months and evaluated serial ESR, CRP, WBC, and procalcitonin. CRP, WBC, and procalcitonin had returned to near-normal levels by 1 week, but ESR remained elevated in patients with bone infection. The authors recommend following ESR in patients with bone infection.

12. Douraiswami B, Dilip PK, Harish BN, Jagdish M: C-reactive protein and interleukin-6 levels in the early detection of infection after open fractures. *J Orthop Surg (Hong Kong)* 2012;20(3):381-385.

    The authors followed 30 patients with open fractures; postoperative wound infections developed in 11 patients. They determined elevated serum IL-6 and CRP aid in the early diagnosis of infection after open fractures, even before clinical signs of infection develop.

13. Stucken C, Olszewski DC, Creevy WR, Murakami AM, Tornetta P: Preoperative diagnosis of infection in patients with nonunions. *J Bone Joint Surg Am* 2013;95(15):1409-1412.

    The authors performed preoperative laboratory tests (WBC, ESR, and CRP) as well as combined WBC/sulfur colloid scan on 93 patients with 95 nonunions. Thirty nonunions were ultimately diagnosed as infected. The risk of infection increased with each additional positive test: with zero to all four of the tests considered "positive" the predicted probability of infection was 18%, 24%, 50%, and 86%, respectively. Considering only the serum WBC, ESR, and CRP, the predicted values were 20%, 19%, 56%, and 100%. Among the tests evaluated, the authors concluded that nuclear imaging was the most expensive and least valuable test to aid in the diagnosis of an infected nonunion. Level of evidence: III.

14. Agarwal S, Zahid M, Sherwani MK, Abbas M, Huda N, Khan AQ: Comparison of the results of sinus track culture and sequestrum culture in chronic osteomyelitis. *Acta Orthop Belg* 2005;71(2):209-212.

15. Akinyoola AL, Adegbehingbe OO, Aboderin AO: Therapeutic decision in chronic osteomyelitis: Sinus track culture versus intraoperative bone culture. *Arch Orthop Trauma Surg* 2009;129(4):449-453.

16. Wu JS, Gorbachova T, Morrison WB, Haims AH: Imaging-guided bone biopsy for osteomyelitis: Are there factors associated with positive or negative cultures? *AJR Am J Roentgenol* 2007;188(6):1529-1534.

17. Schwotzer N, Wahl P, Fracheboud D, Gautier E, Chuard C: Optimal culture incubation time in orthopedic device-associated infections: A retrospective analysis of prolonged 14-day incubation. *J Clin Microbiol* 2014;52(1):61-66.

    Four hundred ninety-nine tissue biopsy specimens from 117 documented infected cases were retrospectively reviewed; 83% were considered true infections and 17% were "contaminations." The average time to positivity was 1 day and 6 days, respectively, and 96% of the infections were diagnosed within 7 days of incubation. The authors conclude that incubation beyond 7days is generally not productive unless slow-growing organisms are suspected.

18. Palmer MP, Altman DT, Altman GT, et al: Can we trust intraoperative culture results in nonunions? *J Orthop Trauma* 2014;28(7):384-390.

    The authors sought to compare routine intraoperative cultures with advanced molecular techniques including PCR, mass spectrometry and fluorescence in situ hybridization in 34 nonunions. Ultimately, molecular diagnostics were found to be more sensitive than cultures for identifying bacteria in cases of infected nonunion. It is proposed that this is because routine cultures do not generally detect bacteria in biofilms. Level of evidence: I.

19. Trampuz A, Piper KE, Jacobson MJ, et al: Sonication of removed hip and knee prostheses for diagnosis of infection. *N Engl J Med* 2007;357(7):654-663.

    This study evaluated 331 patients who underwent removal of a hip or knee prosthesis for aseptic or septic failure. The authors found that culture of sonication fluid was more sensitive than traditional deep tissue culture for the diagnosis of infection. It is believed that bath sonication dislodges adherent bacteria and biofilms from prostheses, allowing for more accurate diagnosis.

20. Yano MH, Klautau GB, da Silva CB, et al: Improved diagnosis of infection associated with osteosynthesis by use of sonication of fracture fixation implants. *J Clin Microbiol* 2014;52(12):4176-4182.

    The authors evaluated 180 patients with suspected osteosynthesis-associated infection. They compared cultures from sonication fluid from removed implants to traditional tissue specimens. The sensitivity and specificity for detecting infection was 90.4 and 90.9 for the sonication fluid group and 56.8 and 96.4 for the tissue culture group. They concluded that sonication fluid culture from removed implants can aid in the microbiological diagnosis of infection.

21. Portillo ME, Salvadó M, Alier A, et al: Advantages of sonication fluid culture for the diagnosis of prosthetic joint infection. *J Infect* 2014;69(1):35-41.

    The authors evaluated 75 consecutive patients who underwent removal of orthopaedic hardware. For detection of an organism, the sensitivity of sonication fluid inoculated in blood culture bottles (100%) was higher than that of conventional sonication fluid (87%) or intraoperative tissue cultures (59%). In addition, previous treatment with antibiotics did not alter the sensitivity of the sonication fluid inoculated in blood culture bottles, while it significantly altered the results for the other groups (100% versus 77% and 55%).

22. Shemesh S, Kosashvili Y, Groshar D, et al: The value of 18-FDG PET/CT in the diagnosis and management of implant-related infections of the tibia: A case series. *Injury* 2015;46(7):1377-1382.

    Ten patients with tibia fractures and suspected infection were evaluated using both standard serum and imaging modalities as well as positron emission tomography/CT. They found positron emission tomography/CT validated their working diagnosis in nine of 10 patients and may be used to aid in clinical decision making.

23. Chim H, Sontich JK, Kaufman BR: Free tissue transfer with distraction osteogenesis is effective for limb salvage of the infected traumatized lower extremity. *Plast Reconstr Surg* 2011;127(6):2364-2372.

    Patients with osteocutaneous defects were treated with free tissue coverage and distraction osteogenesis; 89% returned to work and independent ambulation.

24. Karger C, Kishi T, Schneider L, Fitoussi F, Masquelet AC; French Society of Orthopaedic Surgery and Traumatology (SoFCOT): Treatment of posttraumatic bone defects by the induced membrane technique. *Orthop Traumatol Surg Res* 2012;98(1):97-102.

    Eighty-four post-traumatic long bone defects were treated with the inducted membrane technique with a 90% union rate. Level of evidence: IV.

25. Megas P, Saridis A, Kouzelis A, Kallivokas A, Mylonas S, Tyllianakis M: The treatment of infected nonunion of the tibia following intramedullary nailing by the Ilizarov method. *Injury* 2010;41(3):294-299.

    Nine infected tibial nonunions after intramedullary nail were treated with resection, soft-tissue coverage, and distraction osteogenesis with a 100% union rate.

26. Prasarn ML, Ouellette EA, Miller DR: Infected nonunions of diaphyseal fractures of the forearm. *Arch Orthop Trauma Surg* 2010;130(7):867-873.

    Fifteen patients with infected nonunion of the forearm were treated with débridement, tricortical iliac crest autograft, and secondary wound healing with 100% union rate and infection eradication.

27. Sala F, Thabet AM, Castelli F, et al: Bone transport for postinfectious segmental tibial bone defects with a combined ilizarov/taylor spatial frame technique. *J Orthop Trauma* 2011;25(3):162-168.

    Twelve patients with atrophic tibial nonunions were treated with resection and bone transport with 100% union rate and infection eradication.

28. Stafford PR, Norris BL: Reamer-irrigator-aspirator bone graft and bi Masquelet technique for segmental bone defect nonunions: A review of 25 cases. *Injury* 2010;41(suppl 2):S72-S77.

    Twenty-five patients with 27 segmental defects (average defect 5.8 cm) in the lower extremity were treated with a staged surgical protocol of débridement of nonviable tissue and placement of an antibiotic impregnated spacer, followed by RIA bone grafting. The authors report 90% union at one year with a single bone grafting.

29. Sun Y, Zhang C, Jin D, et al: Free vascularised fibular grafting in the treatment of large skeletal defects due to osteomyelitis. *Int Orthop* 2010;34(3):425-430.

    Ten patients with bony defects due to osteomyelitis averaging 9.5 cm were treated with vascularized free-fibular grafts with 100% union rate with no recurrences of osteomyelitis.

30. Wu CC: Single-stage surgical treatment of infected nonunion of the distal tibia. *J Orthop Trauma* 2011;25(3):156-161.

Twenty-five infected nonunions of the distal tibia were treated with a single-stage débridement, cancellous bone grafting with antibiotics and Ilizarov application with 100% union rate at 2-year follow-up.

31. Kanakaris N, Gudipati S, Tosounidis T, Harwood P, Britten S, Giannoudis PV: The treatment of intramedullary osteomyelitis of the femur and tibia using the Reamer-Irrigator-Aspirator system and antibiotic cement rods. *Bone Joint J* 2014;96-B(6):783-788.

    Twenty-three of 24 patients treated with RIA and antibiotic cement nails for intramedullary osteomyelitis had no evidence of recurrent infection at average follow-up of 21 months.

32. Arciola CR, Campoccia D, Speziale P, Montanaro L, Costerton JW: Biofilm formation in Staphylococcus implant infections. A review of molecular mechanisms and implications for biofilm-resistant materials. *Biomaterials* 2012;33(26):5967-5982.

    Staphylococci growing in a biofilm enhances the organism's ability to protect itself against host defenses and antimicrobials.

33. Sanchez CJ Jr, Ward CL, Romano DR, et al: Staphylococcus aureus biofilms decrease osteoblast viability, inhibits osteogenic differentiation, and increases bone resorption in vitro. *BMC Musculoskelet Disord* 2013;14:187.

    S aureus biofilms increase bone loss by reducing osteoblast viability and promoting bone resorption through increased osteoclastogenesis.

34. Masini BD, Stinner DJ, Waterman SM, Wenke JC: Bacterial adherence to high-tensile strength sutures. *Arthroscopy* 2011;27(6):834-838.

    Bacteria adherence to braided high-tensile sutures was evaluated. Adherence decreased in descending order, from MaxBraid to FiberWire, Ethibond, Orthocord, and silk.

35. Osmon DR, Berbari EF, Berendt AR, et al; Infectious Diseases Society of America: Diagnosis and management of prosthetic joint infection: Clinical practice guidelines by the Infectious Diseases Society of America. *Clin Infect Dis* 2013;56(1):e1-e25.

    The 2012 guidelines from the Infectious Diseases Society of America for the diagnosis and management of prosthetic joint infection are discussed.

36. Berkes M, Obremskey WT, Scannell B, Ellington JK, Hymes RA, Bosse M; Southeast Fracture Consortium: Maintenance of hardware after early postoperative infection following fracture internal fixation. *J Bone Joint Surg Am* 2010;92(4):823-828.

    A multicenter retrospective study demonstrated a 71% union rate with debridement, hardware retention, and culture-specific antibiotics for deep wound infections within 6 weeks of fracture internal fixation; a history of open fracture (42% failure rate) or presence of an intramedullary nail (54% failure rate) substantially increased the risk for failure with implant retention. Level of evidence: IV.

37. Bhadra AK, Roberts CS: Indications for antibiotic cement nails. *J Orthop Trauma* 2009;23(5suppl):S26-S30.

38. Selhi HS, Mahindra P, Yamin M, Jain D, De Long WG Jr, Singh J: Outcome in patients with an infected nonunion of the long bones treated with a reinforced antibiotic bone cement rod. *J Orthop Trauma* 2012;26(3):184-188.

    Sixteen patients with long bone infected nonunions were treated with systemic antibiotics and a reinforced antibiotic nail, with 14 patients experiencing union around the antibiotic nail without recurrence of infection. Level of evidence: IV.

39. Liporace FA, Yoon RS, Frank MA, et al: Use of an "antibiotic plate" for infected periprosthetic fracture in total hip arthroplasty. *J Orthop Trauma* 2012;26(3):e18-e23.

    A case report of a periprosthetic hip fracture infection successfully treated with an antibiotic cement coated plate is presented.

40. McKee MD, Li-Bland EA, Wild LM, Schemitsch EH: A prospective, randomized clinical trial comparing an antibiotic-impregnated bioabsorbable bone substitute with standard antibiotic-impregnated cement beads in the treatment of chronic osteomyelitis and infected nonunion. *J Orthop Trauma* 2010;24(8):483-490.

    A prospective, randomized controlled trial comparing antibiotic loaded calcium sulfate and PMMA antibiotics beads from chronic osteomyelitis and infected nonunion showed no difference in infection eradication and fewer surgeries for the group treated with a bioabsorbable carrier for antibiotics.

41. Penn-Barwell JG, Murray CK, Wenke JC: Local antibiotic delivery by a bioabsorbable gel is superior to PMMA bead depot in reducing infection in an open fracture model. *J Orthop Trauma* 2014;28(6):370-375.

    There was a significantly lower infection rate for a bioabsorbable gel carrier for local antibiotics in a rat model compared to PMMA antibiotic beads.

42. Stinner DJ, Noel SP, Haggard WO, Watson JT, Wenke JC: Local antibiotic delivery using tailorable chitosan sponges: The future of infection control? *J Orthop Trauma* 2010;24(9):592-597.

    A goat model of musculoskeletal infections showed lower infection rates with antibiotic-loaded bioabsorbable chitosan sponges versus irrigation and débridement alone.

43. Guelcher SA, Brown KV, Li B, Guda T, Lee BH, Wenke JC: Dual-purpose bone grafts improve healing and reduce infection. *J Orthop Trauma* 2011;25(8):477-482.

    Bioabsorbable polyurethane scaffolds loaded with BMP-2 and vancomycin showed a more sustained release of BMP-2 and a modest reduction of infection in a rat model as compared to a collagen sponge.

44. Rathbone CR, Cross JD, Brown KV, Murray CK, Wenke JC: Effect of various concentrations of antibiotics

on osteogenic cell viability and activity. *J Orthop Res* 2011;29(7):1070-1074.

Local antibiotics can decrease in vitro osteoblast viability and affect osteogenesis activity. Amikacin, tobramycin, and vancomycin are the least cytotoxic antibiotics.

45. Stinner DJ, Hsu JR, Wenke JC: Negative pressure wound therapy reduces the effectiveness of traditional local antibiotic depot in a large complex musculoskeletal wound animal model. *J Orthop Trauma* 2012;26(9):512-518.

Negative-pressure wound therapy over PMMA antibiotic beads had increased bacterial counts when compared with a bead pouch in an animal infection model.

46. Lalliss SJ, Stinner DJ, Waterman SM, Branstetter JG, Masini BD, Wenke JC: Negative pressure wound therapy reduces pseudomonas wound contamination more than Staphylococcus aureus. *J Orthop Trauma* 2010;24(9):598-602.

Negative pressure wound therapy decreased Pseudomonas contamination when compared with wet-to-dry dressings in a goat model. This benefit was not seen for *S aureus* with NPWT.

47. Stinner DJ, Waterman SM, Masini BD, Wenke JC: Silver dressings augment the ability of negative pressure wound therapy to reduce bacteria in a contaminated open fracture model. *J Trauma* 2011;71(1suppl):S147-S150.

The addition of silver impregnated gauze to NPWT reduces bacterial contamination when compared with negative pressure wound therapy alone in a goat model of open fractures.

48. Krueger CA, Wenke JC, Ficke JR: Ten years at war: Comprehensive analysis of amputation trends. *J Trauma Acute Care Surg* 2012;73(6suppl 5):S438-S444.

There were increased numbers of amputation in the final years of the Iraq and Afghanistan conflicts with lower extremity amputations more common than upper extremity amputations. Multiple amputations were also more common in these conflicts as compared with prior wars. Level of evidence: IV.

49. Hutson JJ Jr, Dayicioglu D, Oeltjen JC, Panthaki ZJ, Armstrong MB: The treatment of gustilo grade IIIB tibia fractures with application of antibiotic spacer, flap, and sequential distraction osteogenesis. *Ann Plast Surg* 2010;64(5):541-552.

Treatment of type IIIB and IIIC open tibia fractures with radical resection, flap coverage, antibiotic spacer, and bone transport via circular ring external fixation resulted in 18 of 19 healing without infection or osteomyelitis. Average time of reconstruction was more than 2 years.

50. Parmaksizoglu F, Koprulu AS, Unal MB, Cansu E: Early or delayed limb lengthening after acute shortening in the treatment of traumatic below-knee amputations and Gustilo and Anderson type IIIC open tibial fractures: The results of a case series. *J Bone Joint Surg Br* 2010;92(11):1563-1567.

Type IIIC tibial injuries, including five traumatic amputations, were treated with débridement, vascular reconstruction, acute shortening, and delayed distraction osteogenesis, with all 13 patients achieving the ability to do light work and walk with a slight limp.

51. Blum AL, BongioVanni JC, Morgan SJ, Flierl MA, dos Reis FB: Complications associated with distraction osteogenesis for infected nonunion of the femoral shaft in the presence of a bone defect: A retrospective series. *J Bone Joint Surg Br* 2010;92(4):565-570.

A retrospective review of 50 patients treated with distraction osteogenesis for femoral shaft defects showed high rates of decreased range of motion in the knee and residual limb-length discrepancy and pin site infections in all patients.

52. Prokuski L: Prophylactic antibiotics in orthopaedic surgery. *J Am Acad Orthop Surg* 2008;16(5):283-293.

53. Haidar R, Der Boghossian A, Atiyeh B: Duration of post-surgical antibiotics in chronic osteomyelitis: Empiric or evidence-based? *Int J Infect Dis* 2010;14(9):e752-e758.

A review article of the level of evidence for recommendations of postoperative antibiotics for chronic osteomyelitis is presented.

54. Teterycz D, Ferry T, Lew D, et al: Outcome of orthopedic implant infections due to different staphylococci. *Int J Infect Dis* 2010;14(10):e913-e918.

A retrospective comparative study of 163 implant-related infections with coagulase-negative staphylococci, MSSA, and MRSA showed the least virulent organism as coagulase-negative staphylococci with the highest cure rates and the most virulent organism MRSA with the lowest cure rates.

55. Kim BN, Kim ES, Oh MD: Oral antibiotic treatment of staphylococcal bone and joint infections in adults. *J Antimicrob Chemother* 2014;69(2):309-322.

A review article of the evidence of oral antibiotic therapy for staphylococcal bone and joint infections in adults is presented.

56. Darley ES, Bannister GC, Blom AW, Macgowan AP, Jacobson SK, Alfouzan W: Role of early intravenous to oral antibiotic switch therapy in the management of prosthetic hip infection treated with one- or two-stage replacement. *J Antimicrob Chemother* 2011;66(10):2405-2408.

Seventeen patients undergoing two-stage revision total hip arthroplasty were treated with 10 to 14 days of intravenous antibiotic followed by 3 to 4 months of oral antibiotic therapy. Four patients had one-stage revision total hip arthroplasty with a similar antibiotic protocol. There were no recurrences at minimum of 24 months after revision.

57. Samuel J, Gould F: Prosthetic joint infections: Single versus combination therapy. *J Antimicrob Chemother* 2010;65(1):18-23.

2: Nonunions, Malunions, and Infections

The effectiveness of several antibiotic agents, single or combination, was evaluated

58. Klouche S, Sariali E, Mamoudy P: Total hip arthroplasty revision due to infection: A cost analysis approach. *Orthop Traumatol Surg Res* 2010;96(2):124-132.
A retrospective costs analysis demonstrated the cost of revision for infected THA was 3.6 times greater than the cost of a primary THA. Level of evidence: IV.

59. Tice AD, Rehm SJ, Dalovisio JR, et al; IDSA: Practice guidelines for outpatient parenteral antimicrobial therapy. IDSA guidelines. *Clin Infect Dis* 2004;38(12):1651-1672.

Section 3

Soft-Tissue Injury and the Polytrauma Patient

SECTION EDITOR

Robert V. O'Toole, MD

Evaluation and Management of Soft-Tissue Injury and Open Fractures

Theodore T. Manson, MD Raymond A. Pensy, MD

Abstract

Open fractures can be devastating injuries that have the potential for infection, nonunion, neurovascular injury, and long-term debilitating dysfunction of the limb. Knowledge about the initial management of open fractures, including antibiotic choice, débridement, and adjuncts to closure, is important. For wounds that do not close primarily, the surgeon should be aware of the latest advances in skin grafting and techniques for rotational and free tissue transfer.

Keywords: soft-tissue injury; open fractures; Gustilo-Anderson classification; antibiotic prophylaxis; timing of closure; skin grafting

Classification

Open fractures are classified by the Gustilo-Anderson classification system.[1] A Gustilo-Anderson type I fracture exhibits a laceration of less than 1 cm in length and no substantial soft-tissue or periosteal stripping. A type II fracture has a laceration longer than 1 cm but is a lower-energy injury with minimal periosteal stripping. The type III fracture is a high-energy injury with substantial soft-tissue injury and periosteal stripping. Type IIIA injuries have substantial stripping of the periosteum, but the wound can be closed primarily at some point during the initial hospitalization. Segmental open fractures typically are considered to be type III fractures regardless of the soft-tissue wound because of the high energy necessary to cause such an injury. Type IIIB injuries have substantial soft-tissue and periosteal stripping and cannot be closed primarily; they require rotational or free tissue transfer for closure. Type IIIC fractures include vascular injury that requires repair to maintain the distal perfusion of the limb.

Systemic Antibiotic Prophylaxis for Open Fractures

The intravenous administration of antibiotics after open fracture reduces the incidence of secondary infection. Early administration of antibiotics is preferable. A 2015 retrospective analysis of type III open tibial fractures observed a substantial benefit for intravenous administration of antibiotics within 66 minutes of injury.[2] The authors found that late infection was markedly higher in patients who received later antibiotic coverage, with a progressive increase in late infection directly correlating with the progressive time from injury to first antibiotic dose. Clearly, 1 hour from injury to administration of antibiotics is not possible much of the time, but making an effort at rapid administration is warranted.

The ideal choice of antibiotic agent is thought to depend on the severity of the open fracture and the environment in which the fracture occurred. Type I and II open fractures are managed effectively with a first-generation cephalosporin alone. For patients with an allergy to cephalosporins, clindamycin is an acceptable alternative. The treatment of type III fractures remains controversial. Many orthopaedic and trauma surgeons advocate adding an agent with gram-negative coverage

Dr. Manson or an immediate family member has received royalties from Stryker; serves as a paid consultant to Stryker; has received research or institutional support from DePuy and Synthes; and serves as a board member, owner, officer, or committee member of the American Academy of Orthopaedic Surgeons and the American Association of Hip and Knee Surgeons. Neither Dr. Pensy nor any immediate family member has received anything of value from or has stock or stock options held in a commercial company or institution related directly or indirectly to the subject of this chapter.

such as gentamicin; that guideline was based on a single retrospective study that did not assess the addition of gram-negative coverage specifically.[3]

A contrary opinion holds that the addition of aminoglycosides to the regimen for open fractures might increase the incidence of resistant bacteria if infection does develop. The necessity of adding aminoglycosides to the antibiotic regimen is not supported by any comparative study. Also, if an additional agent for gram-negative coverage is desired, aminoglycosides might not be the optimal choice because of concerns regarding nephrotoxicity and ototoxicity.

Similarly, clostridial infection is rare in the modern era of open fracture management, even in combat injuries.[4] The historic recommendation to use penicillin G for heavily contaminated wounds might no longer be applicable because of the rarity of clostridial infection and the sensitivity of *Clostridium perfringens* and group A streptococci to first-generation cephalosporins.[4]

Timing of Open Fracture Débridement

Historically, open fractures were thought of as surgical emergencies that required débridement within 6 hours of injury to reduce infection rates.[1] That strategy is supported by basic science research showing lower infection rates with earlier débridement.[5,6] In an open femoral fracture model in rats, the authors of a 2012 study concluded that a delay in antibiotic administration of longer than 2 hours after injury or a delay in surgical débridement of longer than 6 hours resulted in substantially higher infection rates.[6]

Conversely, clinical studies of the effect of timing on open fracture débridement have not shown reduced infection rates after urgent versus delayed débridement. The Lower Extremity Assessment Project study group was one of the first large prospective studies to show no link between delayed débridement and increased infection rates.[7] A recent systematic review of the existing literature on this subject also reached the same conclusion: that débridement performed before or after 6 hours from injury has no effect on infection rate in open long-bone fractures.[8]

Many surgeons think that early débridement is preferable for type IIIB fractures, especially for those with notable contamination. This thinking is not supported by the literature, however. A 2012 study found no association between a delay in débridement and infection, even when independently analyzing type III fractures.[8] In this study's analysis, type III fractures that underwent débridement late had lower infection rates (11%) than those undergoing débridement early (15%).

A recent prospective study of 736 patients with open fractures showed no association between infection and time to surgery, using before or after 8 hours from injury as the breakpoint.[9] Of the fractures in that multicenter study, 52% were open tibial fractures. Although the timing of surgery was not predictive of infection, type III fractures and tibial fractures had higher infection rates than did other fractures, as expected. Furthermore, in a recent study specifically examining type III open tibial fractures, no association was found between the time to débridement and the infection risk.[2]

Although early débridement remains the preference of some surgeons, the literature clearly supports not treating an open fracture as a surgical emergency. Surgical débridement of an open fracture certainly is not indicated in the case of a physiologically unstable patient or when operating room resources are suboptimal. A delay to allow time for physiologic stabilization, assemblage of the correct operating room team, or even transfer to a specialized center is preferable to a misguided focus on early débridement.

Wound Adjuncts

Wounds that cannot be closed during the first débridement procedure now can benefit from several advances in wound management that aid in dead space management and infection control until subsequent débridement and soft-tissue coverage can be accomplished. These advances include negative-pressure wound therapy (NPWT) and the delivery of antibiotics directly to a wound.

Negative-Pressure Wound Therapy

Historically, open fracture wounds that could not be closed during the first débridement procedure were treated with wet-to-dry gauze dressings several times a day until the patients were returned to the operating room. A 2009 randomized controlled trial showed a dramatic reduction in infection incidence (28% versus 5.4%, respectively) when NPWT was used in lieu of gauze dressings.[10] A more recent nonrandomized study showed an 80% reduction in infection risk when NPWT was used instead of gauze dressings.[11] NPWT should be used only as a temporary wound adjunct. Relying on NPWT to delay rotational or free tissue transfer will increase the wound infection rate.[12]

Interruption of the suction applied to the NPWT sponge should be avoided because it could lead to an increase in wound complications, including infection and the loss of underlying skin graft or skin graft substitute.[13] When performing bedside NPWT sponge changes, the instillation of 1% lidocaine into the sponge before removal dramatically reduces the pain associated with the change of dressing.[14]

Direct Delivery of Antibiotics to the Wound

Antibiotic bead pouches deliver high doses of antibiotics directly to the traumatized tissues local to an open fracture.[15] Usually, polymethyl methacrylate (PMMA) is mixed with any of several heat-stable antibiotics and formed into small beads. The beads are placed into the wound, and the wound is then sealed with a barrier dressing. Extremely high concentrations of local antibiotics, sometimes greater than 100 times the minimum inhibitory concentration, are achieved with this strategy. The bead pouch is used as a temporary adjunct only until the wound can be closed or covered.

A recent meta-analysis[16] reviewed the use of antibiotic-loaded PMMA beads in open tibial fractures. For type III fractures, the overall infection rate using systemic antibiotics alone was 14.4%; using antibiotic-impregnated PMMA beads, the infection rate dropped to 2.4%. A statistically significant difference was shown for type III fractures but not for type I and II fractures, which exhibit low infection rates initially. A clear benefit for type III open tibial fractures was found and antibiotic-loaded PMMA beads was advocated for the treatment of this challenging injury.

Débridement Technique

A systematic débridement technique is a cornerstone of open fracture management. Ideally, the extension of open wounds would proceed. The débridement of skin, subcutaneous tissue, fascia, muscle, and devascularized bone then would be performed in a centripetal fashion down to the base of the wound.[17]

Inadequate débridement can increase the bacterial load that is initially present in the wound and serves as a potential sequestrum leading to the development of late infection. In areas prone to infection such as the tibia, aggressive débridement with removal of all bone that lacks robust muscular attachment serves to provide a robust wound bed but leaves marked bony defects.

Recently, some authors have questioned whether aggressive débridement is necessary for all open fractures. A 2013 retrospective cohort study investigated infection and nonunion rates in open distal femoral fractures treated at two trauma centers.[18] One center used an aggressive débridement protocol with the removal of all devitalized bone, the liberal use of antibiotic spacers, and later grafting. The other center used a less aggressive protocol with the removal of clearly contaminated fragments only and no antibiotic spacer use. The two groups were not equivalent exactly; more patients with diabetes mellitus were included in the more aggressive débridement group. No statistically significant difference was shown in the infection rate between the two groups: 18% in the more aggressive débridement group and 25% in the less aggressive group. The less aggressive group healed without further surgery 92% of the time. In contrast, in the more aggressive group, only 35% of the fractures healed without further surgery. Although the study was not powered to detect a difference in infection rates and the treatment groups were not exactly equal, it remains an important study that started a discussion about the proper level of débridement of open fracture.

A balanced approach, in which aggressive débridement is deemed more appropriate for type IIIB fractures and less aggressive débridement is reserved for less severe soft-tissue injuries, probably is the most appropriate strategy. Further research into the level of débridement performed in a randomized multicenter study likely is needed.

A pilot multicenter randomized controlled trial called the Fluid Lavage of Open Wounds Trial found lower reoperation rates when open fracture irrigation used normal saline solution rather than castile soap. Performing low-pressure versus high-pressure irrigation did not affect reoperation rates.[19]

Timing of Closure of Open Fracture Wounds

Historically, open fracture wounds were left open after the first débridement and then closed at a subsequent débridement or allowed to close by secondary intention. This practice was a byproduct of the attempt to limit clostridial myonecrosis (gas gangrene) in combat casualties in World War I.[20] An open wound would limit anaerobic bacterial proliferation in necrotic material that had not undergone débridement because of wartime logistical conditions.

Whether clostridial myonecrosis remains a concern in modern civilian injuries is questionable, but the timing of wound closure remains controversial. The infection rate is low in type I and II open fractures, and evidence suggests that they should be closed at the first débridement if the surgeon thinks the wound is clean and the tissues are viable.[8,9,21]

Infections that develop in open fractures most frequently are acquired from nosocomial pathogens and not from the original injury environment. In patients in whom infection develops after open tibial fracture, the pathologic organism is present during the first débridement only 18% of the time. Therefore, it could be advantageous to seal the wounds earlier to shield the underlying tissues from nosocomial bacteria.[22]

The authors of a 2014 study instituted a protocol of immediate closure of all type IIIA open fracture wounds at the first débridement as long as the wound could be closed without tension.[23] In that study, 77% of type IIIA open tibial fractures could be closed definitively at the first débridement. The deep infection rate of type IIIA open tibial fractures was only 9%, which compares favorably with historical controls.

A 2010 study reported a diametrically opposite strategy of taking cultures at the first débridement, returning the patient to the operating room every 48 hours for further débridement, and closing the open fracture wound only when the cultures from the previous débridement were negative.[24] For type IIIA lower extremity fractures, the infection rate using this protocol was 2.2%. For type IIIB fractures, it was 4.2%. The infection rates were low, but a subgroup analysis of open tibial fractures was not reported, rendering direct comparison difficult. Although not specifically tested in this study, serial débridement procedures performed while waiting for negative cultures might be an appealing strategy for open fracture wounds that develop gross evidence of infection.

In a study specifically of type IIIB tibial fractures requiring flap coverage, the timing of flap coverage did not predict later infection as long as the definitive coverage was accomplished within 7 days.[25] After 7 days, the odds of infection increased 16% per day with each day of delay to flap coverage.

Ideally, the deep tissues would be sealed off from the nosocomial environment as soon as possible. Waiting for negative wound cultures before closure is an intriguing concept that should be tested in a prospective manner and stratified by fracture location and severity. Flap coverage of type IIIB tibial shaft fractures should ideally be accomplished within 1 week of injury.

Reconstruction of Soft-Tissue Deficits

The Skin

The skin provides the primary mode of defense against pathogens and desiccation. From deep to superficial, the muscle, fascia, dermis, and epidermis are critical in maintaining a moist, nourished, and infection-free environment to the underlying skeleton and deep tissue. The skin provides a static passive barrier through the keratin and epithelial layer and an active, immunocompetent host of cells such as macrophages, mast cells, and lymphocytes that form a resilient bastion against the pathogens of the environment. A healthy, robust layer of dermal and epidermal tissue is irreplaceable in its ability to not only provide a protective barrier but also a means for the smooth unhindered gliding of tendons, the suppleness and pliability of the large areas of skin required for joint motion, and important thermoregulatory actions.[26] The physiology and immunology of the skin remain important areas of active research.[27]

Despite current notions, almost any full-thickness wound will heal in a healthy host without surgical intervention. These full-thickness wounds heal only by contracture and fibroblast activity, the deposition of nonspecific collagen, resultant scarification, and cicatrix. Obviously, in some cases, healing by secondary intention is preferable. Furthermore, allowing a wound to mature, equilibrate, or "declare" often is preferred before definitive methods of skin closure are attempted.

Recent investigations of natural disasters and war provide important contemporary data regarding the management of complex upper extremity and lower extremity wounds in austere conditions and focus on the principles of débridement, irrigation, wound dressings, and limb salvage.[28,29] Notable rates of contracture, stiffness, and chronic osteomyelitis ensue in these environments. Nonetheless, these results provide valuable experience to the trauma surgeon faced with complex wounds of the extremities and further support early soft-tissue coverage to minimize complications, the hospital stay, and the time to return to work and to maximize overall functional outcomes. These studies provide contemporary evidence that bolsters the rationale behind the reconstructive surgeon's attempts to achieve early wound closure, utilizing healthy, robust, normal muscle, fascia, and/or skin.[30]

Finally, when a soft-tissue defect is untreatable by primary intent and primary closure or by secondary intent, multiple factors should be considered during the decision about the best way to handle a particular defect. These factors include the size, configuration, and location of the defect; the degree of contamination; the health and skeletal status of the host; the planned treatment of the skeletal fracture (to include the bone defect); the resources and capability of the treating physician and the hospital; and, most importantly, the patient's wishes.

The Reconstructive Ladder

Reconstruction of the soft-tissue envelope historically has been likened to a ladder, wherein the most basic and noninvasive measures to obtain closure comprise the bottom rungs. Rung 1 is represented by primary closure, rung 2 by secondary intention, and rung 3 is delayed primary closure. Rung 4 is a split-thickness skin graft, and rung 5 is a full-thickness graft. Rung 6 stands for tissue expansion. Rungs 7, 8, and 9 signify the random flap, the axial flap, and the free flap, respectively. A revised ladder incorporating the use of dermal substitutes/matrices and NPWT has been proposed (**Figure 1**).[31]

Some authors have noted that the concept of the reconstructive ladder is not ideal. Just because secondary intention or a split-thickness skin graft might succeed in obtaining closure, is perhaps the easiest technique, and sits on a lower rung does not mean that it is optimal in terms of overall outcomes or success in restoring function to a limb. For example, the burn surgeon faced with an axillary or antecubital contracture and the orthopaedic surgeon treating a skeletal defect under a friable layer of skin graft over the mid or distal tibia know the critical importance of a pliable healthy layer of skin.

For this reason, some prefer the term "reconstructive elevator," in which each of the rungs is envisioned as a level. Thus, in the perfect scenario, the treating physician can choose the ideal level representing the best means to achieve skin closure while maximizing and optimizing outcome. Perhaps the new concept has become more acceptable despite the accordant risks because the more complex methods of soft-tissue management such as free tissue and pedicled flaps have become increasingly reliable. The complexity of the decision cannot be understated, considering the factors mentioned previously. These factors must be balanced and weighed carefully before embarking on a treatment plan.

According to some authors, the separation between skeletal surgery and soft-tissue surgery is arbitrary and may do a disservice to the patient and surgeon. Those surgeons faced with the combined skeletal and soft-tissue defect understand this point entirely and have coined the term "orthoplastics." This term is taken to mean that the surgeon faced with complex open fractures must address the bone (ortho) and soft tissue (plastics) defects in concert, as the methods of treatment for each defect are often tied together and cannot be considered separately.[32,33]

For example, the requisite reconstructive efforts during the management of a tibia with bone loss are obviously much different from those of an anterior knee wound with no underlying skeletal involvement. Thus, careful and deliberate communication must occur between the surgeons charged with the skeletal and soft-tissue reconstructions. More specifically, a degloved knee that requires no skeletal fixation will be managed differently from an exposed tibia, which might require an external fixator for bone transport or repeated flap elevation for planned bone grafting. Thus, the management of the skin and bone defects are tied inextricably.[34] Using "like tissue" for transfer is an important concept; for example, a thin, pliable skin flap will likely be ideal for replacing the skin over the dorsum of the foot, where a three-dimensional cavity overlying a complex tibia might best be served by a composite myocutaneous anterolateral thigh flap.

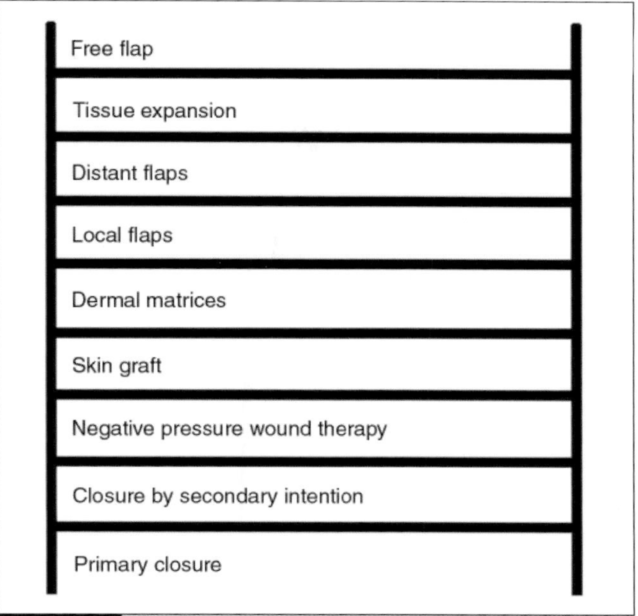

Figure 1 Modified reconstructive ladder as proposed by Janis et al. (Reproduced with permission from Janis JE, Kwon RK, Attinger CE: The new reconstructive ladder: Modifications of the traditional model. *Plast Reconstr Surg* 2011;127[suppl]:205S-212S.)

Critical Areas of Soft-Tissue Loss

It is readily apparent that some areas of the lower and upper extremities are prone to difficulties and require special consideration and advanced techniques. These areas include the axilla, the posterior elbow, the popliteal fossa, and the tibia.

The Axilla

Soft-tissue loss after massive upper extremity trauma is uncommon but is difficult to treat. Open injuries about the axilla occur with the severe displacement of humeral surgical neck fractures and occasionally result in large wounds not treatable by primary closure. Hyperabduction is the suspected mechanism and often results after ejection from a motor vehicle. Another obvious cause is a massive burn injury.

Regardless of the etiology, the loss of the redundant and pliable skin of the axilla, which is necessary for functional abduction and elevation of the shoulder girdle, invariably results in some degree of adduction contracture beyond that inherent to concomitant nerve and muscle tendon loss.[35] Cases in which the defect of skin and muscle involves the exposure of the brachial plexus, axillary and proximal brachial artery, and proximal humerus are covered insufficiently by skin graft or dermal substitute.

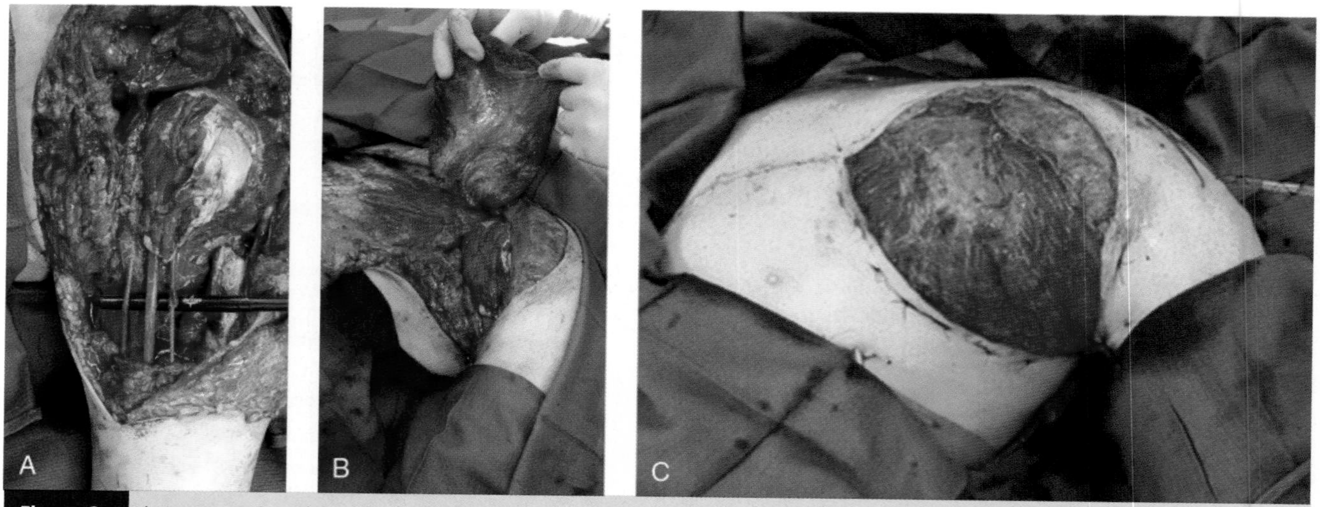

Figure 2 Intraoperative photographs demonstrate the use of temporizing pectoralis flaps. **A**, The exposed proximal humerus, proximal brachial artery, and brachial plexus are shown in a critically ill patient with an open proximal humeral fracture. **B**, Harvest of the pectoralis major flap is shown. The pectoralis insertion was avulsed during the original injury, facilitating harvest. **C**, The pectoralis major pedicle flap has been rotated approximately 120° counterclockwise, covering the exposed proximal humerus plate, plexus, and vascular structures.

Fasciocutaneous free flaps often provide ideal soft-tissue coverage and the redundancy necessary for optimized outcome. Additionally, rotational flaps, including the pedicled latissimus dorsi muscle or myocutaneous flaps, scapular/parascapular flaps, or a variety of propeller flaps, can provide excellent soft-tissue coverage.[36]

Careful selection of soft-tissue coverage is required in the presence of axillary nerve injury; proximal humeral fracture-dislocation; and concomitant rotator cuff or deltoid, axillary nerve, or brachial plexus injuries. The latissimus dorsi or associated neurovascular axis pedicled scapular/parascapular flaps potentially can compromise transfers that might be useful for further reconstructive efforts in shoulder function restoration.[37] In such cases, temporizing pectoralis flaps or dermal matrix substitutes might be suitable in the critically ill patient and can be staged to permit free fasciocutaneous transfer at a later date (**Figure 2**).

The Posterior Elbow

The olecranon process and the proximal ulna are frequent sites of wound complications. The most common mechanisms for severe elbow trauma and soft-tissue loss are direct, blunt blows, strikes from ballistic projectiles, or avulsions to the posterior surface of the ulna. Addressing the spectrum of injuries to the proximal ulna with an orthoplastics mentality requires that the surgeon carefully consider not only the soft-tissue envelope but also the means by which skeletal fixation can be achieved and vice versa, because they are inextricably tied.

Whether the injury is a simple olecranon fracture or an associated transolecranon fracture-dislocation, fixation of the proximal ulna is suited ideally to an intramedullary implant. The proximal ulna, like the mid and distal tibia, does not have a robust soft-tissue envelope. Care must be taken when using large prominent plates along the dorsal surface of the ulna, because this tissue, which already has been compromised by the injury mechanism, does not tolerate prominent fixation devices, particularly after additional dissection. For this reason, several authors have discussed the usefulness of intramedullary implants for fixation.[38,39]

If the soft-tissue envelope about the proximal ulna is compromised—whether from avulsion, infection, hematoma, or decubitus ulcer —several flaps warrant discussion. Excellent options for soft-tissue coverage include the sensate transposition lateral arm flap, the pedicled latissimus dorsi muscle, propeller flaps, the flexor carpi ulnaris turn-down flap, and the reverse pedicle radial forearm flap. Free tissue always remains a viable alternative, depending primarily on the size of the defect, the health status of the patient, and future reconstructions required.

The sensate transposition lateral arm flap has proven to be reliable and easy to harvest. Based on the posterior radial collateral artery within the lateral intermuscular septum, this flap can extend up to 4 to 5 cm distal to the lateral epicondyle, as does the extended lateral arm free flap. As a simple axial pattern transposition flap, this flap can be rotated from the lateral arm and positioned easily

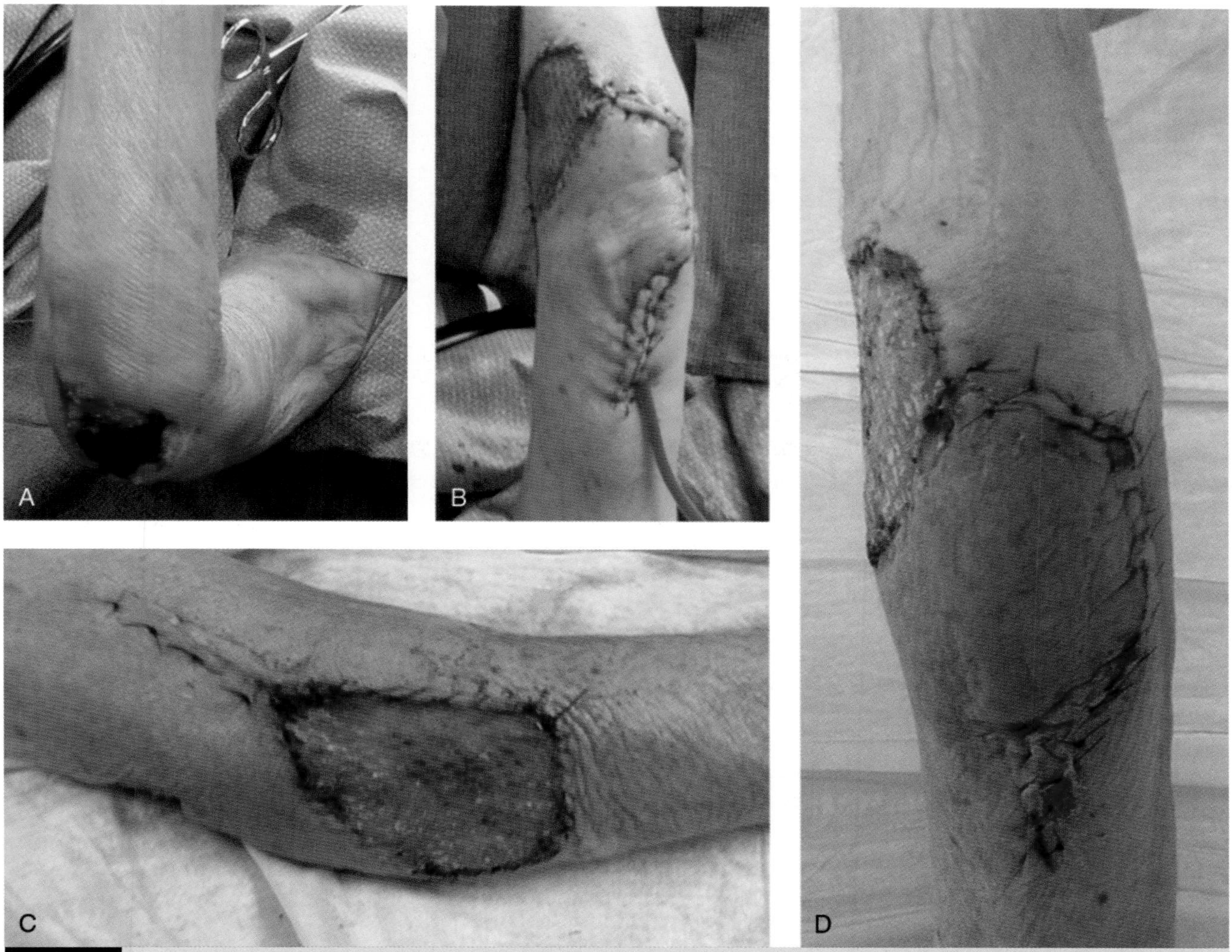

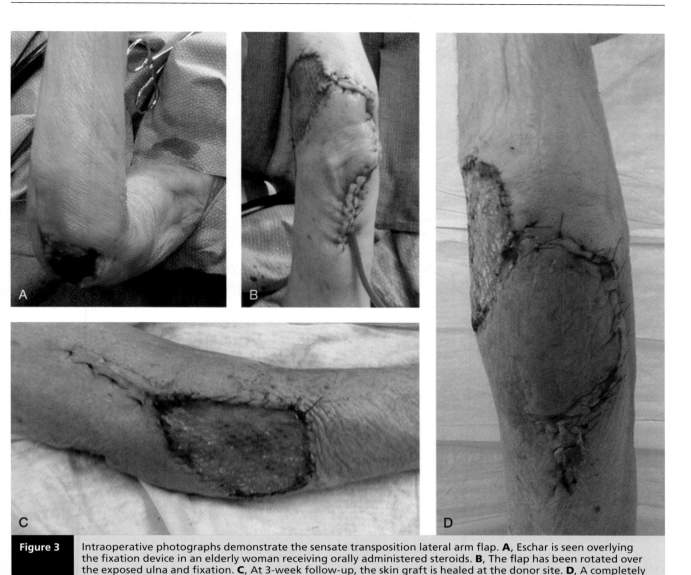

Figure 3 Intraoperative photographs demonstrate the sensate transposition lateral arm flap. **A**, Eschar is seen overlying the fixation device in an elderly woman receiving orally administered steroids. **B**, The flap has been rotated over the exposed ulna and fixation. **C**, At 3-week follow-up, the skin graft is healed at the donor site. **D**, A completely healed posterior soft-tissue envelope is shown.

over the olecranon and proximal ulna, with the resultant donor defect covered with skin graft[40] (**Figure 3**).

The Popliteal Fossa

Massive degloving injuries of the popliteal fossa associated with knee dislocations and proximal tibial fractures frequently are associated with popliteal artery injury and compartment syndrome. The management of these soft-tissue defects can be particularly difficult, with complication rates higher than 50% but overall limb salvage rates at 87%.[41]

Surgery for degloving injuries of the popliteal fossa must involve a team approach from the very start of management. The dislocated knee with associated vascular disruption, with or without fracture, is an injury without well-defined protocols for skeletal stabilization, vascular management, and soft-tissue management. Yet the survivability of the limb and on rare occasion, the patient, depend on the successful completion of each stage of management. During each stage, thought must be given to the next stage.

For patients with a soft-tissue defect without vascular insult, pedicled medial/lateral gastrocnemius flaps are an obvious choice. Frequently used alternatives are propeller flaps based on the inferior lateral geniculate, turn-down vastus lateralis flaps, and turn-down gracilis flaps. In patients with vascular insult and soft-tissue loss, the gastrocnemius flaps often have been compromised by disruption of the medial/lateral sural arteries. In recognition of a large soft-tissue defect, preservation of these pedicles if possible during exposure of the injury and revascularization provides reliable soft-tissue coverage.

Often, the surgeons charged with the vascular reconstruction are not those responsible for covering the exposed plastic conduit or vein graft, which are prone to infection, dehiscence, and rapid exsanguination if not afforded the appropriate healthy and viable soft-tissue surroundings. Soft-tissue coverage often becomes much more problematic, with loss of the gastrocnemius flaps an option, whether secondary to direct trauma, ligation during exposure, or bypass of the sural arteries. In these cases, the overall condition of the patient generally is poor to begin with secondary to massive trauma, myoglobinemia, anasarca, poor respiratory status, and other serious conditions. Thus, free tissue transfer is difficult, if not impossible, to accomplish. Yet, the team is faced with an exposed graft and vascular reconstruction that present a ticking time bomb, rendering coverage a pressing issue. In these cases, the immediate concurrent involvement, if possible, of the orthopaedic surgeon, the vascular surgeon, and the plastic or microvascular surgeon is recommended for the reasons described previously.

When the gastrocnemius flap is not available, local rotation muscle flaps have some usefulness, as do fasciocutaneous perforator flaps. For patients who are critically ill, have no gastrocnemius flap available, and are not candidates for free tissue flap, the lateral superior genicular flap or distal lateral thigh flap can be useful.[42]

Free tissue, if available, is the most robust tissue and the most reliable means of covering large defects of the popliteal fossa in cases of exposed vascular and bony reconstruction. Ideally, full-thickness skin flaps, such as those from the anterolateral thigh, the scapular, parascapular, and latissimus dorsi, would be indicated in such cases.

The Tibia

Coverage of the tibia generally has been achieved over the proximal and middle thirds by the rotational gastrocnemius flaps and soleus flaps, respectively. These flaps are reliable and relatively easy to harvest. Their use for open tibial fractures remains somewhat controversial. Debate continues regarding whether these local muscles reside within the zone of injury and therefore, whether they are suitable for use as flaps. In a retrospective series, the rates of union, infection, and overall limb salvage remained comparable between rotational flaps and free tissue transfer.[43]

For the distal tibia, options are more limited, and free tissue is more frequently required. Limb salvage, infection, union, and complication rates are similar regardless of the free tissue chosen. The gracilis flap provides excellent coverage, is easy and reliable to harvest, permits a two-team approach, and is harvested with the patient in the supine position. For this flap, the donor site almost always is primarily closed[44] (**Figure 4**). The anterolateral thigh flap similarly allows a two-team approach, provides a large and long pedicle, is harvested with the patient in the supine position, and provides a robust, thick skin envelope.[45] The anterolateral thigh flap can provide a larger flap but is more difficult to harvest and potentially is less reliable in its perimeter if the planned flap is large and perforators are not available or multiple perforators are not included.[46]

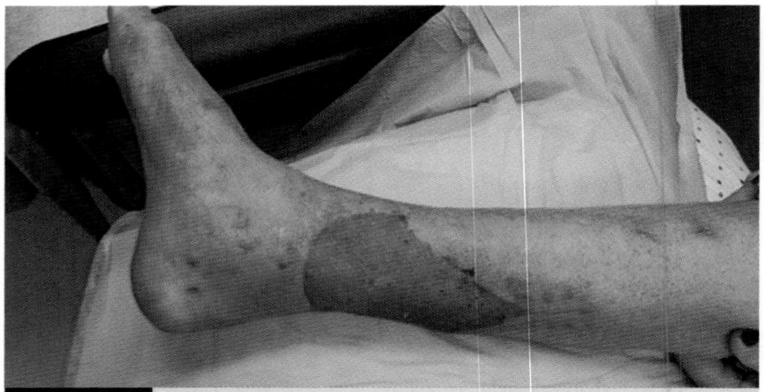

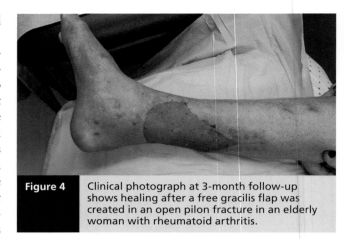

Figure 4 Clinical photograph at 3-month follow-up shows healing after a free gracilis flap was created in an open pilon fracture in an elderly woman with rheumatoid arthritis.

When the decision is made to proceed with free tissue for salvage in the patient with a type IIIB tibial fracture and in consideration of the aforementioned overall salvage rates, flap selection might be based most importantly on surgeon preference, the size of the defect, possible re-elevation requirements, the donor defect location, patient obesity, patient positioning, and the availability of a cosurgeon or assistant to provide a two-team approach. Finally, the resultant flap thickness is an important factor, particularly around the ankle and foot, where shoe wear and fit are an important concern. Well-tailored appropriately inset muscle flaps often atrophy, providing a good cosmetic result (**Figure 4**). For the lateral ankle in a thin patient, the parascapular flap allows the simultaneous harvest and procurement of the peroneal artery (**Figure 5**).

Additional flaps such as the posterior tibial artery perforator propeller flap, the hemisoleus muscle flap, and the anterior tibialis muscle flaps play roles in providing coverage and are useful for the distal third of the tibia in patients with relatively smaller defects and in those who cannot tolerate free tissue transfer.[47] Finally, although inconvenient and cumbersome, cross-leg flaps are still effectively used to provide soft-tissue coverage to the tibia when other methods have failed or are unavailable.

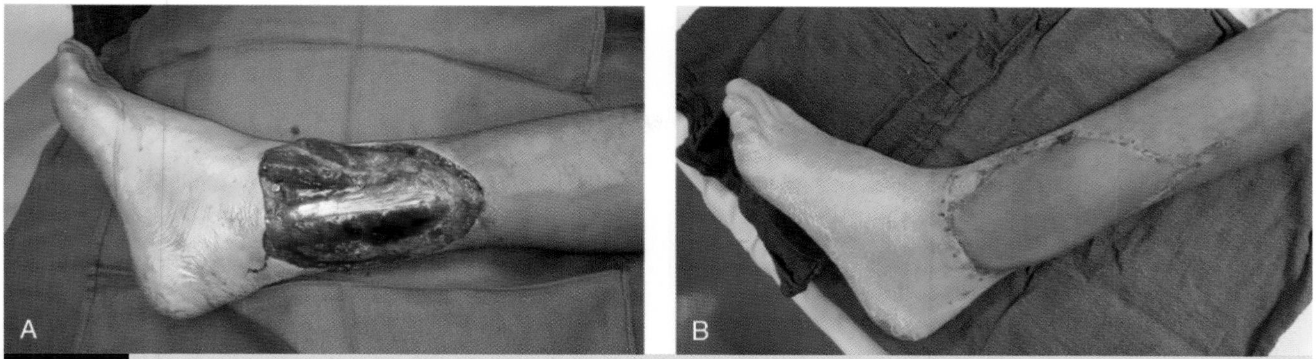

Figure 5 Clinical photographs show a parascapular flap used for a lateral ankle soft-tissue defect **A**, A lateral ankle defect with exposed distal fibula, syndesmotic screws, and peronei is shown. **B**, Healing is shown at 1-month follow-up after the creation of a free parascapular flap with end-to-end anastomosis into the peroneal artery and venae comitantes.

Skin Grafting and Dermal Substitutes

Skin grafting and dermal substitutes play a limited role in the management of open fractures in the areas of concern discussed previously. The surgeon must remember to replace tissues or skin with similar materials. Although it is possible to graft skin or to place dermal matric substitute over the periosteum and achieve closure, doing so generally is not suitable for the patient who requires some form of fixation immediately adjacent to the defect. It also is not suitable for the functional restoration of tendon gliding or the ideal restoration of joint range of motion when performed over exposed tenosynovium, tendon, or extensor/flexor retinaculum. The patient with multiple traumatic injuries does not afford the reconstructive surgeon the best-case scenario, and some compromise of function might be preferable to attempting more complex efforts in a patient not deemed suitable.

Ideally, a skin graft or dermal substitute is used only for replacing defects that involve the epidermis and dermis and not the synovium, periosteum, or joint capsule. Thus, full-thickness or partial-thickness skin loss over healthy, viable muscle bellies away from joint, bone, or tendon can be replaced with dermal substitute or skin grafting when convenient. Allowing time for a degree of swelling to subside can result in less need for total area skin graft coverage and can result in complete adherence and incorporation. Finally, a brief delay before definitive wound coverage can allow sufficient time for nonviable muscle to fully demonstrate that it requires débridement, or 'declare.' Thus, grafting should be delayed for as long as reasonable. In areas where nutrition is of concern, in areas with small portions of exposed tendon, or when the overall health status of the patient is in question, dermal matrix substitutes can be used effectively to increase the overall completeness of skin graft adherence and viability; provide a thicker, more robust dermal substrate; and potentially lessen the contracture inherent in any split-thickness skin graft.

Full-thickness skin grafts ideally are suited for any region with full-thickness loss, but supply is limited. The antecubital fossa, the groin, and the flexion crease of the wrist can be used, but only to a certain degree, for large areas of loss such as the axilla and popliteal fossa.

For these reasons, particularly in the unstable patient, using dermal matrix substitutes over multiple layers has proven effective. Dermal matrix substitutes are bovine collagen and glycosaminoglycan composites placed on a semipermeable silicon layer and are commercially available for application to traumatic wounds. After application, the dermal matrix is colonized with host dermal cells and fibroblasts and eventually undergoes remodeling and neovascularization, with the host capillaries providing a suitable bed for skin grafting. The wound bed treated with dermal matrix is less prone to desiccation and has a thicker, dermal-like substrate than that achieved by granulation and skin grafting alone. The period of neovascularization, which is the period between application and skin grafting, can be shortened with negative or subatmospheric pressure dressings[48,49] using the original manufacturer's recommendation of 21 days to 10 days. Dermal matrix substitutes have been used for the coverage of degloving injuries, donor sites for large fasciocutaneous flaps, oncologic reconstruction, and burns.

Although dermal matrices provide an easy-to-use and fairly reliable means of coverage, a dermal matrix is not suitable for the coverage of large areas of exposed bone, particularly when involved with open fracture with concomitant fixation devices. It also is not suitable for large areas of exposed tendon where tendon gliding is necessary, because the resultant coverage is similar in property to an area of tissue that has been allowed to granulate and then is skin grafted. These areas remain friable and unworkable for any subsequent procedures, such as hemolysis, fixation revision, fixation removal, capsulectomy, and bone grafting, all of which frequently are necessary in the posttraumatic extremity.

In general, a nonadherent dressing that does not allow shearing yet permits effluent release is ideal for immediate placement on a graft. In many cases, vacuum-assisted closure is appropriate. A well-prepared bolstered dressing in a wound with few concavities can be equally effective and less expensive. For large areas of grafting, such as circumferentially degloved extremities, vacuum-assisted closure has been shown to be effective in securing the graft, reducing shear, and improving graft survival.[50]

Summary

The salvage of limbs with open fractures has become increasingly possible due to advances in basic science, temporizing wound coverage techniques, skeletal fixation methods, and increasing capability in both rotational and free tissue transfer. Despite the above, however, important work remains regarding the optimization of the carefully orchestrated balance between antimicrobial prophylaxis, débridement, fixation methods, and the choice and timing of soft-tissue coverage.

Key Study Points

- Optimizing soft-tissue coverage of open fractures requires a thorough understanding of the complex interplay of patient-associated comorbidities, the nature of the wound, and the capabilities of the treating hospital and surgeon.
- A coordinated orthoplastics approach is often required, where careful and deliberate communication between those charged with the skeletal reconstruction and soft-tissue reconstruction exists.

Acknowledgment

Special thanks to Dori Kelly, MA, senior editor and writer at the University of Maryland School of Medicine, for professional manuscript editing and figure formatting.

Annotated References

1. Gustilo RB, Anderson JT: Prevention of infection in the treatment of one thousand and twenty-five open fractures of long bones: Retrospective and prospective analyses. *J Bone Joint Surg Am* 1976;58(4):453-458.

2. Lack WD, Karunakar MA, Angerame MR, et al: Type III open tibia fractures: Immediate antibiotic prophylaxis minimizes infection. *J Orthop Trauma* 2015;29(1):1-6.

   Timing of antibiotic prophylaxis is the main driver of later infection rates, not time of débridement. Level of evidence: II (prognostic).

3. Vasenius J, Tulikoura I, Vainionpää S, Rokkanen P: Clindamycin versus cloxacillin in the treatment of 240 open fractures. A randomized prospective study. *Ann Chir Gynaecol* 1998;87(3):224-228.

4. Murray CK, Obremskey WT, Hsu JR, et al; Prevention of Combat-Related Infections Guidelines Panel: Prevention of infections associated with combat-related extremity injuries. *J Trauma* 2011;71(2suppl 2):S235-S257.

   Methods to prevent infection in combat-related extremity injuries are discussed. Level of evidence: III.

5. Brown KV, Walker JA, Cortez DS, Murray CK, Wenke JC: Earlier debridement and antibiotic administration decrease infection. *J Surg Orthop Adv* 2010;19(1):18-22.

   In a rat femur defect model, there was less infection with earlier débridement and antibiotic administration.

6. Penn-Barwell JG, Murray CK, Wenke JC: Early antibiotics and debridement independently reduce infection in an open fracture model. *J Bone Joint Surg Br* 2012;94(1):107-112.

   In a rat femur defect model, early antibiotic administration was more important than early surgical débridement in preventing later infection.

7. Pollak AN, Jones AL, Castillo RC, Bosse MJ, MacKenzie EJ; LEAP Study Group: The relationship between time to surgical debridement and incidence of infection after open high-energy lower extremity trauma. *J Bone Joint Surg Am* 2010;92(1):7-15.

   In this subset of the LEAP study group patients, neither the time from injury to débridement nor the time from injury to soft-tissue coverage had an effect on infection rates. Level of evidence: III.

8. Schenker ML, Yannascoli S, Baldwin KD, Ahn J, Mehta S: Does timing to operative debridement affect infectious complications in open long-bone fractures? A systematic review. *J Bone Joint Surg Am* 2012;94(12):1057-1064.

   In this meta-analysis, there was little support for the historic "6-hour rule" as the window for débridement of open fractures. The data did not indicate that time to débridement had an effect on infection rates. Level of evidence: I.

9. Weber D, Dulai SK, Bergman J, Buckley R, Beaupre LA: Time to initial operative treatment following open fracture does not impact development of deep infection: A

prospective cohort study of 736 subjects. *J Orthop Trauma* 2014;28(11):613-619.

Infection after open fracture was not associated with the time from injury to surgical débridement; rather, Gustilo grade and location in the tibia drove infection rates. Level of evidence: I (prognostic).

10. Stannard JP, Volgas DA, Stewart R, McGwin G Jr, Alonso JE: Negative pressure wound therapy after severe open fractures: A prospective randomized study. *J Orthop Trauma* 2009;23(8):552-557.

11. Blum ML, Esser M, Richardson M, Paul E, Rosenfeldt FL: Negative pressure wound therapy reduces deep infection rate in open tibial fractures. *J Orthop Trauma* 2012;26(9):499-505.

    In this study of 229 open tibia fractures, lower infection rates were seen in those patients in whom negative pressure wound therapy was used rather than standard dressings. Level of evidence: III (therapeutic).

12. Bhattacharyya T, Mehta P, Smith M, Pomahac B: Routine use of wound vacuum-assisted closure does not allow coverage delay for open tibia fractures. *Plast Reconstr Surg* 2008;121(4):1263-1266.

13. Collinge C, Reddix R: The incidence of wound complications related to negative pressure wound therapy power outage and interruption of treatment in orthopaedic trauma patients. *J Orthop Trauma* 2011;25(2):96-100.

    Increased complications including return to the operating room for graft loss and infection were more common in patients who had interruption in the negative pressure component of their wound therapy. Level of evidence: III (retrospective).

14. Christensen TJ, Thorum T, Kubiak EN: Lidocaine analgesia for removal of wound vacuum-assisted closure dressings: A randomized double-blinded placebo-controlled trial. *J Orthop Trauma* 2013;27(2):107-112.

    Topical lidocaine injected into the vacuum-assisted closure sponge resulted in less pain and narcotic requirements than not using lidocaine. Level of evidence: I (therapeutic).

15. Ostermann PA, Seligson D, Henry SL: Local antibiotic therapy for severe open fractures. A review of 1085 consecutive cases. *J Bone Joint Surg Br* 1995;77(1):93-97.

16. Craig J, Fuchs T, Jenks M, et al: Systematic review and meta-analysis of the additional benefit of local prophylactic antibiotic therapy for infection rates in open tibia fractures treated with intramedullary nailing. *Int Orthop* 2014;38(5):1025-1030.

    This meta-analysis supports the practice of including locally delivered antibiotics in the treatment of open tibia fracture in addition to systemic therapy. Level of evidence: III.

17. No authors listed: A report by the British Orthopaedic Association/British Association of Plastic Surgeons Working Party on the management of open tibial fractures. September 1997. *Br J Plast Surg* 1997;50(8):570-583.

18. Ricci WM, Collinge C, Streubel PN, McAndrew CM, Gardner MJ: A comparison of more and less aggressive bone debridement protocols for the treatment of open supracondylar femur fractures. *J Orthop Trauma* 2013;27(12):722-725.

    In this study of open distal femur fractures, fewer reoperations were seen in patients treated with less aggressive bony débridement. Although there was no statistical difference in infection rates, the study was admittedly underpowered to detect a difference. Level of evidence: II (therapeutic).

19. Petrisor B, Sun X, Bhandari M, et al; FLOW Investigators: Fluid lavage of open wounds (FLOW): A multicenter, blinded, factorial pilot trial comparing alternative irrigating solutions and pressures in patients with open fractures. *J Trauma* 2011;71(3):596-606.

20. Trueta J: The treatment of war fractures by the closed method. *Proc R Soc Med* 1939;33(1):65-74.

21. DeLong WG Jr, Born CT, Wei SY, Petrik ME, Ponzio R, Schwab CW: Aggressive treatment of 119 open fracture wounds. *J Trauma* 1999;46(6):1049-1054.

22. Patzakis MJ, Bains RS, Lee J, et al: Prospective, randomized, double-blind study comparing single-agent antibiotic therapy, ciprofloxacin, to combination antibiotic therapy in open fracture wounds. *J Orthop Trauma* 2000;14(8):529-533.

23. Moola FO, Carli A, Berry GK, Reindl R, Jacks D, Harvey EJ: Attempting primary closure for all open fractures: The effectiveness of an institutional protocol. *Can J Surg* 2014;57(3):E82-E88.

    In this study of 297 open fractures, a deep infection rate of 4.7% was observed despite the fact that an attempt was made to close all wounds at the initial débridement rather than leave the wound open and return to the operating room for "a second look" and closure. Level of evidence: III (retrospective).

24. Lenarz CJ, Watson JT, Moed BR, Israel H, Mullen JD, Macdonald JB: Timing of wound closure in open fractures based on cultures obtained after debridement. *J Bone Joint Surg Am* 2010;92(10):1921-1926.

    This article outlined a strategy of serial cultures of open fractures with closure only if the cultures were negative. They also reported a deep infection rate of 4.3%. Like the study by Moola et al, there was no comparison group so definitive recommendations cannot be made from this article alone. Level of evidence: IV (therapeutic).

25. D'Alleyrand JC, Manson TT, Dancy L, et al: Is time to flap coverage of open tibial fractures an independent predictor of flap-related complications? *J Orthop Trauma* 2014;28(5):288-293.

Time to flap coverage in Gustilo 3B tibia fractures was an independent predictor of flap complications and infection with the breakpoint for worse outcomes being 7 days following injury. Level of evidence: III (therapeutic).

26. Romanovsky AA: Skin temperature: Its role in thermoregulation. *Acta Physiol (Oxf)* 2014;210(3):498-507.

    This review article provides a comprehensive examination of the components of each skin type and their respective roles in thermoregulation. Level of evidence: IV (therapeutic).

27. Wulff BC, Wilgus TA: Mast cell activity in the healing wound: More than meets the eye? *Exp Dermatol* 2013;22(8):507-510.

    This review provides an examination of the specific actions of the mast cells with the skin layer, which have been demonstrated to produce anti-inflammatory mediators, release mediators with degranulations, and have the ability to change phenotype. Level of evidence: IV (therapeutic).

28. Liu L, Tan G, Luan F, et al: The use of external fixation combined with vacuum sealing drainage to treat open comminuted fractures of tibia in the Wenchuan earthquake. *Int Orthop* 2012;36(7):1441-1447.

    Information is provided regarding treatment of severe open fractures in austere environments with simple negative pressure dressings. Level of evidence: IV (therapeutic).

29. Wuthisuthimethawee P, Lindquist SJ, Sandler N, et al: Wound management in disaster settings. *World J Surg* 2015;39(4):842-853.

    An expert panel opinion and systematic review of 62 papers dealing with wound care in disaster situations is presented, with the focus on appropriate wound débridement, dressing, and wound preparation in an austere environment. Level of evidence: IV (therapeutic).

30. Liu DS, Sofiadellis F, Ashton M, MacGill K, Webb A: Early soft tissue coverage and negative pressure wound therapy optimises patient outcomes in lower limb trauma. *Injury* 2012;43(6):772-778.

    The experience of a tertiary trauma center with free flap reconstruction for lower extremity reconstruction is presented; increased rates of complications delays in soft-tissue reconstruction beyond 3 days were reported. The authors recommend the use of negative pressure wound therapy as an important adjunct in managing soft-tissue defects. Level of evidence: IV (therapeutic).

31. Janis JE, Kwon RK, Attinger CE: The new reconstructive ladder: Modifications to the traditional model. *Plast Reconstr Surg* 2011;127(suppl 1):205S-212S.

    Expert opinion is presented regarding contemporary methods of achieving wound closure, adding the newer reconstructive adjuncts of dermal matrix substitutes and negative pressure wound therapy dressings. Level of evidence: V (therapeutic).

32. Levin LS: The reconstructive ladder. An orthoplastic approach. *Orthop Clin North Am* 1993;24(3):393-409.

33. Beltran MJ, Blair JA, Rathbone CR, Hsu JR: The gradual expansion muscle flap. *J Orthop Trauma* 2014;28(1):e15-e20. A series of patients were treated with the novel technique of acute deformity induction with external fixation devices and rotational flaps to achieve wound closure in severe open tibia fractures where more standard wound closure methods are ineffective. Level of evidence: IV (therapeutic).

34. Sommar P, Granberg Y, Halle M, Skogh AC, Lundgren KT, Jansson KÅ: Effects of a formalized collaboration between plastic and orthopedic surgeons in severe extremity trauma patients; a retrospective study. *J Trauma Manag Outcomes* 2015;9:3.

    The authors present the clinical experience of a tertiary referral center before and after the implementation of a formalized collaboration between the orthopaedics and reconstructive plastic surgery services. They report increased numbers of flaps, shorter hospital stays, and fewer revisions/re-operations in the years following the implementation of this combined service. Level of evidence: IV (therapeutic).

35. Karki D, Mehta N, Narayan RP: Post-burn axillary contracture: A therapeutic challenge! *Indian J Plast Surg* 2014;47(3):375-380.

    Outcomes of a retrospective series of 44 patients treated with a variety of resurfacing techniques used in post-burn axillary contractures are discussed. Level of evidence: IV (therapeutic).

36. Schmidt M, Dunst-Huemer KM, Lazzeri D, Schoeffl H, Huemer GM: The versatility of the islanded posterior arm flap for regional reconstruction around the axilla. *J Plast Reconstr Aesthet Surg* 2015;68(7):953-959.

    The authors review their experience with 35 posterior arm flaps and their clinical results in resurfacing the axilla. Level of evidence: IV (therapeutic).

37. El-Azab HM, Rott O, Irlenbusch U: Long-term follow-up after latissimus dorsi transfer for irreparable posterosuperior rotator cuff tears. *J Bone Joint Surg Am* 2015;97(6):462-469.

    The authors present a series of 108 patients treated with latissimus transfer for the treatment of irreparable rotator cuff tears. They report significant improvement in shoulder Constant Scores with relatively low requirements to proceed to shoulder prosthetic replacement. Level of evidence: IV (therapeutic).

38. Selvam P, Wilkerson J, Dubina A, Eglseder WA, Pensy R: Comparison of intramedullary fixation techniques in the maintenance of functional anatomy of the elbow after fixation of the proximal ulna. *J Surg Orthop Adv* 2015;24(1):18-21.

    The authors present clinical outcomes of two different intramedullary techniques for fixation of the proximal ulna and radiographic parameters for assessing maintenance of reduction. Level of evidence: IV (therapeutic).

39. Rodriguez EK, Eglseder A: A technique for low-profile intramedullary fixation of intraarticular proximal ulnar fractures. *J Surg Orthop Adv* 2008;17(4):252-261.

40. Mears SC, Zadnik MB, Eglseder WA: Salvage of functional elbow range of motion in complex open injuries using a sensate transposition lateral arm flap. *Plast Reconstr Surg* 2004;113(2):531-535.

41. Meyer A, Goller K, Horch RE, et al: Results of combined vascular reconstruction and free flap transfer for limb salvage in patients with critical limb ischemia. *J Vasc Surg* 2015;61(5):1239-1248.

    The authors report on complex lower extremity salvage utilizing combined vascular reconstruction and free tissue transfer. Thirty-three patients underwent both vascular reconstruction and free tissue transfer, demonstrating preservation of the limb at a rate of 75% at 5 years' follow-up. Level of evidence: IV (therapeutic).

42. Zheng X, An HB, Chen T, Wang HB: [The lateral superior genicular artery perforator iliotibial band flap for the treatment of scar contraction of popliteal fossa][in Chinese]. *Zhongguo Gu Shang* 2013;26(2):128-130.

    This case series of 11 patients reviews the utility of the lateral superior genicular artery and the associated iliotibial band for coverage of defects of the posterior knee. Level of evidence: IV (therapeutic).

43. Choudry U, Moran S, Karacor Z: Soft-tissue coverage and outcome of Gustilo grade IIIB midshaft tibia fractures: A 15-year experience. *Plast Reconstr Surg* 2008;122(2):479-485.

44. Redett RJ, Robertson BC, Chang B, Girotto J, Vaughan T: Limb salvage of lower-extremity wounds using free gracilis muscle reconstruction. *Plast Reconstr Surg* 2000;106(7):1507-1513.

45. Wei FC, Jain V, Celik N, Chen HC, Chuang DC, Lin CH: Have we found an ideal soft-tissue flap? An experience with 672 anterolateral thigh flaps. *Plast Reconstr Surg* 2002;109(7):2219-2226, discussion 2227-2230.

46. Yang JF, Wang BY, Zhao ZH, Zhou P, Pang F, Sun WD: Clinical applications of preoperative perforator planning using CT angiography in the anterolateral thigh perforator flap transplantation. *Clin Radiol* 2013;68(6):568-573.

    Evidence is presented that suggests that CT angiography can be a useful adjunct to identifying the location, size, and type (septal versus muscular) of perforators in the harvest of the anterolateral thigh flap. Level of evidence: IV (therapeutic).

47. Dong KX, Xu YQ, Fan XY, et al: Perforator pedicled propeller flaps for soft tissue coverage of lower leg and foot defects. *Orthop Surg* 2014;6(1):42-46.

    Twenty patients were reviewed, demonstrating the utility of lower extremity reconstruction using perforator propeller flaps for coverage of small- to medium-sized defects. Color ultrasonography was found to be a useful adjunct in preoperative planning. Level of evidence: IV (therapeutic).

48. Molnar JA, DeFranzo AJ, Hadaegh A, Morykwas MJ, Shen P, Argenta LC: Acceleration of Integra incorporation in complex tissue defects with subatmospheric pressure. *Plast Reconstr Surg* 2004;113(5):1339-1346.

49. Jeschke MG, Rose C, Angele P, Füchtmeier B, Nerlich MN, Bolder U: Development of new reconstructive techniques: Use of Integra in combination with fibrin glue and negative-pressure therapy for reconstruction of acute and chronic wounds. *Plast Reconstr Surg* 2004;113(2):525-530.

50. Scherer LA, Shiver S, Chang M, Meredith JW, Owings JT: The vacuum assisted closure device: A method of securing skin grafts and improving graft survival. *Arch Surg* 2002;137(8):930-933, discussion 933-934.

Chapter 15

The Mangled Lower Extremity

Bryan W. Ming, MD   Michael Bosse, MD

Abstract

Limb-threatening injuries to the lower extremity are challenging to treat, in both civilian and military settings. Advances in orthopaedic and plastic surgery over the past 25 years have made reconstruction a possibility over amputation. Successful management of these complicated injuries must include a multifactorial examination. Whether treatment with limb salvage or amputation is pursued, long-term studies continue to show that patients with these injuries suffer significant disability.

Keywords: mangled extremity; limb salvage; amputation

Introduction

Limb-threatening injuries to the lower extremity continue to pose a challenge to orthopaedic surgeons in both civilian and military settings. Thousands of civilians experience limb-threatening injuries annually,[1] and more than one-half of the combat-related injuries in recent conflicts in Iraq and Afghanistan involved extremity injuries.[2] Advances in orthopaedic and plastic surgery have made reconstruction a possibility for extremities that would have been more amenable to amputation only 25 years ago. Successful management of these complicated injuries goes beyond initial treatment of the injured extremity and must include a multifactorial examination and treatment of the total patient. To the authors' knowledge through 2015, no data exist that support definitive recommendations in regard to limb salvage versus amputation. Regardless of which treatment is pursued, or whether limb salvage or amputation is undertaken, long-term studies indicate that patients with limb-threatening injuries suffer significant disability.

Neither Dr. Ming nor any immediate family member has received anything of value from or has stock or stock options held in a commercial company or institution related directly or indirectly to the subject of this chapter. Dr. Bosse or an immediate family member has stock or stock options held in The Orthopaedic Implant Company.

Patient Characteristics

Much of the understanding of the mangled extremity has come from civilian research as well as more recent information coming out of the conflicts in Iraq and Afghanistan. The mangled lower extremity in a civilian patient is typically caused by high-energy blunt trauma and involves complex fractures (Gustilo type IIIB or IIIC), dysvascular limbs, major soft-tissue injuries (severe degloving, crush), severe foot and ankle injuries, or a combination of these injuries.[3] Within the military population, open fractures caused by blast injuries predominate.[2] Whereas the mechanisms of injury often differ between civilian and military populations, there is a significant amount of crossover in regard to risk factors and patient outcomes.

In a study of civilian National Trauma Data Bank records from 2007 through 2009, researchers identified 1,354 patients with a mangled lower extremity.[4] The patients' mean age was 41 years, 82% were men, and motor vehicle crash was the most common mechanism of injury (49%). Most patients (81%; n = 1,096) had a crush injury diagnosis; the remainder (19%; n = 258) were identified as having severe fracture with severe soft-tissue (n = 258), arterial (80%; n = 207), or nerve (50%; n = 129) injury. The median Injury Severity Score was 8, and the in-hospital mortality rate was 11% (n = 29) for this patient group.

A comparison of open tibial fractures in military combat casualties (n = 103) with those from a civilian Level I trauma center (n = 850) revealed military combat patients were more severely injured, more likely to have hypotension, and were more likely to have experienced fractures as a result of a blast mechanism the majority of the time as compared with the civilian population. Civilian patients with IIIB fractures had a 3.7% rate of amputation (n = 8 of 216), which was found to be not significant compared with 12.5% (n = 5 of 40) in the military group. Civilian patients with IIIC fractures had a 28.8% (n = 23 of 80) amputation rate compared with 71 % (n = 20 of 28) in the military group.[5]

Classification

The decision to amputate rather than perform limb salvage is difficult. An ideal classification scheme would allow universal communication among medical providers, be descriptive, provide guidance regarding the decision to amputate versus salvage the limb, and be prognostic. Patients with mangled lower extremities often have concurrent trauma, preexisting comorbid conditions, and socioeconomic considerations that can affect the final functional outcomes.

Many classification systems have attempted to quantify the severity of limb trauma and assign numerical parameters for the decision to amputate or salvage the limb. These classifications include the Mangled Extremity Severity Score (MESS)[6,7] (**Table 1**); the Predictive Salvage Index (PSI);[7] the Limb Salvage Index (LSI);[8] the Nerve Injury, Ischemia, Soft Tissue Injury, Skeletal Injury, Shock, and Age of Patient (NISSSA) Score;[9] and the Hannover Fracture Scale-97 (HFS-97).[10,11] The scoring systems vary in terms of items scored (hypotension, neurologic status, vascular status, etc.) and timing of scoring (emergency department versus operating room). Each classification purports to have high sensitivity and specificity for predicting limb salvage, but independent studies have not been able to re-create the results reliably.[12-15]

In the only known prospective analysis of these classifications studies, the Lower Extremity Assessment Project (LEAP) group was unable to validate the clinical utility of any of the injury-severity scores.[16] The ideal index would be 100% sensitive (all amputated limbs would have scores at or above the threshold) and 100% specific (all salvaged limbs would have scores below the threshold). Overall, the Injury Severity Scores lacked sensitivity, but they were quite specific in some cases. The utility of these scores could not be established, and the group recommended against using injury severity scores as the sole criterion for the decision to amputate.

The most well-known classification, MESS, was recently evaluated for predicting outcomes in soldiers sustaining all type III Gustilo open tibial fractures. A total of 155 patients who had type III open tibial fractures were treated; 110 limbs were salvaged and 45 were amputated. The mean MESS values for patients whose limbs were salvaged and those whose limbs were amputated were 5.3 and 5.8 ($P = 0.057$), respectively. The sensitivity and specificity of a MESS ≥ 7 predicting amputation were 35% and 88%, respectively. A MESS ≥ 7 had a positive predictive value of only 50%.[17] Additionally, another research team evaluated the prognostic factors predicting secondary amputations in 93 type III open tibial fractures.[18] Seven patients underwent primary amputation; initial limb salvage was attempted in 72 patients, and 10 required secondary amputation. The MESS was found to be significantly higher in the amputation group than in the limb-salvage group. However, 20% of the patients with successful limb salvage had a MESS ≥ 7. The authors also cautioned against the use of the MESS in daily clinical decision making. Two of the original authors of the MESS tool addressed concerns regarding its use for the early assessment of severely injured lower extremities. In their opinion, the biologic and clinical principles underlying the MESS remain relevant, but the clinical application of a MESS value of 7 fails to reflect current leading-edge trauma care. Using contemporary injury management techniques not available in 1990 (when the MESS study was published) might lead to a functional, viable limb that would have otherwise received primary amputation solely on the basis of MESS scores.[19]

Table 1

Mangled Extremity Severity Score

Patient Variable	Points
Extremity Injury	
Low energy	0
Medium energy	1
High energy	2
Massive crush	3
Shock	
Normotensive	0
Transient hypotension	1
Prolonged hypotension	2
Ischemia	
None	0
Diminished pulses	1
No pulses as measured via Doppler	2
Pulseless, Cool	3
Age	
<30 years	0
30-50 years	1
>50 years	2

Antibiotic Prophylaxis

There is much literature available regarding the efficacy of prophylactic antibiotics in treating open fractures, but controversy exists regarding the optimal timing, duration, and type of antimicrobials given.[20-25] Prior studies have shown ideal timing of antibiotic prophylaxis to be within 3 hours of injury,[20] but a more recent evaluation of deep infection in type IIIA tibial fractures showed that prophylactic antibiotics given later than 66 minutes of injury independently predicted infection.[22] Guidelines for the prevention of infections associated with combat-related injuries recommend systemic antimicrobials be administered as soon as possible after injury, ideally within 3 hours.[23] Antimicrobial selection should focus on providing the narrowest spectrum of activity required for common early infectious complications, not for established infections. For extremity injuries, cefazolin 2 g administered intravenously every 6 to 8 hours was recommended, with clindamycin as an alternate agent for documented anaphylaxis to β-lactam antimicrobials. Local delivery of antimicrobials in the form of antibiotic beads or pouches was recommended as long as the emphasis of wound care was still firmly placed on surgical débridement and irrigation.[24,25]

Decision Making

Patients with a mangled lower extremity are by definition patients who have sustained high-energy trauma. As such, the tenets of Advanced Trauma Life Support—including controlling massive hemorrhage and securing an airway, breathing, and circulation—take precedence during the initial evaluation.[26] Any life-threatening injuries should be addressed and stabilized before management of the severely injured limb begins. Secondary evaluation should not only focus on the mangled lower extremity but also include a thorough evaluation to assess for concurrent injuries that might affect the treatment of the lower extremity in question. Specifically, a detailed neurologic and vascular examination of the patient is mandatory. Soft-tissue status and contamination are also assessed and documented.

After the patient has been thoroughly evaluated, the surgical team can begin the process of treating the mangled extremity. Often the patient has significant concurrent traumas that require active management. In these situations, expeditious débridement and temporization according to the tenets of damage-control orthopaedics are advised (**Figures 1** and **2**).

A limb-salvage attempt is predicated on a perfused extremity. If meaningful perfusion cannot be obtained or maintained, the patient requires an amputation. In patients with a perfused and reconstructible extremity (unlike the foot injury in the patient shown in **Figure 1**, which is not reconstructible), a decision-making pathway is started to determine the final treatment strategy. This should involve frank discussions with the patient and his or her family regarding potential advantages and disadvantages of each treatment. Patient factors in addition to the mangled extremity also should be considered (**Figures 3** and **4**). In the LEAP study,[27] injury characteristics were not significantly correlated with patient outcomes. Risk factors in all patients for worse outcomes at 2 years included being rehospitalized for a major complication, having less than a high-school education, having a household income below the federal poverty level, being nonwhite, having no insurance or having Medicaid, having a poor social-support network, having a low level of self-efficacy (confidence in one's ability to resume

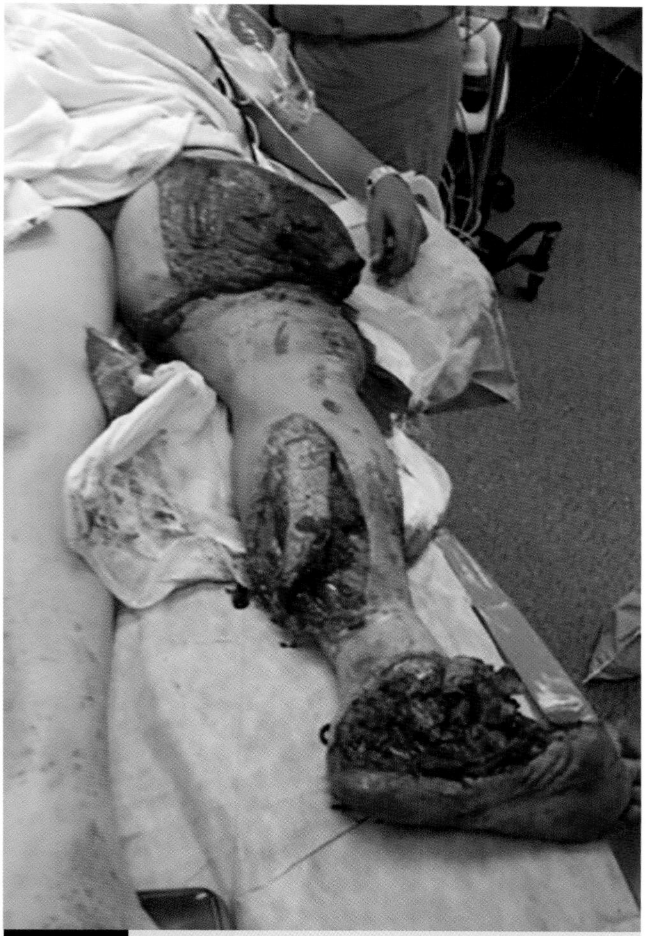

Figure 1 Preoperative photograph of a mangled lower extremity after a motorcycle collision: open femoral, tibial, and foot fractures with significant soft-tissue injury and contamination.

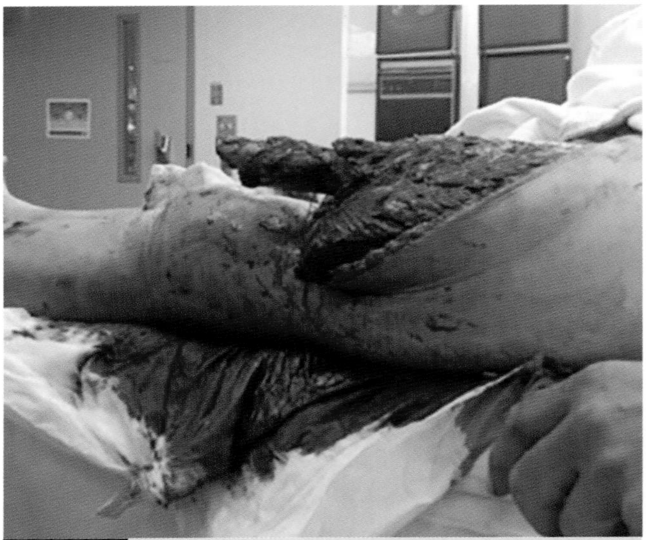

Figure 2 Preoperative photograph of an open femoral fracture with gross contamination.

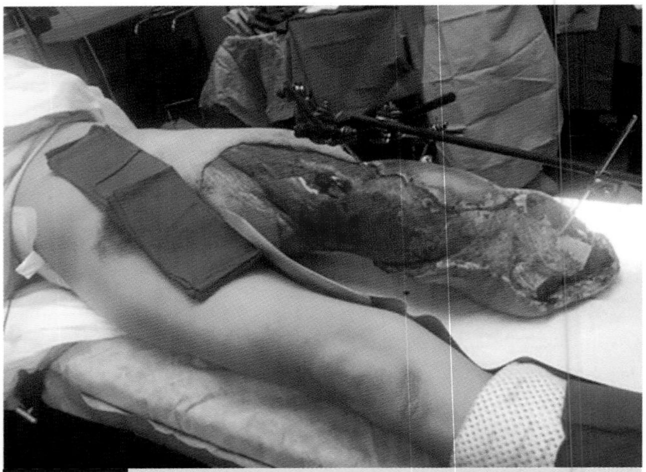

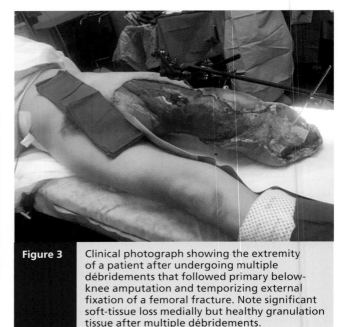

Figure 3 Clinical photograph showing the extremity of a patient after undergoing multiple débridements that followed primary below-knee amputation and temporizing external fixation of a femoral fracture. Note significant soft-tissue loss medially but healthy granulation tissue after multiple débridements.

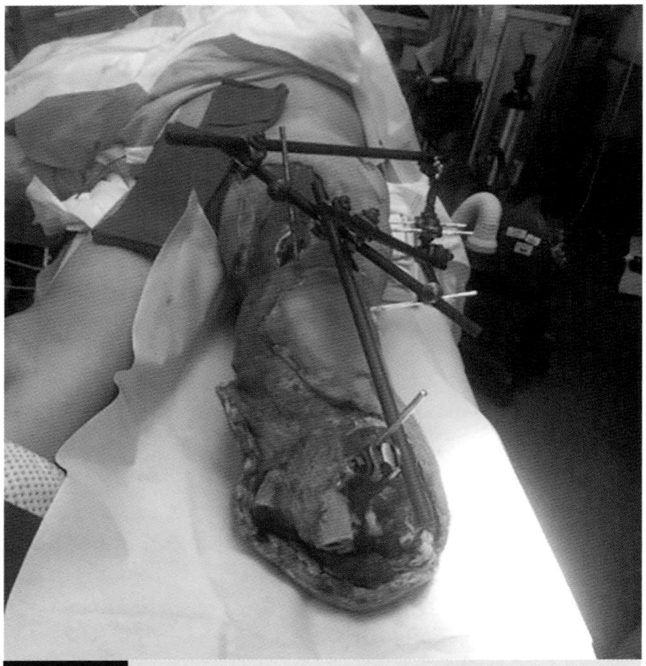

Figure 4 Clinical photograph of the extremity of a patient after undergoing multiple débridements that followed primary below-knee amputation and external fixation of femoral fracture. Healthy granular tissue is noted but the distal end of the amputation required additional revision to cover the tibial osteotomy. Note significant soft-tissue loss after serial débridements.

one's chief life activities), smoking, and involving the legal system for injury compensation. Long-term follow-up of LEAP study patients beyond 2 years confirmed that poor outcomes were associated with the aforementioned risk factors.[27] These influencers of outcome, however, applied to both treatment arms; in other words, they diminished the final expected outcome of patients regardless of whether they underwent amputation or reconstruction.

No definitive criteria have been validated for amputation of the mangled extremity. Relative strong indications for amputation include near-total amputation, nonreconstructible vascular injury, ischemia of longer than 6 hours' duration, nonreconstructible soft-tissue loss, or life-threatening hemorrhage. Loss of plantar sensation was previously considered an indication for amputation; however, the LEAP study showed no significant difference in outcomes when plantar sensation was impaired. Also, initially insensate salvage group recovered intact sensation 67% of the time.[28]

In 2012, the Western Trauma Association presented a comprehensive algorithm to address mangled extremities seen in civilian practice. In the absence of prospective randomized controlled trials, the algorithm is based on expert opinion and published observational trials. The association advocated that hemodynamically unstable patients who failed to respond to initial resuscitation be taken directly to the operating room for exploration and vascular control. For stable patients, the association recommended thorough vascular and neurologic evaluation with a comprehensive evaluation of factors that may help predict appropriateness of limb salvage such as degree of soft-tissue loss, level of potential amputation, and systemic disease.[29]

Researchers characterized the contemporary management of mangled extremities by evaluating 1,354 patients with mangled extremities from 222 centers. Of these, 278 patients (21%) underwent amputations and 124 (9%) underwent early amputation. Limb injury mechanism (such as proximal crush injury), experiencing shock in the emergency department, and severe head injury were all associated with performing early amputation. In contrast, age, comorbidity level, and insurance status were not associated with the decision to amputate early.[4]

Deciding in favor of limb salvage versus amputation is challenging in the face of a mangled lower extremity. Ultimately, the decision, when possible, must be based on a multifactorial assessment of the patient's clinical picture, preinjury functionality, and patient preferences.

Limb Salvage Versus Amputation

Outcomes

The LEAP study has provided outcomes of a large cohort of prospectively followed patients who were treated by means of either amputation or limb salvage.[27] The initial hypothesis was that after adjustments for injury severity and other patient characteristics, those undergoing amputation would have better outcomes than those undergoing limb salvage. The primary outcome measured was scores on the Sickness Impact Profile (SIP), a self-reported health status tool (scores range from 0 to 100; scores for the general population average 2 to 3, and scores greater than 10 represent severe disability). Secondary outcomes included limb status and presence or absence of major complications resulting in rehospitalization. At 2 years, there was no significant difference in SIP scores between the amputation and reconstruction groups. At 2 years, both groups showed high levels of disability, with only one-half of all patients returning to work. The limb-salvage group did have higher rates of hospitalization and complications, including nonunion (31%), wound infection (23%), and osteomyelitis (9%).

Some surgeons have misinterpreted the LEAP study as advocating for limb salvage in all cases, if possible, as the functional outcomes were similar to those in amputation and the cost significantly less over the life of the patient. The LEAP study was not a randomized study. It was an observational study performed in major trauma centers where the care was provided by seasoned orthopaedic trauma surgeons.

Subsequent follow-up studies of the LEAP population showed similar poor results at 7 years. SIP scores among 50% of the patients remained at ≥ 10, indicating significant disability. Only 58% of patients who were working before their injury were working at 7 years postinjury, with the majority of these patients requiring significant limitations in their work duties.[30,31] A research team evaluated a subset of LEAP patients with mangled foot and ankle injuries treated with below-knee amputation or complex limb salvage requiring free flaps, ankle fusion, or both. When compared with patients who underwent standard below-knee amputation, patients in the limb-salvage group had significantly worse 2-year outcomes. Overall SIP scores were 2.5 points higher in the limb-salvage group than in the amputation group, with psychosocial SIP scores that were 8.4 points higher than in the amputation group.[32] An additional study of the LEAP population examined functional outcomes after trauma-related lower extremity amputation according to the level of amputation. Researchers evaluated 161 patients who had undergone above-the-ankle amputation within 3 months of injury, following them prospectively for 24 months. There was no significant difference in SIP scores between patients treated with above-knee amputation and those treated with below-knee amputation. Patients who had undergone below-knee amputation had the best timed-test results for walking speed compared with those who had undergone above-knee or through-knee amputation. Patients who had undergone through-knee amputations had the worst regression-adjusted SIP and the slowest walking speeds, resulting in the recommendation that through-knee amputation be critically evaluated when deciding on level of amputation in patients with a traumatic injury.[33]

Researchers in the Military Trauma Amputation/Limb Salvage (METALS) study investigated functional outcomes for major lower-extremity trauma after amputation versus limb salvage in wounded warriors. The retrospective cohort study included 324 service members who underwent either amputation or limb salvage involving revascularization, bone graft or bone transport, local or free-flap coverage, repair of a major nerve injury, or treatment of a complete compartment injury or compartment syndrome. The Short Musculoskeletal Function Assessment (SMFA) questionnaire was used to measure overall function, and other standardized instruments were used to measure depression, posttraumatic stress disorder (PTSD), chronic pain, and engagement in sports and leisure activities. The researchers compared outcomes between amputation and limb salvage by using regression analysis with adjustment for age, time until interview, military rank, upper limb and bilateral injuries, social support, and intensity of combat experiences. Patients scored significantly worse than population norms in all SMFA domains except arm/hand function, with 38.3% screening positive for depressive symptoms and 17.9% for PTSD. One-third were not working, on active duty, or in school at an average of 38 months postinjury. After adjustment for variables, patients with an amputation had significantly better scores in all SMFA domains compared with those who had undergone limb salvage as well as lower likelihood of PTSD and high likelihood of being engaged in vigorous sports.[34] These findings were counter to the LEAP findings in the civilian study. Possible reasons for these different conclusions include higher levels of postoperative rehabilitation and support networks available to military personnel than to their civilian counterparts. Also, as limb-salvage techniques have continued to improve, the postoperative rehabilitation protocols and attention paid to military patients with salvaged limbs have also improved, whereas the level of care and rehabilitation for patients with amputations has been excellent for quite some time now. A long-term follow-up study of the METALS group is ongoing.

Return to duty after an open tibial fracture was also investigated in the military population. Researchers retrospectively reviewed records for 115 soldiers who had sustained battle-related type III open tibial fractures. The overall return to duty rate was 18%; among those with salvaged extremities it was 21%, and among those with amputations it was 13%. Older age and higher rank were significant factors identified in increasing the likelihood of return to duty. Those with amputations had disability ratings significantly higher than those of patients with salvaged extremities. The return-to-duty rates were noted to be lower in the military population than in the literature about the civilian population, likely because of more significant injuries and more physically demanding jobs in the military than in the civilian population.[35]

A meta-analysis of patients with mangled lower extremities compared quality of life after limb salvage versus after amputation. Inclusion criteria included English language, posttraumatic amputations, unilateral amputations, outcomes measurements via Short Form-36 or Sickness Impact Profile, minimum of 20 cases in each study, minimum follow-up of 2 years, and studies published between 1990 and 2007. Eleven studies met inclusion criteria. No statistical differences were noted regarding physical outcomes, but psychological outcomes indicated that limb-salvage patients had better outcomes than did amputation patients, with a P value of 0.008 (SF-36) and 0.05 (SIP).[36]

Costs

Costs of patient treatment and effects on healthcare systems are becoming increasingly important considerations in the healthcare landscape. The best outcomes for patients is paramount, but in working with limited healthcare resources in modern medicine, one must make evidence-based and fiscally sound decisions. The LEAP group performed a cost analysis of amputation or reconstruction of limb-threatening injuries, looking at 2-year direct healthcare costs and projected lifetime healthcare costs.[37] Included in the calculation were costs related to the initial hospitalization, all rehospitalizations for acute care related to the limb injury, inpatient rehabilitation, outpatient physician visits, outpatient therapy, and purchase and maintenance of prosthetic devices. At 2 years, the costs for reconstruction and amputation were similar when compared with costs for initial hospitalization, rehospitalizations and postacute care. However, once prosthesis-related costs were added, there was substantial difference between the two groups at 2 years. Projected lifetime healthcare costs were approximately three times higher for patients who underwent amputation than for those treated with reconstruction, something explained by the cost of ongoing maintenance of prostheses.

Researchers performed a cost-utility analysis of amputation versus salvage for type IIIB and IIIC open tibial fractures by using data derived from LEAP.[38] Relevant data regarding projected lifetime costs were extracted and analyzed by means of discounting and sensitivity analysis. Amputation was found to be more expensive than salvage independent of varied ongoing prosthetic needs, discount rate, and patient age at presentation. Salvage was considered to be the dominant cost-saving strategy, with amputation yielding fewer quality-adjusted life-years.

Summary

Limb-threatening injuries continue to present a significant challenge to both patients and surgeons. Mid- to long-term outcomes show patients have persistently poor outcomes regardless of amputation or limb salvage, with significant disability reported. The ultimate choice of management should be made in consultation with the patient, family, surgeon, and other medical practitioners. No treatment option is without potential complications, cost, or challenges. However, a multidisciplinary team approach to the management of these life-changing injuries involving physicians, physical therapists, and behavioral therapists will give the patient the best chance regardless of treatment choice.

Key Study Points

- Patients with a mangled extremity have significant disability and poor SIP profiles long term, regardless of whether amputation or limb salvage is performed.
- Amputation is more expensive than salvage independent of varied ongoing prosthetic needs, discount rate, and patient age at presentation.
- There is no ideal soft-tissue scoring model for mangled extremities that accurately predicts need for amputation versus limb salvage.
- The decision for amputation versus limb salvage should be made with the patient, family, and other medical practitioners when the situation allows.

Annotated References

1. Finkelstein EA, Corso PS, Miller TR, Fiebelkorn IA, Zaloshnja E, Lawrence BA: *Incidence and Economic Burden of Injuries in the United States* , New York, Oxford University Press, 2006.

2. Owens BD, Kragh JF Jr, Macaitis J, Svoboda SJ, Wenke JC: Characterization of extremity wounds in Operation Iraqi Freedom and Operation Enduring Freedom. *J Orthop Trauma* 2007;21(4):254-257.

3. Prasarn ML, Helfet DL, Kloen P: Management of the mangled extremity. *Strategies Trauma Limb Reconstr* 2012;7(2):57-66.

   The authors review current strategies regarding management of mangled extremities. The hierarchy of importance regarding injuries is noted to be soft tissues, nerve, bone, and then artery. No clear cutoff is noted for any scoring systems in regard to salvage versus amputation. The authors recommend that an experienced multidisciplinary team care for these complex injuries at a trauma center. Level of evidence: V.

4. de Mestral C, Sharma S, Haas B, Gomez D, Nathens AB: A contemporary analysis of the management of the mangled lower extremity. *J Trauma Acute Care Surg* 2013;74(2):597-603.

   The authors conducted a retrospective cohort study of patients in the National Trauma Data Bank, identifying 1,354 patients with mangled extremities from 2007 through 2009. Of those patients, 21% underwent amputation and 9% underwent amputation within one day of admission. Level of evidence: IV.

5. Doucet JJ, Galarneau MR, Potenza BM, et al: Combat versus civilian open tibia fractures: The effect of blast mechanism on limb salvage. *J Trauma* 2011;70(5):1241-1247.

   The authors compared open-tibial fractures in civilian and military patients. They identified 850 open-tibial fractures with 45 amputations among civilian patients and 115 open-tibial fractures with 21 amputations among military patients. Prospects of salvage for limbs with fractures of Gustilo-Anderson IIIB and IIIC grades were significantly worse for open tibial fractures that resulted from blast injury than for fractures resulting from typical mechanisms responsible for civilian injuries. Mangled Extremity Severity Scores (MESS) did not adequately predict likelihood of limb salvage in combat or civilian open tibia fractures. Level of evidence: IV.

6. Helfet DL, Howey T, Sanders R, Johansen K: Limb salvage versus amputation. Preliminary results of the Mangled Extremity Severity Score. *Clin Orthop Relat Res* 1990;256:80-86.

7. Johansen K, Daines M, Howey T, Helfet D, Hansen ST Jr: Objective criteria accurately predict amputation following lower extremity trauma. *J Trauma* 1990;30(5):568-572, discussion 572-573.

8. Howe HR Jr, Poole GV Jr, Hansen KJ, et al: Salvage of lower extremities following combined orthopedic and vascular trauma. A predictive salvage index. *Am Surg* 1987;53(4):205-208.

9. Russell WL, Sailors DM, Whittle TB, Fisher DF Jr, Burns RP: Limb salvage versus traumatic amputation. A decision based on a seven-part predictive index. *Ann Surg* 1991;213(5):473-480, discussion 480-481.

10. Seekamp A, Köntopp H, Tscherne H: Hannover Fracture Scale '98—reevaluation and new prospects for an established score system. *Unfallchirurg* 2001;104(7):601-610.

11. Tscherne H, Oestern HJ: A new classification of soft-tissue damage in open and closed fractures (author's transl). *Unfallheilkunde* 1982;85(3):111-115.

12. McNamara MG, Heckman JD, Corley FG: Severe open fractures of the lower extremity: A retrospective evaluation of the Mangled Extremity Severity Score (MESS). *J Orthop Trauma* 1994;8(2):81-87.

13. Bonanni F, Rhodes M, Lucke JF: The futility of predictive scoring of mangled lower extremities. *J Trauma* 1993;34(1):99-104.

14. Durham RM, Mistry BM, Mazuski JE, Shapiro M, Jacobs D: Outcome and utility of scoring systems in the management of the mangled extremity. *Am J Surg* 1996;172(5):569-573, discussion 573-574.

15. Lange RH: Limb reconstruction versus amputation decision making in massive lower extremity trauma. *Clin Orthop Relat Res* 1989;243:92-99.

16. Bosse MJ, MacKenzie EJ, Kellam JF, et al: A prospective evaluation of the clinical utility of the lower-extremity injury-severity scores. *J Bone Joint Surg Am* 2001;83-A(1):3-14.

17. Sheean AJ, Krueger CA, Napierala MA, Stinner DJ, Hsu JR; Skeletal Trauma and Research Consortium (STReC): Evaluation of the mangled extremity severity score in combat-related type III open tibia fracture. *J Orthop Trauma* 2014;28(9):523-526.

The authors evaluated data for 155 patients who had type III open tibial fractures; 110 of them had salvaged limbs and 45 had undergone amputation. MESS values for amputees and limb salvage were 5.8 and 5.3, respectively. A MESS value of ≥7 was found to have a positive predictive value of 50%. Thirty-three percent of patients treated with amputation had an associated vascular injury versus 12.7% of patients treated with limb salvage ($P < 0.0026$). The authors concluded that MESS was not accurate in predicting need for amputation in type III open tibia fractures. Level of evidence: IV.

18. Fochtmann A, Mittlböck M, Binder H, Köttstorfer J, Hajdu S: Potential prognostic factors predicting secondary amputation in third-degree open lower limb fractures. *J Trauma Acute Care Surg* 2014;76(4):1076-1081.

The authors evaluated 93 patients with type III open tibial fractures, 72 of whose limbs were salvaged, 7 of whom underwent primary amputations, and 10 of whom underwent secondary delayed amputations. MESS was noted to be significantly higher in the groups that underwent amputation versus the group whose limbs were salvaged. The authors indicate that MESS is highly prognostic but should be used with caution in daily clinical decision making. Level of evidence: III.

19. Johansen K, Hansen ST Jr: MESS (Mangled Extremity Severity Score) 25 years on: Time for a reboot? *J Trauma Acute Care Surg* 2015;79(3):495-496.

Two of the original authors of the MESS grading system discussed the current clinical implications of the MESS score. With current improvements in technology and modern limb salvage techniques, a MESS score of 7 is thought to not accurately represent current management techniques and may doom certain lower extremity injuries to primary amputation when aggressive salvage techniques may result in a viable and functional extremity. Level of evidence: V.

20. Patzakis MJ, Wilkins J: Factors influencing infection rate in open fracture wounds. *Clin Orthop Relat Res* 1989;243:36-40.

21. Melvin JS, Dombroski DG, Torbert JT, Kovach SJ, Esterhai JL, Mehta S: Open tibial shaft fractures: I. Evaluation and initial wound management. *J Am Acad Orthop Surg* 2010;18(1):10-19.

In a review article, the authors outlined evaluation and initial wound management of open tibial shaft fractures. Guidelines for prophylactic antibiotic include use of first-generation cephalosporins as soon as possible. Data for the routine use of gram-negative coverage is not directly supported by the data. Use of local antibiotic delivery systems (ie, bead pouches) and negative-pressure wound therapy has been shown to be efficacious in the management of open tibia fractures. Level of evidence: IV.

22. Lack WD, Karunakar MA, Angerame MR, et al: Type III open tibia fractures: Immediate antibiotic prophylaxis minimizes infection. *J Orthop Trauma* 2015;29(1):1-6.

The authors conducted a retrospective review of 137 type III open tibial fractures. Time from injury to administration of antibiotics and to wound coverage independently predicted infection of type III open tibial fractures. Prehospitalization administration of antibiotics may improve outcomes in severely open wounds. Level of evidence: II.

23. Hospenthal DR, Murray CK, Andersen RC, et al; Infectious Diseases Society of America; Surgical Infection Society: Executive summary: Guidelines for the prevention of infections associated with combat-related injuries: 2011 update: endorsed by the Infectious Diseases Society of America and the Surgical Infection Society. *J Trauma* 2011;71(2suppl 2):S202-S209.

The authors made recommendations regarding timing, type, duration of antibiotic use, and surgical management of combat-related wounds. Recommendations made in regard to extremity fractures for high-dose cefazolin every 6 to 8 hours, against the routine use of enhanced gram-negative coverage, and the use of local antimicrobial delivery systems such as bead pouches. Level of evidence: V.

24. Obremskey W, Molina C, Collinge C, et al; Evidence-Based Quality Value and Safety Committee Orthopaedic Trauma Association, Writing Committee: Current practice in the management of open fractures among orthopaedic trauma surgeons. Part A: Initial management. A survey of orthopaedic trauma surgeons. *J Orthop Trauma* 2014;28(8):e198-e202.

The authors conducted a survey of 379 orthopaedic trauma surgeons in regard to open-fracture management. Eighty-six percent of respondents reported administration of antibiotics within 1 hour to be optimal. Despite concerns for efficacy and toxicity, 24% to 76% reported use of aminoglycosides in management of open fractures. Level of evidence: V.

25. Hoff WS, Bonadies JA, Cachecho R, Dorlac WC; East Practice Management Guidelines Work Group: East Practice Management Guidelines Work Group: Update to practice management guidelines for prophylactic antibiotic use in open fractures. *J Trauma* 2011;70(3):751-754.

Systemic antibiotic coverage directed at gram-positive organisms should be initiated as soon as possible after injury; additional gram-negative coverage should be added for type III fractures. High-dose penicillin should be added when there is fecal or potential clostridial contamination (eg, with farm-related injuries). Fluoroquinolones offer no benefit over cephalosporin/aminoglycoside regimens. Furthermore, use of fluoroquinolones may unfavorably affect fracture healing and may result in higher infection rates in type III open fractures. In type III fractures, antibiotic use should be continued for 72 hours after injury or not more than 24 hours after soft-tissue coverage has been achieved. Once-daily dosing with aminoglycoside is safe and effective for fractures of types II and III. Level of evidence: V.

26. American College of Surgeons Committee on Trauma: *Advanced Trauma Life Support Program for Doctors* , 7th ed. Chicago, American College of Surgeons, 2004.

27. Bosse MJ, MacKenzie EJ, Kellam JF, et al: An analysis of outcomes of reconstruction or amputation after leg-threatening injuries. *N Engl J Med* 2002;347(24):1924-1931.

28. Bosse MJ, McCarthy ML, Jones AL, et al; Lower Extremity Assessment Project (LEAP) Study Group: The insensate foot following severe lower extremity trauma: An indication for amputation? *J Bone Joint Surg Am* 2005;87(12):2601-2608.

29. Scalea TM, DuBose J, Moore EE, et al: Western Trauma Association critical decisions in trauma: Management of the mangled extremity. *J Trauma Acute Care Surg* 2012;72(1):86-93.

    A review of current literature was performed by the Western Trauma Association to develop an evidence-based algorithm to help with decision making regarding management of the mangled lower extremity. No adequate scoring was identified to predict limb salvage versus amputation. Level of evidence: IV.

30. MacKenzie EJ, Bosse MJ: Factors influencing outcome following limb-threatening lower limb trauma: Lessons learned from the Lower Extremity Assessment Project (LEAP). *J Am Acad Orthop Surg* 2006;14(10 Spec No.):S205-S210.

31. MacKenzie EJ, Bosse MJ, Pollak AN, et al: Long-term persistence of disability following severe lower-limb trauma: Results of a seven year follow-up. *J Bone Joint Surg Am* 2005;87(8):1801-1809.

32. Ellington JK, Bosse MJ, Castillo RC, MacKenzie EJ; LEAP Study Group: The mangled foot and ankle: Results from a 2-year prospective study. *J Orthop Trauma* 2013;27(1):43-48.

    The authors of this therapeutic study investigated outcomes of patients with mangled feet and ankles who underwent limb salvage with or without free tissue flaps for wound coverage compared with similar patients who underwent early below-knee amputation (BKA). The Sickness Impact Profile (SIP) was the principal outcome measure. SIP scores for patients who underwent salvage with free tissue transfer were significantly worse than scores for those who underwent BKA with typical skin flap design closure. Patients who underwent salvage with standard soft-tissue coverage had statistically significantly better SIP scores than those who underwent BKA, emphasizing the importance of handling delicate soft tissue. Level of evidence: II.

33. MacKenzie EJ, Bosse MJ, Castillo RC, et al: Functional outcomes following trauma-related lower-extremity amputation. *J Bone Joint Surg Am* 2004;86-A(8):1636-1645.

34. Doukas WC, Hayda RA, Frisch HM, et al: The Military Extremity Trauma Amputation/Limb Salvage (METALS) study: Outcomes of amputation versus limb salvage following major lower-extremity trauma. *J Bone Joint Surg Am* 2013;95(2):138-145.

    The authors conducted a retrospective cohort study of 324 service members with lower-limb injury requiring amputation or limb salvage. Patients scored significantly lower than population norms in all Short Musculoskeletal Function Assessment domains except arm/hand function. Thirty-eight percent screened positive for depressive symptoms and 17% for post-traumatic stress syndrome. Patients who had undergone amputation scored better in all SMFA domains than did those who had undergone limb salvage and had lower likelihood of PTSD. Level of evidence: III.

35. Cross JD, Stinner DJ, Burns TC, Wenke JC, Hsu JR; Skeletal Trauma Research Consortium (STReC): Return to duty after type III open tibia fracture. *J Orthop Trauma* 2012;26(1):43-47.

    Researchers retrospectively reviewed data regarding 115 soldiers who sustained battle-related type III open tibial fractures. The overall return to duty (RTD) rate was 18%; those with isolated open fractures had a RTD rate of 22%, those with salvaged extremities had a RTD rate of 20.5%, and those who underwent amputation had a RTD rate of 12.5%. Older age and higher rank were both significant factors in increasing the likelihood of RTD, and amputees had significantly higher disability ratings than did those with salvaged extremities. Level of evidence: IV.

36. Akula M, Gella S, Shaw CJ, McShane P, Mohsen AM: A meta-analysis of amputation versus limb salvage in mangled lower limb injuries—the patient perspective. *Injury* 2011;42(11):1194-1197.

    The authors conducted a meta-analysis of 214 studies of quality of life in patients who underwent post-traumatic amputation versus patients whose limbs were salvaged. Inclusion criteria included English language, post-traumatic amputations, unilateral amputees, outcomes measurements via Short Form-36 or SIP, minimum cases of 20 in each study, minimum follow-up of 2 years, and studies between 1990 and 2007. Eleven studies met the inclusion criteria. No statistical differences were noted regarding physical outcomes, but psychological outcomes indicated that patients whose limbs were salvaged had better outcomes than did patients who underwent amputation (P = 0.008 [SF-36] and 0.05 [SIP]). Level of evidence: I.

37. MacKenzie EJ, Jones AS, Bosse MJ, et al: Health-care costs associated with amputation or reconstruction of a limb-threatening injury. *J Bone Joint Surg Am* 2007;89(8):1685-1692.

38. Chung KC, Saddawi-Konefka D, Haase SC, Kaul G: A cost-utility analysis of amputation versus salvage for Gustilo type IIIB and IIIC open tibial fractures. *Plast Reconstr Surg* 2009;124(6):1965-1973.

Chapter 16

Amputations in Patients With Trauma

Benjamin K. Potter, MD, FACS

Abstract

Improved medical care of patients with diabetes, peripheral vascular disease, cancer, or trauma requiring limb salvage has led to a decrease in amputation rates during the past several decades. Concurrent advances in surgical, prosthetic, and rehabilitation treatment have led to improved functional outcomes for many patients. Nonetheless, the amputation of a major extremity sometimes is necessary. Amputation is a devastating event for many affected patients, and it is a life-changing event for all patients. Novel techniques such as osseointegration and targeted muscle reinnervation are evolving and hold promise in the near future for improving many patients' functional potential. Most patients continue to be treated with conventional surgery, however. Careful attention to sound surgical principles, detailed patient counseling, and complication prevention and management are critical to optimal functional and psychosocial outcomes.

Keywords: amputation; heterotopic ossification; osseointegration; residual limb; targeted muscle reinnervation; trauma

Introduction

Amputation of a damaged or diseased limb is one of the oldest major surgical procedures. Amputation may be required because of trauma, cancer, infection, congenital malformation, or vascular disease, and often it is lifesaving. Despite the long and detailed history of amputation and the great improvement in patient survival rates that occurred after the introduction of antiseptic and antibiotic regimens, amputation generally remains an overlooked component of the practicing orthopaedic surgeon's procedural armamentarium. The surgery is by definition ablative, but it should not be maligned as representing a treatment failure or the inevitable undesirable sequela of a severe injury. Instead, amputation is a reconstructive procedure, and it should be understood as one. The surgical principles are simple, but the complexity of the common pitfalls as well as patient- and limb-specific variables often require both creativity and attention to detail. A successful amputation must provide the patient with the best possible residual limb, which will form a robust foundation for the fitting of a prosthesis and the return of optimal function. Recent advances in amputation surgery techniques, limb prostheses, rehabilitation, and complication management are leading to improved functional outcomes.

General Principles of Amputation

There has been little change to the basic principles of amputation surgery. Adherence to these principles offers patients the best opportunity to achieve optimal functional recovery and offers the surgeon the best opportunity to avoid complications or an unplanned reoperation. The initial amputation after trauma usually is performed through or adjacent to the zone of injury in an open, length-preserving manner, with no attempt to fashion conventional flaps. Guillotine and open-circular amputations are antiquated techniques that sacrifice important residual limb length and soft tissue for only minimal improvement in surgical time. In contrast, preservation of viable tissues during the initial amputation provides options for coverage, closure, and length or level salvage if a subsequent débridement procedure is required because of infection or wound necrosis. Except for an amputation well proximal to the zone of injury, such as an immediate transtibial amputation of a pristine leg above a mangled foot, amputation closure should be delayed until both

Dr. Potter or an immediate family member serves as a board member, owner, officer, or committee member of the Society of Military Orthopaedic Surgeons and the American Academy of Orthopaedic Surgeons (Board of Subspecialty Societies–Research and Quality Committee).

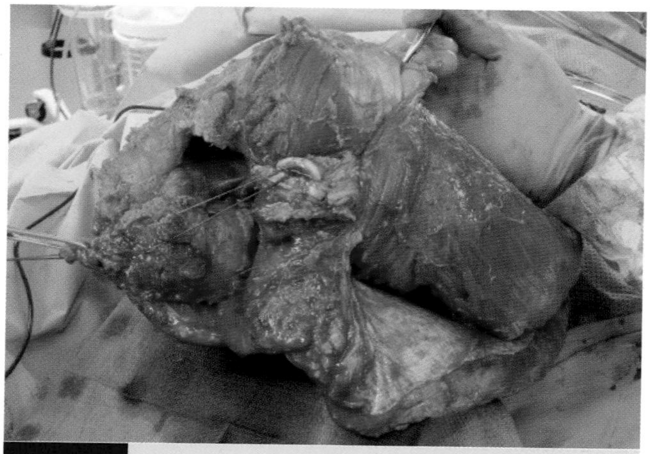

Figure 1 Intraoperative photograph of a trauma-related left transfemoral amputation shows serial myodeses to achieve a myodesis by proxy of all involved muscle groups and maximize stability of the soft-tissue envelope and volitional residual limb control. An adductor magnus myodesis has been secured with braided nonabsorbable sutures on both the medial and lateral distal femoral cortices to reinforce the myodesis and stabilize it from anterior or posterior subluxation, resulting in loss of tension. Sutures placed in the semimembranosus and semitendinosus muscles for subsequent medial hamstring myodesis augment the adductor myodesis and further anchor the terminal muscles to bone. The biceps muscles are subsequently sewn to the medial hamstrings, and the quadriceps apron is sewn to the posteromedial and lateral hamstring fasciae to create a myodesis by proxy of all terminal muscle groups, to anchor the distal padding to prevent symptomatic hypermobility, and to prevent deep bursa formation.

the wound and the patient's general condition are stable. Repeated débridement and wound reassessment for viability should be performed within 24 to 28 hours of injury, if feasible. Open packing, negative pressure wound therapy, and antibiotic bead pouches are acceptable for interim use. The use of negative pressure wound therapy or antibiotic bead pouches allows painful bedside dressing changes to be avoided and soft-tissue tension to be maintained with provisional fasciocutaneous reapproximation through temporary sutures or vessel loops. These methods of preventing skin and soft-tissue retraction have largely supplanted skin traction techniques.

Novel or extra-long amputation levels generally should be avoided because of suboptimal soft-tissue coverage, and they may obligate patients to the prosthetic limitations of both the more proximal and distal described amputation levels without affording the full benefits of either (for example, an extra-long transtibial amputation may limit prosthetic options and leave inadequate distal padding while also lacking the benefits of a Syme ankle disarticulation). A transfemoral amputation length and level salvage for a patient who will not be able to ambulate can improve sitting comfort and balance. Preservation of a functional or salvageable major joint, even with a short residual limb, almost always is desirable.

It is crucial to retain or form a robust soft-tissue envelope. The soft-tissue envelope determines the quality of the final residuum at least as much as the underlying osseous platform, and it is the final determinant of residual limb length. Myocutaneous and fasciocutaneous flaps are preferred, but so-called flaps of opportunity are completely acceptable to facilitate robust coverage of a long residuum. The edges of the transected bone should be carefully smoothed with a saw or rasp to prevent pain, soft-tissue erosion, or myodesis failure. Extensive periosteal stripping should be avoided to preserve the blood supply to the bone, but excess periosteum should be excised to avoid bone spur formation. A myodesis or tenodesis affecting a muscle group critical for terminal padding or residual limb control of the proximal joint should be performed using heavy sutures through drill holes in the bone or the adjacent periosteum. This principle remains true regardless of amputation level. For example, a myodesis anchors and prevents migration of the heel pad or gastrocnemius muscle required for padding in a Syme or transtibial amputation, respectively; restores adduction and hip extension strength in a transfemoral amputation; and anchors padding and improves myoelectric device control after a transradial or transhumeral amputation. Myoplasty performed by suturing antagonist muscle groups to each other is a less stable technique that can be used for secondary muscles. Alternatively, muscle closure can be done in layers beginning with myodesis and suturing of each subsequent muscle layer to the preceding layer, thus effectively creating a proxy myodesis of all groups (**Figure 1**).

Coverage and closure with native innervated skin is preferable because it is more robust than grafted skin, is more resistant to skin breakdown and shear, and provides terminal residuum sensation and prosthetic proprioception. Skin grafting may be acceptable if robust, mobile, and healthy muscle and fat are available to receive the graft. A skin graft directly over bone, periosteum, tendon, or fascia often quickly fails, or it breaks down in the prosthetic socket after initial healing. Major vessels should be individually securely ligated at the level of the bone transection.

All transected nerves will form neuromas. Although neuroma formation is inevitable, persistent symptoms are not. All major nerves must be identified at the time of definitive amputation to prevent formation of symptomatic neuromata. In the trauma setting, identification can be facilitated by avoiding aggressive nerve transection during the open, length-preserving index amputation. A traction neurectomy should be performed on each nerve; the nerve is isolated, proximally dissected, placed under gentle tension, and sharply transected. Deinnervation of functionally important proximal muscle groups should be avoided, particularly in the upper extremity. Usually the resulting neuromas will be relatively deep, well padded, and away from the terminal residual limb that bears most of the load from a prosthetic socket. Alternative approaches, such as burying the nerve in muscle, fat, or bone, are not reliably successful, although acute targeted muscle reinnervation (TMR) may become a reasonable option in the near future.

Amputation Epidemiology and Prevention

Some progress has been made in the prevention of dysvascular and diabetic amputation. Improved preventive care was believed to be partly responsible for the decline in the number of foot amputations in patients with diabetes during a 10-year period, which was accompanied by a 140% increase in the orthopaedic treatment of foot conditions.[1] Approximately one-sixth of all amputations in the United States are necessitated by trauma.[2] Almost half of all surviving people with amputation in the United States have a trauma-related amputation, however, because most such patients are relatively young and have few medical comorbidities. An assessment of amputation rates in the National Trauma Data Bank found almost 9,000 people with amputation, representing 1% of all patients with trauma.[2] Most of these amputations (77%) involved a digit rather than a major extremity. A lower extremity amputation was most likely to require discharge to a skilled nursing facility. The presence of multiple limb amputations was an independent risk factor for death; this finding is especially noteworthy because multiple extremity injuries or amputations are not adequately captured by the Injury Severity Score.

Advances in orthopaedic and plastic surgical techniques in the future may make limb salvage a realistic alternative for many patients with traumatic injury. However, amputation rates after limb-threatening trauma in general have remained stable during the past decade. No reliable scoring system is available for use in deciding whether to amputate a limb immediately after injury.

Recent Advances in Amputation Surgery

Osseointegration

Osseointegration is the direct skeletal attachment of a prosthesis using osseous fixation and a transcutaneous interface. Osseointegration originated as an extrapolation to terminal amputations of dental implant and major joint arthroplasty principles and technologies. The putative subjective benefits of osseointegration include avoidance of socket- and skin-related complications, increased patient comfort, and improved residual limb control and sense achieved through osseoproprioception. Two major osseointegrated devices have gained popularity in Europe and recently in Australia. The Osseointegrated Prosthesis for Rehabilitation of Amputees (OPRA) was developed in Sweden and has been in use for two decades. An 18% infection rate within 3 years of OPRA implantation was reported in 39 patients with upper or lower extremity amputation.[3] In a separate but overlapping study, a 55% rate of superficial infection was found in 51 patients with a transfemoral OPRA.[4] Superficial infection usually could be managed with oral antibiotics, however, and the implant survivorship rate at 2 years was 92%. This study was the first to objectively find improved patient function when an osseointegrated implant was used rather than a conventional socket; significantly better scores were reported on the Questionnaire for Persons With Transfemoral Amputation and the Medical Outcomes Study 36-Item Short Form (SF-36) physical function scale.

A study of 55 transfemoral amputations using the OPRA found no significant migration or rotation of the intraosseous fixture at 7-year follow-up.[5] Three implants had been removed because of loosening, and one was removed because of a deep infection. Changes in cortical thickness and porosity caused by stress shielding were minimal; this finding may bode well for long-term implant longevity and possible eventual revision.

The endo-exo prosthesis for the femur, also called the integral leg prosthesis, was developed in Germany and has been used there since 1999. A study of 74 lower extremity amputations performed between 1999 and 2013 found only four verified intramedullary infections requiring implant removal.[6] Initially a high rate of unplanned surgical revisions was necessitated by soft-tissue infection, but the issue was largely resolved after the implant's transcutaneous abutment was changed from a porous to a polished design. No implants were removed because of infection during the first 3 years after the design was modified. However, caution is warranted until longer-term follow-up results are available.

Several implants currently are under development in the United States, and US FDA early feasibility studies began in 2015. The FDA recently granted a humanitarian device exemption for use of the OPRA in patients with a transfemoral amputation. At least seven custom osseointegrated implants have been used in patients in the United States, and large-scale use should begin in the next few

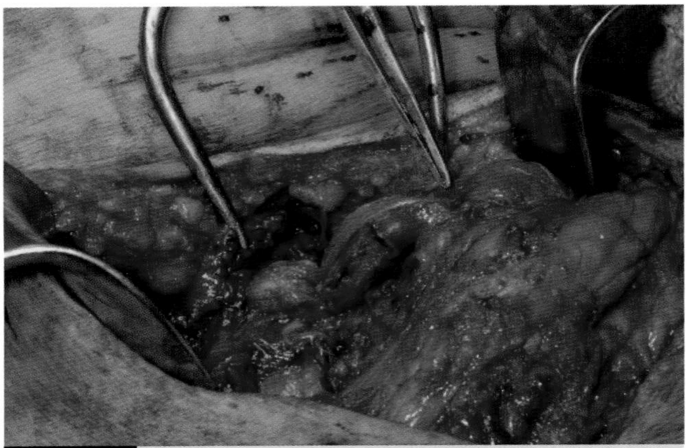

Figure 2 Intraoperative photograph demonstrates an advanced lower extremity targeted muscle reinnervation procedure to relieve neuroma-related pain in a left transfemoral amputation. The patient is prone. The tibial division of the sciatic nerve has been coapted to a motor branch to the semimembranosus muscle, and the peroneal division is sewn to a motor branch to the short head of the biceps to separate and bury the neuromas as well as reduce their size and symptoms. The symptoms were completely resolved 1 year later.

years. If initial US results related to safety and longevity equal or exceed European results, osseointegration technology soon may become available for a broad range of patients who currently struggle with the effects of a short residual limb or an untenable socket that impedes or prevents ambulatory function.

TMR and Advanced Pattern Recognition

Originally, TMR was described for patients with a transhumeral amputation or shoulder disarticulation and until recently was primarily used for these patients. In the TMR surgical technique, unused nerves in the residuum are transposed into the motor branches of expendable muscle groups to improve intuitive myoelectric terminal device control; for example, the median nerve is transferred to the biceps to achieve hand closing, and the terminal radial nerve is transferred to the lateral triceps for hand opening. The TMR technique has been highly successful in achieving functional myoelectric signals. Reinnervation takes place during the first 4 to 6 months after the procedure. Patients with a successful outcome are tested, trained, and fitted with a specialized myoelectric prosthesis interface (Coapt LLC) that uses an advanced pattern recognition algorithm to harness the power of TMR. The Coapt system is compatible with most commercially available myoelectric upper extremity prostheses. A recent study using a generic grid array (rather than site-specific electrodes, which may be more susceptible to sweat interference and require precise placement in relation to the residual limb) found improvement in the real-time performance of multi–degree-of-freedom myoelectric prostheses.[7] This grid array and pattern recognition approach may improve the reliability of terminal device control, regardless of whether the patient has undergone TMR surgery, and it may eliminate the need for the complex, site-specific electrode placement process.

Recently, TMR surgery has been used in the lower extremity for relief of neuroma-related pain, in addition to control of prototype lower extremity myoelectric prostheses (**Figure 2**). A rabbit model study found that the effectiveness of TMR for neuroma-related pain depends on providing a functional purpose for the transected nerve.[8] In transferred nerves, myelinated fiber counts were decreased, fascicle diameter was increased, and neuroma size was decreased. A study of pain in 28 patients who underwent TMR to improve function found that 14 of 15 patients with preoperative neuroma-related pain had complete resolution of pain, and the final patient had some improvement.[9] In a related technique called targeted nerve implantation (TNI), no direct nerve coaptation is performed; instead, transected nerves are implanted into muscle near the area of greatest sensitivity to stimulation. At short-term follow-up, 92% of patients who underwent primary TNI and 87% of those who underwent secondary TNI were found to be free of palpation-induced neuroma pain.[10]

Traditional Surgical Techniques

Advances in conventional surgical techniques have been reported during the past several years. In the presence of an ipsilateral fracture proximal to a traumatic amputation, the surgeon must decide whether to revise the amputation proximally through the fracture site in an effort to simplify the patient's injury and surgical burden. However, the more proximal amputation can lead to an unacceptably short residual limb or the loss of a functional knee or elbow joint. In 37 such combat-related fractures, conventional intramedullary or plate-and-screw fixation was used after serial irrigation and débridement of open injuries.[11] All the fractures healed despite an extremely high infection rate in the terminal residual limbs, no implants were removed because of infection, and amputation length and level salvage was successful in all the patients. Amputation of convenience through the proximal fracture site was not recommended.

The modified Ertl procedure is a distal tibiofibular synostosis done as part of a so-called osteomyoplasty for transtibial amputation. The putative aim is to improve function, but the procedure continues to be controversial. Several studies compared the results of bone bridge and conventional transtibial amputation and found generally mixed and inconclusive results. A comparison of the results of 27 synostosis procedures and 38 conventional modified Burgess transtibial amputations found that patients who underwent synostosis had a longer residual limb, but there was no between-group difference in functional outcomes on any SF-36 or Prosthesis Evaluation Questionnaire subsection.[12] The two techniques were found to have similar functional outcomes in the young active-duty military patient population. A related study evaluated complication and reoperation rates in 37 patients who underwent a modified Ertl synostosis procedure compared with 100 patients who underwent a modified Burgess transtibial amputation.[13] Patients who underwent synostosis had a significantly greater risk of reoperation in general and specifically for a noninfectious complication, and 32% required surgery for a bone bridge–specific complication such as nonunion, fracture, or a need for implant removal. Tibiofibular synostosis did not reduce the risk of postoperative infection, although patients who underwent synostosis creation were more likely to be further from injury and undergoing a revision procedure or late amputation. Real-time in-socket weight-bearing fluoroscopy was used in a small comparison study of patients after synostosis or conventional transtibial amputation.[14] There was no between-group difference in residual limb in-socket displacement or platform stability in total surface–bearing sockets, which are the most commonly used type of transtibial socket; however, these were not end-bearing, Ertl-specific sockets. These findings suggest that the end-bearing potential of the bridge synostosis is theoretical only and/or is not often harnessed. Collectively, these findings suggest that the modified Ertl procedure has no clear functional benefit and an increased risk of complications. However, this procedure continues to have strong advocates. Careful patient selection and counseling are necessary before a bridge synostosis is performed. A current prospective randomized study of the Major Extremity Trauma Research Consortium is attempting to evaluate the functional benefits of the bridge synostosis procedure, and its findings may definitively resolve the issue.

Apart from surgeon and patient preference, the indication for a bridge synostosis procedure is injury-caused overt proximal tibiofibular joint instability or its late symptoms. A percutaneous proximal suture bridge construct, such as the TightRope (Arthrex), can be used to stabilize the dislocated tibiofibular joint after indirect reduction under fluoroscopy.[15] This technique is an alternative to a distal synostosis and is suitable for patients in whom a synostosis is not feasible because of bone loss or asymmetry.

Traction neurectomy is desirable for all major, named nerves to decrease the potential for symptomatic neuroma formation. Management of the sural nerve in the posterior calf is problematic. This nerve normally lies just deep to the subcutaneous fascia after transtibial amputation, and a typical traction neurectomy with a classic posterior myofasciocutaneous flap places the nerve directly under or just posterior to the terminal tibia. A method of anterior resection of the sural nerve has been described in which dissection is within the median raphe of the soleus and between the two heads of the gastrocnemius muscle.[16] Proximal traction neurectomy can be performed away from the terminal residuum in the posterior calf or popliteal fossa. By delivering the identified nerve from distal to proximal through the muscle split, the surgeon can ensure that the fibular communicating branch of the sural nerve proper is not missed and can avoid placing the eventual sural neuroma directly in the distal, weight-bearing soft tissues (**Figure 3**).

The results of a Gritti-Stokes long transfemoral amputation, in which the femur is transected at the supracondylar level to maintain the native insertion of the adductor magnus and subsequently is fused to the patella, were compared with those of a conventional transfemoral amputation.[17] The 14 patients treated with the Gritti-Stokes procedure were less likely to use a nonprosthetic assist device and had better Sickness Impact Profile scores than the 15 patients who underwent conventional amputation. There was some selection bias in this study in that one of the outcome measures was residual limb length, which was greater after the Gritti-Stokes procedure because the procedure requires a more distal bone cut. Nonetheless, the results suggest that further study of this transfemoral amputation technique is warranted.

Recent Advances in Prostheses and Rehabilitation

Oxygen consumption and the metabolic demands of ambulating after lower extremity amputation have been extensively studied. In general, the more proximal the amputation level, the greater the oxygen consumption and metabolic equivalents required for ambulating; historical data revealed a 10% to 40% increase after transtibial amputation and a more than 100% increase after proximal transfemoral or hip disarticulation amputation. A simple alternative for some patients with low physical demands, particularly those with a painful residual limb or a problematic socket, is to ambulate without a prosthesis by using crutches. A study of 30 patients who underwent a transtibial amputation found a 21% increase in energy expenditure during ambulation using crutches and without a prosthesis compared with ambulation using a prosthesis.[18] Ambulating with crutches, therefore, is not

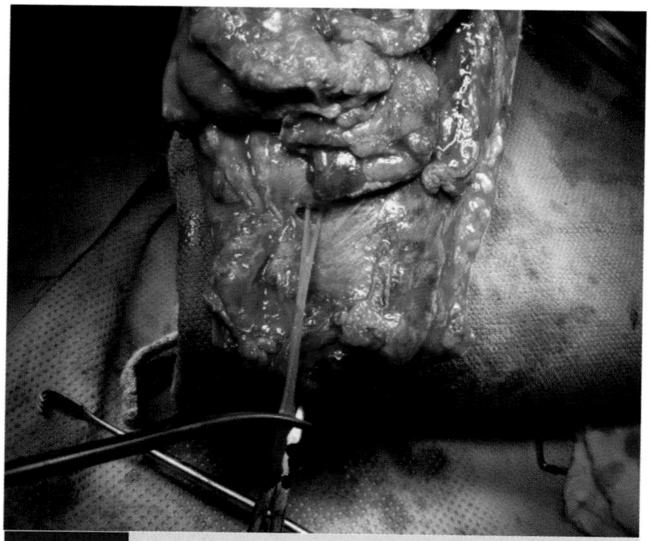

Figure 3 Intraoperative photograph shows the technique for a proximal sural neurectomy using a recently described technique to prevent sural neuroma formation in the terminal soft tissues of the residual limb and ensure that the fibular communicating branch to the nerve has been concurrently addressed. The confluence of the medial sural and lateral (fibular) communicating branches is shown. A split is made in the median raphe of the soleus muscle, and blunt dissection is performed between the medial and lateral gastrocnemius muscles. The sural nerve is identified by palpation and gentle tension on the distal nerve, and it is delivered anteriorly through the incision using a right-angle hemostat.

an energy-efficient solution for a patient who has cardiovascular disease, is severely deconditioned, or has neurologic deficits preventing ambulation with a prosthesis.

Despite continuing advancements in upper extremity prostheses, including the multiple–degree-of-freedom myoelectric devices that are now widely available, prosthesis rejection is common after upper extremity amputation. A survey of 307 patients in Korea who had undergone upper extremity amputation found that more than 80% wore a prosthesis primarily for cosmetic purposes, and only 45% wore a prosthesis longer than 8 hours a day.[19] Although higher rates of prosthetic device use and acceptance have been reported in other studies in different patient populations, this study highlights the need for further advances in upper extremity prosthetic technology to improve patient comfort, function, and acceptance.

During the past two decades, several generations of microprocessor-powered lower extremity prostheses have been developed. Proving the functional benefit of these devices is necessary not only so that improvement in patient function will continue but also so that third-party payers will approve the purchase of an expensive new device. A small study compared the use of a powered knee device and a standard microprocessor knee prosthesis on inclines and stairs.[20] When the powered knee was used during stair ascent, the normal contralateral knee generated less power and the prosthesis generated more power compared with the standard prosthesis. Few other gait differences or benefits were found, however. Another study found that the use of a powered prosthetic ankle decreased the metabolic cost of walking by 8%, decreased biologic leg work by 10%, and increased patient-selected preferred walking velocity by 23% compared with the use of a passive elastic ankle.[21] Although further study is needed, eventually all lower extremity prostheses may become truly bionic—powered prostheses controlled volitionally by the user via myoelectric interfaces similar to modern upper extremity prostheses—as issues related to cost, weight, battery life, and function gradually are resolved.

Complication Management and Patient Outcomes

Functional and Psychosocial Outcomes

Validated and reliable outcome measures are necessary for objective evaluation, reporting, and comparison of outcomes in people with limb loss. Forty-four patients with a unilateral lower extremity amputation were examined on two separate occasions using a battery of tests, including the Prosthetic Evaluation Questionnaire, the SF-36 for Veterans, the Orthotics and Prosthetics Users' Survey, the Patient-Specific Functional Scale, the 2-minute walk test, the 6-minute walk test, and the timed up-and-go test.[22] The results yielded strong reliability and intraclass correlation coefficients between 0.83 and 0.97. Any clinically important differences related to these test findings remain to be determined, however.

A retrospective cohort study of 324 military patients found that after adjustment for covariates and confounders, those with amputation had better scores in all the domains of the Short Musculoskeletal Function Assessment questionnaire and several other outcome measures than those with limb salvage.[23] Another study evaluated the mental health outcomes of patients with a limb-threatening injury or amputation sustained in military conflict between 2001 and 2008.[24] Significantly lower rates of psychologic diagnoses were found in patients who underwent early amputation than in those who had limb salvage, but those who underwent late amputation had higher rates of psychologic diagnoses and pain than those with early amputation or limb salvage. Although selection bias may have been a factor in these studies, the findings provide generally encouraging news for patients with

23. Doukas WC, Hayda RA, Frisch HM, et al: The Military Extremity Trauma Amputation/Limb Salvage (METALS) study: Outcomes of amputation versus limb salvage following major lower-extremity trauma. *J Bone Joint Surg Am* 2013;95(2):138-145.

    A retrospective cohort study of 324 military service members who sustained an extremity injury had a poor response rate (55% for those requiring limb salvage and 64% for those requiring amputation). After adjustment for covariates, participants with an amputation had better scores in all domains of the Short Musculoskeletal Function Assessment and a lower incidence of posttraumatic stress disorder, and they were more likely to engage in vigorous sports. Outcomes in favor of amputation may have been influenced by selection bias, but the superior outcomes are striking. Level of evidence: III.

24. Melcer T, Sechriest VF, Walker J, Galarneau M: A comparison of health outcomes for combat amputee and limb salvage patients injured in Iraq and Afghanistan wars. *J Trauma Acute Care Surg* 2013;75(2, suppl 2):S247-S254.

    A 2001 to 2008 evaluation of patients with combat-related limb-threatening injury or major extremity amputation found significantly lower rates of psychologic diagnoses in those who underwent amputation within 90 days of injury compared with those who had limb salvage. Patients who underwent late amputation had higher rates of mental health diagnoses and pain compared with the other patients. Level of evidence: III.

25. Sansam K, Neumann V, O'Connor R, Bhakta B: Predicting walking ability following lower limb amputation: A systematic review of the literature. *J Rehabil Med* 2009;41(8):593-603.

    A literature review of predication and ambulatory and functional status after lower extremity amputation suggested that a short time from surgery to rehabilitation, avoidance of residual limb complications, young age, and unilateral distal amputation predicted successful ambulation. The available evidence was often weak and heterogeneous.

26. Tintle SM, Baechler MF, Nanos GP, Forsberg JA, Potter BK: Reoperations following combat-related upper-extremity amputations. *J Bone Joint Surg Am* 2012;94(16):e1191-e1196.

    A review of 100 consecutive major upper extremity amputations found that 42% of residual limbs underwent repeated surgical intervention to treat complications or persistent symptoms. Patients increased their regular prosthesis use and acceptance from 19% before revision surgery to 87% after revision. These findings suggest that aggressive management of complications and surgical treatment of persistently symptomatic residual limbs can have a dramatic positive effect on prosthesis use and outcomes. Level of evidence: IV.

27. Tintle SM, Shawen SB, Forsberg JA, et al: Reoperation after combat-related major lower extremity amputations. *J Orthop Trauma* 2014;28(4):232-237.

    A 53% reoperation rate was found in a study of 300 combat-related major lower extremity amputations. The most common indications were infection (27%), HO (24%), and neuroma excision (11%). Pain and prosthesis tolerance were consistently improved after surgical treatment of identifiable complications and pain generators in persistently symptomatic residual limbs after nonsurgical management. Level of evidence: IV.

28. Singh R, Venkateshwara G: Effect of fluid collections on long-term outcome after lower limb amputation. *Arch Phys Med Rehabil* 2012;93(3):509-511.

    Seventy living amputees from a cohort of 105, of whom 30% had fluid collections postoperatively, were surveyed at 3 years' follow-up. The authors found no difference in survival, complications, or prosthetic use between patients with or without early postoperative fluid collections.

29. Polfer EM, Hoyt BW, Senchak LT, Murphey MD, Forsberg JA, Potter BK: Fluid collections in amputations are not indicative or predictive of infection. *Clin Orthop Relat Res* 2014;472(10):2978-2983.

    A review of 300 major lower extremity amputations found that 55% of limbs had a fluid collection within 3 months of residual limb closure; this percentage fell to 11% after 3 months. In the absence of clinical indicators of infection specific to the residual limb (erythema, warmth, drainage), there was no relationship between the presence of a fluid collection and infection. Asymptomatic fluid collections within residual limbs should be ignored. Level of evidence: III.

30. Polfer EM, Tintle SM, Forsberg JA, Potter BK: Skin grafts for residual limb coverage and preservation of amputation length. *Plast Reconstr Surg* 2015;136(3):603-609.

    A review of 300 lower and 100 upper extremity combat-related amputations compared the results of delayed primary closure and STSG. Rates of early wound failure, HO excision, and soft-tissue revision were higher after STSG. In approximately half of the patients, STSG essentially represented a successful staging procedure intended to salvage residual limb length. For patients receiving STSG over robust muscle not on the terminal residuum, STSG can be a durable definitive coverage alternative. Level of evidence: IV.

31. Pavey GJ, Polfer EM, Nappo KE, Tintle SM, Forsberg JA, Potter BK: What risk factors predict recurrence of heterotopic ossification after excision in combat-related amputations? *Clin Orthop Relat Res* 2015;473(9):2814-2824.

    A review of 172 HO excisions in residual limbs after major extremity amputation found that 6.5% of patients underwent reexcision of symptomatic HO. Persistent symptoms more commonly represented partially excised HO than a true recurrence. Risk factors for reexcision were found to be incomplete initial excision or an initial excision performed within 180 days of injury. Complete excision of symptomatic HO performed more than 6 months after injury was unlikely to lead to radiographic and/or symptomatic recurrence of HO. Complications of HO excision were common and required surgery in 31% of patients. Level of evidence: III.

32. Matsumoto ME, Khan M, Jayabalan P, Ziebarth J, Munin MC: Heterotopic ossification in civilians with lower limb amputations. *Arch Phys Med Rehabil* 2014;95(9):1710-1713.

    A review of 158 civilian lower extremity amputations identified symptomatic HO in 36 patients (23%), of whom 4 (11%) required surgical resection of HO. There was no identified relationship between trauma as the indication for amputation and the incidence of HO. Level of evidence: IV.

33. Pet MA, Ko JH, Friedly JL, Smith DG: Traction neurectomy for treatment of painful residual limb neuroma in lower extremity amputees. *J Orthop Trauma* 2015;29(9):e321-e325.

    Of 38 patients with 63 symptomatic neuromata treated with traction neurectomy, 16 patients (42%) had recurrent or persistent neuroma-related pain at mean 37-month follow-up, and 8 patients (21%) underwent further surgical treatment of persistent or recurrent symptoms.

Chapter 17

Disaster and Mass Casualty Preparedness

Roman Hayda, MD   Philip McClure, MD

Abstract

Recent events such as the Boston Marathon bombings and the Haiti earthquake have provided important lessons for disaster and mass casualty preparedness. The most modern principles of disaster management planning and execution have been modified and influenced by events in the past 5 years (Incident Command System, tourniquet use, international preparation).

Keywords: disaster; mass casualty; preparedness; terrorism

Introduction

The key role of orthopaedic surgery in disaster response has been highlighted in the responses to the Haiti earthquake of 2010 and the Boston Marathon bombings. In part because of these high-profile events, disasters and disaster response have gained increasing attention in the medical community. Recognizing the need for an effective response, government entities and nongovernmental organizations have devoted substantial resources to the planning, coordination, and exercise of disaster response. Among these organizations, the American Academy of Orthopaedic Surgeons (AAOS), the Orthopaedic Trauma Association (OTA), the Society of Military Orthopaedic Surgeons, and the Pediatric Orthopaedic Society of North America have been instrumental in organizing the orthopaedic community.

The response to recent disasters such as the Haiti earthquake and the Boston Marathon bombings has been analyzed closely and has generated important recommendations for improvement, which are described in the following sections. The overriding lesson of these events was the key role of preparedness in limiting the human cost of disasters. A recent review of disaster preparedness in the European Union, however, yielded somewhat discouraging results in this regard. Although at least 73% of European Union countries have had recent natural or human disasters, large differences in perceived preparedness were apparent among the countries. Overall preparation was deemed "acceptable" but varied widely across nations. Areas of weakness were observed in hospital preparedness and education and training.[1] It would not be a surprise if similar variability was found across regions and hospitals in the United States.

Disasters vary in cause and scope but always overwhelm the usual resources for protection and care of the population. Whether natural or manmade, the disaster can be local, regional, or national in scope. The burden on medical resources in general and orthopaedic surgery in particular can vary greatly depending on the cause, location, and timing of the event. Earthquakes in urban areas that may have inadequate building codes, such as the earthquake in Haiti, and terrorist bombings in areas with a high density of people, such as the Boston Marathon bombings, are examples of incidents known to generate the largest number of orthopaedic injuries.

Further emphasis on disaster preparedness with the ability to manage not only blunt injury but also less familiar, complex war-type injury is highlighted by the terrorist attack in Paris in November 2015. In the Paris

Dr. Hayda or an immediate family member is a member of a speakers' bureau or has made paid presentations on behalf of AO North America and Synthes, serves as an unpaid consultant to BioIntraface, and serves as a board member, owner, officer, or committee member of the American Academy of Orthopaedic Surgeons, the Orthopaedic Trauma Association, and METRC (Major Extremity Trauma Research Consortium). Neither Dr. McClure nor any immediate family member has received anything of value from or has stock or stock options held in a commercial company or institution related directly or indirectly to the subject of this chapter.

attack, the terrorists used a complex multicentric tactic including suicide bombers and high-velocity military-style weapons that caused 129 immediate deaths. More than 300 injured survivors were triaged to 16 hospitals, with only 4 deaths (2 were essentially dead on arrival). A preliminary analysis cited the early activation of the recently rehearsed city disaster plan, which placed particular emphasis on military-type injuries, as a key component in the successful response.[2] Clinicians interested in disaster response should prepare themselves and their hospital systems to ensure a successful response in natural and manmade disasters and terrorist acts.

Principles of Disaster Response

Disasters are inherently chaotic, straining both medical and nonmedical resources. An effective medical disaster response requires changes to the usual medical care processes. During disasters, providers strive to provide the most good for the highest number of casualties.

Disaster planners have defined four phases of disaster management: mitigation, preparation, response, and rehabilitation.[3] Mitigation consists of taking steps to limit the potential of a disaster to put lives and property at risk. Examples include seawalls to protect against hurricanes and barriers to limit vehicle access to potential terrorist targets. The preparation phase involves planning for potential disasters and includes resourcing, education, and coordination among various constituents. In many ways, planning is the most important phase, but it often is underemphasized. In the response phase, often shown in the media, action is taken to limit any further threat to lives and property while rescuing the injured. Critical elements of this phase include identifying the scope of the disaster, defining needs, and ensuring that responders are not placed at undue risk. The rehabilitation phase involves the process of returning to normalcy by rebuilding structures and rehabilitating those with severe injuries. During this time, it is important to analyze the response to the disaster while attending to the physical needs and mental stresses of the casualties and the responders.

The chaos associated with any disaster is addressed best by an organizational structure that can respond to needs while managing limited resources. The Incident Command System (ICS) provides a structure for the response to a disaster. By centralizing organizational activities, resources (including manpower and supplies, security, food, shelter, water, and other essentials) can be distributed optimally. The ICS model, otherwise known as the "all hazards approach," is scalable and adaptable to various circumstances. Common components of the command structure include positions such as incident commander, safety officer, liaison officer, public relations official, logistics manager, and additional technical specialists as dictated by the disaster. The incident commander should be well versed in disaster response and resource management and should have previous experience in the field. Typically, the commander is not a medical person. The medical/surgical response—including orthopaedic surgery—is a critical element of a proper response, and clear communication between the orthopaedic component and other groups is essential. The organization of an orthopaedic response is similar to the organization of the ICS[3] (**Figure 1**).

The principles of disaster response include the limitation of disaster progression, triage, and evacuation, while simultaneously conserving resources. Triage requires the careful evaluation of individuals and the categorization of injuries by acuity to optimize care for the largest number of casualties. The categories of triage are (1) immediate (urgent, lifesaving treatment), (2) delayed (the walking wounded), (3) expectant (extensive injuries requiring considerable time and resources), and (4) dead. The expectant category represents the highest difficulty of disaster care. Resources often are focused on this group in typical emergency care; however, high resource consumption by these cases adversely affects the delivery of care to a larger number of patients. The categorization of expectant injury will vary based on the scale of the disaster and the availability of resources. It is generally accepted that overtriage, or inappropriate placement of casualties into the immediate category, negatively affects the overall mortality rates.

Domestic Disaster Response: Boston Marathon Bombings

The response to the Boston Marathon bombings largely has been considered a success.[4-10] Aside from the immediate deaths from overwhelming injury, no other casualties died, reflecting an efficient response to the event. The successful management of the bombing was credited to advance planning and a fortunate combination of circumstances. Throughout the Boston Trauma System, numerous drills were conducted in preparation for potential mass casualty events.[8,11] The centralized command center was able to make optimal use of its resources to include the medical personnel immediately available at the scene who were already mobilized to provide medical care to the marathon runners. Three level I trauma centers were located nearby, facilitating transport. Additionally, the hospitals receiving casualties were undergoing a shift change, doubling the personnel available to render care.[8,10] Regardless of the fortuitous circumstances,

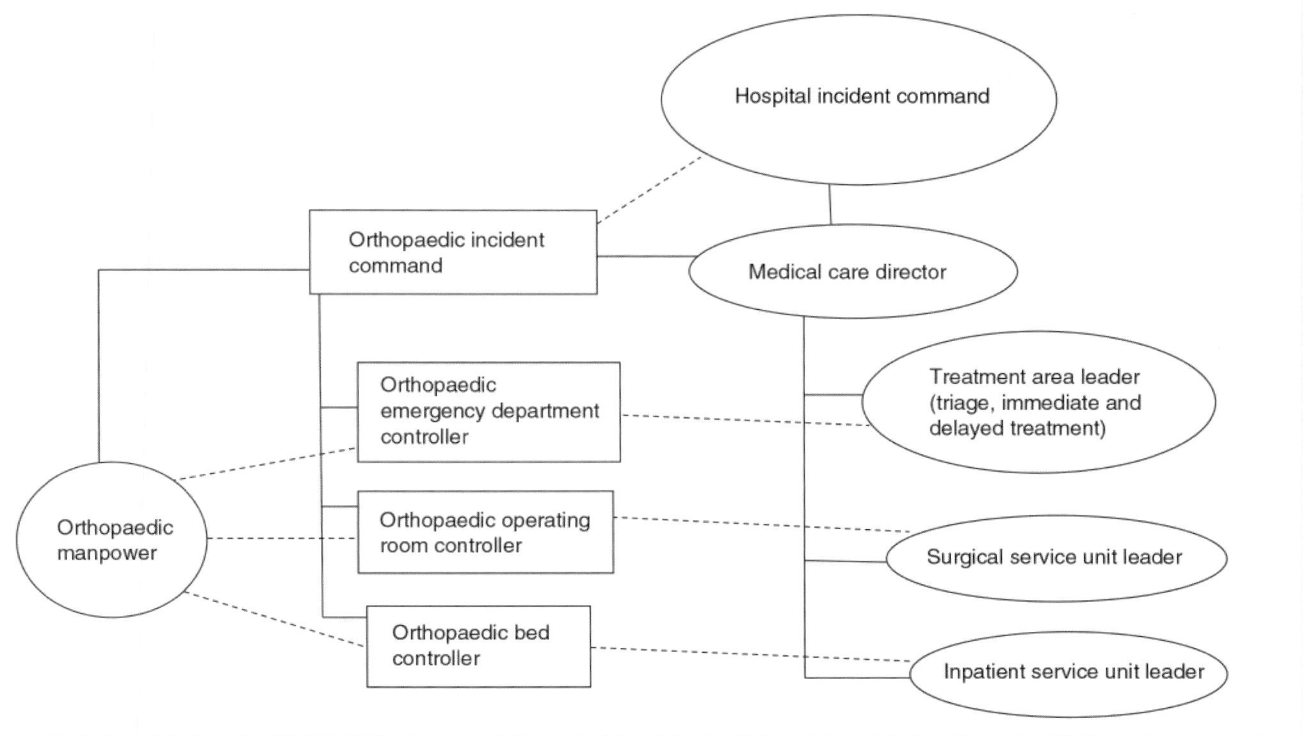

Figure 1 Schematic drawing of the orthopaedic Incident Command System. In the hospital setting, orthopaedic surgery disaster response falls under the direction of the hospital disaster plan, with its hospital incident command and the medical care director. (Adapted with permission from Born CT, Mamczak C, Pagenkopf E, et al: Disaster management response guidelines for departments of orthopaedic surgery. *JBJS Reviews* 2016;4[1]:e1.)

it must be emphasized that the planning and rehearsal by the system were crucial in the effective response. Such planning and rehearsal should be performed in all communities.

The Boston Trauma Center Chiefs' Collaborative reported several important aspects of the Boston Marathon bombings response.[10] The group emphasized that maintaining a state of readiness and avoiding complacency are key. They recommended regular disaster training, with considerations for limited personnel. Other crucial elements include developing a robust and modern communication system and having a backup of personal radio communication in the event that the cellular technology system fails. Although well managed in the Boston Marathon incident, triage and casualty disposition were identified as other areas that require specific attention. At the Boston Marathon, emergency medical services (EMS) were readily available, and prehospital triage and disposition were completed through direct feedback mechanisms. If communication is compromised, hospitals must develop a plan to triage adequately within the facility because a large number of patients may show up unannounced. This situation is more likely to occur in underdeveloped countries or during very large disasters. A summary of the recommendations is provided in **Table 1**.

Despite the success of the Boston Marathon bombings response, reviewers noted a major potential flaw: no system for resource sharing or patient sharing had been developed among the multiple trauma centers involved.[10] They noted that a plan should be in place to adequately care for emergencies, such as acute abdomen, myocardial infarction, or stroke, that are not related to the disaster, possibly including transfer or diversion. Equipment suppliers should be included in the overall disaster planning. Difficulties in obtaining radiographic studies should be expected during a mass casualty event, and preparation by the department of radiology should be incorporated into the hospital disaster plan. Increased use of blood products should be anticipated. Blood supply chains should be verified and their procedures should be rehearsed.[7,12,13]

The bombing incident also highlighted the potential importance of tourniquets in civilian disaster response.[4,6] Commercial and improvised tourniquets

3: Soft-Tissue Injury and the Polytrauma Patient

Table 1

Boston Trauma Center Chiefs' Collaborative Recommendations

Issue	Primary Action	Secondary Action
Preparedness	Yearly drills with limited personnel	Resist complacency
Communication	Cellular communication	Backup systems or personal radio
Field triage	May not be possible; hospital triage plan required	Feedback from hospitals to EMS to avoid overload or underuse of facilities
Tourniquets	Train response personnel in use	Military tourniquets stocked in EMS system
System-based care	Develop system for patient sharing	Develop a system for human/medical resource sharing

EMS = emergency medical services.
Data from Boston Trauma Center Chiefs' Collaborative: Boston marathon bombings: An after-action review. *J Trauma Acute Care Surg* 2014;77(3):501-503.

Table 2

Seven Sins of Humanitarian Medicine

Error	Example
Leaving a mess behind	Creating complications of care without having a plan to address them
Failing to match technology to needs	Having insufficient basic supplies; using useless advanced technology that cannot be supported
Failing to cooperate	Solo missions or unaffiliated volunteers attempting to render care without training, experience, or support becoming a burden to responders; military/nongovernmental organizations not working or communicating with one another
Losing patients to follow-up	Performing a complex reconstruction process not sustainable locally; amputations without prostheses
Misplacing priorities	Using the disaster as a training area; emphasizing politics or personal gain
Offering a superfluous response	Providing unwanted or unneeded aid
Having a wrong motivation	Participating to gain prestige or status

Data from Welling DR, Ryan JM, Burris DG, Rich NM: Seven sins of humanitarian medicine. *World J Surg* 2010;34(3):466-470.

prevented life-threatening exsanguination in casualties with mangled extremities, capitalizing on recent military experience.[14] Planners should consider training and equipping responders with tourniquets to address this need.[6]

International Disaster Response: Haiti Earthquake

Orthopaedic surgeons have a strong tradition of international service through organizations such as Doctors Without Borders, Health Volunteers Overseas, and a variety of other groups. International service trips can be very productive, but volunteers incur substantial associated costs. Interestingly, in reviewing the cost of elective relief missions versus those occurring after a disaster provided through Operation Smile, disaster relief was found to have higher cost efficiency in cost per patient.[15]

In planning a disaster response, assessment of the available infrastructure is critical. In the Haiti earthquake disaster of 2010, an overall lack of systems organization led to a suboptimal response in an overwhelmed system. Faced with more than 200,000 injured people, any system would have been overwhelmed; however, previous infrastructure inadequacy in Haiti compounded the problem. Local infrastructure needs should be anticipated and evaluated before departure to minimize unforeseen needs that can exacerbate difficulties in delivering care.[16]

Volunteers should remember that international relief efforts are vastly different from routine medical practice. Although the international need for humanitarian efforts in medicine remains great, it is important to remember to avoid making errors when attempting to help others in an unfamiliar and potentially undeveloped location. Optimizing patient care, both immediately and over the long term, is an important responsibility. Common pitfalls of humanitarian medicine that were identified and reviewed in a 2010 study are summarized in **Table 2** and can be applied to disaster relief missions.[17]

The spectrum of injury should be expected to vary considerably with the mechanism of the disaster. Earthquakes in particular are capable of producing an extreme number of casualties and a very high percentage of orthopaedic injuries.[18,19] A 2011 study identified opportunities to improve the response to large disaster events, particularly earthquakes, including planning additional operating room capability, adding plastic surgery capability, and planning peritoneal dialysis capability for the management of crush syndrome.[19] When coordinating a disaster response, it is essential to remember that basic human needs are often unmet. Providing early support that includes shelter, food, and water can help limit the magnification of the disaster. Planners should be mindful that during many international responses, nongovernmental and military groups often are not functioning until 2 to 4 days after the event, unless they were present before the event occurred. Surgical capability and planning should be adjusted to the realities of the situation. Open fractures often are infected already, muscle affected by compartment syndrome may already be beyond the point of salvage, and only limited prosthetic resources may be available for amputees. Proposed guidelines for the response to an international mega–mass casualty event are outlined in **Table 3**.

Communication

A 2014 study reviewed the telecommunications experience of Israeli field hospitals during disasters in Haiti, Japan, and Turkey.[20] The authors concluded that a variety of telecommunication methods should be available to provide backup, communication systems should operate independently of local infrastructure, and participants should take advantage of a wide variety of radiofrequencies. In addition, mass media should be used when appropriate. Direct interpersonal communication should be sought whenever possible, and digital photographs are helpful in maintaining patient records and identities.

Modifying a disaster response system will be necessary for areas without appropriate infrastructure. Deploying specialty teams to the casualty site and distributing casualties to other facilities may need to be sacrificed because of poor communication networks. Prehospital care may be inadequate or nonexistent, and triage should be managed at the site.[21]

Information Technology

Medical record keeping in disaster responses is often difficult, but it is a critical component of optimal care. The advent of mobile technology available to many volunteers offers a potential solution. One group evaluated the implementation of a mobile phone–based record system in postearthquake Haiti.[22] A three-phase implementation was used: needs assessment and tool selection, feasibility testing with high-risk patients, and widespread use. The group tracked 617 patients in the electronic system.

Table 3

Response to an International Mega–Mass Casualty Event

Issue	Primary Principle	Secondary Principle
Extremity injury priority	Life-threatening infection requires emergency débridement/amputation	Limb salvage secondary
Closed fractures	Treated nonsurgically generally (minimize chronic infection and limit resource use)	Surgically stabilize adult closed femur when resources allow
Open fractures	Débridement and external fixation (especially adult femur)	Perform acute shortening as needed after débridement of devitalized bone to limit need for flaps and amputations
Amputations	For nonviable or unreconstructible limbs; poorly controlled infection	Use open technique to allow sequential débridement and delayed closure
Compartment syndrome	No fasciotomies for chronic compartment syndrome because of infection risk	Consider only if limb is pulseless
Radiology	Single AP view for diagnosis of fractures	Use postoperative radiographs judiciously

Data from Bar-On E, Lebel E, Kreiss Y, et al: Orthopaedic management in a mega mass casualty situation: The Israel Defence Forces Field Hospital in Haiti following the January 2010 earthquake. *Injury* 2011;42(10):1053-1059.

They noted many anecdotal and verified adverse effects before implementation of a mobile phone–based system, including missed surgery appointments for patients who could not be located, a failure to identify unaccompanied minors, suboptimal prosthetic care, unrecorded surgical dates, and fragmented care plans. In a setting with many handoffs to other workers, providers thought that the electronic handheld record improved care and eased the workload.

Pediatric Disaster Victims

Pediatric patients often are involved in disaster situations, but the focus of disaster response often has been centered on adult patients. This focus is unlikely to be conscious, but the oversight has resulted in the erroneous use of adult orthopaedic trauma care in children, who require different equipment and a special understanding. The authors of a 2007 study distributed a survey to 42 Disaster Medical Assistance Teams in the United States to gain an understanding of their training protocols and preparation.[23] According to their report, pediatric equipment, including airway supplies, cervical collars, and backboards, often was missing. Deficiencies were noted in pediatric-based topics in the training curricula, missing pediatric equipment, and the omission of children from disaster drills in 37% of cases.

The pediatric care experience of the personnel on the US Navy hospital ship *Comfort* during the earthquake in Haiti is of particular interest.[24] Of the patients aboard, 27% were children, similar to the figures from the Gujarat earthquake. Of the procedures performed in children, 71% were orthopaedic in nature. Of all the pediatric admissions, 43% needed surgery. Children were less likely than adults to have pelvis or spine fractures requiring surgery. After the mission was complete, the phases of response to trauma were reviewed, with specific pediatric considerations (**Table 4**). Considerable difficulty occurred when many of the children were discharged because they had no remaining family to care for them. The deficiency of care services upon discharge likely limited further admissions or delivery of care to more acute and severe pediatric cases.

Table 4

Pediatric Disaster Response

Phase	Priority	Pediatric Considerations
Phase I: Mass casualty response	Life- or limb-saving procedures	Conservation of growth potential
Phase II: Subacute response	Optimization of functional outcomes	Conservation of growth potential
Phase III: Rehabilitation	Rehabilitation or transition back to daily life for patients	Creation of a secondary facility for long-term care of orphaned children to decompress acute hospital census

Data from Sonshine DB, Caldwell A, Gosselin RA, Born CT, Coughlin RR: Critically assessing the Haiti earthquake response and the barriers to quality orthopaedic care. *Clin Orthop Relat Res* 2012;470(10):2895-2904.

Credentialing

After the response to the Haiti earthquake in 2010, a survey was distributed to responders, and key responders were interviewed.[25] Most responders arrived in Haiti after the start of the second week. Of the responders, 32 were trained in disaster response, and 96 were untrained. The authors concluded that a robust credentialing process was needed. The authors asserted that the AAOS/OTA should be involved in personnel distribution. They also recommended that nontraumatologists and noncredentialed volunteers should be limited and that volunteers should have disaster experience, predisaster training, and resource self-sufficiency. Local contacts are needed before arrival. Overall, disaster-trained physicians reported less difficulty in transporting equipment and in keeping the equipment secure.

In 2011, the Society of Military Orthopaedic Surgeons, the AAOS, the Pediatric Orthopaedic Society of North America, and the OTA developed a disaster response course to address the concerns about surgeon preparedness for disaster response. They also introduced a credentialing process for orthopaedic surgeons interested in disaster response. This process has continued to gain traction in the effort to optimize disaster response in the field of orthopaedics. Further information regarding courses and certification can be requested by emailing disasterprep@aaos.org. Other sources for information and training include the websites of federal agencies such as the Federal Emergency Management Agency and nongovernmental organizations such as the American Red Cross.

Three levels of orthopaedic disaster responders have been defined, depending on their level of preparation and training. Level I includes surgeons trained in orthopaedic trauma who are prepared for immediate deployment.

Level II represents acute-phase responders prepared for the aftermath of a disaster. Level III includes responders prepared for the reconstruction and maintenance phases. Two pathways for credentialing are available. Civilian surgeons may volunteer through a nongovernmental agency, and temporary government employees may volunteer through a branch of the military such as the Department of Defense or the Department of Health and Human Services. Completion of the Disaster Response Course is required for certification through the AAOS and for entry into the academy volunteer list.

Summary

Disaster response remains a substantial aspect of orthopaedic trauma care. Multiple recent disasters have been reviewed in the literature, identifying areas for potential improvement in telecommunications, patient tracking, credentialing, volunteer databases, prehospital care or first response, and pediatric care. Orthopaedic trauma surgeons and other subspecialists planning to serve on disaster response teams should be aware of the differences between disaster care and routine medical practice and should use the most up-to-date protocols for disaster response to provide optimal care. Because of the inherent nature of disasters, a perfect response to a disaster will never occur; however, preparation, cooperation, communication, and flexibility will serve to limit the extent of the disaster.

Key Study Points

- An effective medical disaster response is dependent on up-to-date preparedness protocols.
- Areas for improvement in the disaster response include communications, education, and sharing of resources.

Annotated References

1. Djalali A, Della Corte F, Foletti M, et al: Art of disaster preparedness in European Union: A survey on the health systems. *PLoS Curr* 2014;6.

   This survey of health system disaster preparedness in the European Union found that areas of weakness included education and training. Preparedness varied widely between nations. The study was limited by its design, surveying three specialists from each country, with a 79% response rate.

2. Hirsch M, Carli P, Nizard R, et al; Health Professionals of Assistance Publique-Hôpitaux de Paris (APHP): The medical response to multisite terrorist attacks in Paris. *Lancet* 2015;386(10012):2535-2538.

   The preliminary review of the Paris terrorist attack of 2015 emphasized early implementation of a disaster/terrorist response plan. On-site triage to multiple hospitals and preparation of providers to treat war-type injuries allowed for effective treatment of more than 300 casualties. Level of evidence: IV.

3. Born CT, Mamczak C, Pagenkopf E, et al: Disaster management response guidelines for departments of orthopaedic surgery. *JBJS Reviews* 2016;4(1):e1.

   The ICS has been adapted to medical disasters to enable a coordinated administration of disaster response through a hierarchy of command. The system is scalable and adaptable.

4. Biddinger PD, Baggish A, Harrington L, et al: Be prepared: The Boston Marathon and mass-casualty events. *N Engl J Med* 2013;368(21):1958-1960.

   Physicians helped EMS personnel distribute 30 critically injured patients efficiently to associated trauma centers during the Boston Marathon bombings. The workflow was improved by expeditiously admitting patients undergoing workup to make room for new patients, holding all pending elective cases, and mobilizing additional operating room staff. Level of evidence: IV.

5. Gates JD, Arabian S, Biddinger P, et al: The initial response to the Boston marathon bombing: Lessons learned to prepare for the next disaster. *Ann Surg* 2014;260(6):960-966.

   The Boston Level I Trauma Center Collaborative reviewed the factors that facilitated an excellent outcome to the Boston Marathon bombings disaster response. Preparation, a rapid logistical response, immediate access to operating rooms, multidisciplinary care, and fortunate circumstance played key roles in the successful response. Level of evidence: V.

6. King DR, Larentzakis A, Ramly EP; Boston Trauma Collaborative: Tourniquet use at the Boston Marathon bombing: Lost in translation. *J Trauma Acute Care Surg* 2015;78(3):594-599.

   Tourniquet use is not a common part of the civilian EMS protocol. During the Boston Marathon bombings, tourniquets were used, but many were improvised. The authors acknowledge that commercial tourniquets have higher success rates and lower morbidity rates than improvised tourniquets, and the commercial tourniquets should be made more widely available. Level of evidence: V.

7. Quillen K, Luckey CJ: Blood and bombs: Blood use after the Boston Marathon bombing of April 15, 2013. *Transfusion* 2014;54(4):1202-1203.

   An increased need for transfusion should be expected at all mass casualty events. To optimize the response, the increased need should be anticipated, and supply chains should be verified. Practice events can help identify weaknesses in the chain. Level of evidence: V.

8. Walls RM, Zinner MJ: The Boston Marathon response: Why did it work so well? *JAMA* 2013;309(23):2441-2442.

   Planning contributed to the successful response to this mass casualty event. In the year leading up to the disaster, 14 hospitals had conducted disaster drills. EMS assignment to the marathon enabled a rapid EMS response, and the fortuitous timing of a change of shift facilitated increased staffing at area hospitals. Level of evidence: IV.

9. The Boston Marathon bombings: A post-event review of the robust emergency response. *ED Manag* 2013;25(7):73-78.

   This review found that the response of inpatient units was critical in helping the emergency department make room for incoming casualties during this mass casualty event in Boston. The establishment of a secure work zone helped limit potential threats. Extra staff that had come in to help required plans and organization to optimize the response. Level of evidence: IV.

10. Boston Trauma Center Chiefs' Collaborative: Boston marathon bombings: An after-action review. *J Trauma Acute Care Surg* 2014;77(3):501-503.

   Of 40 Boston Marathon bombing patients who arrived at a trauma center alive, none died. This success was attributed to the work of individual healthcare workers and the overall coordination of multiple distinct entities, including EMS and individual trauma centers. Preparation played a key role in the successful execution. Level of evidence: IV.

11. Goralnick E, Gates J: We fight like we train. *N Engl J Med* 2013;368(21):1960-1961.

   The Brigham and Women's Hospital had conducted 78 disaster-response activations during the 8 years before the Boston Marathon bombings. This preparation was evident in the presentation of the timeline of treatment of the 39 bombing survivors. Of the total, nine required surgery. Level of evidence: IV.

12. Raja AS, Propper BW, Vandenberg SL, et al: Imaging utilization during explosive multiple casualty incidents. *J Trauma* 2010;68(6):1421-1424.

   This review examined the responses to three mass casualty events managed by the US Air Force Theater Hospital in Iraq between February and April 2008. Fifty patients with Injury Severity Scores greater than 18 were managed, with mortality of 8%. Of the total, 46 patients (92%) underwent imaging procedures, 45 (90%) underwent CT, 35 (70%) underwent radiography, and 19 (38%) received focused abdominal sonography for trauma ultrasound examinations. The authors concluded that increased imaging use should be anticipated during mass casualty events. Level of evidence: III.

13. Kimberly HH, Stone MB: Clinician-performed ultrasonography during the Boston marathon bombing mass casualty incident. *Ann Emerg Med* 2013;62(2):199-200.

   Standard imaging procedures were rapidly overwhelmed in the Boston Marathon event. Bedside ultrasound was used to decompress protocols and facilitate rapid diagnosis. The authors recommended that procedures and protocols be modified to include bedside ultrasound in mass casualty events. Level of evidence: IV.

14. Kragh JF Jr, Littrel ML, Jones JA, et al: Battle casualty survival with emergency tourniquet use to stop limb bleeding. *J Emerg Med* 2011;41(6):590-597.

   A prospective cohort in the battlefield environment demonstrated that prehospital application of tourniquets was associated with increased survival rates (89% versus 78% when applied at the hospital). Tourniquet application before the onset of shock also improved survival (96% versus 4% after the onset of shock). A low rate of tourniquet-related morbidity was observed. Level of evidence: II.

15. Gosselin RA, Gialamas G, Atkin DM: Comparing the cost-effectiveness of short orthopedic missions in elective and relief situations in developing countries. *World J Surg* 2011;35(5):951-955.

   The cost-effectiveness of emergency disaster care in Haiti before and after the earthquake provided by the nongovernmental organization Operation Rainbow was compared with that of its usual elective missions. Despite the emergency nature of the disaster relief, the costs were lower, and thus more cost-effective, in disaster relief as measured in disability-adjusted life-years. Level of evidence: III.

16. Lorich DG, Jeffcoat DM, MacIntyre NR, Chan DB, Helfet DL: The 2010 Haiti earthquake: Lessons learned? *Tech Hand Up Extrem Surg* 2010;14(2):64-68.

   The assessment of available infrastructure is critical in planning a disaster response. Failure to anticipate infrastructure problems can lead to a suboptimal disaster response. Some infrastructure failures may prevent satisfactory responses. Level of evidence: V.

17. Welling DR, Ryan JM, Burris DG, Rich NM: Seven sins of humanitarian medicine. *World J Surg* 2010;34(3):466-470.

   Well-intentioned international humanitarian missions to provide disaster assistance may be marred by a failure to understand local need and the inability to integrate modern technology and procedures. Care provided must maintain ethical standards and take into account sustainability following mission completion. Level of evidence: V.

18. Lebel E, Blumberg N, Gill A, Merin O, Gelfond R, Bar-On E: External fixator frames as interim damage control for limb injuries: Experience in the 2010 Haiti earthquake. *J Trauma* 2011;71(6):E128-E131.

   The experience of the Israeli Defense Forces Field Hospital in Haiti included performing orthopaedic procedures that represented 90%of the surgical procedures performed (221 of 244). The field hospital was not operational until day 4 and was closed after 10 days. Most patients with torso or head injuries already were dead. The number of fractures that were stabilized with an external fixator was 73. The authors concluded that using external fixator frames for bone stabilization and soft-tissue care is a viable approach during a mass casualty scenario. Level of evidence: IV.

19. Bar-On E, Lebel E, Kreiss Y, et al: Orthopaedic management in a mega mass casualty situation: The Israel Defence Forces Field Hospital in Haiti following the January 2010 earthquake. *Injury* 2011;42(10):1053-1059.

 The effect of the Haiti earthquake included a high proportion of musculoskeletal injuries and suboptimal conditions in the field hospital, compounded by a lack of preexisting infrastructure. Potential areas to improve included preplanning two to three operating rooms, adding plastic surgery capabilities, and adding peritoneal dialysis capabilities to treat crush syndrome. Level of evidence: V.

20. Finestone AS, Levy G, Bar-Dayan Y: Telecommunications in Israeli field hospitals deployed to three crisis zones. *Disasters* 2014;38(4):833-845.

 A variety of telecommunication systems should be available during a crisis. These systems should be independent of local infrastructure and should take advantage of a wide variety of radiofrequencies. Mass media should be used when appropriate. Level of evidence: V.

21. Shah AA, Rehman A, Sayyed RH, et al: Impact of a predefined hospital mass casualty response plan in a limited resource setting with no pre-hospital care system. *Injury* 2015;46(1):156-161.

 Modification of a disaster-response system is often necessary. The state of communication networks must be considered in the prehospital assessment. Prehospital care may be inadequate or nonexistent, and triage should be managed at the site. Level of evidence: V.

22. Callaway DW, Peabody CR, Hoffman A, et al: Disaster mobile health technology: Lessons from Haiti. *Prehosp Disaster Med* 2012;27(2):148-152.

 Multiple mobile technologies are available to aid in record keeping. Patient location and identity should be recorded to avoid lost productivity. Providers thought that the mobile technology used in this situation improved the flow of care. Level of evidence: V.

23. Mace SE, Bern AI: Needs assessment: Are Disaster Medical Assistance Teams up for the challenge of a pediatric disaster? *Am J Emerg Med* 2007;25(7):762-769.

24. Walk RM, Donahue TF, Sharpe RP, Safford SD: Three phases of disaster relief in Haiti: Pediatric surgical care on board the United States Naval Ship Comfort. *J Pediatr Surg* 2011;46(10):1978-1984.

 The authors described three phases of response in Haiti: (1) mass casualty response, including triage and the saving of life and limb; (2) subacute response, including optimization of the outcomes of those without life- or limb-threatening conditions; and (3) humanitarian response, including rehabilitation. The discharge of casualties is difficult, especially the discharge of children who are orphaned or whose families cannot be located. Level of evidence: IV.

25. Sonshine DB, Caldwell A, Gosselin RA, Born CT, Coughlin RR: Critically assessing the Haiti earthquake response and the barriers to quality orthopaedic care. *Clin Orthop Relat Res* 2012;470(10):2895-2904.

 The authors conducted a postdisaster survey to determine the barriers to care faced by surgeons during mass casualty disasters. They found that media involvement did not affect patient care, an improved credentialing process was needed, and the AAOS and OTA should be involved in personnel distribution. They also found that nontraumatologists and noncredentialed volunteers should be limited and volunteers should have disaster experience or predisaster training.

Evaluation of the Polytrauma Patient

Greg E. Gaski, MD   Todd O. McKinley, MD

Abstract

Orthopaedic injuries in patients with polytrauma present unique diagnostic and therapeutic challenges. The orthopaedic traumatologist must coordinate with the general surgery trauma team and other consultants to formulate an appropriate, individualized plan of care. Multiply injured patients can follow multiple, often unpredictable, clinical trajectories and continuous reevaluation of the patient's physiology is critical to guiding treatment. There are several advantages and limitations of current trauma scoring systems, in addition to advances in the evaluation of region-specific injuries (head, lung, kidney, liver, spleen). The importance of early control of pelvic-related hemorrhage has been further substantiated. Geriatric patients represent a unique, growing population of trauma patients with increased risks of complications. Substantial strides have been made in the comprehension of postinjury immune dysfunction and this field is on the forefront of trauma research.

Keywords: polytrauma; trauma scoring systems; geriatric trauma; pelvic hemorrhage; postinjury immune dysfunction

Introduction

The appropriate evaluation and treatment of a multiply injured patient depends on the collection and interpretation of a large volume of data in a relatively short time. Care is primarily driven by the general surgery trauma service, but multidisciplinary input from neurosurgery, emergency medicine, anesthesiology, vascular surgery, radiology, and orthopaedic surgery is often vital to ensure prompt prioritization of treatment strategies. Initial care of the multiply injured patient continues to evolve, as does the definition of a patient with polytrauma.[1] Although the anatomically based Injury Severity Score (ISS) is most commonly used to estimate a patient's injury burden, the lack of a uniformly accepted trauma scoring system makes it difficult to compare injury profiles and outcomes across different trauma centers. Endorsed by the American College of Surgeons, the Advanced Trauma Life Support (ATLS) protocol outlines the most widely accepted best-practice guidelines for the initial care of the trauma patient.[2]

Dr. McKinley or an immediate family member serves as a paid consultant to Bioventus. Neither Dr. Gaski nor any immediate family member has received anything of value from or has stock or stock options held in a commercial company or institution related directly or indirectly to the subject of this chapter.

Advanced Trauma Life Support

Since its inception in 1978, the ATLS course has been the most comprehensive training program for the initial assessment and care of the trauma patient. The course is taught in more than 60 countries and the content is commonly regarded as the standard of care for early treatment of the trauma patient.[3] Although initial teaching was rooted in expert opinion, the process of content modification has evolved, and the ninth edition incorporates only evidence-based changes.

The ninth edition of ATLS was published in 2012 and incorporates few content changes from an orthopaedic perspective. The eighth edition of ATLS outlined content changes surrounding pelvic fracture such as advocating external fixation or compression devices (binder or sheet) for pelvic injuries in hemodynamically compromised patients. The indications for angioembolization in hemodynamically unstable patients with pelvic fractures were explored in the seventh edition of ATLS. Although the ninth edition does not embrace substantial alteration in the treatment of patients with pelvic injuries, recognizing the potential for exsanguination in this population is emphasized.

The concept of balanced resuscitation has replaced aggressive resuscitation in the setting of uncontrolled hemorrhage and promotes early administration of platelets and plasma in patients requiring massive transfusion and less crystalloid solution (1 L versus 2 L).[3] Controversy persists regarding the ideal ratio of fluid to blood product administration, but a trend toward the avoidance of early aggressive crystalloid hemodilution remains in favor of more judicious use of packed red blood cells, fresh frozen plasma, and platelets.

Measuring Injury

Current trauma scoring systems fall into three categories: anatomic, physiologic, and combined anatomic and physiologic. Originally described to classify injury severity among different institutions for research, generalized outcomes, and triage, many are now used for treatment strategies, quality improvement, and specific outcome prediction. Each scoring system has unique advantages and limitations. An ideal scoring system would encompass anatomic injury, physiologic insult, and patient-specific characteristics with reproducible methods and accurate prediction of clinical trajectory and outcome.[4]

Anatomic Injury Scoring Systems

The Abbreviated Injury Severity (AIS) score was described in 1971 and has undergone multiple revisions. The most recent AIS-90 has more than 1,300 injuries and categorizes nine body regions (head, face, neck, thorax, abdomen, spine, upper extremity, lower extremity, and external) with an increasing severity index score (1, minor; 2, moderate; 3, serious; 4, severe; 5, critical; 6, unsurvivable). The AIS score alone is not designed to predict outcome, but provides the foundation for other anatomic scoring systems such as the ISS.

The ISS, developed in 1974, is calculated by squaring the worst AIS score in each respective region (consolidated into six regions: head/neck, face, chest, abdomen, extremities including pelvis, external) and summing the three highest scores.[5] Higher ISS scores are correlated with an increased risk of mortality and longer hospital stays. Although the ISS is the most frequently reported measure of trauma severity, its ubiquitous use has many criticisms. The ISS typically is not calculated at the time of injury and often is tabulated after discharge, thus limiting its patient-specific predictive capacity on admission. The ISS accounts for the physiologic insult and individualized resuscitation response of the patient. In addition, by only integrating one injury per region into the overall score, it dilutes severe injuries in the same area (such as bilateral hemopneumothoraces and thoracic aortic transection) in favor of incorporating minor remote injuries (such as metatarsal fracture). The ISS can also underestimate the severity of injury in patients with multiply injured extremities. In a combat setting, the ISS diminished the severity of upper extremity amputations with respect to intensive care unit (ICU) length of stay, blood product requirements, and resource utilization.[6]

The New Injury Severity Score (NISS) was proposed to eliminate the regional bias of the ISS by squaring the three worst AIS scores and summing them irrespective of bodily region.[7] The NISS has been found to be a better predictor of postinjury length of stay and ICU admission than ISS, especially in patients with multiple orthopaedic injuries.[8] The NISS is also based on the AIS, and is thus subjected to similar criticisms as the ISS.

The Trauma Mortality Prediction Model (TMPM) was recently described to supplant the ISS and the NISS and showed improved discrimination and calibration in predicting mortality to previous models.[9,10] TMPM is based on the AIS lexicon and the International Classification of Diseases, Ninth Edition (ICD-9), and although enhanced mortality prediction is offered over current anatomic scoring systems, it also lacks incorporation of physiologic components of injury.

Physiologic Injury Scoring Systems

The Revised Trauma Score (RTS) was drafted in 1981 and subsequently revised in 1989 to assimilate three measures of physiologic derangement: Glasgow Coma Scale (GCS), systolic blood pressure, and respiratory rate.[11] Each category is scored 0 (most severe) through 4 (normal) and summed to yield an overall RTS. When used for triage purposes, an RTS of 11 or less identified 97% of patients requiring trauma center care.[11,12] Overall, the RTS has not been well validated in the prediction of outcome or mortality, although improved RTS accuracy in predicting survival has been reported with the use of complex statistical modeling (fractional polynomial models).[13]

The reported limitations of the RTS are related to its weighting of GCS scores. Intubated patients (for neurologic injury and/or other physiologic reasons) and those who are obtunded (drugs, alcohol) present challenges in accurately assessing neurologic response. In addition, the RTS is a static representation of the injury at random times, although polytrauma patients typically exhibit dynamic fluctuation of vital signs (heart rate, blood pressure, respiratory rate) and consciousness, depending on the volume of insult over time, resuscitation, and medications administered.

The Acute Physiology and Chronic Health Evaluation (APACHE), described in the early 1980s, has undergone three revisions (APACHE II in 1985, APACHE III in 1991, and APACHE IV in 2006).[14] The APACHE II is the physiologic scoring system most frequently used in

ICUs to assess the severity of disease within 24 hours of admission (using a scale of 0 to 71). The APACHE II is based on age, chronic health status, and 12 physiologic measurements (FiO_2/PaO_2, temperature, mean arterial pressure, pH, heart rate, respiratory rate, sodium, potassium, creatinine, hematocrit, white blood cell count, and GCS). Although not specifically designed for use in a trauma population, APACHE II has been used in this population to predict mortality and guide treatment.[15] APACHE III and IV offer refined variables and more complex statistical computation, thus limiting its usefulness. Resuscitation and treatment before ICU admission and data acquisition can undervalue the severity of injury. As with the RTS, the APACHE II has no anatomic component, and one study concluded it was invalid in an otherwise healthy trauma population because of its lack of injury magnitude quantification.[16]

Combined Injury Scoring Systems

To improve the predictive capacity of trauma scoring for survival probability and outcomes research, the Trauma and Injury Severity Score (TRISS) was devised.[17] The TRISS integrates age, mechanism of injury, an anatomic measure of injury (ISS), and a physiologic component (RTS) to calculate the probability of survival (P_s) by using the equation $P_s = 1 / 1+e^{-b}$, where b = b0 + b1 (RTS) + b2 (ISS) + b3 (age index).[17,18] This formula has become the most commonly used tool in evaluating trauma outcomes, mortality rates, and hospital performance evaluation.[19] Although several recent studies consider the TRISS an effective means of comparing outcomes and predicting survival, the studies also question its accuracy and recommend refinement and/or replacement by other prediction models.[19,20] The shortcomings of TRISS are well characterized, including utilization of outdated coefficients leading to inaccurate modeling, lack of incorporation of a patient's comorbidities, and the inherent inadequacies of the ISS and RTS.[20]

A Severity Characterization of Trauma (ASCOT) was proposed as an improvement over TRISS in the early 1990s. It encompasses physiologic (RTS) and anatomic (Anatomic Profile) variables but has shown minimal to no benefit over TRISS with a more complex score derivation, thus limiting its acceptance.

No current globally accepted trauma scoring system exists. As the comprehension of the complex immunology and pathophysiology of trauma improves, future instruments to estimate patient-specific injury burden will be proposed. Literature reviews emphasize the importance of incorporating anatomic quantification of mechanical tissue injury, physiologic insult and response to ischemic tissue injury, immunologic reaction, genetic predisposition, and other patient-specific variables such as age and comorbidities into future prediction models.[4,20]

Region-Specific Injury in Polytrauma and Orthopaedic Implications

A paradigm shift has occurred over the past four decades in the evaluation and treatment of patients with polytrauma including pelvic and long bone fractures. Early total care was undertaken in the 1970s and 1980s. In the 1990s and early 2000s, the term "damage control orthopaedics" was introduced and studies demonstrated an improved survival in severely injured and underresuscitated patients initially treated with external fixation of femoral fractures in contrast to primary intramedullary nailing.[21,22] More recently, early appropriate care has been advocated and refers to preferential definitive fixation of femur fractures when feasible, immobilization of other long bone injuries, and attention given to appropriate resuscitation.[23] Although somewhat controversial, literature supports early definitive fixation in stable resuscitated polytrauma patients, damage control measures in physiologically unstable patients, and consideration of early definitive femur fixation in resuscitated borderline patients.[24,25]

Head Injury

The evaluation of and the timing of treatment in patients with head injuries and concomitant orthopaedic injuries continues to be debated. The high mortality rate in multiply injured patients with a traumatic brain injury (TBI) is attributed not only to the initial mechanical force, but also to secondary insults to the injured brain.[26] Secondary injury is a result of systemic inflammation, hypoxia, acidosis, fat embolization from a fracture site, and coagulopathy.[27] Evaluation of neurologic status using the GCS is an important consideration in planning orthopaedic intervention. A review of current literature endorsed the following principles outlined in **Table 1** in patients with head injuries and femur fractures.[28]

Ongoing research is focused on minimizing the second inflammatory insult in TBI. Remote ischemic conditioning is a process by which normal tissue (such as in the arm) is subjected to short cycles of ischemia and reperfusion.[29] Systemic anti-inflammatory mediators are released in response to the remote site of ischemic injury (such as in the arm) and potentially negate pathologic inflammation in the region of interest (in the brain). A prospective comparative study of patients with TBI (GCS up to 8) demonstrated decreased levels of biomarkers of brain injury (S-100B and neuron-specific enolase) at 6 and 24 hours in the remote ischemic conditioning group (four

Table 1

Treatment Recommendations in Patients With Head Injuries and Femur Fractures

TBI	GCS	CT Scan/Physiology	Treatment Principle
Mild	14–15	Normal CT	Early total care
Moderate	9–13	Minor intracranial pathology (small SAH)	Consider damage control measures
Severe	<9 or	Significant intracranial pathology (edema, midline shift, sub-/epidural bleeding)	Damage control
Moderate/ Severe	>11 or	Stable intracranial pressure (<20 mmHg) and cerebral perfusion pressure (>80 mmHg) for >48 hours	Conversion from external to internal fixation

TBI, traumatic brain injury; GCS, Glasgow Coma Scale; CT, computed tomography; SAH, subarachnoid hemorrhage; ICP, intracranial pressure; CPP, cerebral perfusion pressure.

Data from Flierl MA, Stoneback JW, Beauchamp KM, et al: Femur shaft fracture fixation in head-injured patients: When is the right time? *J Orthop Trauma* 2010;24(2):107-114.

Table 2

Acute Respiratory Distress Syndrome: The Berlin Definition

	Acute Respiratory Distress Syndrome	
Timing	Within 1 week of insult or worsening symptoms	
Chest Imaging	Bilateral opacities (not explained by effusions, lung collapse, or nodules)	
Origin of Edema	Respiratory failure not explained by cardiac failure or fluid overload	
Oxygenation	**PaO_2/FiO_2**	**PEEP**
Mild	200–300 mm Hg	≥5 cm H20 (or CPAP)
Moderate	100–200 mm Hg	≥5 cm H20
Severe	≤100 mm Hg	≥5 cm H20

PaO_2, partial pressure of arterial oxygen; FiO_2, fraction of inspired oxygen; PEEP, positive end-expiratory pressure; CPAP, continuous positive airway pressure.

Data from Ranieri VM, Rubenfeld GD, Thompson BT, et al; ARDS Definition Task Force: Acute respiratory distress syndrome: The Berlin Definition. *JAMA* 2012;307(23):2526-2533.

cycles of blood pressure cuff elevation on the arm for 5 minutes) compared with the control group.

Lung Injury

The timing of definitive fixation of femur fractures in trauma patients with lung injuries has been extensively studied over the past two decades. Although some studies have reported higher complication rates in patients with lung injuries when early definitive femoral fixation strategies were used, other investigations have showed no difference in outcome with early total care.[22,25,30] One study demonstrated a lower incidence of acute respiratory distress syndrome (ARDS) than historically reported (2% versus more than 25%) and endorsed primary intramedullary nail fixation of femur fractures in multiply injured patients who respond to resuscitation.[30]

The wide spectrum of acute lung injury and subjectivity encompassing the diagnosis of posttraumatic ARDS compounds the debate on femoral fixation. Since the American-European Consensus Conference defined ARDS in 1994, issues regarding the diagnostic reliability and validity of ARDS have arisen.[31] A refined Berlin Definition has recently been drafted by an international panel, the ARDS Definition Task Force. The revised definition describes inclusive criteria and different degrees of ARDS: timing within 1 week of an insult; bilateral opacities on chest imaging not explained by effusions, nodules, or lung collapse; respiratory failure not explained by cardiac failure or fluid overload (echocardiogram to exclude cardiogenic etiology when necessary); and hypoxemia (**Table 2**). Compared with the American-European Consensus Conference definition, the Berlin definition had improved predictive validity for mortality.

As research continues to refine the definition of post-traumatic lung injury, the rationale for the optimal timing of osseous stabilization using a patient-centered approach will become more transparent. The Eastern Association for the Surgery of Trauma recently published practice management guidelines on the specific injury pattern of pulmonary contusion and flail chest,[32] which is recognized as a complex injury pattern with little improvement in morbidity and mortality over the past three decades. No benefit was reported for fluid restriction, and the use of mechanical ventilation in the absence of respiratory failure was cautioned against.

Kidney Dysfunction

When considering fracture stabilization in patients with polytrauma, consideration of renal dysfunction is vital to avoid secondary insults. Hemorrhagic shock and global hypoperfusion are implicated in the development of acute kidney injury (creatinine > 1.8), which has been found to be a driving factor in the development of multiple organ failure (MOF).[33] Although a patient can be hemodynamically stable and cleared for the orthopaedic stabilization of open lower extremity fractures, the volume of insult resulting from blood loss (ischemia and reperfusion) must be considered to prevent further deterioration of renal function. Early acute kidney injury (by day 2) is associated with a 78% incidence of MOF and a 27% incidence of mortality.

Hepatic and Splenic Injury

The Eastern Association for the Surgery of Trauma practice management guidelines of hepatic and splenic injuries provide historical background pertaining to the current trend toward nonsurgical management when feasible and summarize the best available evidence for treatment.[34,35] Nonsurgical management of blunt hepatic and splenic injuries is advocated in hemodynamically stable patients, irrespective of injury grade. Peritonitis and hemodynamic compromise are indications for laparotomy, and angiography is an adjunct imaging tool in select hepatic and splenic injuries. Clinical status is closely monitored for nonsurgical management by means of serial abdominal examination and serial hematocrit tests. Nonurgent orthopaedic interventions with the potential for high-volume blood loss should be avoided in this patient population, especially in those with higher grade injuries.

Pelvic Vascular Injury

Pelvic ring injuries are associated with uncontrolled hemorrhage, potentially leading to hemodynamic instability, shock, and death. Advances have been made in hemorrhage control with these injuries.

A contrast blush seen on a CT angiogram indicates bleeding related to pelvic fracture and has been shown to have 90% sensitivity.[36] Diagnosis is more definitively made by using visualization of contrast extravasation during pelvic angiography. Delayed diagnosis and management of pelvic exsanguination has life-threatening consequences and was found to be the most common cause of preventable hemorrhagic death in a trauma population.[37]

Rapid identification of the patients at highest risk of pelvic bleeding and subsequent hemodynamic compromise is of great interest to the treating clinician. The initial evaluation of a patient with polytrauma is fairly uniform, as outlined by recommendations set forth by ATLS. Evaluation begins with the primary survey (airway, breathing, circulation, disability, exposure), followed by laboratory testing to measure hypoperfusion (base deficit, pH, lactate), and electrolyte and serum abnormalities. Simultaneous imaging, such as the Focused Assessment with Sonography in Trauma (FAST) scan is performed to identify regional injury. Hemodynamically unstable patients with positive FAST scans are typically moved to the operating room for laparotomy before or after undergoing CT. Algorithms for the management of hemodynamically unstable patients in the absence of obviously mangled limbs or intraperitoneal or thoracic injury seen on FAST or CT vary by institution.

Base deficit, frequently used as a measure of metabolic derangement, is defined as the amount of strong base required per liter of fully oxygenated blood to restore pH to 7.40. Physiologic measurements such as base deficit up to 6, decrease in base deficit greater than 2, systolic blood pressure less than 104 mm Hg, and the need for transfusion are risk factors for arterial bleeding related to pelvic fracture, especially in the absence of major abdominal, chest, or extremity hemorrhage.[38] Although it seems intuitive that earlier diagnosis and control of pelvic bleeding can result in better outcomes, it was not well described until 2014[39]: 191 patients with pelvic fracture who required transfusion and met the indications for interventional radiology evaluation were studied. Compared with patients who presented during the day (n = 45), patients who presented at night (n = 146) experienced profound delays in interventional radiology treatment (3 hours from admission versus 5 hours), and a 100% increase in mortality after controlling for age and injury severity.

The lifesaving benefits of angioembolization outweigh potential side effects, but subsequent decision-making should account for its ischemic effect. A risk of infection greater than tenfold was characterized for patients undergoing acetabular open reduction and internal fixation after pelvic arterial embolization.[40] As with other reports, selective arterial embolization was advocated for instead of occlusion of the entire internal iliac artery when possible to avoid potential infection and wound complications.

Spine Fractures

No consensus exists on the chronology of spine stabilization in patients with polytrauma. Proponents of delayed fixation cite a higher risk of infectious complications and potential aggravation of pulmonary dysfunction in critically ill patients in the ICU. Advocates of early spine fixation contend that earlier mobilization can prevent secondary complications such as pressure sores, deep vein thrombosis, and hospital-acquired infection. A review of the German Trauma Registry concluded that fixation of unstable spinal column injuries in less than 72 hours can result in shorter hospital stays and a lower incidence of complications in patients who are medically suitable.[41] Prolonging the time to spine stabilization often delays other definitive orthopaedic interventions and can preclude lateral, beach chair, or prone positioning, and thus require a multidisciplinary approach to provide optimal care.

Geriatric Trauma

Elderly patients with multiple traumatic injuries have higher mortality rates and an increased risk of complications compared with a younger population.[42] Geriatric trauma patients are often undertriaged and studies have demonstrated lower mortality rates and fewer adverse events when treated at designated trauma centers.[43,44] The Eastern Association for the Surgery of Trauma published practice management guidelines in 2012 to address several questions: lower thresholds should be used for trauma activation in patients 65 years or older, including an AIS score of 3 or higher in one body region or a base deficit of −6 or less; patients undergoing therapeutic anticoagulation should undergo international normalized ratio reversal to 1.6 or as soon as possible (ideally within 2 hours), especially in those whose head CT shows evidence of intracranial hemorrhage; patients with a GCS score less than 8 after 72 hours should be considered for limited further aggressive care because of high mortality rates.[45]

The long-term survival of geriatric trauma patients was examined and an early (within 5 days) mortality rate of 33% was reported.[46] Patients who survived hospitalization had a median survival of 3 years (with a severe head injury) to 4 years (with minimal or no head injury). The 5-year survival rate was 20%, which is comparable to the prognosis for many types of cancer. As epidemiologic data and the natural history of this disease entity become clear, questions remain not only regarding initial treatment regimens, but also the location of treatment. Data extracted from the National Trauma Data Bank showed that geriatric trauma patients had 34% lower mortality if they presented to a trauma center that typically manages a higher volume of elderly patients.[47] The study questioned whether dedicated geriatric trauma centers can provide clinical benefit.

Immunologic Dysfunction

Although a detailed synopsis of the pathophysiology of trauma is beyond the scope of this chapter, considerable advances have been made in the past decade toward understanding trauma on a molecular basis. On the forefront of current research endeavors is the topic of immune dysregulation in trauma. Inflammatory cytokines, chemokines, free radicals, and damage-associated molecular patterns drive the host inflammatory response. An exaggerated inflammatory response can result in the systemic inflammatory response syndrome and subsequent MOF. It is unknown why some patients with similar demographics, injury profiles, and severity recover uneventfully and others experience complicated clinical trajectories. A new syndrome, persistent inflammation, immunosuppression, and catabolism syndrome, has been described as the predominant phenotype in patients requiring extended stays (longer than 10 days) in the ICU.[48,49]

The investigation of the magnitude and chronicity of inflammatory biomarkers following trauma could help predict clinical trajectory and outcomes. A case-control study of trauma patients with similarly matched injury profiles and demographics reported specific magnitude and temporal differences in biomarker patterns among patients who acquired nosocomial infection compared with those who did not.[50]

Multiple Organ Failure

Trauma is the leading cause of death for people younger than 45 years.[51] The most common cause of death for patients who survive the initial traumatic insult is MOF.[52,53] The incidence of MOF has decreased over the past 15 years, but MOF-related complications, ICU length of stay, and mortality have remained relatively constant.[53,54] As polytrauma research focuses on injury patterns and therapeutic interventions, the importance of applying standardized outcome instruments increases. In addition to reporting demographics and mortality, the

Table 3

Denver MOF Score and SOFA Score

Denver MOF Score

Organ System	Measure of dysfunction	Grade 0	Grade 1	Grade 2	Grade 3
Cardiac	Inotrope support*	None	Minimal	Moderate	High
Pulmonary	PaO_2/FIO_2 ratio (mmHg)	>250	200–250	100–199	<100
Hepatic	Bilirubin (mg/dL)	<1.0	1.0-4.0	4.1–8.0	>8.0
Renal	Creatinine (mg/dL)	<1.8	1.8–2.5	2.6–5.0	>5.0

SOFA Score

Organ System	Measure of dysfunction	Grade 0	Grade 1	Grade 2	Grade 3	Grade 4
Cardiovascular	MAP or vasopressors	None	MAP < 70 mmHg	Dopamine ≤ 5 or dobutamine (any dose)	Dopamine > 5 or epinephrine ≤ 0.1 or norepinephrine ≤ 0.1	Dopamine > 15 or epinephrine > 0.1 or norepinephrine > 0.1
Respiratory	PaO_2/FIO_2 ratio (mmHg)	>400	301–400	201–300	101–200 (with respiratory support)	≤ 100 (with respiratory support)
Hepatic	Bilirubin (mg/dL)	<1.2	1.2–1.9	2.0–5.9	6.0–11.9	≥12.0
Renal	Creatinine (mg/dL)	<1.2	1.2–1.9	2.0–3.4	3.5–4.9	≥5.0
Hematologic	Platelets x $10^3/\mu L$	>150	101–150	51–100	21–50	≤20
Neurologic	Glasgow Coma Scale	15	13–14	10–12	6–9	≤5

Greater scores are indicative of increasing organ dysfunction; MOF is defined as a score of ≥4 with involvement of two or more organ systems; inotrope support definitions: minimal = one agent at a small dose; moderate = any agent at a moderate dose or more than one at a small dose; high = any agent at large dose or more than two at moderate doses.

MAP, mean arterial pressure; MOF, multiple organ failure; SOFA, Sequential Organ Functional Assessment; MAP, mean arterial pressure; PaO_2, partial pressure of arterial oxygen; FiO_2, fraction of inspired oxygen.

Data from Antonelli M, Moreno R, Vincent JL, et al: Application of SOFA score to trauma patients. Sequential Organ Failure Assessment. *Intensive Care Med* 1999;25(4):389-394 and Sauaia A, Moore EE, Johnson JL, Ciesla DJ, Biffl WL, Banerjee A: Validation of postinjury multiple organ failure scores. *Shock* 2009;31(5):438-447.

application of validated outcome measures is encouraged. Currently, the Denver MOF score and the Sequential Organ Failure Assessment score, detailed in **Table 3**, are the most frequently used instruments to assess organ dysfunction and both have been validated in a trauma population.[55,56]

Summary

The evaluation and treatment of multiply injured patients requires a coordinated, multidisciplinary approach. Even with the development of several trauma scoring systems over the past four decades using anatomic regions of injury and physiologic variables, the ISS is the most commonly used system. Although the shortcomings of the ISS are well known, it is easy to use. Investigative capacity exists to refine current scoring instruments or to develop novel patient-specific measures that accurately represent mechanical tissue injury, ischemic insult, and patient reserve.

Patients with head injury or severe chest injury represent specific populations in which temporizing versus definitive orthopaedic treatment should be determined by the severity of region-specific injury and resuscitation parameters. Improved comprehension of posttraumatic immunologic dysregulation could result in the discovery of biomarkers that better predict the clinical trajectory of critically injured patients. Geriatric trauma patients are often undertriaged and display substantially higher rates of morbidity and mortality than patients younger than 65 years.

Key Study Points

- The evaluation and ongoing care of multiply injured patients requires a multidisciplinary approach, close coordination with the general surgery trauma team, and continuous reassessment of evolving pathophysiology.
- Current trauma scoring systems provide outcome analyses but are limited in their prospective ability to guide treatment decisions.
- The assessment of resuscitation in patients with polytrauma is critical in planning definitive, staged orthopaedic interventions.
- The management of long bone fractures and injuries to the axial skeleton in patients with head injuries requires coordination with neurosurgery and ongoing assessment of GCS and intracranial pressure.
- Substantial advances have been achieved in postinjury immunologic dysfunction. A better understanding of immune dysregulation after injury could allow improved stratification of clinical trajectories.

Annotated References

1. Pape HC, Lefering R, Butcher N, et al: The definition of polytrauma revisited: An international consensus process and proposal of the new 'Berlin definition'. *J Trauma Acute Care Surg* 2014;77(5):780-786.

   This expert panel in Germany was convened to develop a uniform definition of the term "polytrauma." Based on an extensive literature review, the panel defined polytrauma patients with a predicted mortality of greater than 30% by an ISS greater than 15, AIS *greater than*3 in at least two body regions, and any one of the following: hypotension (systolic blood pressure < 90 mm Hg), unconsciousness (GCS ≤ 8), acidosis (base excess ≤ -6), coagulopathy (partial thromboblastin time ≥ 40 seconds or international normalized ratio ≥ 1.4), and age *older than* 70 years.

2. Committee on Trauma: *American College of Surgeons. Advanced Trauma Life Support (ATLS)*, ed 9. Chicago, IL, Student Course Manual, 2012.

   Updated approximately every four years, the ninth edition of ATLS continues to rely on evidence to support changes in ATLS content. Balanced resuscitation principles are outlined and there is a heightened emphasis placed on potential exsanguination from pelvic injuries.

3. The ATLS Subcommittee: American College of Surgeons' Committee on Trauma, and the International ATLS working group: Advanced trauma life support (ATLS): The ninth edition. *J Trauma Acute Care Surg* 2013;74(5):1363-1366

   This special report summarizes the content and format changes in the ninth edition of ATLS. The concept of balanced resuscitation is described and levels of evidence are provided for content changes.

4. Chawda MN, Hildebrand F, Pape HC, Giannoudis PV: Predicting outcome after multiple trauma: Which scoring system? *Injury* 2004;35(4):347-358.

5. Baker SP, O'Neill B, Haddon W Jr, Long WB: The injury severity score: A method for describing patients with multiple injuries and evaluating emergency care. *J Trauma* 1974;14(3):187-196.

6. Shin E, Evans KN, Fleming ME: Injury severity score underpredicts injury severity and resource utilization in combat-related amputations. *J Orthop Trauma* 2013;27(7):419-423.

   This study reviewed 109 amputations from 2007 to 2010 in the Combat Trauma Registry. This population is much more likely to undergo another extremity amputation, has increased hospital length of stay, blood product requirements, and overall worse burden of injury than what would be predicted using ISS or NISS. Severe combat-related injury resource use cannot be extrapolated by using current scoring systems, and the group proposed development of a more specific military-based ISS. Level of evidence: II.

7. Osler T, Baker SP, Long W: A modification of the injury severity score that both improves accuracy and simplifies scoring. *J Trauma* 1997;43(6):922-925, discussion 925-926.

8. Balogh ZJ, Varga E, Tomka J, Süveges G, Tóth L, Simonka JA: The new injury severity score is a better predictor of extended hospitalization and intensive care unit admission than the injury severity score in patients with multiple orthopaedic injuries. *J Orthop Trauma* 2003;17(7):508-512.

This prospective cohort study of 3,100 patients reported that the NISS had improved predictive capacity over ISS in estimating patient length of stay and ICU admission. Multiple orthopaedic injuries are underrepresented with the regional restrictions of the ISS and the NISS better characterizes outcomes in this population.

9. Cook A, Weddle J, Baker S, et al: A comparison of the Injury Severity Score and the Trauma Mortality Prediction Model. *J Trauma Acute Care Surg* 2014;76(1):47-52, discussion 52-53.

This diagnostic study evaluated over 337,000 patients from the National Trauma Data Bank to determine the best scoring system in mortality prediction. The TMPM demonstrated superior performance to the ISS, NISS, and ICD-9-Based ISS for mortality prediction. The TMPM inputs data from ICD-9 or AIS-based lexicons to calculate prediction models. Level of evidence: I.

10. Haider AH, Villegas CV, Saleem T, et al: Should the IDC-9 Trauma Mortality Prediction Model become the new paradigm for benchmarking trauma outcomes? *J Trauma Acute Care Surg* 2012;72(6):1695-1701.

This prognostic study retrospectively examined mortality prediction in three scoring systems for more than 533,000 patients in the National Trauma Data Bank. The TMPM based on ICD-9 diagnoses outperformed the ISS and NISS in predicting mortality for all injury severity ranges. TMPM has the potential to become the benchmark for trauma outcomes. Level of evidence: III.

11. Champion HR, Sacco WJ, Carnazzo AJ, Copes W, Fouty WJ: Trauma score. *Crit Care Med* 1981;9(9):672-676.

12. Champion HR, Sacco WJ, Copes WS, Gann DS, Gennarelli TA, Flanagan ME: A revision of the Trauma Score. *J Trauma* 1989;29(5):623-629.

13. Moore L, Lavoie A, LeSage N, et al: Statistical validation of the Revised Trauma Score. *J Trauma* 2006;60(2):305-311.

14. Knaus WA, Zimmerman JE, Wagner DP, Draper EA, Lawrence DE: APACHE-acute physiology and chronic health evaluation: A physiologically based classification system. *Crit Care Med* 1981;9(8):591-597.

15. Beck DH, Taylor BL, Millar B, Smith GB: Prediction of outcome from intensive care: A prospective cohort study comparing Acute Physiology and Chronic Health Evaluation II and III prognostic systems in a United Kingdom intensive care unit. *Crit Care Med* 1997;25(1):9-15.

16. McAnena OJ, Moore FA, Moore EE, Mattox KL, Marx JA, Pepe P: Invalidation of the APACHE II scoring system for patients with acute trauma. *J Trauma* 1992;33(4):504-506, discussion 506-507.

17. Champion HR, Sacco WJ, Hunt TK: Trauma severity scoring to predict mortality. *World J Surg* 1983;7(1):4-11.

18. Boyd CR, Tolson MA, Copes WS: Evaluating trauma care: The TRISS method. Trauma Score and the Injury Severity Score. *J Trauma* 1987;27(4):370-378.

19. Schluter PJ: The Trauma and Injury Severity Score (TRISS) revised. *Injury* 2011;42(1):90-96.

Almost 900,000 patients with all TRISS variables in the New Zealand National Trauma Data Bank were reviewed (97% had blunt trauma). With redefined variables and improved statistical computation, the authors recommended replacing current TRISS models with the proposed TRISS computational software.

20. Rogers FB, Osler T, Krasne M, et al: Has TRISS become an anachronism? A comparison of mortality between the National Trauma Data Bank and Major Trauma Outcome Study databases. *J Trauma Acute Care Surg* 2012;73(2):326-331, discussion 331.

This study suggests that the current form of TRISS is inaccurate because its survival predictions are based on coefficients derived from data from the 1980s and updated once in the early 1990s. The authors suggested replacing TRISS with a modern statistical trauma prediction model as more productive than updating TRISS. Level of evidence: II.

21. Rotondo MF, Schwab CW, McGonigal MD, et al: 'Damage control': An approach for improved survival in exsanguinating penetrating abdominal injury. *J Trauma* 1993;35(3):375-382, discussion 382-383.

22. Scalea TM, Boswell SA, Scott JD, Mitchell KA, Kramer ME, Pollak AN: External fixation as a bridge to intramedullary nailing for patients with multiple injuries and with femur fractures: Damage control orthopedics. *J Trauma* 2000;48(4):613-621, discussion 621-623.

23. Nahm NJ, Como JJ, Wilber JH, Vallier HA: Early appropriate care: Definitive stabilization of femoral fractures within 24 hours of injury is safe in most patients with multiple injuries. *J Trauma* 2011;71(1):175-185.

Early (less than 24 hours) versus delayed (longer than 24 hours) stabilization of 750 patients with femur fractures was retrospectively reviewed; 492 patients had an ISS of 18 or higher. Lower complication rates (pneumonia, ARDS, DVT, PE, ARF, sepsis, MOF, infection, death) were reported with early definitive stabilization of femur fractures ($n = 408$) than in those with delayed fixation ($n = 84$). Severe abdominal injury (AIS ≥ 3) was the strongest predictor of complications irrespective of the timing of surgery, followed by head injury (GCS ≤ 8) and chest injury (AIS ≥ 3). However, patients receiving delayed fixation were older (44 versus 35 years) and had a higher mean ISS (37 versus 29). After adjusting for age and ISS, a higher complication rate was reported in those undergoing delayed fixation. ISS may not be an accurate representation of actual injury severity, especially in those with an ISS greater than 16.

24. D'Alleyrand JC, O'Toole RV: The evolution of damage control orthopedics: Current evidence and practical

applications of early appropriate care. *Orthop Clin North Am* 2013;44(4):499-507.

This review chronicles the evolution of early total care to damage control orthopaedics to early appropriate care with an evidence-based discussion. Practical applications of treatment are emphasized with special considerations noted in borderline patients and an emphasis on appropriate resuscitation before definitive management.

25. Pape HC, Hildebrand F, Pertschy S, et al: Changes in the management of femoral shaft fractures in polytrauma patients: From early total care to damage control orthopedic surgery. *J Trauma* 2002;53(3):452-461, discussion 461-462.

26. Bayir H, Clark RS, Kochanek PM: Promising strategies to minimize secondary brain injury after head trauma. *Crit Care Med* 2003;31(1suppl):S112-S117.

    In this review of 83 studies on the treatment of TBI, the high mortality rate in multiply injured patients with a TBI is attributed not only to the initial mechanical force, but also to secondary insults to the injured brain. The pathophysiology of secondary brain damage is described, including ischemia, neuronal death cascades, cerebral swelling, and inflammation. Current treatment protocols are summarized.

27. Jeremitsky E, Omert L, Dunham CM, Protetch J, Rodriguez A: Harbingers of poor outcome the day after severe brain injury: Hypothermia, hypoxia, and hypoperfusion. *J Trauma* 2003;54(2):312-319.

28. Flierl MA, Stoneback JW, Beauchamp KM, et al: Femur shaft fracture fixation in head-injured patients: When is the right time? *J Orthop Trauma* 2010;24(2):107-114.

    The authors of this study reviewed the best available literature on the pathophysiology of TBI with the effect of orthopaedic injury and subsequent surgery.

29. Joseph B, Pandit V, Zangbar B, et al: Secondary brain injury in trauma patients: The effects of remote ischemic conditioning. *J Trauma Acute Care Surg* 2015;78(4):698-703, discussion 703-705.

    This prospective, comparative study of 40 patients reported on the management of TBI, focusing on the prevention of secondary brain insults. Level of evidence: III.

30. O'Toole RV, O'Brien M, Scalea TM, Habashi N, Pollak AN, Turen CH: Resuscitation before stabilization of femoral fractures limits acute respiratory distress syndrome in patients with multiple traumatic injuries despite low use of damage control orthopedics. *J Trauma* 2009;67(5):1013-1021.

31. Ranieri VM, Rubenfeld GD, Thompson BT, et al; ARDS Definition Task Force: Acute respiratory distress syndrome: The Berlin Definition. *JAMA* 2012;307(23):2526-2533.

    The ARDS Definition Task Force proposed a revised definition of ARDS that describes inclusive criteria and different degrees of ARDS. When compared with the American-European Consensus Conference definition in 1994, the Berlin definition had improved predictive validity for mortality.

32. Simon B, Ebert J, Bokhari F, et al; Eastern Association for the Surgery of Trauma: Management of pulmonary contusion and flail chest: An Eastern Association for the Surgery of Trauma practice management guideline. *J Trauma Acute Care Surg* 2012;73(5suppl 4):S351-S361.

    In this review of 129 articles, six level 2 and eight level 3 recommendations were made. Important recommendations include: patients with this injury complex should not be excessively fluid restricted but should be resuscitated to adequate levels of tissue perfusion; obligatory mechanical ventilation in the absence of respiratory failure is not indicated; epidural catheter is the preferred mode of analgesia in severe flail chest; high frequency oscillatory ventilation should be considered for patients failing conventional ventilatory modes; surgical fixation of flail chest may be considered in severe flail chest in patients that fail to wean from the ventilator; and steroids should not be used for pulmonary contusion.

33. Wohlauer MV, Sauaia A, Moore EE, Burlew CC, Banerjee A, Johnson J: Acute kidney injury and posttrauma multiple organ failure: The canary in the coal mine. *J Trauma Acute Care Surg* 2012;72(2):373-378, discussion 379-380.

    Over 17 years, 2,157 severely injured patients from a database were reviewed (ISS > 15 for those who survived 48 hours); the incidence of early acute kidney injury (creatinine > 1.8 on day 2) was found to be 2%. Early acute kidney injury was a stronger predictor of eventual MOF (78%) and mortality (27%) than hepatic, cardiac, or pulmonary failure by using the Denver MOF score. Level of evidence: I.

34. Stassen NA, Bhullar I, Cheng JD, et al; Eastern Association for the Surgery of Trauma: Nonoperative management of blunt hepatic injury: An Eastern Association for the Surgery of Trauma practice management guideline. *J Trauma Acute Care Surg* 2012;73(5suppl 4):S288-S293.

    In this study, 94 articles were reviewed to suggest practice management guidelines regarding blunt hepatic injury.

35. Stassen NA, Bhullar I, Cheng JD, et al; Eastern Association for the Surgery of Trauma: Selective nonoperative management of blunt splenic injury: An Eastern Association for the Surgery of Trauma practice management guideline. *J Trauma Acute Care Surg* 2012;73(5suppl 4):S294-S300.

    In this study, 125 reports were reviewed to substantiate practice management guidelines pertaining to blunt splenic injury.

36. Pereira SJ, O'Brien DP, Luchette FA, et al: Dynamic helical computed tomography scan accurately detects hemorrhage in patients with pelvic fracture. *Surgery* 2000;128(4):678-685.

37. Tien HC, Spencer F, Tremblay LN, Rizoli SB, Brenneman FD: Preventable deaths from hemorrhage at a level I Canadian trauma center. *J Trauma* 2007;62(1):142-146.

38. Toth L, King KL, McGrath B, Balogh ZJ: Factors associated with pelvic fracture-related arterial bleeding during trauma resuscitation: A prospective clinical study. *J Orthop Trauma* 2014;28(9):489-495.

In this prospective cohort of 143 consecutive trauma patients, the incidence of arterial bleeding related to pelvic fracture was 10%. Several risk factors were identified for pelvic hemorrhage. Level of evidence: I.

39. Schwartz DA, Medina M, Cotton BA, et al: Are we delivering two standards of care for pelvic trauma? Availability of angioembolization after hours and on weekends increases time to therapeutic intervention. *J Trauma Acute Care Surg* 2014;76(1):134-139.

In this study, 191 patients with pelvic fracture who underwent transfusion and met the criteria for evaluation by interventional radiology were studied over 3 years. After adjusting for age and injury severity, patients presenting at night had a 100% increased risk of mortality. The authors suggested that two standards of care are being delivered in the treatment of pelvic trauma, depending on the time of admission. Level of evidence: II.

40. Manson TT, Perdue PW, Pollak AN, O'Toole RV: Embolization of pelvic arterial injury is a risk factor for deep infection after acetabular fracture surgery. *J Orthop Trauma* 2013;27(1):11-15.

This retrospective study evaluated patients with surgically treated acetabular fractures, comparing those who underwent angiography with pelvic arterial embolization (n = 12) and without embolization (n = 14). Infection developed in 7 of 12 patients (58%) who underwent arterial embolization and in 2 of 14 patients (14%) who did not undergo embolization. A high percentage of patients with deep infection underwent embolization of the entire internal iliac artery. The authors highlighted the importance of surgeon awareness of potential complications in treating acetabular fractures surgically following embolization and recommended selective embolization whenever possible. Level of evidence: II.

41. Bliemel C, Lefering R, Buecking B, et al: Early or delayed stabilization in severely injured patients with spinal fractures? Current surgical objectivity according to the Trauma Registry of DGU: Treatment of spine injuries in polytrauma patients. *J Trauma Acute Care Surg* 2014;76(2):366-373.

In this study, more than 2,300 patients from the Trauma Registry of German Trauma Society with thoracolumbar spine injuries (AIS ≥ 3) were analyzed retrospectively: 70% of patients underwent early spine fixation (< 72 hours), 30% underwent late fixation (> 72 hours). Despite greater degrees of spinal injury severity noted in the early fixation group, the early group had shorter ICU and hospital stays, required fewer days of mechanical ventilation, and had lower rates of sepsis. Although some patients may require delay in fixation for medical reasons, every reasonable effort should be made treat patients with unstable spine injuries as early as possible. Level of evidence: III.

42. Hashmi A, Ibrahim-Zada I, Rhee P, et al: Predictors of mortality in geriatric trauma patients: A systematic review and meta-analysis. *J Trauma Acute Care Surg* 2014;76(3):894-901.

This systematic review pooled data from 17 studies and reported an overall mortality rate of 15% for trauma patients age 65 years or older with an ISS of 16 or greater. Increased injury severity using ISS was associated with a higher risk of death (9.5-fold increase for ISS of 16 to 24; and 52-fold increase for ISS > 25). Low systolic blood pressure alone doubled the odds of mortality. Level of evidence: IV.

43. Chang DC, Bass RR, Cornwell EE, Mackenzie EJ: Undertriage of elderly trauma patients to state-designated trauma centers. *Arch Surg* 2008;143(8):776-781, discussion 782.

44. MacKenzie EJ, Rivara FP, Jurkovich GJ, et al: A national evaluation of the effect of trauma-center care on mortality. *N Engl J Med* 2006;354(4):366-378.

45. Calland JF, Ingraham AM, Martin N, et al; Eastern Association for the Surgery of Trauma: Evaluation and management of geriatric trauma: An Eastern Association for the Surgery of Trauma practice management guideline. *J Trauma Acute Care Surg* 2012;73(5suppl 4):S345-S350.

In this report, 90 studies were reviewed to generate recommendations surrounding geriatric trauma patients.

46. Grossman MD, Ofurum U, Stehly CD, Stoltzfus J: Long-term survival after major trauma in geriatric trauma patients: The glass is half full. *J Trauma Acute Care Surg* 2012;72(5):1181-1185.

In this 10-year retrospective review, 145 geriatric trauma patients older than 65 years underwent head injury analysis: one-third of all patients died within 1 week, the median survival for patients with head injury (AIS > 3) was 3 years, and the median survival for those without a substantial head injury (AIS ≤ 3) was 4 years. The overall survival rate at 5 years was 20%, similar to that of many aggressive malignancies. Most patients who survived for several years returned home. Level of evidence: III.

47. Zafar SN, Obirieze A, Schneider EB, et al: Outcomes of trauma care at centers treating a higher proportion of older patients: The case for geriatric trauma centers. *J Trauma Acute Care Surg* 2015;78(4):852-859.

48. Gentile LF, Cuenca AG, Efron PA, et al: Persistent inflammation: A common syndrome and new horizon for surgical intensive care. *J Trauma Acute Care Surg* 2012;72(6):1491-1501.

This review identified an increasing population of patients in surgical ICUs who survive initial sepsis or trauma but have extended ICU stays (>10 days). The patients had a moderate amount of organ dysfunction, are discharged to long-term care facilities, and never regain independence and meaningful function. The authors proposed a new entity termed "persistent inflammation, immunosuppression, and catabolism syndrome" as the dominant pathophysiology and phenotype of chronic critical illness that has replaced late MOF and results in poor outcomes.

49. Vanzant EL, Lopez CM, Ozrazgat-Baslanti T, et al: Persistent inflammation, immunosuppression, and catabolism syndrome after severe blunt trauma. *J Trauma Acute Care Surg* 2014;76(1):21-29, discussion 29-30.

In this report, 1,989 patients from the Inflammation and Host Response to Injury Glue Grant database were divided into two cohorts defined as complicated (time to recovery from organ dysfunction > 14 days; $n = 785$) and uncomplicated (time to recovery from organ dysfunction < 5 days; $n = 369$). Patients in the complicated group were older, sicker, and mechanically ventilated for longer periods of time than those in the uncomplicated group. Complicated patients also had persistent leukocytosis and lower lymphocyte counts and albumin levels, as well as substantial downregulation of adaptive immunity and upregulation of inflammatory genes on days 7 and 14, compared with uncomplicated patients. Level of evidence: III.

50. Namas RA, Vodovotz Y, Almahmoud K, et al: Temporal patterns of circulating inflammation biomarker networks differentiate susceptibility to nosocomial infection following blunt trauma in humans. *Ann Surg* 2014;00:1-8.

This case-control study of 472 blunt trauma patients had 1:1 matching that compared serum biomarkers and outcomes in 44 patients with nosocomial infection and 44 without. Groups were matched based on ISS, age, sex, mechanism of injury, and transfusion requirements: 26 serum inflammatory biomarkers were collected within 24 hours of injury and daily for 7 days. Circulating inflammatory biomarkers exhibited four distinct dynamic patterns, two of which were predictive of the development of nosocomial infection independent of mechanism of injury, injury severity, age, or sex. Level of evidence: II.

51. Centers for Disease Control and Prevention: 2015. Available at: http://www.cdc.gov/injury/wisqars/leadingcauses.html. Accessed March 2015.

This website published by the Centers for Disease Control and Prevention lists the leading causes of mortality among various age groups.

52. Moore FA, Sauaia A, Moore EE, Haenel JB, Burch JM, Lezotte DC: Postinjury multiple organ failure: A bimodal phenomenon. *J Trauma* 1996;40(4):501-510, discussion 510-512.

53. Ciesla DJ, Moore EE, Johnson JL, Burch JM, Cothren CC, Sauaia A: A 12-year prospective study of postinjury multiple organ failure: Has anything changed? *Arch Surg* 2005;140(5):432-438, discussion 438-440.

54. Sauaia A, Moore EE, Johnson JL, et al: Temporal trends of postinjury multiple-organ failure: Still resource intensive, morbid, and lethal. *J Trauma Acute Care Surg* 2014;76(3):582-592, discussion 592-593.

55. Antonelli M, Moreno R, Vincent JL, et al: Application of SOFA score to trauma patients. Sequential Organ Failure Assessment. *Intensive Care Med* 1999;25(4):389-394.

56. Sauaia A, Moore EE, Johnson JL, Ciesla DJ, Biffl WL, Banerjee A: Validation of postinjury multiple organ failure scores. *Shock* 2009;31(5):438-447.

Chapter 19

Management of the Polytrauma Patient and Damage Control Orthopaedic Care

Heather A. Vallier, MD

Abstract

Patients with multiple-system injury and unstable fractures are managed best in a collaborative fashion. In some severely injured patients, damage control orthopaedics, consisting of provisional fixation, reduces the risks of morbidity and mortality. Expeditious resuscitation optimizes patients for the skeletal stabilization of major axial and femoral injuries on an urgent basis. Fracture reduction and fixation contributes to the control of hemorrhage, pain relief, and improved mobility. Simple laboratory parameters, including venous lactate, indicate the readiness for definitive fixation rather than damage control orthopaedics. Recent evidence suggests that most patients are resuscitated adequately and are served best with definitive care within approximately the first 36 hours after injury.

Keywords: damage control; fixation timing; resuscitation; polytrauma

Introduction

In the United States, trauma is the leading cause of death and disability in individuals younger than 45 years, accounting for 200,000 deaths each year and annual medical expenses totaling more than $400 billion.[1] Most deaths are associated with closed head injuries or exsanguination immediately after injury. Trauma care has evolved to reduce later mortality and to mitigate other complications. In some severely injured patients, the provisional treatment of fractures, known as damage control orthopaedics (DCO), reduces the risks of morbidity and mortality. Expeditious and iterative patient assessment determines the response to resuscitation so that the optimal musculoskeletal treatment plan, including the type and timing of fracture care, may be undertaken.

Dr. Vallier or an immediate family member serves as a board member, owner, officer, or committee member of the American Academy of Orthopaedic Surgeons, the Center for Orthopaedic Trauma Advancement, and the Orthopaedic Trauma Association.

Treatment Goals for the Polytrauma Patient

The essential goals of treatment include resuscitation, pain relief, improved fracture alignment and stability, enhanced mobility, and the restoration of function. The American College of Surgeons Committee on Trauma has developed Advanced Trauma Life Support algorithms for initial evaluation and treatment.[2] The primary survey identifies the location and severity of most injuries and determines the physiologic status, including the presence of shock. Musculoskeletal injuries are associated with hemorrhage, and hypovolemic shock is most frequently encountered after trauma, especially in patients with pelvic ring injury, long bone fractures, and/or multiple open fractures (**Table 1**). Shock results in tissue hypoperfusion, hypoxemia, activation of the inflammatory cascade, and immune dysfunction.[3,4] The reduction and fixation of fractures helps to control hemorrhage, aiding in resuscitation.

Pain from injury also induces sympathetic discharge, which can contribute to a hyperinflammatory response, increasing the risks of morbidity and mortality. Chest wall splinting and impaired ventilation caused by pain can contribute to atelectasis, which may result in hypoxemia or pneumonia. Uncontrolled and constant pain likewise

Table 1

Classification of Hemorrhagic Shock

Indication	Class 1	Class 2	Class 3	Class 4
Blood loss (mL)	Up to 750	750-1,500	1,500-2,000	>2,000
Blood loss (% of volume)	Up to 15%	15%-40%	30%-50%	>40%
Heart rate	<100	>100	>129	>140
Blood pressure	Normal	Normal	Decreased	Decreased
Pulse pressure (mm Hg)	Normal	Decreased	Decreased	Decreased
Respiratory rate (/min)	14-20	20-30	30-40	>35
Urine output (mL/hr)	>30	20-30	5-15	Negligible
Mental status	Slightly anxious	Mildly anxious	Confused	Lethargic

Data from American College of Surgeons: *Advanced Trauma Life Support Student Manual*, ed 9. Chicago, IL, American College of Surgeons, 2012.

contributes to continued immobility, which can lead to thromboembolic events, decreased motion, pulmonary complications, and death. Fracture stabilization reduces pain and narcotic use, potentially resulting in less respiratory depression and other adverse effects.[5]

The early reduction and fixation of fractures is an essential step in the resuscitation and pain relief of trauma patients. Unstable pelvis, acetabulum, and femur fractures often are managed definitively within the first 24 hours after injury.[6-12] The urgency and type of stabilization vary, depending on the injuries and the overall patient status. General principles for long bone fractures include the correction of longitudinal, angular, and rotational deformities. Articular fractures, involving joint surfaces, demand strict attention to accurate reduction. These procedures usually are undertaken on a delayed basis several days or even weeks after injury to allow swelling around the fracture to subside, reducing the risks of wound healing problems and infections. Provisional external fixation frequently is performed within 48 hours to control alignment and provide acute pain relief for complex intra-articular fractures. After fractures are stabilized, mobility improves. An upright posture in bed enhances ventilation and reduces the risks of pulmonary and thromboembolic complications as well as pressure ulceration of the skin.

Timing of Musculoskeletal Care

Prioritization of Systemic and Musculoskeletal Injuries

The selection of the type and timing of treatment in a patient with multiple-system trauma and fractures should be undertaken in a collaborative fashion, including all members of the multidisciplinary team. Life- and limb-threatening injuries, including massive hemorrhage from a pelvic fracture or multiple long bone fractures, complete arterial injury in an extremity, and compartment syndrome, are addressed emergently. In these situations, orthopaedic management contributes to resuscitation and promotes the survival of life and limb. Certain other musculoskeletal injuries ideally are managed on an urgent basis, provided the patient has been adequately resuscitated. These injuries include open fractures, which should be débrided within the first 24 hours, and mechanically unstable spine, pelvis, acetabulum, and proximal and diaphyseal femur fractures, which benefit from provisional or definitive stabilization within the first 36 hours after injury.

Benefits of Early Fixation

Most multiply-injured patients have musculoskeletal injuries. Orthopaedic injuries place the patient at risk for various complications, including fat embolism, pneumonia, deep vein thrombosis, and sepsis. Many studies have documented the benefits of early stabilization in reducing morbidity and mortality.[6-20] Early definitive long bone fixation and external fixation methods have evolved and are considered an integral part of the initial care. Recent attention has been placed on the adequate resuscitation of patients before they undergo definitive fixation. In resuscitated patients, early definitive fracture care is associated with low rates of pulmonary complications, and hospital and intensive care unit stays are minimized.[19-24]

Risks of Early Definitive Fixation

When developing a treatment plan for patients with multiple-system injuries and unstable fractures, an important consideration is whether the patient's physiologic state has been optimized to tolerate surgery. The injury itself is considered the first hit to the systemic status. Surgery to stabilize the fractures provides control of bony bleeding, pain relief, and pulmonary benefits; however, the surgery also causes further hemorrhage, the so-called second hit. When the second hit exceeds a threshold level, severe systemic inflammation may occur. In this model, systemic inflammatory response syndrome, which has been associated with multiple-organ failure and death, may develop in severely injured patients.[4,25,26] Fracture fixation contributes to this secondary response and can result in systemic inflammatory response syndrome in underresuscitated patients, depending on the amount of blood loss generated by surgery. An adequate level of resuscitation is crucial in minimizing the effect of the second hit and its adverse consequences.[18,20,24-26]

In the 1980s, the benefits of early stabilization were described, with an emphasis on femoral shaft fractures. The concept of early total care (ETC) led many providers to address various other extremity fractures as well, including more peripheral injuries, which initially could be splinted. The practice of ETC was questioned by some in the 1990s, as more pulmonary complications and mortality were reported in severely injured patients with chest trauma who underwent intramedullary nailing of the femur within 24 hours of injury. Shortly thereafter, the practice of DCO was proposed as an alternative to definitive fixation of femoral shaft fractures in patients deemed too severely injured to tolerate early definitive surgery.[27] The application of an external fixator to the femur provides provisional skeletal stability and pain relief and facilitates nursing care and upright posture while eliminating the need for skeletal traction. Using external fixation minimizes the second hit of early surgery, thereby promoting expeditious fracture stabilization without adversely affecting the systemic status of the patient.

Damage Control Orthopaedics

DCO is a means of providing early fracture stabilization while minimizing the second hit caused by prolonged surgical procedures. This tactic generally involves avoiding longer definitive procedures with large blood loss in favor of shorter surgical procedures. The aforementioned stabilization of a femur with provisional external fixation instead of an intramedullary nail is one example.[26-28] Many unstable pelvis fractures cannot be provisionally stabilized with external fixation, however.[29] Acetabulum fractures and spine fractures also cannot be stabilized with external fixation, limiting the applicability of the damage control concept.[30] Furthermore, the need for additional definitive surgery on a delayed basis, such as the conversion of a femoral external fixator to an intramedullary nail, and the potential for greater complications and costs make this practice controversial.[31,32] Currently, it is unclear which patients benefit from a damage control strategy. Recent studies suggest that definitive fixation of femoral shaft, pelvis, and acetabulum fractures is well tolerated in most patients without using damage control tactics when adequate resuscitation has occurred.[10,16,18,21,23,24,33] The exact timing of surgical intervention depends on the magnitude and duration of acidosis and the response to resuscitation. Injury complexity and underlying factors such as patient age and cardiac function are also important to consider. The orthopaedic surgeon, trauma critical care team, and anesthesiologist must work together to determine the appropriate timing of fixation.

Management of the Polytrauma Patient

Treatment Based on Physiologic and Laboratory Assessment

The identification and characterization of shock are based on factors that include heart rate, blood pressure, temperature, respiratory rate, urine output, and mental status (**Table 1**). Several laboratory parameters routinely obtained during care of the multiply-injured patient are crucial. Combined with physiologic parameters and physical examination findings, these factors are usually sufficient for estimating blood loss and performing resuscitation. Severe musculoskeletal trauma and its associated hemorrhage results in tissue hypoperfusion, which leads to acidosis. The extent of acidosis is measured with pH, base excess, or lactate levels. Normalization of these values within 24 hours of injury is predictive of survival.[23,34] The pH and base excess are less specific and more subject to confounders such as alcohol ingestion and renal disease; thus, lactate level is considered the most reliable indicator of resuscitation.[23,34] Guidelines for the adequacy of resuscitation have been proposed to provide objective measurements with which to guide the timing of definitive fracture fixation. Early results suggest that a patient with improving acidosis, as measured by pH of 7.25 or greater, base excess of −5.5 mmol/L or greater, or lactate level less than 4.0 mmol/L, will benefit from definitive fracture care as long as a severe head injury or other medical pathology does not preclude it. These parameters have been termed Early Appropriate Care, and they recommend the surgical stabilization of all spine, pelvis, acetabulum, and femur fractures within 36 hours of injury.[23,24]

In patients presenting with class 1 or 2 shock (**Table 1**), intravenous access is established, and 2 L of crystalloid is administered. The initial laboratory assessment is performed, including complete blood cell count, electrolytes, international normalized ratio, and venous lactate. Other laboratory tests may be obtained, depending on the patient and the severity of injury. Patients with greater or ongoing hemorrhage require transfusions. To assess the response to resuscitation, the vital signs are measured continuously, and laboratory tests are repeated every 4 to 8 hours until they improve. Critically ill patients in class 4 shock warrant initiation of a massive transfusion protocol.

Coagulopathy also is present in patients who sustain massive hemorrhage after injury. Providing resuscitation with fluid and blood products restores tissue oxygenation, normalizing acidosis. Massive resuscitation without specific attention to clotting factors and platelets may accentuate coagulopathy via dilution. Transfusion ratios for platelets and fresh frozen plasma have been proposed, with initial studies supporting 1:1:1 administration of packed red blood cells, platelets, and fresh frozen plasma in extreme cases.[35,36] Thromboelastography to identify individual factors warranting repletion recently also has shown promise in providing factor-specific replacement.[37,38]

Associated Soft-Tissue Injury

Many high-energy injuries are associated with severe soft-tissue damage or destruction. Open fractures and unstable femoral and pelvic fractures are managed urgently, but extremity fractures often are stabilized provisionally with splints or external fixation until the soft tissues have healed sufficiently to tolerate additional surgery. This protocol minimizes wound healing problems and infections.

Adequate nutrition is essential for the healing of wounds and fractures. Trauma increases caloric needs, making it difficult to maintain body weight and protein stores during the healing period. The burden of multiple trauma combined with the inability to take food by mouth, possibly because of associated injuries that may necessitate ventilatory support, lead to a catabolic state after injury. Inadequate nutrition is associated with increased risks of infection, wound and fracture healing problems, and decubitus ulcers. Trauma also produces stress, which leads to more gastric acid production and the increased intestinal translocation of bacteria. Early enteral nutrition mitigates these issues in trauma patients. Recent work demonstrated more infections, other complications, and readmissions in malnourished patients.[39] Some clinicians argue that it is prudent to delay reconstructive procedures associated with fractures until nutrition has been optimized.

Head Injury

Concurrent head injuries are common in orthopaedic trauma patients. Most head injuries are minor, with presenting Glasgow Coma Scale (GCS) scores higher than 12[2] (**Table 2**). The postresuscitation GCS score correlates with functional outcome.[40] In less than 3% of patients with mild head injury, progressive deterioration of the mental status develops; thus, CT of the head is performed liberally in new trauma patients. Patients with severe head injury (GCS score ≤8) are comatose, requiring mechanical ventilation and intensive care unit monitoring.

The timing of fracture fixation in patients with severe head injury has been a long-standing topic of debate. Most previous studies have focused on femoral shaft fractures and support a strategy of DCO for patients with elevated intracranial pressure (ICP) and limited cerebral perfusion pressure (CPP). The monitoring of ICP is initiated in patients at risk for intracranial hypertension[41] (**Table 3**). CPP is calculated as the mean arterial pressure minus the ICP. It indicates the adequacy of blood flow to the brain. Ischemia with CPP less than 70 mm Hg for several hours can cause permanent brain damage. To proceed with the definitive management of axial and femoral fractures, ICP should be 20 mm Hg or less and CPP should be greater than 70 mm Hg.[41] For patients with a higher ICP, various measures, including ventriculostomy,

Table 2

Glasgow Coma Scale

Clinical Parameter	Points
Best Eye Response (E)	
Spontaneous	4
To speech	3
To pain	2
None	1
Best Motor Response (M)	
Obeys commands	6
Localizes pain	5
Normal flexion (withdrawal)	4
Abnormal flexion (decorticate)	3
Extension (decerebrate)	2
None (flaccid)	1
Best Verbal Response (V)	
Fully oriented	5
Disoriented/confused conversation	4
Inappropriate words	3
Incomprehensible words	2
None	1

Glasgow Coma Scale score = E+M+V: 14 to 15 points = mild, 9 to 13 points = moderate, and 3 to 8 points = severe.

Table 3

Indications for Intracranial Pressure Monitoring

Severe TBI (GCS score of 3-8 after resuscitation) and abnormal findings on CT of the head, including hematoma, contusion, swelling, herniation, and/or compression.

Severe TBI and normal findings on CT of the head if two or more of the following parameters are noted at admission: age >40 years, motor posturing, and systolic blood pressure <90 mm Hg.

GCS = Glasgow Coma Scale, TBI = traumatic brain injury.
Data from Healey C, Osler TM, Rogers FB, et al: Improving the Glasgow Coma Scale score: Motor score alone is a better predictor. *J Trauma* 2003;54(4):671-678, discussion 678-680.

craniotomy, mannitol infusion, and hypothermia, may be undertaken. The judicious use of DCO with external fixation of femur and pelvis fractures is appropriate. Previous studies are limited by the very small numbers of patients studied and the heterogeneity of injuries. For femoral shaft fractures, the literature suggests that early definitive fixation is safe in hemodynamically stable patients who are well oxygenated and have a CPP greater than70 mm Hg.[42-44]

Chest Injury

Chest injuries are also very common in multiply-injured orthopaedic trauma patients. Even minor chest injuries are problematic because they increase the risk of pulmonary complications. Chest injuries are painful and cause splinting and poor inspiratory effort in conscious patients. Narcotic medications suppress the respiratory drive, and recumbency contributes to poor ventilation; both accentuate the risk of adverse sequelae in patients with chest trauma. Direct parenchymal lung damage in patients with pulmonary contusions and other severe chest trauma further diminishes oxygenation in the first several days after injury. Fracture reduction and stabilization promotes pain relief, upright posture, and mobility from bed, all of which reduce the risks of pulmonary and other complications.

Previously, the ETC of femur and other fractures was associated with pulmonary complications in some studies.[3,4,19] More recent studies have shown that although major chest injury is a risk factor for pulmonary complications, the early definitive fixation of axial and femoral fractures in resuscitated patients is associated with fewer complications than delayed surgery, even in the presence of severe chest injury.[7-10,15,17,21,24] If definitive fixation is not possible within the first 2 days after injury, it may be safer to wait until more than 5 days after injury for pulmonary status to improve.[7]

Abdominal Injury

Abdominal injuries occur commonly, and during the past 10 years, a steady decrease in the number of patients requiring exploratory laparotomy has been observed. The increased availability of high-quality diagnostic imaging has facilitated the rapid and specific characterization of abdominal injuries. Selective angiography and embolization for solid-organ injury is also more common, again reducing the number of patients who undergo surgery. Some of the most severe abdominal injuries remain life threatening, however, and are often present concurrently with musculoskeletal trauma. According to numerous studies, patients with these injury combinations have been shown to have some of the highest morbidity and mortality rates.[11,16,23,45]

Multidisciplinary management in such patients requires algorithm-based care. Life-threatening injuries are addressed first. In the presence of combined pelvic ring and abdominal injury, it is recommended that provisional reduction and external fixation of the pelvic ring be performed in amenable fracture patterns before laparotomy. This protocol provides better venous tamponade in the pelvis and prevents further enlargement of the pelvic diameter. In critically ill patients with persistent hemodynamic instability and/or acidosis, DCO should be used in the initial setting. The expeditious débridement of open fractures and the application of external fixation or splints may be the only procedures appropriate until further resuscitation has taken place.

Spinal Column Injury and Spinal Cord Injury

Most spinal column injuries are mechanically stable. Unstable injuries to the thoracolumbar spine pose a similar physiologic burden to the patient as do fractures of the acetabulum, hip, or femoral shaft in that these injuries relegate a patient to bed rest and recumbency until stabilized. Thus, an increasing body of literature has reported fewer complications and shorter hospital stays with fewer days of mechanical ventilation when these injuries are stabilized early.[12,23,24,46,47] The surgical stabilization of spinal column injury is advocated within 36 hours in resuscitated patients.[23,24] A spine damage control strategy also has been described in which the first of two stages of surgery occurs early, affording mechanical stability, pain relief, and better posturing.[30]

The American Spinal Injury Association Impairment Scale is used to classify spinal cord injuries (**Table 4**). In the presence of spinal cord injury, most surgeons advocate decompressive surgery for the neurologic elements. Surgical timing remains controversial. Decompression may entail the reduction of fractures and dislocations because the neural elements may be under pressure from bone,

Table 4

American Spinal Injury Association Impairment Scale

A = Complete	No motor or sensory function is preserved in sacral segments S4-5.
B = Incomplete	Sensory function, but not motor function, is preserved below the neurologic level and includes sacral segments S4-5.
C = Incomplete	Motor function is preserved below the neurologic level and more than half of the key muscles below the neurologic level have a muscle grade <3.
D = Incomplete	Motor function is preserved below the neurologic level and at least half of the key muscles below the neurologic level have a muscle grade of ≥3.
E = Normal	Motor and sensory function are normal.

disk material, hematoma, or foreign material. Incomplete injuries are decompressed in an emergent or urgent manner because improvement in neurologic function is possible.

Principles of DCO

Reduction of Fractures and Dislocations

When patients are critically ill, damage control strategies are used to address musculoskeletal injuries. Closed reduction of fractures and dislocations should be undertaken, and splints should be applied for peripheral extremity fractures. Provisional skeletal traction is recommended for femur fractures and for acetabulum fractures that have an associated dislocation and/or have retained osteochondral fragments. Pelvic ring injuries with cephalad displacement also may benefit from skeletal traction. Certain authors have debated the benefit of provisional external fixation versus skeletal traction for femoral shaft fractures.[48] Their study was underpowered to detect a difference in pulmonary complications, however, and all patients underwent intramedullary nailing within 24 hours. Thus, DCO with external fixation of femoral shaft fractures is considered appropriate in patients too unstable to tolerate definitive surgery within 24 to 36 hours. Care should be taken to maintain healthy pin hygiene to minimize infection risk. External fixation should be converted to definitive internal fixation within 2 weeks.[31,32]

Débridement of Wounds

The recent emphasis on administering intravenous antibiotics to patients with open fractures at the time of presentation has contributed to lower infection rates.[49] Yet, most clinicians believe that the quality of the surgical débridement remains the most important determinant in reducing risk of later infection. Although open fractures ideally would be addressed within several hours after injury to minimize bacterial adherence and glycocalyx production, newer studies demonstrate acceptable rates of infection in patients who undergo surgical débridement of open fractures within 12 to 24 hours.[50] Open fractures and dislocations are treated urgently and should be given priority in critically ill patients who are stable enough to tolerate short surgical procedures. If fracture complexity, soft-tissue injury, and/or the systemic status of the patient prevent definitive care, then surgical débridement and irrigation followed by splinting or external fixation are appropriate.

Summary

Patients with multiple-system injury and unstable fractures are managed best in a collaborative fashion. Attention to expeditious resuscitation results in patients being optimized for the skeletal stabilization of major axial and femoral injuries. Fracture reduction and fixation contributes to the control of hemorrhage, pain relief, and improved mobility on an acute basis. Simple laboratory parameters, including venous lactate, indicate the readiness for definitive fixation versus DCO. Recent evidence suggests that most patients are resuscitated adequately and are served best with definitive care within approximately the first 36 hours after injury.

Key Study Points

- Multiply-injured patients are best managed with a collaborative, multidisciplinary approach.
- Fixation of axial and femoral fractures reduces pain, controls bleeding, and promotes mobility.
- Most patients are resuscitated adequately, as measured by correction of metabolic acidosis, and are best served with definitive fixation within 36 hours after injury.
- Damage control tactics afford safe provisional stability in patients who are not adequately resuscitated or are otherwise medically too unstable to tolerate definitive surgery.

Annotated References

1. Centers for Disease Control and Prevention: Key injury and violence data. Available at: http://www.cdc.gov/injury/overview/leading_cod.html. Updated September 30, 2015. Accessed December 19, 2015.

2. American College of Surgeons: *Advanced Trauma Life Support, Student Manual* ,ed 9. Chicago, IL, American College of Surgeons, 2012.

3. Pape HC, Giannoudis PV, Krettek C, Trentz O: Timing of fixation of major fractures in blunt polytrauma: Role of conventional indicators in clinical decision making. *J Orthop Trauma* 2005;19(8):551-562.

4. Pape HC, Schmidt RE, Rice J, et al: Biochemical changes after trauma and skeletal surgery of the lower extremity: Quantification of the operative burden. *Crit Care Med* 2000;28(10):3441-3448.

5. Barei DP, Shafer BL, Beingessner DM, Gardner MJ, Nork SE, Routt ML: The impact of open reduction internal fixation on acute pain management in unstable pelvic ring injuries. *J Trauma* 2010;68(4):949-953.

   In this study, 38 patients treated surgically for pelvic ring fracture were examined. Visual analog scale pain scores declined 48% after fixation, and narcotic requirements decreased 25% postoperatively. Level of evidence: III.

6. Bone LB, Johnson KD, Weigelt J, Scheinberg R: Early versus delayed stabilization of femoral fractures: A prospective randomized study. *J Bone Joint Surg Am* 1989;71(3):336-340.

7. Gandhi RR, Overton TL, Haut ER, et al: Optimal timing of femur fracture stabilization in polytrauma patients: A practice management guideline from the Eastern Association for the Surgery of Trauma. *J Trauma Acute Care Surg* 2014;77(5):787-795.

   The practice management guidelines from the Eastern Association for the Surgery of Trauma were developed after meta-analysis and systematic review. Conditional recommendation was made for the fixation of open or closed femoral shaft fractures within 24 hours after injury based on a trend toward lower risks of infection, mortality, and venous thromboembolism. Level of evidence: III.

8. Lefaivre KA, Starr AJ, Stahel PF, Elliott AC, Smith WR: Prediction of pulmonary morbidity and mortality in patients with femur fracture. *J Trauma* 2010;69(6):1527-1535, discussion 1535-1536.

   This retrospective study showed that patients treated with definitive fixation of femoral shaft fractures 8 to 24 hours after injury had the lowest morality compared with those treated within 8 hours or after 24 hours. When fixation was delayed more than 24 hours, a trend toward more acute respiratory distress syndrome was noted. Level of evidence: II.

9. Nahm NJ, Como JJ, Wilber JH, Vallier HA: Early appropriate care: Definitive stabilization of femoral fractures within 24 hours of injury is safe in most patients with multiple injuries. *J Trauma* 2011;71(1):175-185.

   This retrospective study demonstrated that multiply-injured patients with femoral shaft fractures treated definitively within 24 hours after injury had fewer pulmonary and other complications and a shorter length of stay overall than patients treated on a delayed basis. Complications were associated with severe chest injury or severe abdominal injury, regardless of the timing of fixation. Level of evidence: II.

10. Nahm NJ, Vallier HA: Timing of definitive treatment of femoral shaft fractures in patients with multiple injuries: A systematic review of randomized and nonrandomized trials. *J Trauma Acute Care Surg* 2012;73(5):1046-1063.

    This systematic review of 38 studies showed that early definitive fixation of femoral shaft fractures in multiply-injured patients appears safe in most patients and may be associated with fewer pulmonary complications and shorter hospital stays. Level of evidence: III.

11. Vallier HA, Cureton BA, Ekstein C, Oldenburg FP, Wilber JH: Early definitive stabilization of unstable pelvis and acetabulum fractures reduces morbidity. *J Trauma* 2010;69(3):677-684.

    This retrospective review of 645 patients with pelvic ring and/or acetabulum fractures treated surgically reported fewer complications and shorter hospital stays when fixation occurred within 24 hours after injury. Severe chest injury or transfusion greater than 10 units of packed red blood cells was associated with higher complication rates. Level of evidence: II.

12. Vallier HA, Super DM, Moore TA, Wilber JH: Do patients with multiple system injury benefit from early fixation of unstable axial fractures? The effects of timing of surgery on initial hospital course. *J Orthop Trauma* 2013;27(7):405-412.

    In this review, 1,005 patients with Injury Severity Scores of 18 or greater treated surgically for high-energy fractures of the pelvis, acetabulum, thoracolumbar spine, and/or proximal or diaphyseal femur were reviewed. Definitive fracture management within 24 hours resulted in shorter intensive care unit and hospital stays, fewer complications, and fewer cases of acute respiratory distress syndrome after adjusting for age and the type and severity of other system injuries. Level of evidence: III.

13. Frangen TM, Ruppert S, Muhr G, Schinkel C: The beneficial effects of early stabilization of thoracic spine fractures depend on trauma severity. *J Trauma* 2010;68(5):1208-1212.

    This retrospective review of 160 patients with thoracolumbar fractures showed that fixation within 72 hours after injury was associated with shorter intensive care unit and hospital stays than those of patients treated on a more delayed basis. No adverse effects on pulmonary function were noted with early surgery. Level of evidence: II.

14. Han G, Wang Z, Du Q, et al: Damage-control orthopedics versus early total care in the treatment of borderline high-energy pelvic fractures. *Orthopedics* 2014;37(12):e1091-e1100.

In this study, of 72 patients with high-energy pelvic ring fracture, 33 underwent early fixation, or ETC, and 39 underwent provisional damage control external fixation. For Tile B fractures, no significant difference was seen in the overall rates of postoperative complications. In patients with Tile C fractures, however, especially in those 40 years and older, the damage control external fixation group had a lower rate of acute lung injury and lower Acute Physiology and Chronic Health Evaluation II scores than did the ETC group. Level of evidence: III.

15. Harvin JA, Harvin WH, Camp E, et al: Early femur fracture fixation is associated with a reduction in pulmonary complications and hospital charges: A decade of experience with 1,376 diaphyseal femur fractures. *J Trauma Acute Care Surg* 2012;73(6):1442-1448, discussion 1448-1449.

This retrospective review of 1,376 patients treated for femur fracture compared early fixation performed within 24 hours at a mean of 7.4 hours with delayed fixation performed at a mean of 31 hours. After controlling for Injury Severity Score, a 57% decrease in the risk of pulmonary complications was noted with early fixation, as well as a shorter ventilation time, a shorter hospital stay, and lower hospital charges. Level of evidence: IV.

16. Morshed S, Miclau T III, Bembom O, Cohen M, Knudson MM, Colford JM Jr: Delayed internal fixation of femoral shaft fracture reduces mortality among patients with multisystem trauma. *J Bone Joint Surg Am* 2009;91(1):3-13.

17. Nicholas B, Toth L, van Wessem K, Evans J, Enninghorst N, Balogh ZJ: Borderline femur fracture patients: Early total care or damage control orthopaedics? *ANZ J Surg* 2011;81(3):148-153.

A prospective evaluation of 66 patients with stable or borderline status and femoral shaft fracture was reported. Early definitive fixation of stable (98%) and borderline (86%) patients resulted in fewer intensive care unit and ventilator days and fewer complications than in the randomized controlled trial, which had 57% overall utilization of ETC. Level of evidence: II.

18. O'Toole RV, O'Brien M, Scalea TM, Habashi N, Pollak AN, Turen CH: Resuscitation before stabilization of femoral fractures limits acute respiratory distress syndrome in patients with multiple traumatic injuries despite low use of damage control orthopedics. *J Trauma* 2009;67(5):1013-1021.

19. Pape HC, Rixen D, Morley J, et al, EPOFF Study Group: Impact of the method of initial stabilization for femoral shaft fractures in patients with multiple injuries at risk for complications (borderline patients). *Ann Surg* 2007;246(3):491-499, discussion 499-501.

20. Steinhausen E, Lefering R, Tjardes T, Neugebauer EA, Bouillon B, Rixen D,Committee on Emergency Medicine, Intensive and Trauma Care (Sektion NIS) of the German Society for Trauma Surgery (DGU): A risk-adapted approach is beneficial in the management of bilateral femoral shaft fractures in multiple trauma patients: An analysis based on the trauma registry of the German Trauma Society. *J Trauma Acute Care Surg* 2014;76(5):1288-1293.

This review of the German trauma registry of bilateral femoral fractures reported no difference in mortality between DCO and ETC groups when adjusting for injury severity. The authors suggested a risk-adapted approach when considering DCO for patients deemed clinically unstable. Level of evidence: IV.

21. Nahm NJ, Moore TA, Vallier HA: Use of two grading systems in determining risks associated with timing of fracture fixation. *J Trauma Acute Care Surg* 2014;77(2):268-279.

This comparison of two grading systems, the Clinical Grading System (CGS) and the Early Appropriate Care (EAC) system, suggested that EAC effectively can identify patients at risk for complications with early definitive fixation, whereas the CGS differentiates unstable patients who may benefit from DCO. Borderline patients also may benefit from early definitive fixation, but further study is required. Level of evidence: III.

22. Paladino L, Sinert R, Wallace D, Anderson T, Yadav K, Zehtabchi S: The utility of base deficit and arterial lactate in differentiating major from minor injury in trauma patients with normal vital signs. *Resuscitation* 2008;77(3):363-368.

23. Vallier HA, Wang X, Moore TA, Wilber JH, Como JJ: Timing of orthopaedic surgery in multiple trauma patients: Development of a protocol for early appropriate care. *J Orthop Trauma* 2013;27(10):543-551.

Statistical modeling of 1,443 patients with surgical spine, pelvis, acetabulum, and/or femur fractures was used to predict the probability of pulmonary and other complications. Acidosis on presentation is associated with complications, lactate being most specific. Resuscitation with correction of pH to 7.25 or greater, base excess to −5.5 or greater, or lactate level to less than 4.0 mmol/L is associated with fewer pulmonary complications. Other significant variables to include in a predictive model and in algorithm development for the Early Appropriate Care protocol are the presence and severity of chest injury, the number of fractures, and the timing of fixation. Level of evidence: III.

24. Vallier HA, Moore TA, Como JJ, et al: Complications are reduced with a protocol to standardize timing of fixation based on response to resuscitation. *J Orthop Surg Res* 2015;10(1):155-164.

This prospective evaluation of the Early Appropriate Care protocol in 335 patients, which defined adequate resuscitation to recommend the definitive fixation of spine, pelvis, acetabulum, and femur fractures within 36 hours after injury, showed that early fixation was associated with fewer complications and a shorter length of stay. Level of evidence: I.

25. Harwood PJ, Giannoudis PV, van Griensven M, Krettek C, Pape HC: Alterations in the systemic inflammatory response after early total care and damage control procedures for femoral shaft fracture in severely injured patients. *J Trauma* 2005;58(3):446-452, discussion 452-454.

26. Tuttle MS, Smith WR, Williams AE, et al: Safety and efficacy of damage control external fixation versus early definitive stabilization for femoral shaft fractures in the multiple-injured patient. *J Trauma* 2009;67(3):602-605.

27. Scalea TM, Boswell SA, Scott JD, Mitchell KA, Kramer ME, Pollak AN: External fixation as a bridge to intramedullary nailing for patients with multiple injuries and with femur fractures: Damage control orthopedics. *J Trauma* 2000;48(4):613-621, discussion 621-623.

28. Mathieu L, Bazile F, Barthélémy R, Duhamel P, Rigal S: Damage control orthopaedics in the context of battlefield injuries: The use of temporary external fixation on combat trauma soldiers. *Orthop Traumatol Surg Res* 2011;97(8):852-859.

This case series of damage control external fixation for battlefield lower extremity injuries reported successful early conversion to internal fixation but for one case with late infection, in which external fixation was converted after 3 months. Level of evidence: IV.

29. Tai DK, Li WH, Lee KY, et al: Retroperitoneal pelvic packing in the management of hemodynamically unstable pelvic fractures: A level I trauma center experience. *J Trauma* 2011;71(4):E79-E86.

This retrospective review described two periods of treatment of hemodynamically unstable pelvis fracture. Pelvic packing with or without angiography seems as effective in controlling hemorrhage as does angiography alone. Level of evidence: III.

30. Stahel PF, VanderHeiden T, Flierl MA, et al: The impact of a standardized "spine damage-control" protocol for unstable thoracic and lumbar spine fractures in severely injured patients: A prospective cohort study. *J Trauma Acute Care Surg* 2013;74(2):590-596.

This prospective cohort study of single-stage delayed thoracolumbar fixation (n = 70) compared with posterior-only damage control posterior fixation within 24 hours (n = 42) showed fewer complications, shorter stays, and less mechanical ventilation in the damage control group. Level of evidence: III.

31. Mody RM, Zapor M, Hartzell JD, et al: Infectious complications of damage control orthopedics in war trauma. *J Trauma* 2009;67(4):758-761.

32. Nowotarski PJ, Turen CH, Brumback RJ, Scarboro JM: Conversion of external fixation to intramedullary nailing for fractures of the shaft of the femur in multiply injured patients. *J Bone Joint Surg Am* 2000;82(6):781-788.

33. Kerwin AJ, Griffen MM, Tepas JJ III, Schinco MA, Devin T, Frykberg ER: Best practice determination of timing of spinal fracture fixation as defined by analysis of the National Trauma Data Bank. *J Trauma* 2008;65(4):824-830, discussion 830-831.

34. Guyette F, Suffoletto B, Castillo JL, Quintero J, Callaway C, Puyana JC: Prehospital serum lactate as a predictor of outcomes in trauma patients: A retrospective observational study. *J Trauma* 2011;70(4):782-786.

Prehospital lactate level was measured in 1,168 patients, and a median value of 2.4 mmol/L was observed. An elevated lactate level was associated with organ failure, mortality, and a need for surgery. Level of evidence: III.

35. Brakenridge SC, Phelan HA, Henley SS, et al, Inflammation and the Host Response to Injury Investigators: Early blood product and crystalloid volume resuscitation: Risk association with multiple organ dysfunction after severe blunt traumatic injury. *J Trauma* 2011;71(2):299-305.

This multicenter observational study of 1,366 blunt trauma patients showed that a massive packed red blood cell transfusion within the first 12 hours is associated with multiple-organ dysfunction, whereas FFP and crystalloid are not. Level of evidence: II.

36. Pidcoke HF, Aden JK, Mora AG, et al: Ten-year analysis of transfusion in Operation Iraqi Freedom and Operation Enduring Freedom: Increased plasma and platelet use correlates with improved survival. *J Trauma Acute Care Surg* 2012;73(6suppl 5):S445-S452.

Coagulopathy on presentation with an international normalized ratio of 1.5 or greater was associated with mortality. Massive transfusion with high FFP and platelet ratios correlated with higher survival. Level of evidence: IV.

37. Driessen A, Schäfer N, Bauerfeind U, et al: Functional capacity of reconstituted blood in 1:1:1 versus 3:1:1 ratios: A thrombelastometry study. *Scand J Trauma Resusc Emerg Med* 2015;23:2.

Rotational thromboelastometry evaluation of whole blood donors in 1:1:1 and 3:1:1 ratios of packed red blood cells, FFP, and platelets showed better clot formation and lower international normalized ratio in the 1:1:1 group, suggesting better functionality of the 1:1:1 ratio for massive resuscitation.

38. Cotton BA, Faz G, Hatch QM, et al: Rapid thrombelastography delivers real-time results that predict transfusion within 1 hour of admission. *J Trauma* 2011;71(2):407-414, discussion 414-417.

Prospective evaluation of 583 consecutive trauma patients showed rapid thromboelastography to be predictive of early transfusions of packed red blood cells, plasma, and platelets. Level of evidence: IV.

39. Lee JH, Hutzler LH, Shulman BS, Karia RJ, Egol KA: Does risk for malnutrition in patients presenting with fractures predict lower quality measures? *J Orthop Trauma* 2015;29(8):373-378.

A malnutrition screening tool was applied to all trauma patients for 2 years, retrospectively. Malnutrition was associated with a substantially higher rate of readmissions and an 8.0% rate of complications compared with 2.8% ($P = 0.001$) in patients without malnutrition. Level of evidence: II.

40. Healey C, Osler TM, Rogers FB, et al: Improving the Glasgow Coma Scale score: Motor score alone is a better predictor. *J Trauma* 2003;54(4):671-678, discussion 678-680.

41. Brain Trauma Foundation, American Association of Neurological Surgeons, Congress of Neurological Surgeons: Guidelines for the management of severe traumatic brain injury. [published correction appears in J Neurotrauma 2008;25(3):276-278.]. *J Neurotrauma* 2007;24(suppl 1):S1-S106.

42. Flierl MA, Stoneback JW, Beauchamp KM, et al: Femur shaft fracture fixation in head-injured patients: When is the right time? *J Orthop Trauma* 2010;24(2):107-114.

The systemic physiology associated with head injury was reviewed. Clinical recommendations regarding the timing of fixation of fractures were explored. Level of evidence: III.

43. Scalea TM, Scott JD, Brumback RJ, et al: Early fracture fixation may be "just fine" after head injury: No difference in central nervous system outcomes. *J Trauma* 1999;46(5):839-846.

44. Wang MC, Temkin NR, Deyo RA, Jurkovich GJ, Barber J, Dikmen S: Timing of surgery after multisystem injury with traumatic brain injury: Effect on neuropsychological and functional outcome. *J Trauma* 2007;62(5):1250-1258.

45. Nahm NJ, Como JJ, Vallier HA: The impact of major operative fractures in blunt abdominal injury. *J Trauma Acute Care Surg* 2013;74(5):1307-1314.

This article reported a retrospective review of patients with severe abdominal injury with (n = 106) and without (n = 91) associated fixation of a femur, pelvis, or spine fracture. Surgical treatment of fracture increased the odds of a complication developing (odds ratio, 2.88; $P = 0.006$) after controlling for the presence of chest injury and the type of abdominal injury. Level of evidence: III.

46. Cengiz SL, Kalkan E, Bayir A, Ilik K, Basefer A: Timing of thoracolomber spine stabilization in trauma patients: Impact on neurological outcome and clinical course. A real prospective (rct) randomized controlled study. *Arch Orthop Trauma Surg* 2008;128(9):959-966.

47. Giorgi H, Blondel B, Adetchessi T, Dufour H, Tropiano P, Fuentes S: Early percutaneous fixation of spinal thoracolumbar fractures in polytrauma patients. *Orthop Traumatol Surg Res* 2014;100(5):449-454.

Early percutaneous fixation may reduce perioperative morbidity in multiply-injured patients compared with traditional open methods. Level of evidence: IV.

48. Scannell BP, Waldrop NE, Sasser HC, Sing RF, Bosse MJ: Skeletal traction versus external fixation in the initial temporization of femoral shaft fractures in severely injured patients. *J Trauma* 2010;68(3):633-640.

This article is a retrospective review of 205 patients with polytrauma and femoral shaft fracture; 19 had provisional external fixation and 60 had temporary skeletal traction. All patients underwent intramedullary nailing within 24 hours. No differences in pulmonary or other complications were reported, suggesting that skeletal traction is a reasonable temporary option. Level of evidence: III.

49. Lack WD, Karunakar MA, Angerame MR, et al: Type III open tibia fractures: Immediate antibiotic prophylaxis minimizes infection. *J Orthop Trauma* 2015;29(1):1-6.

This observational study showed that shorter time to both administration of intravenous antibiotics (<66 minutes) and soft-tissue coverage (≤5 days) is associated with a lower risk of infection after type 3 open tibial shaft fracture. Level of evidence: III.

50. Pollak AN, Jones AL, Castillo RC, Bosse MJ, MacKenzie EJ, LEAP Study Group: The relationship between time to surgical debridement and incidence of infection after open high-energy lower extremity trauma. *J Bone Joint Surg Am* 2010;92(1):7-15.

This Lower Extremity Assessment Project Study Group review of 315 patients with open fractures demonstrated that the time between injury and admission to the definitive trauma center is an independent predictor of the risk of infection. Level of evidence: II.

Chapter 20

Acute Compartment Syndrome

Christopher Doro, MD

Abstract

Acute compartment syndrome is a clinical emergency that occurs often in current orthopaedic practice. Acute compartment syndrome continues to present orthopaedic surgeons and other clinicians with diagnostic and treatment challenges and can lead to increased costs of care.

Keywords: acute compartment syndrome; fasciotomy; compartment pressure

Introduction

Acute compartment syndrome (ACS) remains a well-recognized clinical emergency that is relatively prevalent in current orthopaedic trauma practice. Despite being first described nearly 150 years ago,[1] ACS continues to present orthopaedic surgeons and other clinicians with diagnostic and treatment challenges. In addition to its clinical importance, a diagnosis of ACS has recently been identified to increase cost of care. Studies have shown that ACS more than doubles hospital stay and charges.[2,3]

Current Incidence Rates and Risk Factors

Risk factors for ACS continue to be analyzed in an effort to alert clinicians to patients who are more likely to develop this syndrome. Patients with tibial fractures have long been known to be at risk of experiencing ACS, and although studies have shown that the rate has varied, according to a 2009 study it was noted to be as high as 10.4% in 386 tibial fractures at a level I trauma center.[4] The rate of ACS in pediatric tibial fractures is thought to be similar (11.6%), with the highest risk in children 14 years and older.[5] A total of 414 tibial fractures were retrospectively reviewed and the highest rate of ACS was found in diaphyseal fractures (8.1%; $P < 0.05$) followed by proximal (1.6%) and distal (1.4%) tibial fractures (P value nonsignificant).[6] However, this finding contradicts existing dogma that proximal fractures have higher rates of ACS, perhaps because the study was retrospective and all-inclusive regardless of injury energy level. The study authors acknowledged that if they had been able to include all risk factors in their analysis, they might have been able to identify other trends. The multivariate analysis of this group showed younger age as the only independent predictor for ACS ($P = 0.006$),[6] as also has been shown in other studies.[7,8] One recent retrospective analysis of 160 patients with diaphyseal tibial fractures diagnosed with ACS also demonstrates the effect of age. In the multivariate analysis, age 12 to 29 years was the strongest predictor of ACS ($P < 0.001$).[8] Also of note, previously recognized risk factors such as sex, treatment with intramedullary nails, open fracture, and sport-related injury were not significant in multivariate analysis.[8]

In contrast to the retrospective data on 414 tibial fractures regardless of injury energy level, investigators in a series involving higher-energy tibial plateau fractures (Schatzker VI or medial condyle fracture-dislocations) found a 27% rate of ACS in 67 fractures.[9] Radiographic risk factors predicting ACS in plateau fractures were examined in a 2013 study.[10] Femoral translation with respect to the tibia and the width of the plateau was measured in relation to the femoral condyles on the AP radiograph.[10] An increased risk of experiencing ACS in plateau fractures with increased femoral translation ($P = 0.004$) was shown in the multivariate model; however, the width of the plateau was a significant predictor only in the univariate calculations.[10] In a study of 938 civilian ballistic skeletal injuries, fractures of the tibia and fibula had a rate of ACS more than four times higher ($P < 0.001$) than that of all the other fractures.[11] ACS in these ballistic injuries was also significantly more common in those with proximal tibia and fibula fractures,[11] perhaps alerting clinicians that these injuries should require increased vigilance for ACS. A recent analysis involving information from the

Neither Dr. Doro nor any immediate family member has received anything of value from or has stock or stock options held in a commercial company or institution related directly or indirectly to the subject of this chapter.

National Trauma Data Bank identified 364 patients with isolated ACS of the foot.[12] The highest incidence of ACS of the foot was noted in patients with a forefoot injury plus a crush injury (18%) and patients with a midfoot injury plus a crush injury (21%).[12] This was followed by patients with a crush injury alone (14%).[12] Also of note was that only 1% of isolated calcaneus fractures in the cohort of 2,481 were managed with fasciotomy for ACS of the foot.[12] Because of the overall higher volume of forefoot injuries among the patients who underwent fasciotomies, one-third had isolated forefoot injuries, and this increased to almost two-thirds when nonisolated forefoot injuries were considered.[12]

Updates in Diagnosis

Many surgeons consider clinical examination, when possible, to be the benchmark for diagnosis of ACS. Clinicians also commonly use intracompartmental pressure readings alone or as an adjunct for diagnosis.[13] However, concerning discrepancies exist with these current diagnostic methods. One study reported on a group of seven orthopaedic surgeons at a high-volume level I trauma center who treated 386 tibial fractures across 2 years. The rate of fasciotomies varied from 2% to 24% among surgeons ($P < 0.005$),[4] perhaps indicating wide variation in diagnostic criteria between clinicians even though they were all operating in the same practice environment. Another study in a cadaver model demonstrating the ability to identify the elevated compartment pressure via palpation had a sensitivity of only 24% and a specificity of 55%, thus bringing into question another component of the physical examination.[14] Few rigorous data exist regarding the efficacy of various aspects of the clinical examination. The sequelae of fasciotomies include sensory changes, swelling, muscle herniation, tethered scars, cosmetic issues,[15] and increased infection when combined with tibial plateau open reduction and internal fixation (odds ratio, 3.81; $P = 0.01$).[16] Given the morbidity of fasciotomies and the desire to avoid unnecessary emergency surgery, there is great interest in identifying better diagnostic methods for ACS.

Intracompartmental Pressure Measurements

Typical modern invasive methods for determining compartment pressure include a slit catheter,[13] a solid-state transducer intracompartmental catheter (STIC), a transducer-tipped catheter, and an 18-gauge needle with an arterial-line transducer.[17] The authors of a 2010 study compared the three of these methods prospectively in 97 muscle compartments (26 patients) suspected to have ACS. They reported an intraclass correlation coefficient of 0.83 (range, 0.77–0.88) with differences between pressure measurements exceeding 10 mm Hg 27% of the time. Their conclusion was the "methods were similar but not completely reliable."[17] In contrast to previous reports,[18] 2012 data demonstrated that in a controlled laboratory setting, an 18-gauge needle was as accurate as other terminal devices (side-port needle and slit catheters).[19] Adding more ambiguity to the use of hand-held pressure monitors, one study using a cadaver model showed wide interobserver variability.[20] Using an indwelling slit catheter as a control, 38 physicians measured lower-leg compartments using a hand-held monitor. When proper technique was used, only 60% of the measurements were within 5 mm Hg of the control measurement. Thirty percent of the participants made catastrophic technique errors (anatomic errors, improper setup, improper zeroing) that led to only 22% of the measurements in this group being within 5 mm Hg of the control.[20] In a 2014 study, there was improvement in the error rate among residents comparing measurements they made before and after receiving educational instruction when using a STIC device in a cadaver model.[21] This has obvious implications for resident training.

Change in Pressure Threshold

The use of measured intracompartmental pressure as a threshold for fasciotomy was first reported in 1975.[22] A more recent classic study in 1996[23] reported on a series of patients showing that a difference of less than 30 mm Hg between the diastolic pressure and the intracompartmental pressure (change in pressure [ΔP] <30) could be considered a safe threshold for fasciotomy. In 2013, a retrospective review was published on continuous monitoring in 850 patients, of whom 152 underwent fasciotomy. A sensitivity of 94% and a specificity of 98% using the ΔP <30 threshold were reported.[13] However, these findings must be interpreted with some caution, as the authors proposed a new, subjective preferred gold standard for their analysis. Their diagnosis was considered correct if the surgeon noted escape of muscles during fasciotomy with discoloration or necrosis, which is, of course, difficult to determine in a retrospective review. The diagnosis was considered incorrect if the wound was able to be closed in 48 hours. The latter definition awaits validation, and it may be problematic for clinicians who do not routinely take ACS patients back to the operating room at 48 hours. This may also be problematic in other situations in which closure is not possible because of swelling or soft-tissue conditions unrelated to ACS.

Recent literature questions the ΔP <30 threshold dogma. Single intracompartmental pressure was prospectively measured in 48 consecutive patients who had tibial fractures and no clinical signs of ACS on presentation or after being followed prospectively for 6 months. The authors reported a 35% false-positive rate of diagnosing ACS if a preoperative pressure measurements threshold of ΔP <30 had been used alone.[24] Similarly, compartment pressure was measured in 41 children with forearm fractures. Twenty-nine of these patients had ΔP <30 and six had ΔP <10, although none of these patients was found to have any signs or symptoms of ACS.[25] Another interesting finding in this study was that in the control, uninjured arm, 21 patients had a ΔP <30 in at least one compartment.[25] These findings raise concern for a significant false-positive rate associated with the practice of relying on the ΔP <30 threshold alone, particularly for a single measurement in time. However, it appears that the ΔP <30 threshold is likely conservative, in that patients outside it are unlikely to have ACS at that time.

Continuous Versus Single Pressure Measurements

The recommendations regarding continuous or single pressure measurements continue to conflict. In the classic 1996 study,[23] given the authors' findings of high reported sensitivity and specificity in ACS diagnosis, it was recommended that continuous intracompartmental monitoring be performed for all patients with tibial fractures who are at risk for ACS.[13] However, several authors have disagreed with this conclusion.[26-28]

The authors of another study randomized 200 consecutive patients with tibial fractures into groups receiving either continuous pressure monitoring or routine clinical care.[26] Interestingly, all five cases of ACS were in the nonmonitored group. Three were diagnosed preoperatively and two postoperatively. There were no cases of late sequelae or missed cases of ACS in either group at 6-month follow-up. The authors concluded that continuous monitoring was not cost-effective and did not improve outcomes.[26] A second research group had a similar conclusion. One hundred nine consecutive patients with tibial fractures were enrolled and evaluated prospectively with continuous monitoring.[27] They were compared to a historical control group of the 109 patients seen previously. No significant differences were found in fasciotomy rate, time to fasciotomy, or complications.[27] There is not enough evidence to definitively recommend continuous monitoring, and the topic remains controversial.[28]

Near-Infrared Spectroscopy

Near-infrared spectroscopy (NIRS) relies on the difference in absorption of near-infrared wavelengths of light (600–1,000 nm) in biologic tissue. The wavelengths can pass through skin, soft tissue, and bone but are absorbed by hemoglobin. The absorption characteristics differ between oxyhemoglobin and deoxyhemoglobin and can be used to estimate oxygenation 2 to 3 cm below the skin surface.[29] This technology is FDA-approved for noninvasive monitoring of cerebral and somatic tissue perfusion.[30] Although NIRS has been described in the literature for use in ACS evaluation since the late 1990s,[30] it still has not gained clinical acceptance. Several reasons may account for this. In a normal response to trauma, a limb usually becomes hyperemic and has a corresponding increase in oxygenation that is seen with NIRS evaluation.[29] Therefore, a lack of hyperemia on NIRS may indicate ACS or lack of a significant injury. In other words, when a normal NIRS reading is obtained in a clinical setting, ACS can be missed because of the blunted normal hyperemia. Other issues may include effects of skin pigmentation, subcutaneous fat, calibration of the device, and depth of penetration with the NIRS sensor. Nonetheless, NIRS has the potential to be an excellent noninvasive tool for ACS evaluation. NIRS was used to evaluate 14 patients in whom ACS was diagnosed (pressure readings within 30 mm Hg of diastole).[31] In compartments with a perfusion gradient less than or equal to 10 mm Hg, average decreases in perfusion of 10.1%, 10.1%, 9.4%, and 16.3% were found in the anterior, lateral, deep posterior, and superficial deep compartments, respectively, as compared with the uninjured contralateral leg. The difference in NIRS values in the injured leg minus those in the uninjured leg was found to positively correlate to compartment perfusion gradient. This finding was statistically significant ($r = 0.82$ anterior, 0.65 lateral, 0.67 deep posterior, 0.62 superficial posterior; $P < 0.05$). The authors concluded that NIRS may be capable of aiding in diagnosis of ACS. Further work is needed and is under way to define the role of NIRS in diagnosing ACS.

Biomarkers

The use of biomarkers in ACS is another area that could provide an objective and accurate diagnosis. In a retrospective analysis, 58 patients who had isolated tibial and fibular fractures without ACS were compared with 39 patients who had extremity ACS. The authors analyzed blood urea nitrogen, bicarbonate, calcium, chloride, creatine kinase (CK), glycopeptide, lactate, potassium, and sodium serum values in each group. In the multivariate analysis, maximum levels of CK >4,000 U/L, chloride >104 mg/dL, and blood urea nitrogen <10 mg/dL had an odds ratio of 49.4 ($P = 0.0061$) for ACS. This study was limited by its retrospective nature and missing data; however, it demonstrated the need to study these markers more closely to determine if they might aid in ACS diagnosis.[32]

The authors of a 2014 study evaluated lactate levels in the femoral vein in 55 patients who had acute femoral artery embolism. The samples were taken before and after re-perfusion. The patients were followed up postoperatively, and 13 had a diagnosis of ACS. Although this was a vascular injury and not a typical orthopaedic injury, the authors were able to show a statistical difference in lactate levels between the patients in whom ACS developed and those in whom it did not ($P < 0.001$).[33]

In a canine model, intracompartmental glucose was measured after an ACS was created. In this study, intramuscular glucose concentration rapidly identified muscle ischemia with high sensitivity and specificity after compartment syndrome was experimentally created in this animal model,[34] demonstrating yet another potential marker that could be used in diagnosing ACS.

Other Diagnostic Tools

MRI, scintigraphy, and laser Doppler flowmetry are some of the diagnostic tools used for ACS diagnosis.[35] Drawbacks related to these modalities include decreased specificity, limited availability, and increased time required to evaluate patients. Ultrasonography has also been used in an attempt to evaluate ACS.[36] Pulsed phase-locked loop ultrasound uses reflection off fascial planes to identify ACS. This method relies on a characteristic waveform from local arterial pulsation that is altered in ACS. In a porcine model, authors using this ultrasound technique were able to correlate fascial displacement to compartment perfusion pressure.[37] A relationship between the pressure and fascial displacement was reproduced in an in vitro model.[38] A research group used this technique in healthy adults.[39] The intracompartmental pressure was elevated with blood pressure cuffs covering the leg from the knee to the ankle. Although this model was not ideal, sensitivity and specificity were reportedly as high as 0.77 and 0.93, respectively.[39] This technology offers many advantages: It is noninvasive and can monitor four compartments simultaneously. More research will be needed to define the role and efficacy of this promising technique in ACS diagnosis.

Updates in Treatment

Current treatment of ACS requires a rapid fasciotomy to restore perfusion to the injured compartment. A typical example of this is shown in **Figure 1**. For the lower leg, both a dual-incision[40] and a single-incision technique have been described.[41] The authors of a 2013 study evaluated 141 patients at a level I trauma center who had tibial fractures that were treated for ACS. Ninety-five patients had single-incision fasciotomies and 46 had dual incisions. The authors were not able to show any difference in infection or nonunion rates; they concluded that either technique was safe and that the choice should be based on the patient's condition, the surgeon's comfort, or both.[42] Unfortunately, the authors of this study did not evaluate or compare any functional parameters in these patients.[42]

Recommendation for treatment of ACS in the foot has traditionally been surgical decompression.[43,44] More recently, delayed treatment of ACS of the foot has been suggested as a possible alternative to immediate decompression.[45] This concept theoretically minimizes the soft-tissue coverage issues and possible infections after decompression and instead deals with the resulting lesser toe deformities, cavus deformities, neuropathic pain, and secondary ulcerations.[45] However, there are no studies in which researchers have compared these treatment methods. Surgeons should use caution in purposely delaying treatment. In their review of ACS in the foot, the authors concluded that complications of decompression "pale in comparison to complications of delayed treatment."[43] Another group of investigators prospectively followed, for an average of 24 months, 14 patients who had ACS of the foot and decompression.[46] They found no infections; in addition, they found that the time to fasciotomy was 4.6 hours in the patients with no complications and 8 hours in the patients with complications ($P = 0.05$).[46] Because of the lack of data, purposeful delay in treatment is not recommended. Finally, several authors have advocated for dermal fenestration or "pie crusting" the dorsal foot.[47,48] This technique has obvious merits in that additional closure methods are not needed and closed underlying fractures are not converted to exposed fractures. Again, follow-up studies are needed to show how this technique compares with traditional fasciotomies.

Ultrafiltration is another proposed treatment of ACS that has been described.[49] This technique requires inserting a catheter into the concerning compartment and applying negative pressure. Removal of excess fluid theoretically could improve perfusion and decrease fasciotomy rates. Initially, in a porcine model, the authors showed decreased pressure and improved histology in the ACS-affected limbs treated with ultrafiltration.[49] Later, in a pilot study of 10 patients with tibial fractures treated with intramedullary nails, the authors showed the safety of the device in human use.[50] They were able to show reasonable correlation between their ultrafiltration catheter pressure readings and conventional pressure measurement.[50] Another feature of this technique is its allowance for analysis of the ultrafiltrate. The authors found significant increases in levels of CK and lactate from the intracompartmental filtrate over serum levels. This feature could also prove to be a useful diagnostic tool.[50]

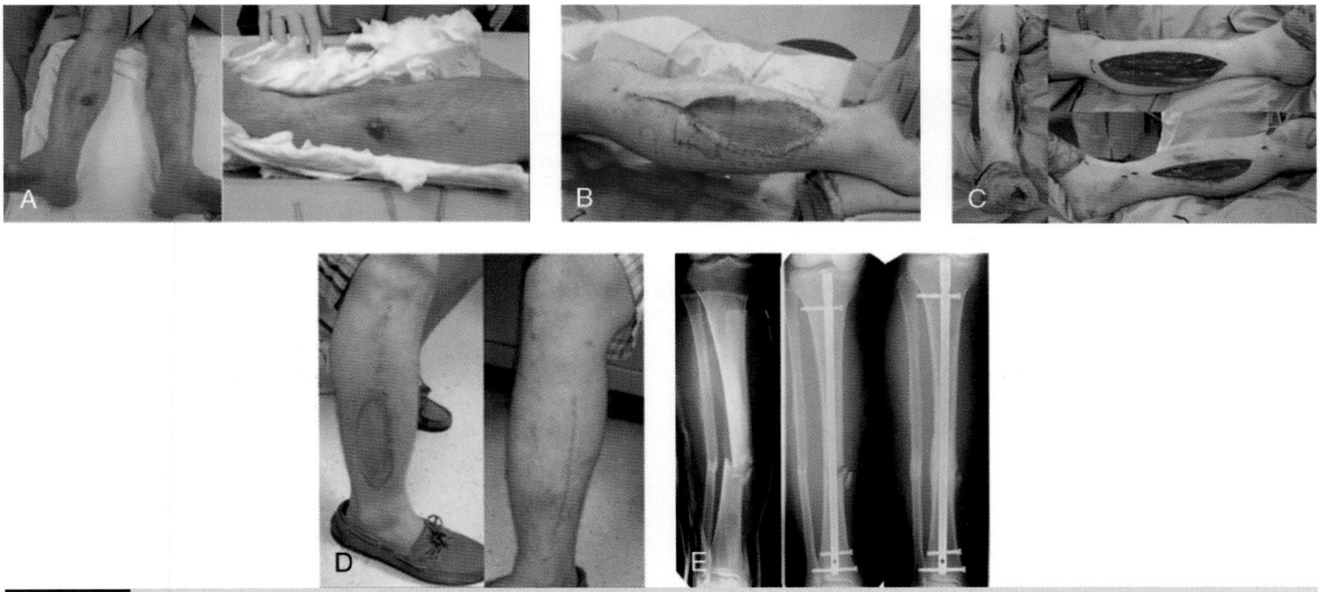

Figure 1 Clinical photographs and radiographs depict a typical case of acute compartment syndrome. The patient is a middle-aged man who sustained a sports-related diaphyseal tibia and fibula fracture. **A**, Clinical photographs demonstrate the evolving fracture blisters, swollen limb, and taut skin compared to the contralateral side. The closure of the wounds required split-thickness skin grafting laterally and delayed primary closure medially (**B**). The postoperative images show the appearance of the limb after adequate two-incision fasciotomy (**C**). The final images show the limb 1 year after the injury (**D**). The radiographs of the case are provided showing the injury films, postoperative films, and the 1-year follow-up films (**E**). (Photographs and images courtesy of Gerald Lang, MD)

Although ACS is often thought to be predominantly a result of perfusion and ischemia, there may also be an important inflammatory component to the disease process. Although re-perfusion is known to play a role in propagating cellular damage and apoptosis, it is unclear to what extent these processes affect ACS patients. In a rat model, the authors elevated intracompartmental pressures, and they used videomicroscopy to quantify inflammatory response and microcirculation.[51] A substantial increase in activated leukocytes and a decrease in the continuously perfused capillaries was seen.[51] These studies were repeated with this model, and the animals were administered indomethacin at time points after the ACS creation. The authors were able to detect significantly less cellular damage and improved perfusion in the indomethacin group. The apoptosis rate, however, was not affected.[52] These studies are limited to rat models, and the ACS was created for 90 minutes or less. Typically, clinically significant muscle damage occurs in humans after 6 to 8 hours; it is unclear if there are any relevant changes at the cellular level in subclinical ischemic time. Although it is unknown what effects indomethacin would have in true ACS, these preliminary reports suggest that this treatment warrants additional investigation.

Summary

The diagnosis and treatment of ACS continues to challenge clinicians. More research is needed for reliable, affordable, and rapid methods of obtaining an objective diagnosis of ACS. An important limitation of current clinical research is that there is yet no validated objective measure of the diagnosis of compartment syndrome, which makes it difficult to validate any diagnostic tools. Controversy continues to exist regarding the use of intracompartmental pressures in CS diagnosis. Some researchers have cautioned against the use of single intracompartmental measurement of $\Delta P < 30$ as a threshold for diagnosis, as this may lead to unnecessary fasciotomies. There is still no definitive evidence that continuous monitoring is superior to noncontinuous monitoring or other techniques. NIRS, biomarkers, and ultrasound all have potential advantages and could improve diagnosis of ACS, although more research is required. Ultrafiltration and anti-inflammatory agents may play a treatment role in the future, but for now the benchmark standard of ACS treatment is still emergent fasciotomy for the lower leg through either single or dual fasciotomies. Although most of the data and current studies relate to the lower leg, it is reasonable to apply these principles of diagnosis and treatment to all of the body's osteofascial compartments, including the foot, at this time.

Key Study Points

- ACS is a clinical emergency that requires urgent decompression.
- Using an intracompartmental pressure measurement is still the current standard for evaluation in patients where an adequate clinical exam is not possible.
- The reader should understand the limitations of relying on the $\Delta P < 30$ threshold.
- Newer diagnostic and therapeutic agents are currently being evaluated; however, none have shown superiority over clinical examination, pressure measurements (when applicable), or fasciotomies at this time.

Annotated References

1. Volkmann R: Die Krankheiten der Bewegungsorgane [Diseases of the musculoskeletal system], in von Pitha FR, Billroth T, eds: Handbuch der allgemeinen und speziellen Chirurgie. Stuttgart, Germany: Ferdinand Enke, 1865, vol 2, pp 234–920.

2. Crespo AM, Manoli A III, Konda SR, Egol KA: Development of Compartment Syndrome Negatively Impacts Length of Stay and Cost After Tibia Fracture. *J Orthop Trauma* 2015;29(7):312-315.

   The authors performed a retrospective review of New York State hospital admissions from 2001 to 2011. They identified 33,629 patients with tibial shaft fractures, 692 in whom ACS eventually developed. ACS more than doubled the length of stay and hospital charges. Level of evidence: IV (economic and diagnostic).

3. Schmidt AH: The impact of compartment syndrome on hospital length of stay and charges among adult patients admitted with a fracture of the tibia. *J Orthop Trauma* 2011;25(6):355-357.

   The author performed a retrospective review of admissions to a Level I trauma center. Forty-six patients with tibial shaft fractures were identified; ACS developed in five of them. ACS tripled the length of stay and more than doubled hospital charges. Level of evidence: III (therapeutic).

4. O'Toole RV, Whitney A, Merchant N, et al: Variation in diagnosis of compartment syndrome by surgeons treating tibial shaft fractures. *J Trauma* 2009;67(4):735-741.

5. Shore BJ, Glotzbecker MP, Zurakowski D, Gelbard E, Hedequist DJ, Matheney TH: Acute compartment syndrome in children and teenagers with tibial shaft fractures: Incidence and multivariable risk factors. *J Orthop Trauma* 2013;27(11):616-621.

   The authors reviewed 212 pediatric patients with 216 tibial shaft fractures. The rate of pediatric tibial fractures with ACS was 11.6%, with the highest risk in children 14 years and older. The other independent predictor for ACS, besides age, was a motor vehicle accident. Level of evidence: III (prognostic).

6. Park S, Ahn J, Gee AO, Kuntz AF, Esterhai JL: Compartment syndrome in tibial fractures. *J Orthop Trauma* 2009;23(7):514-518.

7. Shadgan B, Pereira G, Menon M, Jafari S, Darlene Reid W, O'Brien PJ: Risk factors for acute compartment syndrome of the leg associated with tibial diaphyseal fractures in adults. *J Orthop Traumatol* 2015;16(3):185-192.

   The authors retrospectively reviewed 1,125 adult patients with tibial fractures. They found that younger patients were at a significantly higher risk of developing ACS after a tibial diaphyseal fracture. Male sex, open fracture, and intramedullary nailing were not shown to be risk factors for ACS. Level of evidence: IV (prognostic).

8. McQueen MM, Duckworth AD, Aitken SA, Sharma RA, Court-Brown CM: Predictors of compartment syndrome after tibial fracture. *J Orthop Trauma* 2015;29(10):451-455.

   The authors performed a retrospective analysis of 1,407 patients with diaphyseal tibial fractures, of whom 160 had ACS. As this group has published in the past, univariate analysis showed age, sex, blue-collar occupation, sporting injury, treatment with intramedullary nails, and fracture classification all were predictive of ACS. However, in the multivariate analysis, patient age of 12 to 29 years was the strongest predictor of ACS ($P < 0.001$). Level of evidence: II (prognostic).

9. Stark E, Stucken C, Trainer G, Tornetta P III: Compartment syndrome in Schatzker type VI plateau fractures and medial condylar fracture-dislocations treated with temporary external fixation. *J Orthop Trauma* 2009;23(7):502-506.

10. Ziran BH, Becher SJ: Radiographic predictors of compartment syndrome in tibial plateau fractures. *J Orthop Trauma* 2013;27(11):612-615.

    The authors retrospectively analyzed radiographic parameters in 158 patients with 162 plateau fractures. They measured femoral translation and tibial width in these injuries. ACS was associated with increased femoral translation. Tibial plateau width and ACS was correlated only in the univariate analysis. Level of evidence: II (prognostic).

11. Meskey T, Hardcastle J, O'Toole RV: Are certain fractures at increased risk for compartment syndrome after civilian ballistic injury? *J Trauma* 2011;71(5):1385-1389.

    The authors retrospectively reviewed 650 patients with 938 fractures resulting from gunshot wounds. In ballistic skeletal injuries among civilian patients, tibial or fibular fractures had risk factor of 4.1 and 4.2, respectively ($P < 0.001$) of developing ACS compared to all the other ballistic fractures. The study also showed fractures of the proximal third of the tibia or fibula were more likely to develop ACS when compared to respective middle and distal fractures ($P < 0.03$ fibula and $P < 0.01$ tibia). Level of evidence: II (prognostic).

12. Thakur NA, McDonnell M, Got CJ, Arcand N, Spratt KF, DiGiovanni CW: Injury patterns causing isolated foot compartment syndrome. *J Bone Joint Surg Am* 2012;94(11):1030-1035.

    The authors in this study used the National Trauma Data Bank to identify 364 patients who had an isolated foot ACS. The highest incidence of foot ACS was noted in patients with a forefoot injury plus a crush injury (18%) and patients with a midfoot injury plus a crush injury (21%). This was followed by patients with a crush injury alone (14%). Only 1% of isolated fractures of the calcaneus in their cohort of 2,481 underwent fasciotomy for foot ACS. In patients who underwent fasciotomies, one-third had isolated forefoot injuries; this increased to almost two-thirds when non-isolated forefoot injuries were considered. Level of evidence: II (prognostic).

13. McQueen MM, Duckworth AD, Aitken SA, Court-Brown CM: The estimated sensitivity and specificity of compartment pressure monitoring for acute compartment syndrome. *J Bone Joint Surg Am* 2013;95(8):673-677.

    The authors retrospectively reviewed 850 patients with tibial fractures, 152 of whom underwent fasciotomies to treat ACS. The sensitivity of continuous pressure monitoring for ACS was 94%, with an estimated specificity of 98%. Level of evidence: I (diagnostic).

14. Shuler FD, Dietz MJ: Physicians' ability to manually detect isolated elevations in leg intracompartmental pressure. *J Bone Joint Surg Am* 2010;92(2):361-367.

    The authors created an artificially elevated compartment pressure in cadaver lower legs. After this, clinicians were asked to palpate the limbs to determine if there was elevated pressure. They found the manual detection of the compartment firmness pressure was poor.

15. Fitzgerald AM, Gaston P, Wilson Y, Quaba A, McQueen MM: Long-term sequelae of fasciotomy wounds. *Br J Plast Surg* 2000;53(8):690-693.

16. Morris BJ, Unger RZ, Archer KR, Mathis SL, Perdue AM, Obremskey WT: Risk factors of infection after ORIF of bicondylar tibial plateau fractures. *J Orthop Trauma* 2013;27(9):e196-e200.

    This was a retrospective review of 302 AO/OTA 41-C fractures. Revision surgery became necessary for 14% of patients in whom deep infections developed and 28% after undergoing definitive fixation. Risk factors for infection were open fracture (odds ratio [OR]), 3.44; $P = 0.003$); smoking (OR, 2.40; $P = 0.02$); fractures requiring two incisions and two plates (OR, 3.19; $P = 0.01$); and finally compartment syndrome requiring fasciotomy (OR, 3.81; $P = 0.01$). Level of evidence: II (prognostic).

17. Collinge C, Kuper M: Comparison of three methods for measuring intracompartmental pressure in injured limbs of trauma patients. *J Orthop Trauma* 2010;24(6):364-368.

    The authors compared a solid-state transducer intracompartmental catheter, a transducer-tipped catheter, and an 18-gauge needle with an A-line transducer prospectively in 97 muscle compartments (26 patients) suspected to have ACS. They reported an interclass correlation correction coefficient of 0.83 (range, 0.77–0.88), with differences between ratings exceeding 10 mm Hg 27% of the time. Level of evidence: I (diagnostic).

18. Boody AR, Wongworawat MD: Accuracy in the measurement of compartment pressures: A comparison of three commonly used devices. *J Bone Joint Surg Am* 2005;87(11):2415-2422.

19. Hammerberg EM, Whitesides TE Jr, Seiler JG III: The reliability of measurement of tissue pressure in compartment syndrome. *J Orthop Trauma* 2012;26(9):e166, author reply e166.

    The authors created an in vitro ACS model and tested several terminal devices. The side-ported needle, slit catheter, and 18-gauge bevel-tipped needle were found to measure equivalent pressure when compared statistically.

20. Large TM, Agel J, Holtzman DJ, Benirschke SK, Krieg JC: Interobserver variability in the measurement of lower leg compartment pressures. *J Orthop Trauma* 2015;29(7):316-321.

    The authors used a cadaver model to demonstrate a wide interobserver variability. An indwelling slit catheter served as a control; 38 physicians measured lower leg compartments by means of a handheld monitor. With the use of proper technique, only 60% of the measurements were within 5 mm Hg of the control measurement. Nearly one-third—30%—of the participants made catastrophic technique errors that led to only 22% of the measurements in this group being within 5 mm Hg of the control. Common errors included anatomic errors, improper set-up, and improper zeroing.

21. Morris MR, Harper BL, Hetzel S, et al: The effect of focused instruction on orthopaedic surgery residents' ability to objectively measure intracompartmental pressures in a compartment syndrome model. *J Bone Joint Surg Am* 2014;96(19):e171.

    The authors compared pressure measurements performed by residents before and after receiving educational instruction when using a STIC device in a cadaver model. They showed an improvement in the resident error rates.

22. Whitesides TE, Haney TC, Morimoto K, Harada H: Tissue pressure measurements as a determinant for the need of fasciotomy. *Clin Orthop Relat Res* 1975;113:43-51.

23. McQueen MM, Court-Brown CM: Compartment monitoring in tibial fractures. The pressure threshold for decompression. *J Bone Joint Surg Br* 1996;78(1):99-104.

24. Whitney A, O'Toole RV, Hui E, et al: Do one-time intracompartmental pressure measurements have a high false-positive rate in diagnosing compartment syndrome? *J Trauma Acute Care Surg* 2014;76(2):479-483.

The authors measured compartment pressures in 48 patients with tibial fractures who had no signs of ACS. They found a 35% false-positive diagnosis rate in patients who were not thought to have compartment syndrome by using a pressure-measurement criterion of $\Delta P < 30$ mm Hg. Level of evidence: II (diagnostic).

25. Tharakan SJ, Subotic U, Kalisch M, Staubli G, Weber DM: Compartment pressures in children with normal and fractured forearms: A preliminary report. *J Pediatr Orthop* 2015. [Epub ahead of print].

The authors prospectively studied 41 children aged 16 or younger who had forearm fractures that needed reduction with or without surgery. The patients' compartment pressures were measured by means of needle manometry. None of the patients had any signs of acute compartment syndrome. Some children tolerated absolute pressures of >30 mm Hg and 29 patients had a $\Delta P < 30$ mm Hg without clinical signs of ACS. Level of evidence: I (prognostic).

26. Harris IA, Kadir A, Donald G: Continuous compartment pressure monitoring for tibia fractures: Does it influence outcome? *J Trauma* 2006;60(6):1330-1335, discussion 1335.

27. Al-Dadah OQ, Darrah C, Cooper A, Donell ST, Patel AD: Continuous compartment pressure monitoring vs. clinical monitoring in tibial diaphyseal fractures. *Injury* 2008;39(10):1204-1209.

28. Giannoudis PV, Tzioupis C, Pape HC: Editorial: Early diagnosis of tibial compartment syndrome. Continuous pressure measurement or not? *Injury* 2009;40(4):341-342.

29. Shuler MS, Reisman WM, Whitesides TE Jr, et al: Near-infrared spectroscopy in lower extremity trauma. *J Bone Joint Surg Am* 2009;91(6):1360-1368.

30. Harvey EJ, Sanders DW, Shuler MS, et al: What's new in acute compartment syndrome? *J Orthop Trauma* 2012;26(12):699-702.

The authors provide a review of newer developments regarding acute compartment syndrome. Topics covered include anti-inflammatory agents, ultrafiltration, near-infrared spectroscopy, and radiofrequency identification chips.

31. Shuler MS, Reisman WM, Kinsey TL, et al: Correlation between muscle oxygenation and compartment pressures in acute compartment syndrome of the leg. *J Bone Joint Surg Am* 2010;92(4):863-870.

The authors used NIRS to evaluate 14 patients diagnosed with ACS. The authors found that compartments with a perfusion gradient of ≤10 mm Hg had less perfusion than did compartments in the uninjured contralateral leg. They also showed that difference in NIRS value in the injured leg minus that in the uninjured leg was positively correlated to compartment perfusion gradient ($P < 0.05$). Level of evidence: IV (diagnostic).

32. Valdez C, Schroeder E, Amdur R, Pascual J, Sarani B: Serum creatine kinase levels are associated with extremity compartment syndrome. *J Trauma Acute Care Surg* 2013;74(2):441-445, discussion 445-447.

In this retrospective analysis, 58 patients with isolated tibial and fibular fractures without ACS were compared with 39 patients who had extremity ACS. The authors analyzed blood urea nitrogen, bicarbonate, calcium, chloride, creatine kinase, glycopeptide, lactate, potassium, and sodium serum values in each group. In their multivariate analysis, maximum levels of CK >4,000 U/L, chloride > 104 mg/dL, and blood urea nitrogen <10 mg/dL had an odds ratio of 49.4 (3.0–802.6) ($P = 0.0061$) for predicting ACS. This study was limited by its retrospective nature and missing data; however, it demonstrated the need to study these markers more closely to determine if they might aid in ACS diagnosis. Level of evidence: III (diagnostic).

33. Mitas P, Vejrazka M, Hruby J, et al: Prediction of compartment syndrome based on analysis of biochemical parameters. *Ann Vasc Surg* 2014;28(1):170-177.

The authors studied lactate levels in the femoral vein in 55 patients who had acute femoral artery embolism. The samples were taken before and after re-perfusion. The patients were followed up postoperatively, and ACS was diagnosed in 13. A statistical difference in lactate levels was shown in the patients in whom ACS versus those in whom ACS did not develop. Level of evidence: II (diagnostic).

34. Doro CJ, Sitzman TJ, O'Toole RV: Can intramuscular glucose levels diagnose compartment syndrome? *J Trauma Acute Care Surg* 2014;76(2):474-478.

The authors used a canine ACS model to measure intracompartmental glucose concentration. The results showed that intramuscular glucose concentration rapidly identified muscle ischemia with high sensitivity and specificity in experimentally created compartment syndrome.

35. Shadgan B, Menon M, O'Brien PJ, Reid WD: Diagnostic techniques in acute compartment syndrome of the leg. *J Orthop Trauma* 2008;22(8):581-587.

36. Wiemann JM, Ueno T, Leek BT, Yost WT, Schwartz AK, Hargens AR: Noninvasive measurements of intramuscular pressure using pulsed phase-locked loop ultrasound for detecting compartment syndromes: A preliminary report. *J Orthop Trauma* 2006;20(7):458-463.

37. Garabekyan T, Murphey GC, Macias BR, Lynch JE, Hargens AR: New noninvasive ultrasound technique for monitoring perfusion pressure in a porcine model of acute compartment syndrome. *J Orthop Trauma* 2009;23(3):186-193, discussion 193-194.

38. Sellei RM, Hingmann SJ, Kobbe P, et al: Compartment elasticity measured by pressure-related ultrasound to determine patients "at risk" for compartment syndrome: An experimental in vitro study. *Patient Saf Surg* 2015;9(1):4.

The authors used an in vitro ACS model to test ultrasound elastography. A relationship between the compartment pressure and displacement was found.

39. Lynch JE, Lynch JK, Cole SL, Carter JA, Hargens AR: Noninvasive monitoring of elevated intramuscular pressure in a model compartment syndrome via quantitative fascial motion. *J Orthop Res* 2009;27(4):489-494.

40. Mubarak SJ, Owen CA: Double-incision fasciotomy of the leg for decompression in compartment syndromes. *J Bone Joint Surg Am* 1977;59(2):184-187.

41. Maheshwari R, Taitsman LA, Barei DP: Single-incision fasciotomy for compartmental syndrome of the leg in patients with diaphyseal tibial fractures. *J Orthop Trauma* 2008;22(10):723-730.

42. Bible JE, McClure DJ, Mir HR: Analysis of single-incision versus dual-incision fasciotomy for tibial fractures with acute compartment syndrome. *J Orthop Trauma* 2013;27(11):607-611.

The authors evaluated 141 patients who had tibial fractures that were treated for ACS. Ninety-five had single-incision fasciotomies and 46 had dual incisions. The authors were not able to show any difference in infection or nonunion rates and concluded that either technique was safe and should be based on the patient's condition, the surgeon's comfort, or both. Level of evidence: III.

43. Ojike NI, Roberts CS, Giannoudis PV: Foot compartment syndrome: A systematic review of the literature. *Acta Orthop Belg* 2009;75(5):573-580.

44. Fulkerson E, Razi A, Tejwani N: Review: Acute compartment syndrome of the foot. *Foot Ankle Int* 2003;24(2):180-187.

45. Dodd A, Le I: Foot compartment syndrome: Diagnosis and management. *J Am Acad Orthop Surg* 2013;21(11):657-664.

The authors review the pathophysiology, anatomy, diagnosis, and management of foot compartment syndrome.

46. Han F, Daruwalla ZJ, Shen L, Kumar VP: A prospective study of surgical outcomes and quality of life in severe foot trauma and associated compartment syndrome after fasciotomy. *J Foot Ankle Surg* 2015;54(3):417-423.

The authors prospectively followed, for an average of 24 months, 14 patients who had ACS of the foot and decompression. They had no infections and were able to show that the time to fasciotomy was 4.6 hours in patients with no complications, and 8 hours in patients with complications ($P = 0.05$). Two (14%) patients had claw-toe deformities and three (21%) had sensory defects directly attributable to ACS. Finally, the authors showed improved scores on the American Orthopaedic Foot and Ankle Society scale and Medical Outcomes Study: 36-Item Short Form, with decreased time to fasciotomy. Level of evidence: III (therapeutic).

47. Dunbar RP, Taitsman LA, Sangeorzan BJ, Hansen ST Jr: Technique tip: Use of "pie crusting" of the dorsal skin in severe foot injury. *Foot Ankle Int* 2007;28(7):851-853.

48. Poon H, Le Cocq H, Mountain AJ, Sargeant ID: Dermal fenestration with negative pressure wound therapy: A new technique for managing soft tissue injuries associated with high-energy complex foot fractures. *J Foot Ankle Surg* 2016;55(1):161-165.

The authors describe a novel technique of dermal fenestrations in a foot followed by negative pressure wound therapy in 2 patients. The authors suggest that this technique may obviate the need for formal fasciotomies and prevent fracture blisters in injured feet. Level of evidence: V (therapeutic).

49. Odland R, Schmidt AH, Hunter B, et al: Use of tissue ultrafiltration for treatment of compartment syndrome: A pilot study using porcine hindlimbs. *J Orthop Trauma* 2005;19(4):267-275.

50. Odland RM, Schmidt AH: Compartment syndrome ultrafiltration catheters: Report of a clinical pilot study of a novel method for managing patients at risk of compartment syndrome. *J Orthop Trauma* 2011;25(6):358-365.

The authors report a pilot study of 10 patients with tibial fractures treated with an intramedullary nail. An ultrafiltration catheter was placed in these patients. The authors were able to show reasonable correlation between their ultrafiltration catheter pressure readings and conventional pressure measurements. There were no adverse events using their device. They were also able to detect markedly elevated CK and lactate dehydrogenase levels compared with serum levels. Level of evidence: IV (therapeutic).

51. Lawendy AR, Sanders DW, Bihari A, Parry N, Gray D, Badhwar A: Compartment syndrome-induced microvascular dysfunction: An experimental rodent model. *Can J Surg* 2011;54(3):194-200.

The authors used a rat ACS model. Videomicroscopy was used to quantify inflammatory response and microcirculation. They were able to show a significant increase in activated leukocytes and a decrease in the continuously perfused capillaries.

52. Manjoo A, Sanders D, Lawendy A, et al: Indomethacin reduces cell damage: Shedding new light on compartment syndrome. *J Orthop Trauma* 2010;24(9):526-529.

The authors used a rat ACS model. The animals were administered indomethacin at time points after the ACS creation. The authors were able to detect significantly less cellular damage and improved perfusion in the indomethacin group. The apoptosis rate, however, was not affected.

Section 4

Upper Extremity

SECTION EDITOR

Melvin P. Rosenwasser, MD

Chapter 21

Fractures of the Clavicle and Scapula

Matthew J. Furey, MD, MSc, FRCS(C) Michael D. McKee, MD, FRCS(C)

Abstract

During the past decade, the classification and treatment of fractures of the clavicle and scapula have significantly changed. These injuries historically were treated nonsurgically, but a recent focus on patient-rated outcomes has led to a substantially increased interest in surgical management. Fractures of the middle third of the clavicle have been the subject of rigorous prospective randomized studies defining clear surgical indications, whereas medial- and lateral-third clavicle fractures have not benefited from such investigations. Research concerning the treatment of scapula fractures continues to rapidly expand and is leading to the development of evidence-based surgical indications.

Keywords: clavicle fracture; glenopolar angle; plating; intramedullary pinning; scapula fracture

Introduction

Although both scapula and clavicle fractures have historically been treated with "benign neglect," the past decade has seen a shift toward surgical management of displaced fractures of the shoulder girdle. This shift is likely caused by a variety of factors, including improved surgical technique and implants, enhanced understanding of fracture characteristics, and advancement of the scientific literature related to functional and patient-rated outcomes. Recent developments in the imaging, classification, and treatment of both clavicle and scapula fractures have helped optimize outcomes.

Clavicle Fractures

Clavicle fractures are common, accounting for as many as 9% of upper extremity fractures and 4% of all fractures.[1] These fractures are categorized by their medial-, middle-, or lateral-third anatomic location.[2] Middle-third (midshaft) fractures account for 80% to 85% of all clavicle fractures; lateral- and medial-third fractures account for 15% to 20% and zero to 5%, respectively.[3]

Middle-Third Fractures

The treatment of nondisplaced clavicle fractures primarily is nonsurgical. Treatments such as figure-of-8 bandaging and plaster casting have largely been abandoned as they are associated with pain or discomfort and have no functional or radiographic benefit over treatment with a simple sling.[4] Displaced fractures now are primarily treated surgically, in contrast to the former universally held paradigm of closed treatment. Meta-analyses of randomized studies found that surgical treatment led to significantly lower rates of nonunion, malunion, and other complications compared with nonsurgical treatment. In addition, surgical treatment led to an earlier functional return compared with nonsurgical treatment of displaced midshaft clavicle fractures.[5,6]

The evidence-based indications for surgical fixation of a midshaft clavicle fracture include at least 2 cm of radiographic shortening, displacement in a caudal-cephalad plane of at least 100% (one bone width), and significant

Dr. McKee or an immediate family member has received royalties from Elsevier and Stryker; serves as a paid consultant to or is an employee of Acumed LLC, Olympus Biotech, Synthes, and Zimmer; has received research or institutional support from Olympus Biotech, Wright Medical Technology, and Zimmer; and serves as a board member, owner, officer, or committee member of the American Shoulder and Elbow Surgeons, Orthopaedic Trauma Association, and Canadian Orthopaedic Association. Neither Dr. Furey nor any immediate family member has received anything of value from or has stock or stock options held in a commercial company or institution related directly or indirectly to the subject of this chapter.

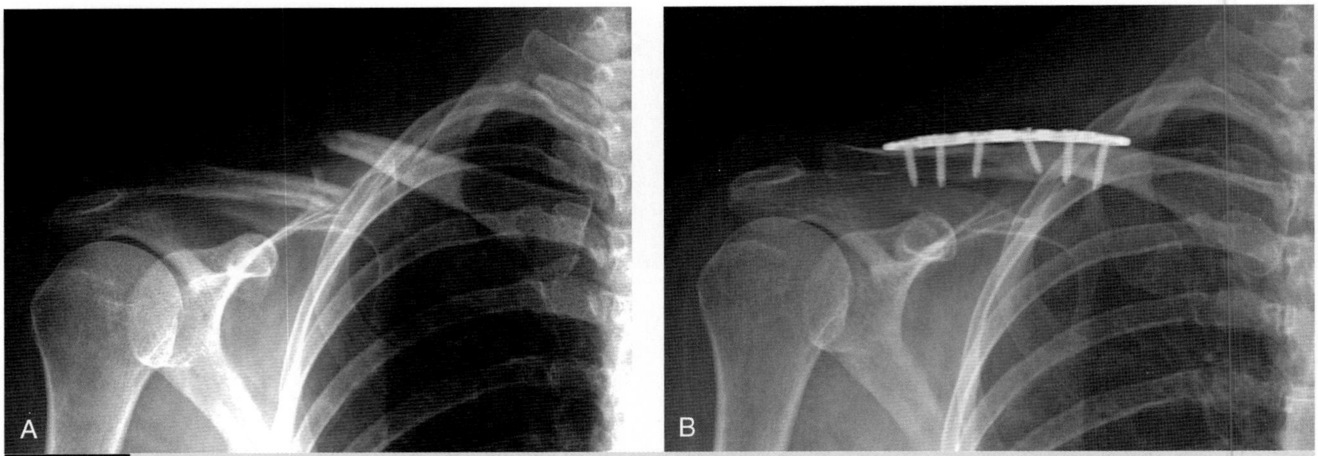

Figure 1 Upright AP clavicle radiographs showing a more than 100%-displaced middle-third clavicle fracture (**A**) and the fracture after surgical fixation with a precontoured clavicular plate (**B**).

comminution.[7,8] This amount of displacement typically appears as an asymmetric or drooping shoulder, which is an obvious clinical deformity. Surgical intervention also is indicated for an open fracture, a fracture with an underlying neurovascular injury, or a floating shoulder injury.[9]

Imaging

Radiographic imaging of the clavicle should be obtained with the patient upright and the arm positioned at the side. Positioning was found to dramatically affect measured displacement in a study in which 41% of patients had more than 100% displacement on upright but not on supine radiographs.[10] The size of this discrepancy has important implications for fracture management.

Despite good interrater and intrarater reliability of displacement and comminution measurement, radiographic measurement of shortening in midshaft clavicle fractures was found to be difficult to accurately assess.[11] Assessing the amount of shortening as a percentage of the contralateral side has been suggested; shortening of 9.7% was associated with patient-rated failure of nonsurgical treatment.[12] Although comparative methods for assessing shortening probably yield an accurate result in most patients, a demographic study found that 7% of patients had more than 1 cm of clavicular asymmetry.[13] Thus, a combination of comparative and direct methods should be used to ensure the accuracy of the diagnosis and guide fracture management. It is important to measure the length both clinically and radiographically.

Treatment

Fixation of a displaced fracture of the clavicle can be done by open plate or intramedullary pinning. Intramedullary fixation of clavicle fractures has had a resurgence in popularity. A meta-analysis of five randomized controlled studies that compared plate and intramedullary fixation found that intramedullary fixation led to fewer complications such as prominent hardware and superficial infection than open plate fixation, and Constant shoulder scores were similar (93.8 for patients who received intramedullary fixation, 89.3 for those who received plate fixation).[14] Intramedullary fixation was found to be inferior to plate fixation in terms of rotational control and axial rigidity, and it may not be sufficient in comminuted fracture patterns requiring restoration of rotatory control and axial stability.[15]

The anatomic location of plate application has been the subject of recent interest. The use of anteroinferior plating was recommended as an alternative to superior plating as well as an alternative to anterosuperior plating to decrease the risk of neurovascular injury and hardware prominence.[16] These theoretical benefits have not been substantiated by research, however. A cadaver study found no significant difference between the two techniques in hardware prominence or the distance from screw tips to neurovascular structures.[17] No association was found between plate position and reoperation rate in midshaft clavicle fractures; the overall rate of reoperation for hardware irritation was 17%.[18]

The use of precontoured clavicular plates has led to a significant reduction in hardware prominence compared with the earlier standard use of straight compression or reconstruction plates[19] (**Figure 1**). Precontoured 2.7-mm plates were found to be biomechanically superior to reconstruction plates in both load to failure and bending failure stiffness.[20,21]

Anterior chest numbness caused by injury to the branches of the suprascapular nerve during the surgical

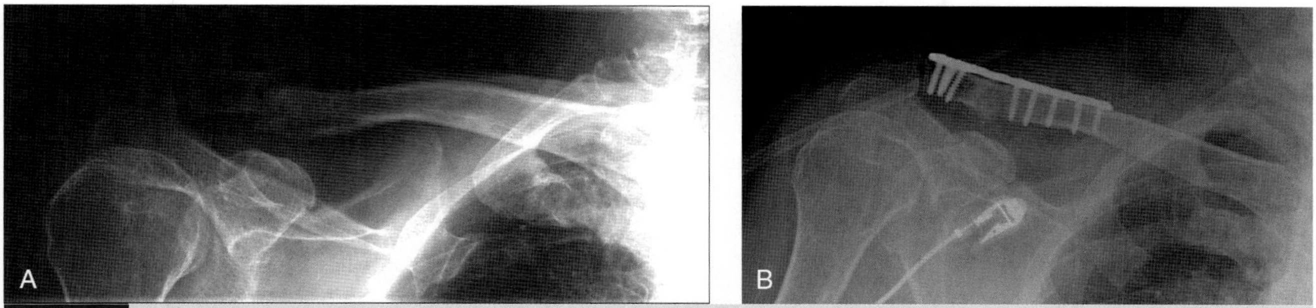

Figure 2 Upright AP clavicle radiographs showing a lateral-third clavicle nonunion in a patient with symptoms 12 months after injury (**A**) and the fracture after surgical fixation with a precontoured clavicular plate and bone grafting (**B**).

approach is a commonly reported complication of surgical fixation.[22] More than 50% of patients were found to have numbness 1 year after surgery.[23] The surgical dissection should include identifying and protecting these nerves if they were not concomitantly injured with the clavicle fracture. The functional significance of cutaneous numbness is uncertain because no correlation has been found between chest numbness and patient-rated outcomes. The risk of this complication should be included in the informed consent discussion before surgery. It remains to be seen whether patients' awareness of the risk of sensory deficit will lead to acceptance.

Medial-Third Fractures

Medial-third clavicle fractures often are not fully appreciated on plain radiographs. A case study found that 22% of patients had a fracture that could be identified only on CT; this finding suggests that these fractures often are unrecognized.[24] The research literature on the treatment of medial-third clavicle fractures is substantially less robust than that on midshaft fractures because medial-third fractures are less common. Most of these fractures can be treated without surgery despite a nonunion rate as high as 14%.[25] Although surgical fixation was found to dramatically decrease the risk of nonunion, nonunion is not correlated with a poor outcome.[26]

There are no clear indications for acute surgical treatment of a medial-third fracture. Osteosynthesis for displaced periarticular fractures has led to excellent postoperative Disabilities of the Arm, Shoulder and Hand scores.[27] Open or displaced fractures with neurovascular compromise should be surgically fixed, but other indications for internal fixation are less clear.

Lateral-Third Fractures

Despite a nonunion rate of 11% to 44% for Neer type II fractures (unstable medial-segment fractures due to either separation from or disruption of coracoclavicular ligaments), many patients with nonunion are minimally symptomatic.[25,28] Evidence-based indications are lacking for acute surgical intervention in lateral-third clavicle fractures. Reported functional outcomes of closed or open treatment are equivocal. It is prudent to treat the fracture with a sling and observation; surgery is indicated if a symptomatic nonunion develops (**Figure 2**).

Despite the lack of high-level evidence for acute surgical fixation, retrospective studies have described surgical techniques for the fixation of Neer type II lateral-third fractures.[29] Most techniques recommend anatomic reduction of the fracture and coracoclavicular ligament augmentation. A meta-analysis of surgical techniques for treatment of displaced lateral-third clavicle fractures reported an overall 98% union rate and Constant shoulder scores greater than 90.[29] Use of a hook plate was found to significantly increase the risk of complications (other than obligatory hardware removal), including acromial osteolysis, refracture, and implant failure.

Scapula Fractures

Scapula fractures occur less often than clavicle fractures, accounting for fewer than 1% of all fractures and approximately 3% to 5% of all upper extremity fractures.[2,30] The low incidence of injury to the scapula probably is attributable to the protection afforded by the surrounding musculature and the mobility of the scapula along the thoracic wall, which allows force to be dispersed, especially with a low-energy mechanism of injury.

Scapula fractures often occur with a high-energy mechanism such as a motor vehicle crash, a pedestrian–motor vehicle crash, or a fall from a height. As many as 94% of patients with a scapula fracture have associated injuries, commonly including regional thoracic injuries (rib fracture, flail chest, pneumothorax, pulmonary contusion), clavicle or pelvis fracture, or injury to the central nervous system.[31-33] One study found a concomitant brachial plexus injury in 2% of patients.[34]

Table 1

Indications for Surgical Treatment of a Scapula Fracture

Indication	Criterion
Intra-articular fracture	
Articular step-off	≥4 to 5 mm
Percentage of glenoid affected	≥20%
Glenohumeral articulation	Unstable despite closed reduction
Extra-articular fracture	
Glenopolar angle	≤20°
Lateral border offset	≥20 mm
Angulation	≥45°
Translation	≥100%

Classification

There is no universally accepted classification of scapula fractures. Two new systems, the AO Foundation–Orthopaedic Trauma Association (AO/OTA) scapula fracture classification and the New International Classification for Scapula Fractures, have been developed recently.[35,36] Earlier classification systems primarily were based on the radiographic characterization of glenoid fractures. In contrast, the AO/OTA and New International systems use advanced imaging, including CT and three-dimensional CT, and emphasize the distinction between intra-articular and extra-articular scapula fractures.

The AO/OTA system classifies a scapula fracture as extra-articular (A), partial articular (B), or total articular (C). Each of these classes has subgroups 1 through 3. A median surgeon classification accuracy of 94% was reported in the initial published description of the AO/OTA system.[35] The New International system similarly classifies a scapula fracture as glenoid fossa (F), body (B), or process (P).[36] Glenoid fossa and body fractures are subclassified from simple to complex, and process fractures are subclassified as coracoid (P1), acromion (P2), or both (P3). These classification systems are useful for improving communication and the understanding of common scapula fracture patterns, but they have not yet been found to provide reliable guidance for clinical fracture management.

Treatment

The current recommendations for surgical treatment of a scapula fracture are summarized in **Table 1**. Most scapula fractures are treated without surgery, but during the past decade interest has increased in internally fixing displaced injuries. This trend stems from improved diagnoses attributable to advanced imaging techniques and research reports of poor functional outcomes after closed treatment of some displaced scapula fractures.[37] The current treatment guidelines largely are based on level IV and V evidence. There is a dearth of randomized studies of scapula fractures. Several single-cohort studies found that surgical fixation of displaced scapula fractures led to good to excellent functional results.[31,38,39] A single level III comparative study of extra-articular scapula fractures found no significant difference in return to work, pain, or complications based on whether patients were treated surgically or nonsurgically.[40] There was an inherent bias in this study, however, in that the fractures treated with surgical reduction and fixation were the fractures with the greatest preoperative displacement.

A single retrospective comparative study documented better functional outcomes after surgical than nonsurgical treatment of displaced intra-articular scapula fractures (Constant shoulder scores, 87 and 59, respectively).[41] The presence of a brachial plexus injury or a glenohumeral fracture-dislocation predicted a poor outcome. The baseline characteristics of patients in the two groups were significantly different in that those treated nonsurgically were believed to be medically unfit to undergo surgery. It is unclear how this variable affected the reported outcomes, but it precludes drawing any strong conclusions from this study.

The current recommendations for surgical intervention in articular and extra-articular scapula fractures are largely based on quantification of five common measures: glenopolar angle, articular step-off, lateral border offset, translation, and angulation. The use of three-dimensional CT was found to be the most sensitive and specific method for detection of scapula fractures, and it has the highest

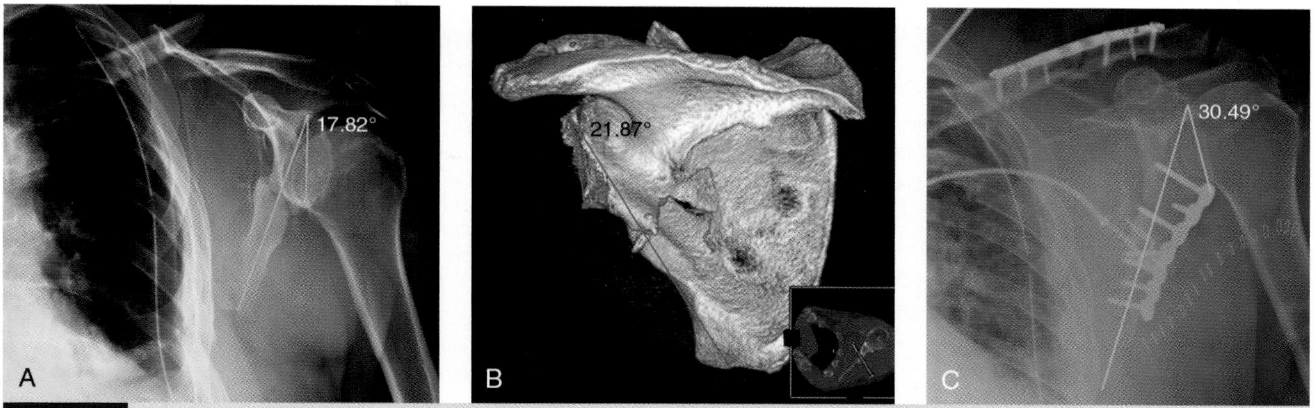

Figure 3 **A,** AP shoulder radiograph showing a combined fracture of the midshaft clavicle and the scapular neck and body. The depressed glenopolar angle (blue lines) was measured at 17.82°. **B,** Three-dimensional CT showing the scapula fracture with coronal CT landmarking (inset). The glenopolar angle (red lines) was measured at 21.87°. **C,** AP shoulder radiograph showing clavicle fixation with a precontoured plate and scapula fixation with a reconstruction plate. The glenopolar angle (blue lines) was restored to 30.49°.

interobserver and intraobserver reliability for measurement of glenopolar angle and angulation.[42,43] Three-dimensional CT with subtraction of the thoracic cage, clavicle, and humerus should be used if possible and can replace the use of radiographs.

The glenopolar angle, originally described in relation to recurrent shoulder dislocations, is one of the most important measures in scapula fracture assessment.[44] The glenopolar angle is measured as the angle between a line drawn from the most cranial to the most caudal portion of the glenoid and a line drawn from the most cranial portion of the glenoid to the most caudal portion of the scapula (**Figure 3**). Restoration of the glenopolar angle correlated with improved functional outcomes.[9] A glenopolar angle of 20° or less correlated with a poor functional outcome and may be an indication for surgical intervention[45] (**Figure 3**).

Normal glenopolar angle values have been defined as 30° to 46°.[46] Comparison with the uninjured scapula is the benchmark for a normal value and is useful to the surgeon in fracture reduction and fixation. Side-to-side variation is negligible (1° to 2°).[47] The glenopolar angle was found to be most accurately measured on three-dimensional CT; measurements from a chest or shoulder radiograph were less accurate (5° to 6° lower).

An articular step-off of approximately 4 to 5 mm or a fragment size of 20% or more of the glenoid has been suggested as an indication for surgical intervention. Osteosynthesis has had good to excellent functional results for return to preinjury work and activity.[38,39,41] Any intra-articular glenoid fracture with residual glenohumeral subluxation or instability after a closed reduction should be surgically repaired.

Lateral border offset, angulation, and translation have not been directly correlated with patient outcomes. The terms lateral border offset and medial displacement often are used interchangeably for medial to lateral shortening of the scapula. A combination of medialization of the proximal fragment (the glenoid) and lateralization of the distal fragment (the body) occurs.[46,48] Lateralization and distal migration of the distal fragment result from the force of muscles acting on the scapula, including the deltoid, rotator cuff, and long head of the triceps. A lateral border offset of 20 mm or more has been proposed as an indication for surgical intervention in extra-articular scapula fractures.[31,49]

Angular deformity and translation are parameters of displacement in the sagittal plane that affect scapular glide on the thoracic wall. An angular deformity of more than 45° or 100% translation with no cortical contact are other indications for surgical intervention in extra-articular fractures.[31,49]

Nonsurgical treatment continues to be preferred for nondisplaced intra- and extra-articular fractures. Routine weekly radiographs are obtained for 3 weeks to ensure the stability of the fracture during nonsurgical treatment. Progressive displacement of an extra-articular fracture has been documented, occurring most frequently within the first 2 weeks after injury.[50] Continued fracture displacement beyond acceptable norms warrants consideration for conversion to surgical treatment.

Summary

Investigation into surgical treatment of displaced clavicle and scapula fractures has dramatically increased during the past decade, primarily because of an emphasis on patient-oriented outcomes and the development of advanced imaging modalities that have improved the understanding of fracture characteristics. Surgical treatment of middle-third clavicle fractures is well supported by high-quality clinical studies, but treatment recommendations for medial- and lateral-third clavicle fractures as well as scapula fractures are based on lower-level research and expert opinion. As the research literature evolves, so too will injury treatment pathways that will lead to improved patient outcomes.

Key Study Points

- In a healthy, active adult, a midshaft clavicle fracture should be surgically stabilized if it is significantly displaced (2 cm of shortening, 100% displacement, or significant comminution).
- The use of a precontoured plate facilitates the surgical treatment of a clavicle fracture by decreasing hardware prominence and the need for secondary surgery.
- Parameters for the treatment of distal and medial clavicle fractures remain unclear and should be assessed on a case-by-case basis. Fracture displacement or nonunion, in isolation, may not affect the outcome.
- The treatment of scapula fractures continues to evolve. The evidence-based parameters include a glenopolar angle of no more than 20° or intra-articular step-off of at least 4 to 5 mm. The decision to operate on a displaced scapula fracture is based on criteria such as angulation and translation and should be made on a case-by-case basis.

Annotated References

1. Karl JW, Olson PR, Rosenwasser MP: The epidemiology of upper extremity fractures in the United States: 2009. *J Orthop Trauma* 2015;29(8):e242-e244.

   The 2009 incidence of fractures of the upper extremity in the United States was derived from census and state databases related to emergency department visits and inpatient stays. Distal radius, hand, proximal humerus, and clavicle fractures were most common.

2. Court-Brown CM: The epidemiology of fractures and dislocations, in Tornetta P III, Court-Brown CM, Heckman JD, McKee M, McQueen M, Ricci W, eds: *Rockwood and Green's Fractures in Adults*, ed 8. Philadelphia, PA, Walters Kluwer Health, 2015, pp 59-108.

   This chapter outlined the epidemiology of fractures and dislocations in adult patients. Based largely on epidemiologic data from the Royal Infirmary of Edinburgh, Scotland, it addressed factors affecting fracture distribution, including age, sex, and socioeconomic status.

3. McKee M: Clavicle fractures, in Tornetta P III, Court-Brown CM, Heckman JD, McKee M, McQueen M, Ricci W, eds: *Rockwood and Green's Fractures in Adults*, ed 8. Philadelphia, PA, Walters Kluwer Health, 2015, pp 1427-1473.

   This chapter detailed midshaft, medial, and lateral clavicle fracture clinical assessment, classification, pathoanatomy, and treatment options. Common injury and treatment complications are discussed.

4. Lenza M, Belloti JC, Andriolo RB, Faloppa F: Conservative interventions for treating middle third clavicle fractures in adolescents and adults. *Cochrane Database Syst Rev* 2014;5:CD007121.

   A systematic review included three studies with 594 patients. Two studies compared the use of a sling and a figure-of-8 bandage. Figure-of-8 bandages were associated with increased pain and discomfort.

5. McKee RC, Whelan DB, Schemitsch EH, McKee MD: Operative versus nonoperative care of displaced midshaft clavicular fractures: A meta-analysis of randomized clinical trials. *J Bone Joint Surg Am* 2012;94(8):675-684.

   In a meta-analysis of six studies including 412 patients, the nonunion rate after a displaced midshaft clavicle fracture was significantly higher in the 200 patients treated nonsurgically than in the 212 treated surgically (29 versus 3 patients), as was the rate of symptomatic malunion (17 versus 0 patients).

6. Xu J, Xu L, Xu W, Gu Y, Xu J: Operative versus nonoperative treatment in the management of midshaft clavicular fractures: A meta-analysis of randomized controlled trials. *J Shoulder Elbow Surg* 2014;23(2):173-181.

   An updated meta-analysis reported on seven studies. Surgery was found to lead to a lower rate of nonunion, fewer overall complications, and fewer symptomatic malunions than nonsurgical treatment.

7. Hill JM, McGuire MH, Crosby LA: Closed treatment of displaced middle-third fractures of the clavicle gives poor results. *J Bone Joint Surg Br* 1997;79(4):537-539.

8. Nowak J, Holgersson M, Larsson S: Sequelae from clavicular fractures are common: A prospective study of 222 patients. *Acta Orthop* 2005;76(4):496-502.

9. Lin TL, Li YF, Hsu CJ, et al: Clinical outcome and radiographic change of ipsilateral scapular neck and clavicular shaft fracture: Comparison of operation and conservative treatment. *J Orthop Surg Res* 2015;10(1):9.

   A randomized study compared fixation of the scapular neck and clavicle, the clavicle alone, and nonsurgical treatment. Glenopolar angle was significantly improved in those who underwent scapular neck and clavicle fixation and was associated with significantly improved function.

10. Backus JD, Merriman DJ, McAndrew CM, Gardner MJ, Ricci WM: Upright versus supine radiographs of clavicle fractures: Does positioning matter? *J Orthop Trauma* 2014;28(11):636-641.

    Standardized clavicle radiographs were obtained in both the supine and upright positions in 46 patients with acute clavicle fracture. Three traumatologists and one resident measured displacement and shortening and found an 89% increase in displacement on upright films.

11. Jones GL, Bishop JY, Lewis B, Pedroza AD; MOON Shoulder Group: Intraobserver and interobserver agreement in the classification and treatment of midshaft clavicle fractures. *Am J Sports Med* 2014;42(5):1176-1181.

    In a cohort study of intraobserver and interobserver agreement in clavicle measurement, surveys were sent to shoulder and sports medicine orthopaedic surgeons. Moderate interrater agreement was found for displacement and comminution, and weak agreement was found for shortening.

12. De Giorgi S, Notarnicola A, Tafuri S, Solarino G, Moretti L, Moretti B: Conservative treatment of fractures of the clavicle. *BMC Res Notes* 2011;4:333.

    Twenty of 71 patients with clavicle fracture (61 middle-third, 8 lateral-third, and 3 medial-third) were dissatisfied; these patients had mean clavicular shortening of 9.7%. Dissatisfaction also was associated with diaphyseal location and female sex.

13. Cunningham BP, McLaren A, Richardson M, McLemore R: Clavicular length: The assumption of symmetry. *Orthopedics* 2013;36(3):e343-e347.

    The authors report on a cohort of 102 skeletally mature adults who underwent a chest CT for unrelated reasons. Clavicle length was compared bilaterally. There were 71.5% of patients who were symmetric (<5 mm difference), and 7% of all clavicles measured had a difference of greater than 10 mm

14. Zhu Y, Tian Y, Dong T, Chen W, Zhang F, Zhang Y: Management of the mid-shaft clavicle fractures using plate fixation versus intramedullary fixation: An updated meta-analysis. *Int Orthop* 2015;39(2):319-328.

    In this updated meta-analysis of five studies including 128 plated and 157 nailed fractures, nail fixation required less surgical time than plate fixation, and fewer complications occurred in patients who received nail fixation. There was a nonsignificant trend toward better function at 1-year follow-up.

15. Renfree T, Conrad B, Wright T: Biomechanical comparison of contemporary clavicle fixation devices. *J Hand Surg Am* 2010;35(4):639-644.

    Biomechanical data were reported on a synthetic bone model of transverse clavicle fractures fixed with precontoured clavicle plates or intramedullary clavicle pins. Intramedullary pins failed at a lower maximum load and were unable to resist any torsional load.

16. Collinge C, Devinney S, Herscovici D, DiPasquale T, Sanders R: Anterior-inferior plate fixation of middle-third fractures and nonunions of the clavicle. *J Orthop Trauma* 2006;20(10):680-686.

17. Hussey MM, Chen Y, Fajardo RA, Dutta AK: Analysis of neurovascular safety between superior and anterior plating techniques of clavicle fractures. *J Orthop Trauma* 2013;27(11):627-632.

    The authors present a cadaver study (n=17) on the anatomic relationships of neurovascular structures to the clavicle following superior versus anterior plating techniques. There was no significant difference in distance to the subclavian vein/artery and the brachial plexus between the two groups.

18. Ashman BD, Slobogean GP, Stone TB, et al: Reoperation following open reduction and plate fixation of displaced mid-shaft clavicle fractures. *Injury* 2014;45(10):1549-1553.

    A retrospective study of 143 patients undergoing clavicle fixation found no association between reoperation and age, fracture class, plate type, or plate location. Twenty percent of patients underwent reoperation for hardware prominence, nonunion, or hardware failure.

19. VanBeek C, Boselli KJ, Cadet ER, Ahmad CS, Levine WN: Precontoured plating of clavicle fractures: Decreased hardware-related complications? *Clin Orthop Relat Res* 2011;469(12):3337-3343.

    In a retrospective review of 42 patients, 14 were treated using a noncontoured plate and 28 received a precontoured plate. Prominent hardware occurred significantly less often after precontoured plate fixation (nine patients in each group), as did hardware removal (three patients in each group).

20. Celestre P, Roberston C, Mahar A, Oka R, Meunier M, Schwartz A: Biomechanical evaluation of clavicle fracture plating techniques: Does a locking plate provide improved stability? *J Orthop Trauma* 2008;22(4):241-247.

21. Iannotti MR, Crosby LA, Stafford P, Grayson G, Goulet R: Effects of plate location and selection on the stability of midshaft clavicle osteotomies: A biomechanical study. *J Shoulder Elbow Surg* 2002;11(5):457-462.

22. Nathe T, Tseng S, Yoo B: The anatomy of the supraclavicular nerve during surgical approach to the clavicular shaft. *Clin Orthop Relat Res* 2011;469(3):890-894.

    A cadaver study documented the branches of the supraclavicular nerve. Wide variability in branch location was found; most of the 37 cadavers had both a medial and a lateral branch, and 50% also had an intermediate branch.

23. Christensen TJ, Horwitz DS, Kubiak EN: Natural history of anterior chest wall numbness after plating of clavicle fractures: Educating patients. *J Orthop Trauma* 2014;28(11):642-647.

A study of 25 patients after clavicle plate fixation found that 21 (84%) had numbness at 2 weeks and 13 (52%) had numbness at 1 year. No correlation between numbness and functional outcome was found.

24. Throckmorton T, Kuhn JE: Fractures of the medial end of the clavicle. *J Shoulder Elbow Surg* 2007;16(1):49-54.

25. Robinson CM, Court-Brown CM, McQueen MM, Wakefield AE: Estimating the risk of nonunion following nonoperative treatment of a clavicular fracture. *J Bone Joint Surg Am* 2004;86(7):1359-1365.

26. Low AK, Duckworth DG, Bokor DJ: Operative outcome of displaced medial-end clavicle fractures in adults. *J Shoulder Elbow Surg* 2008;17(5):751-754.

27. Oe K, Gaul L, Hierholzer C, et al: Operative management of periarticular medial clavicle fractures: Report of ten cases. *J Trauma Acute Care Surg* 2012;72(2):540-548.

A retrospective study of eight patients who underwent locking T-plate fixation and two patients who underwent nonlocking plate fixation found a 90% union rate.

28. Rokito AS, Zuckerman JD, Shaari JM, Eisenberg DP, Cuomo F, Gallagher MA: A comparison of nonoperative and operative treatment of type II distal clavicle fractures. *Bull Hosp Jt Dis* 2002-2003;61(1-2):32-39.

29. Stegeman SA, Nacak H, Huvenaars KH, Stijnen T, Krijnen P, Schipper IB: Surgical treatment of Neer type-II fractures of the distal clavicle: A meta-analysis. *Acta Orthop* 2013;84(2):184-190.

A meta-analysis of surgical technique included 21 studies with an overall union rate of 98%. Hook plating was associated with an 11-fold increase in complications compared with intramedullary fixation and a 24-fold increase compared with suture anchoring.

30. Goss TP: Scapular fractures and dislocations: Diagnosis and treatment. *J Am Acad Orthop Surg* 1995;3(1):22-33.

31. Cole PA, Gauger EM, Herrera DA, Anavian J, Tarkin IS: Radiographic follow-up of 84 operatively treated scapula neck and body fractures. *Injury* 2012;43(3):327-333.

In a retrospective review of 84 patients with a scapula fracture that met at least one surgical criterion, all patients underwent fixation through a posterior approach, and 5 patients required a combined anterior-posterior approach. Union was achieved in all patients.

32. Coimbra R, Conroy C, Tominaga GT, Bansal V, Schwartz A: Causes of scapula fractures differ from other shoulder injuries in occupants seriously injured during motor vehicle crashes. *Injury* 2010;41(2):151-155.

Differences in demographic and crash characteristics were investigated in patients with scapula fracture and shoulder injury not involving the scapula. Patients with scapula fracture were three times as likely to be male, and they were taller and weighed more than patients with another shoulder injury.

33. Baldwin KD, Ohman-Strickland P, Mehta S, Hume E: Scapula fractures: A marker for concomitant injury? A retrospective review of data in the National Trauma Database. *J Trauma* 2008;65(2):430-435.

34. Chamata E, Mahabir R, Jupiter D, Weber RA: Prevalence of brachial plexus injuries in patients with scapular fractures: A National Trauma Data Bank review. *Plast Surg (Oakv)* 2014;22(4):246-248.

The National Trauma Data Bank from 2007 to 2011 had 68,118 scapula fractures, including 1.7% with a brachial plexus injury and 49% with a radial nerve injury.

35. Jaeger M, Lambert S, Südkamp NP, et al: The AO Foundation and Orthopaedic Trauma Association (AO/OTA) scapula fracture classification system: Focus on glenoid fossa involvement. *J Shoulder Elbow Surg* 2013;22(4):512-520.

A new classification system was developed by seven experienced shoulder surgeons using a consensus process.

36. Harvey E, Audigé L, Herscovici D Jr, et al: Development and validation of the New International Classification for Scapula Fractures. *J Orthop Trauma* 2012;26(6):364-369.

A new classification system was based on radiography and CT with four iterations of feedback. The classification was found to be more reliable when CT images were added.

37. Ada JR, Miller ME: Scapular fractures: Analysis of 113 cases. *Clin Orthop Relat Res* 1991;269:174-180.

38. Anavian J, Gauger EM, Schroder LK, Wijdicks CA, Cole PA: Surgical and functional outcomes after operative management of complex and displaced intra-articular glenoid fractures. *J Bone Joint Surg Am* 2012;94(7):645-653.

A review of functional outcomes of 33 patients with a surgically treated intra-articular glenoid fracture found that 30 (91%) had returned to their preinjury level of work and activity at 2-year follow-up.

39. Hu C, Zhang W, Qin H, et al: Open reduction and internal fixation of Ideberg IV and V glenoid intra-articular fractures through a Judet approach: A retrospective analysis of 11 cases. *Arch Orthop Trauma Surg* 2015;135(2):193-199.

A retrospective review of 11 patients who underwent surgical fixation for a complex intra-articular glenoid fracture found union in all patients and an average Constant shoulder score of 92.

40. Jones CB, Sietsema DL: Analysis of operative versus nonoperative treatment of displaced scapular fractures. *Clin Orthop Relat Res* 2011;469(12):3379-3389.

In a comparative retrospective review of 62 patients with a displaced scapula fracture, 31 patients were treated surgically and 31 were treated nonsurgically. There was no between-group difference in return to work, pain, or complications. More patients had displacement after surgical treatment.

41. Sen RK, Sud S, Saini G, Rangdal S, Sament R, Bachhal V: Glenoid fossa fractures: Outcome of operative and nonoperative treatment. *Indian J Orthop* 2014;48(1):14-19.

 In a retrospective review of 21 patients with glenoid fracture, those who underwent surgical fixation had a Constant shoulder score of 87.25 at 7.3-year follow-up. Those who did not undergo surgical fixation because of critical illness had a score of 58.55.

42. Tadros AM, Lunsjo K, Czechowski J, Corr P, Abu-Zidan FM: Usefulness of different imaging modalities in the assessment of scapular fractures caused by blunt trauma. *Acta Radiol* 2007;48(1):71-75.

43. Anavian J, Conflitti JM, Khanna G, Guthrie ST, Cole PA: A reliable radiographic measurement technique for extra-articular scapular fractures. *Clin Orthop Relat Res* 2011;469(12):3371-3378.

 Three observers (one orthopaedic surgeon, one resident, and one clinical research fellow) measured 45 fractures for medial or lateral displacement, angulation, translation, glenopolar angle, and glenoid version. Measurements of angulation and glenopolar angle were most accurate on three-dimensional CT.

44. Bestard EA, Schvene HR, Bestard EH: Glenoplasty in the management of recurrent shoulder dislocations. *Contemp Orthop* 1986;12:47-55.

45. Romero J, Schai P, Imhoff AB: Scapular neck fracture: The influence of permanent malalignment of the glenoid neck on clinical outcome. *Arch Orthop Trauma Surg* 2001;121(6):313-316.

46. Zuckerman SL, Song Y, Obremskey WT: Understanding the concept of medialization in scapula fractures. *J Orthop Trauma* 2012;26(6):350-357.

 A retrospective review of 70 patients with scapula fracture found an average 6-mm lateralization of the glenoid relative to the midline on CT compared with the uninjured side.

47. Tuček M, Naňka O, Malík J, Bartoníček J: The scapular glenopolar angle: Standard values and side differences. *Skeletal Radiol* 2014;43(11):1583-1587.

 A study of glenopolar angle measured anatomically and on radiography and three-dimensional CT found that the anatomic average angle was 42.3°, with a side-to-side difference of 1.6°. On the Neer I radiographic view, the angle was 40.6°, and on three-dimensional CT it was 43°.

48. Patterson JM, Galatz L, Streubel PN, Toman J, Tornetta P III, Ricci WM: CT evaluation of extra-articular glenoid neck fractures: Does the glenoid medialize or does the scapula lateralize? *J Orthop Trauma* 2012;26(6):360-363.

 On CT of 18 patients admitted with an isolated scapular neck fracture, the glenoid was lateralized an average of almost 1 cm. In most patients the scapula was shortened an average of 6 mm.

49. Cole PA, Freeman G, Dubin JR: Scapula fractures. *Curr Rev Musculoskelet Med* 2013;6(1):79-87.

 The authors present a review of the current understanding of scapula fractures, including anatomy, imaging, fracture characterization including current accepted measurement values, and treatment.

50. Anavian J, Khanna G, Plocher EK, Wijdicks CA, Cole PA: Progressive displacement of scapula fractures. *J Trauma* 2010;69(1):156-161.

 Eight patients initially treated nonsurgically later required reconstruction because of progressive displacement in angulation, translation, glenopolar angle, or lateral boarder offset. Mean time between the initial and follow-up radiographs showing displacement was 11 days.

Chapter 22

Proximal Humerus Fracture

Xavier Simcock, MD William H. Seitz Jr, MD

Abstract

Proximal humerus fractures are one of the most common osteoporotic fractures and present a clinical challenge for orthopaedic surgeons because of their heterogeneity. There is a low degree of interobserver agreement with current classification schemes. Unlike other fractures, fixation of both the surrounding soft tissue in addition to the bone fragments in proximal humerus fractures is critical to the ultimate functional outcome. Several surgical fixation methods, with their own benefits and complications, are available to address these fractures and related fracture pathology. The goal of surgical fixation should be to optimize function with minimal soft-tissue disruption. The large amount of outcomes data for different surgical techniques coincides with the overall increase in surgical management. Ultimately these results have helped maximize functional outcomes, particularly for fractures in elderly patients and when shoulder reconstruction is considered. Retrospective studies have recently reported improved forward elevation with reverse total shoulder arthroplasty compared with humeral head replacement hemiarthroplasty, but with higher complication rates.

Neither Dr. Simcock nor any immediate family member has received anything of value from or has stock or stock options held in a commercial company or institution related directly or indirectly to the subject of this article/chapter. Dr. Seitz or an immediate family member serves as a paid consultant to Kapp Surgical Instruments, Materialise, and Stryker, and serves as a board member, owner, officer, or committee member of the American Academy of Orthopaedic Surgeons, the Academy of Medicine Foundation, the Academy of Medicine of Northern Ohio, the American Orthopaedic Association, and the American Society for Surgery of the Hand.

Keywords: proximal humerus fractures; reverse total shoulder arthroplasty reconstruction; fracture specific hemiarthroplasty reconstruction; locking plate fixation with and without bone augmentation

Introduction

Fractures involving the proximal humerus account for 4% to 6% of all fractures. These fractures occur in a bimodal distribution, with three-fourths occurring in patients older than 60 years. Younger individuals tend to sustain a fracture from a high-energy mechanism. The majority of fractures are fragility factures resulting from low-energy mechanisms and predominantly occur in women (85%). Overall, proximal humeral fractures are considered the third most common osteoporotic fragility fracture.[1]

Based on the most recent epidemiology data, the prevalence of proximal humerus fractures has remained constant, and there has been a substantial increase in surgical treatment. This increase in surgical treatment has coincided with the widespread availability of proximal humeral locking plates. A comparison of Medicare data from 1999 to 2000 and 2004 to 2005 showed a 25.6% rise in surgical treatment of proximal humerus fractures.[2] Furthermore, there was a relative increase in open reduction and internal fixation (ORIF) of 29% compared to only a 20% increase in humeral head arthroplasties. During the same period the revision rates of ORIF also increased at 90 days and 1 year with an odds ratios of 3.3 and 3.9, respectively.

Indications and rates of intervention have a geographic variability ranging from 0 to 68%, with an overall surgical rate of 15.7% in 2005.[2] There is no clear consensus regarding which patients or fracture patterns benefit from surgery.[3,4] The heterogeneity of outcomes is likely associated with the poor interobserver reliability of the current fracture classifications. Orthopaedic surgeons are more inclined to recommend surgical fixation for a displaced proximal humerus fracture. Studies analyzing surgeon decision making have revealed that surgeons are more likely to offer surgical intervention when looking at radiographs alone than when patient age and mechanism of injury are taken into consideration.[5] Some studies have suggested that upper extremity fellowship-trained specialists are more likely to offer surgical intervention; however, more recent studies failed to reproduce this result.[5,6] Patients are also living longer with active lifestyles, and therefore may increase demand for a rapid return to function, which influences surgeon decision making.

The various forms of internal fixation include percutaneous pins and screws, tension bands, nonabsorbable sutures, locking plates, external fixation, and intramedullary devices. Humeral head arthroplasty has continued to advance, with an increase in both fracture-specific implants and reverse total shoulder arthroplasty. Each technique has specific indications, learning curves, and complications.

Presentation, Anatomy, and Classification

After sustaining a high- or low-energy mechanism of injury, the patient most commonly presents with a painful shoulder and ecchymosis along the pectoralis and biceps muscles. Nerve deficits may be present in 70% of fractures, including those with low-energy mechanisms.[7] Standard radiographs often include anteroposterior, true anteroposterior (Grashey), axillary lateral, and scapular-Y views. Internal and external rotation views can help distinguish subtle tuberosity fractures. CT can provide more detail especially with comminuted fracture patterns, articular or glenoid involvement, and when considering surgical intervention. There are clear advantages to CT axial imaging, with plain radiographs underestimating the number of fragments in comminuted fractures by 60%.[8]

Overcoming the deforming forces around the proximal humerus is essential in obtaining reduction during surgery. The supraspinatus, infraspinatus, and teres minor muscles attach to the greater tuberosity and exert abduction and external rotation forces. The subscapularis attached to the lesser tuberosity exerts adduction and internal rotation. The deltoid and pectoralis insert more distally on the shaft and provide deforming forces displacing the shaft component into flexion, and internal rotation.

Older case series suggested that osteonecrosis resulted in almost one-third of three- or four-part humeral head fractures. Subsequently, the vascularity of the proximal humerus has been emphasized and has even influenced classification schemes. It was previously suggested that the anterior humeral circumflex artery was the predominant blood supply to the humeral head.[9] Recent studies have brought the importance of the anterior humeral circumflex artery into question. Arteriography studies found the anterior humeral circumflex artery was disrupted in 80% of fractures, whereas the posterior humeral circumflex artery was normal in 85% of these same fracture cases.[10] In 2011, a new investigation using gadolinium-enhanced MRI to assess flow in the humeral head of fresh-frozen cadavers revealed that the posterior humeral circumflex artery was responsible for the majority (64%) of blood flow to the humeral head.[11] This finding correlates with the relatively low rates of humeral head osteonecrosis. The posterior humeral circumflex artery anastomoses with the arcuate artery at the epiphyseal line and provides collateral blood flow to the humeral head when the anterolateral branch of the anterior humeral circumflex artery is disrupted during fracture.

Fracture patterns that disrupt the posteromedial neck were correlated with a higher risk of humeral head ischemia using intraoperative laser Doppler flowmetry. Higher rates of ischemia were observed with fracture extension into the metaphysis greater than 2 mm and less than 8 mm.[12] At surgery, the diminished blood flow was noted in 78% of fractures with a disrupted medial hinge, whereas only 20% of perfused heads had a disrupted medial cortex. It is important to note that intraoperative blood flow does not predict osteonecrosis, because in a subsequent study with 5-year follow-up osteonecrosis had not developed in 8 of 10 initially avascular heads.[13]

Since its publication in 1970, the Neer classification system for proximal humerus fractures has been widely used. In this system four fracture segments were defined: the greater tuberosity, the lesser tuberosity, the humeral shaft, and the humeral articular surface (**Figure 1**). Displacement was defined as angulation of 45° or translation of 1 cm.[14] Additional categories such as valgus impacted and head splits were subsequently recognized.

The AO classification was defined in 1988 and identified 27 categories (**Figure 2**). The classification system recognized the blood flow to the humeral head. It is organized into three main groups that are further subdivided based on comminution, impaction, and alignment. The main groups are A, extra-articular unifocal; B, extra-articular bifocal; and C, intra-articular. Despite the added level of detail, less interobserver reliability is found with this classification scheme, perhaps because of its complexity.

All classification schemes for proximal humerus fractures exhibit poor interobserver reliability. At best, interobserver values with proximal humerus classification represent slight to moderate agreement. The AO system has the lowest values (κ 0.11) and the Neer and Codman-Hertel classifications are only mildly better (κ 0.33 and κ 0.44).[3] Widespread agreement remains elusive

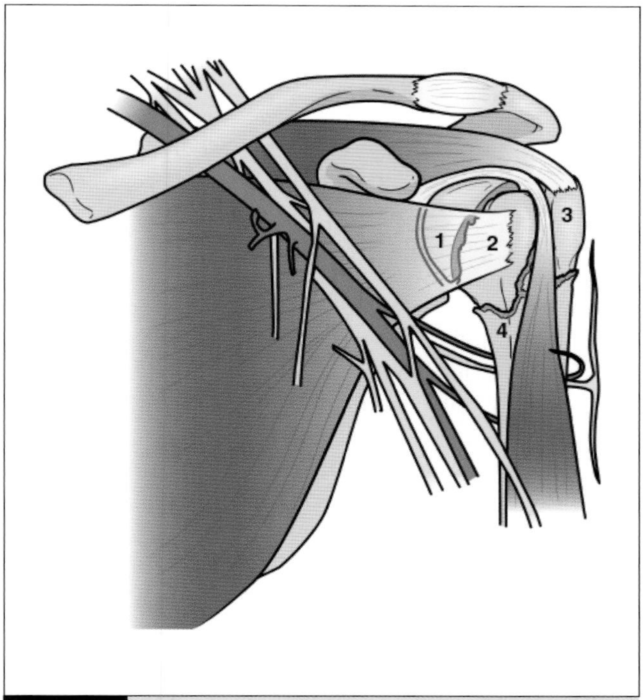

Figure 1 Fracture anatomy as identified by Neer. 1, Articular surface. 2, Lesser tuberosity. 3, Greater tuberosity. 4, Humeral shaft.

even with more sophisticated imaging such as two-dimensional and three-dimensional CT.[4] It is a widely held belief that the lack of reliability in classification likely confounds clinical trials for proximal humerus fractures.

Nonsurgical Treatment

Most (50% to 85%) proximal humerus fractures are osteoporotic fragility fractures that are nondisplaced or minimally displaced. As a group these fractures are managed by closed means with good outcomes.[15-18] Although closed treatment of these fractures is not controversial, there is a substantial effect on morbidity, mortality, disability, and health-related quality of life. The Disabilities of the Arm, Shoulder and Hand (DASH) score averages 26.6 ± 27.7. A retrospective study of 912 nondisplaced proximal humerus fractures revealed 67.3% of patients had significant pain and limitations of function, predominantly in self-care (44.5%), daily life activities (56.5%), and anxiety and depression 32.7%.[1]

In stable fractures, mobilization of the injured arm should occur as soon as the patient is comfortable and the initial sling use can be discontinued. Patients are instructed in pendulum exercise, finger and hand mobilization, and ways to minimize swelling, especially in the hand. Supervised physical therapy should begin by 2 weeks. Prospective randomized data revealed that waiting more than 3 weeks for the resolution of pain before initiating formal therapy prolongs recovery for patients who experience more pain during the rehabilitation period.[19] No increase in nonunion rate has been observed, even when initiating formal therapy within 3 days after fracture.[20]

Results of surgical versus nonsurgical interventions in two retrospective cohorts of matched proximal humerus fractures yielded surprising conclusions. At 1 year the nonsurgical group's American Shoulder and Elbow Surgeons score was better than that of the surgical group, 82.5 versus 71.6.[16] Moreover, the nonsurgical shoulder range of motion was better in all categories except for internal rotation. This study, like many others, is limited by clinician bias and the lack of prospective randomization. However, the studies agreed that the nonsurgical treatment group had fewer complications that presented early after treatment.

The primary complication encountered with nonsurgical treatment of fracture is settling of the fracture fragments, which can have a varied effect on shoulder function depending on the fracture pattern and alignment. A prospective study of 89 patients treated conservatively was conducted using CT and radiographs to measure the amount of settling at 1 year.[17] Posteromedial (varus) impaction patterns settled an additional 9° in varus and 7° retroversion. Lateral (valgus) impaction patterns were more stable, and usually resulted in a decrease in valgus tilt with increased anteversion of the articular surface. Greater tuberosity fractures were seen to displace more than 5 mm 20% of the time. Malunions of proximal humeral fractures may be tolerated depending on the age and physical demands of the patient.

Surgical Treatment

Although most proximal humerus fractures do not require surgery, it is recognized that significant displacement and resultant malunions do result in poor functional outcomes. There is no clear consensus on specific indications for surgical intervention. Malunion of the tuberosities as well as neck shaft displacement with angulation can lead to poor functional outcomes. ORIF is considered for patients with greater tuberosity fracture displacement of more than 5 mm, displaced lesser tuberosity fractures contiguous with the articular surface, displaced or unstable surgical neck fractures, and displaced and reconstructible three- and four-part fractures in younger patients. Surgical indications are preferable in the patient younger than 55 years with good bone stock. Surgical goals are the restoration of the proximal humeral anatomy, especially the neck- shaft angle, version of the humeral head, and

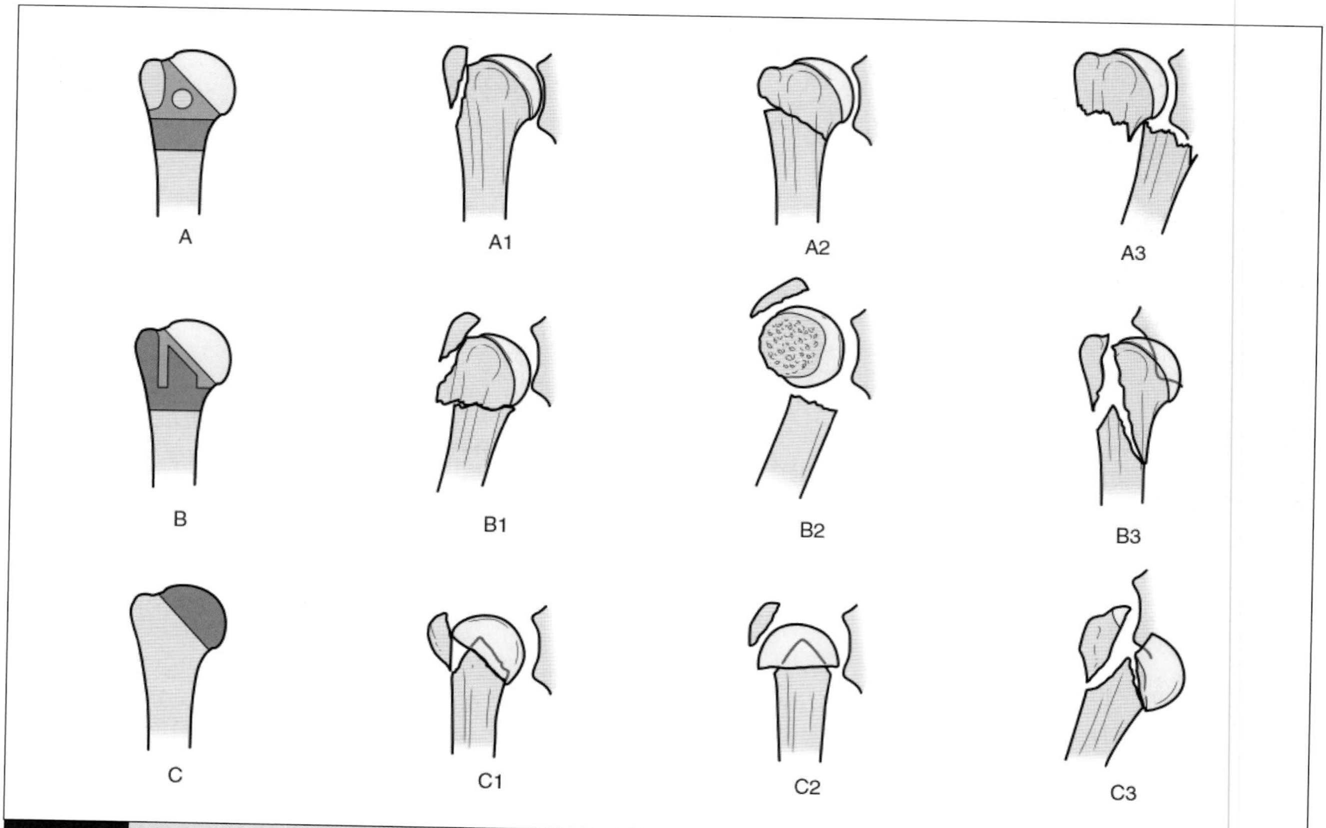

Figure 2 AO classification of proximal humerus fractures. The main groups are A, extra-articular unifocal; B, extra-articular bifocal; and C, intra-articular.

tuberosity position. These goals can be achieved through either minimally invasive techniques or open techniques augmented with intercalary allograft. Head-splitting fractures may require a humeral head replacement.

Minimally Invasive Techniques

Minimally invasive techniques require good bone quality, minimal comminution, and an intact medial calcar. Isolated tuberosity fractures and displaced two part surgical neck fractures are usually treated with minimally invasive techniques. Closed reduction and percutaneous pinning, minimally invasive osteosynthesis, and intramedullary locked nails have all been used with success and with caveats.

Intramedullary nails have evolved along with an improved understanding of failures of fixation. Previous generations of intramedullary nailing have been criticized for the frequency of shoulder pain, ranging from 25% to 56%, and union rates of 70%.[21] The most recent design of angular stable locked nails were retrospectively reviewed in a multicenter study. In 38 displaced two-part fractures of the surgical neck that underwent intramedullary nailing, all but one maintained a neck-shaft angle greater than 125°, and all fractures united.[22] Eleven percent of patients required a secondary procedure, including nail removal, heterotopic bone resection, and manipulation. The authors of the most recent review advocate for an articular starting point to minimize hardware pain and rotator cuff injury at the nail entry point.

Closed reduction and percutaneous pinning in the right patient can be equivalent to treatment with intramedullary nails (**Figure 3**). This technique requires good bone stock and an intact medial calcar; the obvious appeal is minimal dissection and maintenance of the fracture hematoma for early consolidation. Complications associated with this technique include infection, nonunion, malunion, nerve injury, articular injury, and stiffness in a patient in whom this minimally invasive technique is poorly indicated. It is essential to protect the axillary nerve when placing the retrograde pins. Adequate closed reduction must be demonstrated before percutaneous fixation is elected. Despite all precautions, pin migration occurs in 30% of patients, and malunion rates range

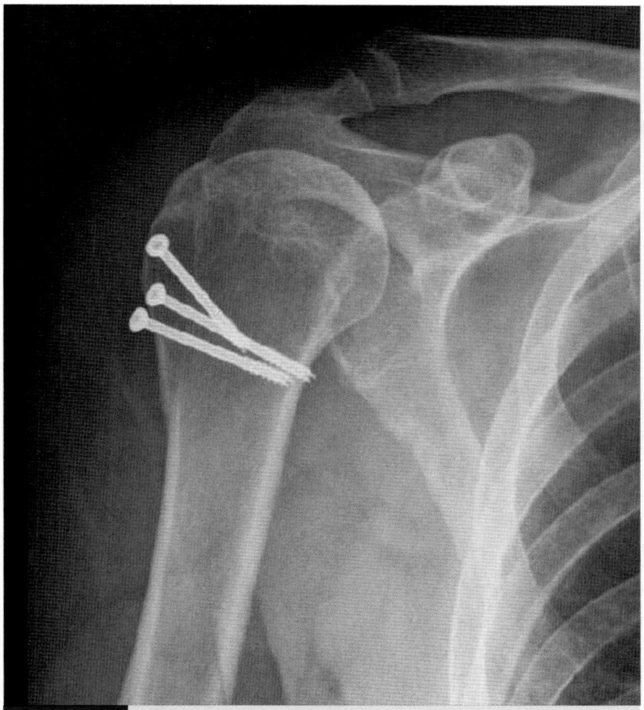

Figure 3 Radiograph shows closed reduction and percutaneous fixation.

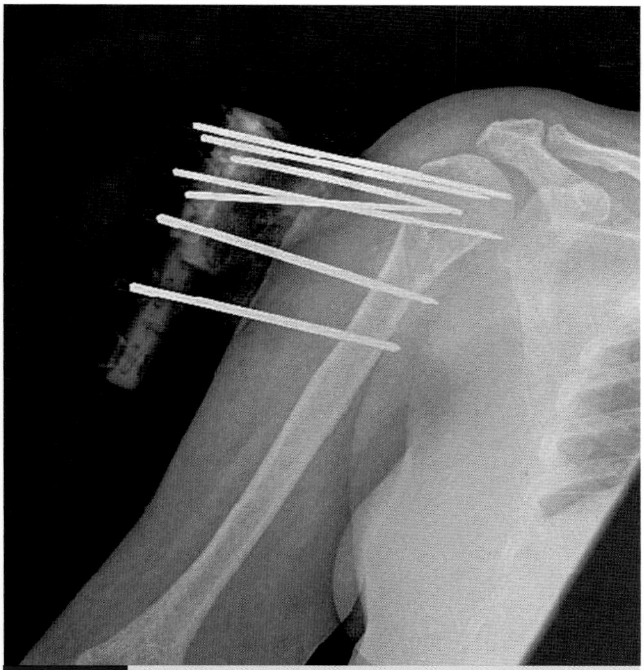

Figure 4 Radiograph shows external fixation.

from 11% to 30%.[23] Percutaneous pins connected to an external fixator decrease the risk of pin migration (**Figure 4**). In a retrospective review of 62 cases using 5-mm external fixation screws, 82% of patients achieved good or excellent results.[24]

Transosseous suturing is another minimally invasive technique with retrospective support. In a review of 188 consecutive patients, 94% had good or excellent outcomes at 5 years, with only 2 nonunions within 5 months after fixation.[25] A nonabsorbable robust suture (No. 5) was used via a transdeltoid approach (**Figure 5**). A 9% incidence of heterotopic ossification was the most common complication. Certain fracture patterns and poor bone quality preclude transosseous suturing as sole fixation, but it can be used on three-part fractures and four-part valgus impacted fractures in addition to greater tuberosity and displaced subcapital fractures.

Locked plates are being used more often for the more complex fractures, especially those with poor bone stock, with good results.[26] The deltopectoral and deltoid splitting approaches provide easier and more direct access to the greater tuberosity. There is obvious risk to the axillary nerve with the deltoid splitting approach and identification and protection of the nerve is paramount. Loss of reduction and malunion have decreased with locked plating and have been replaced by other complications such as stiffness. Thus, minimally invasive techniques should be a treatment option in the properly selected patient.[27]

Open Reduction and Internal Fixation

The advent of locked plates focus has led to primary osteosynthesis of three- and four-part proximal humerus fractures instead of hemiarthroplasty. Rates of failure of fixation range from 8.6% to 22%.[28-30] Common errors are inadequate or loss of reduction with locked screw cutout, which occurs in 13% to 23.7%. The utilization of pegs instead of screws does not decrease this rate.[31]

The most common cause of fixation failure is loss of medial calcar buttress support. Several studies have highlighted the biomechanical significance of medial cortical integrity. Locked plate designs incorporate a medial calcar screw support called the kick-stand, which resists varus displacement and locked screw cutout in the head (**Figure 6**). Loss of reduction is mediated by the bending and rotational moments from rotator cuff activity. Independent risk factors for loss of reduction include osteoporosis, varus displacement of the head fragment (angle less than 110°), medial calcar comminution (more than one fragment), and lack of cortical contact or screw support on the medial calcar.[28,32,33] The combination of these risk factors increases the likelihood of failure. Fractures displaced into

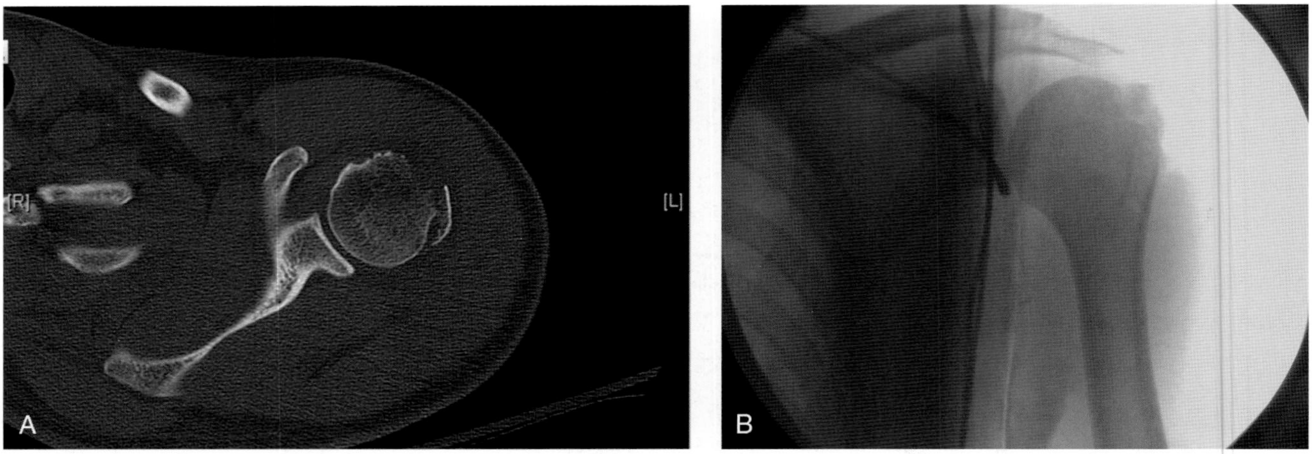

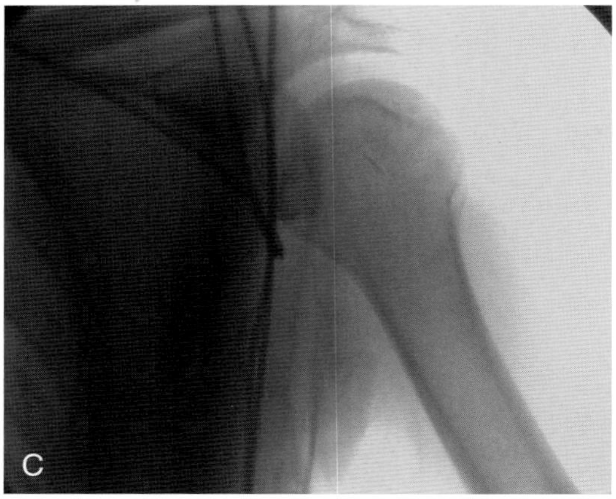

Figure 5 **A**, CT of displaced greater tuberosity fracture. **B**, AP view of transosseous suture fixation. **C**, Lateral view of transosseous suture fixation.

varus have a much higher complication rate compared to valgus patterns (79% versus 19%).[34,35] Adequacy of tuberosity reduction will ensure a good functional outcome.

Multiple strategies have emerged to augment plate fixation to preserve reduction and prevent redisplacement of the fracture. Securing the rotator cuff to the plate with sutures will support tuberosity fixation.[36] The use of intramedullary cortical struts, or quadricortical fixation, can prevent collapse in osteoporotic bone and has been demonstrated to enhance fixation in the laboratory and in clinical applications.[37,38] In a retrospective review of 71 patients grouped older and younger than 65 years, no difference in outcomes were seen after ORIF except for mildly decreased flexion in the older group.[39] Bone substitute augmentation was reported. In a retrospective review of 92 patients using calcium phosphate, decreased fracture subsidence and screw penetration were seen compared to cancellous autograft.[40]

Overall, locked plating has allowed stable reconstruction of a greater number of proximal humerus fractures.[30] This option has changed surgeon behavior to attempt internal fixation instead of humeral head replacement especially in the younger and more active patient. A decreased rate of osteonecrosis and relatively good DASH and Constant scores were seen in a retrospective review of 16 patients younger than 55 years who underwent ORIF for a head-splitting fracture.[41] The overall rate of complications for patients undergoing surgical intervention remains high. In a prospective study of elderly patients with three-part fractures randomized to ORIF versus nonsurgical intervention, no difference in outcomes was found in DASH and Constant scores at 2 years.[33] The patients in the surgical group had better range of motion and a 30% complication rate.

Arthroplasty for Fracture

Patients with an articular surface head split greater than 40%, comminuted fracture patterns involving the tuberosities, and concern for viability of the humeral head such as in a fracture-dislocation have been indicated for humeral head replacement. Hemiarthroplasty has predictably provided pain relief in elderly patients with fracture, but restoration of mobility has been inconsistent (**Figure 7**).

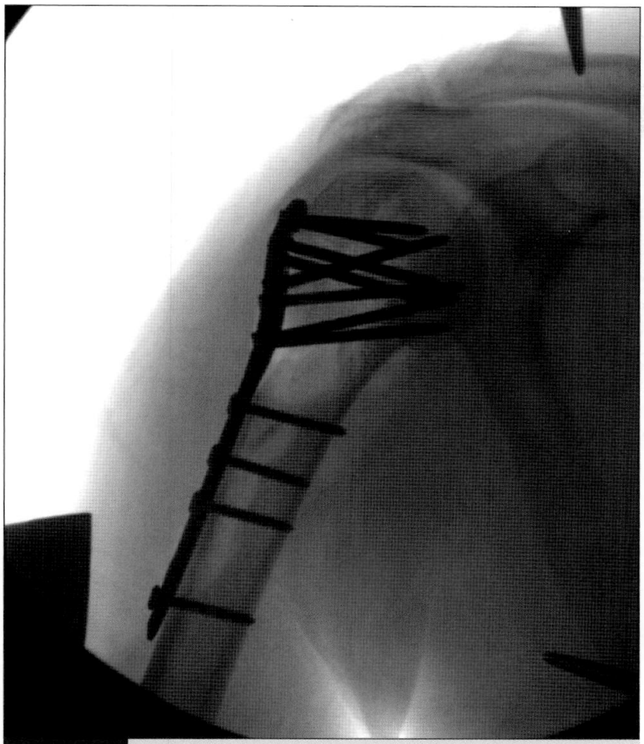

Figure 6 Radiograph shows plate fixation using a "kick-stand" screw.

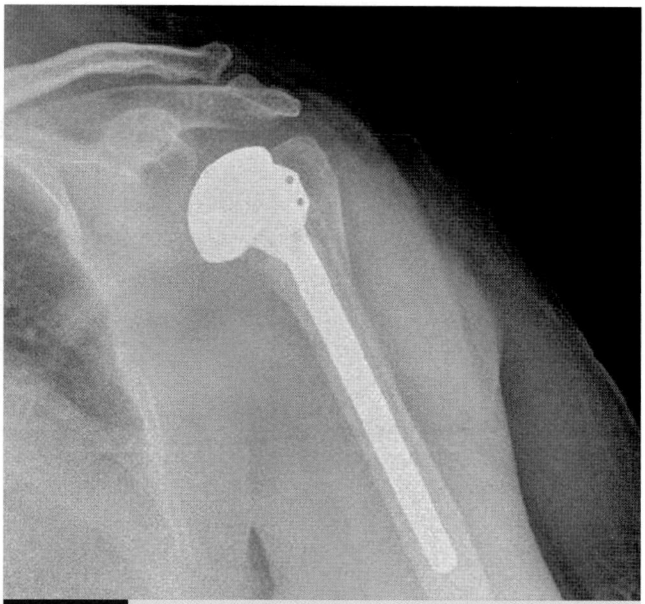

Figure 7 Radiograph shows hemiarthroplasty for fracture.

Poor outcomes after nonunion of the tuberosity and rotator cuff dysfunction occur in 11.2% of patients, with an additional 6.8% having tuberosity migration. Incorrect tuberosity positioning is seen in as many as 50% of patients undergoing hemiarthroplasty.[42] The insertion of the pectoralis tendon on the shaft can act as a reliable anatomic marker to adjust the height of the humeral head. Two level I studies have failed to show clear benefit with hemiarthroplasty over nonsurgical treatment of four-part fractures in elderly patients.[33,43] Because of the mixed results with hemiarthroplasty, a lot of attention has been placed on the functional outcomes following reverse total shoulder arthroplasty (rTSA) (**Figure 8**). The theoretical benefits are twofold. First, healing of osteoporotic tuberosities is not essential for functional outcome. Second, replacing the glenoid removes the potential of progressive wear and subsequent pain.

A retrospective cohort study reviewed the New Zealand joint registry comparing 55 rTSA patients versus 313 hemiarthroplasty patients for acute proximal humerus fractures. The 5-year functional outcomes were superior in the rTSA using the Oxford Shoulder Score.[44] Another retrospective cohort study reviewed patient outcomes of three- and four-part fractures following rTSA, hemiarthroplasty, or ORIF. The rTSA group had more patients achieving 90% forward elevation and a significant cost saving for the overall treatment.[45] The cost savings were realized in fewer physical therapy visits, and implant costs were equivalent between locked implants and reverse total shoulder procedures and less than fracture-specific hemiarthroplasty. A Cochrane meta-analysis of retrospective outcomes also found rTSA to have statistically improved range of motion. One-year clinical assessment demonstrated forward flexion improved by an average of 20° without an increase in overall complication rate.[46] The management of the greater tuberosity during rTSA affects final external rotation. If the greater tuberosity is excised or not repaired, there is an average loss of external rotation of 10°.[47]

rTSA for a fracture indication has a higher complication rate than for reconstruction of an arthritic shoulder. Revision rates range from 5% to 15% even among experienced surgeons.[47,48] Dislocation is the most common complication for rTSA at 11%.[49] Survivorship of rTSA is greater than 90% at 10 years for rotator cuff arthropathy; however, these data are not available for patients with proximal humerus fractures. Based on aggregate retrospective data, the clinical complication rates for those undergoing rTSA remains higher than hemiarthroplasty (9.6% versus 4.1%), and the overall surgical revision rate is lower for the hemiarthroplasty group than rTSA (1.7% versus 4%).[47]

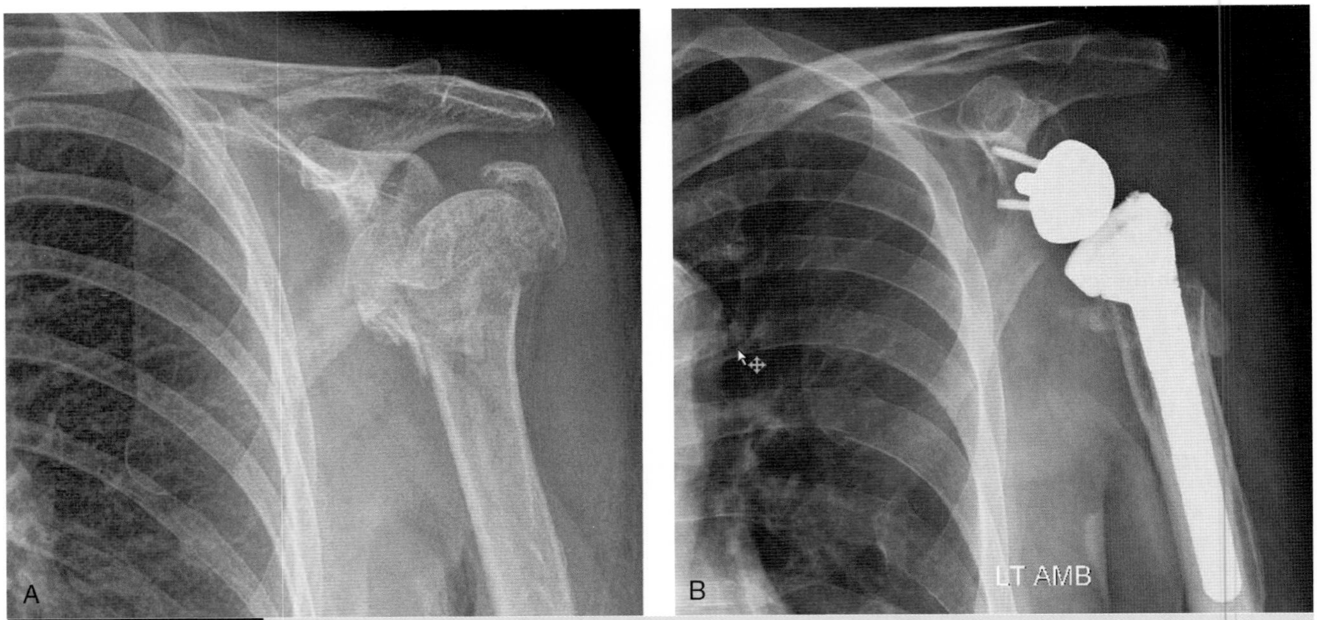

Figure 8 Radiographs show reverse total shoulder arthroplasty for fracture.

Summary

Although there has been a recent increase in enthusiasm for surgical management of proximal humerus fractures, most (50% to 85%) are best treated via closed reduction and immobilization. When considering nonsurgical management it is essential to monitor patients closely. Twenty percent of initially nondisplaced greater tuberosity fractures will displace, and fracture patterns involving varus displacement (posterior medial) have shown the largest degree of subsidence. Proximal humerus fractures affect self-care and activities of daily life. Even with appropriate physical therapy, 67% of patients will experience functional limitations and some pain.

Several options exist for implants and approaches to fixation of proximal humerus fractures. These include percutaneous pins and screws, tension bands, nonabsorbable sutures, locking plates, external fixation, and intramedullary devices. Moreover, humeral head replacing techniques have been refined with increased utility of fracture-specific hemiarthroplasty and rTSA. Each technique has specific indications, learning curves, and complications.

Key Study Points

- Despite an increase in proximal humerus fractures undergoing surgical intervention, there is no clear consensus regarding which fracture patterns benefit from surgical intervention partly because of low interobserver reliability rates and heterogeneity of current classification systems.
- Several surgical fixation methods to address proximal humerus fractures exist, each with its own benefits and complications. The goal of surgical fixation should be to optimize function with minimal soft-tissue injury.
- When compared with humeral head replacement hemiarthroplasty, retrospective studies have recently reported improved forward elevation with rTSA, but with a higher complication rate.

Annotated References

1. Calvo E, Morcillo D, Foruria AM, Redondo-Santamaría E, Osorio-Picorne F, Caeiro JR; GEIOS-SECOT Outpatient Osteoporotic Fracture Study Group: Nondisplaced proximal humeral fractures: High incidence among outpatient-treated osteoporotic fractures and severe impact on upper extremity function and patient subjective health perception. *J Shoulder Elbow Surg* 2011;20(5):795-801.

This retrospective study of 912 nondisplaced proximal humerus fractures revealed 67.3% of patients had substantial pain and limitations in function. Specifically, functional limitations in self-care 44.5%, daily life activities 56.5%, and anxiety and depression 32.7%. Level of evidence: IV.

2. Bell JE, Leung BC, Spratt KF, et al: Trends and variation in incidence, surgical treatment, and repeat surgery of proximal humeral fractures in the elderly. *J Bone Joint Surg Am* 2011;93(2):121-131.

   Although the incidence and demographics of proximal humerus fractures did not increase from 1999 to 2005 the rate of operative intervention increased by 25.6%. Level of evidence: II (therapeutic).

3. Majed A, Macleod I, Bull AM, et al: Proximal humeral fracture classification systems revisited. *J Shoulder Elbow Surg* 2011;20(7):1125-1132.

   The interobserver values with proximal humerus classification represent slight to moderate agreement. The AO system has the lowest values at κ 0.11 and the Neer and Codman-Hertel classifications are only mildly better at κ 0.33 and κ 0.44, respectively.

4. Bruinsma WE, Guitton TG, Warner JJ, Ring D; Science of Variation Group: Interobserver reliability of classification and characterization of proximal humeral fractures: A comparison of two and three-dimensional CT. *J Bone Joint Surg Am* 2013;95(17):1600-1604.

   Even with widespread use of two-dimensional and three-dimensional CT, current proximal humerus classifications have poor interobserver reliability. The lack of reliability likely confounds clinical trials for proximal humerus fractures.

5. Hageman MG, Jayakumar P, King JD, Guitton TG, Doornberg JN, Ring D; Science of Variation Group: The factors influencing the decision making of operative treatment for proximal humeral fractures. *J Shoulder Elbow Surg* 2015;24(1):e21-e26.

   Older age is associated with a surgeon recommending nonsurgical treatment. The surgeon specialization, years in practice, and number of proximal humerus fractures treated per year did not influence the decision to operate.

6. Okike K, Lee OC, Makanji H, Harris MB, Vrahas MS: Factors associated with the decision for operative versus non-operative treatment of displaced proximal humerus fractures in the elderly. *Injury* 2013;44(4):448-455.

   In a retrospective review of 229 displaced proximal humerus fractures, younger patients, presence of associated orthopaedic injuries, severity of fracture, and/or glenohumeral dislocation were associated with surgical intervention. In addition, treatment by a shoulder or upper extremity specialist was associated with a higher likelihood of surgical intervention (49.1% versus 26.1%).

7. Visser CP, Coene LN, Brand R, Tavy DL: Nerve lesions in proximal humeral fractures. *J Shoulder Elbow Surg* 2001;10(5):421-427.

8. Haapamaki VV, Kiuru MJ, Koskinen SK: Multidetector CT in shoulder fractures. *Emerg Radiol* 2004;11(2):89-94.

9. Gerber C, Schneeberger AG, Vinh TS: The arterial vascularization of the humeral head. An anatomical study. *J Bone Joint Surg Am* 1990;72(10):1486-1494.

10. Coudane H, Fays J, De La Salle H, Nicoud C, Pilot L: Arteriography after complex fractures of the upper extremity of the humerus bone (a prospective study— preliminary results). *J Shoulder Elbow Surg* 2000;9:548.

11. Hettrich CM, Boraiah S, Dyke JP, Neviaser A, Helfet DL, Lorich DG: Quantitative assessment of the vascularity of the proximal part of the humerus. *J Bone Joint Surg Am* 2010;92(4):943-948.

    Assessment of 24 fresh frozen cadavers with gadolinium-enhanced MRI revealed the posterior humeral circumflex artery provides 64% of the blood flow to the humeral head.

12. Hertel R, Hempfing A, Stiehler M, Leunig M: Predictors of humeral head ischemia after intracapsular fracture of the proximal humerus. *J Shoulder Elbow Surg* 2004;13(4):427-433.

13. Bastian JD, Hertel R: Initial post-fracture humeral head ischemia does not predict development of necrosis. *J Shoulder Elbow Surg* 2008;17(1):2-8.

14. Neer CS II: Displaced proximal humeral fractures. I. Classification and evaluation. *J Bone Joint Surg Am* 1970;52(6):1077-1089.

15. Gaebler C, McQueen MM, Court-Brown CM: Minimally displaced proximal humeral fractures: Epidemiology and outcome in 507 cases. *Acta Orthop Scand* 2003;74(5):580-585.

16. Sanders RJ, Thissen LG, Teepen JC, van Kampen A, Jaarsma RL: Locking plate versus nonsurgical treatment for proximal humeral fractures: Better midterm outcome with nonsurgical treatment. *J Shoulder Elbow Surg* 2011;20(7):1118-1124.

    This retrospective review of nonsurgical versus operative outcomes at one year revealed no significant difference in American Shoulder and Elbow Surgeons scores. Except in internal rotation, an increased range of motion was found in the nonsurgical group. Level of evidence: IV.

17. Foruria AM, Martí M, Sanchez-Sotelo J: Proximal humeral fractures treated conservatively settle during fracture healing. *J Orthop Trauma* 2015;29(2):e24-e30.

    In a prospective comparison, 89 patients were evaluated radiographically and with CT to measure the amount of settling at 1 year. The greater tuberosity displaced more than 5 mm in less than 20% of patients. Varus patterns settled 9° and 7° retroverted on CT. Head shaft displacement increased over time. Level of evidence: IV (prognostic).

18. Murray IR, Amin AK, White TO, Robinson CM: Proximal humeral fractures: Current concepts in classification, treatment and outcomes. *J Bone Joint Surg Br* 2011;93(1):1-11.

    This review article explored the greater number of complex surgical patterns that may benefit from surgical intervention.

19. Hodgson SA, Mawson SJ, Saxton JM, Stanley D: Rehabilitation of two-part fractures of the neck of the humerus (two-year follow-up). *J Shoulder Elbow Surg* 2007;16(2):143-145.

    The authors report 2-year results of a prospective randomized controlled trial of minimally displaced proximal humeral fractures treated either by immediate physiotherapy or after 3 weeks of immobilization. Delayed rehabilitation by 3 weeks of shoulder immobilization produces a slower recovery, which continues for at least 2 years after injury. Level of evidence: I.

20. Lefevre-Colau MM, Babinet A, Fayad F, et al: Immediate mobilization compared with conventional immobilization for the impacted nonoperatively treated proximal humeral fracture. A randomized controlled trial. *J Bone Joint Surg Am* 2007;89(12):2582-2590.

21. Ajmal M, O'Sullivan M, McCabe J, Curtin W: Antegrade locked intramedullary nailing in humeral shaft fractures. *Injury* 2001;32(9):692-694.

22. Hatzidakis AM, Shevlin MJ, Fenton DL, Curran-Everett D, Nowinski RJ, Fehringer EV: Angular-stable locked intramedullary nailing of two-part surgical neck fractures of the proximal part of the humerus. A multicenter retrospective observational study. *J Bone Joint Surg Am* 2011;93(23):2172-2179.

    Thirty-eight patients with displaced surgical neck fractures were retrospectively reviewed after intramedullary nailing. New angular stable locked nails were used with an articular starting point avoiding the rotator cuff insertion. All but one fracture healed with neck shaft angle > 125° and minimal persistent shoulder pain. Level of evidence: IV.

23. Keener JD, Parsons BO, Flatow EL, Rogers K, Williams GR, Galatz LM: Outcomes after percutaneous reduction and fixation of proximal humeral fractures. *J Shoulder Elbow Surg* 2007;16(3):330-338.

24. Martin C, Guillen M, Lopez G: Treatment of 2- and 3-part fractures of the proximal humerus using external fixation: A retrospective evaluation of 62 patients. *Acta Orthop* 2006;77(2):275-278.

25. Dimakopoulos P, Panagopoulos A, Kasimatis G: Transosseous suture fixation of proximal humeral fractures. *J Bone Joint Surg Am* 2007;89(8):1700-1709.

26. Zhu Y, Lu Y, Shen J, Zhang J, Jiang C: Locking intramedullary nails and locking plates in the treatment of two-part proximal humeral surgical neck fractures: A prospective randomized trial with a minimum of three years of follow-up. *J Bone Joint Surg Am* 2011;93(2):159-168.

    A prospective trial of 51 patients with two-part proximal humerus fractures is presented. There was no difference in American Shoulder and Elbow Surgeons and visual analog scale scores between locked plates and intramedullary nails. Level of evidence: I.

27. Karataglis D, Stavridis SI, Petsatodis G, Papadopoulos P, Christodoulou A: New trends in fixation of proximal humeral fractures: A review. *Injury* 2011;42(4):330-338.

    This review article proposes a treatment algorithm given the heterogeneous classification systems and data available for each surgical intervention.

28. Krappinger D, Bizzotto N, Riedmann S, Kammerlander C, Hengg C, Kralinger FS: Predicting failure after surgical fixation of proximal humerus fractures. *Injury* 2011;42(11):1283-1288.

    Several parameters had a significant influence on the failure rate of surgical fixation: age, local bone mineral density, anatomic reduction, and restoration of the medial cortical support. The failure rate significantly increased with the number of risk factors. Level of evidence: IV.

29. Aaron D, Shatsky J, Paredes JC, Jiang C, Parsons BO, Flatow EL: Proximal humeral fractures: Internal fixation. *J Bone Joint Surg Am* 2012;94(24):2280-2288.

    This review article focused on the indications for each potential surgical option for proximal humerus fractures and their corresponding complications.

30. Lescheid J, Zdero R, Shah S, Kuzyk PR, Schemitsch EH: The biomechanics of locked plating for repairing proximal humerus fractures with or without medial cortical support. *J Trauma* 2010;69(5):1235-1242.

    In this prospective randomized study, at 3 years postoperatively, no significant difference could be found in terms of any parameter between the two groups. Significant improvement in the visual analog scale pain scores, American Shoulder and Elbow Surgeons scores, and Constant-Murley scores were found between the 1-year and 3-year follow-up examinations in each group. Level of evidence: I.

31. Schumer RA, Muckley KL, Markert RJ, et al: Biomechanical comparison of a proximal humeral locking plate using two methods of head fixation. *J Shoulder Elbow Surg* 2010;19(4):495-501.

    Although locking plates for proximal humerus fractures have emerged as the preferred method in open reduction internal fixation, no benefit in biomechanics are seen with smooth pegs versus threaded screws in this biomechanical study of 16 cadavers.

32. Jung SW, Shim SB, Kim HM, Lee JH, Lim HS: Factors that influence reduction loss in proximal humerus fracture surgery. *J Orthop Trauma* 2015;29(6):276-82.

In a retrospective review of 252 patients undergoing locking plate fixation, multivariable regression analysis revealed that osteoporosis (less than -2.5 bone mineral density, $P = 0.015$), displaced varus fracture (less than 110° of neck-shaft angle, $P = 0.025$), medial comminution (more than one fragment, $P = 0.018$), and insufficient medial support (no cortical or screw support, $P = 0.001$) were independent risk factors for reduction loss in the proximal humerus fractures surgery. Level of evidence: II (prognostic).

33. Olerud P, Ahrengart L, Ponzer S, Saving J, Tidermark J: Internal fixation versus nonoperative treatment of displaced 3-part proximal humeral fractures in elderly patients: A randomized controlled trial. *J Shoulder Elbow Surg* 2011;20(5):747-755.

The authors performed a prospective randomized study of 60 patients with an average age of 74 years. Although all patients improved in range of motion, there was no statistical difference in pain or Constant and DASH scores at 2 years. Thirty percent of the surgical group required further surgery. Level of evidence: I.

34. Solberg BD, Moon CN, Franco DP, Paiement GD: Locked plating of 3- and 4-part proximal humerus fractures in older patients: The effect of initial fracture pattern on outcome. *J Orthop Trauma* 2009;23(2):113-119.

35. Solberg BD, Moon CN, Franco DP, Paiement GD: Surgical treatment of three and four-part proximal humeral fractures. *J Bone Joint Surg Am* 2009;91(7):1689-1697.

36. Ricchetti ET, Warrender WJ, Abboud JA: Use of locking plates in the treatment of proximal humerus fractures. *J Shoulder Elbow Surg* 2010;19(2suppl):66-75.

In a review of 54 cases of proximal humeral fractures that underwent ORIF, a 20.4 % complication rate was reported. The case series focuses on the surgical principles and technique involved in proximal humeral ORIF. Level of evidence: IV.

37. Osterhoff G, Baumgartner D, Favre P, et al: Medial support by fibula bone graft in angular stable plate fixation of proximal humeral fractures: An in vitro study with synthetic bone. *J Shoulder Elbow Surg* 2011;20(5):740-746.

In a biomechanical study, an intramedullary strut used with a locked plate increased overall stiffness of the construction and reduced migration of the humeral head fragment.

38. Gardner MJ, Weil Y, Barker JU, Kelly BT, Helfet DL, Lorich DG: The importance of medial support in locked plating of proximal humerus fractures. *J Orthop Trauma* 2007;21(3):185-191.

39. Hinds RM, Garner MR, Tran WH, Lazaro LE, Dines JS, Lorich DG: Geriatric proximal humeral fracture patients show similar clinical outcomes to non-geriatric patients after osteosynthesis with endosteal fibular strut allograft augmentation. *J Shoulder Elbow Surg* 2015;24(6):889-96.

In a retrospective review, 71 patients were divided into two cohorts based on age of 65 years. Despite decreased forward flexion, there was no overall difference in functional outcome between both groups. Level of evidence: IV.

40. Egol KA, Sugi MT, Ong CC, Montero N, Davidovitch R, Zuckerman JD: Fracture site augmentation with calcium phosphate cement reduces screw penetration after open reduction-internal fixation of proximal humeral fractures. *J Shoulder Elbow Surg* 2012;21(6):741-748.

In a retrospective study of 91 patients, augmentation with calcium phosphate cement in the treatment of proximal humeral fractures with locked plates decreased fracture settling and intra-articular screw penetration when compared with no augmentation and cancellous chips. Level of evidence: III.

41. Gavaskar AS, Tummala NC: Locked plate osteosynthesis of humeral head-splitting fractures in young adults. *J Shoulder Elbow Surg* 2015;24(6):908-14.

A retrospective case series of head splitting fractures in 16 patients younger than 55 years undergoing locked plate ORIF is presented. DASH and Constant scores were significantly better in simple fractures with a lower rate of osteonecrosis. Level of evidence: IV.

42. Boileau P, Krishnan SG, Tinsi L, Walch G, Coste JS, Molé D: Tuberosity malposition and migration: Reasons for poor outcomes after hemiarthroplasty for displaced fractures of the proximal humerus. *J Shoulder Elbow Surg* 2002;11(5):401-412.

43. Boons HW, Goosen JH, van Grinsven S, van Susante JL, van Loon CJ: Hemiarthroplasty for humeral four-part fractures for patients 65 years and older: A randomized controlled trial. *Clin Orthop Relat Res* 2012;470(12):3483-3491.

In a randomized controlled trial, of 50 patients with four-part humeral head fractures underwent hemiarthroplasty versus nonsurgical intervention. No significant difference was found in strength, function, and pain in patients older than 65 years between surgical and nonsurgical intervention. Level of evidence: I.

44. Boyle MJ, Youn S-M, Frampton CM, Ball CM: Functional outcomes of reverse shoulder arthroplasty compared with hemiarthroplasty for acute proximal humeral fractures. *J Shoulder Elbow Surg* 2013;22(1):32-37.

A retrospective cohort review of New Zealand joint registry compared 55 rTSA patients versus 313 hemiarthroplasty patients for acute proximal humerus fractures. The 5-year functional outcomes were superior in the rTSA using the Oxford Shoulder Score. Level of evidence: III.

45. Chalmers PN, Slikker W III, Mall NA, et al: Reverse total shoulder arthroplasty for acute proximal humeral fracture: Comparison to open reduction-internal fixation and hemiarthroplasty. *J Shoulder Elbow Surg* 2014;23(2):197-204.

In a retrospective cohort study, 27 patients with three- and four-part fractures underwent rTSA, hemiarthroplasty, or ORIF. The rTSA group had a substantial increase in patients achieving 90% of forward elevation and a significant cost-saving benefit to Medicare. Level of evidence: III.

46. Mata-Fink A, Meinke M, Jones C, Kim B, Bell JE: Reverse shoulder arthroplasty for treatment of proximal humeral fractures in older adults: A systematic review. *J Shoulder Elbow Surg* 2013;22(12):1737-1748.

    A Cochrane meta-analysis of 15 retrospective studies compared 377 rTSA to 504 hemiarthroplasties for proximal humerus fractures. Overall functional outcomes were improved with the rTSA group and an average increase of 20° in forward flexion. Systematic review.

47. Ferrel JR, Trinh TQ, Fischer RA: Reverse total shoulder arthroplasty versus hemiarthroplasty for proximal humeral fractures: A systematic review. *J Orthop Trauma* 2015;29(1):60-68.

    When reverse total shoulder to hemiarthroplasty for fracture was compared in a systematic review, an increase in forward elevation by 10° with a corresponding decrease in external rotation by 10° on average was found. Level of evidence: IV.

48. Sirveaux F, Roche O, Molé D: Shoulder arthroplasty for acute proximal humerus fracture. *Orthop Traumatol Surg Res* 2010;96(6):683-694.

    This review article focused on optimizing the results for hemiarthroplasty in the setting of proximal humeral fracture.

49. Cazeneuve JF, Cristofari DJ: The reverse shoulder prosthesis in the treatment of fractures of the proximal humerus in the elderly. *J Bone Joint Surg Br* 2010;92(4):535-539.

    The radiographic and clinical outcomes for patients with a reverse total shoulder for fracture at an average of 6.6 years are presented. Overall radiographic glenoid baseplate loosening was most common (63%); however, only one patient was symptomatic. Level of evidence: IV.

of nerve injury. Spontaneous recovery occurred in 93% of these patients. The authors advised against primary exploration of the radial nerve in humeral nailing with or without radial nerve palsy.[31] In a systematic review of initial nonsurgical and surgical management of radial nerve palsy associated with acute humeral shaft fractures, there was no improvement in recovery with surgical treatment and increased patient complaints related to surgical management.[32]

A series of six cases of secondary radial nerve palsy after internal fixation of humeral shaft fractures were described.[33] Four cases were treated without surgery and the remaining two were treated with isolated nerve exploration after no recovery at 3 months postoperatively; all recovered near-normal function by 2 years without further intervention.

In a retrospective review of 25 cases of closed humeral shaft fractures with complete radial nerve palsies, 12 patients underwent nerve exploration after a mean period of expectant management of 16.8 weeks, with 2 patients demonstrating complete nerve transection. All intact nerves fully recovered after a mean of 22 weeks, and in 12 weeks in those not requiring exploration. The authors recommend expectant management for a period of 16 to 18 weeks due to the high rate of spontaneous recovery.[34] Complete radial nerve transections were reported in the setting of closed humeral shaft fractures in two patients with high-energy mechanisms of injury.[35]

The Holstein-Lewis fracture is a unique entity involving a spiral fracture of the distal third of the humeral diaphysis, representing 7.5% of all shaft fractures.[36] It is associated with a higher incidence of radial nerve palsy than other types of humeral shaft fractures. In a series of 27 patients with this injury (of whom 6 had radial nerve palsies), the overall outcome regarding fracture healing, radial nerve recovery, and function was very good irrespective of the primary treatment undertaken.[36]

Open Fractures With Radial Nerve Palsy

Radial nerve palsies are more commonly associated with open fractures. In a series of 530 consecutive isolated humeral shaft fractures, there were 117 documented radial nerve palsies. There were 30 open fractures, of which 16 had a radial nerve palsy (12 in Gustilo-Anderson grade I, 4 in Gustilo-Anderson grade II).[37] The authors observed spontaneous nerve recovery in 95% of closed fractures and 94% of grade I and II open fractures and recommended initial nonsurgical treatment of these injuries for a minimum of 10 to 12 weeks. However, surgeons must consider the mechanism of injury, as higher-energy injuries are less likely to result in spontaneous recovery of radial nerve function, and these may warrant early nerve exploration and possible repair or reconstruction.[30]

Multifocal Fractures

Humeral shaft fractures with associated ipsilateral injuries present a more challenging clinical scenario and usually lead to surgical management. A series of 35 patients sustaining a humeral shaft fracture and associated fracture of the proximal humerus that underwent ORIF with plates was described in a 2014 study.[38] The mean time to consolidation was 5 months. Major complications included one case of hardware failure, one case of pseudarthrosis, and one case of iatrogenic radial nerve palsy.[38] A series of floating elbow injuries treated with ORIF was described.[39] There were 15 injuries involving humeral shaft fractures, of which 8 were open and 9 had radial nerve palsies at presentation. Presence of nerve injury and intra-articular involvement negatively affected clinical outcomes.

Pathologic Fractures

Pathologic humeral shaft fractures represent a unique treatment dilemma, with a need for immediate stability and protection of the entire shaft from local disease spread and subsequent fractures. In a biomechanical study using a sawbone model of a completed mid-diaphyseal pathologic fracture, the fracture was treated with three plating and two nailing constructs.[40] Plating combined with cement augmentation of the medullary canal and defect demonstrated superior torsional stiffness and failure torque. Also, the addition of cement improved the torsional stiffness but not failure torque in the nailing groups.

Recent clinical studies have demonstrated positive results with intramedullary nails and plates. A series of five metastatic lesions to the humeral shaft were treated with intramedullary locked nails, curettage, cryosurgery, and cementing with acceptable results.[41] A case control study involving 21 patients who underwent intramedullary nailing for pathologic fractures with cement augmentation compared with 19 patients who underwent intramedullary nailing alone demonstrated less use of analgesics and better functional restoration immediately postoperatively in the former group, without a difference in complication rate.[42] In a series of 214 pathologic humerus fractures, there were 128 fractures involving the humeral shaft that were treated surgically, 117 of which were treated with a nail and 11 of which were fixed with plates. There were two failures with plates (both secondary to stress fractures) and eight failures with nails (five for nonunion, two for infection, one for stress fracture).[43] A series of 57 pathologic fractures were treated with antegrade unreamed intramedullary locked nailing without (9 cases) and with resection and cement augmentation (48 cases).

There were three cases of infection and one case of transient radial nerve palsy. All patients demonstrated improved pain and functional scores postoperatively.[44]

Nonunions

In a retrospective review of 659 surgically treated humeral shaft fractures, the incidence of nonunion was 3.6%.[45] Advanced age, smoking, use of NSAIDs, and American Society of Anesthesiologists score were associated with an increased risk of aseptic nonunion. Several different treatment modalities have proven successful for managing nonunion. A prospective randomized controlled trial compared an intramedullary nail to a locking compression plate for diaphyseal nonunions with 20 patients per group. At 2-year follow up, no differences were demonstrated with respect to union rate, time to union, shoulder and elbow range of motion, and Disabilities of the Arm, Shoulder and Hand scores.[46] In a series of 32 patients with humeral nonunions secondary to failed intramedullary nails, all cases were successfully treated with plating, achieving union in all cases with an average time to union of 3.8 months.[47] Nineteen of the cases were diaphyseal and in seven of these patients, the nail was left in situ. Bone graft was used in 25 cases (23 iliac crest bone grafts and 2 morselized, cryopreserved allografts). In a series of seven humeral shaft nonunions initially treated with intramedullary nails, isolated interfragmentary compression was successful in achieving union in all cases in 3 to 5 months.[48]

Osteoporotic Fractures

Humeral shaft fractures in elderly patients or those with osteoporosis present a technical challenge for surgical fixation when it is required. In a biomechanical study on osteoporotic human cadaver humeri, locked plates were compared to nonlocked plates. Locking constructs demonstrated higher mean cycles survived and stiffness. Catastrophic failure of the constructs occurred at a higher rate in the nonlocking group.[47]

Summary

Humeral shaft fractures account for 1% to 3% of all fractures. Radial nerve palsy occurs 11.8% of the time. Nonsurgical treatment of humeral shaft fractures is preferred, with an initial period in a coaptation splint that is converted to a functional brace. Indications for nonsurgical treatment include AP angulation less than 20°, varus-valgus angulation less than 30°, and less than 3 cm of shortening. Absolute surgical indications include open fracture with substantial soft-tissue injury or contamination, vascular injury, and compartment syndrome. Overall, there is a paucity of evidence favoring surgical over nonsurgical management of isolated humeral shaft fractures. Fixation options include plating, intramedullary nailing, and external fixation. Spontaneous recovery after radial nerve palsy has been demonstrated in 70% to 93% patients. Special consideration should be given to nonunions as well as high-energy, multifocal, pathologic, or osteoporotic fractures involving the humerus.

Key Study Points

- Surgical treatment of humeral shaft fractures may reduce the risk of malunion and nonunion compared with nonsurgical treatment; however, excellent results can often be obtained with initial coaptation splinting followed by functional bracing. Accepted alignment criteria for nonsurgical treatment include AP angulation less than 20°, varus-valgus angulation less than 30°, and less than 3 cm of shortening.
- Risk factors for humeral shaft nonunion include female sex, older age, high-energy mechanism, proximal third location, lack of comminution, smoking, and higher American Society of Anesthesiologists score.
- Radial nerve palsy occurs 12% of the time in humeral shaft fractures. Approximately 88% to 95% of these palsies recover spontaneously, even after iatrogenic injury from closed reduction or surgical fixation.

Annotated References

1. Mahabier KC, Vogels LM, Punt BJ, Roukema GR, Patka P, Van Lieshout EM: Humeral shaft fractures: Retrospective results of non-operative and operative treatment of 186 patients. *Injury* 2013;44(4):427-430.

   In a retrospective study involving 186 patients with humeral shaft fractures, 91 were treated nonsurgically and 95 were treated surgically. There were no differences with respect to consolidation time and complication rates between the groups. Level of evidence: IV.

2. Shao YC, Harwood P, Grotz MR, Limb D, Giannoudis PV: Radial nerve palsy associated with fractures of the shaft of the humerus: A systematic review. *J Bone Joint Surg Br* 2005;87(12):1647-1652.

3. Klenerman L: Fractures of the shaft of the humerus. *J Bone Joint Surg Br* 1966;48(1):105-111.

4. Stedtfeld HW, Biber R: Proximal third humeral shaft fractures — a fracture entity not fully characterized by conventional AO classification. *Injury* 2014;45(suppl 1):S54-S59.

In a retrospective study, 72 patients with proximal third humeral shaft fractures were treated with an intramedullary nail. The authors discuss the differences between proximal third humeral shaft fractures and the distal two-thirds with respect to fracture morphology and outcomes. Level of evidence: IV.

5. Ali E, Griffiths D, Obi N, Tytherleigh-Strong G, Van Rensburg L: Nonoperative treatment of humeral shaft fractures revisited. *J Shoulder Elbow Surg* 2015;24(2):210-214.

   A retrospective review of 207 humeral shaft fractures treated nonsurgically with a functional brace was done. The authors present union rates based on fracture location and morphology, indicating that surgeons should have a lower threshold for surgical intervention in proximal third, two-part spiral-oblique humeral shaft fractures. Level of evidence: IV.

6. Neuhaus V, Menendez M, Kurylo JC, Dyer GS, Jawa A, Ring D: Risk factors for fracture mobility six weeks after initiation of brace treatment of mid-diaphyseal humeral fractures. *J Bone Joint Surg Am* 2014;96(5):403-407.

   Seventy-nine closed, mid-diaphyseal humeral shaft fractures treated with a functional brace were retrospectively reviewed. Risk factors for motion at the fracture site and a persistent fracture line on radiographs at 6 weeks after injury included each millimeter of gap between the main fracture fragments after brace application, female sex, and smoking. Level of evidence: IV.

7. Shields E, Sundem L, Childs S, et al: Factors predicting patient-reported functional outcome scores after humeral shaft fractures. *Injury* 2015;46(4):693-698.

   In a retrospective review of 77 patients with humeral shaft fractures, 45 had surgery and 32 were treated nonsurgically. Patient age, history of psychiatric illness, insurance type, fracture location, and Charlson Comorbidity Index scores demonstrated a statistically significant effect on patient-reported functional outcomes (Disabilities of the Arm, Shoulder and Hand, Simple Shoulder Test, Short Form-12). Level of evidence: IV.

8. Denard A Jr, Richards JE, Obremskey WT, Tucker MC, Floyd M, Herzog GA: Outcome of nonoperative vs operative treatment of humeral shaft fractures: A retrospective study of 213 patients. *Orthopedics* 2010;33(8).

   In a retrospective review, 213 patients with humeral shaft fractures were treated both nonsurgically and surgically with plate fixation. Closed treatment resulted in a substantially higher rate of nonunion and malunion, whereas no differences were found compared with surgical treatment with respect to time to union, infection, and iatrogenic nerve injury. Level of evidence: III.

9. van Middendorp JJ, Kazacsay F, Lichtenhahn P, Renner N, Babst R, Melcher G: Outcomes following operative and non-operative management of humeral midshaft fractures: A prospective, observational cohort study of 47 patients. *Eur J Trauma Emerg Surg* 2011;37(3):287-296.

   A prospective, observational cohort study of 47 patients demonstrated an early benefit in patients treated with a humeral nail at 6 weeks with respect to shoulder abduction strength, elbow flexion strength, functional hand positioning, and return to recreational activities, but these benefits were not present at 1-year follow-up. Level of evidence: II.

10. Singh AK, Narsaria N, Seth RR, Garg S: Plate osteosynthesis of fractures of the shaft of the humerus: Comparison of limited contact dynamic compression plates and locking compression plates. *J Orthop Traumatol* 2014;15(2):117-122.

    The authors performed a retrospective review of 212 patients treated with either compression plates (102) or locking compression plates (110). No significant differences were found with respect to surgical time, time to fracture union, complication rates, or clinical outcome scores. Level of evidence: III.

11. Kim JW, Oh CW, Byun YS, Kim JJ, Park KC: A prospective randomized study of operative treatment for noncomminuted humeral shaft fractures: Conventional open plating versus minimal invasive plate osteosynthesis. *J Orthop Trauma* 2015;29(4):189-194.

    In a prospective, multicenter randomized controlled trial, 68 patients with humeral shaft fractures were treated with either conventional open plating or minimally invasive plate osteosynthesis. There were no significant differences found between groups with respect to surgical time, complications, union rate, or functional outcome. Level of evidence: I.

12. Patel R, Neu CP, Curtiss S, Fyhrie DP, Yoo B: Crutch weightbearing on comminuted humeral shaft fractures: A biomechanical comparison of large versus small fragment fixation for humeral shaft fractures. *J Orthop Trauma* 2011;25(5):300-305.

    A biomechanical study compared nonlocking small-fragment and large-fragment plates for the treatment of humeral shaft fractures with a 1-cm defect in composite humeri. The axial and torsional stiffness, plastic deformation, and yield force were significantly better in the large fragment group. Level of evidence: IV.

13. Kosmopoulos V, Nana AD: Dual plating of humeral shaft fractures: Orthogonal plates biomechanically outperform side-by-side plates. *Clin Orthop Relat Res* 2014;472(4):1310-1317.

    A finite element analysis was used to compare five dual small fragment locking plate construct configurations for mid-diaphyseal humeral shaft fractures. The 90° plate configuration where a nine-hole plate was placed anterior and a seven-hole plate was placed lateral provided the best fixation with respect to torsional and axial stiffness, stress shielding, and strain. Level of evidence: IV.

14. Cheng HR, Lin J: Prospective randomized comparative study of antegrade and retrograde locked nailing for middle humeral shaft fracture. *J Trauma* 2008;65(1):94-102.

15. Patino JM: Treatment of humeral shaft fractures using antegrade nailing: Functional outcome in the shoulder. *J Shoulder Elbow Surg* 2015;24(8):1302-1306.

A retrospective review of 30 patients who underwent antegrade locked intramedullary nailing for humeral shaft fractures was performed. Results were reported as excellent in 40% of patients, good in 20%, fair in 23.3%, and poor in 16.6%. Full shoulder mobility was achieved in 40% of patients and restricted compared with the contralateral unaffected shoulder in the remaining 60% of patients. Avoidance of nail impingement can improve final outcomes. Level of evidence: IV.

16. Baltov A, Mihail R, Dian E: Complications after interlocking intramedullary nailing of humeral shaft fractures. *Injury* 2014;45(suppl 1):S9-S15.

A retrospective review of 111 patients with humeral shaft fractures treated with intramedullary humeral nails was performed. Intraoperative and postoperative complications both occurred in 36% of patients. Intraoperative and postoperative complications were more likely in patients treated with first-generation humeral nails compared with second-generation nails. Level of evidence: IV.

17. Tyllianakis M, Tsoumpos P, Anagnostou K, Konstantopoulou A, Panagopoulos A: Intramedullary nailing of humeral diaphyseal fractures. Is distal locking really necessary? *Int J Shoulder Surg* 2013;7(2):65-69.

A retrospective review of 64 patients with acute humeral shaft fractures treated with antegrade humeral nailing without distal locking screws was performed. After nail impaction into the olecranon fossa, rotational stability was carefully assessed. Patients were instructed to avoid external rotation for 4 weeks postoperatively. Two nonunions were successfully treated with revision procedures. This technique reduces surgical time and radiation exposure, and avoids potential damage to neurovascular structures. Level of evidence: IV.

18. Garnavos C: Diaphyseal humeral fractures and intramedullary nailing: Can we improve outcomes? *Indian J Orthop* 2011;45(3):208-215.

This review article on the use of intramedullary nails for the management of humeral shaft fractures discusses antegrade versus retrograde, reamed versus unreamed, and static versus dynamic locking. Level of evidence: V.

19. Kurup H, Hossain M, Andrew JG: Dynamic compression plating versus locked intramedullary nailing for humeral shaft fractures in adults. *Cochrane Database Syst Rev* 2011;6:CD005959.

A meta-analysis of randomized and quasi-randomized controlled trials compared compression plates and locked intramedullary nail fixation for humeral shaft fractures in adults. Nailing is associated with an increased risk of shoulder impingement, decreased shoulder motion, and increased incidence of hardware removal compared with plating, No differences were found in fracture union. Level of evidence: I.

20. Ouyang H, Xiong J, Xiang P, Cui Z, Chen L, Yu B: Plate versus intramedullary nail fixation in the treatment of humeral shaft fractures: An updated meta-analysis. *J Shoulder Elbow Surg* 2013;22(3):387-395.

A meta-analysis of 10 randomized controlled trials comparing plating and intramedullary nailing for the treatment of humeral shaft fractures was performed. Plating resulted in a lower incidence of shoulder impingement, shoulder motion restriction, and reoperation for hardware removal compared with nailing. Level of evidence: I.

21. Li Y, Wang C, Wang M, Huang L, Huang Q: Postoperative malrotation of humeral shaft fracture after plating compared with intramedullary nailing. *J Shoulder Elbow Surg* 2011;20(6):947-954.

A prospective randomized controlled trial was performed comparing ORIF and antegrade humeral nailing for humeral shaft fractures in 45 patients. Malrotation of 20° or more as measured by postoperative CT scans occurred in 27% of the nail group but did not occur in the ORIF group. Level of evidence: I.

22. Benegas E, Ferreira Neto AA, Gracitelli ME, et al: Shoulder function after surgical treatment of displaced fractures of the humeral shaft: A randomized trial comparing antegrade intramedullary nailing with minimally invasive plate osteosynthesis. *J Shoulder Elbow Surg* 2014;23(6):767-774.

A prospective randomized controlled trial comparing minimally invasive plate fixation to locking intramedullary nails was performed on 41 patients with humeral shaft fractures. No significant differences were found with respect to shoulder and elbow function, union rate, and complications between groups. Level of evidence: I.

23. Chen F, Wang Z, Bhattacharyya T: Outcomes of nails versus plates for humeral shaft fractures: A Medicare cohort study. *J Orthop Trauma* 2013;27(2):68-72.

In a retrospective study of cancer-free Medicare claims derived from a 5% sample during the period from 1993 to 2007, there were 511 individuals identified who underwent surgical fixation. Nail fixation was more prevalent and had shorter anesthesia time by 27 minutes. There were no significant differences with respect to secondary procedures and 1-year mortality. Level of evidence: II.

24. Scaglione M, Fabbri L, Dell' Omo D, Goffi A, Guido G: The role of external fixation in the treatment of humeral shaft fractures: A retrospective case study review on 85 humeral fractures. *Injury* 2015;46(2):265-269.

A retrospective review of 85 humeral fractures (62 of which were shaft, 23 of which were extra-articular distal third fractures) treated with external fixation was performed. Healing occurred in 97.6% of cases with an average consolidation time of 12 weeks. There was one case of delayed union and one case of re-fracture. Level of evidence: IV.

25. Suzuki T, Hak DJ, Stahel PF, Morgan SJ, Smith WR: Safety and efficacy of conversion from external fixation to

plate fixation in humeral shaft fractures. *J Orthop Trauma* 2010;24(7):414-419.

A retrospective review of 17 patients treated with immediate external fixation followed by conversion to internal plate fixation for humeral shaft fractures was performed. Indications included polytrauma (nine patients), massive soft tissue injury (six patients), suspected vascular injury (one patient), and upper arm compartment syndrome (one patient). Fifteen fractures healed at an average of 11 weeks. Two fractures did not heal in the setting of deep infection. Level of evidence: IV.

26. Arora S, Goel N, Cheema GS, Batra S, Maini L: A method to localize the radial nerve using the 'apex of triceps aponeurosis' as a landmark. *Clin Orthop Relat Res* 2011;469(9):2638-2644.

    An anatomic study involving cadaver dissections and intraoperative measurements assessed the distance of the radial nerve from the apex of the triceps aponeurosis during the posterior approach, which demonstrated a mean distance of 2.5 cm. Level of evidence: IV.

27. Seigerman DA, Choung EW, Yoon RS, et al: Identification of the radial nerve during the posterior approach to the humerus: A cadaveric study. *J Orthop Trauma* 2012;26(4):226-228.

    In an anatomic study, cadaver dissections identified the location of the radial nerve at a mean distance 3.9 cm proximal to the intersection of the long and lateral heads of the triceps and the triceps aponeurosis during the posterior approach. Level of evidence: IV.

28. Yin P, Zhang L, Mao Z, et al: Comparison of lateral and posterior surgical approach in management of extra-articular distal humeral shaft fractures. *Injury* 2014;45(7):1121-1125.

    A retrospective study comparing the lateral and posterior approaches for the management of extra-articular distal humerus fractures was performed. The overall complication rate was lower in the lateral approach group. No other statistically significant differences were found. Level of evidence: III.

29. Lee TJ, Kwon DG, Na SI, Cha SD: Modified combined approach for distal humerus shaft fracture: Anterolateral and lateral bimodal approach. *Clin Orthop Surg* 2013;5(3):209-215.

    A retrospective review of 35 patients treated with a combined anterolateral and lateral approach for distal humeral shaft fractures was performed, demonstrating its clinical utility without complications. Level of evidence: IV.

30. Venouziou AI, Dailiana ZH, Varitimidis SE, Hantes ME, Gougoulias NE, Malizos KN: Radial nerve palsy associated with humeral shaft fracture. Is the energy of trauma a prognostic factor? *Injury* 2011;42(11):1289-1293.

    A retrospective review of 18 patients treated surgically for humeral shaft fracture with associated radial nerve palsy was performed. All patients with low-energy trauma experienced full radial nerve recovery. Five of 13 patients with high-energy trauma had intact radial nerves and experienced full recovery, whereas the remaining 13 had severely damaged nerves and no spontaneous recovery. Level of evidence: IV.

31. Grass G, Kabir K, Ohse J, Rangger C, Besch L, Mathiak G: Primary exploration of radial nerve is not required for radial nerve palsy while treating humerus shaft fractures with unreamed humerus nails (UHN). *Open Orthop J* 2011;5:319-323.

    A retrospective review of 38 patients treated with humeral shaft fractures treated with humeral nails was performed. There was a 40% incidence of radial nerve palsy, of which 93% resolved spontaneously. There were no iatrogenic nerve injuries. Level of evidence: IV.

32. Liu GY, Zhang CY, Wu HW: Comparison of initial nonoperative and operative management of radial nerve palsy associated with acute humeral shaft fractures. *Orthopedics* 2012;35(8):702-708.

    A meta-analysis of studies comparing initial nonsurgical and surgical management of radial nerve palsy associated with humeral shaft fractures was performed. One prospective observational study and eight retrospective studies were included. Surgical management showed no improved recovery from radial nerve palsy. Level of evidence: II.

33. Wang X, Zhang P, Zhou Y, Zhu C: Secondary radial nerve palsy after internal fixation of humeral shaft fractures. *Eur J Orthop Surg Traumatol* 2014;24(3):331-333.

    A retrospective review of 125 patients with humeral shaft fractures treated with internal fixation was performed, identifying six patients with secondary radial nerve palsies. Four patients spontaneously recovered, whereas two were found to have no macroscopic nerve damage. These patients recovered as well. Level of evidence: IV.

34. Korompilias AV, Lykissas MG, Kostas-Agnantis IP, Vekris MD, Soucacos PN, Beris AE: Approach to radial nerve palsy caused by humerus shaft fracture: Is primary exploration necessary? *Injury* 2013;44(3):323-326.

    A retrospective review of 25 patients with closed humeral shaft fractures complicated by radial nerve palsy was performed. Surgical exploration of the radial nerve was performed in 12 patients at a mean period of expectant management of 16.8 weeks, of whom 10 had intact radial nerves and 2 had complete radial nerve transections. All intact radial nerves fully recovered. Level of evidence: IV.

35. Leucht P, Ryu JH, Bellino MJ: Radial nerve transection associated with closed humeral shaft fractures: A report of two cases and review of the literature. *J Shoulder Elbow Surg* 2015;24(4):e96-e100.

    The authors found complete radial nerve transections associated with closed humeral shaft fractures in two patients with high-energy mechanisms of injury.

36. Ekholm R, Ponzer S, Törnkvist H, Adami J, Tidermark J: The Holstein-Lewis humeral shaft fracture: Aspects of radial nerve injury, primary treatment, and outcome. *J Orthop Trauma* 2008;22(10):693-697.

37. Bumbasirević M, Lesić A, Bumbasirević V, Cobeljić G, Milosević I, Atkinson HD: The management of humeral shaft fractures with associated radial nerve palsy: A review of 117 cases. *Arch Orthop Trauma Surg* 2010;130(4):519-522.

A retrospective review of 117 consecutive patients with humeral shaft fractures and associated radial nerve palsy was performed. Spontaneous radial nerve recovery occurred at a mean of 6 weeks with full recovery at a mean of 17 weeks in 95% of patients. Level of evidence: IV.

38. Maresca A, Pascarella R, Bettuzzi C, et al: Multifocal humeral fractures. *Injury* 2014;45(2):444-447.

A retrospective review of 35 patients with multifocal fractures of the proximal humerus and humeral shaft treated surgically was performed. A classification system was proposed. Level of evidence: IV.

39. Ditsios K, Boutsiadis A, Papadopoulos P, et al: Floating elbow injuries in adults: Prognostic factors affecting clinical outcomes. *J Shoulder Elbow Surg* 2013;22(1):74-80.

A retrospective review of 19 patients with floating elbow injuries was reviewed. Fractures were open in 10 patients and radial nerve palsy was present in 10 patients. Intra-articular involvement and nerve palsy were correlated with worse clinical outcomes. Level of evidence: IV.

40. Al-Jahwari A, Schemitsch EH, Wunder JS, Ferguson PC, Zdero R: The biomechanical effect of torsion on humeral shaft repair techniques for completed pathological fractures. *J Biomech Eng* 2012;134(2):024501.

A biomechanical study on artificial humeri with a 2-cm hemicylindrical defect comparing five fixation constructs was performed. The construct using a 10-hole 4.5 mm dynamic compression plate with bone cement inserted into the defect and screws inserted into dry cement demonstrated the highest torsional load to failure. Level of evidence: IV.

41. Muramatsu K, Ihara K, Iwanagaa R, Taguchi T: Treatment of metastatic bone lesions in the upper extremity: Indications for surgery. *Orthopedics* 2010;33(11):807.

A retrospective review of 20 patients with metastatic lesions in the upper extremity, of which 12 were in the humerus, was performed. Humeral shaft lesions were treated with curettage, internal fixation, and cementing whereas humeral head lesions or intra-articular distal humerus lesions were treated with endoprostheses. Level of evidence: IV.

42. Laitinen M, Nieminen J, Pakarinen TK: Treatment of pathological humerus shaft fractures with intramedullary nails with or without cement fixation. *Arch Orthop Trauma Surg* 2011;131(4):503-508.

A case control study of 40 patients treated with cemented or uncemented intramedullary nails was performed. Patients in the cemented group had better pain relief, less use of analgesics, and better functional restoration immediately after surgery without an increase in complication rate. Level of evidence: III.

43. Wedin R, Hansen BH, Laitinen M, et al: Complications and survival after surgical treatment of 214 metastatic lesions of the humerus. *J Shoulder Elbow Surg* 2012;21(8):1049-1055.

A retrospective review of 208 patients treated surgically for 214 metastatic lesions of the humerus was performed. There was a total of 128 pathologic humeral shaft fractures treated with either a nail or a plate. The reoperation rate was 7% in the proximal humerus, 8% in the diaphysis, and 33% in the distal humerus. Intramedullary nail failure rate was 7% compared with 22% in the osteosynthesis group. Level of evidence: IV.

44. Piccioli A, Maccauro G, Rossi B, Scaramuzzo L, Frenos F, Capanna R: Surgical treatment of pathologic fractures of humerus. *Injury* 2010;41(11):1112-1116.

A retrospective review of 87 pathologic humeral fractures in 85 patients was performed. Good results were achieved with endoprostheses and locked intramedullary nailing (57 fractures). Level of evidence: IV.

45. Ding L, He Z, Xiao H, Chai L, Xue F: Factors affecting the incidence of aseptic nonunion after surgical fixation of humeral diaphyseal fracture. *J Orthop Sci* 2014;19(6):973-977.

A retrospective review of 659 humeral diaphyseal fractures, of which 24 resulted in aseptic nonunion, was performed. Risk factors for nonunion were advanced age, smoking, use of NSAIDs, and American Society of Anesthesiologists score. Level of evidence: IV.

46. Singh AK, Arun GR, Narsaria N, Srivastava A: Treatment of non-union of humerus diaphyseal fractures: A prospective study comparing interlocking nail and locking compression plate. *Arch Orthop Trauma Surg* 2014;134(7):947-953.

A prospective randomized controlled trial comparing intramedullary nails to locking compression plates for 40 nonunions of humeral diaphyseal fractures was performed. No significant differences were found with respect to union time or rate, shoulder and elbow range of motion and function, and complication rate. Level of evidence: I.

47. Allende C, Paz A, Altube G, Boccolini H, Malvarez A, Allende B: Revision with plates of humeral nonunions secondary to failed intramedullary nailing. *Int Orthop* 2014;38(4):899-903.

A retrospective review of 32 patients with humeral nonunions treated with plating after intramedullary nailing was performed. Union was achieved in all cases at an average of 3.8 months. Level of evidence: IV.

48. Apard T, Ducellier F, Hubert L, Talha A, Cronier P, Bizot P: Isolated interfragmentary compression for nonunion of humeral shaft fractures initially treated by nailing: A preliminary report of seven cases. *Injury* 2010;41(12):1262-1265.

A retrospective review of seven cases of humeral shaft nonunion treated with interfragmentary compression after initial retrograde locked nailing was performed. Union was achieved in all cases without complications. Level of evidence: IV.

Chapter 24

Distal Humerus Fracture

Yaron Sela, MD   Mark E. Baratz, MD

Abstract

Distal humerus fractures are a challenge in diagnosis, surgical intervention, and rehabilitation. Dual plate fixation oriented at 90° or 180° is indicated for most adult fractures involving both columns of the distal part of the humerus. Fixation techniques and failure of adequate reconstruction or fixation are controversial and can be treated with other measures such as incorporation of structural bone grafts, external fixation, and salvage with total elbow arthroplasty (TEA). Acute TEA is the preferred treatment of elderly patients with a displaced, comminuted, intra-articular distal humerus fracture that is not amenable to stable internal fixation. Displaced coronal shear fractures of the distal humerus articular surface require surgical fixation. Advances in the understanding of fracture patterns by means of improved diagnostic imaging, new exposure techniques, improved fixation, and recognition of proper rehabilitation techniques has improved patient outcomes.

Keywords: distal humerus fracture; elderly patients; open reduction internal fixation; ORIF; arthroplasty

Dr. Baratz or an immediate family member has received royalties from Integra; serves as a paid consultant to Elizur and Integra; has stock or stock options held in UPEX; and serves as a board member, owner, officer, or committee member of the American Association for Hand Surgery. Neither Dr. Sela nor any immediate family member has received anything of value from or has stock or stock options held in a commercial company or institution related directly or indirectly to the subject of this chapter.

Introduction and Epidemiology

Fractures of the distal humerus can be challenging to treat. Although the overall incidence of distal humerus fractures in adults has been reported to be only 5.7 cases per 100,000,[1] these fractures can result in considerable long-term impairment. Fractures can range from simple extra-articular fractures to complex fractures with extensive comminution of the metaphysis and articular surface. Surgical intervention is indicated in most cases and is often complicated by difficult exposure, osteoporotic bone, and comminution. Controversy exists regarding the management of distal humeral fractures, including the surgical approach, fixation strategies, the role of total elbow arthroplasty (TEA), and management of the ulnar nerve.

Anatomy

The complex anatomy of the distal humerus reflects its articulation with both the radius and ulna (**Figure 1**) and allows a wide range of motion (ROM) in multiple planes. The trochlea and capitellum comprise the articular component of the distal humerus. The articular surface of the distal humerus articulates with the ulna at the ulnohumeral joint and with the radius at the radiocapitellar joint. Just proximal to the trochlea are the olecranon and coronoid fossae; these concavities are composed of thin cortical bone that articulates with the proximal olecranon in extension and the coronoid process in flexion. The medial epicondyle is the origin of the flexor-pronator muscle group and the medial collateral ligament. The lateral epicondyle is the origin of the extensor-supinator muscle group and the lateral collateral ligament complex. The ulnar nerve lies in a bony groove covered and restrained by the annular ligament posterior to the medial epicondyle.

Evaluation

Clinical Examination

The thorough clinical evaluation of a patient with a distal humeral fracture must include examination of the

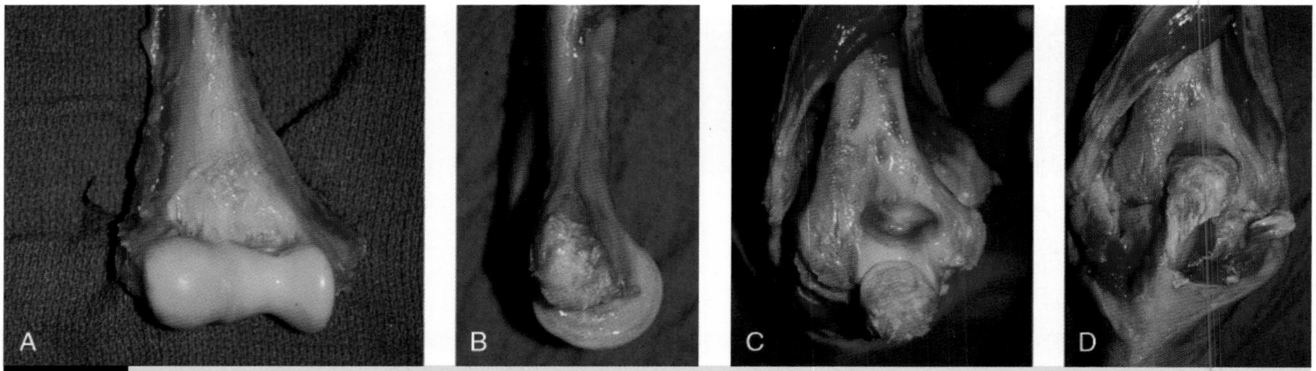

Figure 1 Photographs demonstrate distal humerus anatomy. **A**, View of the articular surface of distal humerus is in 5° to 6° of valgus with respect to the humeral shaft. **B**, View of the articular surface in 30° of flexion. **C** and **D**, Views of the posterior aspect of the distal humerus show a bare area on the posterior aspect of the lateral condyle that permits safe placement of hardware. Screws placed into or across the olecranon fossa can block elbow extension if they impinge against the tip of the olecranon during attempted elbow extension.

ipsilateral shoulder and wrist. Soft-tissue integrity is documented and a detailed neurovascular examination is performed.

Radiographic Evaluation

Conventional radiography should include AP, lateral, and oblique views.[2] Severely unstable fractures should undergo simple realignment and splinting before the radiographs are obtained to minimize any further soft-tissue injury. Contralateral elbow radiographs can help with preoperative planning, especially in selecting the length of implants. Traction films also can help delineate fracture patterns.

CT is a powerful tool for characterizing fractures of the distal humerus.[2] Two-dimensional (2D) CT allows accurate assessment of the fracture in multiple planes and is often useful in surgical planning. Three-dimensional (3D) reconstructions provide a topographic view of the anatomy and use subtraction technology to isolate the distal humerus for a more detailed picture of the fracture complexity (**Figure 2**).

One study compared the use of 3D CT reconstructions with the use of 2D CT and radiographs to classify distal humeral fractures and for preoperative planning.[3] Increased interobserver and intraobserver reliability for fracture classification were reported, as well as increased intraobserver reliability for treatment decisions with the use of 3D CT. A 2012 study reported that 3D CT substantially improved sensitivity but not specificity in diagnosis and did not change the treatment of distal humerus fractures.[4] Despite these contradicting reports, most surgeons find CT helpful when reassembling these fractures.

Classification

Distal humeral fractures include both the supracondylar metadiaphyseal distal humerus often extending to split the articular components. Anatomically, the fractures can be classified as supracondylar, transcondylar, and intercondylar. Further subclassification describes fracture extension: type A includes extra-articular fractures; type B fractures extend from the metaphysis into the articular surface; and type C fractures are the T-type with a transverse extra-articular limb and a vertical intra-articular portion that splits the trochlea and capitellum, which makes fracture reduction and stabilization challenging. These three types are further graded by the extent of comminution using the descriptors 1, 2, and 3.

Coronal shear fractures are confined to articular injuries with displacement of the major osteochondral fragment. These fractures can include just the capitellum, or the entire trochlea in some cases. These injuries are subdivided based on the five possible major articular fragments. No classification scheme has been shown to reliably indicate treatment or predict outcome.

Treatment

Nonsurgical Treatment

In nondisplaced or minimally displaced, stable distal humerus fractures, closed treatment is preferred, consisting of splinting for up to 1 month followed by bracing until clinical union is achieved.[2] The typical patients treated with this approach are the elderly with low demands and multiple medical comorbidities. Careful patient assessment is required because some of the distal transverse fragility fractures often go on to nonunion and can create

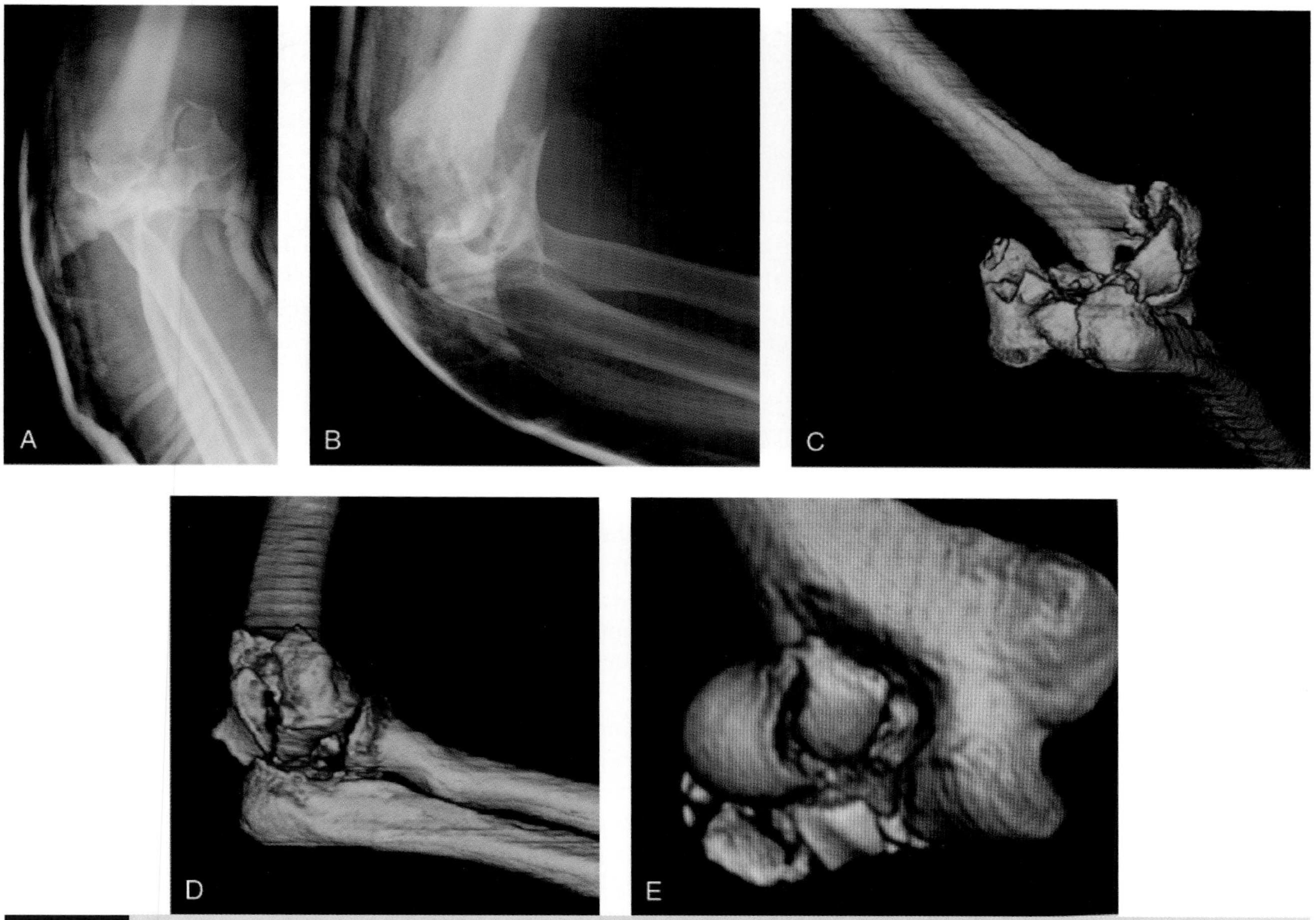

Figure 2 Images demonstrate evaluation of a distal humerus fracture. AP (**A**) and lateral (**B**) radiographs of a 54-year-old who sustained an intra-articular shear fracture. **C** and **D**, Preoperative three-dimensional CT scans. **E**, Preoperative 3D CT scan with subtraction of radius and ulna.

a flail-type extremity with diminished potential for use as an assistive arm.

A 2013 study reviewed the role of nonsurgical treatment in patients older than 65 years.[5] One prospective and one retrospective study reviewed a total of 56 patients with a mean age of 84.7 years. All were treated using a posterior splint for 6 to 8 weeks without fracture reduction: 18 AO type A fractures, 8 type B fractures, and 30 type C fractures were treated. At a mean 20-month follow-up for the retrospective study and a mean 8.6-month follow-up for the prospective series, the mean Mayo Elbow Performance Score (MEPS), satisfaction, and Quick Disabilities of the Arm, Shoulder and Hand (DASH) score were acceptable and roughly equivalent. Three cases of nonunion were reported. In the retrospective series, 70% of patients had extra-articular malunion and 65% had intra-articular malunion; in the prospective series, 16% had intra-articular malunion. The rate of osteoarthritis increased over time, but the mean follow-up of 20 months and advanced patient age may limit the negative consequence of slow progression of arthritis following malunion. Three complications were reported: two hematomas and one skin lesion. Nonsurgical treatment of distal humerus fracture is used infrequently in patients older than 65 years but provides satisfactory clinical results despite a high incidence of malunion.

Osteosynthesis is the preferred treatment of all displaced distal humerus fractures, although some highly comminuted fractures that are extremely distal (as is typical of osteoporotic fragility fractures) may be better managed with immediate TEA. A retrospective study compared the results of 273 patients who underwent osteosynthesis with 47 patients treated using immobilization alone.[1] In the patients undergoing closed treatment, nonunion was six times more likely to develop and delayed union was four times more likely to occur.

Surgical Approach

Several surgical options are available, and selection is based on the fracture type and comminution as well as the surgeon's experience and comfort level. Nonarticular patterns (simple type B articular patterns) can be managed by using either a medial or lateral column approach. The comminuted type C articular fractures need a more extensile approach and tend to be grouped as either "triceps-on" or "triceps-off." The advantages of triceps-on are that continuity of the extensor mechanism is maintained and that another fracture is not created, resulting in additional potential problems of incongruence, nonunion, and hardware intolerance. Described approaches include the paratricipital (Alonso-Llames) and triceps-splitting, which are triceps sparing (triceps-on); and triceps-reflecting (Bryan-Morrey), triceps-reflecting anconeus pedicle, and olecranon osteotomy (triceps-off). The rationale for each approach has been discussed in a study in which triceps-splitting, triceps-reflecting, and olecranon osteotomy were performed on human cadaver elbows. By painting the exposed articular surfaces with methylene blue, the olecranon osteotomy was determined to expose the most articular surface compared with the triceps-splitting and triceps-reflecting techniques, but this difference did not reach significance in the setting of triceps-reflecting exposure.[6] Furthermore, the assistance of the intact olecranon articular surface to reduce the trochlear fragments and help prevent overreduction or malreduction by narrowing the joint through compression of comminuted central fragments or by placing the trochlea into excessive extension to gain bony contact is not accounted for. The triceps-splitting and triceps-reflecting exposures allow adequate visualization for reassembly of the posterior portion of the trochlea.[6] The most common exposure (which could be considered a default) of the olecranon osteotomy provides the best overall view of both the trochlea and capitellum.

The triceps-splitting approach (triceps on) preserves the proximal innervation of the muscle maintaining muscle contractility (**Figure 3, A** through **C**). Most surgeons will limit the exposure to a split that stops at the tip of the olecranon. The exposure can be continued to elevate the triceps off the proximal ulna entirely, but it can still be repaired with a running suture.[7] The proximal 1 cm of the olecranon tip also can be resected to improve visualization of the articular surface.

This technique is most commonly used for fractures without articular comminution (types A and B) because visualization of the articular surface is limited.[2,8] One study reviewed a triceps-splitting approach in 34 fractures.[7] A variation of this approach was performed in which the triceps was peeled off the olecranon and both collateral ligaments were peeled off the distal humerus. This extensile exposure better visualized the anterior trochlea. One case of heterotopic ossification, one transient ulnar nerve palsy, five instances of nonunion, and four cases of varus or valgus instability were reported. There are concerns regarding elbow destabilization with distal elevation of the triceps tendon.

The paratricipital approach avoids violation of the extensor mechanism of the elbow by using medial and lateral windows on either side of the triceps, which makes it amenable to treat extra-articular and intra-articular fractures[9] (**Figure 3, D** and **E**). Increased visualization of the distal and anterior aspects of the articular surface can be obtained by releasing the noncritical posterior ulnar collateral ligament while preserving its critical anterior bundle. This allows the forearm to be subluxated and the anterior trochlea to be visualized. This approach is appealing because it can be converted to the standard olecranon osteotomy at any time. This triceps-sparing approach also allows easy conversion from planned internal fixation to TEA.

A 2012 study reported a median motion arc of 126° and 90% triceps strength using "extensor mechanism-on approach" to treat distal humerus fractures.[10] Indirect methods and fluoroscopy were used to achieve articular fragment fixation. Some highly comminuted fractures required conversion to olecranon osteotomy.

The posterior triceps-sparing approach was initially designed for elbow reconstruction, particularly TEA (**Figure 3, F** and **G**). The procedure elevates the triceps tendon off the olecranon from medial to lateral, being careful to maintain continuity of the triceps tendon with a sliver of proximal ulna to aid in healing and reattachment to the proximal ulna using sutures placed through drill holes. One study reviewed the functional outcome of AO type C fractures following a triceps-sparing approach.[11] Seven patients had good clinical scores, median motion arcs of 90°, and no heterotopic ossification. However, some difficulty fixing lateral condylar fractures was noted using this approach. Another study evaluated triceps tendon strength after triceps-sparing versus triceps-splitting or V-Y approach.[12] All approaches weakened the triceps, but significantly better strength was reported after a triceps-reflecting approach instead of following the division of the tendon. A 2011 study reported on equivalent mobility between the triceps-sparing approach and olecranon osteotomy.[13] Some patients older than 60 years had diminished elbow extension. Care must be taken when retracting the lateral triceps, as during a direct lateral column approach, to not place the radial nerve under traction by overzealous use of a levering retractor, which can result in radial nerve injury.

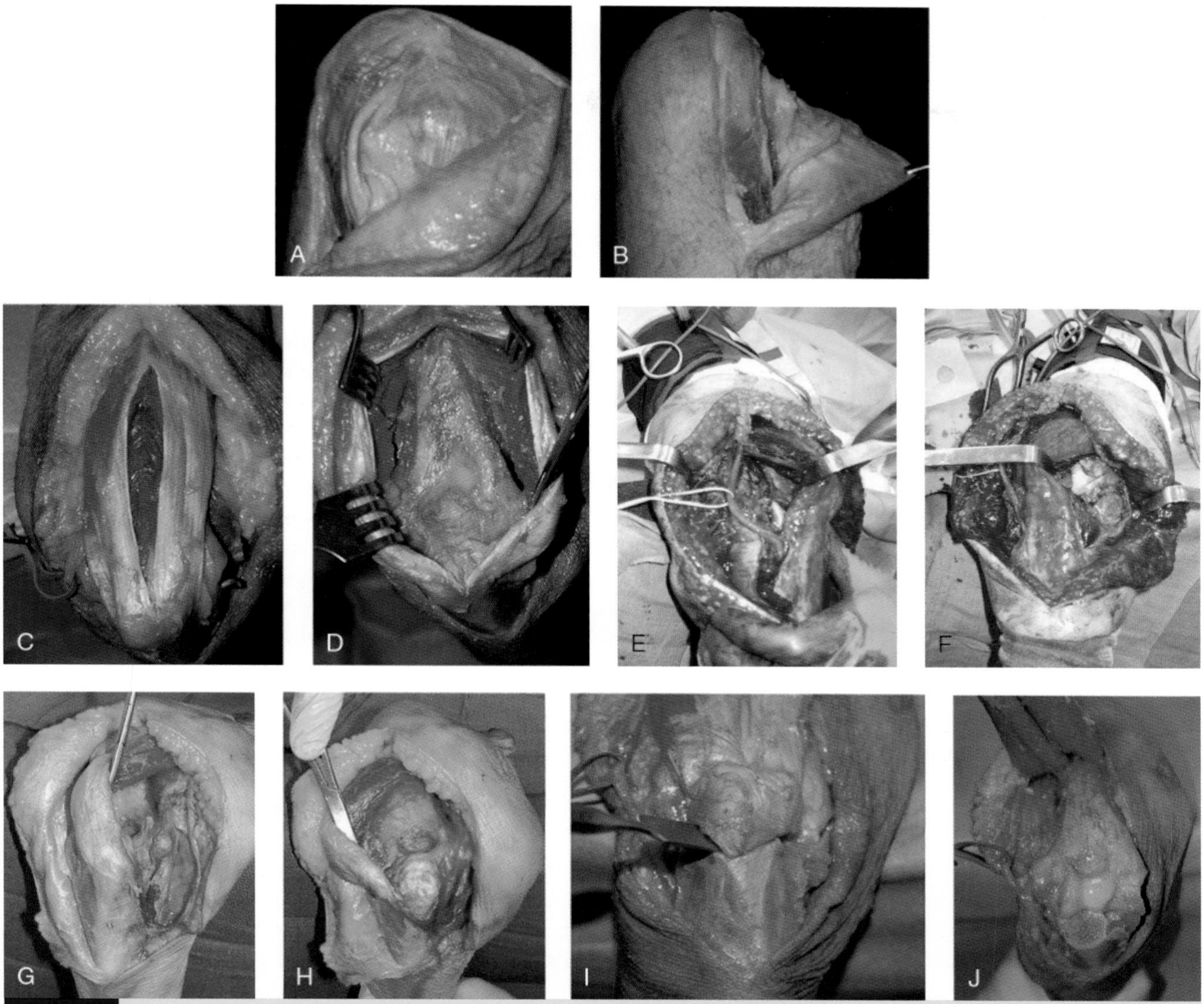

Figure 3 Photographs demonstrate surgical approaches to the distal humerus. **A** and **B**, The ulnar nerve is identified, mobilized, and carefully protected. **C**, Triceps-splitting approach: superficial division of triceps. **D**, Triceps-splitting approach: deep dissection exposing the distal humerus; 1 cm of the olecranon tip can be resected to increase visualization; triceps retraction (paratricipital approach). **E**, The medial border of the triceps is elevated to expose the medial humerus. **F**, The lateral border of the triceps is elevated to expose the lateral humerus, being careful to avoid excessive traction on the radial nerve. **G**, Triceps-reflecting approach: The triceps is elevated from the distal humerus and the triceps tendon is dissected subperiosteally from the olecranon insertion. **H**, Triceps-reflecting approach: The triceps tendon is completely reflected laterally, taking care to preserve continuity with the ulnar periosteum. The tendon is subsequently repaired back to the olecranon using bone tunnels. **I**, Olecranon osteotomy: A chevron-shaped osteotomy provides increased bony healing surface. Completion of the osteotomy through the anterior cortex is completed with an osteotome to avoid damage to articular surface. **J**, Olecranon osteotomy: extensive exposure of the distal humerus, including the articular surface, following elevation of the triceps off the posterior humerus.

The olecranon osteotomy is the utilitarian approach for most distal humeral fractures, especially those with complex intra-articular involvement (**Figure 3, H** and **I**). The olecranon osteotomy technique uses an apex distal chevron osteotomy 2.5 to 3.0 cm from the tip of the olecranon, oriented to intersect the bare area of the proximal ulnar articulation. The osteotomy is begun with an oscillating saw and completed with an osteotome to minimize iatrogenic injury to the adjacent articular cartilage either directly or by thermal necrosis. At the conclusion of the procedure, the osteotomy is repaired with a tension band construct with or without an intramedullary screw, or with a precontoured plate. Proper bone cuts help stabilize the fixation construct and lessen the risk of nonunion or malunion.[2]

A retrospective review of 67 patients with adequate follow-up after olecranon osteotomy for complex distal humerus fractures reported on healing of the osteotomy.[14] All osteotomies healed; however, two required revision secondary to loss of reduction. In most cases, the osteotomy was stabilized with a single intramedullary screw, washer, and dorsal-ulnar figure-of-8 wire construct. Plate fixation was used if initial fixation was deemed inadequate. Implant irritation and patient intolerance to that pain appeared to be major factors for revision surgery: 8% of patients underwent elective implant removal for hardware irritation alone, and an additional 21% had their implants removed with coincident revision procedures.

A 2013 retrospective study on the high number of revision cases suggested a novel fixation device.[15] An olecranon sled was used for fixation of olecranon osteotomies for exposure of intra-articular distal humerus fractures in 14 patients (mean clinical follow-up, 33.5 weeks). No olecranon nonunion was reported. One patient (7%) underwent additional surgery for symptomatic hardware removal, one patient underwent revision open reduction and internal fixation (ORIF) for distal humerus fracture nonunion (7%), and one underwent surgical release for elbow contracture (7%).

Ulnar Nerve

Irrespective of the approach, treatment of distal humerus fractures requires identification and protection of the ulnar nerve.[8] The nerve is at risk from the original injury, including fracture deformity and hemorrhage, as well as during fracture reduction and from the fixation implants, especially the medial column plates. No consensus exists regarding ulnar nerve management.

In a prospective study, 29 patients with distal humeral fracture and preoperative ulnar nerve symptoms were randomized to undergo either anterior subcutaneous transposition of the ulnar nerve or in situ decompression.[16] No patients were lost to follow-up. Patients in the transposition group had significantly improved outcomes, with complete nerve recovery in 12 of 15 patients compared with 8 of 14 patients treated with decompression alone ($P < 0.05$). A 2007 study reported on 12- to 30-year follow-up of surgical treatment of intra-articular distal humerus fractures treated without ulnar nerve transposition.[17] Of 30 patients evaluated, only one ulnar nerve complication was reported: a case of painful ulnar neuropathy that required subsequent anterior ulnar nerve transposition.

A 2010 retrospective analysis studied patients who underwent either in situ release of the ulnar nerve alone or anterior transposition following ORIF.[18] Patients with normal ulnar nerve function on preoperative examination were included, as well as those with preoperative ulnar nerve symptoms. Transposition of the ulnar nerve as an independent variable was associated with the development of ulnar neuritis. In this series, 33% of patients (16 of 48) who underwent transposition reported ulnar nerve symptoms compared with 9% of patients (8 of 89) in the nontransposed group ($P = 0.0003$). These findings were independent of placement of a medial plate. The authors hypothesized that the increased handling, possible devascularization during mobilization, and potential for entrapment in the transposed position as reasons for increased ulnar neuritis.

A 2012 study suggested that columnar fractures are a factor in the development of ulnar neuritis.[19] In coronal shearing fractures of the capitellum or trochlea, the rate of neuritis was lower, irrespective of transposition. In a 2012 retrospective study reporting on ulnar neuropathy following distal humerus fracture,[20] 24 patients underwent ORIF for distal humerus fractures over a 5-year period. A 38% incidence of late ulnar neuropathy following fracture fixation was reported, which included all patients with preoperative symptoms. This supported the first hypothesis that the incidence of late ulnar nerve dysfunction following ORIF is higher than previously reported. The authors also hypothesized that the type of intraoperative nerve management does not substantially affect ulnar nerve dysfunction. Among the patients with persistent ulnar neuropathy at final follow-up, 44% had undergone in situ release and 56% had undergone anterior transposition, but this finding was not significant. Careful handling of the ulnar nerve was recommended during fixation of distal humerus fractures as well as routine disclosure to patients regarding the high incidence of ulnar neuropathy following treatment. In situ release was not favored over anterior transposition of the ulnar nerve. At the start of the procedure, the ulnar nerve can be decompressed and mobilized. At completion of the procedure, the nerve can be transposed anteriorly to avoid contact with hardware. As a result, secondary surgery is made easier and safer with regard to hardware removal or joint release.

The Biomechanics of Fracture Fixation Constructs

The articular surface of the distal humerus is linked to the shaft of the humerus via medial and lateral metaphyseal cortical columns. The central area of the supracondylar region is weak as a result of the thin veneer of bone between

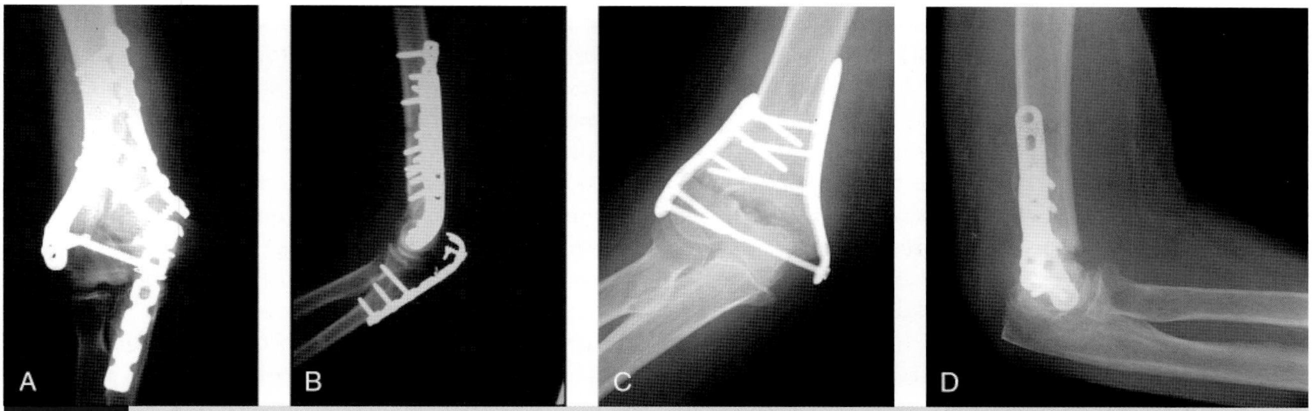

Figure 4 AP (**A**) and lateral (**B**) radiographs of the medial and posterolateral columns of the distal humerus demonstrate the 90-90 plating technique. AP (**C**) and lateral (**D**) radiographs of parallel placement plating technique on the medial and lateral aspects of the distal humerus.

the coronoid and olecranon fossae.[2] This area is especially fragile in patients with osteopenia.[21] Diaphyseal-metaphyseal contact is essential for stability and healing.[2]

The sequence of fracture reduction requires reassembly of articular fragments and reconnection to the humeral shaft without obliterating the required shape, width, and depth of the articulating surfaces. The best fit approach can be used: The humerus is rebuilt at the point with the best interdigitation of fracture fragments, but it is important to remember that some of the bone may be missing and/or impacted, and it is permissible to have voids in the central fossa area. This is especially important so that the trochlea is not excessively narrowed, resulting in mismatch of articular contours. When there is severe comminution of the metaphysis or substantial bone loss, it is acceptable to have shortening at the fracture site with maintenance of appropriate alignment of the articular surface. This scenario can lead to enhanced stability of the fracture, particularly in the presence of osteoporotic bone.[22] Re-creation of the olecranon fossa and/or resection of part of the olecranon tip must be performed carefully to allow full extension during shortening. Bone grafting of the intermediate fragmented trochlear articular surface may be necessary to maintain trochlear width. In higher energy open fractures, bone grafting should be delayed until a clean wound is established.

Many implants have been used in the fixation of distal humerus fractures, such as specialized Y-shaped plates or headless screws for articular fragments.[21,23] Dual plating began with a posterolateral dynamic compression plate and a medial reconstruction plate[24,25] (**Figure 4**). With the advent of precontoured plates there was an initial shift to parallel plating. More recently, precontoured plates can be plates either in an orthogonal or parallel orientation. A 2010 study reported the results of a prospective randomized controlled trial that compared the clinical outcomes in 35 patients with intra-articular distal humerus fractures treated using two different double-plating methods.[26] No substantial difference was reported between the two groups in terms of MEPS, reoperation for complications (3 of 17 versus 3 of 18), elbow motion, or complications. Although the perpendicular plating group had more patients who failed to achieve bony union, both parallel and orthogonal plates provided adequate stability, allowing anatomic reconstruction of distal humerus fractures.

One study reported on the stiffness of perpendicular and parallel constructs using 3.5-mm reconstruction plates on epoxy resin humeri.[27] Plates placed in a parallel orientation were found to have significantly greater strength and stiffness than those placed in a perpendicular orientation. A 2012 study compared the biomechanical properties of 90-90 versus mediolateral parallel plating by creating comminuted, intra-articular, bicolumnar distal humerus fractures in 10 matched pairs of fresh-frozen cadaver elbows.[28] Comparable biomechanical properties for fixation of comminuted intra-articular distal humerus fractures were found with 90-90 and parallel plating, and 90-90 plating had greater resistance to torsional loading.

Placing a plate on the lateral aspect of the distal humerus can be technically difficult and requires stripping soft tissues off the lateral supracondylar ridge.[27] An anatomic study evaluating the intraosseous blood supply of the distal humerus showed that the distal humerus diaphysis is consistently supplied by a single nutrient artery. Distal to this point, blood flow consists of a watershed supply via multiple perforating vessels. The lateral column is perfused by segmental posterior condylar perforating vessels, which can be stripped away with extensive subperiosteal elevation, increasing the risk of delayed union or nonunion.[29]

Simple T-type distal humerus fractures can be treated adequately with almost any form of bicolumnar fixation including Y-type plates, dual reconstruction plates, 3.5-mm dynamic compression plates, and precontoured plates placed in either parallel or orthogonal orientation. The most challenging fracture to treat is the extremely distal transverse humerus fracture with articular comminution. This injury has had the best results using parallel, precontoured plates because these implants alone have the necessary screw density potential to be secure on the distal fragment.[30]

Locking plates provide improved fixation in osteoporotic bone. The indication and necessity for locking plates in the treatment of distal humeral fractures remains uncertain. Cost-effectiveness studies could help clarify their use. According to biomechanical studies, locking plates provided somewhat improved fixation in models of osteoporotic or comminuted distal humeral fractures.[25] Despite the lack of compelling evidence for locking plates, many experts think they are essential in the management of comminuted, osteoporotic fractures.

A 2012 study compared reconstruction plates with precontoured locking plates for fixation of distal humerus fractures.[31] In a cadaver model that simulated metaphyseal comminution, three groups of humeri were compared using biomechanical testing. Groups 1, 2, and 3 used conventional reconstruction plates in a perpendicular configuration, precontoured locking plates in a perpendicular configuration, and precontoured locking plates in a parallel configuration, respectively. Stiffness in anterior bending, posterior bending, axial compression, and torsion was tested in all three groups. The specimens underwent cyclic loading and then single load to failure in posterior bending. No substantial difference was shown among the three groups, and no substantial difference in load to failure was reported. Screw loosening was substantially higher in patients in group 1 after cyclic loading when compared with groups 2 and 3. Immediately after surgery, perpendicular reconstruction plate constructs provide similar stiffness and load-to-failure properties to newer precontoured locking plate systems irrespective of plate configuration.

A 2013 retrospective study assessed the efficacy and limitations of locking compression plates in 46 patients older than 65 years.[32] The patients had a mean age of 80 years; 15 distal humerus fractures were extra-articular and 31 were intra-articular. At a mean follow-up of 25 months, flexion was 127° with an extension deficit of 23°. Functional recovery was routine with a MEPS of 87 (range, 70—100) and patient-mediated outcomes of 95% good and very good results. Postoperative complications were infection (n = 3), metaphyseal nonunion (n = 2), ulnar nerve injury (n = 6), transient radial nerve palsy (n = 1), and periarticular heterotopic ossification (n = 4). Compound fracture and higher grade AO fracture types were associated with poorer functional outcomes.

Irrespective of fixation technique, failed osteosynthesis and nonunion can result from comminution, bone loss, or bone quality.[33] The primary mode of failure is loss of fixation on the distal fragment.[22,34] In this setting, a hinged external fixation device has protected the repair while allowing some elbow motion. One study measured the additional stability of the external fixation construct combined with internal fixation in a cadaver model.[33] The beneficial effects of external fixation were demonstrated in protecting compromised reconstruction plate constructs.

Reconstruction of the articular surface of the distal humerus is fundamental not only to the maximization of mobility and stability but also to mitigate against the progression of posttraumatic osteoarthritis. Although the joint is entirely exposed following olecranon osteotomy overreduction or underreduction of the comminuted articular fracture fragments is probable, and thus, a compression screw should be avoided and a fully threaded cortical screw used instead.[2] In the setting of severe destruction of the distal humerus in a younger, high-demand patient, the articular segment may not be reconstructible using hardware alone and may require intercalary tricortical iliac crest bone grafting.[35] Several authors have used portions of the radial head to reconstruct lateral trochlear defects.[36] In rare instances, the use of osteochondral allografts may be indicated.[2]

Elbow Arthroplasty

Primary TEA is a viable option for the management of distal humerus fractures in the appropriately selected patient[2] (**Figure 5**). Indications include severely comminuted intra-articular fractures that cannot be reassembled in a stable fashion, irrespective of which implant is used. This is certainly true for older, low-demand individuals with poor bone quality, and who may even have preexisting symptomatic elbow arthritis.

Contraindications include previous infection, high-demand and/or noncompliant patients, nonfunctioning biceps muscle, and (according to some authors) open fractures.[37,38] The goal of each case is to fix the distal humerus; however, in older patients with distal fractures and poor bone quality, a TEA implant and a surgeon with the requisite skill should be available.

One study reported the results of a prospective randomized controlled trial that compared the outcomes of TEA versus ORIF in 40 patients.[39] Inclusion criteria were

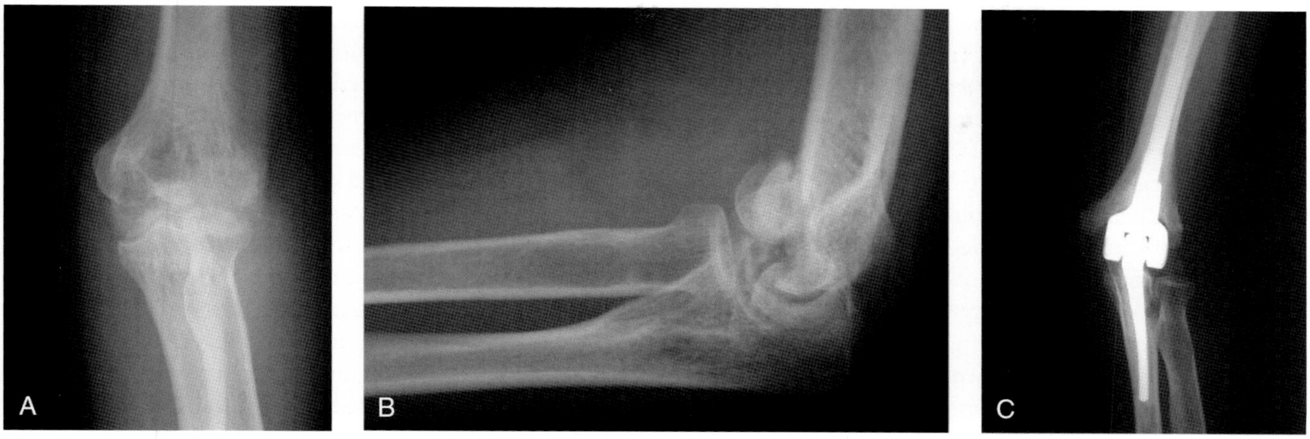

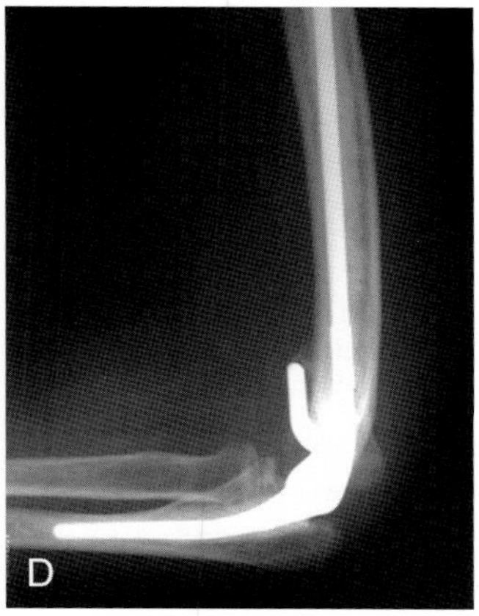

Figure 5 Radiographs demonstrate total elbow arthroplasty for the treatment of intra-articular distal humerus fracture. AP (**A**) and lateral (**B**) presurgical radiographs show a displaced intra-articular distal humerus fracture. AP (**C**) and lateral (**D**) views obtained following total elbow arthroplasty.

patients with closed or Gustilo grade I open comminuted intra-articular fractures in patients older than 65 years. Five of 20 patients in the ORIF group were converted to TEA because of failure to obtain adequate fixation. At 2-year follow-up, superior MEPS rates were reported at almost all time points after TEA, including at final 2-year assessment. Surgical time was 32 minutes less with TEA; ROM was greater at 107° (versus 95°). This study suggests improved outcomes and decreased reoperation rates with TEA for highly comminuted fractures in patients older than 65 years. These results are compelling support for TEA in this patient population; however, follow-up ends at 2 years. TEA survivability is questionable, even in low-demand individuals.

Several studies provide longer term results of TEA following fracture. A 2005 study reported on 43 fractures treated with primary TEA with a mean follow-up of 7 years.[37] These patients achieved a mean flexion arc from 24° to 131°. Thirty-two of 49 elbows underwent no additional surgery and experienced no complications. Five revision arthroplasty procedures were required.

In an extensive 2008 review[40] of 92 elbows that underwent TEA as a salvage procedure for distal humeral nonunion (in contradistinction to the 2009 study[39] on fresh fractures), substantial improvements were reported in most patients: 74% of patients had no pain or mild pain and 85% had satisfactory subjective results.[40] Regarding function, 83% reported that they could use their extremity in four or more activities of daily living. Patients had a mean flexion-extension arc of 113°. A substantial complication rate was reported, with 32 reoperations. Complications included aseptic implant loosening in 12 patients, with increased risk for loosening observed in younger patients (younger than 65 years) and ulnar components that had "Precoat," a process by which the stem of the manufactured implants is coated with polymethyl methacrylate. Five implant fractures occurred. Review of implant failure revealed that the fractures were likely associated with substantial bone loss because failure occurred at the junction of the fixed component and the unsupported segment. Fractures of the implant with extra-small or small titanium implants resulted in the recommendation to use the largest implants possible and strictly adhere to activity restrictions. Additional complications included 4 periprosthetic fractures, 12 soft-tissue and wound complications, 2 transient nerve palsies, 1 C-ring failure,

1 bushing failure, and 1 painful proximal radioulnar joint requiring radial head excision. Implant survival was 96% at 2 years, 82% at 5 years, and 65% at 10 and 15 years. This study emphasized the technical nature and requirements of this procedure.

A 2012 series reported on 16 patients treated with linked TEA who had a comminuted fracture of the distal humerus that was not considered amenable to reliable ORIF.[41] At a mean follow-up of 57 months, mean elbow flexion-extension ROM was from 28° to 117°. Five patients with moderate to severe pain (31%) were not satisfied with the results of the procedure. Three patients had an infection (one underwent implant removal), and eight patients had symptoms of sensory ulnar nerve neuropathy. The authors of the study concluded that elbow arthroplasty may be a solution for highly comminuted osteoporotic fractures. However, the rate of substantial and minor complications such as infection or postoperative ulnar nerve symptoms is probably higher than reported.

A series of 20 cases evaluated the functional recovery and morbidity of complex distal humerus fractures in elderly patients (mean age, 80 years) following treatment with an elbow prosthesis.[42] Fifteen patients were reevaluated at a mean follow-up of 3.6 years: mean elbow ROM was 97° (range, 60° to 130°), with a mean flexion of 130° (range, 110° to 140°) and a mean loss of extension of 33° (range, 0° to 80°); mean MEPS was 83. Radiographs revealed seven cases of radiolucent lines, two of which were progressive. Wear of the polyethylene bushings at the hinge was not noted. Six patients had moderate periarticular heterotopic ossification. Two cases of olecranon osteotomy and one case of olecranon fracture had healed. No surgical site infections were reported. Two cases of ulnar compression were reported, one of which required neurolysis. One case of humeral component loosening after 6 years was reported, but the implant was not exchanged. Elbow ROM was comparable with published data. The functional scores were slightly lower, mainly because of pain.

A 2008 retrospective study compared patients who underwent primary versus delayed TEA for distal humeral fractures with a mean follow-up of 56 months.[43] Patients were found to have no significant difference in MEPS. Implant survival was also similar in the two groups, with survivorship of 93% at 88 months in the early group and 76% in the delayed group. Of the 32 patients in this series, 10 were reported to have complications including aseptic loosening (5 cases), infection (2 cases), heterotopic ossification (1 case), and ulnar nerve palsy (2 cases). Reported risk factors for implant failure include patient age of 65 years or younger, two or more prior surgeries, or prior infection.[40] Although several reports have set forth promising results for this difficult problem, caution should be used in elbow arthroplasty performed in the setting of fracture. Patients must be appropriately counseled regarding the potential for complications and the importance of adherence to restrictions.

A 2008 study reported on the primary treatment of distal humerus fractures using an unlinked TEA prosthesis.[44] Nine elbows in nine patients were followed for a mean of 3.5 years. At final evaluation, all elbows were stable and pain relief was satisfactory.

A 2012 retrospective study reported on 10 patients who underwent distal humeral hemiarthroplasty for comminuted intra-articular distal humerus fractures.[45] This currently is an off-label treatment in the United States and no implants are marketed for this purpose. The short-term clinical outcomes were evaluated at a mean follow-up of 12 months. All patients regained triceps extension strength subjectively similar to their contralateral extremity. All patients had a mean (±SD) flexion of 121° ± 32°, mean extension deficit of 22° ± 16°, mean elbow ROM of 102° ± 25°, mean pronation of 64° ± 11°, and mean supination of 69° ± 6°. Mean Mayo score at follow-up was 77.2 ± 16.0, and mean DASH score was 35.1 ± 24.0. No postoperative elbow subluxation or dislocations were observed. No heterotopic ossification was seen and no superficial or deep infections occurred. No radiographic lucencies were visible around the humeral components at final follow-up. In addition, a 2006 study reported on four patients treated with humeral hemiarthroplasty, all of whom had good or excellent results at short-term follow-up.[46]

Expected Outcomes of Surgical Treatment

Reported outcomes are difficult to interpret given the wide range of injury and treatment. Furthermore, much of the existing literature consists of relatively small series.[43] However, with appropriate, stable, adequate fixation, rates of union are excellent, ranging from 91% to 100%.[1] Several reports have rated outcomes based on patient-reported outcome scales as well as objective outcome measures. In an outcome report following treatment of complex distal humerus fractures with parallel plating (mean follow-up, 2 years), good to excellent outcomes based on the MEPS were found in 79% (27 of 34 patients).[21] This is comparable with other reports, with good to excellent outcomes ranging from 84% to 100%.[11,47] In objectively measured outcomes, mean elbow flexion arcs after fixation are 90° to 106°,[11,17,21] with mean pronation-supination arcs of 150° to 165°.[11,17] Regaining terminal extension is difficult, with a mean extension deficit of 25°. Residual muscle weakness is common, with

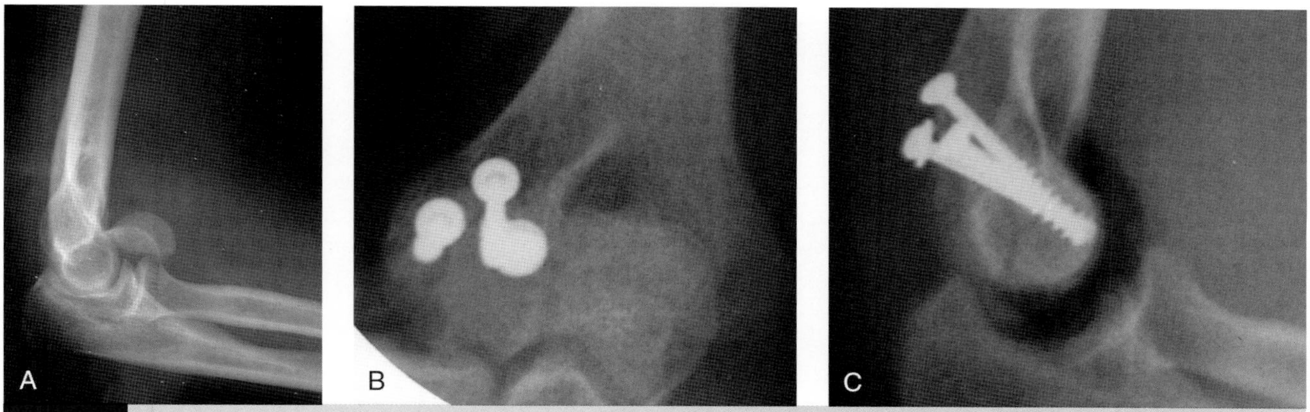

Figure 6 Radiographs demonstrate the double-arc sign in a 48-year-old patient who sustained an intra-articular shear fracture. **A**, Preoperative view. AP (**B**) and lateral (**C**) views obtained following open reduction and internal fixation.

strength measured at 75% of the contralateral healthy side. A 2007 study of 12- to 30-year outcomes after surgical treatment of intra-articular fractures found the short-term reports of success to be durable based on DASH, MEPS, American Shoulder and Elbow Surgeons (ASES) score, and visual analog satisfaction scale, with 87% (26 of 30 patients) good to excellent results.[17] However, the findings also revealed radiographic evidence of post-traumatic arthritis in 80% of patients despite optimal surgical treatment.

Decision-Making Process in the Elderly

Fractures of the distal humerus are challenging in elderly patients with osteopenia. All forms of treatment are associated with a substantial risk of complication and there is no right answer. ORIF seems best suited for fractures with minimal articular comminution and reasonable bone stock. When ORIF is successful, the arm can be used without restriction because late complications are relatively infrequent. Elbow arthroplasty is appropriate for comminuted fractures and patients with poor bone quality. Early results are favorable, but comes with the warning "may not be suitable for long-term use."

Articular Shear Fractures

Articular shear fractures merit a separate discussion given the challenges unique to this injury. These fractures are rare, comprising only 1% of all elbow fractures. They usually result from low-energy trauma, such as a fall from standing height, but also can result from high-energy trauma. Additionally, the capitellum can be injured indirectly. In this instance, a subluxated or dislocated radial head forcefully reduces, applying a shear force to the capitellum.

In shear fractures of the distal humeral surface, a radial head–capitellum view can be helpful. This modified lateral view is obtained by angling the x-ray beam 45° anteriorly to diminish overlap of the humeroradial and humeroulnar articulations. This allows better visualization of small fragments of the capitellum that can be largely composed of articular cartilage. The double arc sign indicates a fracture of the capitellum and lateral trochlear ridge. The double arc represents the increased radiographic density of the subchondral bone of the capitellum and trochlear ridge (**Figure 6**).

Articular shear fractures are separately classified from other distal humeral fractures. Type I fractures, or Hahn-Steinthal fractures, involve the entire capitellum and lateral trochlear ridge. Type II (Kocher-Lorenz) fractures involve only the articular surface of the capitellum with subchondral bone. Type III fractures are comminuted fractures of the capitellum.[2] A type IV fracture has been described, consisting of a coronal shear fracture of the capitellum with extension across much of the trochlea.[48] A more descriptive method of classification exists, based on division of the articular surface into five regions: capitellum and lateral trochlea, lateral epicondyle, posterior aspect of the lateral column, posterior aspect of the trochlea, and medial epicondyle.[49] Accounting for these anatomic regions, five patterns of injury were identified involving various combinations of the five regions.

Many treatment methods have been reported since a capitellar fracture was first described in 1853 based on findings of a palpable prominence at the elbow at autopsy. These include closed reduction and immobilization, excision, ORIF, and arthroplasty. Current literature supports the closed treatment of nondisplaced fractures with a brief period of immobilization.[2] With nonsurgical management, close clinical and radiographic monitoring is

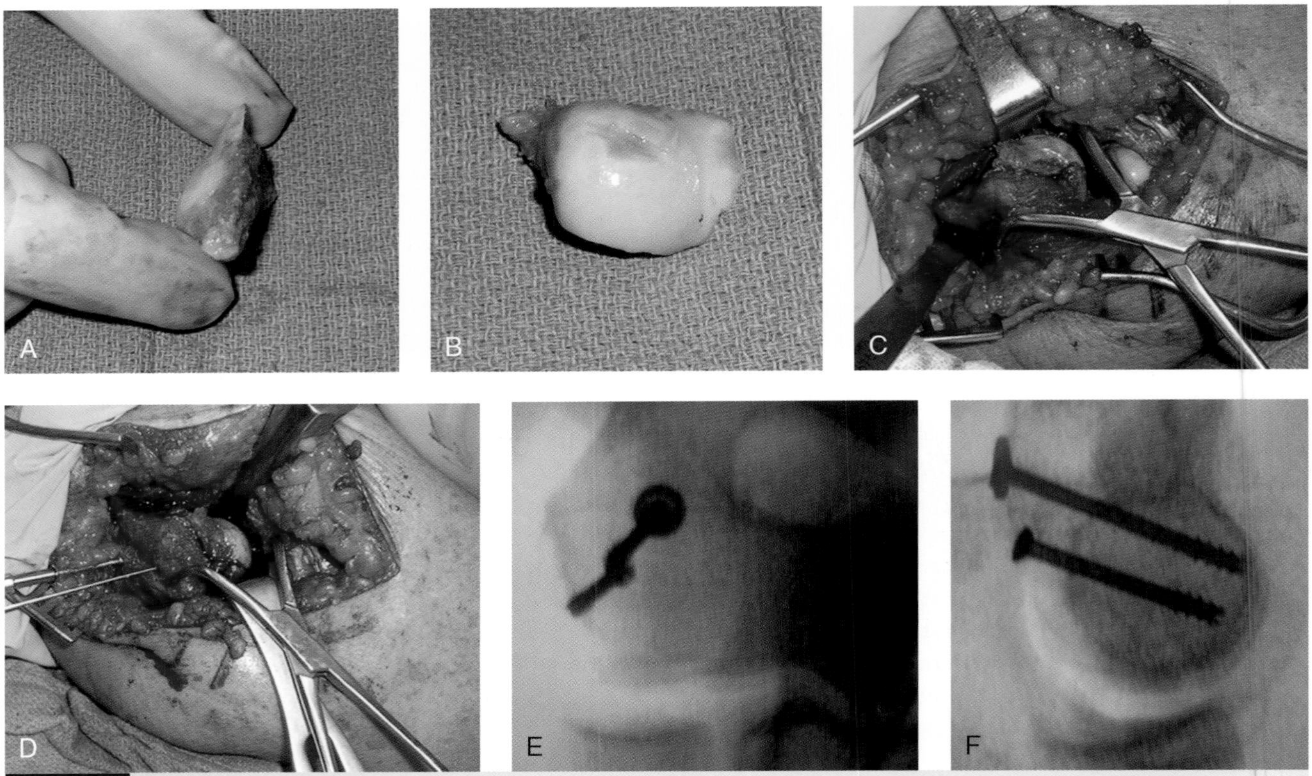

Figure 7 Intraoperative images of a capitellar shear fracture. **A** and **B**, Photographs depict articular fragment. Photographs depict reduction and compression of capitellar fragment with reduction forceps (**C**) and provisional fixation with guidewires for cannulated lag screws (**D**). **E** and **F**, Fluoroscopic views verify anatomic reduction and fixation of fracture.

necessary to ensure maintenance of reduction. However, current literature favors ORIF whenever possible because this restores the lateral buttress of the elbow.

Regarding surgical approach, some authors favor a posterior skin incision over the more common lateral incision.[50-52] A posterior incision facilitates medial and lateral approaches. A lateral approach can be used for types I, II, and III fractures.[50,51] In the setting of a fracture with extensive trochlear involvement, the medial extent of the fracture is often difficult to access. In such instances, it may be necessary to perform a medial approach via a flexor-pronator split, or in some cases an olecranon osteotomy.[49,50,53] The exposure can be started on the lateral condylar ridge and the common extensor split in line with the axis of the radius. If the lateral ulnar collateral ligament (LUCL) is intact, it can be left alone in most cases. An excellent view of the capitellum and lateral half of the trochlea is facilitated by elevating the capsule and the origins of the radial wrist extensors off the anterolateral aspect of the humerus. The LUCL should be reflected off the lateral epicondyle with or without a fleck of bone if necessary to help reduce or fix the fracture. The LUCL is repaired through drill holes in the lateral epicondylar region at the end of the case. If the fracture involves the entire trochlea, an olecranon osteotomy is performed. Reducing the fracture can be complicated by anterior impaction of the posterolateral margin of the lateral epicondyle. The technique of disimpacting this bone has been demonstrated to allow it to hinge on its posterior cortex and bone grafting into the defect to facilitate reduction.[49]

Various fixation methods have been described, reflecting the extensive variability in fracture patterns. Fracture fixation can be accomplished with lag screws, headless compression screws, bioabsorbable screws, plates, and pins, alone or in various combinations (**Figure 7**). It is important to make sure that the articular fragment screws are in different planes to stabilize the fragments.

In a retrospective study of 18 patients with coronal plane fractures of the distal humerus involving the capitellum and trochlea, ORIF was performed with cannulated screws for all cases.[54] According to the Bryan and Morrey classification, seven type 1, five type 3, and six type 4 fractures were reported. Mean follow-up was 43.6 months; mean elbow ROM was 8.9° to 132.8°. The mean MEPS was 86.7 points (range, 60 to 100), with 12 excellent, 2 good, and 4 fair outcomes. The mean DASH score was 15.3 points (range, 17.0 to 35.8). Heterotopic ossification developed in one patient with delayed fixation; 14 patients with excellent or good results returned to their previous activity levels. For coronal plane fractures of the distal humerus, satisfactory results were obtained with ORIF with cannulated screws, which maintains a stable anatomic articular position.

In several studies, the authors appear to favor using a screw placed from the posterolateral column anteriorly into the fragment to minimize articular damage.[50,51,53] However, a 2010 study favored placing screws from lateral to anterior to avoid posterior stripping of the lateral condyle to diminish the risk of capitellar osteonecrosis.[51] However, the risk of osteonecrosis seems to be exceptionally low.[48,52] The 2010 study also described an antiglide plate used in conjunction with screw fixation to resist shearing forces at the capitellum.[51] In this technique, a mini-fragment plate is bent distally to fit the curvature of the superior extra-articular portion of the capitellum. The plate is placed over the anterior surface of the lateral column and only fixed proximally. More complex fractures involving the trochlea may require additional screws placed from the posteromedial column. In the case of posterior comminution, it may be necessary to supplement fixation with additional plates, pins, cannulated screws, or bone graft.[50] In type II fractures, the fragment is often composed primarily of articular cartilage and contains only a thin shell of subchondral bone, making fixation difficult with lag techniques. In these cases it may be necessary to use anterior-to-posterior screws, bioabsorbable screws, or, as a last resort, fragment excision.

Assessing outcomes in current literature is difficult because fixation techniques and fracture types vary among studies; furthermore, most studies are retrospective in design and include relatively few cases. One relatively large series reported on 28 patients after ORIF of capitellar and trochlear fractures.[50] Patients had a mean flexion-extension arc of 119° and supination-pronation arc of 156°. This is equivalent to other studies, which report a flexion-extension arc from 96° to 131°and a pronation-supination arc from 167° to 180°.[48,49,52,53]

Review of patient-reported outcomes have shown similarly promising results. A 2003 study reported 76% good to excellent results (16 of 21 patients) based on MEPS.[49] A 2006 study reported that the mean MEPS corresponded to an excellent outcome.[50] Many other reports have shown that all patients in those series achieved good to excellent outcomes using a variety of outcomes scores.[48,52,53] A 2006 study also reported a correlation between severity of injury and patient outcome based on the MEPS.[50] Type I fractures had a substantially better outcome than types II and III.

Although reported outcomes after surgical treatment of articular shear fractures are generally favorable, it is important to note the substantial rate of complications and need for additional surgery associated with treating these fractures. In the two largest series, 43% (12 of 28 patients)[50] and 48% (10 of 21 patients)[49] required at least one additional procedure. Common reasons for reoperation included removal of symptomatic hardware after olecranon osteotomy, capsulectomy, and hardware removal for inadequate motion and nonunion.[49,50] More infrequently, radiocapitellar arthrosis, heterotopic ossification, and ulnar nerve neuropathy have been reported.[49,52] A 2006 study described two patients with severe type III fractures that required conversion to TEA.[50] In a review of recent studies, no authors reported osteonecrosis of the capitellum.[48-50,52,53]

Complications

Various complications are encountered in the treatment of distal humerus fractures, with rates reported as high as 48%.[55] Risk factors include high-energy injuries, open fractures, and, in some accounts, nonsurgical treatment.[1,21,55,56] Elbow stiffness is the most common of these complications, and most patients lose some degree of elbow extension. Early surgical intervention and stable fixation allowing early and consistent ROM exercises help minimize elbow stiffness. Early failure of fixation is frequently the result of inadequate fracture stabilization, although contributing factors include noncompliance and osteopenia.

Nonunion, especially in the supracondylar region, can occur and is more common after an open fracture. A 2012 study compared surgical treatment of open and closed AO type C fractures of the distal humerus to investigate any differences in outcomes and prognosis.[57] Twenty-eight matched cohort patients were treated using surgical fixation (14 open and 14 closed injuries), with a mean follow-up of 98.9 weeks. The mean time to osseous healing following definitive treatment was 24.7 weeks for open fractures compared with 18.7 weeks for those in the closed group ($P = 0.085$). The mean ROM at final follow-up for open fractures was 82.5° and 108.7° for those in the closed group ($P = 0.03$). Results from the Medical Outcomes Study 12-Item Short-Form Survey were significantly poorer ($P = 0.002$) in the open group (57.9) than in the closed group (79.0). For open distal humerus fractures, functional outcome scores were worse and elbow motion was decreased. Patients with open fractures were more likely to have higher complication rates, prolonged times to union, and higher rates of persistent nerve deficits requiring further surgery. Although most patients experience healing, one author reported delayed union in 9.4% of patients at 12 weeks, with approximately one-half of these patients experiencing healing without additional surgery within 24 weeks.[1] Management of nonunion in the supracondylar region typically involves revised fixation and bone grafting. Intra-articular nonunion can be difficult to manage and usually requires a complete revision of the surgical procedure with adequate joint visualization to restore the articular surface.

Another consistently reported complication is heterotopic ossification. A 2003 study noted clinically significant heterotopic ossification in 13% of patients, with a trend toward decreased incidence in patients who received postoperative prophylaxis with 100 mg of indomethacin twice per day for 24 hours, followed by 25 mg three times daily for 6 weeks.[55] A retrospective study reported on the risk factors for development of heterotopic ossification of the elbow following fracture fixation in 89 patients.[58] Patients with distal humeral fractures were more likely to experience heterotopic ossification ($P = 0.003$), have grade 2 heterotopic ossification or greater ($P < 0.001$), and have more compromised functional outcomes than those with a proximal radius or ulna fracture. Other reports have noted development of heterotopic ossification as the most important complication that limited motion.[21]

Other less commonly reported complications include infection and ulnar nerve neuropathy. Ulnar neuritis can occur as a result of distal humerus fracture because of the surgical procedure, postoperative hardware irritation, or the development of scarring from the healing process in and around the cubital tunnel. The ulnar nerve should be identified and protected throughout the surgical procedure, and excessive traction should be avoided. Transposition of the ulnar nerve following fixation remains controversial and superior results have not been demonstrated with either approach.

Rehabilitation and Postoperative Care

Following fracture stabilization, motion is typically initiated after 5 to 7 days. Extended immobilization is associated with elbow stiffness and should be avoided except in those instances for which stable fixation cannot be achieved. It is easier to manage a stiff elbow with a healed humerus than to manage a nonunited humerus.

Initially, the arm is placed in a well-padded posterior splint to protect the surgical wound and to minimize discomfort. Longer immobilization may be required in patients with posterior open fractures, extensive soft-tissue injuries, or wounds that were difficult to close after a lengthy procedure. If possible and prudent, some active-assisted flexion and gravity-aided extension is initiated within 1 to 2 days of surgery. It is important to allow the wound to seal before moving the elbow, particularly for cases with a large posterior incision.[50] Early motion can promote postoperative seroma. Exercises that allow active extension against resistance are typically avoided until fracture union. Weight bearing following articular injuries is typically delayed for 12 weeks. Adequate repair of the LUCL complex ideally leaves the elbow stable; however, because of concern over lateral ligament instability, splinting is used to keep the forearm in pronation and limit extension within the arc of stability.

Summary

Distal humerus fractures are substantial injuries that require specific diagnosis, surgical planning and execution, and carefully timed rehabilitation to maximize and promote the best patient outcomes. Dual-plate fixation oriented at 90° or 180° is indicated for most adult fractures involving both columns of the distal humerus.

In elderly patients with a displaced, comminuted, intra-articular distal humeral fracture that cannot be repaired, acute TEA is preferable. Surgical fixation, most typically via a lateral approach, is required for displaced coronal shear fractures of the distal humerus articular surface.

Advances in understanding the fracture pattern through improved diagnostic imaging, new exposure techniques, improved fixation, and recognition of proper rehabilitation techniques have improved patient outcomes. Larger clinical trials are necessary for advances in treatment and rehabilitation, especially given the aging population and increased patient expectations.

Key Study Points

- The triceps splitting, triceps reflecting, and paratricipital approaches allow visualization of the posterior portion of the trochlea. The olecranon osteotomy provides the best view of the anterior aspect of the trochlea and capitellum.
- The paratricipital approach avoids violation of the extensor mechanism of the elbow by utilizing medial and lateral windows on either side of the triceps, making it amenable to treating extra-articular fractures. This approach also makes it easy to change plans from open reduction and internal fixation to TEA.
- In cases of severe comminution of the metaphysis or substantial bone loss in that region, some shortening at the fracture site with maintenance of appropriate alignment of the articular surface is acceptable and can substantially enhance the stability of the fracture, particularly in the setting of osteoporotic bone.
- Acute total elbow arthroplasty is indicated as the primary treatment for elderly patients with extensively comminuted intra-articular fracture of the distal humerus with poor bone quality that is not amenable to stable internal fixation.
- Displaced coronal shear fractures of the distal humeral articular surface require surgical fixation, most typically via a lateral approach. Fracture reduction may be complicated by anterior impaction of the posterolateral margin of the lateral epicondyle. Disimpaction of this bone should occur first, allowing it to hinge on its posterior cortex, and then bone-grafting into the defect in order to facilitate reduction.

Acknowledgments

The authors would like to thank Joelle Tighe, BS, for her assistance in preparing this manuscript.

Annotated References

1. Robinson CM, Hill RM, Jacobs N, Dall G, Court-Brown CM: Adult distal humeral metaphyseal fractures: Epidemiology and results of treatment. *J Orthop Trauma* 2003;17(1):38-47.

2. Seth AK, Baratz ME. Fractures of the elbow. In: Trumble TE, Budoff JE, Cornwall R, ed. *Hand, Elbow & Shoulder*. Philadelphia: Mosby, 2006. 522-31.

3. Doornberg J, Lindenhovius A, Kloen P, van Dijk CN, Zurakowski D, Ring D: Two- and three-dimensional computed tomography for the classification and management of distal humeral fractures. Evaluation of reliability and diagnostic accuracy. *J Bone Joint Surg Am* 2006;88(8):1795-1801.

4. Brouwer KM, Lindenhovius AL, Dyer GS, Zurakowski D, Mudgal CS, Ring D: Diagnostic accuracy of 2- and 3-dimensional imaging and modeling of distal humerus fractures. *J Shoulder Elbow Surg* 2012;21(6):772-776.

   This investigation used prospectively recorded intraoperative evaluation as the reference standard for distal humerus fracture type and characteristics to measure the diagnostic performance characteristics of CT and physical models. The addition of 3D CT and the 3D models to 2D CT and radiographs resulted in substantial improvements in sensitivity, but not specificity, in the diagnosis and proposed treatment. There was also improved interobserver agreement with respect to specific fracture characteristics. Level of evidence: I.

5. Pidhorz L, Alligand-Perrin P, De Keating E, Fabre T, Mansat P; Société française de chirurgie orthopédique et traumatologie (SoFCOT): Distal humerus fracture in the elderly: Does conservative treatment still have a role? *Orthop Traumatol Surg Res* 2013;99(8):903-907.

   One prospective and one retrospective study included a total of 56 patients, with a mean age of 84.7 years. All were treated with 6 to 8 weeks of long arm immobilization without fracture reduction. Nonsurgical treatment of distal humerus fracture in patients older than 65 years was acceptable because it provided satisfactory clinical results, with no substantial joint stiffness or elbow instability. Nonanatomic results on radiographs, however, have to be accepted. Level of evidence: IV.

6. Wilkinson JM, Stanley D: Posterior surgical approaches to the elbow: A comparative anatomic study. *J Shoulder Elbow Surg* 2001;10(4):380-382.

7. Ziran BH, Smith WR, Balk ML, Manning CM, Agudelo JF: A true triceps-splitting approach for treatment of distal humerus fractures: A preliminary report. *J Trauma* 2005;58(1):70-75.

8. Anglen J: Distal humerus fractures. *J Am Acad Orthop Surg* 2005;13(5):291-297.

9. Mühldorfer-Fodor M, Bekler H, Wolfe VM, McKean J, Rosenwasser MP: Paratriciptal-triceps splitting "two-window" approach for distal humerus fractures. *Tech Hand Up Extrem Surg* 2011;15(3):156-161.

10. Erpelding JM, Mailander A, High R, Mormino MA, Fehringer EV: Outcomes following distal humeral fracture fixation with an extensor mechanism-on approach. *J Bone Joint Surg Am* 2012;94(6):548-553.

    Distal humeral ORIF was performed with either orthogonal or parallel plate constructs in 79 elbows; 37 elbows were fixed via an extensor mechanism surgical approach, 24 were available for additional evaluation. All 37 fractures

4: Upper Extremity

healed primarily. The median arc of elbow motion was 126°. Open treatment of distal humeral fractures with an extensor mechanism approach resulted in excellent healing, a mean elbow flexion-extension arc exceeding 100°, and maintenance of 90% of elbow extension strength compared with that of the contralateral healthy elbow. Level of evidence: IV.

11. Ek ET, Goldwasser M, Bonomo AL: Functional outcome of complex intercondylar fractures of the distal humerus treated through a triceps-sparing approach. *J Shoulder Elbow Surg* 2008;17(3):441-446.

12. Guerroudj M, de Longueville JC, Rooze M, Hinsenkamp M, Feipel V, Schuind F: Biomechanical properties of triceps brachii tendon after in vitro simulation of different posterior surgical approaches. *J Shoulder Elbow Surg* 2007;16(6):849-853.

13. Chen G, Liao Q, Luo W, Li K, Zhao Y, Zhong D: Triceps-sparing versus olecranon osteotomy for ORIF: Analysis of 67 cases of intercondylar fractures of the distal humerus. *Injury* 2011;42(4):366-370.

    In this study, the triceps-sparing approach was compared with olecranon osteotomy. There were 67 cases of intercondylar distal humerus fractures. All fractures united. Overall, no statistically substantial difference was reported in the mean flexion, extension, arc of flexion/extension, pronation, supination, and arc of pronation/supination between the triceps-sparing group (n = 34) and the olecranon osteotomy group (n = 33). ORIF via the triceps-sparing approach conferred inferior functional outcomes for intercondylar distal humerus fractures in patients older than 60 years. However, for patients younger than 60 years, especially those younger than 40 years, either approach conferred satisfactory outcomes.

14. Coles CP, Barei DP, Nork SE, Taitsman LA, Hanel DP, Bradford Henley M: The olecranon osteotomy: A six-year experience in the treatment of intraarticular fractures of the distal humerus. *J Orthop Trauma* 2006;20(3):164-171.

15. Iorio T, Wong JC, Patterson JD, Rekant MS: Olecranon osteotomy fixation using a novel device: The olecranon sled. *Tech Hand Up Extrem Surg* 2013;17(3):151-157.

    In this study, the olecranon sled was used for fixation of olecranon osteotomies in 14 patients. Mean clinical follow-up was 33.5 weeks. Olecranon nonunion was not reported. One patient underwent additional surgery for symptomatic hardware removal (7.1%). Two additional procedures were performed, one for revision ORIF of distal humerus fracture nonunion (7.1%) and one for release of elbow contracture (7.1%).

16. Ruan HJ, Liu JJ, Fan CY, Jiang J, Zeng BF: Incidence, management, and prognosis of early ulnar nerve dysfunction in type C fractures of distal humerus. *J Trauma* 2009;67(6):1397-1401.

17. Doornberg JN, van Duijn PJ, Linzel D, et al: Surgical treatment of intra-articular fractures of the distal part of the humerus. Functional outcome after twelve to thirty years. *J Bone Joint Surg Am* 2007;89(7):1524-1532.

18. Chen RC, Harris DJ, Leduc S, Borrelli JJ Jr, Tornetta P III, Ricci WM: Is ulnar nerve transposition beneficial during open reduction internal fixation of distal humerus fractures? *J Orthop Trauma* 2010;24(7):391-394.

    The incidence of ulnar neuritis with and without ulnar nerve transposition was compared following ORIF of distal humerus fractures. Patients who underwent ulnar nerve transposition had almost four times the incidence of ulnar neuritis than those without transposition.

19. Wiggers JK, Brouwer KM, Helmerhorst GT, Ring D: Predictors of diagnosis of ulnar neuropathy after surgically treated distal humerus fractures. *J Hand Surg Am* 2012;37(6):1168-1172.

    Ulnar neuropathy was examined in 107 consecutive adults who underwent surgical treatment of a distal humerus fracture followed up for at least 6 months after injury. Fractures were categorized as either columnar fractures or fractures of the capitellum and trochlea. Patients with columnar fractures might be at higher risk for the development of postoperative ulnar neuropathy than patients with capitellum and trochlea fractures, irrespective of whether the ulnar nerve was transposed. Level of evidence: IV.

20. Worden A, Ilyas AM: Ulnar neuropathy following distal humerus fracture fixation. *Orthop Clin North Am* 2012;43(4):509-514.

    A 38% incidence of late ulnar neuropathy following ORIF was identified. No statistical difference was reported between an in situ release and all anterior transpositions, except for submuscular.

21. Luegmair M, Timofiev E, Chirpaz-Cerbat JM: Surgical treatment of AO type C distal humeral fractures: Internal fixation with a Y-shaped reconstruction (Lambda) plate. *J Shoulder Elbow Surg* 2008;17(1):113-120.

22. O'Driscoll SW: Optimizing stability in distal humeral fracture fixation. *J Shoulder Elbow Surg* 2005;14(1suppl S):186S-194S.

23. Russell GV Jr, Jarrett CA, Jones CB, Cole PA, Gates J: Management of distal humerus fractures with minifragment fixation. *J Orthop Trauma* 2005;19(7):474-479.

24. Sanchez-Sotelo J, Torchia ME, O'Driscoll SW: Complex distal humeral fractures: Internal fixation with a principle-based parallel-plate technique. Surgical technique. *J Bone Joint Surg Am* 2008;90(suppl 2 Pt 1):31-46.

25. Schuster I, Korner J, Arzdorf M, Schwieger K, Diederichs G, Linke B: Mechanical comparison in cadaver specimens of three different 90-degree double-plate osteosyntheses for simulated C2-type distal humerus fractures with varying bone densities. *J Orthop Trauma* 2008;22(2):113-120.

26. Shin SJ, Sohn HS, Do NH: A clinical comparison of two different double plating methods for intraarticular distal humerus fractures. *J Shoulder Elbow Surg* 2010;19(1):2-9.

    Outcome was compared for patients with intra-articular distal humerus fractures treated using two different double-plating methods: 17 patients treated by perpendicular plating (group 1) and 18 by parallel plating (group 2). Eleven patients in group 1 recovered full arc of flexion and 13 patients in group 2 achieved full arc of flexion. All patients obtained bone union, except two patients in group 1. Although more patients did not achieve bony union in the perpendicular plating group, both parallel and orthogonal plate positioning can provide adequate stability and anatomic reconstruction of distal humerus fractures. Level of evidence: II.

27. Arnander MW, Reeves A, MacLeod IA, Pinto TM, Khaleel A: A biomechanical comparison of plate configuration in distal humerus fractures. *J Orthop Trauma* 2008;22(5):332-336.

28. Got C, Shuck J, Biercevicz A, et al: Biomechanical comparison of parallel versus 90-90 plating of bicolumn distal humerus fractures with intra-articular comminution. *J Hand Surg Am* 2012;37(12):2512-2518.

    This study compares the biomechanical properties of 90-90 versus mediolateral parallel plating of C-3 bicolumn distal humerus fractures. The researchers created intra-articular AO C-3 bicolumnar fractures in 10 fresh-frozen matched pairs of cadaver elbows. Compared with parallel fixation, 90-90 plate fixation had substantially greater torque-to-failure load. Both techniques had the same mode of failure in torsion, a spiral fracture extending from the medial plate at the metaphyseal-diaphyseal junction. No substantial difference was reported in the stiffness of fixation of the articular fragment or the entire distal segment in anteroposterior loading.

29. Kimball JP, Glowczewskie F, Wright TW: Intraosseous blood supply to the distal humerus. *J Hand Surg Am* 2007;32(5):642-646.

30. Lee SK, Kim KJ, Park KH, Choy WS: A comparison between orthogonal and parallel plating methods for distal humerus fractures: A prospective randomized trial. *Eur J Orthop Surg Traumatol* 2014;24(7):1123-1131.

    The purpose of this study was to compare the clinical and radiographic outcomes in patients with distal humerus fractures who were treated with orthogonal and parallel plating methods using precontoured distal humerus plates. Sixty-seven patients with a mean age of 55.4 years were included in this prospective study. This study concluded that orthogonal plating method may be preferred in cases of coronal shear fractures, where posterior to anterior fixation may provide additional stability to the intra-articular fractures and that parallel plating method may be the preferred technique for fractures that occur at the most distal end of the humerus.

31. Koonce RC, Baldini TH, Morgan SJ: Are conventional reconstruction plates equivalent to precontoured locking plates for distal humerus fracture fixation? A biomechanics cadaver study. *Clin Biomech (Bristol, Avon)* 2012;27(7):697-701.

    Three groups of humerus specimens were compared via biomechanical testing in a cadaver model simulating metaphyseal comminution. Group 1 consisted of conventional reconstruction plates in a perpendicular configuration. Group 2 used precontoured locking plates in a perpendicular configuration. Group 3 used precontoured locking plates in a parallel configuration. Each group was tested for stiffness in anterior bending, posterior bending, axial compression, and torsion. In the early postoperative period, less expensive perpendicular reconstruction plate constructs provided similar stiffness and load-to-failure properties to newer precontoured locking plate systems irrespective of plate configuration.

32. Ducrot G, Bonnomet F, Adam P, Ehlinger M: Treatment of distal humerus fractures with LCP DHP™ locking plates in patients older than 65 years. *Orthop Traumatol Surg Res* 2013;99(2):145-154.

    In this retrospective study, 46 patients were treated with LCP DHP locking plate fixation, with a mean age of 80 years. Forty-three patients were re-evaluated after a mean follow-up of 25 months. Flexion was 127° and loss of extension was 23°, producing a mean ROM of 104°. Functional recovery was highly satisfactory. Postoperative complications consisted of infection (n = 3), metaphyseal nonunion (n = 2), ulnar nerve injury (n = 6), transient radial nerve palsy (n = 1), and periarticular ossification (n = 4). Compound fracture and worse AO fracture type were associated with worse functional outcomes. Level of evidence: IV.

33. Deuel CR, Wolinsky P, Shepherd E, Hazelwood SJ: The use of hinged external fixation to provide additional stabilization for fractures of the distal humerus. *J Orthop Trauma* 2007;21(5):323-329.

34. Korner J, Lill H, Müller LP, et al: Distal humerus fractures in elderly patients: Results after open reduction and internal fixation. *Osteoporos Int* 2005;16(suppl 2):S73-S79.

35. Giannoudis PV, Al-Lami MK, Tzioupis C, Zavras D, Grotz MR: Tricortical bone graft for primary reconstruction of comminuted distal humerus fractures. *J Orthop Trauma* 2005;19(10):741-743.

36. Spang JT, Del Gaizo DJ, Dahners LE: Reconstruction of lateral trochlear defect with radial head autograft. *J Orthop Trauma* 2008;22(5):351-356.

37. Müller LP, Kamineni S, Rommens PM, Morrey BF: Primary total elbow replacement for fractures of the distal humerus. *Oper Orthop Traumatol* 2005;17(2):119-142.

38. Athwal GS, Goetz TJ, Pollock JW, Faber KJ: Prosthetic replacement for distal humerus fractures. *Orthop Clin North Am* 2008;39(2):201-212, vi.

39. McKee MD, Veillette CJ, Hall JA, et al: A multicenter, prospective, randomized, controlled trial of open reduction—internal fixation versus total elbow arthroplasty

for displaced intra-articular distal humeral fractures in elderly patients. *J Shoulder Elbow Surg* 2009;18(1):3-12.

40. Cil A, Veillette CJ, Sanchez-Sotelo J, Morrey BF: Linked elbow replacement: A salvage procedure for distal humeral nonunion. *J Bone Joint Surg Am* 2008;90(9):1939-1950.

41. Antuña SA, Laakso RB, Barrera JL, Espiga X, Ferreres A: Linked total elbow arthroplasty as treatment of distal humerus fractures. *Acta Orthop Belg* 2012;78(4):465-472.

    This review of linked elbow arthroplasty reported on 16 patients with a comminuted fracture of the distal humerus not amenable to ORIF. At a mean follow-up of 57 months, mean ROM was from 28° to 117° of flexion-extension. Five patients with moderate to severe pain (31%) were not satisfied with the results of the procedure. Three patients had an infection, which resulted in implant removal in one patient; eight patients had symptoms of sensory ulnar nerve neuropathy.

42. Ducrot G, Ehlinger M, Adam P, Di Marco A, Clavert P, Bonnomet F: Complex fractures of the distal humerus in the elderly: Is primary total elbow arthroplasty a valid treatment alternative? A series of 20 cases. *Orthop Traumatol Surg Res* 2013;99(1):10-20.

    This study examined the functional recovery and morbidity of complex distal humerus fractures in elderly patients when treated with elbow prosthesis. This series consisted of 20 patients with a mean age of 80 years. Based on AO classification, there were 2 type A2 fractures, 2 type B fractures, 15 type C fractures, and 1 fracture that could not be classified because of previous history of rheumatoid disease in this elbow. Treatment consisted of the implantation of a Coonrad-Morrey, hinge-type TEA prosthesis. Fifteen of 20 patients were available for reevaluation with a mean follow-up of 3.6 years. The clinical ROM results were comparable to published data. The functional scores were slightly lower, mainly because of the pain factor. Level of evidence: IV.

43. Prasad N, Dent C: Outcome of total elbow replacement for distal humeral fractures in the elderly: A comparison of primary surgery and surgery after failed internal fixation or conservative treatment. *J Bone Joint Surg Br* 2008;90(3):343-348.

44. Kalogrianitis S, Sinopidis C, El Meligy M, Rawal A, Frostick SP: Unlinked elbow arthroplasty as primary treatment for fractures of the distal humerus. *J Shoulder Elbow Surg* 2008;17(2):287-292.

45. Argintar E, Berry M, Narvy SJ, Kramer J, Omid R, Itamura JM: Hemiarthroplasty for the treatment of distal humerus fractures: Short-term clinical results. *Orthopedics* 2012;35(12):1042-1045.

    The authors retrospectively evaluated the short-term clinical outcomes of 10 patients who underwent elbow hemiarthroplasty for distal humerus fractures. This short-term review suggests that distal humerus hemiarthroplasty can be an effective treatment of certain distal humerus fractures.

46. Adolfsson L, Hammer R: Elbow hemiarthroplasty for acute reconstruction of intraarticular distal humerus fractures: A preliminary report involving 4 patients. *Acta Orthop* 2006;77(5):785-787.

47. Throckmorton TW, Zarkadas PC, Steinmann SP: Distal humerus fractures. *Hand Clin* 2007;23(4):457-469, vi.

48. McKee MD, Jupiter JB, Bamberger HB: Coronal shear fractures of the distal end of the humerus. *J Bone Joint Surg Am* 1996;78(1):49-54.

49. Ring D, Jupiter JB, Gulotta L: Articular fractures of the distal part of the humerus. *J Bone Joint Surg Am* 2003;85-A(2):232-238.

50. Dubberley JH, Faber KJ, Macdermid JC, Patterson SD, King GJ: Outcome after open reduction and internal fixation of capitellar and trochlear fractures. *J Bone Joint Surg Am* 2006;88(1):46-54.

51. Sen MK, Sama N, Helfet DL: Open reduction and internal fixation of coronal fractures of the capitellum. *J Hand Surg Am* 2007;32(9):1462-1465.

52. Mighell MA, Harkins D, Klein D, Schneider S, Frankle M: Technique for internal fixation of capitellum and lateral trochlea fractures. *J Orthop Trauma* 2006;20(10):699-704.

53. Sano S, Rokkaku T, Saito S, Tokunaga S, Abe Y, Moriya H: Herbert screw fixation of capitellar fractures. *J Shoulder Elbow Surg* 2005;14(3):307-311.

54. Bilsel K, Atalar AC, Erdil M, Elmadag M, Sen C, Demirhan M: Coronal plane fractures of the distal humerus involving the capitellum and trochlea treated with open reduction internal fixation. *Arch Orthop Trauma Surg* 2013;133(6):797-804.

    The researchers reviewed the records of all patients with coronal plane fractures of the distal humerus treated using ORIF. Fractures were classified according to the Bryan and Morrey system. Cannulated screws were used for fixation. All patients were evaluated using the Mayo Elbow Score and DASH scores at least 1 year later. ORIF with cannulated screws, which maintains a stable anatomic articular position, provides satisfactory results in coronal plane fractures of the distal humerus. Level of evidence: IV.

55. Gofton WT, Macdermid JC, Patterson SD, Faber KJ, King GJ: Functional outcome of AO type C distal humeral fractures. *J Hand Surg Am* 2003;28(2):294-308.

56. Jawa A, McCarty P, Doornberg J, Harris M, Ring D: Extra-articular distal-third diaphyseal fractures of the humerus. A comparison of functional bracing and plate fixation. *J Bone Joint Surg Am* 2006;88(11):2343-2347.

57. Min W, Ding BC, Tejwani NC: Comparative functional outcome of AO/OTA type C distal humerus fractures: Open injuries do worse than closed fractures. *J Trauma Acute Care Surg* 2012;72(2):E27-E32.

A case-control comparison of open and closed AO type C fractures of the distal humerus. Outcomes were determined clinically and radiographically. When compared with closed fractures, open distal humerus fractures had worse functional outcome scores and decreased ROM. Patients with open fractures also demonstrated a trend toward having higher complication rates, prolonged times to union, and higher rates of persistent nerve deficits requiring further surgery.

58. Abrams GD, Bellino MJ, Cheung EV: Risk factors for development of heterotopic ossification of the elbow after fracture fixation. *J Shoulder Elbow Surg* 2012;21(11):1550-1554.

A retrospective study assesses the factors associated with heterotopic ossification formation following surgical fixation of elbow trauma in 89 patients. Age, male sex, lateral collateral ligament repair, and dual-incision approach were not associated with increased ectopic bone formation. Distal humerus fractures were an important predictor of heterotopic bone. For patients in whom heterotopic ossification ultimately developed, it was visible on radiographs obtained 2 weeks postoperatively in 86% of cases. Level of evidence: II.

Chapter 25

Fractures of the Proximal Radius and Ulna, and Dislocations of the Elbow

Thomas F. Varecka, MD

Abstract

Injuries of the elbow area, including fractures of the proximal radius and proximal ulna and elbow dislocations and fracture-dislocations, are common and sometimes challenging to treat. An understanding of the etiology of injuries and their influence on elbow, forearm, and wrist function, and current treatment methodologies, such as open repair of the radial head and coronoid fractures, and new technologies for olecranon fracture repair, is important as are techniques for avoiding complications.

Keywords: radial head fractures; radial head prosthesis; olecranon fractures; coronoid fractures; elbow dislocation; elbow fracture-dislocations

Introduction

Following an elbow injury, the restoration of elbow function requires recognition of the unique characteristics of this joint. The elbow consists of the complex articulations of three bones: the humerus, the radius, and the ulna. Critical ligaments, including the anterior bundle of the medial collateral ligament (MCL) and the lateral ulnar collateral ligament (LUCL), as well as dynamic functional stabilizers, including the flexor pronator, the common extensor, the triceps, the biceps, and brachialis muscles, also contribute vitally to proper elbow function.

Bony congruity and stability are provided by three separate articulations: the ulnotrochlear joint, the radiocapitellar joint, and the proximal radioulnar joint. All are important for elbow function and, when injured, each must be assessed and repaired or reconstructed to provide the best clinical outcome for elbow, forearm, and wrist function.

Radial Head Fractures

Incidence and Classification

Radial head fractures are the most common fracture about the elbow. It is estimated that radial head fractures account for 3% of all fractures seen in emergency departments and that approximately 75% of all proximal forearm fractures involve the radial head and/or neck.[1-3] Population studies report an incidence of 28 radial head fractures per 100,000 population per year,[4] with a combined radial head and neck fracture incidence of 55 per 100,000 population per year.[3] Men and women are equally at risk for radial head fractures, but injury in men occurs at an average age of 37 years; in comparison, the average age of women with fracture injury is 52 years.[3] The injury occurs about equally in the right arm and in the left arm. Radial head and/or neck fractures frequently are associated with complex injury patterns, such as elbow fracture-dislocations, which require additional scrutiny to understand the full spectrum of bony and ligamentous injury.

Anatomically, it is important to remember that the radial head is neither completely round nor completely cylindrical.[2,5] Mechanically, this shape permits the proximal-distal pistoning effect of the radius during forearm rotation and guides the supination-pronation arc.

Functionally, the radial head is a secondary stabilizer of the elbow; the primary stabilizer is the MCL. The radial

Neither Dr. Varecka nor any immediate family member has received anything of value from or has stock or stock options held in a commercial company or institution related directly or indirectly to the subject of this chapter.

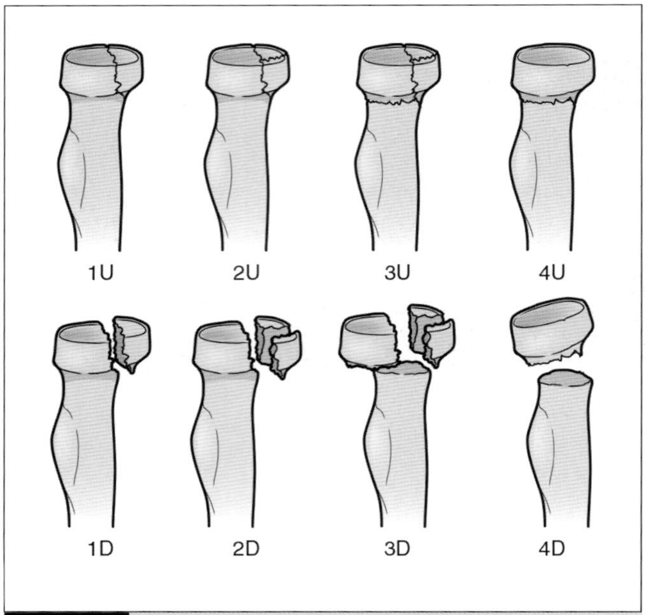

Figure 1 Illustration shows the Charalambous classification, in which fractures are characterized by the degree of displacement.

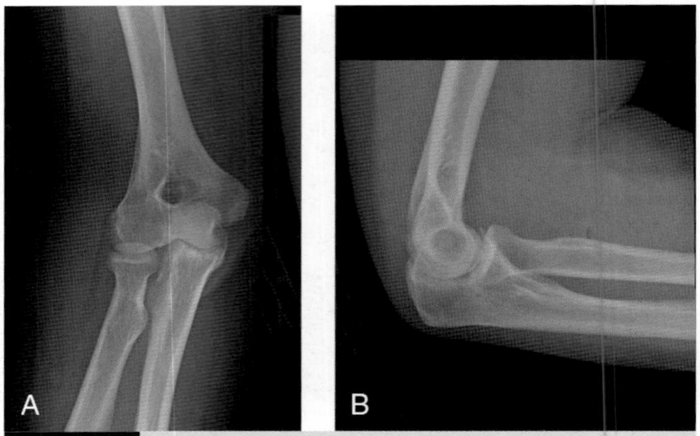

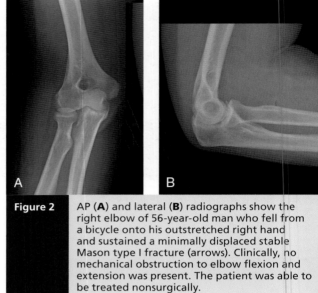

Figure 2 AP (**A**) and lateral (**B**) radiographs show the right elbow of 56-year-old man who fell from a bicycle onto his outstretched right hand and sustained a minimally displaced stable Mason type I fracture (arrows). Clinically, no mechanical obstruction to elbow flexion and extension was present. The patient was able to be treated nonsurgically.

head contributes considerably to the neutralization of the valgus forces across the elbow, which occur in the axially loaded fully extended elbow. An intact radial head or its substitute can unload an injured MCL, allowing the ligament to heal without formal repair in most instances. The radial head along with the LUCL can prevent posterolateral rotatory instability. In addition, the buttressing effect of the radial head prevents the proximal migration of the radius when interosseous membrane injury is present, as seen in Essex-Lopresti type injuries, which can be subtle and may not be obvious at the initial presentation.[6,7]

The classification of radial head fractures is based on the size, location, and displacement of the fracture fragments. The first widely used classification described three general types. Type 1 is a nondisplaced or fissure fracture of the articular rim. Type 2 is a marginal fracture with less than 2 mm of displacement and 25° of angulation. Type 3 is a comminuted fracture involving the entire head.[8,9] A fourth type was subsequently added to include any radial head fracture associated with an elbow dislocation.[10] A 2011 study offered a simplified classification based solely on displacement[11] (**Figure 1**).

Treatment

Radial head fracture treatment options include nonsurgical management, fragment excision, radial head excision, open reduction and internal fixation (ORIF), and radial head arthroplasty.

Nonsurgical treatment is reserved for minimally displaced fractures in which no block to elbow flexion or forearm rotation exists (**Figure 2**). Importantly, the stability of the elbow should be verified by physical examination and imaging, and no evidence of joint laxity or subluxation should be present. No consensus exists regarding the best method of immobilization, or the optimum position or duration of immobilization. Immobilization should be brief, however, and for comfort and protection, usually is achieved in a simple sling, allowing some active-assisted flexion as pain permits.[1] Aspiration of the hemarthrosis has been suggested as a means of encouraging elbow motion.[12]

Surgical treatment is indicated when fragment displacement or malalignment is sufficient to block elbow motion. Fragment excision has been recommended for fragments representing less than 25% of the articular surface, without elbow instability.[1] If such treatment is chosen, the surgeon must ensure that the radial head defect does not engage the proximal radioulnar joint, because this position can cause pain and promote stiffness.

The greatest controversy exists over the treatment of comminuted fractures. The debate over whether to use excision, ORIF, or replacement as the most appropriate management is an old one and, despite many reports, no consensus exists.

Excision of the radial head was first proposed more than 100 years ago[13] and still garners much support in the right clinical setting.[14-17] In the presence of elbow stability, good long-term outcomes have been reported for excision. If ligament instability is ignored or underestimated, then

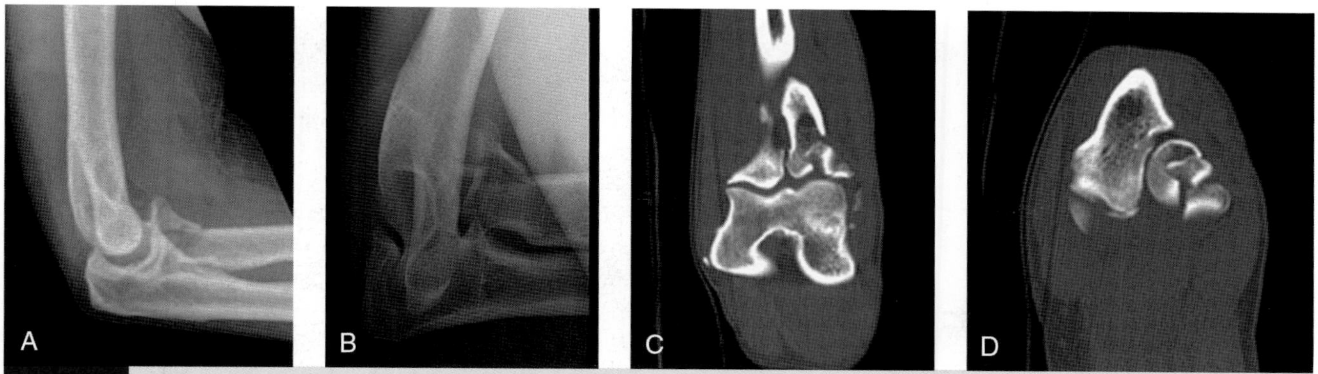

Figure 3 AP (**A**) and lateral (**B**) radiographs show a comminuted radial head and neck fracture pattern in a 60-year-old man who fell from a 13-foot height onto his outstretched right hand. AP (**C**) and lateral (**D**) CT scans of the elbow show a multifragmented configuration.

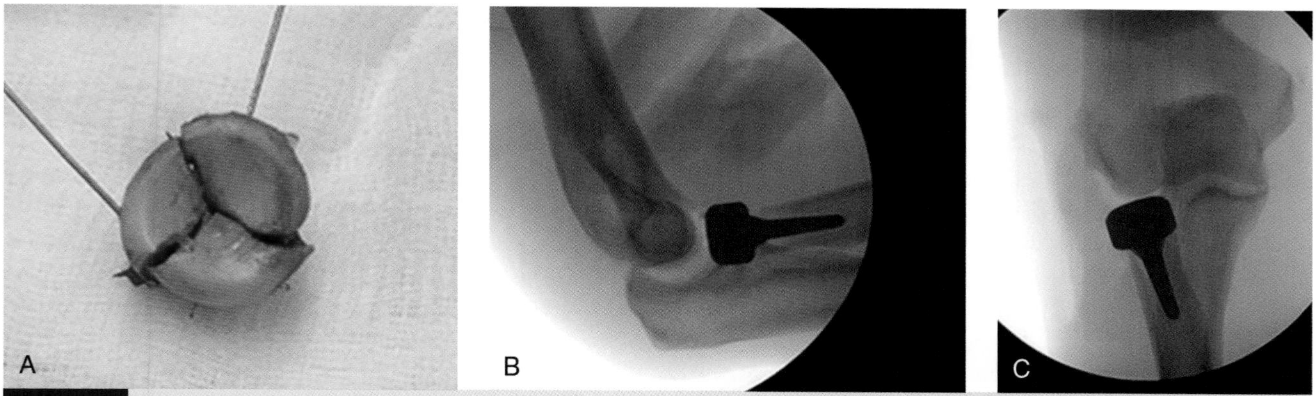

Figure 4 Clinical photograph (**A**) shows an excised, fractured radial head consisting of three large articular fragments. Because of the loss of some articular surface material and comminution of the neck portion, reassembly was not indicated. **B,** Intraoperative image intensifier lateral radiograph shows a noncemented prosthesis with a loose-fitting stem in place. **C,** AP projection from the same patient taken intraoperatively with image intensification showing the noncemented, loose-fitting stem of the radial head prosthesis. Note that the prosthesis is slightly undersized to avoid overstuffing.

radial head excision will potentiate MCL laxity following injury. Radial head-capitellum contact absorbs longitudinal loads, which can protect any interosseous membrane injury, permitting it to heal instead of enabling the dreaded proximal radial migration, with concomitant ulnar abutment syndrome.[1,2,7,18] A higher incidence of radiographically demonstrated posttraumatic osteoarthritis in the ulnotrochlear joint has been reported after radial head excision, although it is unclear whether this outcome is the result of the radial head excision or the initial cartilage impaction.[13,16,17,19] For the most part, these radiographic arthritic changes do not correlate with clinical symptoms.

ORIF of comminuted radial head fractures gained popularity during the 1990s as the need to restore radiocapitellar congruence was recognized.[6,20,21] Many authors reported satisfactory results in the short-term and midterm range.[22] However, the use of ORIF has decreased because of prior lack of site-specific implants, technical difficulties, posterior interosseous nerve injury, osteonecrosis of fracture fragments, and fixation failure—even with the advent of mini locked plates. One study showed that the fixation of radial head fractures with more than three fragments or of those in which fragment diastasis or severe impaction was present resulted in poor outcomes. The study suggested that, under such circumstances, radial head replacement was preferred[6] (**Figure 3**).

Radial head implant arthroplasty for more comminuted fractures or for those associated with elbow or forearm instability recently has gained more acceptance, because the poorer outcomes from resection arthroplasty and ORIF have demonstrated these latter two methods to be unreliable or unpredictable[1,22] (**Figures 4** and **5**).

Current radial head prostheses are available in cobalt-chromium or titanium materials. Designs range from the simple to the complex, with variation in costs. Monoblock or bipolar designs, as well as cemented and

4: Upper Extremity

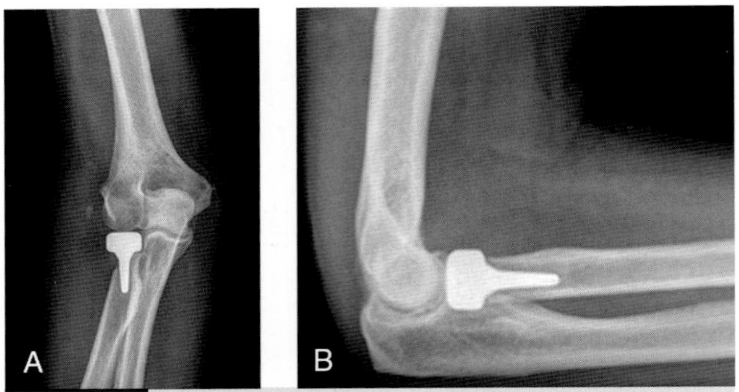

Figure 5 AP (**A**) and lateral (**B**) radiographs of the patient whose images are shown in Figure 4 taken at 4-week follow-up visit. The prosthesis remains well seated, and appropriately aligned. Note the "windshield wiper" effect about the stem, indicating some motion occurring at the bone-stem interface in the absence of cementing. Clinical examination revealed pain-free elbow flexion of 30° to 120° and supination and pronation of 65° and 70°, respectively.

noncemented stem options, are also available. Noncemented stems consist of smooth and press-fit alternatives. A smooth stem allows the prosthesis to rotate and find its best fit, permitting it to loosen or subside into an optimal position. Press-fit and cemented stems require a much more precise initial placement of the prosthesis, because the device then functions as a fixed permanent extension of the radius and tends to be far less forgiving if it is off axis.[7] To date, no evidence has favored one design over another.[23] When an appropriate replacement is unavailable, a hand-fashioned methyl methacrylate spacer reportedly performs almost as well as metallic prostheses, although high rates of failure and the need for secondary removal have been noted.[24]

In the ligament-deficient elbow, the radial column buttress is essential and must be repaired or reconstructed to prevent valgus laxity, posterior instability, and proximal radial migration.[1,2,7,11,22] The same caveat regarding treatment of the radial head component of the injury pattern exists, however. ORIF may be too difficult to perform, and no unique prosthetic design has established itself as being superior.[6,7,9,22-25] In medium-term to long-term follow-up, the performance of radial head prostheses has declined.

Poor motion of the elbow or forearm and progressive pain have resulted in a reported 20% to 30% explantation rate.[26] Metal-on-cartilage capitellar wear is implicated in the delayed onset of elbow pain.[27] Implant loosening also has been implicated as a source of pain.[27,28] The timing of prosthesis insertion has been correlated with the late onset of elbow pain. The performance of radial head implants inserted 6 weeks or more after injury was affected most by symptoms or conditions indicating arthritis.[27] Careful sizing of the radial head prosthesis is critical, because overstuffing of the space left by the radial head excision can result in increased loads on the capitellum and the lesser sigmoid notch of the proximal ulna.[28] This edge loading can cause focal cartilage wear and generate pain. An excessively large radial head prosthesis also can cause a jamming effect on the capitellar cartilage and block elbow flexion as well as forearm rotation. Moreover, it has been shown that simple radiographic evaluation of the prosthetic fit may not be reliable, and undersizing of the prosthesis generally is suggested.[1,7,26,28,29] Heterotopic ossification can occur following elbow fracture-dislocation, especially when the joint has been subluxated for some time or has been manipulated repeatedly because of gross instability and persistent subluxation. Such a development can result in greatly restricted motion.[26,27,30,31]

Proximal Ulnar Fractures

Anatomy and Classification

The proximal ulna is formed by the olecranon and the coronoid process, which together comprise the semilunar or greater sigmoid notch, which in turn forms one side of the main articulation of the elbow, in opposition to the trochlear notch of the distal humerus. The absolute osseous integrity of these two structures is mandatory for ulnohumeral joint stability.[32] The restoration of bony integrity and articular congruity, thus re-establishing joint stability and motion, are the goals of treatment for fractures involving the olecranon or the coronoid process.[32-34]

Fractures of the proximal ulna frequently display the classic bimodal trauma distribution of high-energy injury in younger, typically male patients and lower-energy injury in elderly women and those with osteopenia.[35] It is estimated that fractures of the olecranon area constitute approximately 10% of elbow fractures in adults.[32-34] Most olecranon fractures are isolated injuries, but potential injuries to the radial head, proximal radius, and capsuloligamentous structures must be excluded carefully. Displaced fractures of the olecranon region can be associated with elbow dislocation.

The classification systems for proximal ulnar fractures are mostly simple descriptions of fracture patterns and displacement, with no associated prognostic or mechanistic implications. The two most widely used classification schemes are the Schatzker classification and the Mayo Clinic classification[34] (**Figure 6**). Olecranon fractures result from direct or indirect trauma. The degree of elbow flexion at the time of a direct blow to the olecranon influences the fracture pattern. Direct trauma with the

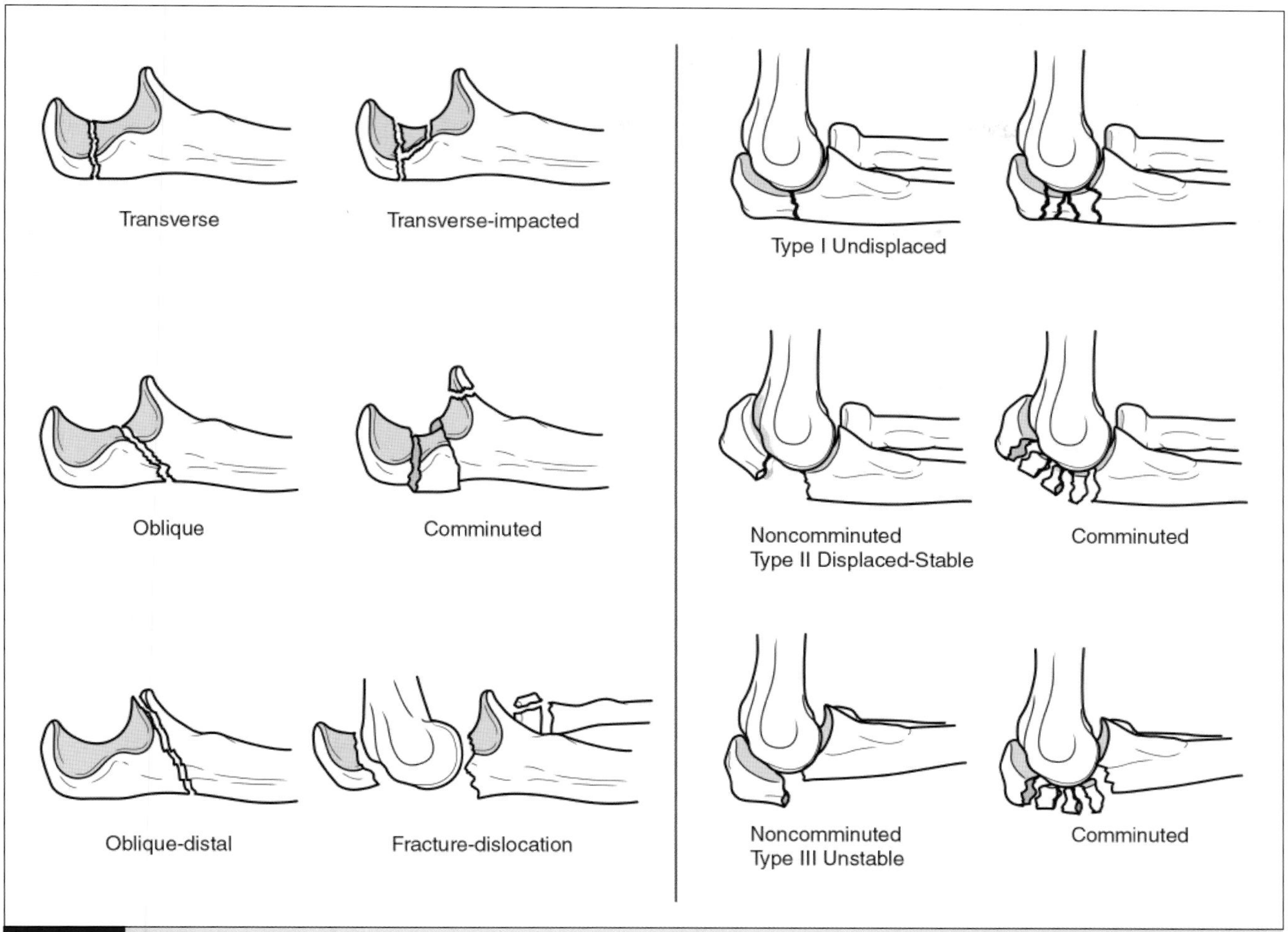

Figure 6 Drawings show the Schatzker classification system (left) and the Mayo Clinic classification system (right) for olecranon fractures.

arm at 90° of elbow flexion results in fractures with substantial comminution and elbow dislocation.[36] Indirect trauma from a fall on the outstretched hand can result in simpler, more transversely oriented fractures as the olecranon fails in tension applied by the forceful contraction of the triceps.[36]

Treatment of Olecranon Fractures

The nonsurgical management of olecranon fractures is reserved for very simple nondisplaced fractures, fractures in children, or fractures in adults who are not surgical candidates because of associated medical comorbidities.

Historically, the goal of treatment has been to internally stabilize the bony injury in most isolated olecranon fractures. The choice of treatment depends on the fracture type, comminution, the obliquity of the fracture line, articular depression, and the displacement of the radial head. Generally, tension band wiring (TBW) is considered the simplest and least invasive fixation method; however, the effective execution of TBW requires that several criteria be met: the cortex opposite the TBW must be intact or securely opposable (ie, having no comminution of the subchondral bone); the fracture orientation should be perpendicular or nearly perpendicular to the long axis of the ulna; and dislocation of the elbow should not have occurred.[37] TBW has been shown to be very reliable, with high patient satisfaction rates when these criteria are met, although the reoperation rates for hardware removal have been reported to range from 46% to 85%.[35,37-39] Using isoelastic cables with a low profile as a substitute for wire may reduce the necessity of hardware removal. Fixation failure and nonunion also have been reported (**Figure 7**).

When the three previously described criteria cannot be met or when bone quality is poor, ORIF with a plate and screws is preferred.[40,41] Fixation with a plate and screws has been demonstrated to be more secure than has TBW, especially in the presence of comminution. In addition, plating allows the width and depth of the

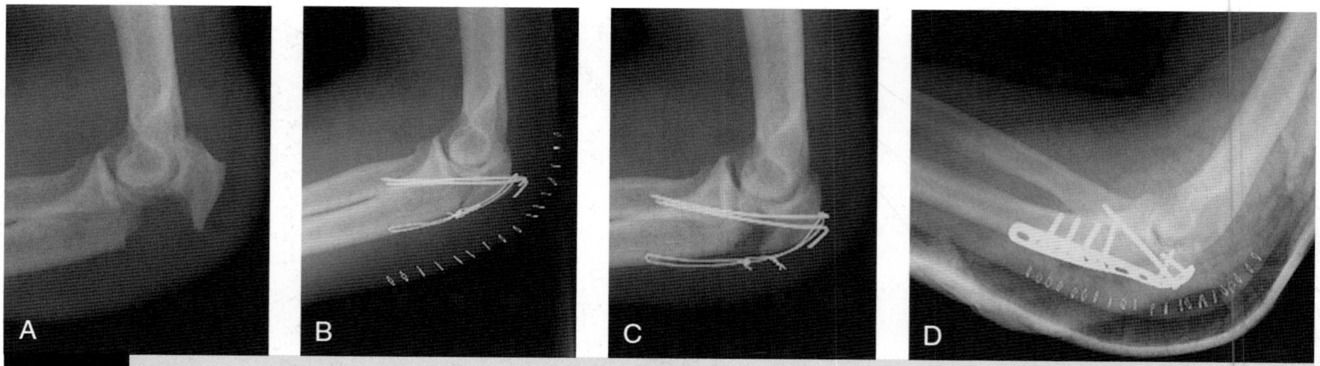

Figure 7 **A** through **D**, A series of lateral radiographs of the proximal ulna showing a displaced, transverse olecranon fracture with initial tension band wire fixation. **A**, The fracture is shown. **B**, The fracture is fixed with tension band wiring. **C**, Failure of the fixation has occurred at 6 weeks. **D**, Fracture fixation has been revised to a plate.

olecranon sulcus to be maintained more readily than does TBW. Alteration in these dimensions has been shown to lead to reduced elbow flexion and extension, as well as postfixation pain.[37,39,41] In biomechanical testing, no clear advantage was seen for any type of plate system that is used (for example, semitubular versus locking plates), because fixation failure tends to occur at the bone-implant interface.[40] When using locking plates, a particularly disconcerting mode of failure is the escape of the proximal small fragment from the fixation construct despite the use of the locking screws. Clinical experience has confirmed the laboratory observation that such small fragment escape can and does occur whether or not locked screw fixation is used. A long intramedullary screw can be used whenever possible to improve construct rigidity.[41] In comminuted fractures or in the presence of bone deficiency, dual plating should be considered and may reduce catastrophic bone-implant failure.[41,42]

Studies documenting recent experience with modified TBW constructs or fixation with site-specific intramedullary devices has been reported. A 2007 study demonstrated no substantial differences in the mechanical strength or security obtained between fractures fixed with metal tension bands and those fixed with FiberWire (Arthrex) suture material.[43] Alternatively, a 2011 study showed that using a modified tension band technique with Kirschner wires (K-wires) having eyelets, through which a cable can be passed after insertion of the wires along the axis of the olecranon, seems to provide distinct advantages. Not only is the fracture reliably fixed, but the wires also are prevented from backing out by being coupled with the cable.[37] Finally, true intramedullary fixation has been introduced recently as a treatment method (**Figure 8**). Although laboratory studies have shown this type of fixation to be a secure and even stronger method of fixation compared with other options after controlled in vitro osteotomies, confirmatory clinical reports still are limited.[44-46]

In nonreconstructible olecranon fractures, especially those in the elderly or those in which extensive bone loss has taken place, fragment excision and advancement of the triceps insertion have been advocated. Although elbow stability can be restored, limitations in flexion and associated weakness often have resulted and may mitigate the utility of the fragment excision/tendon reinsertion technique.[47]

Complications of olecranon fixation have been reported extensively.[30,32,33,38,48] They include delayed union and nonunion, fixation failure, infection, loss of fixation, and most commonly, symptomatic hardware prominence. The unintended prominence of K-wires, when inserted in transcortical fashion and with distal anterior cortical penetration, has been reported to impinge on the proximal radius, the supinator muscle, or the biceps tendon. This impingement results in a primary loss of forearm rotation, which can be confused with fibrous or bony synostosis of the proximal radioulnar space. Proper orientation and appropriate depth of the wires is emphasized to prevent this complication.[49] It is also necessary to bury the pins into the bone, often aided by predrilling of the intended path of the hooked pins, to ensure that they lie below the triceps tendon and are not impaling it. These simple steps can reduce the potential for proximal migration of the wires.

Fractures of the Coronoid Process

Fractures of the coronoid process are relatively uncommon and can occur as isolated injuries but often occur with elbow dislocation.[49] In a study reporting the significance of coronoid fractures, three types of coronoid lesions, each associated with elbow dislocation and recurrent instability if ignored or neglected, were recognized.

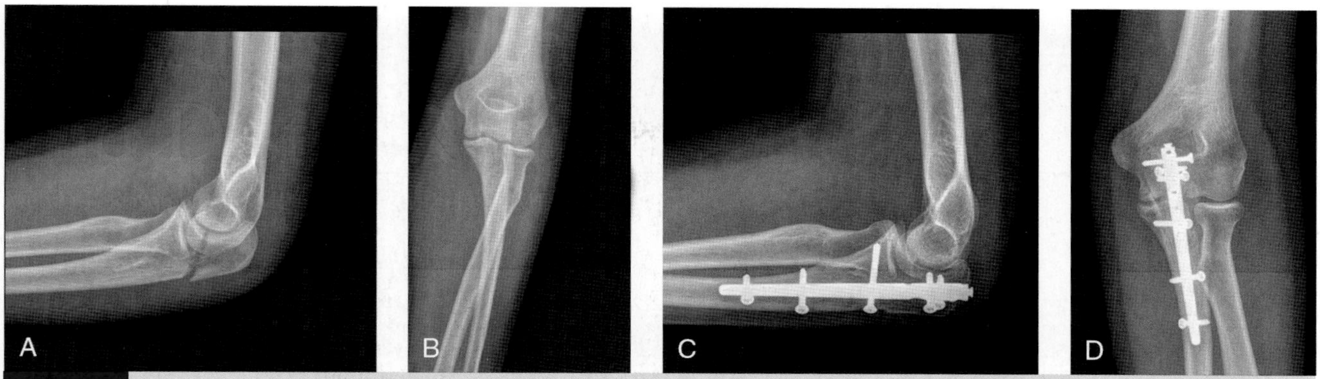

Figure 8 Radiographs show a moderately displaced olecranon fracture in a 20-year-old woman who fell on an outstretched hand. **A**, Lateral view of the injured elbow demonstrating the olecranon fracture. **B**, AP view. **C** and **D**, Lateral and AP radiographic views taken 6 weeks postoperatively after fixation with an intramedullary nail designed for proximal ulnar fracture fixation. Clinical examination showed that almost complete elbow flexion and extension had been restored.

Type I coronoid fractures had a low incidence (16%) of dislocation and instability, whereas type III fractures frequently (80%) were identified with elbow dislocation and subsequent instability.[49] Type II injuries posed an intermediate risk for persistent instability (**Figure 3, Figure 9**).

Studies documenting anatomic subdivision of coronoid fractures recognize that a high potential exists for anterior and medial extension of the fracture plane in type II and type III fractures. This step has added further understanding of fracture patterns that could result in posterior lateral instability and posterior medial instability[50-53] (**Figure 10**).The recognition and treatment of this subset of fractures are essential for avoiding persistent instability, accelerated osteoarthritis, and poor functional outcomes. ORIF of the anteromedial fragment usually is required and should be based not on the size of the fragment but on its displacement and joint congruity, as well as the observed instability during fluoroscopic examination under anesthesia[52] (**Figure 11**).

The surgical approach to the anterior medial slope of the coronoid can be challenging. A variety of exposures have been advocated, including direct anterior exposure and several different medial approaches. The treating surgeon is advised to gain familiarity with the local anatomy before attempting a repair of these fractures, particularly of the locations and courses of the median and ulnar nerves and the brachial artery.

The complications of failing to restore the integrity of the coronoid process include chronic elbow instability, recurrent dislocations, and early degenerative disease. Clearly, recognizing the possible presence of this injury and understanding its significance are paramount in treating any elbow injury.

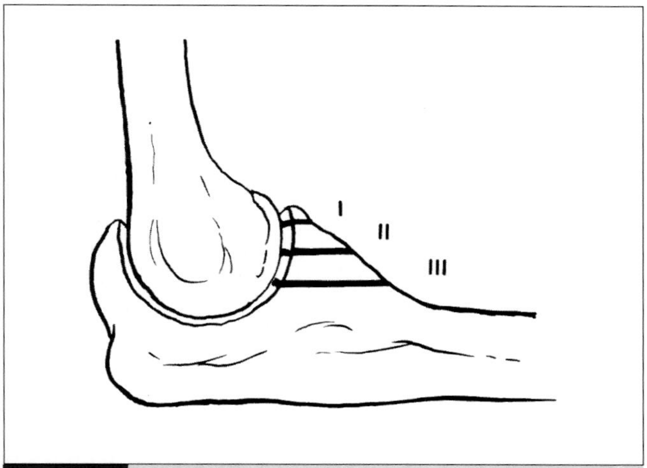

Figure 9 Drawing depicts the locations of coronoid process fractures according to the Regan and Morrey classification of coronoid process fractures. Type I fractures consist of the tip of the coronoid process. It is important to recognize that these are fractures resulting from a shearing injury to the coronoid, and not avulsion injuries. Type III fractures, and to a lesser extent type II, are associated with elbow dislocation and instability. (Reproduced with permission from Regan W, Morrey BF: Fractures of the coronoid process of the ulna. *J Bone Joint Surg Am* 1989;71[9]:1348-1354.)

Elbow Dislocations

Simple dislocations have no associated fracture, whereas complex dislocations are associated with fractures of the distal humerus, radius, olecranon, or coronoid process. The predisposition to elbow dislocation has been correlated with the elbow carrying angle, ligamentous

Fracture	Subtype	Description
Tip	1	≤2 mm of coronoid height
	2	>2 mm of coronoid height
Anteromedial	1	Anteromedial rim
	2	Anteromedial rim and tip
	3	Anteromedial rim and sublime tubercle (± tip)
Basal	1	Coronoid body and base
	2	transolecranon basal coronoid fracture

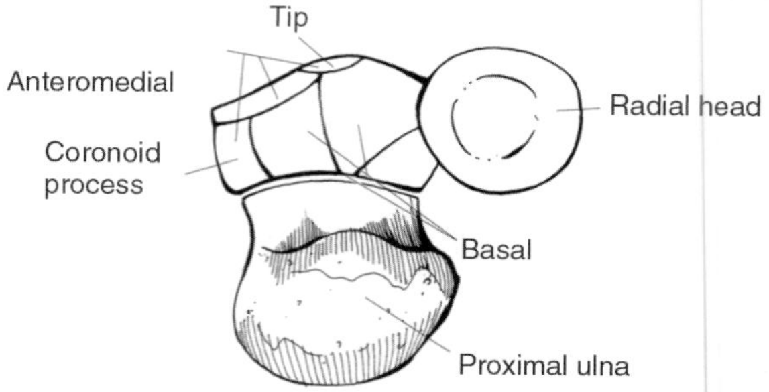

Figure 10 Drawing and chart show the O'Driscoll Modification of the Regan and Morrey coronoid fracture classification. Anteromedial types 1, 2, and 3 are particularly noteworthy for their role in predisposing to anteromedial elbow instability. (Reproduced from O'Driscoll SW, Jupiter JB, Cohen MS, Ring D, McKee MD: Difficult elbow fractures: Pearls and pitfalls. *Instr Course Lect* 2003;52:113-134.)

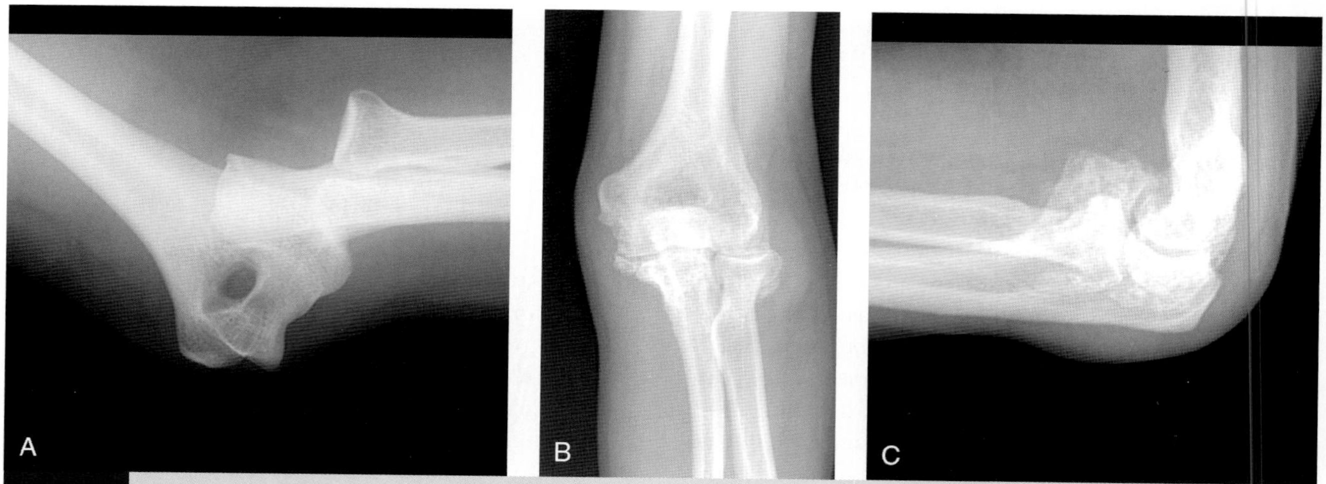

Figure 11 **A,** Plain AP radiograph showing simple dislocation of the elbow in a 27-year-old man after a fall from a height. This injury is considered "simple" because no associated fractures can be identified. **B** and **C,** Follow-up AP and lateral radiographs of the same patient 21 years later demonstrate extensive posttraumatic osteoarthritis. Initial high-energy trauma at the index simple dislocation may have damaged the articular cartilage irreparably, with associated soft-damage predisposing to the patient to extensive heterotopic ossification.

laxity, and the inclination of the trochlea of the humerus.[54] Elbow dislocations are considered to be the second most common major joint dislocation after dislocation of the shoulder. Although the actual incidence of elbow dislocation is unknown, it is estimated that 36,750 elbow dislocations occur in the United States each year.[55] This number represents a calculated rate of 5.2 dislocations per 100,000 lives per year. Males in the second decade of life were most at risk, accounting for 40% of all dislocations. The incidence diminishes with age so considerably that a man in his 20s has a calculated risk of elbow dislocation that is almost eight times that of a 90-year-old individual.[55] The data did not specify the incidence of simple versus complex dislocations.

Simple dislocations are more common than complex dislocations and typically are managed with a closed reduction in the emergency department[56] (**Figure 11**). Based on clinical and laboratory observations, the authors of a 1992 study postulated the sequence of soft-tissue and hard-tissue injury as the elbow dislocates.[50] The injury usually results from a fall from a standing height onto an outstretched hand, forcing the forearm into supination and the elbow into valgus, as an axial load is placed along the length of the arm. This sequence of events results in failure of the LUCL (**Figure 12**), causing the radial head to be driven posteriorly and laterally into the dislocated position. Sequential failure of the anterior joint capsule follows, and the elbow dislocates. The MCL, although at risk, does not always fail in catastrophic fashion.[50,51,56] If the anterior bundle of the MCL has been spared, and the coronoid is intact (stage 3A dislocation) closed reduction usually will result in a stable joint.[56] Immobilization in

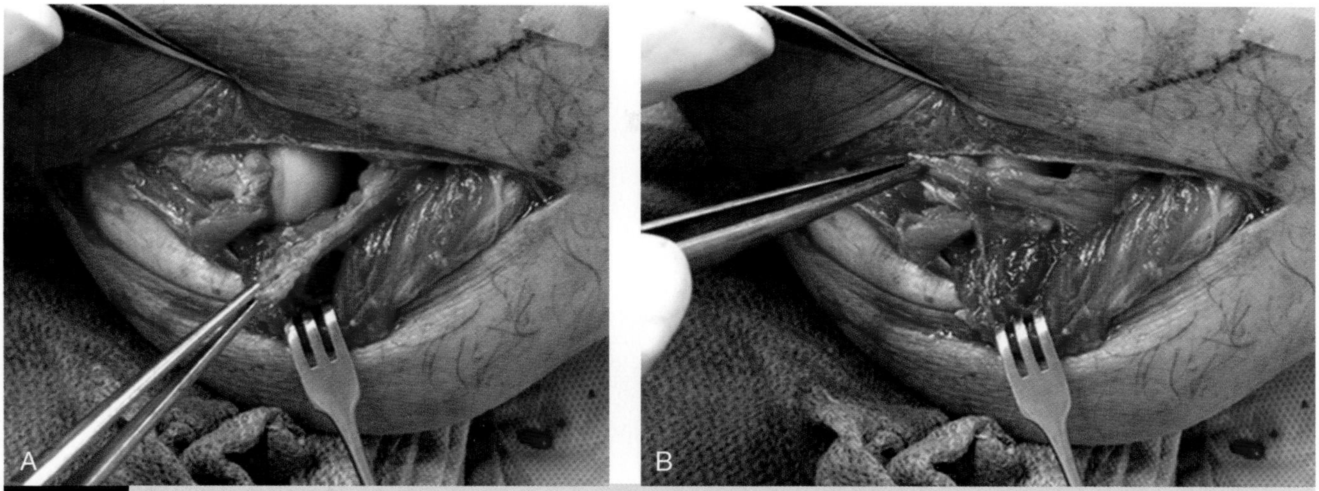

Figure 12 Intraoperative photographs show the lateral ulnar collateral ligament. **A**, The avulsed ligament is shown. **B**, The ligament has been repaired.

a posterior splint for a short period is usually sufficient, with early initiation of elbow flexion exercises preferred. If the MCL is disrupted from the distal humerus (stage 3C dislocation), with degloving of the flexor pronator origin (dynamic stabilizers), residual instability will be more likely.[56] When such extensive soft-tissue disruption has occurred, repair or reconstruction of the LUCL is mandatory if long-term elbow instability is to be avoided.[57] The primary goal in simple dislocation is to achieve a stable reduction that permits early range of motion. Typically, postreduction immobilization is not continued for more than 7 to 10 days, allowing the pain and swelling to subside. Then, range of motion exercises should be initiated.[56] After reduction has been achieved, it is important to assess the stability of the elbow by placing it through a gentle range of motion. The elbow should be able to be fully flexed and brought out to within 30° of full extension, without subluxation or patient apprehension. Elbows that are deemed unstable, signifying a complex dislocation, require surgical repair[58] (**Figure 12**).

With complex dislocations, elbow stability must be restored, and adequate functional motion must be regained if the elbow is to recover its evolutionary mandate of bringing the hand from the peripheral environment to the face and the body midline. As discussed previously, dislocations with radial head fractures (Johnston type IV[10]) are fairly common. Restoring a lateral radial buttress with ORIF or replacement usually results in satisfactory outcomes.[1,2,11,23,58] Transolecranon fracture-dislocations are another subset of complex fractures. Originally considered a variant of Monteggia fractures, these injuries now are recognized as a true disruption of the elbow ulnotrochlear articulation.[59-61] In addition to addressing any concomitant ligamentous or radial head injuries, stable fixation of the ulnar fracture is necessary for the functional restoration of the elbow.[59,61]

The most challenging complex dislocation to manage is the combination of radial head fracture, coronoid process fracture, and multiligamentous disruption, known as the terrible triad of the elbow. This injury dictates an absolute indication for surgical intervention. Transarticular K-wires, static and dynamic external fixators, and traction all have been employed with varying degrees of success.[58] Specifically addressing all elements of the injury has proven to be the most reliable method of restoring elbow stability and function, however.[62,63] The sequence of surgical treatment occurs in the following order: repair of the coronoid process (**Figure 13**), repair or replacement of the radial head, and repair of the LUCL.[63] One study reported that repair of the MCL may not be necessary always and should be undertaken only when the elbow demonstrates posterior medial rotatory instability after the aforementioned three steps have been accomplished.[63] If the coronoid is not repairable, a piece of the radial head or the posterior process of the olecranon may be used as a substitute. Anterior capsulodesis also has been employed. In all instances, a block, or resistance, to the posterior pull of the triceps must be restored to avoid recurrent dislocations. Some authors have questioned the absolute need to repair the anterior structures if adequate stability of the elbow can be restored by addressing the radial head and LUCL injuries alone.[64] This occurrence has led surgeons to begin performing a radial head reassembly or replacement using a lateral approach. Provisionally reattaching the LUCL and assessing overall elbow stability is now possible. If the elbow remains unstable, then

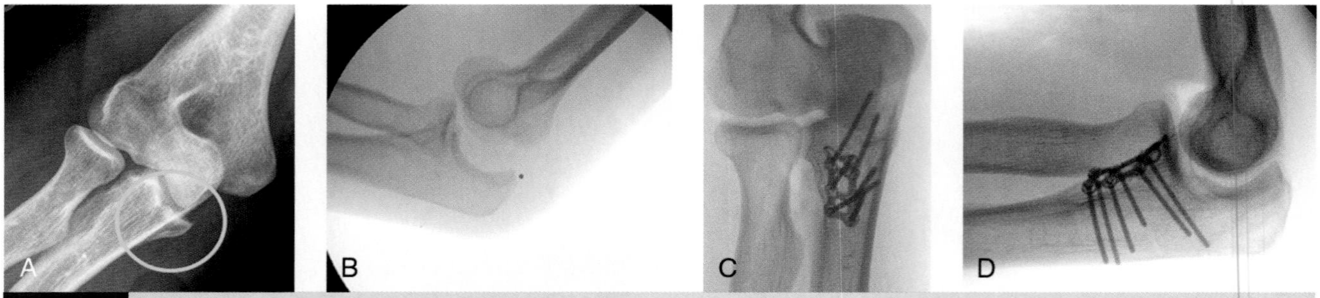

Figure 13 Images show an anterior medial coronoid process fracture in a 27-year-old man who fell onto an outstretched hand during a bicycle crash. **A**, AP radiograph of the injured elbow demonstrating an O'Driscoll type 3 anteromedial coronoid fracture. **B**, Intraoperative lateral radiograph showing tendency toward marked instability of the elbow as evidenced by the ease with which the elbow dislocated with even gentle passive extension. **C** and **D**, Intraoperative AP and lateral radiographs, respectively, showing fixation of the coronoid fracture. The elbow was now stable with stress examination in the operating room.

the coronoid fracture should be addressed. The fracture can be exposed through the lateral incision or through a separate medial approach as previously noted, depending on its size, location, and type.

As with all elbow dislocations, the goal is to restore stability, thereby allowing the early initiation of range of motion, and thus enhancing optimal functional recovery.

Summary

Injuries to the distal side of the elbow joint remain a therapeutic challenge. The occurrence of radial head fractures, their nature, and how they affect elbow function are better understood than previously, but no consensus exists regarding the best treatment. The various opinions regarding treatment choices among the repair of radial head fractures, radial head replacement, or radial head resection when the complexity of these fractures precludes fixation are sometimes controversial. Similarly, an array of treatment options exists for simple olecranon fractures. Treatment options include internal fixation with TBW or plates and screws. For the surgeon treating elbow injuries, a comprehensive and thorough understanding of the complex nature of elbow dislocations and fracture-dislocations issues is paramount for adequate treatment and a satisfactory outcome.

Key Study Points

- Radial head fractures are associated with complex injury patterns, which affect treatment.
- Understanding the significance of coronoid process fractures and their effect on elbow stability will allow better insight into the structure and function of this bony structure, and facilitate selection of appropriate treatment methods.
- The differences between simple elbow dislocations and those with accompanying fractures make these injuries challenging to treat.

Annotated References

1. Yoon A, Athwal GS, Faber KJ, King GJ: Radial head fractures. *J Hand Surg Am* 2012;37(12):2626-2634.

   This article reviewed the mechanism of injury, physical findings, and appropriate imaging studies for establishing the presence of radial head fractures. Treatment alternatives for the various degrees of fracture that can occur were reviewed, including the indications for each option. Level of evidence: V.

2. Lapner M, King GJ: Radial head fractures. *J Bone Joint Surg Am* 2013;95(12):1136-1143.

   This review article summarized radial head fracture treatment. The greatest emphasis was placed on the surgical indications and techniques and the decision-making process. Outcomes of the various techniques were discussed. Level of evidence: IV.

3. Duckworth AD, Clement ND, Jenkins PJ, Aitken SA, Court-Brown CM, McQueen MM: The epidemiology of radial head and neck fractures. *J Hand Surg Am* 2012;37(1):112-119.

The authors conducted this prognostic study of 6,872 patients encountered over 1 calendar year to establish the incidence of radial head and neck fractures. Of the total, 285 patients had radial head and neck fractures. Age, sex, mechanism of injury, and socioeconomic status were reported. Level of evidence: IV.

4. Kaas L, van Riet RP, Vroemen JP, Eygendaal D: The epidemiology of radial head fractures. *J Shoulder Elbow Surg* 2010;19(4):520-523.

   This retrospective review conducted over a 3-year period identified 322 radial head fractures, representing an incidence of 2.8 fractures per 10,000 population per year. The male to female ratio was 2:3, with females being considerably older at the time of injury. The role of osteoporosis was discussed. Level of evidence: IV.

5. van Riet RP, Van Glabbeek F, Neale PG, Bortier H, An KN, O'Driscoll SW: The noncircular shape of the radial head. *J Hand Surg Am* 2003;28(6):972-978.

6. Ring D, Quintero J, Jupiter JB: Open reduction and internal fixation of fractures of the radial head. *J Bone Joint Surg Am* 2002;84-A(10):1811-1815.

7. Stuffmann E, Baratz ME: Radial head implant arthroplasty. *J Hand Surg Am* 2009;34(4):745-754.

8. Mason ML: Some observations on fractures of the head of the radius with a review of one hundred cases. *Br J Surg* 1954;42(172):123-132.

9. Broberg MA, Morrey BF: Results of treatment of fracture-dislocations of the elbow. *Clin Orthop Relat Res* 1987;216:109-119.

10. Johnston GW: A follow-up of one hundred cases of fracture of the head of the radius with a review of the literature. *Ulster Med J* 1962;31:51-56.

11. Charalambous CP, Stanley JK, Mills SP, et al: Comminuted radial head fractures: Aspects of current management. *J Shoulder Elbow Surg* 2011;20(6):996-1007.

    A new radial head fracture classification was proposed, with fracture types distinguished principally on the basis of fragment displacement. Four fracture patterns were described and stratified as displaced or nondisplaced. Level of evidence: V.

12. Ditsios KT, Stavridis SI, Christodoulou AG: The effect of haematoma aspiration on intra-articular pressure and pain relief following Mason I radial head fractures. *Injury* 2011;42(4):362-365.

    In this study, 16 patients with Mason I radial head fractures underwent aspiration of an intra-articular hematoma. Intra-articular pressures declined from a mean of 76.5 mm Hg to a mean of 17 mm Hg. Visual analog scale pain scores declined from 5.5 to 2.5. Both measurements were statistically significant. Level of evidence: IV.

13. Kocher T: *Textbook of Operative Surgery* ,ed 3. London, Adam and Charles Black, 1911.

14. Janssen RP, Vegter J: Resection of the radial head after Mason type-III fractures of the elbow: Follow-up at 16 to 30 years. *J Bone Joint Surg Br* 1998;80(2):231-233.

15. Ikeda M, Oka Y: Function after early radial head resection for fracture: A retrospective evaluation of 15 patients followed for 3-18 years. *Acta Orthop Scand* 2000;71(2):191-194.

16. Karlsson MK, Herbertsson P, Nordqvist A, Hasserius R, Besjakov J, Josefsson PO: Long-term outcome of displaced radial neck fractures in adulthood: 16-21 year follow-up of 5 patients treated with radial head excision. *Acta Orthop* 2009;80(3):368-370.

17. Goldberg I, Peylan J, Yosipovitch Z: Late results of excision of the radial head for an isolated closed fracture. *J Bone Joint Surg Am* 1986;68(5):675-679.

18. Essex-Lopresti P: Fractures of the radial head with distal radio-ulnar dislocation; report of two cases. *J Bone Joint Surg Br* 1951;33B(2):244-247.

19. Iftimie PP, Calmet Garcia J, de Loyola Garcia Forcada I, Gonzalez Pedrouzo JE, Giné Gomà J: Resection arthroplasty for radial head fractures: Long-term follow-up. *J Shoulder Elbow Surg* 2011;20(1):45-50.

    This study examined 51 patients with radial head excision over 14 years. The average Mayo Elbow Performance Score was 96.4, and the mean Disabilities of the Arm, Shoulder and Hand score was 4.89. Pronation averaged 83°, and supination averaged 79°. Of the total, 88% (44 patients) had strength greater than 80% of the opposite arm. Overall, 96% had satisfactory outcomes. Level of evidence: IV.

20. Esser RD, Davis S, Taavao T: Fractures of the radial head treated by internal fixation: Late results in 26 cases. *J Orthop Trauma* 1995;9(4):318-323.

21. Geel CW, Palmer AK, Ruedi T, Leutenegger AF: Internal fixation of proximal radial head fractures. *J Orthop Trauma* 1990;4(3):270-274.

22. Lindenhovius AL, Felsch Q, Doornberg JN, Ring D, Kloen P: Open reduction and internal fixation compared with excision for unstable displaced fractures of the radial head. *J Hand Surg Am* 2007;32(5):630-636.

23. Hartzler RU, Morrey BF, Steinmann SP, Llusa-Perez M, Sanchez-Sotelo J: Radial head reconstruction in elbow fracture-dislocation: Monopolar or bipolar prosthesis? *Clin Orthop Relat Res* 2014;472(7):2144-2150.

    In this terrible triad cadaver model consisting of 10 fresh-frozen specimens, no substantial difference in varus-valgus laxity was measured with a monopolar versus a bipolar prosthesis in place. Associated coronoid fixation did improve varus laxity. Level of evidence: V.

24. Clembosky G, Boretto JG: Open reduction and internal fixation versus prosthetic replacement for complex fractures of the radial head. *J Hand Surg Am* 2009;34(6):1120-1123.

25. Ring D: Radial head fracture: Open reduction-internal fixation or prosthetic replacement. *J Shoulder Elbow Surg* 2011;20(2suppl):S107-S112.

This article discussed the advantages, disadvantages, possibilities, and limitations of radial head fixation versus prosthetic replacement for all types of radial head fractures. Emphasis was placed on the technical difficulties of fixing the multiply fragmented radial head. Level of evidence: V.

26. Duckworth AD, Wickramasinghe NR, Clement ND, Court-Brown CM, McQueen MM: Radial head replacement for acute complex fractures: What are the rate and risks factors for revision or removal? *Clin Orthop Relat Res* 2014;472(7):2136-2143.

Of 105 patients undergoing radial head prosthetic replacement, 29 required revision (3) or removal (26) at a mean of 6.7 years. Independent risk factors for additional surgery included a younger age (mean = 45 years) at time of the index procedure or the use of a Silastic prosthesis. Level of evidence: IV.

27. van Riet RP, Sanchez-Sotelo J, Morrey BF: Failure of metal radial head replacement. *J Bone Joint Surg Br* 2010;92(5):661-667.

In this retrospective review of 47 removed radial head prostheses, painful loosening in 31 patients was the most common indication for revision surgery. Infection was present in only two patients. All but one patient showed substantial degenerative changes at examination. Level of evidence: IV.

28. Popovic N, Lemaire R, Georis P, Gillet P: Midterm results with a bipolar radial head prosthesis: Radiographic evidence of loosening at the bone-cement interface. *J Bone Joint Surg Am* 2007;89(11):2469-2476.

29. Shors HC, Gannon C, Miller MC, Schmidt CC, Baratz ME: Plain radiographs are inadequate to identify overlengthening with a radial head prosthesis. *J Hand Surg Am* 2008;33(3):335-339.

30. Hong CC, Nashi N, Hey HW, Chee YH, Murphy D: Clinically relevant heterotopic ossification after elbow fracture surgery: A risk factors study. *Orthop Traumatol Surg Res* 2015;101(2):209-213.

In 38 of 122 patients studied (30.6%), heterotopic ossification developed after elbow trauma, with 26 (21%) of these patients having clinically significant heterotopic ossification. Risk factors included fracture-dislocation and a delayed time to surgery. Both factors reached statistical significance. Age, sex, and head injury did not correlate. Level of evidence: IV.

31. Delclaux S, Lebon J, Faraud A, et al: Complications of radial head prostheses. *Int Orthop* 2015;39(5):907-913.

This meta-analysis of 34 studies reported on radial head prosthetic replacement. Overstuffing of the radial head void with the prosthesis and capitellar erosion from the prosthesis are two critical modes of failure; prosthetic loosening was the primary mode of failure. Level of evidence: II.

32. Veillette CJ, Steinmann SP: Olecranon fractures. *Orthop Clin North Am* 2008;39(2):229-236, vii.

33. Wiegand L, Bernstein J, Ahn J: Fractures in brief: Olecranon fractures. *Clin Orthop Relat Res* 2012;470(12):3637-3641.

Olecranon fractures comprise about 10% of upper extremity fractures, displaying the typical dichotomy between a high-energy mechanism and young male patients and a lower-energy mechanism and older female patients. The treatment goal is to restore functional elbow flexion, usually with internal fixation. Level of evidence: V.

34. Newman SD, Mauffrey C, Krikler S: Olecranon fractures. *Injury* 2009;40(6):575-581.

35. Chalidis BE, Sachinis NC, Samoladas EP, Dimitriou CG, Pournaras JD: Is tension band wiring technique the "gold standard" for the treatment of olecranon fractures? A long term functional outcome study. *J Orthop Surg Res* 2008;3:9.

36. Amis AA, Miller JH: The mechanisms of elbow fractures: An investigation using impact tests in vitro. *Injury* 1995;26(3):163-168.

37. Sadri H, Stern R, Singh M, Linke B, Hoffmeyer P, Schwieger K: Transverse fractures of the olecranon: A biomechanical comparison of three fixation techniques. *Arch Orthop Trauma Surg* 2011;131(1):131-138.

This study compared three cadaver groups of eight specimens each for ulnar osteotomies fixed with a standard tension band, a tension band with intramedullary wires having eyelets through which the tension band can be looped, and staples with tension bands. The staple-tension band construct proved to be superior

38. Duckworth AD, Court-Brown CM, McQueen MM: Isolated displaced olecranon fracture. *J Hand Surg Am* 2012;37(2):341-345.

39. Rommens PM, Schneider RU, Reuter M: Functional results after operative treatment of olecranon fractures. *Acta Chir Belg* 2004;104(2):191-197.

40. Buijze GA, Blankevoort L, Tuijthof GJ, Sierevelt IN, Kloen P: Biomechanical evaluation of fixation of comminuted olecranon fractures: One-third tubular versus locking compression plating. *Arch Orthop Trauma Surg* 2010;130(4):459-464.

This study biomechanically tested five matched cadaver specimens with simulated comminuted olecranon fractures fixed with locking plates including an intramedullary screw or a one-third tubular plate including a screw capturing the coronoid cortex. Failure in all specimens occurred in the bone, not in the plates. No substantial differences in plate performance were noted.

41. Gordon MJ, Budoff JE, Yeh ML, Luo ZP, Noble PC: Comminuted olecranon fractures: A comparison of plating methods. *J Shoulder Elbow Surg* 2006;15(1):94-99.

42. Wilkerson JA, Rosenwasser MP: Surgical techniques of olecranon fractures. *J Hand Surg Am* 2014;39(8):1606-1614.

    A review of the surgical anatomy of olecranon fractures was presented. Various surgical options for fixing olecranon fractures were discussed, with an emphasis on technique pearls to help achieve exceptional outcomes and avoid complications. Level of evidence: V.

43. Carofino BC, Santangelo SA, Kabadi M, Mazzocca AD, Browner BD: Olecranon fractures repaired with FiberWire or metal wire tension banding: A biomechanical comparison. *Arthroscopy* 2007;23(9):964-970.

44. Nowak TE, Mueller LP, Burkhart KJ, Sternstein W, Reuter M, Rommens PM: Dynamic biomechanical analysis of different olecranon fracture fixation devices—tension band wiring versus two intramedullary nail systems: An in-vitro cadaveric study. *Clin Biomech (Bristol, Avon)* 2007;22(6):658-664.

45. Argintar E, Martin BD, Singer A, Hsieh AH, Edwards S: A biomechanical comparison of multidirectional nail and locking plate fixation in unstable olecranon fractures. *J Shoulder Elbow Surg* 2012;21(10):1398-1405.

    This study biomechanically compared simulated comminuted olecranon fractures fixed with standard plates with those fixed with intramedullary nails; eight specimens were placed in each group. Both devices showed similar resistance to the prevention of fracture gapping. The nail was stronger, although not to a statistically significant degree.

46. Argintar E, Cohen M, Eglseder A, Edwards S: Clinical results of olecranon fractures treated with multiplanar locked intramedullary nailing. *J Orthop Trauma* 2013;27(3):140-144.

    In this multicenter retrospective review of 28 patients with unstable olecranon fractures treated with a multiplanar interlocking intramedullary nail, all fractures healed. All patients had returned to full activity by 1 year. One patient required additional surgery for the removal of a prominent screw. Level of evidence: IV.

47. Imhofe PD, Howard TC: The treatment of olecranon fractures by excision of fragments and repair of the extensor mechanism: Historical review and report of 12 fractures. *Orthopedics* 1993;16(12):1313-7.

48. Davies M, King C, Stanley D. Complications of tension band wire fixation of olecranon fractures. *J Bone Joint Surg Br* 2005;87-B(SuppII):160.

49. Regan W, Morrey B: Fractures of the coronoid process of the ulna. *J Bone Joint Surg Am* 1989;71(9):1348-1354.

50. O'Driscoll SW, Morrey BF, Korinek S, An KN: Elbow subluxation and dislocation. A spectrum of instability. *Clin Orthop Relat Res* 1992;280:186-197.

51. O'Driscoll SW: Classification and evaluation of recurrent instability of the elbow. *Clin Orthop Relat Res* 2000;370:34-43.

52. Park SM, Lee JS, Jung JY, Kim JY, Song KS: How should anteromedial coronoid facet fracture be managed? A surgical strategy based on O'Driscoll classification and ligament injury. *J Shoulder Elbow Surg* 2015;24(1):74-82.

    This article reports the results of a retrospective review of 11 patients treated for coronoid anteromedial facet fractures. Type I fractures had lateral collateral ligament injuries and were satisfactorily treated with repair of this injury alone. Type II and III fractures required a repair of the coronoid fragment and medial collateral ligament. Level of evidence: IV.

53. O'Driscoll SW, Jupiter JB, Cohen MS, Ring D, McKee MD: Difficult elbow fractures: Pearls and pitfalls. *Instr Course Lect* 2003;52:113-134.

54. Habernek H, Ortner F: The influence of anatomic factors in elbow joint dislocation. *Clin Orthop Relat Res* 1992;274:226-230.

55. Stoneback JW, Owens BD, Sykes J, Athwal GS, Pointer L, Wolf JM: Incidence of elbow dislocations in the United States population. *J Bone Joint Surg Am* 2012;94(3):240-245.

    This population and epidemiologic study reported on the National Electronic Injury Surveillance System database. A total of 1,066 acute elbow dislocations were identified, which extrapolated to 36,751 dislocations nationwide, for a calculated incidence of 5.21 dislocations per 100,000 persons per year. Level of evidence: II.

56. Ahmed I, Mistry J: The management of acute and chronic elbow instability. *Orthop Clin North Am* 2015;46(2):271-280.

    This study reviewed the concepts of elbow instability and associated bony and soft-tissue pathology. It emphasized the goals of re-establishing a stable pain-free elbow with a functional arc of motion. The methods of treatment are reviewed, based on the underlying injury. Level of evidence: V.

57. Schneeberger AG, Sadowski MM, Jacob HA: Coronoid process and radial head as posterolateral rotatory stabilizers of the elbow. *J Bone Joint Surg Am* 2004;86-A(5):975-982.

58. Wyrick JD, Dailey SK, Gunzenhaeuser JM, Casstevens EC: Management of complex elbow dislocations: A mechanistic approach. *J Am Acad Orthop Surg* 2015;23(5):297-306.

    As reported in this article, approximately 26% of elbow dislocations have accompanying fractures. The methods of detecting all components of an injured elbow are reviewed, and the stepwise development and implementation of appropriate surgical tactics for addressing all aspects of the injury are discussed. Level of evidence: V.

59. Ring D, Jupiter JB, Sanders RW, Mast J, Simpson NS: Transolecranon fracture-dislocation of the elbow. *J Orthop Trauma* 1997;11(8):545-550.

60. Gereli A, Nalbantoğlu U, Dikmen G, Seyhan M, Türkmen M: Fracture-dislocations of the proximal ulna. *Acta Orthop Traumatol Turc* 2015;49(3):233-240.

    This article reported on a retrospective analysis of 15 patients with elbow dislocations accompanied by transolecranon fractures. Concomitant fractures of the radial head or trochlear notch were found in all patients. Posterior fracture-dislocations did more poorly, with lower MEPS scores and poorer motion. Level of evidence: IV.

61. Ring D, Jupiter JB: Fracture-dislocation of the elbow. *J Bone Joint Surg Am* 1998;80(4):566-580.

62. Ring D, Jupiter JB, Zilberfarb J: Posterior dislocation of the elbow with fractures of the radial head and coronoid. *J Bone Joint Surg Am* 2002;84-A(4):547-551.

63. Pugh DM, Wild LM, Schemitsch EH, King GJ, McKee MD: Standard surgical protocol to treat elbow dislocations with radial head and coronoid fractures. *J Bone Joint Surg Am* 2004;86-A(6):1122-1130.

64. Papatheodorou LK, Rubright JH, Heim KA, Weiser RW, Sotereanos DG: Terrible triad injuries of the elbow: Does the coronoid always need to be fixed? *Clin Orthop Relat Res* 2014;472(7):2084-2091.

    In this study, 14 patients with Regan and Morrey type I fractures (2 patients) or type II fractures (12 patients) are reviewed. The criteria for determining which patients do not require coronoid repair were defined using a specific intraoperative assessment protocol following radial head repair/replacement and ligament repair. The patients were followed for 24 months and had a mean Disabilities of the Arm, Shoulder and Hand score of 14. 64. Level of evidence: IV.

Chapter 26

Fractures of the Forearm and Distal Radius

Melvin P. Rosenwasser, MD David W. Zeltser, MD

Abstract

The goals of treatment of forearm fractures include re-creation of the anatomic bow of the radial shaft and stability of the forearm "ring" to allow full pronation and supination. Although isolated ulnar shaft fractures often can be treated with splinting, isolated radial shaft fractures and fractures of both bones typically must be managed with rigid internal fixation. Distal radius fractures represent a diverse group of injuries for which proper treatment requires careful consideration of many important variables, including patient age, activity, and expectations; fracture pattern; associated injuries; and bone quality. The technical ability to repair distal radius fractures continues to improve with advancements in implants and surgical techniques, and so awareness of the complications associated with such treatments is expanding. As the focus on patient outcomes after treatment shifts from anatomic metrics toward functional capacity, the understanding of what constitutes successful treatment is being refined. In some demographics, satisfactory functional outcomes may not correspond with radiographic indices.

KEYWORDS: Galeazzi fracture; radial shaft fracture; ulnar shaft fracture; distal radius fracture; volar locked plate

Dr. Rosenwasser or an immediate family member has received royalties from Biomet; is a member of a speakers' bureau or has made paid presentations on behalf of Stryker; has stock or stock options held in CoNexions and Radicle Orthopaedics; and serves as a board member, owner, officer, or committee member of The Foundation for Orthopedic Trauma. Neither Dr. Zeltser nor any immediate family member has received anything of value from or has stock or stock options held in a commercial company or institution related directly or indirectly to the subject of this chapter.

Introduction

Fractures of the distal radius represent the most common upper extremity fracture, yet the understanding of the optimal treatment strategy for different fracture types and patient demographics continues to evolve. Advances in surgical techniques and implant design have improved the orthopaedic surgeon's ability to treat this highly heterogeneous group of injuries. Although less common and limited to a narrow demographic of younger patients, fractures of the forearm must be managed properly to avoid loss of rotation. It is important for the orthopaedic surgeon to be knowledgeable about the diagnosis, management, and outcomes associated with these upper extremity injuries and the current controversies surrounding management of distal radius fractures in older patients.

Forearm Fractures

The evaluation of a patient with a forearm fracture begins with a thorough history and physical examination. A history of trauma, often high energy, should be elicited. Pain, deformity, and swelling are typical. Careful examination of the radial, ulnar, median, posterior interosseous, and anterior interosseous nerves is critical. Examination of the radial and ulnar pulses at the wrist should be performed. A high index of suspicion for forearm compartment syndrome is essential both preoperatively and postoperatively. Forearm compartment fasciotomies are required for the diagnosis of compartment syndrome to avoid irreversible muscle ischemia, muscle fibrosis, and contracture. In obtunded patients, percutaneous compartment pressure measurements can be used to aid in diagnosis. Associated open wounds should be noted. Physical examination and imaging of the wrist and elbow are paramount to avoid missing associated injuries.

Galeazzi Fractures

An isolated radial shaft fracture is uncommon in adults. Because the forearm functions as a ring, an associated injury should be suspected. The concept is similar to pelvic ring injuries, in which a single fracture of a ring structure is unlikely. Traditionally, fractures within 7.5 cm of the radiocarpal joint are more likely to represent a Galeazzi fracture (radial shaft fracture with associated distal radioulnar joint [DRUJ] injury). Galeazzi fractures generally require surgical fixation. After open reduction and internal fixation (ORIF), the DRUJ is examined intraoperatively to determine range of motion (ROM), laxity, and the need for additional treatment.

Examination may reveal a prominent ulnar head in cases of dorsal DRUJ subluxation or dislocation, and DRUJ injury should be suspected. Radiographic evaluation includes AP and lateral views of the forearm, wrist, and elbow. A true lateral view of the wrist, in which the pisiform overlies the volar third of the scaphoid, is required to assess DRUJ alignment. If the diagnosis is uncertain, contralateral radiographs may be obtained. In cases of complex injury patterns, CT may be necessary. Traditional radiographic parameters suggesting disruption of the DRUJ include fracture of the base of the ulnar styloid; widening of the DRUJ on the AP wrist radiograph; dislocation of the ulna relative to the radius on a true lateral wrist radiograph; and more than 5 mm of shortening of the radius relative to the ulna (ulnar positive variance) when compared to the contralateral wrist. In a 2014 retrospective study, 52% of radial shaft fractures with injury radiographs showing ulnar variance >4 mm had an unstable DRUJ after radial shaft fixation.[1]

Nonsurgical management in adults results in poor outcomes and should be reserved for patients who are too ill for surgery or who have limited functional demands. Surgery is indicated for all Galeazzi fractures to restore the structural integrity of the forearm ring. The goal of surgery is anatomic reduction of the radial shaft, especially the radial bow, and restoration of a stable DRUJ. Typically, ORIF is performed through a volar approach with a 3.5-mm dynamic compression plate, although a dorsal approach can be used for more proximal radial shaft fractures. Although intramedullary fixation is an option, it is rarely used. Nailing requires interlocking to avoid malrotation and shortening.

In assessing the DRUJ after radial shaft fixation, it is helpful to compare it with the contralateral normal wrist to recognize the normal degree of translation possible. If the DRUJ is deemed stable after translational stress testing, the extremity is immobilized with a long arm splint or cast in the position of greatest stability (most often supination in the case of dorsal instability of the ulnar head) for 6 weeks. A 2012 retrospective study of 10 patients found that postoperative immobilization in supination for 4 weeks conferred no advantage over immobilization for 2 weeks in neutral.[2] However, if the ulna can be dislocated from the sigmoid notch with the forearm in supination, the DRUJ ligamentous support structures, including triangular fibrocartilage complex (TFCC) attachments, are grossly unstable. There are several ways to maintain reduction of the DRUJ, including the use of two transradioulnar Kirschner wires placed in an extra-articular fashion. Displaced ulnar styloid fractures can be internally fixed; alternatively, the TFCC attachment can be fixed with a suture anchor or transosseous suture to maintain DRUJ alignment. If K-wires are used, two wires lessen the risk of breakage. If the ulnar head cannot be reduced closed, then interposed extensor carpi ulnaris, extensor digitorum communis, or extensor digiti minimi may be the cause. Other structures that can impede closed reduction include a metaphyseal fragment buttonholed through the capsule, the periosteum, or an avulsion styloid fracture fragment from the fovea. After reduction and stabilization, the arm is immobilized in a long arm cast or splint for 4 to 6 weeks. True lateral radiographs should document a reduced DRUJ.

Complications include fracture nonunion, malunion with limited forearm rotation, damage to nerves or vessels, infection, complex regional pain syndrome, and residual DRUJ subluxation with subsequent degenerative changes. When transarticular K-wires are used to maintain reduction of the DRUJ, traversing four cortices may facilitate later removal in the event of wire breakage or bending. Patients with a healed Galeazzi fracture in one study demonstrated weakness in forearm rotation at 2 years, and weakness in supination was correlated with lower functional outcomes.[3]

Ulnar Shaft Fractures

Isolated ulnar shaft fractures, known as nightstick fractures, frequently result from a direct blow to the ulna. Soft-tissue inspection is mandatory to rule out an open injury. Nonsurgical management is appropriate for most ulnar shaft fractures. According to a 2013 systematic review, no form of immobilization is superior, although the best functional results occur with early mobilization.[4] Surgery is indicated for angulation >10° and translation >50%, proximal radioulnar joint or DRUJ instability, or proximal ulnar fractures (**Figure 1**).

The diagnosis of Monteggia fracture-dislocation (ulnar shaft fracture associated with dislocation of the proximal radioulnar joint) is frequently missed. To avoid overlooking this diagnosis, the evaluation of every ulnar shaft fracture must include careful scrutiny of elbow radiographs to ensure that the radiocapitellar joint is properly aligned on all views. If any radiographic view indicates that a projected line through the radial neck does not

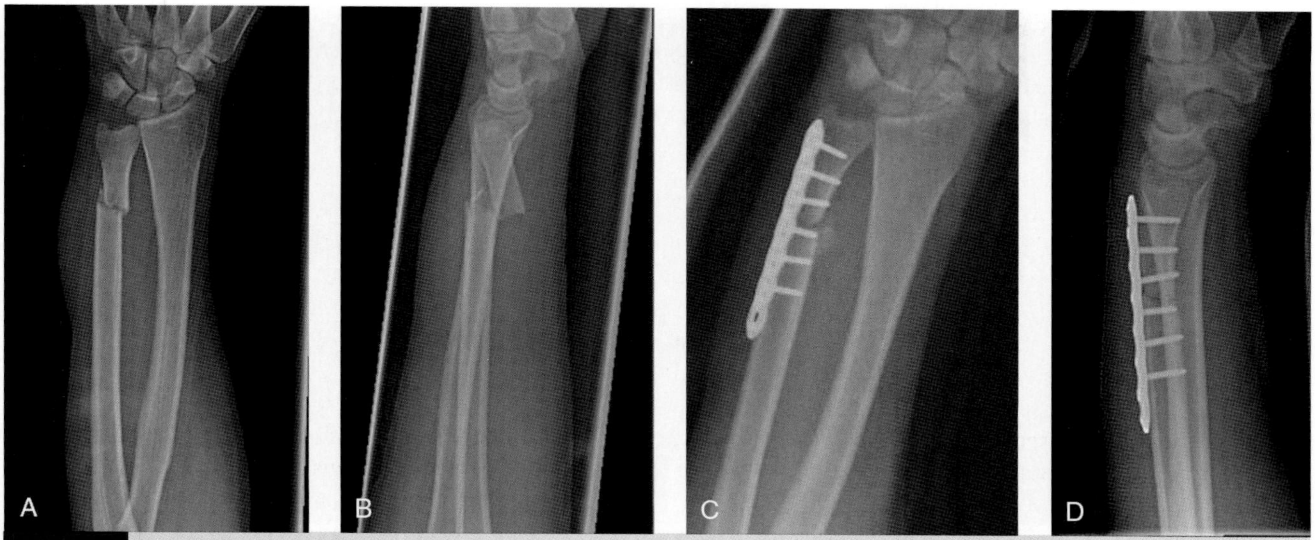

Figure 1 Radiographs of the forearm of a 28-year-old man with an isolated closed distal ulnar shaft fracture. **A**, AP radiograph shows a well-aligned fracture. **B**, Lateral radiograph shows 100% displacement that could not be closed reduced in the emergency department. The patient was lost to follow-up until several weeks later, at which time fracture callus developed and the patient experienced limited forearm rotation. **C**, AP and **D**, Lateral radiographs show open reduction and internal fixation with a 2.7-mm titanium plate; uneventful union was eventually achieved. Photographs courtesy of Robert Strauch, MD.

center on the capitellum, a Monteggia fracture-dislocation should be considered.

Fixation of Forearm Fractures

Fixation of displaced both-bone forearm fractures in adults is mandatory and accomplished with 3.5-mm limited-contact dynamic compression plates and bicortical screws. For very distal or proximal periarticular fractures, additional implants—such as 2.7-mm compression locking plates or precontoured periarticular plates—are helpful in the reassembly of comminuted fractures, especially in patients with osteopenia. To ensure security of the construct until union is achieved, balanced fixation with six cortices on either side of the fracture site is required, with even more screws needed if there is comminution. For longer fracture patterns or segmental fractures, anatomic plates with a built-in physiologic bow of the radius can be used. Alternatively, two orthogonal and overlapped plates can be used; these are preferred to abutting implants to lessen the stress riser effect at the junction.

The use of locking plates for fixation of forearm fractures was compared with standard dynamic compression plating in a retrospective review of 42 diaphyseal forearm fractures. At a mean follow-up of 21 months, no difference was found between groups with regard to time to union or scores on the Disabilities of the Arm, Shoulder and Hand (DASH) questionnaire.[5] This reflects the reality that most diaphyseal fractures have sufficient cortical integrity to provide stable fixation by the use of bicortical screws and standard compression plating and that locking screw fixation, or hybrid fixation with both locking and nonlocking screws, should be reserved for patients with poor bone quality (**Figure 2**).

Intramedullary fixation in adult forearm fractures is reserved for pathologic, segmental, ballistic, and very proximal fractures, and for protection of healed diaphyseal fractures after plate removal (especially in athletes returning to play in a contact sport). Theoretical advantages of intramedullary fixation include reduced exposure and devascularization, decreased rate of refracture after hardware removal, and reduced reports of palpable hardware, especially in subcutaneous locations. A prospective study of 67 patients with fractures of both forearm bones randomly assigned to receive standard ORIF or intramedullary nailing (IMN) found that IMN was associated with decreased surgical time, increased fluoroscopic time, increased risk of nonunion, and a poorer quality of reduction radiographically evident despite equivalent long-term ROM and functional scores.[6] This highlights the difficulty in restoring the anatomic radial bow and maintaining axial length and rotation with an intramedullary device. In short, the radius is not a tibia.

External fixation may be used as temporary stabilization in cases of grossly contaminated open fractures or severe soft-tissue injury and in polytrauma when damage-control principles are used to reduce surgical stressors.

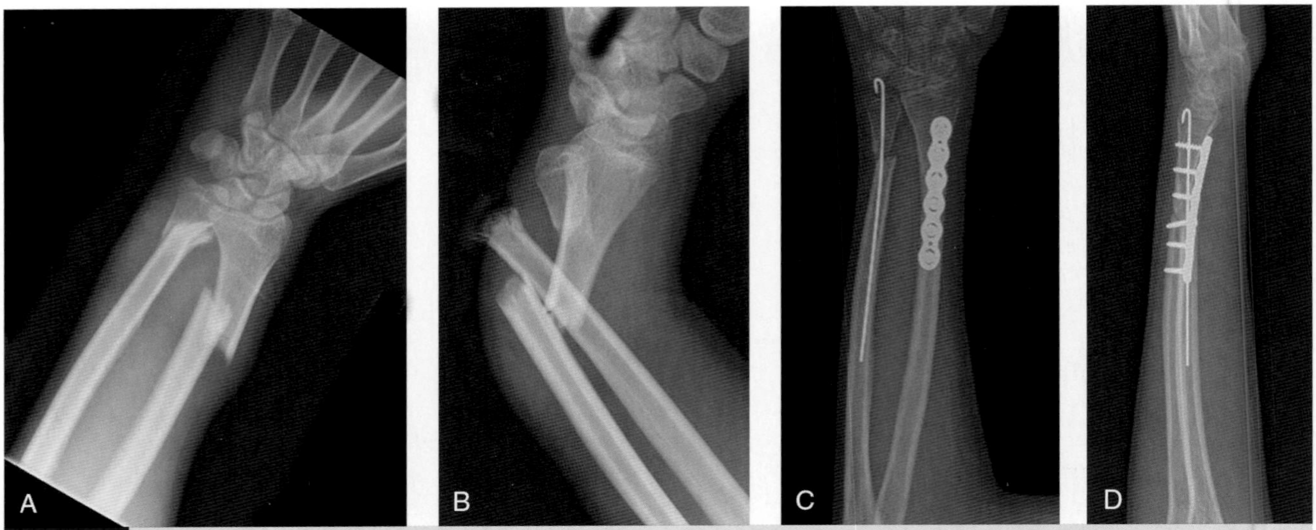

Figure 2 A 16-year-old boy sustained an open left distal both-bone forearm fracture with the proximal fragment of the ulna exposed in the open wound. **A**, AP view. **B**, Oblique view. Treatment was with single-staged open reduction and internal fixation of the radius and ulna through separate incisions. The radial shaft was fixed with a 3.5-mm dynamic compression plate. A 1.6-mm intramedullary Kirschner wire was placed in an antegrade-retrograde fashion across the fracture and supplemented with 0 resorbable cerclage suture. The distal aspect of the wire was left buried. **C**, AP view. **D**, Lateral view.

Outcomes

Healing rates of forearm fractures are typically excellent. A recent retrospective study reported the long-term outcomes of patients across the age spectrum for both-bone forearm fractures.[7] One-half of the patients were skeletally immature and were treated with reduction and immobilization, and the other one-half were skeletally mature and treated with open reduction at the time of injury. At an average of 21 years after surgery, DASH scores correlated more with pain and pain catastrophizing than with objective measures, including ROM and grip strength.[7]

Rehabilitation

Immobilization in an above-elbow splint for 2 weeks allows soft-tissue healing, after which elbow motion can begin immediately. Forearm motion can also be initiated if the DRUJ is stable. In cases of DRUJ instability treated with positioning in supination, DRUJ pinning, or repair of the ulnar styloid or TFCC, above-elbow casting in a position of stability is continued for an additional 4 weeks. Physiotherapy assists with regaining forearm rotation as necessary.

Complications

Nonunion

Nonunion of diaphyseal forearm fractures is rare (<5% with modern techniques).[8] A complex injury pattern, infection, bone defect, or inadequate fixation can result in nonunion. Most nonunions are atrophic and associated with higher energy open injuries, infection, and fracture-dislocations. Treatment of nonunion requires biologic management and eradication of any current infection with serial débridement and, later, reconstitution with bone graft coupled with stable compression plating to restore the radius-ulna relationship with regard to length and shape. The biology of the nonunion site will dictate whether the reconstruction is staged with a temporary antibiotic spacer and a spanning external fixator. After appropriate antibiotic treatment, it may be prudent to obtain a biopsy to ensure a sterile nonunion site before final reconstruction. Bone graft is reserved for atrophic nonunions and compression plating for hypertrophic nonunions.

Malunion

Malunion results when the proper length, alignment, or rotation of the forearm is not restored. Intraoperative imaging can be used to avoid malreduction of the radius. On the AP projection in supination, the bicipital tuberosity should be 180° from (opposite) the radial styloid. Also, the radial shaft has a characteristic apex radial and dorsal bow. Failure to reestablish this anatomic bow will reduce forearm rotation. This can happen when the radial plate is not sufficiently contoured to reconstruct the bow and, when applied, results in straightening of the bow. After fixation of the forearm, rotation must be assessed in the operating room and, if asymmetric, should be corrected. Malunion with a 20° malreduction or straightening magnifies the functional deficit.[9]

Refracture

The rate of refracture after plate removal is between 16% and 26%.[10] Refracture occurred more often when bigger and stiffer plates such as 4.5-mm compression plates were used. Union and remodeling must be confirmed, and a CT scan may be required. After plate removal, all patients should be restricted from participation in contact collision sports for up to 2 months.

Plates are removed most often because of local irritation, usually on the ulna. However, in young patients it may be prudent to remove plates electively; consensus recommends waiting at least 1 year after surgery to do so. A 2014 study suggested waiting until 18 months after initial surgery to minimize the risk of refracture.[10]

Bone Defects

The indications for bone grafting in radial and ulnar shaft fractures are poorly defined or documented in the literature. Despite recommendations for use of autogenous bone graft in forearm fractures with comminution >33% to 50% of the diameter of the shaft, contrarian studies have demonstrated equivalent union rates without grafting.[9]

The Future

The optimal time interval from surgery to hardware removal after fixation of diaphyseal forearm fractures is not clear. The precise role of acute bone grafting has not been established. Future studies may further elucidate the relationship between forearm rotational function and the three- dimensional bony and ligamentous anatomy, with the aim of improving treatment of dysfunction of the forearm ring structure.

Distal Radius Fractures

Since Colles' first description in 1814, the management of distal radius fractures has been one of the most controversial topics in fracture surgery, mainly because of the heterogeneity of fracture patterns and patient presentations, which constitute a broad spectrum of possible injuries. Distal radius fractures occur in a bimodal distribution with peaks for two major demographics: high-energy injuries in young patients and low-energy injuries (fall from standing height) in elderly patients. To provide appropriate and effective care, the treating physician must practice an individualized, patient-specific approach which, to be successful, requires a thorough understanding of the treatment options, their relative merits and disadvantages, and the patient's priorities and expectations.

As the treatment outcomes of distal radius fractures receive more careful scrutiny, treatment goals should be considered. Most would agree that for the young patient, restoration of bony anatomy should be the priority. However, for the elderly patient, mounting evidence suggests that restoring height, tilt, and inclination—the historical radiographic metrics of success—is not necessary or sufficient to achieve pain relief and good function.[11-14]

In an effort to decrease the incidence of fragility fractures of the distal radius through prevention, the focus has been on detection and treatment of osteoporosis. Osteoporosis confers an 8.9 times higher risk of distal radius fracture.[15] Results of a comprehensive osteoporosis program at Kaiser Permanente in Southern California showed that patients who received pharmacologic intervention and patients who were screened for osteoporosis were 48% and 83% less likely, respectively, to sustain a distal radius fracture than patients who did not receive such measures.[15]

In 2007, Medicare spent $170 million on treatment of distal radius fractures in more than 85,000 elderly patients.[16] Seventeen percent of patients were treated with internal fixation. If the current trend toward increasing utilization of internal fixation (using current cost figures) were to reach 50%, Medicare expenditures on distal radius fractures would reach a projected $240 million. As the population ages and the incidence of low-energy distal radius fractures in osteopenic bone increases, health-care payers will require evidence of cost effectiveness of various treatments.[17] The net result could be a profound effect on treatment patterns. In the United Kingdom, a recent large randomized trial conducted by the National Health Service concluded that percutaneous pinning is significantly more cost effective than volar plating and is equally efficacious.[17]

Unfortunately, high-level evidence is lacking. This fact was emphasized by the American Academy of Orthopaedic Surgeons (AAOS) clinical practice guidelines for management of distal radius fractures, published in 2009. Of 29 recommendations, only 5 carried a "moderate" strength of recommendation. All others were weak, inconclusive, or consensus expert opinion statements. Although the AAOS suggested surgery for fractures with postreduction "radial shortening >3 mm, dorsal tilt >10 degrees, or intra-articular displacement or step-off >2 mm," the committee was "unable to recommend for or against operative treatment for patients over age 55."[18] Without conclusive evidence of the superiority of one treatment method over another, an individualized, thoughtful patient-focused and shared decision-making approach will help to inform selection of the right treatment.

Evaluation

All patients with a distal radius fracture must undergo a careful clinical evaluation. The mechanism of injury (high or low energy) should be appreciated. An assessment of the patient's medical comorbidities, functional requirements, activity level, hand dominance, and expectations is essential for treatment planning. A detailed physical examination includes the joints above and below the injury. Particular attention must be paid to nerve function (especially the median nerve), vascular status, swelling, and skin condition.

The initial treatment should include closed reduction with local anesthesia (hematoma block), procedural sedation, or both. Ligamentotaxis—hanging the limb from finger traps for 15 to 20 minutes—can be helpful. For dorsally displaced fractures, an effective manual reduction maneuver includes axial traction, anterior translation, pronation of the hand relative to the forearm, and ulnar deviation. Early reduction of deformity relieves pressure on soft tissues, especially nerves and skin (**Figure 3**). After closed reduction, the wrist should be immobilized in a splint or split cast. Deterioration in median nerve function after closed reduction requires urgent decompression.

High-quality radiographs in AP, lateral, and oblique projections should be obtained before and after reduction. In a correctly aligned lateral view, the pisiform overlies the volar one-third of the scaphoid. Contralateral wrist radiographs may be helpful to determine a patient's normal anatomy. Special views have become widely used, especially the tilted lateral view, which eliminates the overlap of the radial styloid and enhances the view of the articular facets. Commonly measured radiographic indices include radial height and inclination, volar tilt, and articular displacement (**Table 1**). Another important radiographic parameter is sagittal alignment. Carpal translation is seen on the lateral radiograph when the capitolunate axis has translated volar or dorsal to the radial shaft axis, such as in volar or dorsal Barton fractures. This denotes fracture instability and is correlated with poor outcomes if not corrected. Radiographs should be carefully assessed for associated injuries such as intercarpal ligamentous injury with scapholunate or lunotriquetral instability patterns, dorsal intercalated segment instability, volar intercalated segment instability, and carpal diastasis or incongruence.

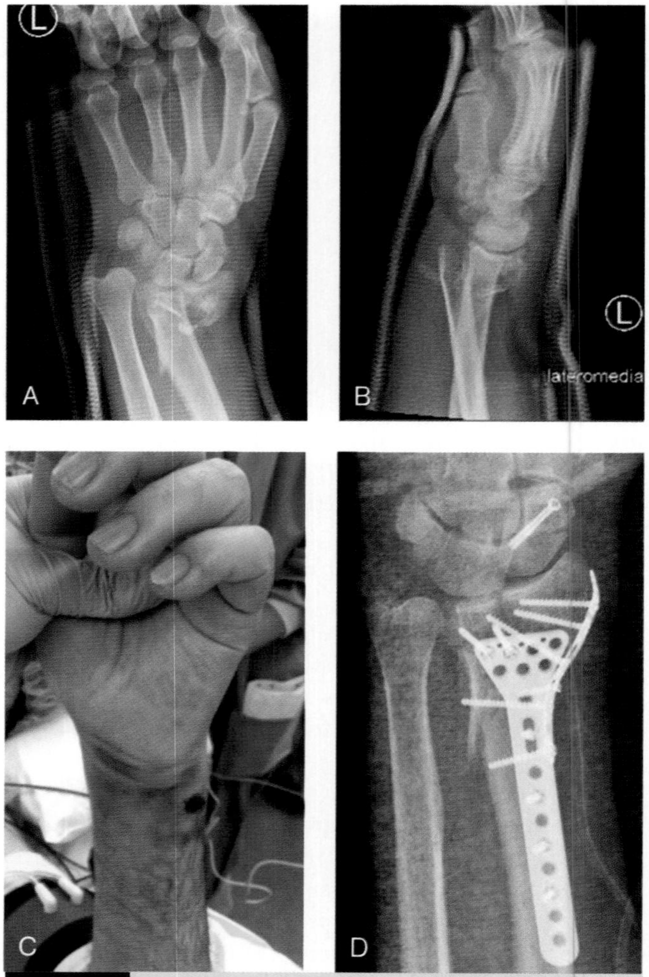

Figure 3 Radiographs of the left wrist of a 74-year-old man show significant fracture comminution and displacement. **A**, AP view. **B**, Lateral view. Surgical treatment was delayed for 5 days, at which point he developed symptoms of median nerve dysfunction. Additionally, prolonged fracture displacement resulted in necrosis of skin overlying the ulnar head. **C,** Clinical photograph of the ulnar aspect of the wrist immediately prior to surgery, demonstrating skin necrosis over displaced ulnar head. **D,** Postoperative AP radiograph shows distal radius fixation with both a volar locking plate and radial column plate. Scaphoid fixation was achieved with a cannulated screw. A carpal tunnel release was performed simultaneously. Images courtesy of R. Kumar Kadiyala, MD.

Coronal translation is another radiographic parameter recently described.[19,20] Residual radial translation of the distal radius (or ulnar translation of the radial shaft) has been associated with DRUJ instability. The anatomic explanation is related to the distal interosseous membrane (DIOM), which connects the ulna to the dorsal rim of the sigmoid notch. Failure to correct ulnar translation of the

Table 1

Classic Radiographic Parameters for Normal Distal Radius Anatomy and Acceptable Values After Closed Reduction or Surgical Intervention[a]

Characteristic	Measurement	Normal	Acceptable Postreduction Value	
			Literature	Author's Opinion[b]
Volar tilt	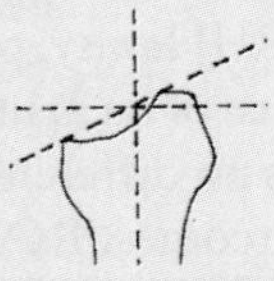	11°	0°-15° dorsal	10° dorsal tilt
Ulnar variance[c]	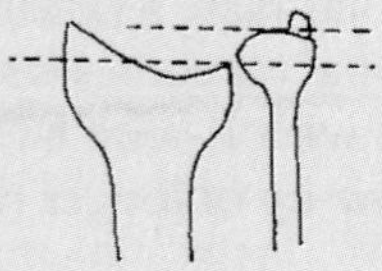	Equal to other side or ± 2 mm	2-4 mm shortening	3 mm shortening
Radial inclination	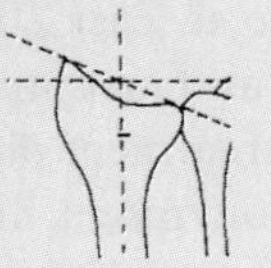	22°	10°-17°	15°
Articular displacement	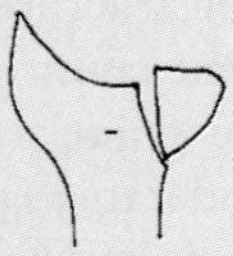	Congruous	1-2 mm step or gap	2-mm step 1-mm gap[d]

[a]The senior author's preferences are presented in bold. The goal of surgical intervention is anatomic restoration of the distal end of the radius. The acceptable postreduction values vary widely by report and opinion and are also related to the functional demands of the individual patient. This is noted in recent literature that shows increased tolerance to malunions in elderly patients.
[b]Predicting fracture stability is more important than minding any specific parameters, in the authors' belief. If the fracture is unstable, no cast will maintain reduction.
[c]Lunate facet to ulnar head, as compared with the contralateral side.
[d]Although preventing point contact is important, the authors believe that containing the lunate is paramount for achieving a good outcome. As such, they accept only 1 mm of gap.

radial shaft may unload and relax the DIOM, which may contribute to DRUJ instability in the setting of a concomitant ulnar-sided soft-tissue injury.[19] This parameter can be quantified on the PA wrist radiograph. Two lines are drawn: one along the transverse axis of the lunate, the other along the ulnar cortex of the radial shaft. The percentage of lunate sitting radial to the point of intersection correlates with radial translation of the distal radius.[20] A cadaver model demonstrated increased DRUJ instability in distal radius osteotomies repaired with a residual 2 mm of ulnar translation if a distinct dorsal oblique bundle (DOB) of the DIOM was present.[21]

CT may be useful in pattern recognition of complex intra-articular distal radius fractures as well as in the assessment of displacement. This is especially true with regard to fragment rotation at the sigmoid notch and the DRUJ. CT is more helpful after a closed reduction is obtained. Three-dimensional CT reconstructions have increased sensitivity and specificity for identifying fracture patterns and appreciating injury severity.[22] Although CT has been shown to alter treatment plans and can be useful for preoperative planning, it has not been shown to affect outcome. Thus, CT should be obtained when there is concern about the adequacy of closed reduction.

Associated Injuries

Clinical and anatomic studies have shown that injuries to adjacent soft-tissue structures occur in approximately one-half of distal radius fractures and in almost all intra-articular fractures. The most common causes of persistent symptoms include injuries to the ulnocarpal ligaments or the TFCC. Concomitant scapholunate

Section 3: Upper Extremity

in young patients require surgery to restore stable radiocarpal and distal radioulnar joints. The most controversial clinical scenario is whether or not to operate on low-energy fractures in elderly patients. Increasing evidence indicates that this population has equivalent functional outcomes with cast treatment, even with malunion, compared with operative treatment and anatomic reduction despite residual cosmetic deformity at the wrist. Thus, restoration of radiographic parameters (tilt, inclination, and height) do not translate into improvement in functional outcome in this demographic.[11,12,30] Although acceptable displacements for this population have not yet been defined, shortening of >5 mm weakens the wrist and substantially limits rotation. The treating surgeon must personalize the care of each patient and not rely on any specific measurements in offering treatment options.

Closed Treatment

Studies comparing below- and above-elbow immobilization after closed reduction have shown equivalent maintenance of reduction. Two clinical studies showed equivalent outcomes for elderly patients who were treated with cast immobilization versus surgery.[12,13] Researchers randomly assigned 73 patients age 65 years or older who presented with unstable fractures (AO type A or C) to treatment with cast immobilization or surgery involving VLP. Although functional scores (DASH and Patient-Rated Wrist Evaluation) favored surgery at 3 months, there was no difference between groups at 6 and 12 months. Surgically treated patients had better grip strength, better radiographic outcomes, and higher complication rates. The conclusion of this large, level I study was that radiographic outcome (quality and maintenance of reduction) did not correlate with functional outcome in patients age 65 years or older.[12] In a retrospective case-control study of patients older than 65 years, another research group compared surgically treated patients with those treated nonsurgically and found equivalent functional outcomes (DASH scores) and complication rates at 12 months despite higher grip strength in surgically treated patients.[13]

Closed Reduction With Percutaneous Pinning

The indications for closed reduction and percutaneous pinning (CRPP) are uncertain, but the results of case series are generally favorable. Biomechanical testing has shown that the greatest rigidity can be achieved with cross-pinning of at least three 0.062 K-wires, two from the radial styloid and one from the dorsal ulnar corner of the distal radius. Researchers from the United Kingdom recently reported a large multicenter randomized trial of CRPP versus ORIF for extra-articular and simple intra-articular (AO/OTA types A and C1) distal radius fractures.[17] They found no significant difference in functional outcomes or complication rates between groups at 1 year. Their conclusion was that CRPP is equally efficacious as and much cheaper than VLP, thereby making it significantly more cost effective and the preferred treatment in the United Kingdom.[17] Other randomized trials of CRPP compared with internal fixation have demonstrated similar functional outcomes when compared with VLP at 1 year,[30,31] although at earlier (3- and 6-month) time points, there is a tendency for better function, probably due to earlier rehabilitation, in patients who underwent plating.[32,33] However, when compared to cast immobilization alone, CRPP achieved equivalent functional outcomes despite worse radiographic parameters in elderly patients with extra-articular fractures.[14]

External Fixation

Spanning of the wrist (bridging external fixation) is the traditional method of providing and maintaining a gentle distraction force across the radiocarpal joint through ligamentotaxis. This force can counteract the forces of compression that accompany gripping exercises, but will in most instances be inadequate to reduce and maintain depressed articular segments without adjunctive K-wire fixation. The fact that the wrist capsule is equally tensioned by the bridging frame also precludes restoration of the anatomic volar tilt of 10° even with adjunctive intrafocal pinning. Neutral tilt, however, is satisfactory, and that is why many studies have demonstrated equivalent results compared to plating when reductions are equivalent.[34] In a 2014 retrospective study of 35 patients with both intra- and extra-articular distal radius fractures treated with bridging external fixation, fracture reduction at final follow-up was deemed acceptable in 83% despite a rate of secondary displacement of 48.5%, primarily involving volar tilt.[35]

In a meta-analysis of 12 studies comparing bridging external fixation with internal fixation, investigators found that ORIF provided overall better functional outcomes, supination, and volar tilt.[36] Interestingly, patients treated with external fixation had better grip strength and wrist flexion. In a similar meta-analysis of 10 studies, researchers found lower DASH scores, higher infection rates, and poor maintenance of radial length in patients treated with external fixation compared with those who underwent ORIF.[37]

Nonbridging external fixation is a powerful but seldom-used technique for controlling distal radius fracture fragments and allowing wrist motion. Even intra-articular fractures can be treated in this manner if the fragments are big enough to accommodate 3-mm threaded half-pins. These joysticks can be manipulated to restore volar tilt,

Table 3

Surgical Indications According to AO/ASIF Fracture Type[a]

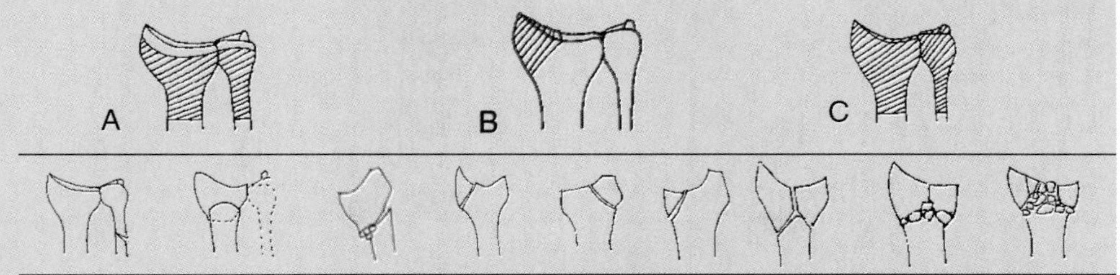

Intervention	A1	A2	A3	B1	B2	B3	C1	C2	C3
Closed Reduction	-	+	+	+/–	+/–	+/–	+	+	+
Closed Reduction Percutaneous Pinning (CRPP)	-	+	+	+	+/–	-	+	+	+
Bridging External Fixation	-	+/–	+/–	-	-	-	+/–	-	-
Bridging External Fixation with CRPP	-	+	+	-	-	-	+	+	+
Bridging External Fixation with Volar Locked Plating	-	+	+	-	-	-	+	+	+
Nonbridging External Fixation	-	++	++	-	-	-	+	+/–	-
Standard Volar Plating	-	+	+	-	-	++	+	+/–	-
Volar Locked Plating	-	+	+	-	-	+	+	+	+
Dorsal Plating	-	+	+	-	++	-	+	+/–	+/–
Radial Column Plating	-	+	+	++	-	-	+	+/–	+/–
Fragment-Specific Fixation	-	+	+	+	+	+	+	+	+
Intramedullary Nailing	-	+	+	-	-	-	+	-	-
Arthroscopy	-	-	-	-	+	+	+	+	+

[a]This classification system was chosen because it is the most commonly reported in the literature and is the most reproducible. Note that there is general agreement on treatment of type B fractures. Fractures of types A2, A3, and C1 are amenable to most treatment options. This chart will change, as many more iterations with the evolution of care are anticipated.

but care must be taken to avoid overtranslation of the articular fragment if the volar cortex is unstable. This can be prevented by placing an intramedullary K-wire to block palmar translation. Both external fixation techniques may use adjunctive fixation, joystick K-wires, and metaphyseal void filling bone grafts or substitutes (**Table 3**).

As a modification of bridging external fixation, a dynamic external fixator both spans the wrist joint and allows wrist motion. In a randomized trial of dynamic versus static external fixation of both intra-articular and extra-articular fractures, dynamic external fixation maintained better length at the expense of more pin-tract infections. Function and volar tilt were equivalent at final follow-up.[38] In general, careful patient selection is critical to avoid complications with any technique.

Internal Fixation

In the past decade, many clinical reports have extolled the virtues and efficacy of VLP and variable-axis locking screws. Clearly, the ability to confidently place screws in a buttressing plate over severely osteoporotic bone has revolutionized the care of distal radius fractures. The concept of axial-stable, fixed-angle implants with screws functioning as a raft to support the articular surface has been affirmed in both the biomechanical and the clinical domains. Enthusiasm for the technique has spawned commercial development of dozens of designs with various precontours, bone fit, and screw trajectories.

Although VLP has been shown to be biomechanically stable, the surgeon must be prepared to apply additional implants through various approaches in certain fracture

Table 4

Summary of Recent Level 1 Evidence Comparing Different Types of Fixation

Comparison	N	F/u (mo.)	Outcome Measures	Results
Cast versus VLP[a] (Arora et al 2011[11])	73	52	ROM, VAS, DASH, PRWE, str, rad	No differences
Cast versus CRPP (Wong et al 2010[14])	60	52	Mayo, rad	Rad better for CRPP; no difference in function
Dynamic versus Static Ex Fix (Hove et al 2010[38])	70	52	DASH, VAS, rad	Rad better for Dynamic Ex Fix; no difference in function
Ex Fix versus VLP[a] versus RCP (Wei et al 2009[34])	46	52	DASH, str, rad	Str better for VLP; rad better for RCP; no difference in function or str
Ex Fix versus VLP[a] (Wilcke et al 2011[42])	63	52	DASH, PRWE	No difference in function
Ex Fix versus VLP (Jeudy 2012)[44]	75	26	PRWE, rad, str	Str better for VLP; no difference in function or rad
Ex Fix versus VLP (Williksen et al 2015[40])	104	260	*Quick*DASH, Mayo, VAS, str, rad, ROM	VLP better supination; no difference in *Quick*DASH; 21% plates removed due to complications
Ex Fix versus VLP (Shukla 2014)[45]	110	52	G+O, ROM, str, VAS	Ex Fix better G+O, ROM, str; no difference in VAS
Ex Fix versus VLP[a] (Roh et al 2015[43])	74	52	MHQ, ROM, str, rad	VLP better ulnar variance; no differences in MHQ, ROM, rad
IMN versus VLP (Gradl et al 2014[39])	152	104	G+W, Castaing, ROM, VAS, rad	No differences
CRPP versus VLP[a] (Rozental et al 2009[31])	45	52	DASH, ROM	No differences
CRPP versus VLP[a] (Marcheix et al 2010[32])	103	26	DASH, Herzberg, rad	Function better for VLP
CRPP versus ORIF[b] (Grewal et al 2011[41])	53	52	DASH, PRWE, ROM, rad	No differences
CRPP versus VLP[a] (McFadyen et al 2011[33])	56	26	DASH, G+W, rad	DASH, G+W, rad better for VLP
CRPP versus VLP[a] (Karantana et al 2013[30])	130	52	*Quick*DASH, PEM, EQ-5D, rad, str	VLP better rad, str; no differences in function
CRPP versus VLP (Costa et al 2015[17])	461	52	PRWE, DASH	No differences; reported only functional outcomes
IMN versus VLP (Plate 2015)[46]	60	104	*Quick*DASH, MHQ, rad, narcotic usage	No difference functional outcome at 2 yr; IMN group used fewer narcotics

CRPP = closed reduction and percutaneous pinning; DASH = Disabilities of the Arm, Shoulder and Hand survey; EQ-5D = EuroQol-5D;Ex Fix = External Fixation; G+O = Green and O'Brien scoring system; G+W = Gartland and Werley point system; IMN = intramedullary nailing; Mayo = Mayo Wrist Score; MHQ = Michigan Hand Questionnaire; ORIF = open reduction and internal fixation (volar or dorsal plating); PEM = Patient Evaluation Measure; PRWE = Patient-Rated Wrist Evaluation; rad = radiographic parameters; RCP = radial column plating; ROM = range of motion; str = strength measurements; VAS = Visual Analog Pain Score; VLP = volar locked plating.

[a] These studies showed some benefit for this treatment at 3 or 6 months but showed no benefit at longer time points, or did not include longer time points.

[b] Either volar or dorsal plate, by surgeon preference.

patterns and clinical scenarios. Comparative level I evidence[11,14,17,30-34,38-46] is presented in **Table 4**.

As the use of VLPs has become widespread, the accompanying common technical errors and associated complications have become well known. Recent reports of delayed flexor tendon rupture range from 0.5%[47] to 2.8%.[48] Delayed extensor tendon rupture has been reported in 1.7% to 8.6% of VLP fixation, compared with

1.3% to 4.0% in dorsal plate fixation.[49,50] The etiology of this particular complication may include plate design and metallurgy, residual malunion, and screw penetration from inaccurate measurement

To adequately support the distal radius articular surface, the temptation is to maximize subchondral screw length. However, any prominence of screw tips beyond the dorsal cortex places the extensor tendons at risk. Thus, accurate measurement of screw lengths is of utmost importance. Commonly, the appropriateness of screw lengths is verified radiographically. However, owing to the irregular contour of the dorsal cortex, the lateral projection can provide inaccurate information. The Lister tubercle projects more dorsal than the rest of the distal radius. Thus, a screw that is too long can appear within bone if it is shadowed by the Lister tubercle. Some authors have advocated alternative radiographic views to judge screw length, including the dorsal horizon view, which requires wrist flexion to project a view tangential to the dorsal cortex.[51] Investigators studied axial MRI images to determine a surrogate marker for accurate screw length and found that the depth of the distal radius at the Lister tubercle is, on average, 116% of the lunate depth (as measured on a lateral radiograph). They suggested using the lunate depth as an estimate of the longest subchondral screw.[52]

Another avoidable technical error is intra-articular screw placement. To provide support to the joint surface, screws may need to be placed within 1 to 2 mm of the subchondral surface without penetrating the joint. This task can be challenging when using plates with fixed-angle screw trajectories, as screw position will be dictated by plate position. Articular facet malreduction may complicate accurate placement as well. Additional radiographic views should be used to evaluate joint-surface penetration. Lateral tilt views (15° to 23°) provide a view tangential to the articular surface by adjusting for radial inclination. The advent of variable-axis locking screws has allowed the surgeon to adjust the trajectory of locking screws within a defined cone. Excellent outcomes have been reported with variable-axis technology, although the surgeon should be aware of potential complications, such as failure of the locking mechanism or screw head prominence if the screw is angled beyond the maximum allowable for that system.

Traditionally, the surgical approach for volar plating of the distal radius involves a modified Henry or flexor carpi radialis sheath-splitting approach that exploits the interval between the radial artery and the flexor carpi radialis tendon. However, when the fracture pattern demands reduction and fixation of a volar ulnar facet fragment, an alternative approach can be used to improve exposure. By biasing the skin incision more midline, the interval between the digital flexors and ulnar neurovascular bundle can be developed. Retracting the carpal tunnel contents radially provides excellent visualization of the lunate facet fragment and theoretically minimizes traction on the median nerve. Although separate incisions can be used, the approach is extensile with an open carpal tunnel release (**Figure 4**).

The complication of flexor tendon rupture after VLP of distal radius fractures deserves attention. Authors of a 2013 meta-analysis found that flexor tendon rupture was diagnosed at a median of 9 months after plate fixation (interquartile range of 6 to 26 months), although ruptures as early as 3 months and as late as 10 years have been reported[53] (**Figures 5** and **6**). Fifty-seven percent of cases involved the flexor pollicis longus (FPL) muscle, and 15% involved the flexor digitorum profundus muscle to the index finger. Although the rate of flexor tendon rupture is only 2% to 4%, avoiding the need for flexor tendon reconstruction is desirable. The current understanding of the etiology of tendon rupture is incomplete. However, plate and screw-head prominence at the watershed line, discussed in more detail in the next paragraphs, is thought to be a major contributing factor over which the surgeon has control. Hardware prominence occurs when the plate is placed too distal, fracture reduction is lost or never obtained, or screws are not fully seated.

The Soong et al system was developed for grading plate prominence by noting the degree of extension of hardware volar to a line drawn tangential to the most volar extension of the volar rim and parallel to the volar cortex of the radial shaft on a true lateral radiograph of the wrist.[48] Plates that do not extend volar to this line are grade 0, plates volar to the line are grade 1, and those on or distal to the volar rim are grade 2. In a series of 73 patients, the prevalence of flexor tendon ruptures was 4%. Plate prominence was grade 2 in two of three ruptures and in 63% of all patients.[48]

Investigators in a case-control study compared volar plate position between cases of flexor tendon rupture and matched control participants without rupture. A higher Soong grade was associated with rupture. Seventy-five percent of ruptures were classified as grade 2. The authors also noted that plates >2 mm beyond the volar critical line or within 3 mm of the volar rim were risk factors for tendon rupture. All ruptures occurred later than 6 months after surgery.[54]

A surgical anatomic landmark for distal plate position is the so-called watershed line. In a 2012 cadaver study, its anatomy was elucidated. One salient feature described was that the ulnar one-half of the watershed line is composed of two separate transverse bony ridges.

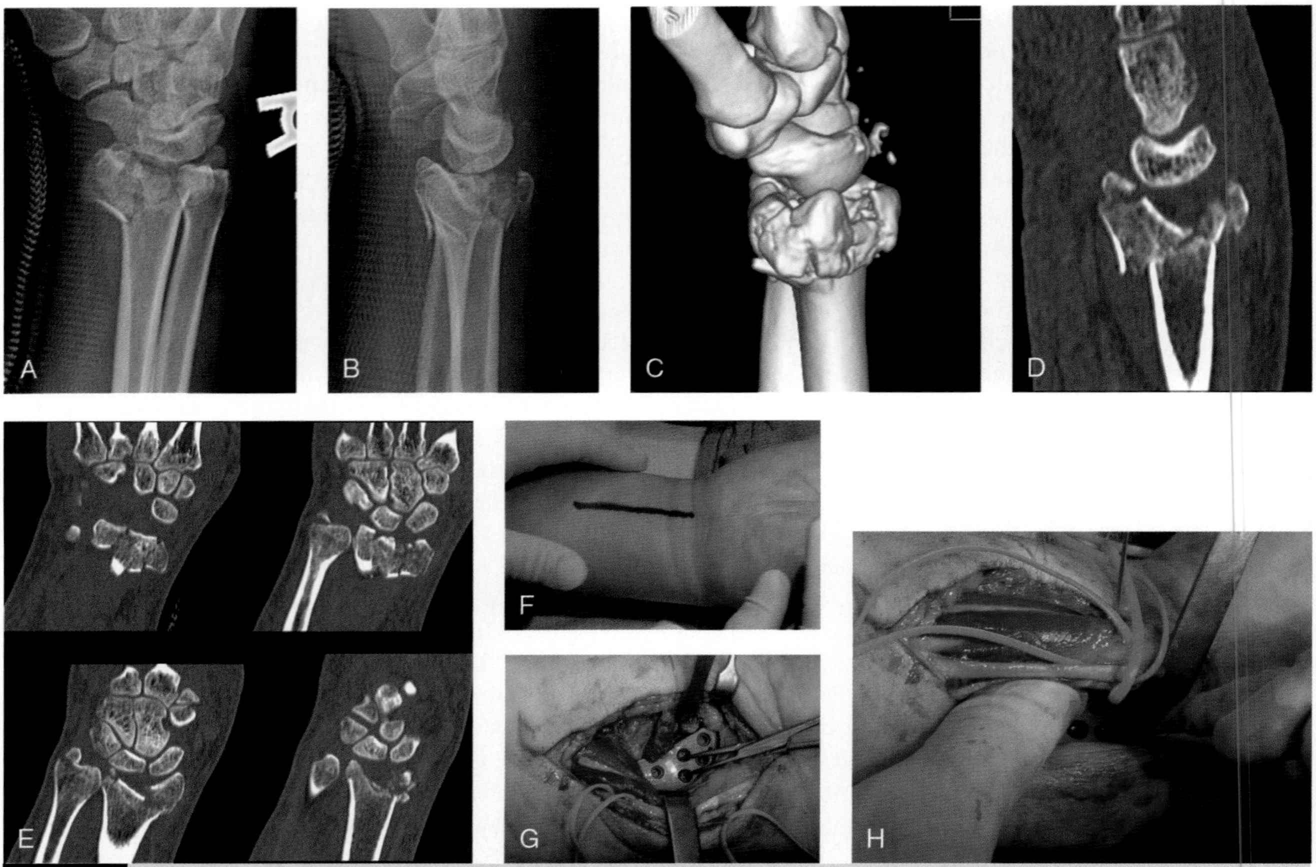

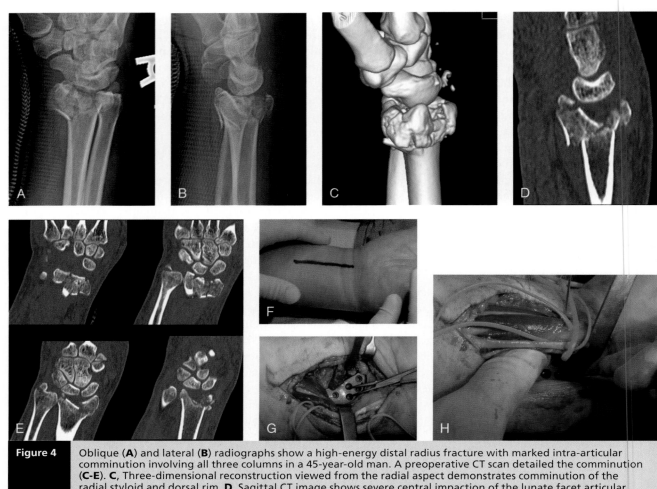

Figure 4 Oblique (**A**) and lateral (**B**) radiographs show a high-energy distal radius fracture with marked intra-articular comminution involving all three columns in a 45-year-old man. A preoperative CT scan detailed the comminution (**C-E**). **C**, Three-dimensional reconstruction viewed from the radial aspect demonstrates comminution of the radial styloid and dorsal rim. **D**, Sagittal CT image shows severe central impaction of the lunate facet articular surface with widening of the anteroposterior distance. **E**, Series of coronal CT images shows marked articular comminution. Top right image shows dorsal ulnar facet fragment whereas bottom left image shows central impaction of the lunate facet. To reduce and fix the fracture fragments, three approaches were required: a volar midline approach by using windows radial and ulnar to the carpal tunnel contents (**F-H**), a midaxial radial column approach, and a dorsal approach. **F**, Intraoperative photograph showing planned incision. The hand is to the right. Note the incision is more midline than the incision used for a standard flexor carpi radialis approach. **G**, Intraoperative photograph shows positioning of the volar plate while the carpal tunnel contents are retracted ulnarly (bottom of picture). The hand is to the right. A red vessel loop is protecting the median nerve. **H**, Intraoperative photograph demonstrates exploitation of the ulnar window by retracting the carpal tunnel contents radially. The surgeon's gloved finger is in the interval between the digital flexor tendons and ulnar neurovascular bundle. Cancellous allograft bone chips were used to support depressed and impacted fragments dorsally.

The authors recommended plate placement proximal to the more proximal ridge.[55] Another study investigated the relationship between several commercially available volar plates and the FPL tendon, which crosses the midpoint (radial to ulnar) of the distal radius. Every plate design used in their study resulted in increased pressure in the path in which the FPL would glide over the distal edge of the plate. It was concluded that future plate designs with lower profiles at the intercarpal sulcus could minimize the risk of FPL rupture.[56]

Plating the dorsal distal radius is the more traditional approach to open treatment, because the comminution and shortening in common dorsally displaced fractures occurs on the dorsal surface. Furthermore, a dorsal approach lends itself to filling a metaphyseal void with bone graft or substitute. However, enthusiasm for dorsal plating waned as a result of extensor tendon complications, including irritation and rupture, which resulted in high rates of hardware removal. More recently, newer designs with better contours and less reactive metals have reduced the rate of tendon rupture.

Specific fracture patterns may require a dorsal

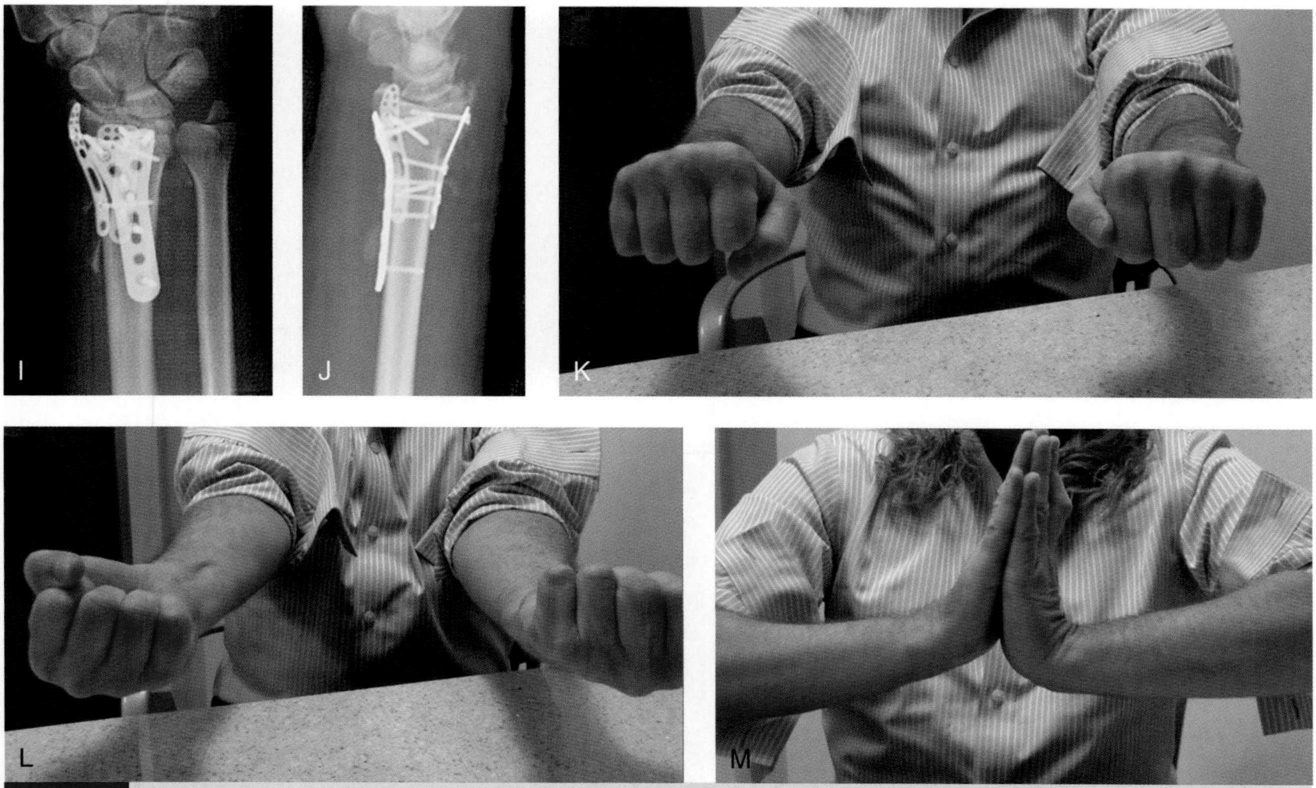

Figure 4 (*Continued*) Postoperative AP (**I**) and lateral (**J**) radiographs show final internal fixation including volar and dorsal distal radius plates and a radial column plate. Overall radiographic parameters have been restored. The patient went on to achieve union with excellent range of motion at his 6-month follow-up visit. **K** through **M**, Clinical photographs show excellent wrist and forearm range of motion.

approach, such as the dorsal die-punch fracture with an intact volar cortex. Also, a dorsal approach may be necessary to reduce and stabilize the dorsal ulnar facet fragment, which cannot be held with screws through a volar plate, owing to poor bone quality (**Figure 7**). It may also be useful when treating a radial styloid fracture associated with a perilunate instability pattern requiring ligament repair.

Other Fixation Techniques

Fragment-specific fixation, intramedullary nailing, and dorsal bridge plating are other treatment methods with specific indications. Nailing is useful for the less comminuted AO/ASIF type A and C1 fractures. In a prospective study of 151 extra-articular (AO/ASIF type A) fractures randomly assigned to either intramedullary nail fixation or volar plate fixation, no significant difference was found between groups in terms of functional scores (Gartland-Werley and Castaing), ROM, pain, radiographic parameters of volar tilt and ulnar variance, and complications at 2-year follow-up.[39] Transient neuritis of the superficial branch of the radial nerve was seen in 11% of patients in a 2015 systematic review.[57]

In some complex fracture patterns, traditional volar and dorsal plates may not provide adequate fixation of small articular facet fragments or periarticular shearing fractures. In these situations, fragment-specific fixation can be used. These smaller plates are placed through more limited approaches with less dissection and require meticulous attention to detail. Achieving adequate fixation of the volar ulnar fragment deserves special attention. Researchers identified fracture characteristics that predicted loss of reduction after fixation of 53 volar shearing fractures (AO B3) with a VLP. Those fractures with a separate volar ulnar fragment, <15 mm of lunate facet available for fixation, or initial lunate subsidence >5 mm were at risk of fixation failure. The authors recommended supplemental fragment-specific fixation for these fracture patterns[58] (**Table 4**).

Dorsal bridge plating can be considered an internal external fixator. The wrist-spanning plate is passed beneath the second dorsal compartment tendons and fixed to the radial shaft and second or third metacarpal shaft. The main indications include severe metaphyseal

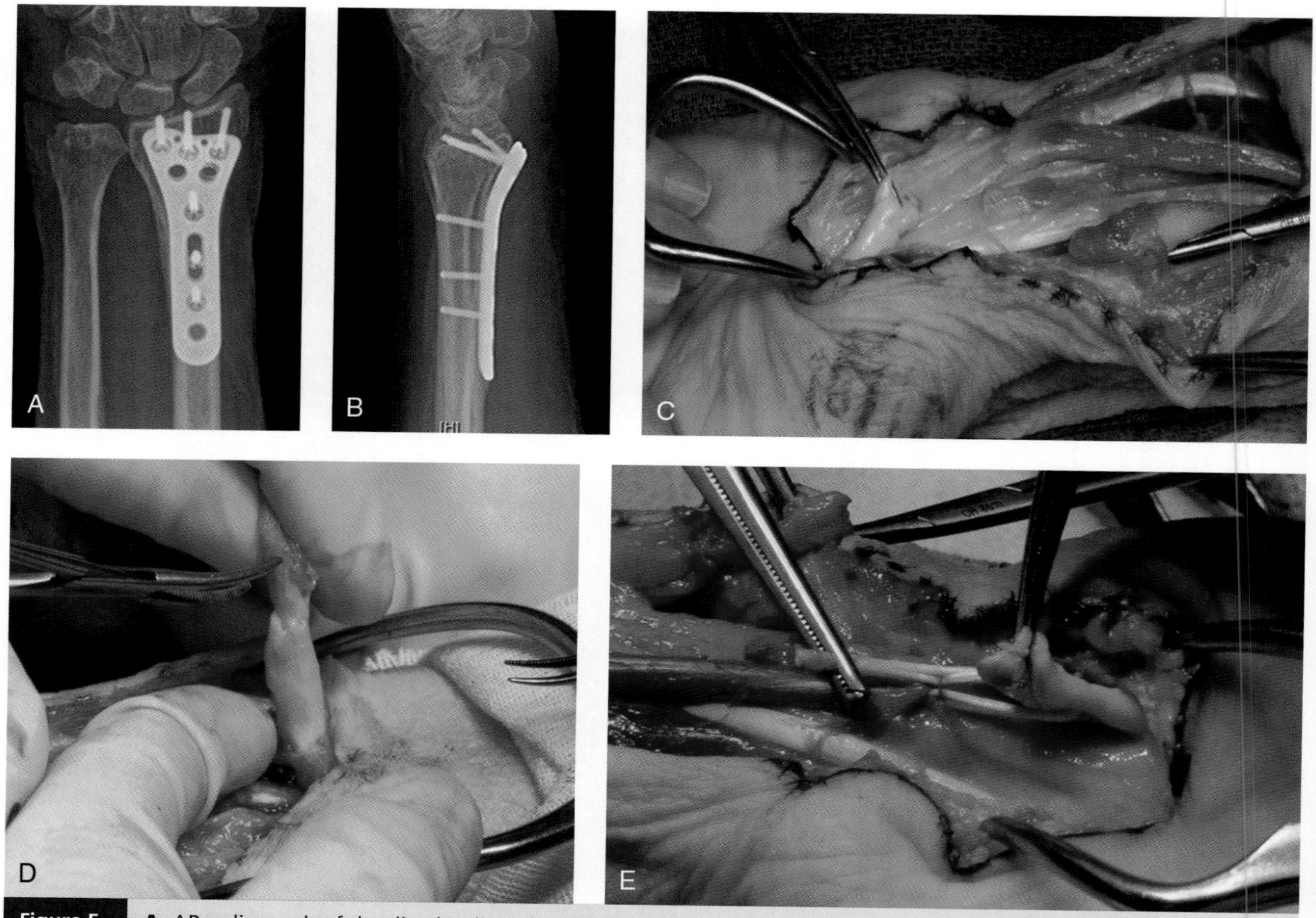

Figure 5 **A,** AP radiograph of the distal radius of an 84-year-old woman with a low-energy fracture treated with volar locked plating. The plate position is Soong grade 2 as seen on the lateral view (**B**). More than 6 years after that surgery, the patient lost the ability to flex her thumb interphalangeal joint, consistent with atraumatic flexor pollicis longus tendon rupture. The plate was removed, and the flexor pollicis longus tendon was reconstructed with a tendon transfer of the flexor digitorum superficialis tendon to the small finger using an intratendinous weave (**C-E**). **C,** Intraoperative photograph shows volar approach to the carpal tunnel contents. The hand is to the left. The clamp to the left is holding the distal stump of the flexor pollicis longus tendon. **D,** Intraoperative photograph of the proximal stump of the ruptured flexor pollicis longus tendon. Evaluation revealed the tendon to be of poor quality. **E,** Intraoperative photograph of the transferred flexor digitorum superficialis tendon. Hand is now to the right. Kocher clamp is on the flexor digitorum superficialis tendon (left) and curved clamp (right) is holding the flexor pollicis longus stump.

comminution due to high energy or osteoporosis as well as polytrauma, because dorsal bridge plating can allow earlier weight-bearing with crutches. Supplemental percutaneous fixation or volar plating can be used to reduce and fix articular comminution. The dorsal bridge plate is removed after approximately 3 months.

The Role of Arthroscopy

Wrist arthroscopy has become an important tool for the diagnosis and treatment of intra-articular pathology, both bony and ligamentous. The arthroscope can be used safely and effectively to directly visualize joint surfaces for articular cartilage injuries as well as associated intercarpal ligament tears and ulnocarpal injuries to the TFCC. Relying on fluoroscopy, which has a resolution of only 2 mm, to confirm adequate articular reduction can be difficult in certain fracture patterns. Fractures such as dorsal die-punch, radial styloid, and chauffeur can be well visualized and the reductions finely tuned with joystick K-wires or elevators (**Figure 8**). As most fractures are approached volarly (where a direct articular read is not possible, owing to the volar radiocarpal ligaments), adjunctive arthroscopy to assist with reduction or confirm the reduction is quite useful.

The natural history of unrepaired complete TFCC tears after distal radius fractures has been reported. At

13 to 15 years after injury, patients with complete tears showed a trend toward decreased functional scores compared with those who had partial tears, although this difference did not reach statistical significance.[59] Immediate identification of associated ligament injuries, especially in the TFCC, has led to acute direct repairs with good early and long-term results.

Bone Grafting

Given the very low nonunion rate for distal radius fractures, the utility of bone grafting is questionable. In both young patients with high-energy mechanisms and elderly patients with osteopenia and lower energy mechanisms, axial loading of the distal radius by the carpus may impact fragments of the articular surface into the metaphysis, leaving a metaphyseal void after the articular surface has been reduced. A VLP is designed to support the articular surface despite this loss of bony support. However, if other fixation is elected, such as spanning external fixation or a nonlocking dorsal plate, then a metaphyseal bone graft or bone substitute may be used instead. By

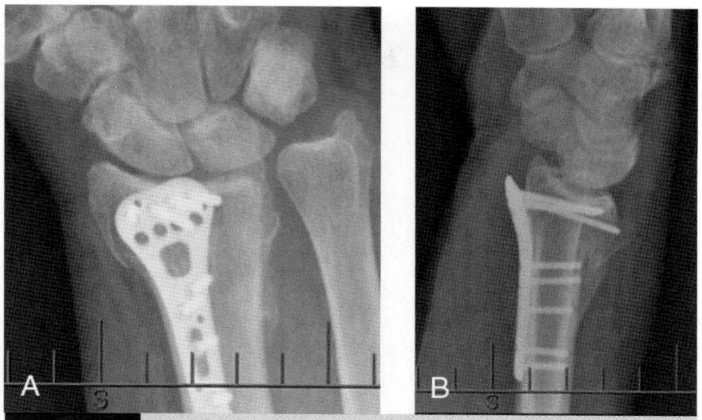

Figure 6 A 52-year-old man had undergone volar plating of a distal radial fracture 9 years ago and was experiencing the sudden inability to flex the index finger after using a door handle. Current AP (**A**) and lateral (**B**) radiographs are shown. The patient was found to have tendinal ruptures of the flexor digitorum profundus and the flexor digitorum superficialis of the right index finger. Treatment was plate removal and intercalary grafting of each ruptured tendon by using tripled palmaris longus and one-half of the flexor carpi radialis.

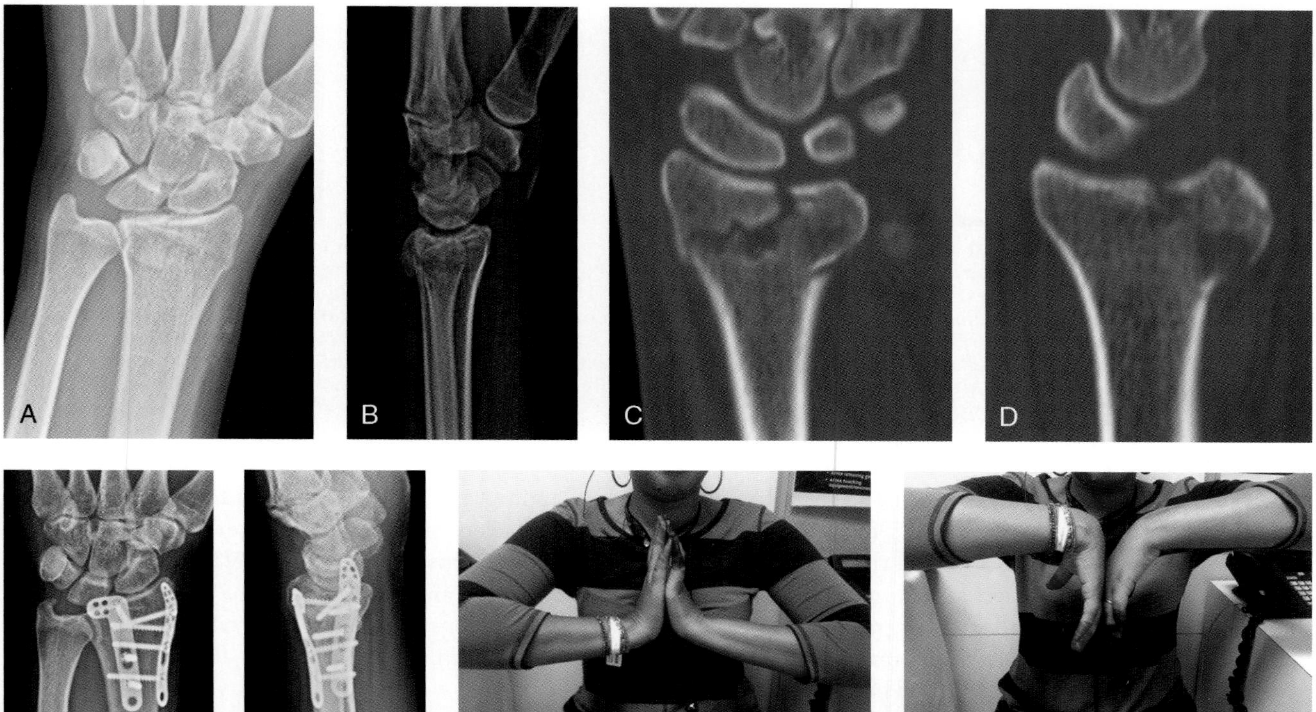

Figure 7 Radiographs show a distal radius fracture in a 35-year-old woman. **A**, AP and **B**, lateral views demonstrate minimal displacement with overall acceptable alignment. **C** and **D**, Coronal and sagittal CT images, respectively, show intra-articular displacement involving primarily the dorsal ulnar facet. A dorsal buttress plate was used to support the dorsal lunate facet, which was supported with impaction grafting of cancellous allograft chips. A radial column plate was placed through a separate incision. AP (**E**) and lateral (**F**) radiographs show fracture union with hardware in place. Clinical photographs (**G** and **H**) obtained 8 months after surgery show excellent wrist flexion and extension.

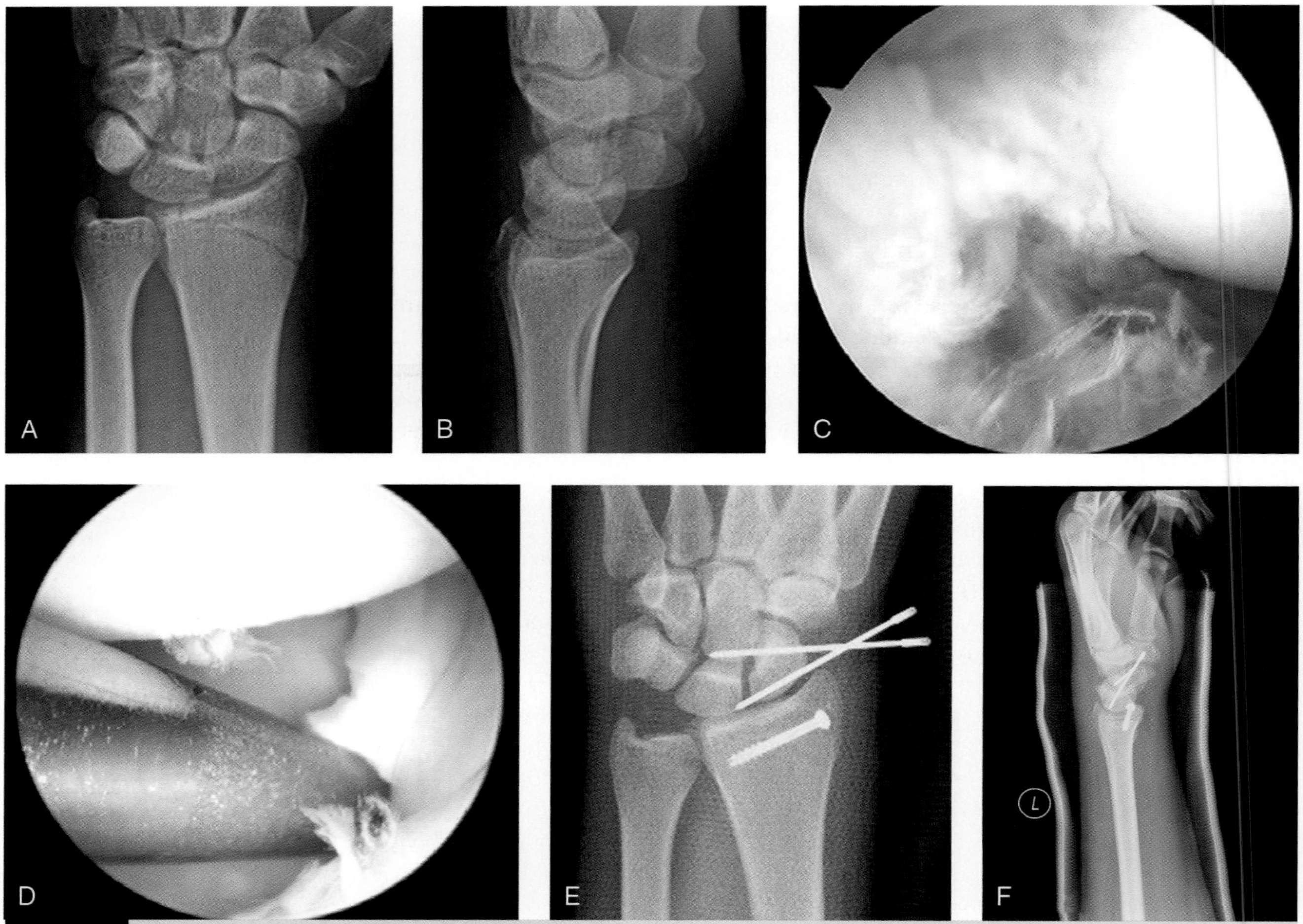

Figure 8 Imaging studies of the wrist of a 21-year-old man with a displaced intra-articular radial styloid fracture. **A,** AP and **B,** lateral radiographs show the radial styloid fracture without obvious carpal malalignment. Arthroscopy revealed the intra-articular extent of the distal radius fracture as well as partial injury (Geissler 2) to the scapholunate interosseous ligament. **C,** Arthroscopic image of scapholunate gap (scaphoid seen on the right). **D,** Arthroscopic image showing instrument approaching fracture of articular surface. The radial styloid fracture was treated with arthroscopically assisted reduction and internal fixation with a cannulated lag screw. The intercarpal ligament injury was treated with arthroscopic reduction and percutaneous Kirschner wire placement. **E** and **F,** Postoperative AP and lateral radiographs of the wrist.

placing a metaphyseal bone graft or bone substitute, it is possible to reduce the natural tendency for subsidence and loss of radial length after removal of the fixator at bony union. There are many types of graft material, including the reference standard of iliac crest graft, which has its own morbidity. Popular options for graft material include freeze-dried cancellous allograft and calcium phosphate cement. These materials support the subchondral articular facets during the healing and remodeling phases and limit subsidence.

In a recent prospective randomized study of 50 patients treated with percutaneous pinning of distal radius fractures, no difference was found between patients treated with a calcium-based demineralized bone matrix allograft and those with no graft in terms of DASH scores, radiographic parameters, and rate of union. Surgical times were significantly higher in the bone graft group.[60] In a retrospective study of VLP with or without hydroxyapatite bone graft substitute in elderly patients, ulnar variance increased in those who did not receive graft augmentation.[61]

Treatment Summary

Despite the current enthusiasm for VLP, it is important to carefully consider the patient's requirements and expectations in devising a treatment plan. Not every fracture needs fixation, and some minimally displaced osteoporotic fractures may not require a formal reduction. The characteristics of the patient and the personality of the fracture should be assessed. The surgical anatomy should be mastered, including all the approaches to the various surfaces of the distal radius that are available for plate fixation (volar, dorsal, and midaxial radial column). Modern implants are available and sized for the patient's anatomy and have both fixed- and variable-axis trajectories, enabling stable fixation in even the patient with the most severe osteopenia. The most frequent complications of screw penetration are avoidable with attention to detail and proper radiographs. The surgeon has various implants, techniques, and approaches at his or her disposal. However, the success of surgery depends on the surgeon, not on the implant. Patient outcome does not rest solely on the reassembly of fracture fragments, but more importantly on the maintenance of a mobile and sensate hand.

Outcomes

Modern studies comparing treatment results have focused on functional outcomes (subjective or patient-reported) rather than traditional surgeon-reported outcomes. As a result of this paradigm shift in evaluation of outcomes, it has become clear that functional outcome may not be related to objective measures of treatment success. For example, the restoration of proper anatomy had been considered essential to obtain good outcomes. However, studies have demonstrated that excellent outcomes can be achieved despite a failure to restore radiographic indices. This is especially true for the elderly population.[11,12]

Few long-term (longer than 10 years) studies have compared posttraumatic arthrosis with patient-based outcomes, and these do not indicate that arthritis inevitably leads to a bad outcome.[62]

In an effort to determine what factors influence functional outcomes, in a 2012 analysis 190 patients from a prospectively gathered registry who underwent surgical treatment of a distal radius fracturewere reviewed.[63] The most important determinants of patient-reported outcomes (DASH scores) were pain, grip strength, and supination. Improvement in supination reached a plateau after 3 to 6 months, whereas pain and grip strength continued to improve for up to 2 years.[63] Given the important role that supination plays in functional outcomes, how best to maximize supination becomes an important question. Presumably, failure to restore the sigmoid notch anatomy after intra-articular fractures could contribute. In one study, at 5-year follow-up patients were randomly assigned to receive either external fixation with adjuvant pins or VLP.[64] Although functional scores were similar at long-term follow-up, supination was significantly better among AO/ASIF type C2 fractures treated with volar plating compared with external fixation.[64]

Many studies show that functional recovery occurs more rapidly in patients treated with VLP. However, in almost all cases, this early difference disappears by the 1-year mark, after which functional outcomes between plating and less invasive treatments are equivalent.[12,30-34,41-43] Psychosocial factors also have a deleterious effect on early recovery from distal radius fracture surgery. Patients scoring high for pain catastrophizing and pain anxiety have decreased ROM, gripstrength, and quality-of-life scores at early follow-up, although these differences are insignificant at 6 months.

Rehabilitation

Early mobilization is one of the advantages of stable internal fixation provided by modern locked plating techniques. Is this theoretical advantage realized in the rehabilitation of these patients? In a 2014 study, 81 patients were randomly assigned to either accelerated rehabilitation (beginning at 2 weeks) or standard rehabilitation (beginning at 6 weeks) after volar plating.[65] Patients who underwent accelerated rehabilitation demonstrated better ROM, strength, and DASH scores at early time points, but there was no difference in patient-reported outcomes at 6 months despite better grip strength in the accelerated group.[65] As has been previously mentioned, any associated intercarpal ligament or TFCC injuries could modify early mobilization protocols.

Several studies have evaluated the effect of formal occupational therapy after surgery for distal radius fractures, but no clear benefit of formal therapy has been demonstrated. In a recent prospective randomized study of 94 patients who underwent VLP, independent exercises resulted in significantly better ROM, grip strength, and Mayo Wrist Scores compared with supervised therapy.[64]

Complications

Complications after distal radius fracture occur with or without surgical intervention and include tendon dysfunction and rupture, hand and wrist stiffness, and carpal tunnel syndrome. The types and frequency of complications will depend on the specific treatment and patient characteristics. Overall complication rates after volar plating in recent series have ranged from 6% to 11%.[47] In patients older than 65 years, surgical treatment is associated with a higher risk of complications (29%) compared with nonsurgical treatment (17%).[66] A 2015 study involving data from the Swedish nationwide registry found a higher incidence of revision surgery in patients treated with a plate compared with patients who were treated with pins or external fixation.[67] Patients treated with plates had higher rates of tendon ruptures and carpal tunnel syndrome. Those who were treated with pins or external fixation experienced more loss of reduction requiring revision surgery.[67] Educating the patients so they have a full understanding of the potential for a poor outcome is a critical component of their care.

Malunion remains the most common complication of distal radius fractures. In the elderly population, treatment should address specific complaints, such as loss of supination. In the younger patient, gross anatomic deformity may require osteotomy and correction to realign the carpus and lessen the potential for premature arthritis, as well as to improve strength and mobility. If the patient's flexion and extension arc is good and the limitation is primarily in forearm rotation because of DRUJ incongruence, an ulnar-shortening osteotomy is warranted to match the deformity and reestablish congruence (**Figure 9**).

Fortunately, nonunion and infection are rare complications. Technical challenges in cases of nonunion occur most notably when a short end segment (less than 2 cm) is involved. Bone graft, calcium phosphate cement augmentation, combined dorsal and volar plating, and external fixation have been used separately and in combination. Some distal radius fractures are repaired with grafts and then bridge plated either to the metacarpal or the carpus. Before total wrist fusion, some of these cases may be amenable to salvage with a distal radioscapholunate fusion.

Open distal radius fractures are treated with prompt initiation of intravenous antibiotics and surgical débridement and irrigation. The requirement for surgical débridement in poke-hole open fractures is controversial. A study of open distal radius fractures found no infections among 32 patients with grade I, II, and IIIA open fractures regardless of time to débridement or fixation strategy. However, in those treated with staged external fixation with later conversion to internal fixation, a trend toward more complications (scarring and stiffness) was seen.[68]

Complex regional pain syndrome (CRPS) is a common and often unrecognized complication of distal radius fractures, with an incidence as high as 18%. The symptoms include hyperpathia, swelling, stiffness, and vascular changes out of proportion to the injury and treatment rendered. The incidence of CRPS does not significantly correlate to depression or other psychosocial factors. Although previous randomized trials have found that vitamin C prophylaxis can prevent CRPS in patients with distal radius fractures, a recent randomized controlled trial of 336 patients failed to show a statistically significant difference in rate of CRPS or DASH scores between groups receiving vitamin C and placebo.[69] The exact role of vitamin C in prevention of CRPS is unclear.

Delayed tendon rupture continues to be an ongoing concern with both dorsal and volar plating. However, this may also occur with relatively nondisplaced distal radius fractures that are treated with casting. Rupture of the extensor pollicis longus tendon is the most common attritional rupture recently reported at 1%, although flexor tendon ruptures have been reported in growing numbers. The extensor pollicis longus tendon can be adequately reconstructed with an extensor indicis proprius tendon transfer. A more detailed discussion about tendon rupture with VLP is presented in the preceding section on treatment.

Hardware removal is commonly performed for dorsal plates and increasingly for volar plates. In a recent study at a single institution, 3% to 4% of volar plates were removed. The most common reasons cited for hardware removal were pain, tenosynovitis, plate malposition, and malunion, in that order.[70] In another study, volar plates were removed in 34% of patients.[47]

Initial fracture displacement is an independent risk factor for carpal tunnel syndrome. The role of carpal tunnel release in the context of distal radius fractures remains controversial. There is no evidence for proceeding with prophylactic release in patients in whom plates are used and who have normal results in a neurologic examination. Patients with dense anesthesia after injury require urgent release, as do patients with a history of carpal tunnel syndrome. The obtunded patient presents a diagnostic challenge. Among 665 cases of volar plate fixation, late carpal tunnel syndrome (3 to 6 months after surgery) developed in 3%, making it the most frequent complication in that series.[47] Management of acute carpal tunnel syndrome requires modification of the surgical approach. A more midline incision during both volar plating and carpal tunnel release minimizes risk of injury to the palmar cutaneous branch of the median nerve, which lies between the flexor carpi radialis and palmaris longus tendons.

The Future

As one of the fractures most frequently treated by orthopaedic surgeons, distal radius fractures will continue to command a high level of interest from surgeons and healthcare payers, who increasingly will demand evidence of improved outcomes to justify costlier treatment options. Earlier diagnosis and medical management of osteoporosis may decrease the incidence of fragility fractures of the distal radius. With evidence that functional outcomes in certain demographics are unrelated to traditional radiographic indices, the prevention of complications associated with surgical management will be

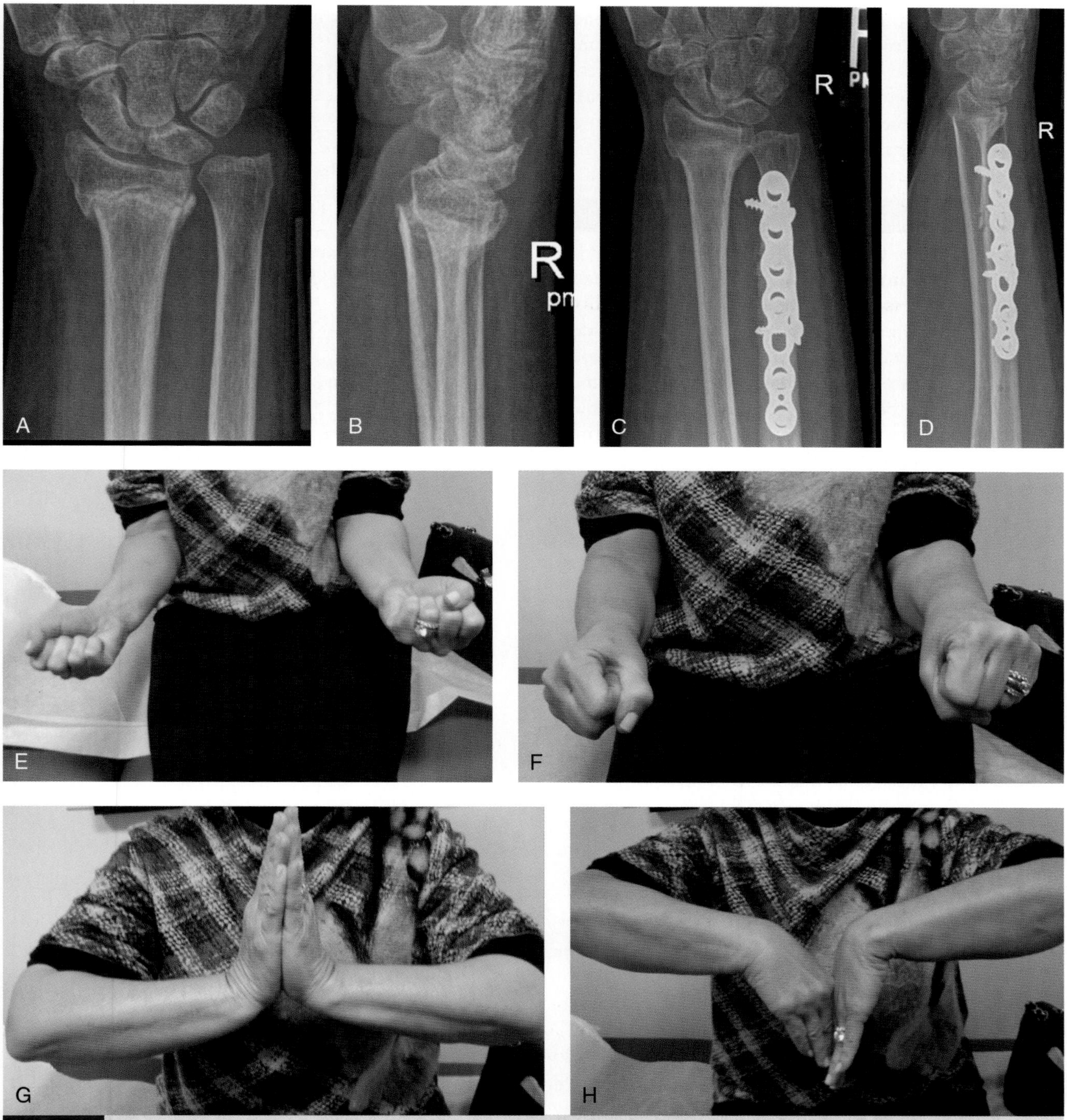

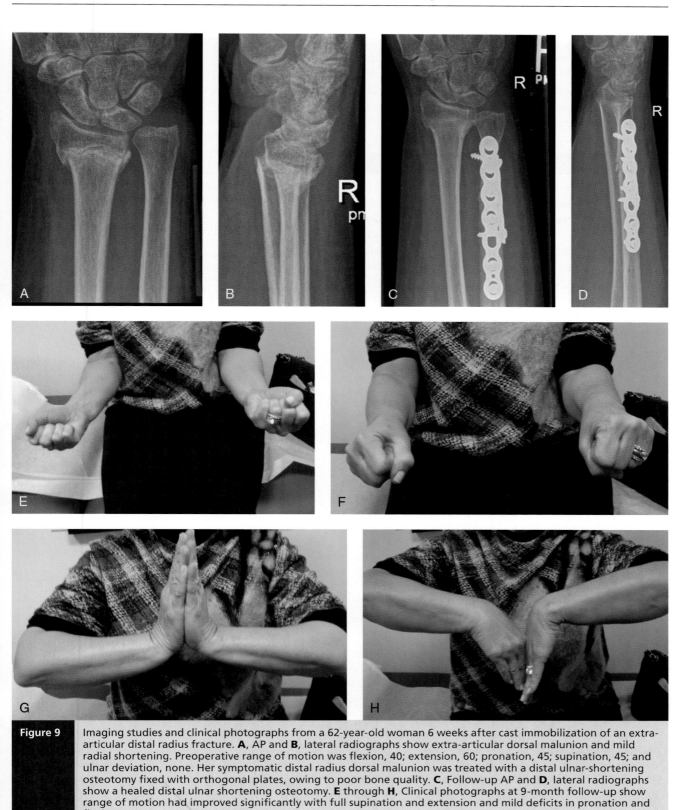

Figure 9 Imaging studies and clinical photographs from a 62-year-old woman 6 weeks after cast immobilization of an extra-articular distal radius fracture. **A**, AP and **B**, lateral radiographs show extra-articular dorsal malunion and mild radial shortening. Preoperative range of motion was flexion, 40; extension, 60; pronation, 45; supination, 45; and ulnar deviation, none. Her symptomatic distal radius dorsal malunion was treated with a distal ulnar-shortening osteotomy fixed with orthogonal plates, owing to poor bone quality. **C**, Follow-up AP and **D**, lateral radiographs show a healed distal ulnar shortening osteotomy. **E** through **H**, Clinical photographs at 9-month follow-up show range of motion had improved significantly with full supination and extension and mild deficits in pronation and flexion.

emphasized. Despite the significant number of studies published on this topic in recent years, the optimal management of distal radius fractures will be influenced by further research on plate design, surgical techniques, and functional outcomes. Carefully designed, larger studies are needed to help clarify these questions.

Summary

Forearm fractures typically occur after trauma and require surgical treatment to restore function. Distal radius fractures are heterogeneous injuries and require individualized treatment. High-energy mechanisms and osteoporosis are associated with these fractures. Although restoration of anatomy is typically the goal of treatment, this seems not to be the case in older patients with distal radius fractures. The surgeon must possess thorough knowledge of the pathoanatomy, instability patterns, and treatment options when treating these injuries.

Key Study Points

- Galeazzi fracture-dislocations and fractures of both forearm bones should be managed with rigid internal fixation to restore stability to the forearm "ring" and allow full rotation.
- Careful attention to surgical technique during VLP fixation of distal radius fractures, such as proper placement proximal to the watershed line, is important to prevent implant prominence and potential complications such as flexor tendon irritation and rupture.
- Although ulnar styloid fractures are commonly associated with distal radius fractures, the surgeon should determine need for fixation on the basis of instability of the DRUJ after distal radius fixation rather than ulnar styloid fracture morphology.
- Long-term patient-reported outcomes in elderly patients with distal radius fractures may not be related to radiographic outcome.
- Reduction of the lunate facet and ensuring DRUJ congruence in the treatment of distal radius fractures are paramount for the restoration of forearm supination, which is directly related to patient satisfaction and function.

Annotated References

1. Takemoto R, Sugi M, Immerman I, Tejwani N, Egol KA: Ulnar variance as a predictor of persistent instability following Galeazzi fracture-dislocations. *J Orthop Traumatol* 2014;15(1):41-46.

   The authors conducted a retrospective analysis of a series of 50 patients with radial shaft fractures to identify factors predictive of DRUJ instability. Although there was no difference with respect to relative distance to the radiocarpal joint, an association was found between ulnar variance and DRUJ instability after fracture fixation.

2. Park MJ, Pappas N, Steinberg DR, Bozentka DJ: Immobilization in supination versus neutral following surgical treatment of Galeazzi fracture-dislocations in adults: Case series. *J Hand Surg Am* 2012;37(3):528-531.

   In a retrospective review of 10 patients treated surgically for a Galeazzi fracture-dislocation, no difference was found between patients immobilized in supination versus neutral rotation with regards to forearm motion and DRUJ stability. Level of evidence: III.

3. Ploegmakers JJ, The B, Brutty M, Ackland TR, Wang AW: The effect of a Galeazzi fracture on the strength of pronation and supination two years after surgical treatment. *Bone Joint J* 2013;95-B(11):1508-1513.

   Ten patients who were treated with plate fixation for Galeazzi fractures were studied at a follow-up of 2 years. Strength of pronation and supination were measured along with functional scores. Loss of supination strength was associated with lower functional scores.

4. Cai XZ, Yan SG, Giddins G: A systematic review of the non-operative treatment of nightstick fractures of the ulna. *Bone Joint J* 2013;95-B(7):952-959 .

   According to a systematic review of published randomized controlled trials and observational studies, it appears that early mobilization is the best treatment of undisplaced or partially displaced nightstick fractures of the ulna.

5. Azboy I, Demirtas A, Uçar BY, Bulut M, Alemdar C, Özkul E: Effectiveness of locking versus dynamic compression plates for diaphyseal forearm fractures. *Orthopedics* 2013;36(7):e917-e922 .

   In a retrospective review of 42 patients, no significant difference in time to union and functional scores was seen between patients whose diaphyseal forearm fractures were treated with locking compression plating and dynamic compression plating. Level of evidence: III (therapeutic).

6. Lee SK, Kim KJ, Lee JW, Choy WS: Plate osteosynthesis versus intramedullary nailing for both forearm bones fractures. *Eur J Orthop Surg Traumatol* 2014;24(5):769-776.

   In this prospective, randomized comparative study, the authors randomly divided 67 patients with fractures of both forearm bones into two treatment groups: ORIF with plate or intramedullary nailing. Plate fixation resulted in improved restoration of the radial bow, although functional scores were similar between groups. Level of evidence: II.

7. Bot AG, Doornberg JN, Lindenhovius AL, Ring D, Goslings JC, van Dijk CN: Long-term outcomes of fractures of both bones of the forearm. *J Bone Joint Surg Am* 2011;93(6):527-532.

   After an average of 21 years after undergoing surgical or nonsurgical treatment of diaphyseal forearm fractures, 71 patients (both skeletally mature and immature) were evaluated. Regardless of age at injury or treatment type, the injured extremity had decreased forearm rotation and wrist motion compared with the other arm. Functional scores correlated with subjective and psychosocial aspects of illness. Level of evidence: IV.

8. Kloen P, Wiggers JK, Buijze GA: Treatment of diaphyseal non-unions of the ulna and radius. *Arch Orthop Trauma Surg* 2010;130(12):1439-1445.

   The authors discuss the history of the treatment of nonunion of the radius and ulna, the rate of which is typically less than 5% although series have reported rates of 2% to 10%. They also presented a series of 47 patients treated for nonunion with average follow-up of 75 months. All nonunions healed.

9. Schulte LM, Meals CG, Neviaser RJ: Management of adult diaphyseal both-bone forearm fractures. *J Am Acad Orthop Surg* 2014;22(7):437-446.

   This review article discusses evaluation, treatment, and complications of fractures of both-bone forearm fractures.

10. Yao C-K, Lin K-C, Tarng Y-W, Chang W-N, Renn J-H: Removal of forearm plate leads to a high risk of refracture: Decision regarding implant removal after fixation of the forearm and analysis of risk factors of refracture. *Arch Orthop Trauma Surg* 2014;134(12):1691-1697.

    The authors retrospectively studied 122 patients treated with fixation of forearm fractures by means of 3.5-mm dynamic compression plates. The rate of refracture was higher in those patients who underwent hardware removal. The authors recommended waiting at least 18 months before considering plate removal. Level of evidence: III.

11. Arora R, Gabl M, Gschwentner M, Deml C, Krappinger D, Lutz M: A comparative study of clinical and radiologic outcomes of unstable Colles type distal radius fractures in patients older than 70 years: Nonoperative treatment versus volar locking plating. *J Orthop Trauma* 2009;23(4):237-242.

12. Arora R, Lutz M, Deml C, Krappinger D, Haug L, Gabl M: A prospective randomized trial comparing nonoperative treatment with volar locking plate fixation for displaced and unstable distal radial fractures in patients sixty-five years of age and older. *J Bone Joint Surg Am* 2011;93(23):2146-2153.

    In a randomized trial comparing nonsurgical treatment and volar locked plating of distal radius fractures in patients 65 years of age or older, no difference was found in functional scores at 6 months despite superior radiographic outcomes with plating. Level of evidence: I.

13. Egol KA, Walsh M, Romo-Cardoso S, Dorsky S, Paksima N: Distal radial fractures in the elderly: Operative compared with nonoperative treatment. *J Bone Joint Surg Am* 2010;92(9):1851-1857.

    Surgical and nonsurgical treatment of displaced distal radial fractures in patients older than 65 years were compared by the authors of this case control study. They found no difference in functional scores at 1 year, although early motion was better in the surgically treated group. Level of evidence: III.

14. Wong TC, Chiu Y, Tsang WL, Leung WY, Yam SK, Yeung SH: Casting versus percutaneous pinning for extra-articular fractures of the distal radius in an elderly Chinese population: A prospective randomised controlled trial. *J Hand Surg Eur Vol* 2010;35(3):202-208.

    Patients older than 65 years who had extra-articular distal radial fractures were randomized to treatment with cast versus percutaneous pinning. Although radiographic outcome was better in the pinning group, there was no difference in functional scores at 1 year. Level of evidence: I.

15. Harness NG, Funahashi T, Dell R, et al: Distal radius fracture risk reduction with a comprehensive osteoporosis management program. *J Hand Surg Am* 2012;37(8):1543-1549.

    In this retrospective cohort study from a large health maintenance organization, authors compared patients 60 years or older with and without distal radius fractures. Risk factors for distal radius fracture included white race, female sex, and osteoporosis. Osteoporosis screening and pharmacologic management significantly decreased the risk of fracture. Level of evidence: III.

16. Shauver MJ, Yin H, Banerjee M, Chung KC: Current and future national costs to medicare for the treatment of distal radius fracture in the elderly. *J Hand Surg Am* 2011;36(8):1282-1287.

    The authors analyzed the Medicare dataset from 2007 to determine costs attributable to care of distal radius fractures.

17. Costa ML, Achten J, Plant C, et al: UK DRAFFT: A randomised controlled trial of percutaneous fixation with Kirschner wires versus volar locking-plate fixation in the treatment of adult patients with a dorsally displaced fracture of the distal radius. *Health Technol Assess* 2015;19(17):1-124, v-vi.

    In this large multicenter study by the British National Health Service known as the Distal Radius Acute Fracture Fixation Trial (DRAFFT), adult patients with operative dorsally displaced distal radius fractures were randomly divided into treatment via plate fixation versus treatment via K-wire fixation. They concluded that percutaneous pinning is more cost effective, because there were no statistically significant differences in functional scores at 12 months. Level of evidence: I.

18. Hammert WC, Kramer RC, Graham B, Keith MW: AAOS clinical practice guideline: Treatment of distal radius fractures. Available at www.aaos.org/research/guidelines/drf-guideline.pdf.

The AAOS recommendations regarding the treatment of distal radius fractures are presented.

19. Moritomo H, Omori S: Influence of ulnar translation of the radial shaft in distal radius fracture on distal radioulnar joint instability. *J Wrist Surg* 2014;3(1):18-21.

In this biomechanical study in cadavers, the authors demonstrated the role of the distal interosseous membrane in distal radioulnar stability. They also studied the effect of coronal plane malreduction on stability.

20. Ross M, Di Mascio L, Peters S, Cockfield A, Taylor F, Couzens G: Defining residual radial translation of distal radius fractures: A potential cause of distal radioulnar joint instability. *J Wrist Surg* 2014;3(1):22-29.

Three orthopaedic surgeons evaluated 100 normal wrist radiographs. High interobserver and intraobserver reliability was found for a novel radiographic parameter that may be useful for measuring coronal translation in distal radial fractures. Level of evidence: II.

21. Dy CJ, Jang E, Taylor SA, Meyers KN, Wolfe SW: The impact of coronal alignment on distal radioulnar joint stability following distal radius fracture. *J Hand Surg Am* 2014;39(7):1264-1272.

In this cadaver study, distal radial osteotomies were created and fixed in various degrees of coronal malreduction. The authors found that 2 mm of coronal shift caused increased DRUJ displacement in specimens with a distinct distal oblique bundle of the intraosseous membrane.

22. Harness NG, Ring D, Zurakowski D, Harris GJ, Jupiter JB: The influence of three-dimensional computed tomography reconstructions on the characterization and treatment of distal radial fractures. *J Bone Joint Surg Am* 2006;88(6):1315-1323.

23. Komura S, Yokoi T, Nonomura H, Tanahashi H, Satake T, Watanabe N: Incidence and characteristics of carpal fractures occurring concurrently with distal radius fractures. *J Hand Surg Am* 2012;37(3):469-476.

A retrospective review of 170 distal radius fractures revealed a 7% rate of associated carpal fracture, most of which were scaphoid fractures. Male sex, young age, high-energy trauma, and AO/ASIF type B fracture pattern raised the risk of concomitant carpal fracture. Level of evidence: III.

24. Kasapinova K, Kamiloski V: Influence of associated lesions of the intrinsic ligaments on distal radius fractures outcome. *Arch Orthop Trauma Surg* 2015;135(6):831-838.

Forty patients treated surgically for distal radial fracture were prospectively studied to determine the effect of arthroscopically identified scapholunate and lunotriquetral ligament injury on outcome. More than one-third (37.5%) of patients had a ligament injury, and those patients had worse functional outcomes.

25. Wijffels MM, Keizer J, Buijze GA, et al: Ulnar styloid process nonunion and outcome in patients with a distal radius fracture: A meta-analysis of comparative clinical trials. *Injury* 2014;45(12):1889-1895.

This systematic review of distal radial fracture outcomes among patients with united and nonunited ulnar styloid process fractures revealed no difference in any outcome measure evaluated (such as patient-reported outcome, functional outcome, grip-strength, pain, and DRUJ instability).

26. Kim JK, Yi JW, Jeon SH: The effect of acute distal radioulnar joint laxity on outcome after volar plate fixation of distal radius fractures. *J Orthop Trauma* 2013;27(12):735-739 .

In this prospective study, 84 patients who had distal radial fractures treated by means of volar locked plating were immobilized for 1 month postoperatively if intraoperative DRUJ testing revealed laxity after fracture fixation. At 1 year, there was no difference in outcomes between those with laxity and those without. Level of evidence: I.

27. Liu J, Wu Z, Li S, et al: Should distal radioulnar joint be fixed following volar plate fixation of distal radius fracture with unstable distal radioulnar joint? *Orthop Traumatol Surg Res* 2014;100(6):599-603.

Patients with intraoperative DRUJ instability after plate fixation of distal radial fractures were treated either with pin fixation in neutral for 6 weeks or with no fixation. In this retrospective review, there was no difference in outcome. Level of evidence: III.

28. Arealis G, Galanopoulos I, Nikolaou VS, Lacon A, Ashwood N, Kitsis C: Does the CT improve inter- and intra-observer agreement for the AO, Fernandez and Universal classification systems for distal radius fractures? *Injury* 2014;45(10):1579-1584.

The authors measured the interobserver and intraobserver agreement in the use of three classification systems for distal radial fractures. Agreement was fair to moderate between observers when using radiographs for all classification systems. Intraobserver reliability did not improve with addition of CT scans.

29. LaMartina J, Jawa A, Stucken C, Merlin G, Tornetta P III: Predicting alignment after closed reduction and casting of distal radius fractures. *J Hand Surg Am* 2015;40(5):934-939.

The authors measured the predictability of the McQueen formula and Lafontaine criteria and found that age was correlated with radial height, radial inclination, ulnar variance, and carpal alignment. A new parameter, volar hook, correlated with dorsal tilt and carpal alignment at healing. Level of evidence: III.

30. Karantana A, Downing ND, Forward DP, et al: Surgical treatment of distal radial fractures with a volar

locking plate versus conventional percutaneous methods: A randomized controlled trial. *J Bone Joint Surg Am* 2013;95(19):1737-1744.

Adult patients with distal radial fractures were randomly assigned to treatment via either volar locked plating or pinning with possible external fixation. Despite better radiographic outcomes with plating, there was no difference in functional scores at 1 year. Level of evidence: I.

31. Rozental TD, Blazar PE, Franko OI, Chacko AT, Earp BE, Day CS: Functional outcomes for unstable distal radial fractures treated with open reduction and internal fixation or closed reduction and percutaneous fixation. A prospective randomized trial. *J Bone Joint Surg Am* 2009;91(8):1837-1846.

32. Marcheix P-S, Dotzis A, Benkö P-E, Siegler J, Arnaud J-P, Charissoux J-L: Extension fractures of the distal radius in patients older than 50: A prospective randomized study comparing fixation using mixed pins or a palmar fixed-angle plate. *J Hand Surg Eur Vol* 2010;35(8):646-651.

    In a randomized controlled trial, patients older than 50 years were treated with volar locked plating or percutaneous pinning. At 6 months, functional scores were better in the plate group. Level of evidence: I.

33. McFadyen I, Field J, McCann P, Ward J, Nicol S, Curwen C: Should unstable extra-articular distal radial fractures be treated with fixed-angle volar-locked plates or percutaneous Kirschner wires? A prospective randomised controlled trial. *Injury* 2011;42(2):162-166.

    After conducting a randomized controlled trial comparing volar plating with percutaneous pinning, the authors concluded that radiographic parameters and functional scores were better at 6 months in patients who underwent plating. Level of evidence: I.

34. Wei DH, Raizman NM, Bottino CJ, Jobin CM, Strauch RJ, Rosenwasser MP: Unstable distal radial fractures treated with external fixation, a radial column plate, or a volar plate. A prospective randomized trial. *J Bone Joint Surg Am* 2009;91(7):1568-1577.

35. Farah N, Nassar L, Farah Z, Schuind F: Secondary displacement of distal radius fractures treated by bridging external fixation. *J Hand Surg Eur Vol* 2014;39(4):423-428.

    In a retrospective study of distal radius fractures treated with bridging external fixation, the rate of secondary displacement was 48.5% and mostly involved loss of palmar tilt.

36. Wei DH, Poolman RW, Bhandari M, Wolfe VM, Rosenwasser MP: External fixation versus internal fixation for unstable distal radius fractures: A systematic review and meta-analysis of comparative clinical trials. *J Orthop Trauma* 2012;26(7):386-394.

    The authors conducted a systematic review and meta-analysis of studies comparing treatment of unstable distal radius fractures with external versus internal fixation. Internal fixation provided better functional outcomes, supination, and volar tilt, whereas external fixation resulted in better grip and flexion. Level of evidence: II.

37. Esposito J, Schemitsch EH, Saccone M, Sternheim A, Kuzyk PR: External fixation versus open reduction with plate fixation for distal radius fractures: A meta-analysis of randomised controlled trials. *Injury* 2013;44(4):409-416.

    In a meta-analysis of studies in which investigators compared external fixation with ORIF of distal radial fractures, the authors found that ORIF was associated with better functional scores, radial length, and reduced infection rates. Level of evidence: II.

38. Hove LM, Krukhaug Y, Revheim K, Helland P, Finsen V: Dynamic compared with static external fixation of unstable fractures of the distal part of the radius: A prospective, randomized multicenter study. *J Bone Joint Surg Am* 2010;92(8):1687-1696.

    In a prospective randomized study, the authors compared dynamic and static external fixation as treatment of distal radial fractures. No differences between groups were seen with regard to functional scores, pain level, tilt, and inclination. However, better radial length and higher rate of pin-tract infection were observed in the dynamic fixator group. Level of evidence: I.

39. Gradl G, Mielsch N, Wendt M, et al: Intramedullary nail versus volar plate fixation of extra-articular distal radius fractures. Two year results of a prospective randomized trial. *Injury* 2014;45(suppl 1):S3-S8.

    Adults with distal radius fractures were randomized to volar plate fixation versus intramedullary nail fixation. At 2 years, there was no difference in functional scores, motion, pain, or complication rate. Level of evidence: I.

40. Williksen JH, Husby T, Hellund JC, Kvernmo HD, Rosales C, Frihagen F: External Fixation and Adjuvant Pins Versus Volar Locking Plate Fixation in Unstable Distal Radius Fractures: A Randomized, Controlled Study With a 5-Year Follow-Up. *J Hand Surg Am* 2015;40(7):1333-1340.

    The authors randomly assigned 111 patients with distal radial fractures to treatment with either volar locked plating or external fixation with adjuvant pins. At 5 years, there was no difference in DASH scores or pain, but patients treated with plating had better supination. Twenty-one percent of plates were removed because of surgical complications. Level of evidence: I.

41. Grewal R, MacDermid JC, King GJ, Faber KJ: Open reduction internal fixation versus percutaneous pinning with external fixation of distal radius fractures: A prospective, randomized clinical trial. *J Hand Surg Am* 2011;36(12):1899-1906.

    In this prospective randomized study, patients were treated either with ORIF or external fixation. Although patients with ORIF had better Patient-Related Wrist Evaluation scores at early time points, there was no difference at 12 months. Level of evidence: I.

42. Wilcke MK, Abbaszadegan H, Adolphson PY: Wrist function recovers more rapidly after volar locked plating than

after external fixation but the outcomes are similar after 1 year. *Acta Orthop* 2011;82(1):76-81.

Patients with distal radius fractures were randomly assigned to undergo treatment with volar locked plating or external fixation. Despite better outcomes scores for the plating group at early time points, there was no difference at 12 months. Level of evidence: I.

43. Roh YH, Lee BK, Baek JR, Noh JH, Gong HS, Baek GH: A randomized comparison of volar plate and external fixation for intra-articular distal radius fractures. *J Hand Surg Am* 2015;40(1):34-41.

In a prospective randomized study of volar locked plating versus external fixation for treatment of distal radius fractures, the authors found no difference in functional scores at 12 months despite results at earlier time points having favored volar locked plating. Level of evidence: I.

44. Jeudy J, Steiger V, Boyer P, Cronier P, Bizot P, Massin P: Treatment of complex fractures of the distal radius: A prospective randomised comparison of external fixation 'versus' locked volar plating. *Injury* 2012;43(2):174-179.

Seventy-five patients with intra-articular distal radius fractures were randomized to treatment with volar locked plate or external fixation with supplemental K-wire fixation. At 6-month follow-up, there was no difference in radiographic parameters or Patient-Related Wrist Evaluation scores, but grip strength was better in the volar plate group.

45. Shukla R, Jain RK, Sharma NK, Kumar R: External fixation versus volar locking plate for displaced intra-articular distal radius fractures: A prospective randomized comparative study of the functional outcomes. *J Orthop Traumatol* 2014;15(4):265-270.

This randomized controlled trial of 110 younger patients (mean age 39) with intra-articular distal radius fractures showed better Green and O'Brien scores at 1-year follow-up in the external fixation group although there was no difference in pain scores or activity level.

46. Plate JF, Gaffney DL, Emory CL, et al: Randomized comparison of volar locking plates and intramedullary nails for unstable distal radius fractures. *J Hand Surg Am* 2015;40(6):1095-1101.

Sixty patients with extra-articular distal radius fractures were randomized to volar plate fixation or intramedullary nail fixation. At 2-year follow-up there was no difference in *Quick*DASH or Michigan Hand Questionnaire. Level of evidence: II.

47. Esenwein P, Sonderegger J, Gruenert J, Ellenrieder B, Tawfik J, Jakubietz M: Complications following palmar plate fixation of distal radius fractures: A review of 665 cases. *Arch Orthop Trauma Surg* 2013;133(8):1155-1162.

In a retrospective review of volar plating of distal radius fractures, the complication rate was 11.3% and revision surgery rate was 10%.

48. Soong M, Earp BE, Bishop G, Leung A, Blazar P: Volar locking plate implant prominence and flexor tendon rupture. *J Bone Joint Surg Am* 2011;93(4):328-335.

In a retrospective comparison of two types of volar locked plates, the authors found that a more prominent plate design had a higher rate of flexor tendon ruptures. They devised a radiographic grading system to evaluate plate prominence as seen on the lateral view. Level of evidence: III.

49. Arora R, Lutz M, Hennerbichler A, Krappinger D, Espen D, Gabl M: Complications following internal fixation of unstable distal radius fracture with a palmar locking-plate. *J Orthop Trauma* 2007;21(5):316-322.

One hundred fourteen patients treated with volar locked plating for distal radius fractures were examined in a prospective observational study. These patients had improved stability but there was a significant incidence of complications with volar locked plates. Level of evidence: IV (therapeutic).

50. Al-Rashid M, Theivendran K, Craigen MA: Delayed ruptures of the extensor tendon secondary to the use of volar locking compression plates for distal radial fractures. *J Bone Joint Surg Br* 2006;88(12):1610-1612.

The authors describe the common complications of volar plating for distal radius fractures and provide three case reports of extensor tendon rupture and volar plating.

51. Brunner A, Siebert C, Stieger C, Kastius A, Link B-C, Babst R: The dorsal tangential X-ray view to determine dorsal screw penetration during volar plating of distal radius fractures. *J Hand Surg Am* 2015;40(1):27-33.

The dorsal tangential view of the distal radius was studied for its reliability in detecting dorsal screw perforation. Reliability was good and compared favorably with postoperative CT scan. Level of evidence: II.

52. Ljungquist KL, Agnew SP, Huang JI: Predicting a safe screw length for volar plate fixation of distal radius fractures: Lunate depth as a marker for distal radius depth. *J Hand Surg Am* 2015;40(5):940-944.

On the basis of axial imaging, the authors determined that the anteroposterior width of the lunate is a good approximation of the depth of the radius. They recommended using the depth of the lunate as the length of the longest screw to avoid dorsal penetration. Level of evidence: III.

53. Asadollahi S, Keith PP: Flexor tendon injuries following plate fixation of distal radius fractures: A systematic review of the literature. *J Orthop Traumatol* 2013;14(4):227-234.

Authors of a systematic review of flexor tendon complications associated with volar plating of the distal radius identified 21 studies. They found the flexor pollicis longus tendon to be the most frequently ruptured tendon.

54. Kitay A, Swanstrom M, Schreiber JJ, et al: Volar plate position and flexor tendon rupture following distal radius fracture fixation. *J Hand Surg Am* 2013;38(6):1091-1096.

The authors compared the lateral radiographs of patients treated with volar locking plates who had tendon ruptures with those of control patients who had no ruptures to measure the sensitivity and specificity of the Soong grading system. They found that Soong grade correlated with risk of rupture. Level of evidence: III.

55. Imatani J, Akita K, Yamaguchi K, Shimizu H, Kondou H, Ozaki T: An anatomical study of the watershed line on the volar, distal aspect of the radius: Implications for plate placement and avoidance of tendon ruptures. *J Hand Surg Am* 2012;37(8):1550-1554.

    The distal radius anatomy, specifically that of the watershed line, was studied in cadavers. The authors made recommendations about proper plate placement with respect to bony landmarks.

56. Limthongthang R, Bachoura A, Jacoby SM, Osterman AL: Distal radius volar locking plate design and associated vulnerability of the flexor pollicis longus. *J Hand Surg Am* 2014;39(5):852-860.

    In a cadaver study, various volar locked plate designs were studied to determine plate prominence at the location of the FPL tendon.

57. Hardman J, Al-Hadithy N, Hester T, Anakwe R: Systematic review of outcomes following fixed angle intramedullary fixation of distal radius fractures. *Int Orthop* 2015;39(12):2381-2387.

    A systematic review identified 14 articles in which investigators discussed fixed-angle intramedullary devices for treatment of distal radius fractures. The most common complication was transient neuritis of the superficial branch of the radial nerve.

58. Beck JD, Harness NG, Spencer HT: Volar plate fixation failure for volar shearing distal radius fractures with small lunate facet fragments. *J Hand Surg Am* 2014;39(4):670-678.

    The authors reviewed a prospective database of AO type B volar shearing fractures to determine risk factors for secondary loss of reduction of the volar lunate facet fragment. Risk factors included AO B3.3, small fragments, and greater initial subsidence. Fragment-specific fixation may be necessary in these cases. Level of evidence: III.

59. Mrkonjic A, Geijer M, Lindau T, Tägil M: The natural course of traumatic triangular fibrocartilage complex tears in distal radial fractures: A 13-15 year follow-up of arthroscopically diagnosed but untreated injuries. *J Hand Surg Am* 2012;37(8):1555-1560.

    In this natural history study of untreated arthroscopically confirmed TFCC tears associated with operatively treated distal radial fractures, the authors found that these untreated tears did not result in negative outcomes at 13- to 15-year follow-up. Level of evidence: I.

60. D'Agostino P, Barbier O: An investigation of the effect of AlloMatrix bone graft in distal radius fracture. A prospective randomised controlled clinical trial. *Bone Joint J* 2013;95-B(11):1514-1520.

    In this prospective randomized study, distal radius fractures treated with K-wire fixation were treated with or without adjunctive demineralized bone matrix allograft. There was no significant difference between groups with respect to functional outcomes, rate of union, or reduction parameters. Level of evidence: I.

61. Goto A, Murase T, Oka K, Yoshikawa H: Use of the volar fixed angle plate for comminuted distal radius fractures and augmentation with a hydroxyapatite bone graft substitute. *Hand Surg* 2011;16(1):29-37.

    The authors compared outcomes between elderly patients with distal radius fractures treated with volar locked plating with or without augmentation with hydroxyapatite bone graft substitute. There were no differences in radiographic parameters except ulnar variance, which was increased in the group that did not receive the graft.

62. Forward DP, Davis TR, Sithole JS: Do young patients with malunited fractures of the distal radius inevitably develop symptomatic post-traumatic osteoarthritis? *J Bone Joint Surg Br* 2008;90(5):629-637.

    In a case series of 106 adults who sustained a distal radius fracture when younger than 40 years of age, the authors followed them clinically at an average of 38 years postoperatively. The degree of radiographic malunion and radiocarpal arthrosis did not correlate with DASH scores.

63. Swart E, Nellans K, Rosenwasser M: The effects of pain, supination, and grip strength on patient-rated disability after operatively treated distal radius fractures. *J Hand Surg Am* 2012;37(5):957-962.

    In this retrospective analysis of prospectively gathered data from a registry of patients undergoing operative fixation of distal radial fractures, pain, grip strength, and supination were significantly correlated with DASH scores. Level of evidence: II.

64. Souer JS, Buijze G, Ring D: A prospective randomized controlled trial comparing occupational therapy with independent exercises after volar plate fixation of a fracture of the distal part of the radius. *J Bone Joint Surg Am* 2011;93(19):1761-1766.

    Patients undergoing volar locked plating of distal radius fractures were randomly assigned to a postoperative therapy program under the supervision of an occupational therapist or to surgeon-directed independent exercises. There were no differences in functional scores at any time point. Level of evidence: I.

65. Brehmer JL, Husband JB: Accelerated rehabilitation compared with a standard protocol after distal radial fractures treated with volar open reduction and internal fixation: A prospective, randomized, controlled study. *J Bone Joint Surg Am* 2014;96(19):1621-1630.

    Patients were prospectively assigned randomly to undergo either an accelerated or a standard rehabilitation protocol after surgical treatment of distal radius fractures with volar locked plating. The accelerated protocol resulted in earlier return to function. Level of evidence: I.

66. Lutz K, Yeoh KM, MacDermid JC, Symonette C, Grewal R: Complications associated with operative versus nonsurgical treatment of distal radius fractures in patients aged 65 years and older. *J Hand Surg Am* 2014;39(7):1280-1286.

In this case-control study, elderly patients with distal radius fractures treated surgically were compared with those treated nonsurgically. The complication rate was higher in the surgically treated group. Median neuropathy was the most common complication. Level of evidence: III.

67. Navarro CM, Pettersson HJ, Enocson A: Complications after distal radius fracture surgery: Results from a Swedish nationwide registry study. *J Orthop Trauma* 2015;29(2):e36-e42.

Using a nationwide prospective registry of operatively treated distal radius fractures, the authors determined the rates of revision surgery for various procedures. The highest rate of revision surgery was for patients who had been treated with a plate. Level of evidence: II.

68. Kurylo JC, Axelrad TW, Tornetta P III, Jawa A: Open fractures of the distal radius: The effects of delayed debridement and immediate internal fixation on infection rates and the need for secondary procedures. *J Hand Surg Am* 2011;36(7):1131-1134.

This retrospective review of open distal radius fractures evaluated the risk factors for infection. There were no infections in grade I or II open fractures, and time to débridement was not a significant factor. Level of evidence: III.

69. Ekrol I, Duckworth AD, Ralston SH, Court-Brown CM, McQueen MM: The influence of vitamin C on the outcome of distal radial fractures: A double-blind, randomized controlled trial. *J Bone Joint Surg Am* 2014;96(17):1451-1459.

In this prospective randomized study, vitamin C had no significant effect on the rate of complex regional pain syndrome. Level of evidence: II.

70. Snoddy MC, An TJ, Hooe BS, Kay HF, Lee DH, Pappas ND: Incidence and reasons for hardware removal following operative fixation of distal radius fractures. *J Hand Surg Am* 2015;40(3):505-507.

The authors retrospectively reviewed the records of patients who underwent removal of a volar plate. The authors addressed the causes of hardware removal, including pain, tenosynovitis, malunion, infection, nonunion, and tendon rupture. Level of evidence: IV.

Chapter 27

Hand Fractures and Dislocations

Michael R. Hausman, MD

Abstract

Hand fractures and dislocations including scaphoid and other carpal fractures, perilunate injuries, and metacarpal and phalangeal fractures and dislocations are among the most common orthopaedic injuries and are associated with significant morbidity. Accurate diagnosis and management are predicated on a thorough physical examination and appropriate imaging.

Keywords: carpal injury; metacarpal fracture; perilunate dislocation; phalanx fracture; scaphoid fracture

Introduction

Fractures of the hand are common injuries that can be treated surgically or nonsurgically. A thorough clinical evaluation will help drive the decision about the most appropriate treatment. Optimal treatment limits joint stiffness and preserves mobilization of joints and ligaments.

Scaphoid Fractures

Scaphoid fractures account for as many as 70% of all carpal bone fractures and are most common in young men.[1]

The specific features of the scaphoid must be recognized for optimal treatment and avoidance of sequelae. The scaphoid has an axial blood supply with a distal-to-proximal orientation. As the only bone that spans the proximal and distal rows of the carpus, the scaphoid is subjected to extreme forces such as cantilever bending and compression. The integrity and the bony and ligamentous attachments of the scaphoid dictate the kinematics of the wrist, and functional and anatomic changes will result if an injury is left untreated. Delayed or unsuccessful treatment increases the risk of nonunion and leads to a predictable pattern of collapse and pancarpal arthritis.

Clinical Examination

Patients with scaphoid fracture have dorsoradial wrist swelling and restricted motion secondary to guarding. Anatomic snuffbox and scaphoid tubercle tenderness to palpation are common. Pain with axial thumb compression may be elicited. A meta-analysis of the clinical predictors of scaphoid fracture found wide variation in the estimated sensitivity and specificity of these tests.[2] The sensitivity of anatomic snuffbox tenderness ranged from 0.87 to 1.00, and that of axial thumb compression ranged from 0.48 to 1.00. Specificity was limited, however, and the lack of specific tests may lead to considerable overtreatment. A prospective study of 223 patients within 2 weeks of a suspected scaphoid fracture found several independent predictors of fracture including male sex, a sports-related injury, anatomic snuffbox tenderness on ulnar deviation within 72 hours after injury, and scaphoid tubercle tenderness 2 weeks after injury.[3] If all four risk factors were positive, the likelihood of fracture was 91%. No patient without anatomic snuffbox tenderness on ulnar deviation within 72 hours of injury had a fracture.

Imaging

The standard radiographic evaluation for a suspected scaphoid fracture begins with the PA, lateral, and PA ulnar deviation views. MRI, CT, and bone scans have been evaluated for their diagnostic usefulness. In a meta-analysis of scaphoid imaging modalities using latent class analysis, sensitivity and specificity were estimated, respectively, at 91.1% and 99.8% for follow-up radiographs, 97.8% and 93.5% for bone scans, 97.7% and 99.8% for MRI, and

Dr. Hausman or an immediate family member has received royalties from Smith & Nephew; is a member of a speakers' bureau or has made paid presentations on behalf of TriMed; serves as a paid consultant to or is an employee of Stryker; serves as an unpaid consultant to Checkpoint Surgical, NDI Medical and SPR Therapeutics, and has stock or stock options held in Checkpoint Surgical, NDI Medical, and SPR Therapeutics.

85.2% and 99.5% for CT.[4] These results are in line with earlier studies that identified MRI as the most accurate modality for identifying scaphoid fracture.[5,6]

A strategy of initial immobilization and reevaluation can minimize missed fractures and the sequelae of delayed treatment, including carpal collapse, nonunion, and osteonecrosis, but at the cost of unnecessary immobilization and productivity loss. A cost-effectiveness study examined diagnostic strategies using a decision tree analysis with a societal perspective.[7] The base model assumed a significant productivity loss. Immediate CT (costing $2,553 per diagnosed scaphoid fracture in 2013) and immediate MRI (with a higher cost) were the most cost-effective diagnostic modalities across most lost-productivity ranges. If immobilization caused only a slight productivity loss, 2-week follow-up radiographs became cost-effective.

Nonsurgical Treatment

Several systems are available for classifying scaphoid fractures, such as the Russe and Herbert and Fisher categories. All classification systems attempt to distinguish between stable and unstable fractures, as this informs the decision for surgical or nonsurgical treatment. Surgical treatment is indicated for a displaced fracture.[8] Considerable debate exists regarding optimal treatment of nondisplaced fractures, however, as shown by two meta-analyses of randomized controlled studies.[9,10] In a meta-analysis of eight studies including 419 patients, the primary outcome metric of standardized functional outcome (in four studies including 247 patients) significantly favored surgical treatment over nonsurgical treatment of nondisplaced scaphoid fractures.[9] Surgical treatment was associated with greater patient satisfaction, increased grip strength, decreased time to union, and earlier return to work. There was no difference in range of motion, nonunion, or treatment cost. Surgical treatment was associated with a nonsignificantly increased rate of complications compared with nonsurgical treatment (23.7% versus 9.1%). A separate meta-analysis of six studies including 363 patients found a nonsignificant 2.36 pooled odds ratio of fracture union, which suggested a higher union rate after surgical treatment than after nonsurgical treatment.[10] Patients who were surgically treated were 6.96 times more likely to have a complication than those who were nonsurgically treated, however. Nonsurgical treatment was recommended as the first-line therapy for a nondisplaced scaphoid waist fracture.

The use of an electrical bone stimulator has been promoted in an effort to reduce the risk of nonunion and the time to union. The efficacy of bone stimulator use in nondisplaced scaphoid fractures was questioned in a randomized controlled study of 102 patients treated with a short arm-thumb spica cast.[11] All patients underwent clinical and radiographic evaluation including CT at 6, 9, 12, 24, and 52 weeks after injury. At 52 weeks, there were no significant differences in time to union, nonunion, or clinical outcome based on bone stimulator use. Post hoc analysis revealed that the time to union was significantly reduced with bone stimulator use in a subset of nondisplaced transverse waist fractures.

The optimal immobilization technique for use in nonsurgical treatment of scaphoid fractures also was a focus of several studies. A prospective multicenter randomized study compared 62 minimally displaced or nondisplaced scaphoid waist fractures immobilized in a short arm cast with or without thumb inclusion.[12] The primary outcome measure was the extent of bony union as determined by CT at 10-week follow-up. Fractures immobilized without thumb inclusion had a significantly greater average extent of bony union than those with thumb inclusion (85% versus 70%, $P = 0.048$). There were no between-group differences in clinical or subjective outcome measures. The overall union rate was 98%, and the only nonunion occurred in a patient who initially was assigned to thumb inclusion but elected to undergo surgical treatment.

Surgical Fixation

A displaced scaphoid fracture typically is defined by more than 1 mm of displacement, although the extent of displacement can be difficult to quantify on plain radiographs alone. In contrast to nondisplaced fractures, displaced scaphoid fractures are widely considered to be unstable injuries with an increased risk of nonunion if managed nonsurgically (**Figure 1**). Surgical treatment of proximal pole fractures is recommended regardless of displacement because the retrograde axial blood supply creates a risk of nonunion. This recommendation was supported by a meta-analysis that found a 7.5-fold increase in the risk of nonunion in proximal pole fractures treated nonsurgically compared with more distal fractures.[13]

Several biomechanical studies of interosseous screw trajectories concluded that central placement allows greater screw length and creates greater fixation strength.[14,15] This recommendation has been questioned, particularly in oblique fracture patterns where an eccentrically placed screw can be directed perpendicular to the fracture line. A biomechanical study compared central and eccentric screw placement in oblique fracture models by cyclically loading fractures to failure.[16] Despite their significantly shorter screw length, eccentric screws perpendicular to the fracture line provided strength equivalent to that of a longer, centrally placed screw. Similarly, eccentric screw placement in distal oblique fractures was found to maximize healing surface area compared with central placement.[17]

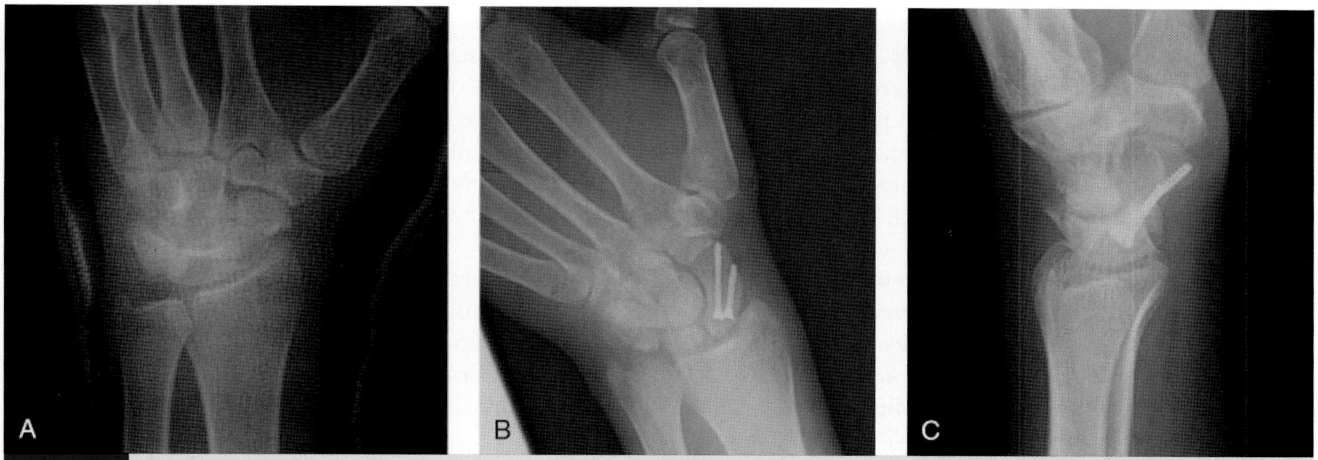

Figure 1 **A,** Preoperative oblique, scaphoid view radiograph showing a minimally displaced scaphoid waist fracture. Follow-up PA (**B**) and lateral (**C**) radiographs showing fracture union after fixation with two screws. Parallel screws are used to ensure rotational stability, as well as resistance to bending forces.

Volar and dorsal, open, percutaneous, and arthroscopically assisted approaches have been described for scaphoid fixation. Central screw trajectory in both proximal and distal poles can be challenging to obtain through a percutaneous approach compared with open techniques, and this is particularly true in a volar percutaneous approach because of obstruction of the trapezium despite hyperextension of the wrist. A dorsal approach avoids the trapezium but requires wrist flexion, which can displace the fracture. A study comparing a percutaneous transtrapezial approach with a standard volar percutaneous approach in simulated transverse waist fractures found that central screw placement in both proximal and distal poles was significantly greater with a transtrapezial approach.[18] In addition, the load to 2 mm of displacement and the load to failure were significantly greater with a transtrapezial approach than with a standard volar percutaneous approach. Although central screw placement can be more accurate through a transtrapezial approach, the required penetration of the scaphotrapezial joint carries a theoretical risk of iatrogenic arthritis. A retrospective review of 34 patients who underwent percutaneous transtrapezial scaphoid fixation found no symptomatic scaphotrapezial osteoarthritis at a mean 6.1-year follow-up.[19] Two patients required removal of six screw protrusions, and one patient had asymptomatic stage II osteoarthritis of the scaphotrapezial joint.

Scaphoid Nonunion

Neglected scaphoid nonunion is associated with osteonecrosis and progressive radiocarpal and midcarpal arthritis; this condition is called scaphoid nonunion advanced collapse. Before surgery for scaphoid nonunion, a thorough assessment is required to establish the extent of bony collapse, osteonecrosis, and carpal malalignment. These factors will guide the choice of surgical approach and bone graft material. A comparison of the carpal height to that of the contralateral wrist allows the extent of collapse and scaphoid shortening to be estimated. A diagnosis of osteonecrosis can be challenging because of the limited sensitivity of imaging modalities, including contrast-enhanced MRI.[20] However, the presence of large cavitary cysts with bone resorption around the midwaist to proximal pole suggests that the bone has a compromised blood supply.

A stable scaphoid nonunion without deformity or osteonecrosis can be successfully managed without bone grafting. Twelve of 14 patients with fibrous scaphoid nonunions treated with screw fixation alone experienced healing at 4.4-month follow-up.[21] The two persistent nonunions occurred in proximal pole fractures more than 1 year after injury.

An unstable nonunion requires bone grafting to restore height and correct carpal malalignment, principally dorsal or volar intercalated segment instability. There is debate as to whether cancellous or compression-tolerant corticocancellous grafts should be used. Twelve scaphoid waist nonunions with humpback deformity were successfully treated with a retrograde screw and ipsilateral distal radius cancellous bone graft.[22] The cited advantages of cancellous graft included technical ease (because of a limited need for intraoperative bone carpentry) and rapid graft incorporation. A systematic review of cancellous and corticocancellous bone grafting found that both techniques led to reliable union (95% or 92%, respectively). Cancellous grafting required less time to union, but corticocancellous grafting led to more consistent deformity correction.[23]

Vascularized bone grafting is recommended for the treatment of nonunion complicated by osteonecrosis. The 1,2 intercompartmental supraretinacular artery commonly is used for a vascularized pedicle bone graft, although there is a wide range of reported union rates. The Mathoulin pedicled graft from the volar distal radius also has been used with good clinical results, and it has the advantage of a corticocancellous component to help maintain the stability of the realigned scaphoid.[24] A novel technique for treating proximal pole scaphoid nonunions uses a free vascularized medial femoral trochlea osteocartilaginous flap.[25] At a minimum 6-month follow-up, a retrospective review found CT-confirmed healing in 15 of 16 scaphoids consecutively treated with a medial femoral trochlea flap. Twelve of the 16 patients were pain free, with maintained preoperative motion and scapholunate alignment. Several cautionary points were included in the report, however. Although the medial femoral trochlea flap has a favorable anatomic similarity to the proximal scaphoid and its use allows aggressive nonunion resection, the scapholunate ligament must be preserved to prevent instability. This technique requires the advanced skills of a microvascular flap surgeon. Donor morbidity of the knee also must be considered.

The method of fixation can affect the union rate, as shown in a review of 132 scaphoid nonunions after fixation with Acutrak (Acumed) or Herbert (Zimmer) screws.[26] Acutrak screw fixation led to a significantly higher union rate than Herbert screw fixation (94% versus 71%, $P = 0.01$) and to more accurate central axis screw placement. The reason for this difference has not been established, but the more extensive interference fit of the non–dumbbell-shaped Acutrak screw may be more resistant to torsional forces.

Nonscaphoid Carpal Bone Fractures

The incidence of fractures of the carpal bones probably is greater than reported because of their complex and overlapping silhouettes, which make radiographic interpretation difficult. Scaphoid fractures represent nearly 70% of carpal fractures, and the remaining seven carpal bones account for the remaining 30%.[1,27]

CT should be considered if persistent focal pain and clinical suspicion of fracture remain after negative radiography. Most nondisplaced carpal bone fractures can be treated with immobilization, but surgical treatment is recommended for a displaced intra-articular fracture to reduce the risk of posttraumatic arthritis.

Triquetral fracture is the most common nonscaphoid carpal bone fracture. This fracture most often occurs at the dorsal ridge at the attachment of the dorsal ligaments and is called a chip fracture. The chip fracture can be successfully treated with a period of immobilization. Persistent ulnar-side wrist pain after a dorsal chip fracture should raise suspicion for a concomitant triangular fibrocartilage complex injury. A CT study of six patients with a triangular fibrocartilage complex injury found confirmed fracture union after successful arthroscopic débridement.[28]

The two distinct structural components of the hamate are the body and the hook. Hook of hamate fractures commonly occur while the patient is playing baseball, a racquet sport, or golf with the bat, racquet, or club resting over the hook. Hamate body fractures occur during a direct impact with a clenched fist, which can also cause a fracture-dislocation of the carpometacarpal joint that may be missed. Hook fractures can be caused by repetitive traction from the pisohamate ligaments during the radial and ulnar deviation required in ball-and-stick sports. Thus, the fracture may represent a stress reaction more than a direct blow. The physical examination should include median and ulnar nerve function as well as the Allen test to rule out ulnar artery thrombosis. The hook of hamate pull test is done with resisted small and ring finger flexion with the hand in ulnar deviation (thus applying an ulnar displacing force on the hook of hamate).[29] The radiographic evaluation should include a carpal tunnel view and a supinated oblique view to define the fracture.

Although a nondisplaced hook of hamate fracture can be treated with immobilization, the risk of chronic painful nonunion or spontaneous tendon rupture makes nonsurgical treatment less appealing than surgical treatment in active patients. The surgical treatment typically consists of excision to allow an early return to sports. The outcomes of hook of hamate fracture excision were reported in 11 high-level athletes who had an average return to sport within 6 weeks; there was only one ulnar nerve paresthesia, which was completely resolved at 6-week follow-up.[30] No evidence of diminished grip strength was found in any patient. Hamate body fractures must be evaluated for a concomitant ring or small finger metacarpal base fracture or dislocation. Open reduction and internal fixation with interfragmentary screws or Kirschner wires often is required to restore carpometacarpal alignment in such injuries.

Trapezoid and trapezial body fractures are rare because of the bony and ligamentous stability of the trapezoid. A review of 11 trapezoid fractures found that many of the diagnoses were delayed, and CT was required particularly for coronal fractures.[31] Most trapezoid fractures did not occur in isolation. Surgery was required only in two patients. Trapezial body fractures can be clinically confused with scaphoid fracture because of their proximity.

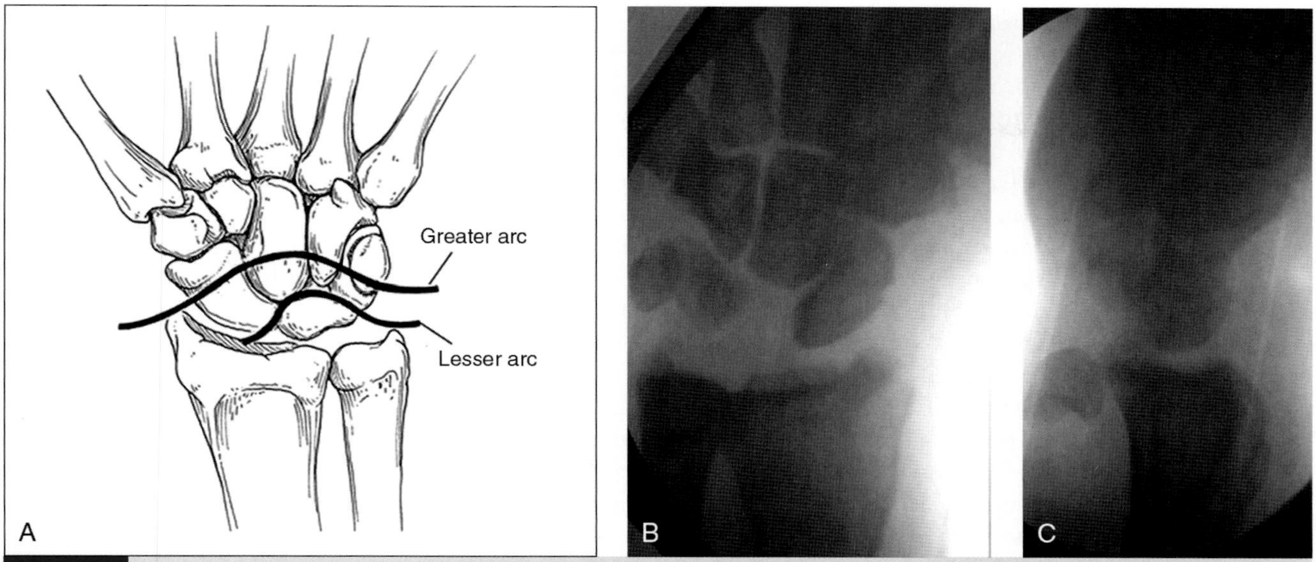

Figure 2 **A,** Schematic drawing showing greater and lesser arc perilunate injury patterns. PA (**B**) and lateral (**C**) radiographs showing stage IV Mayfield perilunate dislocation with a radial styloid fracture. In stage I, the scapholunate ligament is ruptured. Progression of the injury across the capitolunate joint defines a stage II injury, while rupture of the lunatotriquetral ligament and perilunate dislocation characterizes stage III. Finally, the lunate is dislocated palmarly in stage IV. (Adapted from Kozin SH: Perilunate injuries: Diagnosis and treatment. *J Am Acad Orthop Surg* 1998;6[2]:114-120.)

Trapezial body fractures are more common in the geriatric population. Articular incongruity in the trapezium can be reduced and stabilized with an open reduction. Capitate fractures should be closely followed to ensure that union occurs because the retrograde blood supply, like that of the scaphoid, increases the risk of nonunion and osteonecrosis. Fractures of the pisiform occur during resisted sudden hyperextension or a direct impact in an athlete. Displaced fractures of the pisiform can be treated with early excision; nondisplaced fractures are immobilized, with late excision offered if symptoms persist. Isolated fractures of the lunate are rare and most often occur as part of a larger injury. If an isolated fracture is suspected, Kienböck disease should be considered as the true etiology.

Perilunate Dislocations and Fracture-Dislocations

Perilunate dislocation (PLD) and perilunate fracture-dislocation (PLFD) are rare high-energy injuries that usually occur during a motor vehicle crash or a fall from a height with the wrist extended and ulnarly deviated. The result is progressive perilunar instability.[32] The injury can be missed on initial radiologic evaluation, despite external signs of soft-tissue injury. Prompt recognition and treatment are essential because of the risk of acute carpal tunnel syndrome. The dislocation can be broadly categorized as a greater arc injury, in which ligamentous disruption occurs through an associated fracture, or a lesser arc injury, which is purely ligamentous (**Figure 2**). Surgical fixation is recommended for all perilunate injuries, even after anatomic closed reduction, because of the extent of instability.

The surgical approach can be dorsal, volar, or combined. Arthroscopic reduction and percutaneous fixation of PLD and PLFD was found to have satisfactory outcomes.[33] Interposed palmar capsular ligaments were found in all patients surgically treated after unsuccessful closed reduction. At a minimum 10-year follow-up, 18 patients with PLD or PLFD had an average Mayo wrist score of 77 (range, 60 to 90), and 12 (67%) had radiographic evidence of arthritis.[34] Although the intraoperative reduction was considered to be good in more patients with PLFD than PLD, there were no significant differences in long-term clinical or radiographic parameters. These injuries are significant; much of the articular cartilage damage at the time of injury occurs because of shear and compression and cannot be fully mitigated by the reduction. Fortunately, most patients have a satisfactory long-term clinical outcome despite radiologic evidence of osteoarthritis progression.

Metacarpal Fractures and Dislocations

Metacarpal fracture is among the most common upper extremity fractures and typically occurs in patients in their teens and 20s. Most metacarpal fractures can be successfully managed with immobilization for 3 to 4 weeks. The general indications for surgical treatment include rotational malalignment, significant shortening or angulation, and involvement of multiple bones. Not all metacarpal fractures have an equal propensity for displacement. Closed reduction of a metacarpal neck fracture (Boxer fracture) almost always has a satisfactory result. The treatment decision must include the relative risks of deformity and stiffness in the context of the patient's functional requirements as well as the fracture location and pattern. Careful assessment of axial shortening is required because it is correlated with malrotation and extensor lag at the metacarpophalangeal (MCP) joint, and the resulting crossover deformity is poorly tolerated.[35] The standard radiographs include the AP, lateral, and oblique views as well as a 30° pronated view for a ring or small finger injury or a 30° supinated view for an index, middle, or ring finger injury. Fracture location, comminution, angulation, rotation, and shortening must be carefully scrutinized on postinjury and postreduction radiographs.

Metacarpal neck fractures are most common in the ring and small fingers. The initial treatment consists of closed reduction using the Jahss technique, in which dorsal pressure is applied to the metacarpal head using the proximal phalanx, with the MCP joint in 90° of flexion. Immobilization traditionally is done with the MCP joint flexed to 90° (the intrinsic-plus position), but equivalent outcomes were reported with MCP joint extension.[36] The amount of angulation tolerated ranges from 10° in the index finger to more than 50° in the small finger. The presence of pseudoclawing caused by excessive MCP joint hyperextension to counteract excessive metacarpal neck flexion is a relative surgical indication. A prospective comparison study of intramedullary pinning and functional immobilization for treatment of small finger metacarpal neck fractures with 30° to 70° of angulation found no significant difference in range of motion or grip strength at 1-year follow-up. Satisfaction and appearance were superior in the patients who were surgically treated, however, and surgical treatment may offer aesthetic rather than functional improvement.[37]

Metacarpal shaft fractures are identified as transverse, oblique-spiral, or comminuted. As in a metacarpal neck fracture, more angulation can be accepted in a shaft fracture of the mobile fourth and fifth rays than in other rays. Oblique fractures must be clinically assessed for malrotation, which often is not discernable on radiographs. The intermetacarpal ligaments and the interosseous muscles provide relative stability to nonborder digits. Multiple metacarpal fractures inherently have increased instability because of disruption of the secondary soft-tissue stabilizers, and surgical intervention often is indicated. The fixation techniques include the use of Kirschner wires, plates and screws, intramedullary devices, and interfragmentary screw fixation. The type of fracture and its location should inform the surgeon's decision making, but with the caveat that simpler always is better in order to minimize soft-tissue dissection and subsequent scarring and tendon or joint dysfunction. Although plate fixation increases biomechanical strength, complications including nonunion, stiffness, and tendon irritation can occur. Many if not all plates placed near a gliding tendon must be removed during a secondary procedure. Bioabsorbable plates and screws have been used, but a delayed foreign body reaction around these implants may cause osteolysis and or an inflammatory soft-tissue response necessitating surgical débridement.[38] A prospective study of plate fixation in 21 patients with closed multiple metacarpal fractures found fewer complications than previously reported.[39] Eighteen patients (86%) had 100% union with an excellent functional outcome. No hardware or tendon irritation was reported. Five patients had infection that resolved without surgical treatment.

An intra-articular metacarpal base fracture of the thumb is called a Bennett or Rolando fracture. In a Bennett fracture, the shaft is displaced by the intact abductor pollicis longus and adductor pollicis tendons, but the proximal ulnar fragment remains attached by the volar oblique ligament. Surgical treatment typically is required to maintain the reduction. The most commonly used technique after an appropriate reduction is percutaneous Kirschner wire fixation; it is not necessary for the wire to pass through the small palmar fragment because a reduced thumb ray will heal and maintain the thumb–index finger web span and pinch function. A long-term follow-up study of 24 Bennett fractures treated with screw fixation found good clinical results with maintenance of reduction.[40] Seven patients had radiographic signs of arthritis that were not correlated with clinical symptoms or the accuracy of fracture reduction. In a report of arthroscopically assisted fixation, the 1-R and 1-U portals were used for intra-articular visualization and confirmation of reduction.[41] A Rolando fracture is characterized by comminution of the thumb metacarpal base that leaves the shaft without a bony connection to the basal joint. The extent of comminution complicates surgical treatment, but ligamentotaxis provided by monolateral external fixation had encouraging results.[42]

Dislocation can occur in any MCP joint as a result of a hyperextension injury but is most common in the index finger. The initial treatment consists of attempted closed reduction; longitudinal traction and hyperextension must be avoided because they can cause incarceration of the

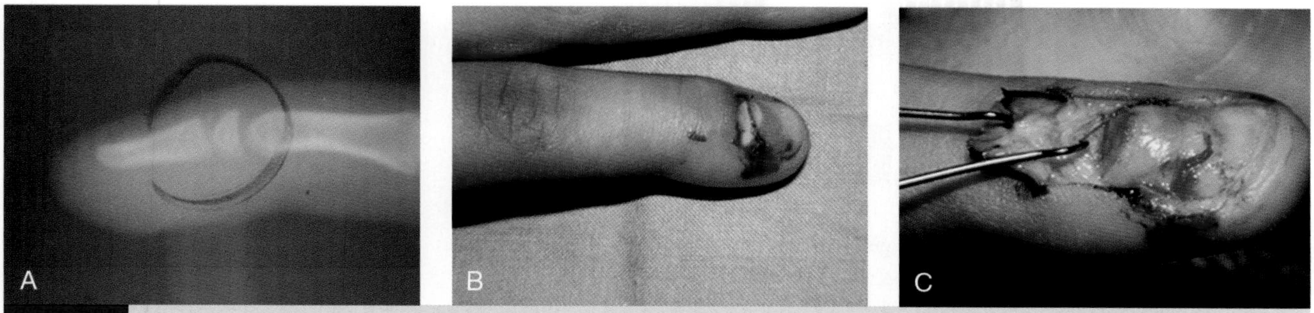

Figure 3 **A**, Lateral radiograph showing subtle distal phalanx physeal widening (circled). **B**, Clinical photograph showing a suspected Seymour fracture. **C**, Intraoperative photograph showing interposition of the germinal matrix.

volar plate in the joint. Postreduction radiographs should be scrutinized for joint space widening, which can indicate interposition of the volar plate. A dislocation may not be reducible because of volar plate or sesamoid interposition, and open reduction may be required using a palmar or dorsal approach. The palmar approach requires care to protect the digital nerves. After reduction the joint must be protected in a splint and may benefit from the use of a transarticular Kirschner wire for several weeks while the capsular injury heals.

Phalangeal Fractures and Dislocations

Phalangeal fractures are common in patients at any age. A careful examination should include assessment for the presence of rotational or angular deformities and wounds. The standard radiographs include the AP, lateral, and oblique views. Because stiffness is common after these injuries, treatment decision making must balance maintaining the reduction with splinting against early mobilization to preserve tendon gliding and joint mobility. A nondisplaced or minimally displaced proximal phalanx fracture can be treated with splinting for 1 to 2 weeks, followed by protected mobilization with buddy taping to an adjacent finger. A displaced fracture often has apex volar angulation because of the deforming flexion forces of the intrinsic muscles on the proximal fragment and the unopposed pull of the extensor tendon on the distal fragment. Displaced fractures can be treated with closed reduction and intramedullary Kirschner wire fixation in an oblique crossed or transarticular pattern (always leaving the proximal interphalangeal [PIP] joint free). A comparison of the two techniques found similar outcomes as well as complications including stiffness and the need for secondary procedures.[43] Spiral and long oblique proximal phalanx fractures are unstable and often require surgical fixation. These fractures lend themselves to lag screw fixation orthogonal to the fracture line. Intramedullary Kirschner wires can be used in a stacked configuration to control length and rotation. Debate remains over the use of two or three screws, despite a biomechanical study that found similar stability in two- and three-screw constructs. The length of the fracture dictates whether it is possible to add a third screw.[44]

Middle phalanx fractures are managed in a fashion similar to that for proximal phalanx fractures. However, either apex volar or dorsal angulation is possible in a middle phalanx fracture. A fracture proximal to the flexor digitorum superficialis typically has apex dorsal angulation because of extension of the proximal fragment through the central slip. Fractures distal to the flexor digitorum superficialis insertion may have an apex volar deformity.

Most distal phalanx fractures are treated with closed reduction and splinting. A distal phalanx fracture must be evaluated for an accompanying nail bed injury requiring nail removal and nail bed repair. In pediatric patients it is important to be aware of a possible Seymour fracture, in which unrecognized incarceration of the germinal matrix at the fracture site can lead to deformity, physeal arrest, or infection (**Figure 3**). A Seymour fracture originally was described as a distal phalanx metaphyseal fracture of skeletally immature patients. The finger typically adopts a flexed posture similar to that of a mallet injury as the extensor tendon inserts on the epiphysis while the flexor tendon inserts on the metaphysis. Closed reduction can be attempted, although interposition of the germinal matrix often necessitates open reduction. A properly treated Seymour fracture typically has a good clinical outcome with a normal range of motion and a cosmetically acceptable nail.[45]

PIP Joint Injuries

The PIP joint is the most commonly injured joint in the hand because of its relatively exposed position and long lever arm. The volar plate and the radial and ulnar

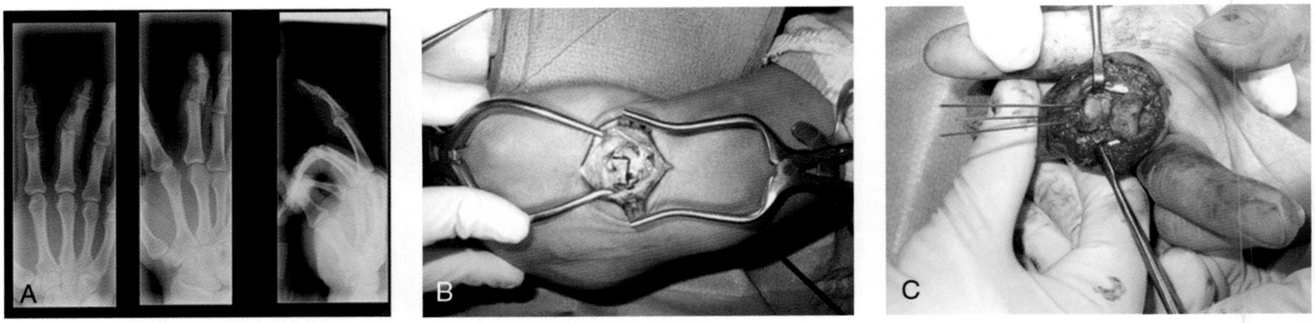

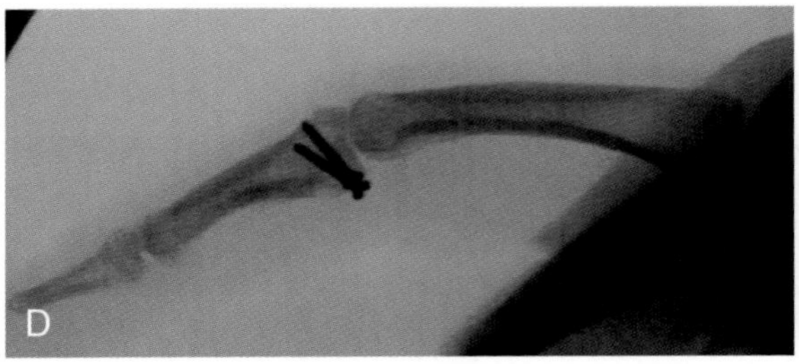

Figure 4 **A,** Preoperative PA (left), oblique (center), and lateral (right) radiographs showing a dorsal PIP joint fracture-dislocation. **B,** Intraoperative photograph showing the harvest of dorsal hamate graft. **C,** Intraoperative photograph showing temporary Kirschner wire fixation in a hemihamate arthroplasty. **D,** Postoperative lateral radiograph showing anatomic reduction of the PIP joint.

collateral ligaments are important stabilizers of the PIP joint, in addition to the bony constraints. PIP joint injuries range from simple ligamentous sprains to comminuted intra-articular fractures and fracture-dislocations. On physical examination all digits must be assessed for deformity, malrotation, and angulation as well as puckering of the skin suggesting soft-tissue interposition. After reduction, stress testing should be used to assess active stability and the integrity of the volar plate, collateral ligaments, and flexor-extensor tendons.

Simple PIP joint dislocations without bony injury can be managed with closed reduction and early protected motion. Care should be taken to avoid interposition of the volar plate, particularly during reduction of a dorsal PIP joint dislocation. Volar PIP joint dislocation is less common than dorsal PIP joint dislocation and can be associated with an injury to the central slip. Volar PIP joint dislocation without fracture can be treated with closed reduction and splinting in extension. A stable fracture-dislocation can be managed nonsurgically, although surgical treatment is required for an incongruous reduction or a fracture with joint involvement greater than 40%. Adequate treatment of a volar PIP joint dislocation is imperative for avoiding a boutonniere deformity because of disruption of the central slip insertion.

Dorsal PIP joint fracture-dislocations can be managed with closed reduction and a dorsal extension blocking splint, provided the joint is congruent and the volar fragment is less than 40% of the articular surface on the lateral radiograph. Several surgical techniques are used for an unstable dorsal PIP joint fracture-dislocation. Percutaneous reduction and pinning through a volar approach was combined with dorsal block pinning in six patients.[46] At minimum 6-month follow-up, the mean PIP joint motion was from 4° to 93°, and the mean Disabilities of the Arm, Shoulder and Hand score was 8. No complications were reported. Because of the anatomic similarities of the dorsal hamate and the volar base of the middle phalanx, hemihamate arthroplasty has been used to treated dorsal PIP joint fracture-dislocations (**Figure 4**). In a retrospective review of 11 patients treated with hemihamate arthroplasty, the average PIP joint motion was 85.4°, grip strength was 94.5% compared with that of the contralateral limb, and the Disabilities of the Arm, Shoulder and Hand score was 4.8 at a mean 38-week follow-up.[47] All patients had radiographic union by 16-week follow-up, and only one patient required reoperation for removal of prominent screws. This procedure is highly technical and requires precise bone cuts to achieve union and adequate stability. Resorption of the graft has been reported.[48] Volar plate arthroplasty is compromised by a high incidence of resubluxation, and tensioning of the volar plate advancement to decrease the risk can lead to flexion contracture. In contrast to PIP joint fracture-dislocations, all pilon fractures, which have a comminuted impaction articular fragment, are unstable injuries because the ligamentous and bony stabilizers of the PIP joint are compromised. Dynamic spanning distraction provided by external fixation is successful for treating both unstable PIP joint fracture-dislocations and pilon injuries.

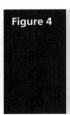

Summary

Despite the prevalence of hand fractures and dislocations, there is no consensus on the optimal treatment to limit joint stiffness. A thorough clinical evaluation guides the differential diagnosis and bolsters the need for further imaging in the setting of negative radiographs. Treatment algorithms must balance fracture stability and immobilization with preservation of tendon gliding and joint mobilization to obtain optimal clinical outcomes. Further research is needed to establish evidence-based indications for surgical and nonsurgical treatment of hand fractures.

Key Study Points

- Displaced scaphoid fractures are poorly tolerated and require surgical fixation.
- Fracture displacement leading to a predictable collapse pattern of carpal instability must be recognized so that appropriate treatment can be provided.
- Percutaneous, limited open, and arthroscopic fixation techniques continue to be developed for treatment of hand and carpal fractures and dislocations.

Annotated References

1. Hove LM: Epidemiology of scaphoid fractures in Bergen, Norway. *Scand J Plast Reconstr Surg Hand Surg* 1999;33(4):423-426.

2. Mallee WH, Henny EP, van Dijk CN, Kamminga SP, van Enst WA, Kloen P: Clinical diagnostic evaluation for scaphoid fractures: A systematic review and meta-analysis. *J Hand Surg Am* 2014;39(9):1683-1691.e2.

   In a systematic review of clinical predictors of scaphoid fracture, anatomic snuffbox tenderness was the most sensitive examination finding. The limited specificity of examination findings could lead to overtreatment. Level of evidence: II.

3. Duckworth AD, Buijze GA, Moran M, et al: Predictors of fracture following suspected injury to the scaphoid. *J Bone Joint Surg Br* 2012;94(7):961-968.

   Independent predictors were identified in a prospective evaluation of 223 suspected scaphoid fractures. The 72 patients without snuffbox tenderness within 72 hours (32%) did not have a fracture. Level of evidence: II.

4. Yin ZG, Zhang JB, Kan SL, Wang XG: Diagnostic accuracy of imaging modalities for suspected scaphoid fractures: Meta-analysis combined with latent class analysis. *J Bone Joint Surg Br* 2012;94(8):1077-1085.

   A meta-analysis of the diagnostic accuracy of scaphoid imaging modalities used latent class analysis to compensate for the absence of a gold standard. The most accurate modality was MRI, with sensitivity of 97.7% and specificity of 99.8%. Level of evidence: II.

5. Foex B, Speake P, Body R: Best evidence topic report. Magnetic resonance imaging or bone scintigraphy in the diagnosis of plain x ray occult scaphoid fractures. *Emerg Med J* 2005;22(6):434-435.

6. Ring D, Lozano-Calderón S: Imaging for suspected scaphoid fracture. *J Hand Surg Am* 2008;33(6):954-957.

7. Yin ZG, Zhang JB, Gong KT. Cost-effectiveness of diagnostic strategies for suspected scaphoid fractures. *J Orthop Trauma* 2015;29(8):e245-52.

   A cost-effectiveness analysis of diagnostic strategies for scaphoid fracture identified immediate CT ($2,553) as the most cost-effective method, assuming significant productivity loss. If productivity loss was minimal, 2-week radiography was the preferred strategy. Level of evidence: II.

8. Buijze GA, Ochtman L, Ring D: Management of scaphoid nonunion. *J Hand Surg Am* 2012;37(5):1095-1100; quiz 1101.

   A review article discussed the natural history, evaluation, imaging, and treatment of scaphoid nonunion. Level of evidence: V.

9. Buijze GA, Doornberg JN, Ham JS, Ring D, Bhandari M, Poolman RW: Surgical compared with conservative treatment for acute nondisplaced or minimally displaced scaphoid fractures: A systematic review and meta-analysis of randomized controlled trials. *J Bone Joint Surg Am* 2010;92(6):1534-1544.

   This review article suggested that the standardized functional outcome of displaced scaphoid fractures was significantly better after surgical treatment than after nonsurgical treatment. A nonsignificantly increased rate of complications was associated with surgical treatment. Level of evidence: II.

10. Ibrahim T, Qureshi A, Sutton AJ, Dias JJ: Surgical versus nonsurgical treatment of acute minimally displaced and undisplaced scaphoid waist fractures: Pairwise and network meta-analyses of randomized controlled trials. *J Hand Surg Am* 2011;36(11):1759-1768.e1.

    With union as the primary outcome, no significant difference was identified between surgical and nonsurgical treatment of scaphoid waist fractures. The risk of complications was significantly increased with surgical treatment. Level of evidence: II.

11. Hannemann PF, van Wezenbeek MR, Kolkman KA, et al: CT scan-evaluated outcome of pulsed electromagnetic fields in the treatment of acute scaphoid fractures: A randomised, multicentre, double-blind, placebo-controlled trial. *Bone Joint J* 2014;96-B(8):1070-1076.

A randomized controlled study did not identify a significant difference in the functional or radiographic outcomes of nonsurgically treated scaphoid fractures, with or without pulse electromagnetic field bone simulation. Level of evidence: I.

12. Buijze GA, Goslings JC, Rhemrev SJ, et al; CAST Trial Collaboration: Cast immobilization with and without immobilization of the thumb for nondisplaced and minimally displaced scaphoid waist fractures: A multicenter, randomized, controlled trial. *J Hand Surg Am* 2014;39(4):621-627.

    A randomized controlled study found no difference in the overall union rate or functional scores in scaphoid fractures treated with or without thumb immobilization. Thumb immobilization appeared to be unnecessary in a nondisplaced fracture. Level of evidence: II.

13. Eastley N, Singh H, Dias JJ, Taub N: Union rates after proximal scaphoid fractures: Meta-analyses and review of available evidence. *J Hand Surg Eur Vol* 2013;38(8):888-897.

    The risk of proximal pole scaphoid fracture nonunion after nonsurgical management was 7.5 times greater than for scaphoid waist fractures. An overall 34% nonunion rate after nonsurgical management of proximal pole fractures was found. Level of evidence: III.

14. McCallister WV, Knight J, Kaliappan R, Trumble TE: Central placement of the screw in simulated fractures of the scaphoid waist: A biomechanical study. *J Bone Joint Surg Am* 2003;85(1):72-77.

15. Chan KW, McAdams TR: Central screw placement in percutaneous screw scaphoid fixation: A cadaveric comparison of proximal and distal techniques. *J Hand Surg Am* 2004;29(1):74-79.

16. Faucher GK, Golden ML III, Sweeney KR, Hutton WC, Jarrett CD: Comparison of screw trajectory on stability of oblique scaphoid fractures: A mechanical study. *J Hand Surg Am* 2014;39(3):430-435.

    A cadaver study found no difference in mechanical testing of central and eccentric screws in an oblique scaphoid fracture pattern. Level of evidence: V.

17. Hart A, Mansuri A, Harvey EJ, Martineau PA: Central versus eccentric internal fixation of acute scaphoid fractures. *J Hand Surg Am* 2013;38(1):66-71.

    Cross-sectional bony apposition was compared in distal oblique, waist, and proximal pole fractures with eccentric and central scaphoid screw placement. Eccentric placement maximized bony surface apposition in distal oblique fractures. Level of evidence: V.

18. Meermans G, Van Glabbeek F, Braem MJ, van Riet RP, Hubens G, Verstreken F: Comparison of two percutaneous volar approaches for screw fixation of scaphoid waist fractures: Radiographic and biomechanical study of an osteotomy-simulated model. *J Bone Joint Surg Am* 2014;96(16):1369-1376.

    A cadaver comparison of volar percutaneous approaches found that a transtrapezial approach offers better central screw position and confers a biomechanical advantage compared with a standard volar approach that avoids the trapezium. Level of evidence: V.

19. Geurts G, van Riet R, Meermans G, Verstreken F: Incidence of scaphotrapezial arthritis following volar percutaneous fixation of nondisplaced scaphoid waist fractures using a transtrapezial approach. *J Hand Surg Am* 2011;36(11):1753-1758.

    A retrospective review of a transtrapezial approach to scaphoid fixation did not identify increased risk of scaphotrapezial osteoarthritis at an average 6.1-year follow-up. Level of evidence: IV.

20. Schmitt R, Christopoulos G, Wagner M, et al: Avascular necrosis (AVN) of the proximal fragment in scaphoid nonunion: Is intravenous contrast agent necessary in MRI? *Eur J Radiol* 2011;77(2):222-227.

    A prospective evaluation of the diagnostic usefulness of contrast-enhanced MRI for osteonecrosis in scaphoid nonunion compared imaging with intraoperative findings. Contrast-enhanced MRI was significantly more sensitive than nonenhanced MRI (76.5% versus 6.3%). Level of evidence: III.

21. Somerson JS, Fletcher DJ, Srinivasan RC, Green DP: Compression screw fixation without bone grafting for scaphoid fibrous nonunion. *Hand (N Y)* 2015;10(3):450-453.

    A retrospective review of 14 patients treated with compression screw fixation alone found an average time to union of 4.4 months. Twelve patients had union, and two required vascular bone grafting. Level of evidence: IV.

22. Cohen MS, Jupiter JB, Fallahi K, Shukla SK: Scaphoid waist nonunion with humpback deformity treated without structural bone graft. *J Hand Surg Am* 2013;38(4):701-705.

    In a retrospective review, 12 scaphoid waist nonunions were treated using a volar approach and screw fixation with ipsilateral distal radius cancellous bone graft. At 2-year follow-up, all patients achieved union. The average Disabilities of the Arm, Shoulder and Hand score was 4. Level of evidence: IV.

23. Sayegh ET, Strauch RJ: Graft choice in the management of unstable scaphoid nonunion: A systematic review. *J Hand Surg Am* 2014;39(8):1500-6.e7.

    A review of graft choice in the treatment of scaphoid nonunion showed that cancellous graft provided the shortest time to union but that corticocancellous graft achieved the most consistent deformity correction. Level of evidence: IV.

24. Mathoulin CL, Haerle M: Vascularized bone grafts from the volar distal radius to treat scaphoid nonunion. *J Am Soc Surg Hand* 2004;4(1):4-10.

25. Bürger HK, Windhofer C, Gaggl AJ, Higgins JP: Vascularized medial femoral trochlea osteocartilaginous flap

reconstruction of proximal pole scaphoid nonunions. *J Hand Surg Am* 2013;38(4):690-700.

A retrospective review of a novel technique to reconstruct chronic proximal pole nonunions with a vascularized medial femoral trochlea flap found that 12 of 16 patients had complete pain relief. Level of evidence: IV.

26. Oduwole KO, Cichy B, Dillon JP, Wilson J, O'Beirne J: Acutrak versus Herbert screw fixation for scaphoid nonunion and delayed union. *J Orthop Surg (Hong Kong)* 2012;20(1):61-65.

A retrospective single surgeon case control series of Acutrak and Herbert screw fixation demonstrated higher union rates with Acutrak screw. However, Acutrak screws were more likely to be placed accurately which also predicted union. Level of evidence: III.

27. Hey HW, Chong AK, Murphy D: Prevalence of carpal fracture in Singapore. *J Hand Surg Am* 2011;36(2):278-283.

A review of all patients treated for carpal fractures at a tertiary referral center in Singapore found that nonscaphoid carpal fractures accounted for 34% of all carpal fractures. Level of evidence: IV.

28. Lee SJ, Rathod CM, Park KW, Hwang JH: Persistent ulnar-sided wrist pain after treatment of triquetral dorsal chip fracture: Six cases related to triangular fibrocartilage complex injury. *Arch Orthop Trauma Surg* 2012;132(5):671-676.

A retrospective review of six patients with persistent ulnar wrist pain after triquetral chip fracture treatment found that débridement for arthroscopic triangular fibrocartilage complex injury led to significant improvement in Mayo wrist scores and grip strength. Level of evidence: V.

29. Wright TW, Moser MW, Sahajpal DT: Hook of hamate pull test. *J Hand Surg Am* 2010;35(11):1887-1889.

A novel physical examination test was described to aid in the diagnosis of hook of hamate fractures. In full ulnar deviation, flexion of the ulnar digits was resisted to create a displacing force on the hook of hamate. Level of evidence: V.

30. Devers BN, Douglas KC, Naik RD, Lee DH, Watson JT, Weikert DR: Outcomes of hook of hamate fracture excision in high-level amateur athletes. *J Hand Surg Am* 2013;38(1):72-76.

Twelve hook of hamate fractures in athletes were treated with excision. All patients returned to sport without functional impairment at an average of 6 weeks. Level of evidence: IV.

31. Kain N, Heras-Palou C: Trapezoid fractures: Report of 11 cases. *J Hand Surg Am* 2012;37(6):1159-1162.

Eleven trapezoid fractures were reviewed. The diagnosis was found to be difficult. CT was recommended if clinical suspicion persisted despite negative radiographs. Level of evidence: IV.

32. Mayfield JK, Johnson RP, Kilcoyne RK: Carpal dislocations: Pathomechanics and progressive perilunar instability. *J Hand Surg Am* 1980;5(3):226-241.

33. Kim JP, Lee JS, Park MJ: Arthroscopic reduction and percutaneous fixation of perilunate dislocations and fracture-dislocations. *Arthroscopy* 2012;28(2):196-203.e2.

A retrospective review of 20 perilunate injuries treated arthroscopically reported a mean Disabilities of the Arm, Shoulder and Hand score of 8 at follow-up. Radiographic evaluation revealed acceptable reduction in 15 patients. Level of evidence: IV.

34. Forli A, Courvoisier A, Wimsey S, Corcella D, Moutet F: Perilunate dislocations and transscaphoid perilunate fracture-dislocations: A retrospective study with minimum ten-year follow-up. *J Hand Surg Am* 2010;35(1):62-68.

At long-term follow-up, 12 of 18 patients with perilunate dislocation or transscaphoid perilunate fracture-dislocation had degenerative changes. There were no between-group differences. Level of evidence: IV.

35. Strauch RJ, Rosenwasser MP, Lunt JG: Metacarpal shaft fractures: The effect of shortening on the extensor tendon mechanism. *J Hand Surg Am* 1998;23(3):519-523.

36. Hofmeister EP, Kim J, Shin AY: Comparison of 2 methods of immobilization of fifth metacarpal neck fractures: A prospective randomized study. *J Hand Surg Am* 2008;33(8):1362-1368.

37. Strub B, Schindele S, Sonderegger J, Sproedt J, von Campe A, Gruenert JG: Intramedullary splinting or conservative treatment for displaced fractures of the little finger metacarpal neck? A prospective study. *J Hand Surg Eur Vol* 2010;35(9):725-729.

A prospective study of 40 patients with a small finger metacarpal neck fracture and volar angulation of 30° to 70° found no functional advantage to intramedullary pinning compared with immobilization, but there was a cosmetic advantage. Level of evidence: II.

38. Givissis PK, Stavridis SI, Papagelopoulos PJ, Antonarakos PD, Christodoulou AG: Delayed foreign-body reaction to absorbable implants in metacarpal fracture treatment. *Clin Orthop Relat Res* 2010;468(12):3377-3383.

A retrospective review of 10 patients with metacarpal fracture treated with a bioabsorbable implant found a delayed foreign body reaction necessitating surgical débridement in 4 patients. Level of evidence: IV.

39. Soni A, Gulati A, Bassi JL, Singh D, Saini UC: Outcome of closed ipsilateral metacarpal fractures treated with mini fragment plates and screws: A prospective study. *J Orthop Traumatol* 2012;13(1):29-33.

A retrospective review of 21 patients with multiple ipsilateral metacarpal fractures treated with plate fixation found a 100% union rate and average Disabilities of the Arm, Shoulder and Hand score of 8.47. Five infections were noted. Level of evidence: IV.

40. Leclère FM, Jenzer A, Hüsler R, et al: 7-year follow-up after open reduction and internal screw fixation in Bennett fractures. *Arch Orthop Trauma Surg* 2012;132(7):1045-1051.

A retrospective review of 24 Bennett fractures at average 83-month follow-up found maintenance of fracture reduction with two lag screws. No correlation was found between the accuracy of the reduction and the development of arthritis. Level of evidence: IV.

41. Culp RW, Johnson JW: Arthroscopically assisted percutaneous fixation of Bennett fractures. *J Hand Surg Am* 2010;35(1):137-140.

A novel technique was described for the treatment of Bennett fractures, in which arthroscopic visualization was used to confirm accurate articular reduction. Level of evidence: V.

42. Marsland D, Sanghrajka AP, Goldie B: Static monolateral external fixation for the Rolando fracture: A simple solution for a complex fracture. *Ann R Coll Surg Engl* 2012;94(2):112-115.

A retrospective review of eight Rolando fractures treated with monolateral external fixation found no evidence of malunion. All patients returned to their preinjury level of activity. Three pin site infections occurred. Level of evidence: IV.

43. Faruqui S, Stern PJ, Kiefhaber TR: Percutaneous pinning of fractures in the proximal third of the proximal phalanx: Complications and outcomes. *J Hand Surg Am* 2012;37(7):1342-1348.

A retrospective case control study of transarticular versus extra-articular pinning of proximal third proximal phalanx fractures found no difference in motion. The overall average PIP joint flexion loss was 27°. Level of evidence: III.

44. Zelken JA, Hayes AG, Parks BG, Al Muhit A, Means KR Jr: Two versus 3 lag screws for fixation of long oblique proximal phalanx fractures of the fingers: A cadaver study. *J Hand Surg Am* 2015;40(6):1124-1129.

A cadaver study found equivalent biomechanical stability in two- and three-screw fixation for proximal phalanx oblique fractures. Two-screw fixation may be more cost- and time-effective. Level of evidence: V.

45. Krusche-Mandl I, Köttstorfer J, Thalhammer G, Aldrian S, Erhart J, Platzer P: Seymour fractures: Retrospective analysis and therapeutic considerations. *J Hand Surg Am* 2013;38(2):258-264.

A retrospective review of 24 Seymour fractures found that patients had a normal range of motion and an acceptable nail appearance. Level of evidence: IV.

46. Vitale MA, White NJ, Strauch RJ: A percutaneous technique to treat unstable dorsal fracture-dislocations of the proximal interphalangeal joint. *J Hand Surg Am* 2011;36(9):1453-1459.

Postoperative motion was good, with an average Disabilities of the Arm, Shoulder and Hand score of 8, in six dorsal PIP fracture-dislocations treated with percutaneous fixation. Level of evidence: IV.

47. Yang DS, Lee SK, Kim KJ, Choy WS: Modified hemihamate arthroplasty technique for treatment of acute proximal interphalangeal joint fracture-dislocations. *Ann Plast Surg* 2014;72(4):411-416.

A retrospective review of hemihamate arthroplasty for the treatment of PIP fracture-dislocations found a supple range of motion and an average Disabilities of the Arm, Shoulder and Hand score of 4.8 at a mean 38-month follow-up. Level of evidence: IV.

48. Afendras G, Abramo A, Mrkonjic A, Geijer M, Kopylov P, Tägil M: Hemi-hamate osteochondral transplantation in proximal interphalangeal dorsal fracture dislocations: A minimum 4 year follow-up in eight patients. *J Hand Surg Eur Vol* 2010;35(8):627-631.

A retrospective review of eight hemihamate arthroplasty for PIP fracture dislocation noted mean 67° degree PIP motion. Graft resorption with intra-articular screw migration was noted in one patient. Level of evidence: IV.

Chapter 28

Degloving Injuries in the Upper Extremity

Alexander B. Dagum, MD, FRCS(C), FACS   Mark Gelfand, MD

Abstract

A degloving injury usually is a high-energy injury that results in an avulsion of the skin at the suprafascial level, often with injury to the underlying structures. Degloving injuries are uncommon in the upper extremity. Prompt attention is required. The recommended treatment is based on the most current available evidence. The initial management focuses on evaluation of the extent of injury. Irrigation and débridement are done, with fasciotomy and bony stabilization as needed as well as any appropriate repair of associated injured structures. The avulsed skin flap is assessed for its viability and potential for revascularization. In the palm or digits (the so-called nonexpendable areas), it is important to make every attempt at revascularization. In the so-called expendable areas revascularization is done through arteriovenous shunting and/or proximal venous anastomosis, if possible. Avulsed tissue that cannot be revascularized is excised, and skin that is not severely contused or abraded is defatted and applied as a full-thickness skin graft. Flap coverage of vital structures, bone, tendon, ligament, or hardware is done as soon as the wound is clean and stable. Secondary surgery is often required.

Keywords: avulsion injury; arteriovenous shunt; degloving injury; microsurgery; Morel-Lavallée lesion; ring avulsion injury; skin grafting; upper extremity

Neither of the following authors nor any immediate family member has received anything of value from or has stock or stock options held in a commercial company or institution related directly or indirectly to the subject of this chapter: Dr. Dagum and Dr. Gelfand.

Introduction

A soft-tissue degloving injury involves the tearing away or avulsion of skin and subcutaneous tissue, with or without avulsion or trauma of the underlying muscle, tendon, nerves, or vessels. In general, degloving injuries have a high-energy mechanism. Often there are underlying fractures.[1] These injuries are uncommon in the upper extremity, and no evidence-based guideline or consensus is available to guide treatment.[2] The management of these injuries depends on sound orthopaedic and plastic surgical principles as well as the findings of small case studies.[1,3-10]

Pathophysiology and Mechanism of Injury

Degloving injuries are the result of high-energy compressive, torsional, frictional, and/or shearing force. They were first described as wringer injuries because they were caused by the rollers on the old electric clothes wringer washing machines.[9] This mechanism of injury was low energy, and the incidence of skin injury, underlying soft-tissue injury, or fracture was low.[9,10] Currently, degloving injuries are the devastating result of motor vehicle crashes or high-energy industrial accidents involving rolling or rotatory machines.[1-7,11] The avulsion typically occurs in the suprafascial areolar plane, which is a potential space and a weak link in the soft-tissue envelope. Depending on the direction and amount of energy applied during the incident, degloving can occur through the underlying musculoligamentous structures (**Figure 1**). Injury leads to avulsion of soft tissues with devascularization caused by direct injury to the subcutaneous vascular plexus and perforating vessels.[6,12,13]

Classification and Assessment

Degloving injuries are classified as open or closed.[2,14] A closed injury (a Morel-Lavallée lesion) is uncommon in the upper extremity. Open injuries are classified by the

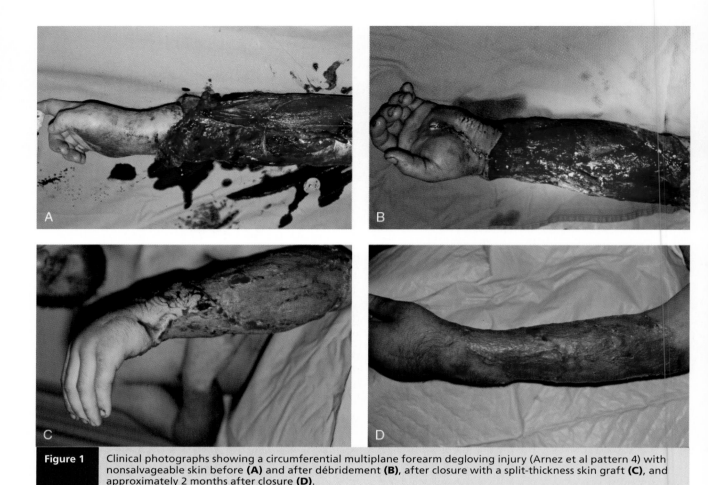

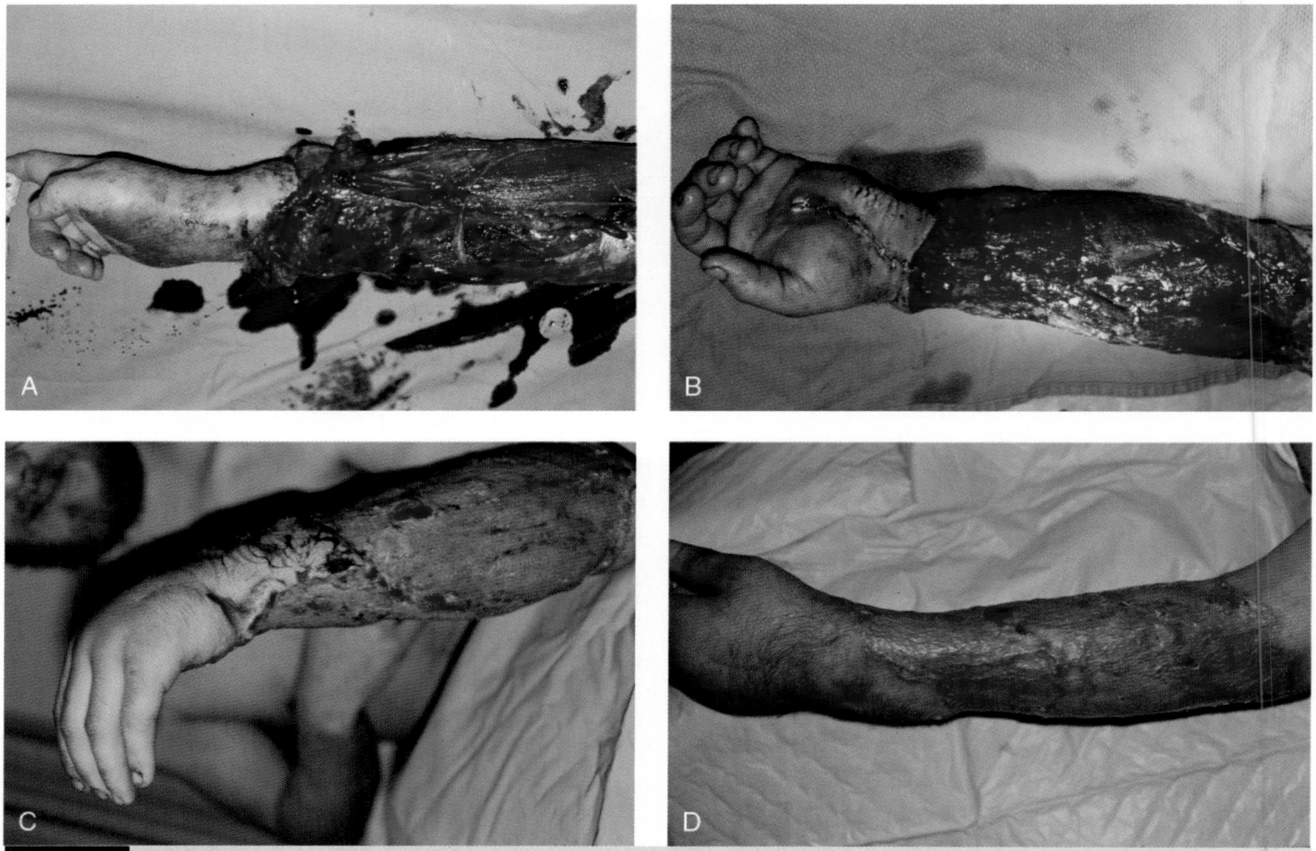

Figure 1 Clinical photographs showing a circumferential multiplane forearm degloving injury (Arnez et al pattern 4) with nonsalvageable skin before **(A)** and after débridement **(B)**, after closure with a split-thickness skin graft **(C)**, and approximately 2 months after closure **(D)**.

pattern of injury, the anatomic location, expendable versus nonexpendable tissue, and whether the degloved tissue is amenable to revascularization.

The classification by Arnez et al is based on injury severity.[5] Pattern 1 is limited degloving with abrasion avulsion (loss of tissue with minimal undermining). Pattern 2 is noncircumferential degloving, in which most of the skin is present as a flap or area of undermining. Pattern 3 is circumferential single-plane degloving, in which the degloving is confined to a single plane, usually at the subcutaneous fascial layer. Pattern 4 is circumferential multiplane degloving that includes a breach of muscle as well as the subcutaneous layer.

The Waikakul classification includes three types distinguished by the feasibility of revascularization of the degloved tissue.[4] In type I, the skin is severely damaged, and the subcutaneous tissue is not amenable to revascularization. In type II, the skin is moderately damaged, and the subcutaneous tissue has identifiable subcutaneous veins without venous back flow. In type III, the skin is not severely crushed, and the subcutaneous veins are intact with venous back flow. Serial débridement and split-thickness skin graft (STSG) closure were recommended for treating a type I injury, arteriovenous shunting with proximal venous anastomosis was recommended for a type II injury, and proximal venous anastomosis was recommended for a type III injury.

Lo et al further expanded on Waikakul's classification by addressing the upper extremity and dividing the area of degloving into nonexpendable (specialized skin of the digits and palm):[6] group 1, palm only; group 2, palm and digits and expendable skin; and group 3, forearm and dorsum of the hand. Treatment recommendations were based on their case series and they recommended proximal venous anastomosis and arteriovenous shunt for group 1, arteriovenous shunt and arterial repair for group 2, and arteriovenous shunt or traditional management for group 3.

None of these classifications is complete, but they are useful for conceptualizing and guiding treatment decisions. It is important to determine the extent of injury, assess the zone of vascular compromise, and determine whether the compromised tissue can be salvaged. The force producing a degloving injury can be severe. The damage to underlying deep structures can be extensive, and it must be assessed and treated. Especially in a patient with multiple traumatic injuries, a soft-tissue degloving injury often is underappreciated by the primary evaluating team. Even if the soft tissue was circumferentially torn and rolled back, emergency stabilization appropriately includes restoring the tissue to its correct position and bandaging the extremity, thus masking the extent of injury during a subsequent cursory examination. A delay in diagnosis is associated with increased morbidity and even mortality. Early complications associated with degloving injuries, in particular in a patient with multiple traumatic injuries, include ongoing blood loss progressing to hypovolemic shock, compartment syndrome, myonecrosis with subsequent acute tubular necrosis, and sepsis.[2,4,5,11,13] A degloving injury should be suspected in a patient with high-energy trauma and significant underlying ecchymosis, crepitus, or overlying laceration.

Evaluation and Management

Initial Evaluation

The initial examination focuses on the extent of the injured tissue, the neurovascular status of the upper extremity, detection of underlying fractures, and compartment syndrome. Multidisciplinary management in accordance with Advanced Trauma Life Support protocols is imperative. In any patient with an open wound, tetanus and early intravenous antibiotic prophylaxis should be administered.[15] The patient is taken to the operating room for evaluation of the extent of injury, débridement, fracture stabilization, and repair of the injured structures. The degloved tissue is evaluated in terms of its anatomic location, extent, and vascularity (capillary refill, temperature, turgor, and color of the skin). Pale, cold skin with no capillary refill and diminished turgor signifies the absence of arterial inflow. Skin that is blue, engorged with rapid capillary refill, and cool signifies venous congestion. The skin is assessed for bleeding by pinprick with a 21-gauge needle: slow, bright red (oxygenated) bleeding signifies well-perfused skin; rapid, dark blue bleeding, a venous outflow issue; and little or no bleeding, an arterial inflow issue.[16]

Clinical examination can be unreliable for assessing degloved tissue, even if done by an experienced surgeon. Adjunctive methods can be used to improve the accuracy of an evaluation of tissue perfusion and predict tissue survival. These methods include the use fluorescein dye and ultraviolet light (a Wood lamp), which are readily available in most hospital operating rooms. In addition, laser Doppler flowmetry and indocyanine green dye angiography (SPY Elite, Novadaq) recently were developed to quantify tissue viability.[7,17,18] The use of fluorescein dye was found to overpredict the area of necrosis by 1 to 3 cm in the degloved flap.[7,18] In a recent prospective study, indocyanine green dye angiography was found to be more accurate for predicting skin flap necrosis than clinical examination or the use of fluorescein dye.[19] The SPY Elite system is expensive and not readily available in most hospitals, but in the future indocyanine green dye angiography probably will be used in most tertiary care institutions to predict tissue survival after injury or revascularization.

Revascularization

The compromised tissue is assessed for its revascularization potential (**Figure 2**). A thrombosed or destroyed venous plexus usually cannot be revascularized, and the skin should be assessed for potential use in grafting. If the skin is not severely contused and abraded, it can be defatted and used to cover the wound bed as a full-thickness skin graft (FTSG) or STSG.[1-7,9-13,20] If the venous plexus is intact, revascularization of the degloved skin flap should be considered.[2,4,6,8,11] The underlying muscle is assessed for viability using the characteristics known as the four Cs: color (bright red versus pale), consistency (firm, does not pull away or easily tear), contractility (when stimulated with a cautery), and capillary bleeding (when cut). Devitalized muscle should be meticulously débrided, fasciotomies should be done as needed, and fractures should be fixed using general orthopaedic principles.

Wound preparation is of the outmost importance. Revascularization is not a substitute for débridement. In an extremely contaminated and or traumatized wound, such as a farm auger injury, serial débridement is required, usually every 24 hours, until all necrotic tissue is excised and a clean wound has been obtained. The goal is to close the wound within 5 days, before significant bacterial colonization has taken place. Early coverage of wounds decreases the risk of infection, edema, stiffness, and flap or graft loss; improves function; and decreases hospital length of stay.[21,22]

If a clean wound is achieved in a nonexpendable area (a Lo et al Group 1 or 2 injury of the palm or digits), every attempt should be made to revascularize the soft tissues (**Figure 3**). The sensate, glabrous skin of the palm and fingers cannot be sufficiently reconstructed using flaps or skin grafts.[6,8] The arterial perforators that supply the skin are perpendicular to the skin, and in a degloving injury the arterial perforators are avulsed and cannot be repaired. In contrast, the venous plexus runs longitudinally in the subcutaneous tissue and therefore is more protected

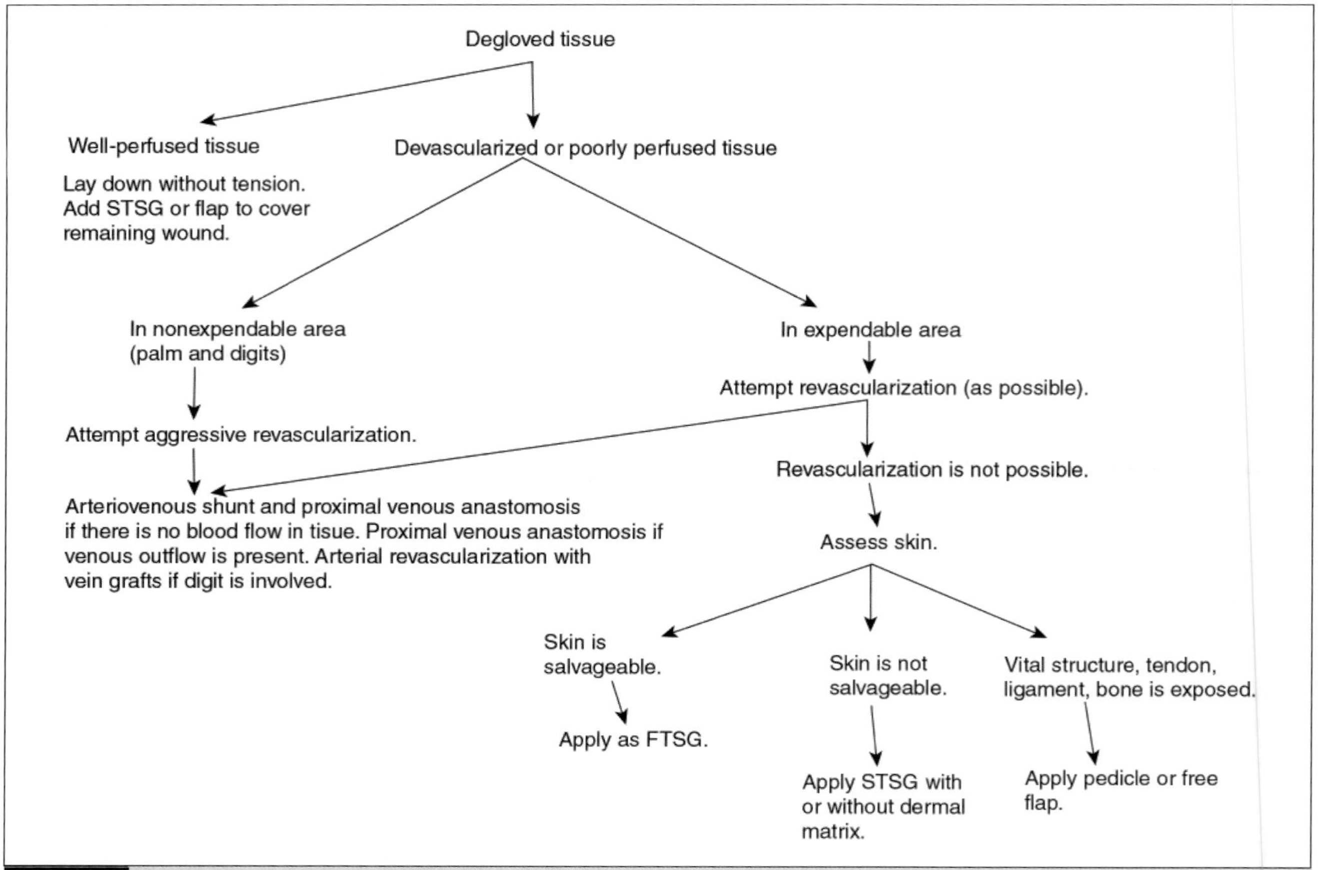

Figure 2 Algorithm for treating a degloving injury. FTSG = full thickness skin graft, STSG = split-thickness skin graft.

from injury. Arteriovenous shunting is used to revascularize the degloved tissue. The concept of arteriovenous shunting to perfuse a flap first was proposed and proved experimentally in 1981. Clinical success subsequently was reported.[23-25] Arteriovenous shunting entails anastomosing a distal vein on the degloved tissue to an artery and anastomosing at least one, preferably two, proximal veins.[6,8,26-28] In the palm the palmar veins are connected proximally to the digital arteries, and the proximal palmar vein is anastomosed to an intact subcutaneous vein with the use of a vein graft if necessary. If possible, two proximal and distal repairs should be performed at the palmar level. If the degloving injury has caused devascularization of the palmar skin and digits, arteriovenous shunting of the palmar skin alone will not revitalize the fingertips, and the digits should be separately revascularized with vein grafts to the digital arteries[6] (**Figure 3**).

In an expendable area such as the dorsum of the hand, forearm (a Lo et al Group 3 injury) or upper arm, revascularization should be considered if the venous plexus is intact.[4,6] Arteriovenous shunting is recommended for a Waikakul type II injury, in which there is no venous outflow. An end-to-side anastomosis is done between the distal cephalic vein and the radial artery, or an end-to-end anastomosis is done with an expandable arterial side branch. Proximally, a venous repair usually is done with the proximal cephalic vein. In a Waikakul type III injury, in which there is some venous outflow, a venous repair is done proximally, often with a vein graft (**Figure 4**). If a vein graft cannot be done proximally in a Waikakul type III injury, often there is progressive congestion and significant necrosis of the degloved flap[4] (**Figure 3, D**). Experimental evidence supports the use of anticoagulation therapy in degloving injuries.[29] After surgery, heparin should be administered (unless contraindicated) to achieve a partial thromboplastin time 1.5 to 2 times normal. Particularly in patients with a hand and digit degloving injury, this step is useful to improve the patency of the anastomosis in the injured small vessels.

Wound Débridement and Closure

The degloved flap tissue is laid down and repaired without tension. Usually an STSG is needed for coverage of a proximal wound and vein graft, if used (**Figure 4** C, D). An

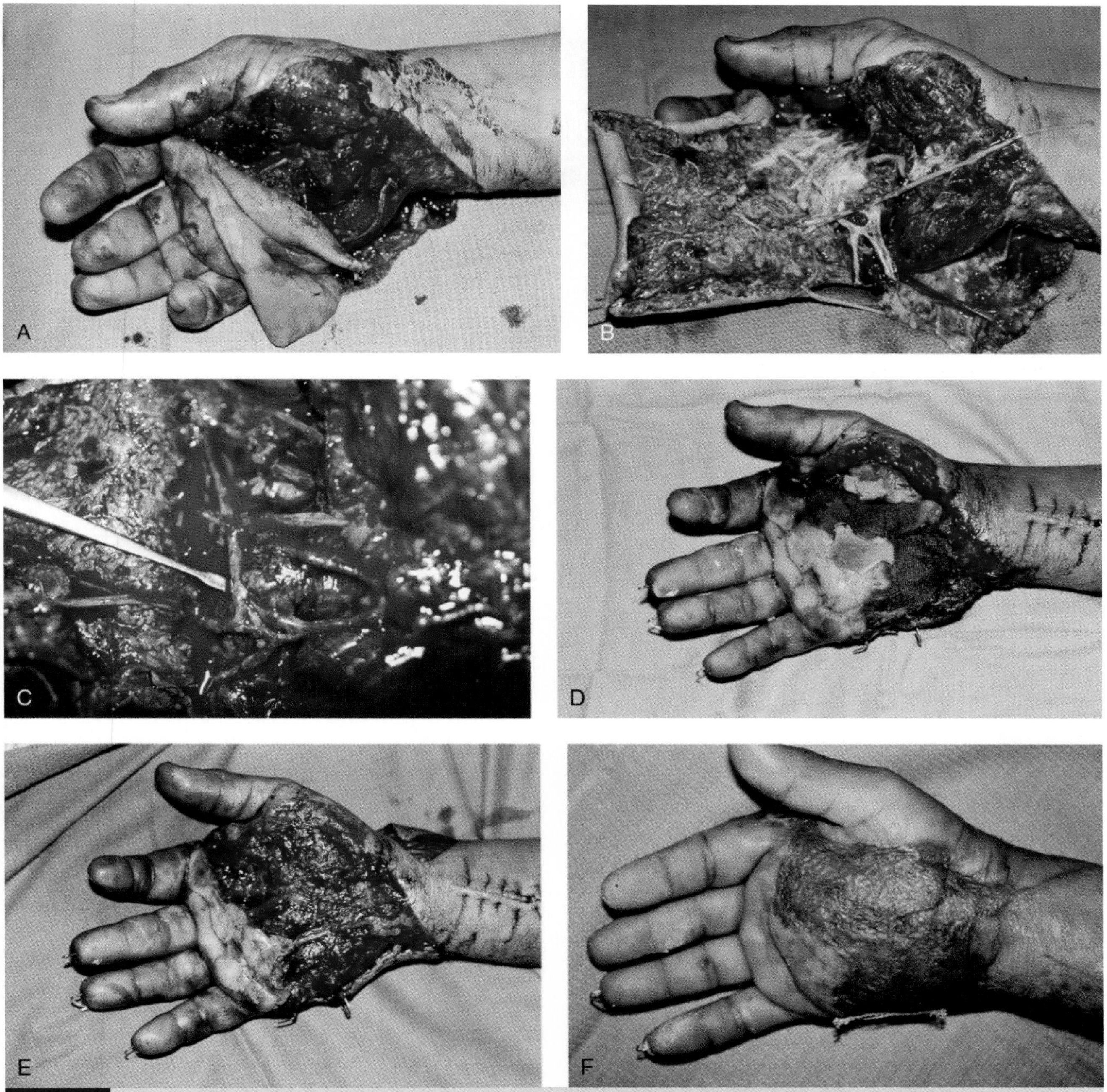

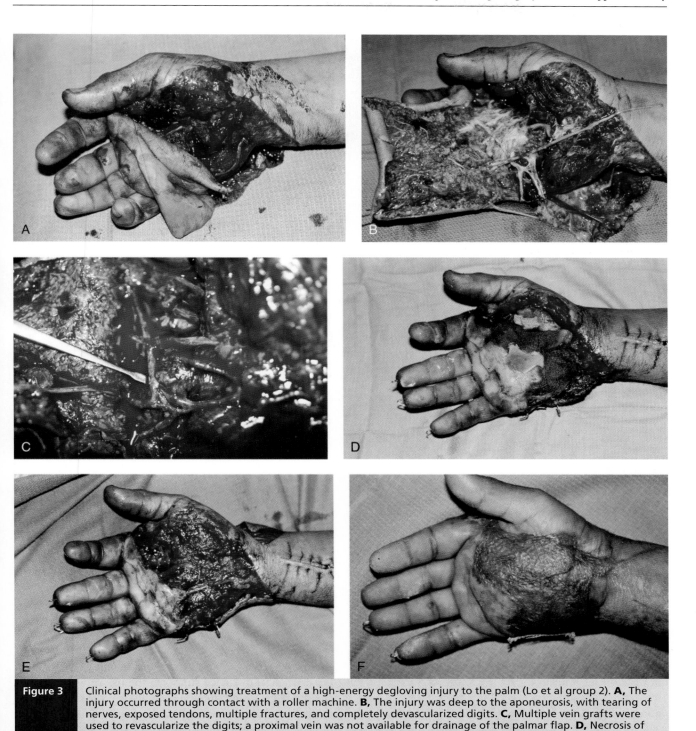

Figure 3 Clinical photographs showing treatment of a high-energy degloving injury to the palm (Lo et al group 2). **A,** The injury occurred through contact with a roller machine. **B,** The injury was deep to the aponeurosis, with tearing of nerves, exposed tendons, multiple fractures, and completely devascularized digits. **C,** Multiple vein grafts were used to revascularize the digits; a proximal vein was not available for drainage of the palmar flap. **D,** Necrosis of the proximal palmar flap is shown. The vein grafts, nerve grafts, and exposed tendons **(E)** were covered by a rectus free flap **(F)**.

attempt at primary closure with tension usually increases the necrosis of the degloved tissue. Any skin that is not amenable to revascularization but has not been severely crushed or abraded is defatted and applied as an FTSG.

In many patients revascularization is not possible, or significant underlying muscle and bone injuries necessitate serial débridement. In Arnez et al pattern 2, 3, and 4 injuries the vascularity of the degloved skin

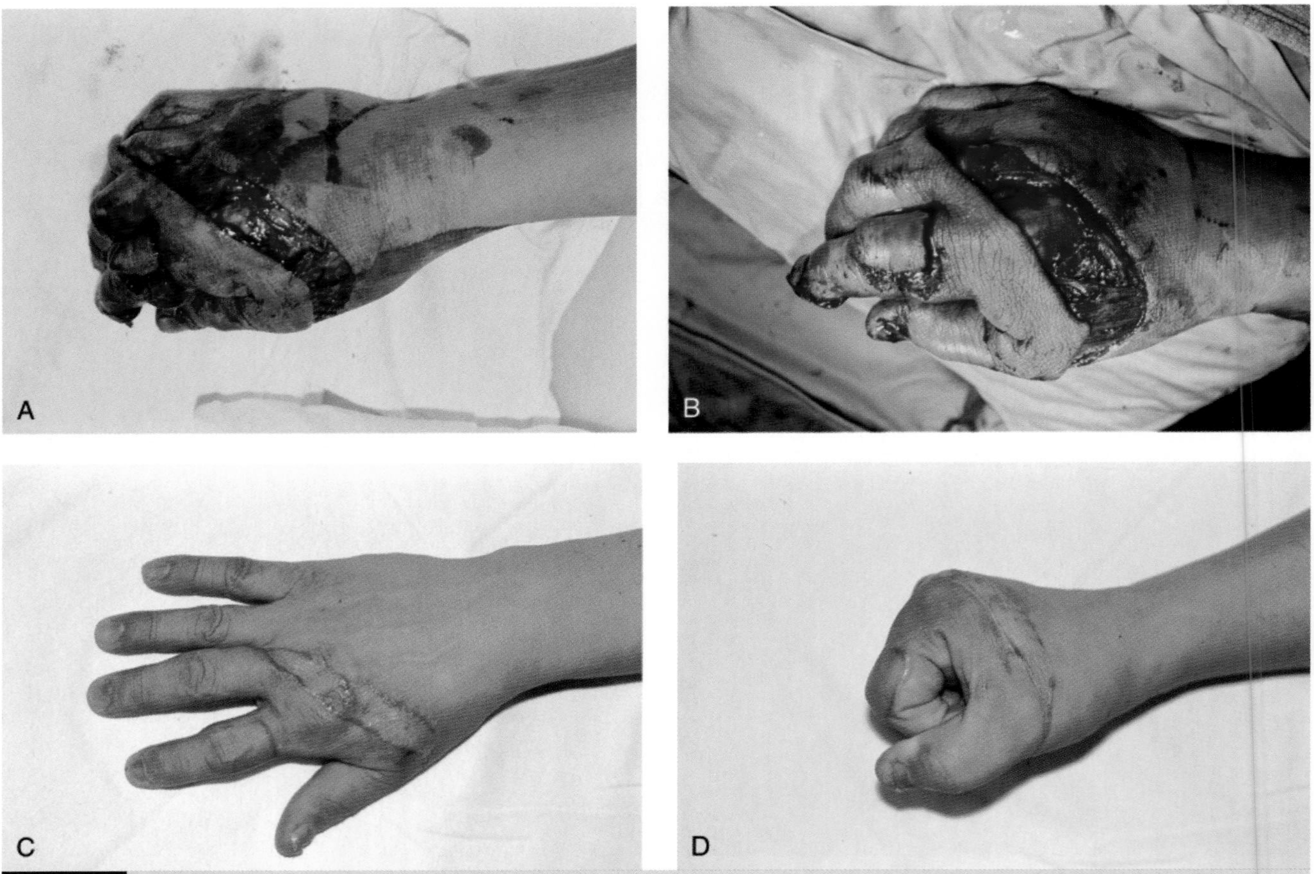

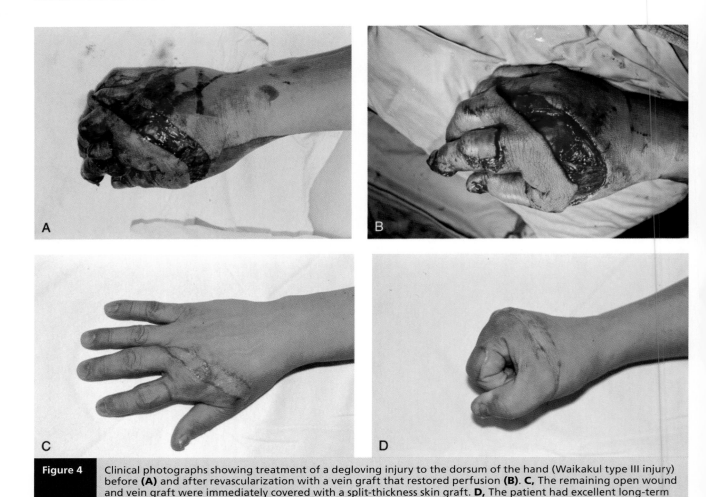

Figure 4 Clinical photographs showing treatment of a degloving injury to the dorsum of the hand (Waikakul type III injury) before **(A)** and after revascularization with a vein graft that restored perfusion **(B)**. **C,** The remaining open wound and vein graft were immediately covered with a split-thickness skin graft. **D,** The patient had excellent long-term restoration of hand function with survival of the degloved flap.

segment is assessed, and it is débrided to viable tissue. If the débrided skin is not severely injured, it is defatted for use as an FTSG. Defatted skin that is not immediately needed for coverage should be maintained for use after further débridement. The defatted skin is wrapped in sterile saline-soaked gauze, placed in a sterile container, and refrigerated at 4°C. The skin can be banked for as long as 2 weeks, but the graft is less likely to be successful after 1 week.

Sequential débridement is necessary in wounds from degloving injuries, and early closure is recommended. The wound must not become desiccated between débridements. After débridement the wound is dressed with a wet-to-dry or negative pressure wound dressing. If vital structures are exposed, a biologic dressing such as a xenograft is preferred. The timing of definitive closure depends on various factors including a stable patient with a clean wound with no evidence of infection or ongoing tissue necrosis. It is helpful to consider the plastic surgical concept of the reconstructive ladder in determining the mode of closure.[30]

An STSG is used, preferably with the patient's banked skin, in an Arnez et al pattern 1 or 2 injury that does not have extensive crossing of a joint surface, exposed vital structures, or exposed bone, ligament, or tendon.[31] If a vital structure, bone, tendon, ligament, or hardware is exposed, a fasciocutaneous or muscle flap is used for closure of the defect. A muscle flap is preferred in wounds with a large dead space, complex geometry, exposed bone, hardware, or heavy contamination (**Figure 5**). A muscle flap adheres well to bone and easily closes the dead space. In addition, a muscle flap is believed to provide a robust blood supply that combats infection by the humoral mechanism and increases antibiotic presence. Early animal studies found better outcomes in the presence of infection when muscle flaps were used compared with random or fasciocutaneous flaps.[32,33] Whether the use of muscle flaps is advantageous in comparison with axial septocutaneous

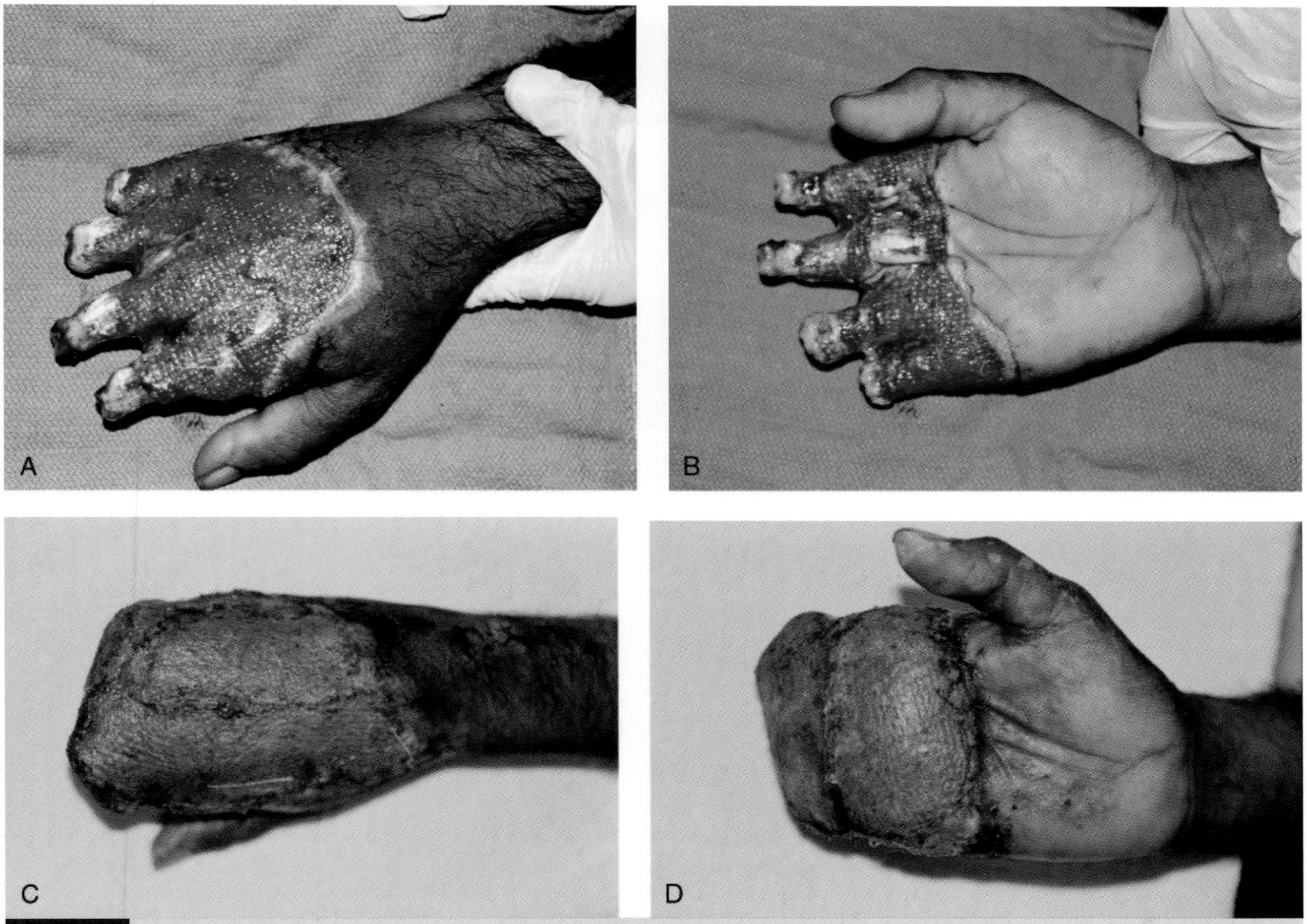

Figure 5 Clinical photographs showing a nonreplantable, multilevel degloving amputation in the dorsal **(A)** and palmar **(B)** views. **C,** A rectus free flap was used to cover the proximal phalanges to preserve length and some grip. **D,** The patient underwent subsequent syndactyly release and debulking.

or perforator flaps has come into question.[34] It is important to note that flaps are not placed in a wound that is infected but only in a wound that has been débrided and has no clinical evidence of an ongoing infection. The latissimus dorsi is the standard muscle for upper extremity muscle flap coverage. As a pedicle flap, the latissimus dorsi can reliably cover the shoulder, upper arm, and elbow as far as 8 cm distal to the olecranon.[22] For coverage of a forearm and hand degloving injury, a free flap with microvascular anastomosis usually is required. The latissimus dorsi, rectus abdominis, and gracilis are preferred for this purpose because they are reliable and lead to minimal donor deficits.

A fasciocutaneous flap is preferred for a defect that is simple, circumferential, or over a joint, tendon, or ligament. Fasciocutaneous flaps cause fewer adhesions and allow better tendon gliding and motion than muscle flaps (**Figure 6**). In an Arnez et al pattern 3 circumferential single-plane degloving injury that cannot be revascularized, with a defect deep to the fascia and degloved skin that cannot be used as an FTSG, the recommended coverage is with a large fasciocutaneous free flap (from the anterolateral thigh, scapula, or parascapula), which provides more stable coverage over the muscle and less distal edema, adhesion, and contraction than an STSG. A large pedicle thoracoabdominal flap always is an option but has the disadvantages of requiring at least two surgical stages and hindering limb elevation and motion at affected joints, thus increasing limb edema and stiffness. A pedicle thoracoabdominal flap is best used in the setting of limb salvage when no other reasonable option is available. When a flap surgery is not possible, a dermal matrix with a subsequently applied STSG is preferable to an STSG alone. The dermal matrix will not be effective if the wound bed is infected or heavily colonized with bacteria.

Many dermal substitutes have been developed over the past decade, including biologic dressings such as Integra

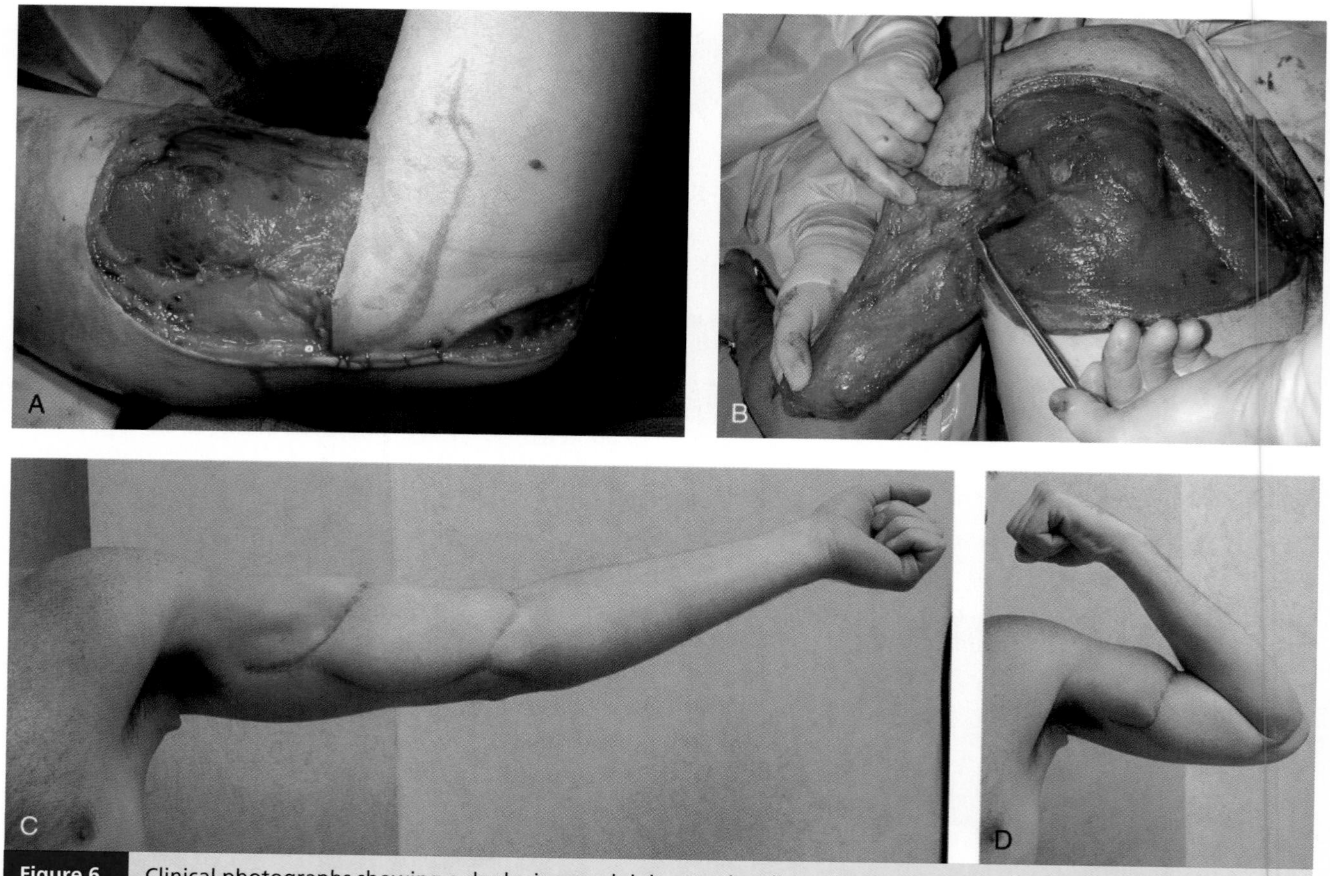

Figure 6 Clinical photographs showing a degloving crush injury to the elbow (Arnez et al pattern 2) in a 23-year-old man. **A,** The injury after débridement with a skin flap tacked proximally and the elbow in flexion to temporarily cover exposed neurovascular structures. **B,** A parascapular free flap was used to cover this large soft-tissue defect. Eight months after surgery, the patient had stable coverage and excellent elbow range of motion in extension **(C)** and flexion **(D)**. (Reproduced with permission from Dagum AB: Soft tissue coverage about the elbow, in Lee DH, Steinmann SP, eds: *Elbow Trauma: A Master Skills Publication.* Chicago, IL, American Society for Surgery of the Hand, 2015, pp 357-370.)

Bilayer Matrix Wound Dressing (Integra LifeSciences). Integra is composed of cross-linked bovine collagen and glucosaminoglycan protected by a layer of silicone. This dermal layer substitute is applied over the wound and allowed to revascularize over the next 3 weeks, after which the silicone layer is removed and a thin STSG is applied over the dressing. Application of a fibrin sealant such as Tisseel (Baxter) or negative pressure wound therapy improves the adherence as well as the incorporation (take or adherence) and decreases the time to revascularization.[35] Integra is more resistant to contracture and appears to cause fewer adhesions than an STSG. However, a wound resurfaced with Integra lacks subcutaneous fat, which serves as an important gliding plane. Integra can be applied over small areas of exposed nonfractured bone, tendon, or ligament. Although this technique was reported to be successful, particularly in children, it is not ideal.[36-38] Revascularization over bare bone, tendon, or ligament requires additional time because it proceeds from the wound edge rather than the underlying bed, is more subject to breakdown, and may require more than one application. The circumferential multiplane degloving in an Arnez et al pattern 4 injury almost always requires staged reconstruction with a free flap or large pedicle flap. If neither flap can be used, a dermal substitute such as Integra can be used with an STSG. An STSG can be used alone if a dermal substitute is not available or if no bone, tendon, or ligament is exposed (**Figure 1**).

Adjunctive Measures

Experimental evidence suggests that the use of adjunctive measures can improve survival of the degloved tissue. These measures include anticoagulation with low-molecular-weight heparin (enoxaparin), rivaroxaban, pentoxifyline, allopurinol, or hyperbaric oxygen.[29,39-41] Enoxaparin and rivaroxaban are believed to

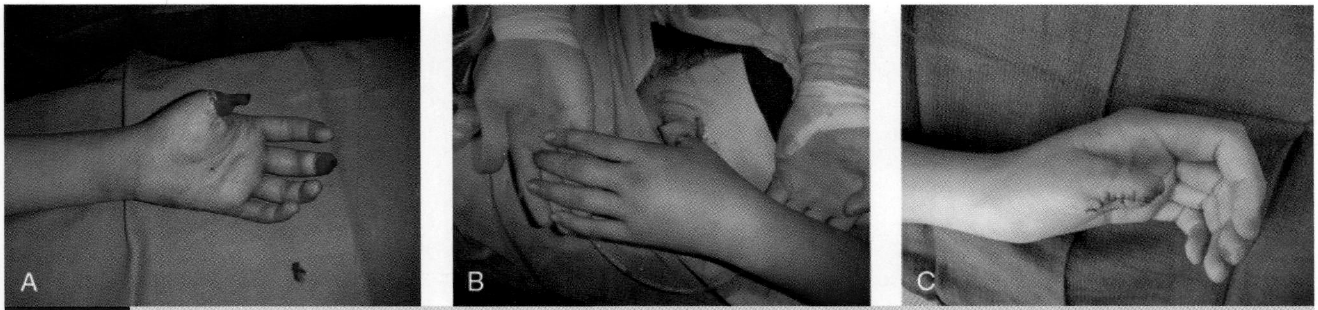

Figure 7 Clinical photographs showing a class 3 ring avulsion injury to the thumb of a 15-year-old boy, which was sustained in a boating accident **(A)**. The thumb part was lost at sea. **B,** A groin flap was used for immediate coverage of the exposed proximal phalanx. **C,** Subsequent debulking created a functional thumb. The patient declined a toe transfer.

act by preventing thrombosis of injured and newly formed vessels and by improving capillary density.[29] Pentoxifylline is believed to improve tissue survival by enhancing erythrocyte flexibility, blood flow, and tissue vascularization.[39,40] Allopurinol is a potent xanthine oxidase that inhibits antioxidants and thus the formation of free radicals, which play an important role in tissue necrosis.[39] Hyperbaric oxygen therapy increases the tolerance of tissue ischemia by increasing oxygenation, decreasing platelet aggregation, and stimulating neoangiogenesis.[41] These adjunctive modalities cannot be recommended for routine clinical use until the results of clinical investigations and studies are available.

Morel-Lavallée Lesions

A closed degloving injury, better known as a Morel-Lavallée lesion, usually occurs in the flank, pelvis, or lower extremity and is rare in the upper extremity. The treatment of a Morel-Lavallée lesion can be challenging.[14,42] The avulsion is most likely to be in the suprafascial plane. The underlying cavity typically fills with liquefying hematoma, lymphatic fluid, and necrotic fat. A pseudocapsule forms around the fluid cavity and may become infected.[14,42] Initially a Morel-Lavallée lesion may be underappreciated. Its clinical features include overlying ecchymosis, a bulge with underlying fluctuance, and loss of sensation. The diagnosis usually is made with ultrasound or MRI. If the lesion is diagnosed acutely, it can be managed nonsurgically with percutaneous aspiration, compression, and occasionally sclerotherapy.[14,43] Surgical management involves evacuation of the hematoma, débridement of the necrotic tissue, and excision of the pseudocapsule. A retrospective study of 79 patients and 87 lesions found that aspiration of more than 50 mL of fluid was a predictor of recurrence, and surgical intervention was recommended.[44] The late complications include delayed infection and soft-tissue contour abnormalities.[14,45]

Ring Avulsion Injuries

Ring avulsion injuries are common and involve a degloving of the skin of the affected finger, with or without the tendons, neurovascular bundles, bone, or joint. These injuries usually occur during a fall, when the patient's motion continues despite a finger ring or other encircling object being caught on a stationary object.[16] The mechanical force is tremendous, and the spectrum of injury ranges from a simple skin tear to a complete amputation. The classification of ring avulsion injuries is based on circulation in the digit, which is important for treatment and prognosis.[46] In class 1, circulation is adequate, with or without tendon or skeletal injury. In class 2, arterial or venous circulation is inadequate, with or without tendon or skeletal injury. In class 3, circulation is entirely absent, and there is complete degloving or amputation (**Figure 7**). The classification has been modified to include amputations proximal to the flexor digitorum superficialis and distal to its insertion.

The treatment depends on the extent of injury as well as the patient's age, sex, cultural background, and occupation. In general, the injured structures are repaired if circulation is adequate. A skin graft usually is required for coverage to avoid venous constriction from a tight closure. If circulation is inadequate, a vein graft usually is required to repair the vein and/or artery (**Figure 8**). The adjacent uninjured digital artery can be used as an alternative to vein grafting. In the past, a complete traumatic amputation was believed to be best treated with a revision amputation; the exceptions involved amputation of a thumb or amputation of any digit in a child (**Figure 9**). More recent studies have shown that amputations distal to the FDS insertion have a better outcome than traditionally thought and are worthy of replantation.[47]

The survival rate of the injured digit after microsurgical revascularization is 78% in a class 2 injury and 66%

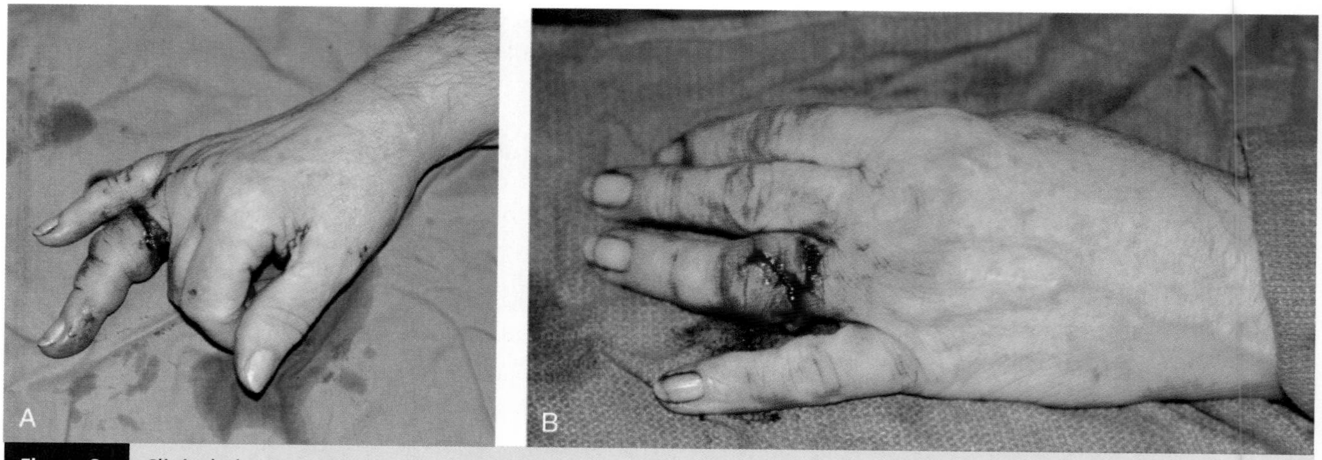

Figure 8 Clinical photographs showing a ring avulsion injury with venous congestion **(A)** and vein graft was used to bridge the injured venous segment **(B)**. Adequate circulation was restored, with subsequent restoration of full digit function.

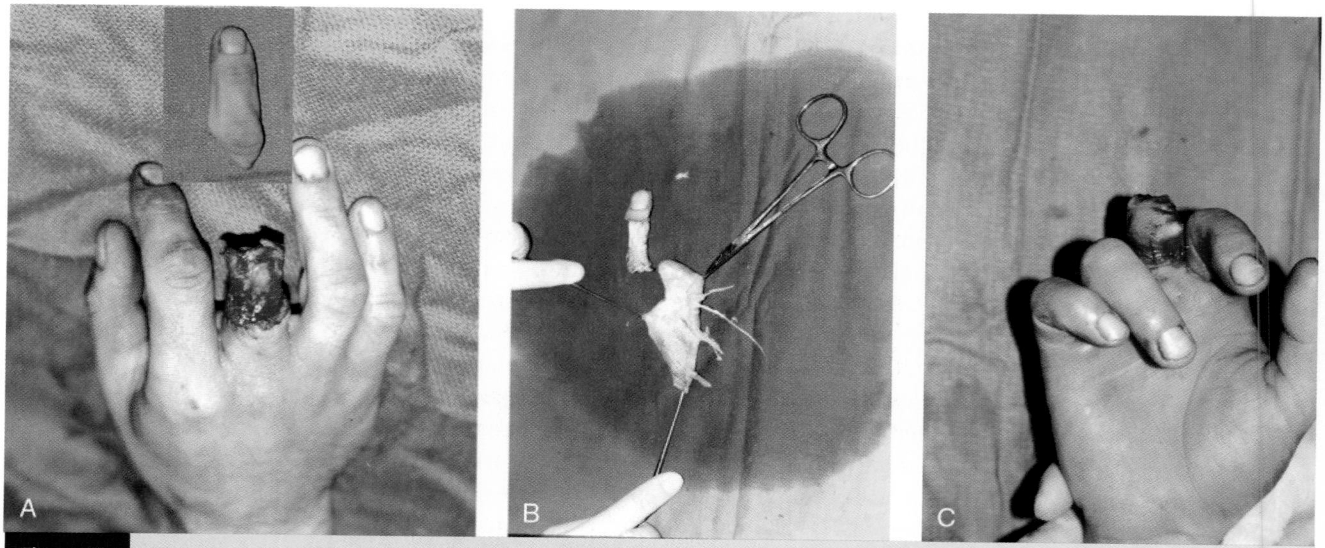

Figure 9 Clinical photographs showing a ring avulsion injury at the proximal interphalangeal joint level, with avulsion of tendons, vessels, and nerves **(A)**. The distal soft tissue and neurovascular structures were salvaged **(B)** and used as an innervated free flap to cover the proximal phalanx **(C)**. (Reproduced with permission from Dagum AB: Replantation: Indications and rationale, in Seitz WH, ed: *Fractures and Dislocations of the Hand and Fingers*. Chicago, IL, American Society for Surgery of the Hand, 2013, pp 260-276.)

in a class 3 injury. Patients are able to return to work an average 6 to 8 weeks after a class 1 injury or a revision amputation and 9 to 12 weeks after revascularization or replantation (class 2 or 3 injury.) Patients with a class 2 injury that is successfully revascularized regain 74% of their range of motion and have 8-mm two-point discrimination. Those with a class 3 injury that is successfully replanted regain an average 64% of range of motion and have 10-mm two-point discrimination.[47] Cold intolerance is a chronic concern for 65% of patients.

Outcomes of Major Degloving Injuries

The outcome of a degloving injury depends on the type of injury, its location, and the presence of associated injured structures. In injuries sustained by 46 patients in a long-term review, the avulsed flap was excised, available skin was used as an FTSG, and the remainder of the wound was closed with an STSG.[7] An average of four operations was required to achieve coverage if only an FTSG initially was used, and three operations were required if an STSG was used. Contractures occurred most often in areas with an STSG, particularly across a joint. Sensitivity was poor in the grafted areas, and distal edema was common after grafting in circumferential injuries. Patients who underwent grafting of a circumferential injury during childhood had an increased incidence of limb-length discrepancy. Contour deformities were a source of significant aesthetic concern for patients. According to one study, 12 of the patients had a circumferentially degloved hand from the wrist and forearm level.[48] These noncrushing roller injuries without bony injury were treated with immediate defatting of the attached distally based flap and its application as an FTSG. The skin graft took (incorporated) in 11 of the wounds (93%), the wound that the FTSG did not take was successfully treated secondarily with a skin graft.[48] It should be noted that these were roller noncrush-type injuries without underlying bony injury. In a retrospective review of 11 patients with high-energy industrial roller injuries to the upper extremity, there were 6 patients with fractures and/or dislocations, with 3 requiring fasciotomies, 3 patients requiring STSG, and 2 immediate amputation.[1] Five patients had nerve injuries, including three with late carpal tunnel syndrome. The development of prolonged edema in all 11 patients complicated recovery. It was concluded that these are severe degloving injuries in which a high percentage of patients have multiple underlying associated injuries. In a retrospective review of 79 degloving injuries, the authors found that primary irrigation, débridement, and closure could be achieved in most injuries, with the exception of Arnez et al pattern 4 injuries, as long as the avulsed skin was not simply resutured.[5] Only 1 of 14 wounds that were initially resutured, 8 of 13 wounds that were initially skin grafted, and 38 of 52 that underwent initial flap reconstruction proceeded to heal by primary intention. It was recommended that in pattern 4 injuries, circumferential multiplane degloving serial débridement and delayed closure be performed. A study of 32 patients with a degloving injury found that revascularization was not possible if the subcutaneous venous plexus was severely injured; the skin, if usable, was reapplied as an FTSG or STSG.[4] In 9 of 13 injuries with a preserved subcutaneous venous plexus, distal arteriovenous shunting and proximal venous anastomosis led to salvage of more than 90% of the degloved flap. In type 2 injuries in which reperfusion was not achieved, débridement of the area that was not reperfused allowed the skin to be used for skin grafting. In all 10 degloving injuries with some venous outflow, proximal venous anastomosis was successful in salvaging more than 95% of the degloved tissue. The remaining small open areas were closed with an STSG. The authors of a 2013 study reviewed 14 major upper extremity degloving injuries where revascularization was attempted;[6] nine involved the forearm or dorsum of the hand (the so-called expendable zone), arteriovenous shunting and proximal venous anastomosis was successful in achieving primary closure in four of nine cases, and in the other five cases there was partial loss of tissue: two required a subsequent groin flap and three a skin graft for closure. The three patients with a palm-only (nonexpendable area) injury were treated with arteriovenous shunting and proximal venous anastomosis; two of them went on to heal primarily and the third patient had a partial loss necessitating a skin graft for subsequent closure. In the two patients with nonexpendable palm, including digits treated with arteriovenous shunting and arterial revascularization, both had fingertip and partial digit losses that were attributed to inadequate revascularization or failure of revascularization of one or more digits. One patient required a subsequent groin flap for closure. The authors concluded that revascularization was necessary in a complete degloving injury of the digits and that arteriovenous shunting alone was insufficient for complete survival of the digits. The expendable areas could be adequately treated with arteriovenous shunting and proximal venous anastomosis, as well as traditional defatting of the avulsed skin and reapplication as an FTSG, or perform a wait-and-see approach with subsequent skin graft or flap coverage as needed.

Secondary Reconstruction

Secondary reconstruction often is needed in a severe degloving injury. Secondary procedures require the wound to be stable and closed. The timing of the reconstruction depends on the involved structures. Nerves are repaired 6 to 12 weeks after injury, and nerve grafting or nerve transfer almost always is required. The zone of nerve injury is clearly delineated approximately 3 weeks after the nerve is torn. It is prudent to wait at least another 3 weeks for a stable closed wound to be suitable for the nerve grafts. Bone grafting can be done after 3 to 6 months but sometimes can be done earlier, depending on the quality of the soft-tissue envelope. Tendon or muscle transfers are done 3 to 9 months after injury, and for success they require soft-tissue equilibrium with a supple mature scar, mobile joints, and a plateau in therapy. Scar revision awaits scar maturation, which requires at least 1 year. Scars are treated earlier if they are causing joint contractures, are unstable and continually break down, or are hypertrophic, pruritic, or painful.

Summary

Upper extremity degloving injuries often are accompanied by extensive blood loss and severe concomitant injuries. These injuries require prompt attention. After irrigation and débridement, the devascularized tissue is assessed for revascularization, especially in the nonexpendable palm and digits. If revascularization is not possible, viable tissue is replaced and sutured without tension, and the nonviable flap of tissue is excised. The skin always is assessed for salvageability as a skin graft, and if acceptable the skin is defatted and placed as an FTSG. If there is significant wound contamination or questionable viability in an underlying muscle injury, the skin is banked and used when a stable clean wound has been obtained. If the skin available for grafting is insufficient or the skin is badly injured, an STSG is applied to the remaining wound. A regional or free flap is used for reconstruction if a vital structure, tendon, ligament, bone, or hardware is exposed.

Key Study Points

- An understanding of the pathophysiology and type of injuries that lead to degloving injuries is necessary.
- The zone of vascular compromise in the degloved tissue should be assessed to determine whether the tissue can be salvaged.
- The method of revascularization necessary to salvage the degloved tissue should be determined.
- Alternative options to close the wound should be proposed when the degloved tissue cannot be salvaged.
- The surgeon should be aware of results of treatment in major degloving injuries and the timing of secondary reconstructive surgery when applicable.

Annotated References

1. Askins G, Finley R, Parenti J, Bush D, Brotman S: High-energy roller injuries to the upper extremity. *J Trauma* 1986;26(12):1127-1131.

2. Latifi R, El-Hennawy H, El-Menyar A, et al: The therapeutic challenges of degloving soft-tissue injuries. *J Emerg Trauma Shock* 2014;7(3):228-232.

   The incidence, clinical appearance, management, and outcomes of degloving soft-tissue injuries were analyzed in general and by specific anatomic region.

3. Farmer AW: Treatment of avulsed skin flaps. *Ann Surg* 1939;110(5):951-959.

4. Waikakul S: Revascularization of degloving injuries of the limbs. *Injury* 1997;28(4):271-274.

5. Arnez ZM, Khan U, Tyler MP: Classification of soft-tissue degloving in limb trauma. *J Plast Reconstr Aesthet Surg* 2010;63(11):1865-1869.

   A retrospective review of 79 injured limbs in 68 patients included a classification into four patterns of injury. Primary irrigation, débridement, and closure could be achieved in most injuries, except pattern 4 injuries. Level of evidence: III.

6. Lo S, Lin YT, Lin CH, Wei FC: A new classification to aid the selection of revascularization techniques in major degloving injuries of the upper limb. *Injury* 2013;44(3):331-335.

   A review of degloving injuries of the hand described injuries, initial management, reconstructive options, and secondary revision procedures.

7. McGrouther DA, Sully L: Degloving injuries of the limbs: Long-term review and management based on whole-body fluorescence. *Br J Plast Surg* 1980;33(1):9-24.

8. Hsu WM, Wei FC, Lin CH, Chen HC, Chuang CC, Chen HT: The salvage of a degloved hand skin flap by arteriovenous shunting. *Plast Reconstr Surg* 1996;98(1):146-150.

9. MacCollum DW: Wringer arm: A report of twenty-six cases. *N Engl J Med* 1938;218:549-554.

10. Golden GT, Fisher JC, Edgerton MT: "Wringer arm" reevaluated: A survey of current surgical management of upper extremity compression injuries. *Ann Surg* 1973;177(3):362-369.

11. Krishnamoorthy R, Karthikeyan G: Degloving injuries of the hand. *Indian J Plast Surg* 2011;44(2):227-236.

    The etiology, pathophysiology, and management of degloving injuries of the hand and digits are discussed.

12. Slack CC: Friction injuries following road accidents. *Br Med J* 1952;2(4778):262-264.

13. Boettcher-Haberzeth S, Schiestl C: Management of avulsion injuries. *Eur J Pediatr Surg* 2013;23(5):359-364.

    A review of the management of degloving injuries in children discussed the role of Integra dermal substitute and negative wound pressure therapy.

14. Dawre S, Lamba S, Sreekar H,Gupta S, Gupta AK: The Morel-Lavallee lesion: A review and a proposed algorithmic approach. *Eur J Plast Surg* 2012;35:489-494.

    A comprehensive review of the management of Morel-Lavallée lesions proposed a simple treatment algorithm.

15. Ross SE: *Prophylaxis Against Tetanus in Wound Management* .Chicago, IL, American College of Surgeons Committee on Trauma, 1995.

16. Dagum AB: Replantation: Indications and rationale, in Seitz WH, ed: *Fractures and Dislocations of the Hand and Fingers* .Chicago, IL, American Society for Surgery of the Hand, 2013, pp 260-276.

17. Fourman MS, Gersch RP, Phillips BT, et al: Comparison of laser Doppler and laser-assisted indocyanine green angiography prediction of flap survival in a novel modification of the McFarlane flap. *Ann Plast Surg* 2015;75(1):102-107.

The use of laser Doppler imaging and laser-assisted indocyanine green angiography was analyzed for predicting flap necrosis using a modified McFarlane flap model. Laser-assisted indocyanine green angiography was found to be superior in its ability to predict necrosis within the first 48 hours after injury.

18. Lim H, Han DH, Lee IJ, Park MC: A simple strategy in avulsion flap injury: Prediction of flap viability using Wood's lamp illumination and resurfacing with a full-thickness skin graft. *Arch Plast Surg* 2014;41(2):126-132.

In a case study of 13 patients with avulsion injuries, a Wood lamp was used to assess viability of avulsed tissue. Nonviable tissue was immediately excised and used for a skin graft. Within preserved flap, tissue necrosis was 8.4% (after exclusion of injury mismanagement in three patients). Level of evidence: IV.

19. Phillips BT, Lanier ST, Conkling N, et al: Intraoperative perfusion techniques can accurately predict mastectomy skin flap necrosis in breast reconstruction: Results of a prospective trial. *Plast Reconstr Surg* 2012;129(5):778e-788e.

A prospective study of intraoperative evaluation of mastectomy skin viability compared clinical assessment, fluorescein dye angiography, and laser-assisted indocyanine green dye angiography. Laser-assisted indocyanine green dye angiography was found to be a superior predictor of skin flap necrosis. Level of evidence: I.

20. McGregor IA: Degloving injuries. *Hand* 1970;2(2):130-133.

21. Godina M: Early microsurgical reconstruction of complex trauma of the extremities. *Plast Reconstr Surg* 1986;78(3):285-292.

22. Dagum AB: Soft tissue coverage about the elbow, in Lee DH, Steinmann SP, eds: Elbow Trauma: A Master Skills Publication. Chicago, IL, American Society for Surgery of the Hand, 2015.pp 357-370.

This comprehensive review chapter outlines the author's approach to the management of soft tissue injury and loss about the elbow and the more common flaps used for reconstruction with the goal being to obtain a stable, closed wound that allows for early motion of the elbow.

23. Nakayama Y, Soeda S, Kasai Y: Flaps nourished by arterial inflow through the venous system: An experimental investigation. *Plast Reconstr Surg* 1981;67(3):328-334.

24. Fukui A, Maeda M, Inada Y, Tamai S, Sempuku T: Arteriovenous shunt in digit replantation. *J Hand Surg Am* 1990;15(1):160-165.

25. Inoue G, Suzuki K: Arterialized venous flap for treating multiple skin defects of the hand. *Plast Reconstr Surg* 1993;91(2):299-302, discussion 303-306.

26. Takeuchi M, Sasaki K, Nozaki M: Treatment of a degloved hand injury by arteriovenous anastomosis: A case report. *Ann Plast Surg* 1997;39(2):174-177.

27. Rodríguez-Lorenzo A, Lin CH, Lin CH, Ching WC, Lin YT: Replantation of a degloved hand with added arteriovenous anastomoses: Report of two cases. *J Hand Surg Am* 2009;34(10):1864-1867.

28. Slattery P, Leung M, Slattery D: Microsurgical arterialization of degloving injuries of the upper limb. *J Hand Surg Am* 2012;37(4):825-831.

In a case study of three patients with degloved tissue in an upper extremity injury, arterialization of the venous system was done by direct arteriovenous anastomosis with or without vein grafts, leading to substantial salvage of avulsed tissue. Level of evidence: IV.

29. Azboy I, Demirtaş A, Bulut M, Alabalik U, Uçar Y, Alemdar C: Effects of enoxaparin and rivaroxaban on tissue survival in skin degloving injury: An experimental study. *Acta Orthop Traumatol Turc* 2014;48(2):212-216.

The effect of the antithrombotic medications enoxaparin and rivaroxaban on tissue survival was evaluated in a rat model. Three groups of eight animals received enoxaparin, rivaroxaban, or placebo after degloving injury to the tail. Both medications significantly improved tissue survival compared with placebo.

30. Mathes SJ, Nahai F: The reconstructive triangle: A paradigm for surgical decision making, in *Reconstructive Surgery: Principles, Anatomy and Technique* .New York, NY, Churchill Livingstone, Quality Medical Publishing, 1997, pp 10-36.

31. Vedder NB, Hanel DP: The mangled upper extremity, in Wolfe SW, Hotchkiss RN, Pederson WC, Kozin SH, eds: *Green's Operative Hand Surgery* ,ed 6. Philadelphia, PA, Elsevier Churchill Livingstone, 2011, pp 1603-1644.

32. Chang N, Mathes SJ: Comparison of the effect of bacterial inoculation in musculocutaneous and random-pattern flaps. *Plast Reconstr Surg* 1982;70(1):1-10.

33. Calderon W, Chang N, Mathes SJ: Comparison of the effect of bacterial inoculation in musculocutaneous and fasciocutaneous flaps. *Plast Reconstr Surg* 1986;77(5):785-794.

34. Guerra AB, Gill PS, Trahan CG, et al: Comparison of bacterial inoculation and transcutaneous oxygen tension in the rabbit S1 perforator and latissimus dorsi musculocutaneous flaps. *J Reconstr Microsurg* 2005;21(2):137-143.

35. Melendez MM, Martinez RR, Dagum AB, et al: Porcine wound healing in full-thickness skin defects using Integra™ with and without fibrin glue with keratinocytes. *Can J Plast Surg* 2008;16(3):147-152.

36. Graham GP, Helmer SD, Haan JM, Khandelwal A: The use of Integra® Dermal Regeneration Template in the reconstruction of traumatic degloving injuries. *J Burn Care Res* 2013;34(2):261-266.

In a retrospective review, 10 patients with degloving injuries to a limb were treated with application of Integra and a subsequent STSG. Nine patients achieved excellent wound healing, even if the injury resulted in exposure of bone or tendon. Level of evidence: IV.

37. Katrana F, Kostopoulos E, Delia G, Lunel GG, Casoli V: Reanimation of thumb extension after upper extremity degloving injury treated with Integra. *J Hand Surg Eur Vol* 2008;33(6):800-802.

38. Herlin C, Louhaem D, Bigorre M, Dimeglio A, Captier G: Use of Integra in a paediatric upper extremity degloving injury. *J Hand Surg Eur Vol* 2007;32(2):179-184.

39. Milcheski DA, Nakamoto HA, Tuma P Jr, Nóbrega L, Ferreira MC: Experimental model of degloving injury in rats: Effect of allopurinol and pentoxifylline in improving viability of avulsed flaps. *Ann Plast Surg* 2013;70(3):366-369.

The effects of allopurinol and pentoxifylline on tissue survival after degloving injury were studied in an experimental rat model. Three groups of 25 rats received saline solution, pentoxifylline (25 mg/kg), or allopurinol (45 mg/kg) after a degloving injury to the hind limb. Both allopurinol and pentoxifylline led to a decrease in the area of necrosis. Allopurinol was found to be slightly more effective, without statistical significance.

40. Oztuna V, Eskandari MM, Unal S, Colak M, Karabacak T: The effect of pentoxifylline in treatment of skin degloving injuries: An experimental study. *Injury* 2006;37(7):638-641.

41. Demirtas A, Azboy I, Bulut M, Ucar BY, Alabalik U, Ilgezdi S: Effect of hyperbaric oxygen therapy on healing in an experimental model of degloving injury in tails of nicotine-treated rats. *J Hand Surg Eur Vol* 2013;38(4):405-411.

The effects of hyperbaric oxygen therapy on tissue survival after degloving injury was studied in nicotine-treated rats. Hyperbaric oxygen therapy positively affected tissue survival even in the presence of nicotine, and it decreased the length of necrosis and the extent of necrosis on histopathologic evaluation.

42. Kim SW, Roh SG, Lee NH, Yang KM: Clinical experience of Morel-Lavallee syndrome. *Arch Plast Surg* 2015;42(1):91-93.

In a case study of three patients with a Morel-Lavallée lesion, *Pseudomonas* infection developed in one patient, requiring multiple débridements and prolonged care. Level of evidence: IV.

43. Zhong B, Zhang C, Luo CF: Percutaneous drainage of Morel-Lavallée lesions when the diagnosis is delayed. *Can J Surg* 2014;57(5):356-357.

In a retrospective review, eight patients with a Morel-Lavallée lesion of more than 1 week's duration underwent percutaneous drainage and débridement. Six patients required a second procedure, and two required a third procedure. Complete healing was achieved in six patients. Skin necrosis requiring skin grafting occurred in two patients. Level of evidence: IV.

44. Nickerson TP, Zielinski MD, Jenkins DH, Schiller HJ: The Mayo Clinic experience with Morel-Lavallée lesions: Establishment of a practice management guideline. *J Trauma Acute Care Surg* 2014;76(2):493-497.

Retrospective evaluation of 79 patients with 87 lesions found that aspiration of more than 50 mL of fluid was a significant predictor of recurrence. Surgical intervention was recommended for such patients. Level of evidence: III.

45. Hudson DA: Missed closed degloving injuries: Late presentation as a contour deformity. *Plast Reconstr Surg* 1996;98(2):334-337.

46. Urbaniak JR, Evans JP, Bright DS: Microvascular management of ring avulsion injuries. *J Hand Surg Am* 1981;6(1):25-30.

47. Sears ED, Chung KC: Replantation of finger avulsion injuries: A systematic review of survival and functional outcomes. *J Hand Surg Am* 2011;36(4):686-694.

A systematic review of the English-language literature on replantation after finger avulsion injuries found a mean survival rate of 66%, with good motion and sensitivity. This outcome was better than previously reported outcomes, and it prompted a challenge to the historical recommendation of revision amputation for a complete finger avulsion injury. Level of evidence: III.

48. Jeng SF, Wei FC: Resurfacing a circumferentially degloved hand by using a full-thickness skin graft harvested from an avulsed skin flap. *Ann Plast Surg* 1997;39(4):360-365.

5. Weber RA, Breidenbach WC, Brown RE, Jabaley ME, Mass DP: A randomized prospective study of polyglycolic acid conduits for digital nerve reconstruction in humans. *Plast Reconstr Surg* 2000;106(5):1036-1045, discussion 1046-1048.

6. Lee JY, Parisi TJ, Friedrich PF, Bishop AT, Shin AY: Does the addition of a nerve wrap to a motor nerve repair affect motor outcomes? *Microsurgery* 2014;34(7):562-567.

   Primary suture repair with and without conduit was compared in a rat injury model. No difference was observed in histologic and functional outcomes at 12 weeks, but less perineural scar tissue formation occurred in the conduit wrapped group.

7. Taras JS, Jacoby SM, Lincoski CJ: Reconstruction of digital nerves with collagen conduits. *J Hand Surg Am* 2011;36(9):1441-1446.

   In this study involving 19 patients, 22 digital nerve lacerations with a 12-mm nerve gap were repaired with collagen conduits. The mean follow-up time was 20 months. Moving and static two-point discrimination measured 5.0 mm and 5.2 mm, respectively. Level of evidence: IV.

8. Rinker B, Liau JY: A prospective randomized study comparing woven polyglycolic acid and autogenous vein conduits for reconstruction of digital nerve gaps. *J Hand Surg Am* 2011;36(5):775-781.

   Digital nerve repair using autogenous vein conduit was compared with polyglycolic acid conduit for a nerve gap of 10 mm. Sensory recovery was equivalent between the two groups and had a similar cost profile. Fewer complications occurred with autogenous vein conduit. Level of evidence: II.

9. Boeckstyns ME, Sørensen AI, Viñeta JF, et al: Collagen conduit versus microsurgical neurorrhaphy: 2-year follow-up of a prospective, blinded clinical and electrophysiological multicenter randomized, controlled trial. *J Hand Surg Am* 2013;38(12):2405-2411.

   Mixed nerves were repaired with conduit or direct suture repair. At 24 months, the sensory and motor functions were equivalent between the two groups when the gap was 6 mm or less. Level of evidence: II.

10. Isaacs J, Mallu S, Yan W, Little B: Consequences of oversizing: Nerve-to-nerve tube diameter mismatch. *J Bone Joint Surg Am* 2014;96(17):1461-1467.

    A 10-mm sciatic nerve gap rat model was repaired with reverse autograft and 3-mm, 2-mm, or 1.5-mm-diameter conduits. At 12 weeks, the muscle contraction force was weakest, and the axon count was lowest in the 3-mm diameter conduit group.

11. Giusti G, Shin RH, Lee JY, Mattar TG, Bishop AT, Shin AY: The influence of nerve conduits diameter in motor nerve recovery after segmental nerve repair. *Microsurgery* 2014;34(8):646-652.

    This study compared autograft repair with 2.0-mm and 1.5-mm diameter conduit reconstructions. At 12 weeks, the autograft performed the best, but 1.5-mm diameter conduit performed better than 2.0-mm conduit as measured by muscle force, muscle weight, and histomorphometry.

12. Taras JS, Amin N, Patel N, McCabe LA: Allograft reconstruction for digital nerve loss. *J Hand Surg Am* 2013;38(10):1965-1971.

    In this study, 14 patients who had 18 digital nerve injuries with an average gap of 11 mm were evaluated at 15 months. Using the Taras outcome criteria, 39% of digits had excellent results, 44% had good results, 17% had fair results, and none had poor results. Level of evidence: IV.

13. Guo Y, Chen G, Tian G, Tapia C: Sensory recovery following decellularized nerve allograft transplantation for digital nerve repair. *J Plast Surg Hand Surg* 2013;47(6):451-453.

    In this study, five patients with an average defect of 22.8 mm underwent repair with decellularized nerve allograft. At 13.2 months, static two-point discrimination was 6 mm, and the average Semmes-Weinstein monofilaments test score was 4.31. Level of evidence: IV.

14. Brooks DN, Weber RV, Chao JD, et al: Processed nerve allografts for peripheral nerve reconstruction: A multicenter study of utilization and outcomes in sensory, mixed, and motor nerve reconstructions. *Microsurgery* 2012;32(1):1-14.

    The authors of this multicenter study reported 76 injuries: 49 sensory, 18 mixed, and 9 motor nerve injuries. The mean graft length was 22 mm (range, 5 to 50 mm). Meaningful recovery (>S3 and >M3) was found in 87%. Level of evidence: III.

15. Cho MS, Rinker BD, Weber RV, et al: Functional outcome following nerve repair in the upper extremity using processed nerve allograft. *J Hand Surg Am* 2012;37(11):2340-2349.

    The authors identified an upper extremity-specific population in the Registry Study of Avance Nerve Graft (AxoGen) Evaluating Outcomes in Nerve Repair program study registry. In all, 51 subjects with 35 sensory, 13 mixed, and 3 motor nerve injuries were examined. The mean gap was 23 mm (range, 5 mm to 50 mm). Overall recovery, S3/M4 and above, was achieved in 86% of all procedures. Level of evidence: III.

16. Whitlock EL, Tuffaha SH, Luciano JP, et al: Processed allografts and type I collagen conduits for repair of peripheral nerve gaps. *Muscle Nerve* 2009;39(6):787-799.

17. Johnson PJ, Newton P, Hunter DA, Mackinnon SE: Nerve endoneurial microstructure facilitates uniform distribution of regenerative fibers: A post hoc comparison of midgraft nerve fiber densities. *J Reconstr Microsurg* 2011;27(2):83-90.

    Nerve fiber density was calculated for a previous study of isograft, conduit, and allograft repairs for a 14-mm and 28-mm rat sciatic nerve defect. The conduit group had less midgraft density than the isograft and allograft groups at both gap sizes.

18. Giusti G, Willems WF, Kremer T, Friedrich PF, Bishop AT, Shin AY: Return of motor function after segmental nerve loss in a rat model: Comparison of autogenous nerve graft, collagen conduit, and processed allograft (AxoGen). *J Bone Joint Surg Am* 2012;94(5):410-417.

A 10-mm nerve defect was repaired with autograft, allograft, or conduit. At 12 weeks, force was equal in the autograft and allograft groups, and worse in the collagen group. At 16 weeks, force was best in the autograft group, and allograft was superior to conduit.

19. Wolfe SW, Strauss HL, Garg R, Feinberg J: Use of bioabsorbable nerve conduits as an adjunct to brachial plexus neurorrhaphy. *J Hand Surg Am* 2012;37(10):1980-1985.

At the 2-year follow-up, 10 transfers performed with nerve conduits demonstrated clinical recovery and electromyographic reinnervation. Of 20 transfers performed using standard end-to-end neurorrhaphy without conduits, 18 demonstrated clinical recovery. Level of evidence: IV.

20. Garg R, Merrell GA, Hillstrom HJ, Wolfe SW: Comparison of nerve transfers and nerve grafting for traumatic upper plexus palsy: A systematic review and analysis. *J Bone Joint Surg Am* 2011;93(9):819-829.

In this review, 31 studies were included. The pooled international data strongly favor dual nerve transfer over traditional nerve grafting for the restoration of improved shoulder and elbow function in traumatic upper brachial plexus injuries of C5-C6. Level of evidence: IV.

21. Wolfe SW, Johnsen PH, Lee SK, Feinberg JH: Long-nerve grafts and nerve transfers demonstrate comparable outcomes for axillary nerve injuries. *J Hand Surg Am* 2014;39(7):1351-1357.

Ten patients treated with nerve grafts for axillary nerve injuries were compared with 14 patients treated with nerve transfer. No differences were observed between the groups as measured by range of motion, deltoid recovery, shoulder abduction, or electromyographic evidence of deltoid reinnervation. Level of evidence: III.

22. Schreiber JJ, Feinberg JH, Byun DJ, Lee SK, Wolfe SW: Preoperative donor nerve electromyography as a predictor of nerve transfer outcomes. *J Hand Surg Am* 2014;39(1):42-49.

This study found that postoperative strength and range of motion was better when donor nerves were graded by preoperative electromyography as normal, than when they were not graded as normal. Level of evidence: Prognostic II.

23. Schreiber JJ, Byun DJ, Khair MM, Rosenblatt L, Lee SK, Wolfe SW: Optimal axon counts for brachial plexus nerve transfers to restore elbow flexion. *Plast Reconstr Surg* 2015;135(1):135e-141e.

Using 10 cadavers, axon counts were taken of median and ulnar fascicles, musculocutaneous biceps, and brachialis branches. Using the published literature the donor-to-recipient nerve axon count ratio was correlated with outcome. A ratio less than 0.7:1 had a less successful outcome.

24. Bertelli JA, Ghizoni MF: Reconstruction of complete palsies of the adult brachial plexus by root grafting using long grafts and nerve transfers to target nerves. *J Hand Surg Am* 2010;35(10):1640-1646.

For total brachial plexus palsy, these authors obtained good results with spinal accessory transfer to the suprascapular nerve, levator scapulae nerve transfer to the triceps long head, and C5 root grafting to the musculocutaneous nerve. Level of evidence: IV.

25. Bertelli JA, Ghizoni MF: Nerve root grafting and distal nerve transfers for C5-C6 brachial plexus injuries. *J Hand Surg Am* 2010;35(5):769-775.

This study examined the results of distal nerve transfer with and without nerve root grafting. Patients treated with nerve root grafting and nerve transfers had the best outcomes. Level of evidence: IV.

26. Yamada T, Doi K, Hattori Y, Hoshino S, Sakamoto S, Arakawa Y: Long thoracic nerve neurotization for restoration of shoulder function in C5-7 brachial plexus preganglionic injuries: Case report. *J Hand Surg Am* 2010;35(9):1427-1431.

This case report discusses intercostal nerves transferred to the long thoracic nerve in addition to spinal accessory nerve transfer to the suprascapular nerve for C5-C7 brachial plexus injuries. The patient obtained excellent shoulder function. Level of evidence: IV.

27. Malungpaishrope K, Leechavengvongs S, Witoonchart K, Uerpairojkit C, Boonyalapa A, Janesaksrisakul D: Simultaneous intercostal nerve transfers to deltoid and triceps muscle through the posterior approach. *J Hand Surg Am* 2012;37(4):677-682.

For C5, C6, and C7 avulsion injuries, these authors performed spinal accessory nerve to the suprascapular nerve combined with third/fourth intercostal nerve to the anterior axillary nerve as well as fifth/sixth intercostal nerve to the radial nerve branch of the triceps. Level of evidence: IV.

28. García-López A, Sebastian P, Martinez F, Perea D: Transfer of the nerve to the brachioradialis muscle to the anterior interosseous nerve for treatment for lower brachial plexus lesions: Case report. *J Hand Surg Am* 2011;36(3):394-397.

In this case report, the motor branch of the brachioradialis muscle was transferred to the anterior interosseous nerve to restore finger flexion in lower brachial plexus lesions. Level of evidence: IV.

29. García-López A, Perea D: Transfer of median and ulnar nerve fascicles for lesions of the posterior cord in infraclavicular brachial plexus injury: Report of 2 cases. *J Hand Surg Am* 2012;37(10):1986-1989.

For this type of injury, these authors recommend (1) the ulnar fascicle to the motor branch of the long triceps, (2) the pronator teres median motor to the extensor carpi radialis longus motor, and (3) the flexor carpi radialis motor to the posterior interosseous nerve. Level of evidence: IV.

30. García-López A, Navarro R, Martinez F, Rojas A: Nerve transfers from branches to the flexor carpi radialis and pronator teres to reconstruct the radial nerve. *J Hand Surg Am* 2014;39(1):50-56.

For radial nerve palsy or posterior cord lesions, the pronator teres motor branch is transferred to the extensor carpi radialis longus motor branch as well as flexor carpi radialis motor branch to the posterior interosseous nerve. The patients had good recovery of finger and wrist extension. Level of evidence: IV.

31. Lin H, Hou C, Chen A, Xu Z: Transfer of the phrenic nerve to the posterior division of the lower trunk to recover thumb and finger extension in brachial plexus palsy. *J Neurosurg* 2011;114(1):212-216.

In this study, the phrenic nerve was transferred to the posterior division of the lower trunk to recover thumb and finger extension. Most patients regained Medical Research Council grade 3 or better extension. Level of evidence: IV.

32. Pet MA, Ray WZ, Yee A, Mackinnon SE: Nerve transfer to the triceps after brachial plexus injury: Report of four cases. *J Hand Surg Am* 2011;36(3):398-405.

This report details nerve transfer to the triceps motor of the radial nerve using an ulnar fascicle to the flexor carpi ulnaris in two patients, a thoracodorsal nerve branch in one patient, and a radial fascicle to the extensor carpi radialis longus branch in one patient. Level of evidence: IV.

33. Soldado F, Ghizoni MF, Bertelli J: Thoracodorsal nerve transfer for elbow flexion reconstruction in infraclavicular brachial plexus injuries. *J Hand Surg Am* 2014;39(9):1766-1770.

The authors found that direct thoracodorsal nerve transfer is a useful technique to restore elbow flexion in patients with infraclavicular brachial plexus injuries. M4 elbow strength was achieved. Level of evidence: IV.

34. Bertelli JA, Ghizoni MF: Nerve transfer from triceps medial head and anconeus to deltoid for axillary nerve palsy. *J Hand Surg Am* 2014;39(5):940-947.

In this study, the branch to the triceps lower medial head and anconeus was transferred to the anterior division of the axillary nerve. All patients recovered deltoid function. Level of evidence: IV.

35. Phillips BZ, Franco MJ, Yee A, Tung TH, Mackinnon SE, Fox IK: Direct radial to ulnar nerve transfer to restore intrinsic muscle function in combined proximal median and ulnar nerve injury: Case report and surgical technique. *J Hand Surg Am* 2014;39(7):1358-1362.

This case report described transferring the radial nerve branches to the abductor pollicis longus, the extensor pollicis brevis, and the extensor indicis proprius to the motor branch of the ulnar nerve end-to-end via an interosseous tunnel. This method restored intrinsic muscle function. Level of evidence: IV.

36. Bertelli JA: Transfer of the radial nerve branch to the extensor carpi radialis brevis to the anterior interosseous nerve to reconstruct thumb and finger flexion. *J Hand Surg Am* 2015;40(2):323-328.e2.

Four patients with a combined high median/ulnar nerve palsy or C7-T1 root avulsion underwent a nerve transfer of the extensor carpi radialis brevis motor to the anterior interosseous nerve. At 13 months, M4 finger and thumb flexion were achieved.

37. Dy CJ, Kitay A, Garg R, Kang L, Feinberg JH, Wolfe SW: Neurotization to innervate the deltoid and biceps: 3 cases. *J Hand Surg Am* 2013;38(2):237-240.

Two patients underwent direct muscle neurotization into the deltoid and one into the biceps. Two recovered M4 strength and one recovered M3 strength. On electrodiagnostic studies, all three patients had evidence of at least partial muscle reinnervation. Level of evidence: IV.

38. Barbour J, Yee A, Kahn LC, Mackinnon SE: Supercharged end-to-side anterior interosseous to ulnar motor nerve transfer for intrinsic musculature reinnervation. *J Hand Surg Am* 2012;37(10):2150-2159.

This study is a review of the anterior interosseous nerve (AIN) end-to-side transfer to the ulnar deep motor branch technique. Although the intact ulnar nerve regenerates, AIN can innervate targets more quickly and "baby-sit" the end plates. If incomplete ulnar nerve recovery is expected, the AIN axons can augment the recovery.

39. Bertelli JA, Ghizoni MF: Very distal sensory nerve transfers in high median nerve lesions. *J Hand Surg Am* 2011;36(3):387-393.

In this study, eight patients with high median nerve injuries underwent radial nerve branch transfers to the palmar nerves at the level of the proximal phalanx to restore fingertip sensation. Protective or better sensation to the fingertips in all patients was restored. Better results were observed for the thumb. Locognosia was acquired in all thumbs and in four of eight index fingers. Level of evidence: IV.

40. Bertelli JA: Distal sensory nerve transfers in lower-type injuries of the brachial plexus. *J Hand Surg Am* 2012;37(6):1194-1199.

To restore ulnar nerve sensation, the cutaneous branches of the median nerve to the palm were used in five patients, and the palmar cutaneous branch of the median nerve was used in three patients. According to the Medical Research Council system of evaluation, five patients scored S3 and three scored S3+. Level of evidence: IV.

41. Chen C, Tang P, Zhang X: Finger sensory reconstruction with transfer of the proper digital nerve dorsal branch. *J Hand Surg Am* 2013;38(1):82-89.

In this study, 21 proper digital nerve defects in 20 fingers were treated with the dorsal branch of the proper digital nerve of the same or adjacent finger. Sensory recovery with this transfer was superior to that observed in sural nerve grafting. Level of evidence: III.

42. Kale SS, Glaus SW, Yee A, et al: Reverse end-to-side nerve transfer: From animal model to clinical use. *J Hand Surg Am* 2011;36(10):1631-1639.e2.

An animal model was used to evaluate an end-to-end and a RETS nerve transfer. The authors found statistically similar regeneration in end-to-end and RETS animals at 5 and 10 weeks. RETS nerve transfer may augment motor recovery when incomplete recovery is expected.

43. Ghosh S, Singh VK, Jeyaseelan L, Sinisi M, Fox M: Isolated latissimus dorsi transfer to restore shoulder external rotation in adults with brachial plexus injury. *Bone Joint J* 2013;95-B(5):660-663.

In this study, 24 patients who lacked shoulder external rotation after plexus injury underwent isolated latissimus dorsi transfer. The mean improvement in active external rotation from neutral was 24°. The mean increase in arc of motion was 52°. Level of evidence: IV.

44. Dodakundi C, Doi K, Hattori Y, et al: Outcome of surgical reconstruction after traumatic total brachial plexus palsy. *J Bone Joint Surg Am* 2013;95(16):1505-1512.

In this study, 36 patients with total brachial plexus injury underwent double free-muscle transfer and had a minimum of follow-up of 24 months. Disabilities of the Arm, Shoulder and Hand and 36-item Short Form Health Survey scores showed significant improvements. The authors concluded that the transfer yielded satisfactory function. Level of evidence: IV.

45. Shah A, Jebson PJ: Current treatment of radial nerve palsy following fracture of the humeral shaft. *J Hand Surg Am* 2008;33(8):1433-1434.

46. Foster RJ, Swiontkowski MF, Bach AW, Sack JT: Radial nerve palsy caused by open humeral shaft fractures. *J Hand Surg Am* 1993;18(1):121-124.

47. Ring D, Chin K, Jupiter JB: Radial nerve palsy associated with high-energy humeral shaft fractures. *J Hand Surg Am* 2004;29(1):144-147.

48. Venouziou AI, Dailiana ZH, Varitimidis SE, Hantes ME, Gougoulias NE, Malizos KN: Radial nerve palsy associated with humeral shaft fracture. Is the energy of trauma a prognostic factor? *Injury* 2011;42(11):1289-1293.

In this study, five patients who had low-energy trauma recovered from radial nerve palsy. Of the 13 who had high-energy trauma, 5 fully recovered, and 8 did not recover—4 had lacerated nerves, and the injuries of 4 were irreparable—despite 4 of the nerves being repaired or reconstructed. Level of evidence: III.

49. Korompilias AV, Lykissas MG, Kostas-Agnantis IP, Vekris MD, Soucacos PN, Beris AE: Approach to radial nerve palsy caused by humerus shaft fracture: Is primary exploration necessary? *Injury* 2013;44(3):323-326.

In this retrospective review of 25 patients, surgery was indicated if nerve recovery was not present after 16 weeks of observation. Of the total, 48% underwent exploration, 10% had complete nerve transection, and the nerves of the remainder were intact. All intact nerves fully recovered after 21.6 weeks. Level of evidence: IV.

Section 5

Axial Skeleton: Pelvis, Acetabulum, and Spine

EDITOR
Paul Tornetta III, MD

Chapter 30

Pelvic Fractures: Evaluation and Acute Management

Milton L. (Chip) Routt, Jr., MD

Abstract

Patients with pelvic ring injuries are challenging to treat for a variety of reasons. The pelvic osteology and its surrounding soft-tissue anatomy can be difficult to understand. The anatomy becomes even more complicated and difficult to decipher after injury. Unstable pelvic ring injuries are uncommon and usually occur after high-energy traumatic events. As a result, they can be potentially life threatening due to pelvic area hemorrhage as well as other primary organ system injuries. Patients with unstable pelvic ring injuries warrant immediate attention and adaptable ongoing clinical care. The initial evaluation and early management are tailored to each patient's dynamic clinical course. Early management decisions can affect patients' overall survivability and eventual outcome.

Keywords: pelvic fractures; pelvic instability; initial management

Introduction

The initial evaluation and management of an injured patient with an unstable pelvic ring injury should be rapid, thorough, and routine. Because death can occur due to pelvis-related hemorrhage, the treating physician must quickly identify open wounds and mechanical pelvic instability. The true pelvic volume expands, allowing for more bleeding as the unstable pelvic ring fragments displace and deform. Like administration of intravenous fluids, emergent pelvic reduction and stabilization maneuvers are essential elements of the overall initial patient resuscitation strategy. Pelvic ring instability is most easily identified on presentation by either obvious deformity on the screening AP radiograph of the pelvis or palpable crepitation and fragment movement on compressive manual examination. Pelvic ring instability patterns have been classified using a variety of schemes so that commonly associated injuries and bleeding potential can be predicted. The orthopaedic surgeon has an important role in the early assessment and management of these patients. The early management decisions can have a substantial effect on patient survivability and final functional result.[1]

Anatomy

The pelvic osteology consists of two innominate bones and the sacrum; all have minimal intrinsic stability and therefore are held together by numerous strong ligaments. The symphysis pubis is stabilized by its surrounding symphyseal ligaments and by the arcuate ligament complex located between the inferior rami. The sacroiliac (SI) joint is an unusual articulation tethered anteriorly by SI ligaments that rim the anterior articular surfaces and posteriorly by strong ligaments located just posterior to the SI articulation. These posterior ligaments span between the medial iliac and the lateral sacral dorsal cortical surfaces and provide most of the posterior pelvic stability, along with the sacrospinous, sacrotuberous, and iliolumbar ligaments. The pelvic floor musculature and other structures also play a role in overall pelvic stability.

The pelvic anatomy is complicated further by the surrounding muscles, the multiple nerves that course through it, the lower genitourinary and intestinal systems, and the vascular network. All of these structures are vulnerable to injury in traumatic pelvic ring disruptions and challenge successful clinical management.

Dr. Routt or an immediate family member is a member of a speakers' bureau or has made paid presentations on behalf of AO North America and Zimmer.

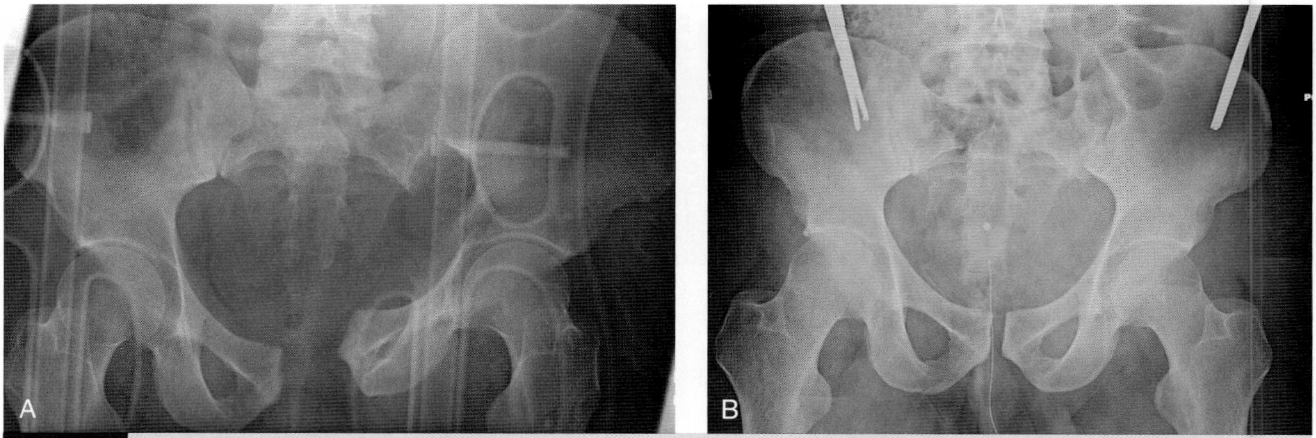

Figure 1 Screening AP plain radiographs of the pelvis demonstrate an unstable pelvic ring injury. **A**, The symphysis pubis and left sacroiliac joint are completely disrupted. Manual traction was applied to the left lower extremity, and a circumferential pelvic sheet was placed around the patient and clamped. **B**, The reduction has been achieved. The injury sites mostly are concealed by the reduction.

Imaging

Good-quality pelvic radiographic imaging is the foundation of the initial evaluation and early management. Such imaging often is difficult to obtain in the chaos that sometimes occurs during patient resuscitation. The screening AP plain radiograph of the pelvis demonstrates the obvious injury sites, fragment displacements, and related deformities. The initial responders at the accident site sometimes apply a circumferential sheet or commercial binder to the pelvis if a pelvic fracture is suspected. Depending on the type of pelvic injury and its application details, the circumferential wrap may conceal or accentuate the injury on the screening radiograph. A 2015 study reported two patients with concealed pelvic ring injuries that had been hidden by a pelvic binder[2] (**Figure 1**).

To see the various injury sites in detail, biplanar inlet and outlet plain radiographs and CT of the pelvis are needed. The importance and variety of imaging studies have been highlighted in numerous studies.[3-17] Modern computer software allows the generation of numerous images from the CT scan's acquired data. CT images reveal details including bone quality, fracture, ligament disruption, deformity, bleeding, hematoma, body habitus, and open wounds, among other features. The value of the screening AP plain radiograph of the pelvis has been questioned recently and has been replaced in some centers by rapid CT scan of the pelvis.[10]

Contrast-enhanced CT adds value by enabling visualization of ongoing hemorrhage of the pelvic area during the evaluation of these patients. The presence of contrast extravasation is associated with the need for pelvic embolization in patients with pelvic fractures, but its absence does not exclude the need for pelvic angiography.[3,11] However, clinicians must remember that a pelvic blush on early contrast-enhanced CT is a frequent finding in patients with pelvic ring fracture, and that many patients with isolated pelvic blushes in particular have stable vital signs and can be managed without surgical or pelvic angiographic embolization (PAE). The need for intervention for a pelvic blush should be determined by the presence of clinical signs of ongoing bleeding.[12]

Routine diagnostic pelvic imaging is more difficult to interpret in elderly patients and others with poor bone quality. One recent study recommended single-photon emission CT for these patients to better identify their occult pelvic ring injuries.[9]

The AP plain radiograph of the pelvis remains the standard initial screening modality for pelvic ring disruptions. CT of the pelvis is recommended to further detail the injury or in those patients for whom clinical concern for occult injuries exists. Other diagnostic studies are obtained as needed to optimize the patient's care.[18-24]

Injury Patterns and Classifications

Various classification systems have been used to categorize pelvic ring disruptions. The Young-Burgess system categorizes pelvic ring disruptions based on load application and resultant instability. The Pennal and Tile classification categorizes these injuries based on their instability patterns, classifying them into focal injuries without ring instability, with rotational instability, and with complex instability. The Denis sacral fracture classification is based on the location of the sacral fracture site relative to the nerve root tunnels and correlates with the incidence of nerve root injury. Many clinicians use the anatomic classification scheme. This descriptive system identifies the injury sites, deformities, and displacements. The anatomic classification system requires no memorization of specific injury patterns. Instead, it details the exact injuries beyond the parameters of the other classifications. Most clinicians prefer the anatomic site scheme because of its site specificity, injury details, and deformity information.

Evaluation

The initial evaluation and early management usually are performed simultaneously, especially in patients with unstable pelvic ring injuries who demonstrate hemodynamic instability. The primary evaluation must be rehearsed and practiced so that it becomes familiar, routine, efficient, and thorough. It is standard to carry out the screening physical examination simultaneously with history taking so that emergent treatment maneuvers are performed as quickly as possible. The accident history is important and can be obtained from the patient, the emergency provider from the accident scene, or other reliable sources. The patient's medical and surgical histories, current medications, and allergies should be obtained whenever possible.

The physical examination has several critical elements. First and foremost, all open traumatic wounds to the pelvic area are sought and identified, because an open wound can provide an easy exit site for pelvic area hemorrhage. These wounds can range from extensive perineal area open wounds that involve the rectum and vagina to small puncture wounds hidden in the gluteal and labial skin folds. All patients with displaced or unstable pelvic fractures require a complete and thorough examination of the perineum, the rectum, and, in women, the vaginal area for open injuries. Obvious debris should be removed, and the wound should be irrigated with saline solution. Intravenous antibiotics and tetanus toxoid are administered in patients with open pelvic fractures. If the patient was exposed to fecal contamination, brackish water, barnyard elements, or other more highly contaminated environments, then the antibiotics should be adjusted accordingly. Using an inside-out technique, open wounds are packed uniformly with a sterile gauze roll, which is readily available in most emergency departments. When unrolled, it provides a sufficient amount of packing material for most traumatic open wounds, and the unrolled sterile gauze packing is difficult to lose within the open wound. Occult open injuries missed on physical examination can be seen on the routine pelvic CT as air densities in atypical locations.[8]

For patients with radiographically obvious displaced fractures that clearly demonstrate instability, no physical assessment of instability is needed. If pelvic stability is in question, then the next portion of the physical examination is a simple pelvic compressive manual maneuver. The examiner applies manual pressure from each iliac crest directed toward the midline. This pelvic compression maneuver reveals gross pelvic instability for a variety of pelvic ring disruption patterns, including distraction open-book injuries, lateral compression injuries, and vertical shear injuries. In awake and alert patients with pelvic mechanical instability, this maneuver can be very painful and therefore does not warrant repeating after the instability has been identified. Misdiagnosed pelvic injuries and chronic pelvic instability and/or malunion may result from an inadequate initial assessment of instability. An examination under anesthesia with dynamic stress fluoroscopy is indicated when the initial examination is inconclusive.[25]

Several other physical examination details are important to remember for patients with pelvic fractures. The urologic examination evaluates for obvious external injuries but also includes inspection for urethral meatal blood, especially in male patients. The rectal examination first is performed visually with inspection to identify any open wounds or anal injury. Next, the digital rectal examination palpates for mucosal abnormalities and defects and assesses the prostate gland's location and surface consistency. The rectal vault stool is examined for obvious blood and tested for occult blood. The neurologic and vascular examinations include the pelvis and lower extremities. The rectal, vaginal, and perineal examinations should be repeated after pelvic stability has been achieved. Early pelvic fixation allows safe placement of the patient in the lithotomy position so that a more thorough evaluation of these anatomic regions can be performed

Initial Management

Resuscitation

The optimal resuscitation method for patients with unstable pelvic ring injuries remains thermoregulation, early stabilization of the pelvic injury, the cessation of obvious bleeding from open wounds, and appropriate intravenous or intraosseous inflow. Numerous algorithms have been produced to appropriately sequence and time these therapeutic interventions and events.[26-30] What remains constant is that each patient warrants principled but tailored treatment. Most pelvic–fracture-specific resuscitation and treatment algorithms recommend some degree of near-excessive fluid resuscitation. Restrained volume resuscitation in the preclinical setting continues to be investigated to assess its effect on the improvement of patient survivability and overall outcomes. The administration of less intravenous fluid should reduce hemodilution and should have a positive effect on concomitant trauma-associated coagulopathy. Low-volume resuscitation remains controversial in practice. Nevertheless, preventing exsanguination and complications such as multiple organ dysfunction syndrome still poses a major challenge in the management of complex pelvic ring injuries.[30]

Recently, whole blood administration has become favored as more clinical studies support its use.[29] The orthopaedic surgeon is an important member of the resuscitation team and must remember that intraosseous access is an option when peripheral or central venous access is limited. The intravenous catheter can be inserted directly into the bone marrow through thin cortical bone in the proximal humerus, distal femur, and proximal tibial areas.

During the initial resuscitation, temporary pelvic stability is achieved using a circumferential pelvic wrap or commercial pelvic binder. The wrap or binder usually is applied from the iliac crests to the greater trochanteric region. Cadaver and clinical studies have shown that the application of pelvic binders at the level of the greater trochanters was optimal.[31,32] The wrap should be smooth and taut to provide a compressive reduction. Wrinkling of the wrap or binder applies focal and occasionally excessive pressure to the skin and certain bony prominences and is avoided. After the circumferential wrap is applied, the awake and alert patient should report improved comfort. An AP plain radiograph of the pelvis is recommended after wrap application to assess the result. For some patients with open-book pelvic injuries, the wrap reduction results can be impressive clinically and radiographically. If the initial screening AP pelvic radiograph is obtained with the patient's pelvis wrapped and the reduction is excellent, the treating physician may miss the diagnosis of an unstable pelvic ring injury[2] (**Figure 1**). In patients with lateral compression instability, the deformity and displacement may be accentuated by the pelvic binder (**Figure 2**). The circumferential pelvic sheet or binder should be adjusted in patients with worsened deformity from the compressive device.[33-35]

When the initial circumferential pelvic sheet application produces an excellent overall reduction, the surgeon may choose to use this opportunity to stabilize the pelvis using the sheet reduction. In these urgent situations, holes are cut in the sheet and are used as working portals to insert percutaneous iliosacral screws or pubic ramus screws or to apply an external fixation device (**Figure 3**).

Circumferential pelvic wrapping continues to be investigated in clinical and cadaver evaluations. It has been shown that patients with unstable pelvic fractures who received pretransfer pelvic compression devices require substantially fewer blood transfusions, shorter intensive care unit stays, and shorter hospital stays compared with patients who do not receive the pretransfer pelvic compression devices.[35] One recent study showed that sheet wrapping for emergent pelvic stabilization was associated with a higher rate of lethal bleeding than pelvic binders and C-clamps.[36] However, cadaver studies have shown that a circumferential pelvic sheet is equally as efficacious at immobilizing the unstable pelvis as a commercial binder. Sheets are more readily available, cost less, and are more versatile than commercial binders, because they can be applied in a variety of ways.[32] In one cadaver study, no statistically significant differences in stability were found when comparing a commercial pelvic binder with anterior pelvic external fixation.[34]

Morbid obesity has been found to affect transfusions for patients with unstable pelvic fractures. A 2015 retrospective review found that morbid obesity represented a substantial risk factor for posttraumatic transfusion in isolated pelvic trauma, even for fracture patterns less likely to receive transfusion.[28]

Angiography

Pelvic angiography allows for the assessment and treatment of pelvic area arterial bleeding sites after trauma. Selective PAE halts ongoing hemorrhage from the injured arterial branch and is recommended whenever possible.[3-6]

In some clinical instances, bilateral or nonselective PAE is performed but is associated with substantial complications. The value of PAE for overall patient survivability must be weighed against its possible adverse consequences.[4] The timing of selective PAE during the resuscitation effort is important to the overall outcome. One recent study showed that earlier pelvic embolization performed within 60 minutes of arrival has a positive effect on the survival rate of hemodynamically unstable patients with pelvic fracture.[6] Also related to PAE timing are the findings of one recent retrospective study showing that two different standards of care were delivered for patients with hemorrhage related to pelvic ring injuries. The authors noted that patients admitted at night and on weekends had a statistically significant increase in time to PAE compared with those arriving during the daytime and during the week. Patients receiving delayed management had an almost 100% increase in mortality.[5]

Aortic Balloon Occlusion

Resuscitative endovascular balloon occlusion of the aorta (REBOA) is another current technique used for managing pelvic related hemorrhage directly. The balloon catheter is inserted using a femoral artery cut-down site and then is positioned within the aorta caudal to the renal and

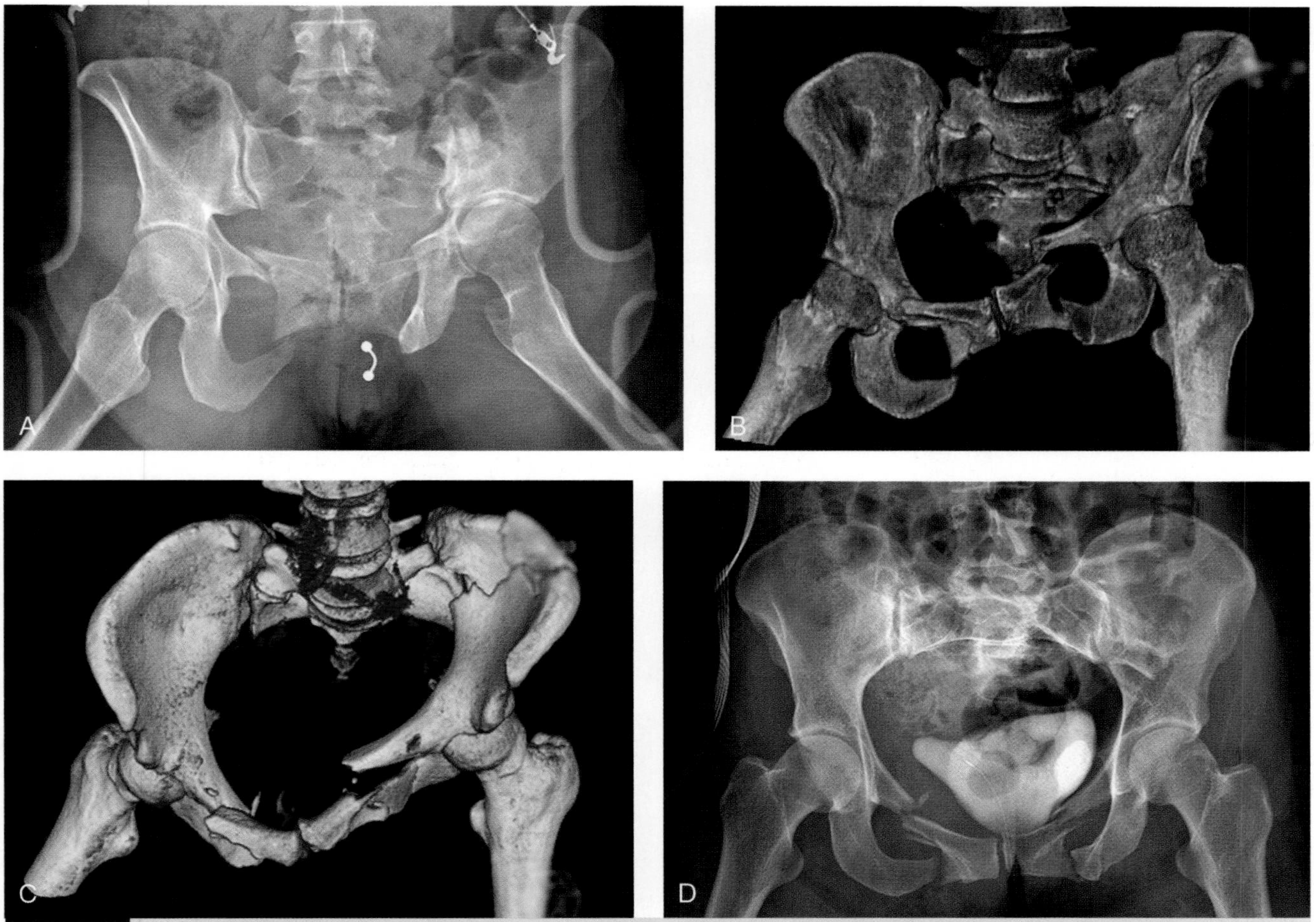

Figure 2 Images show an accentuation of deformity caused by a pelvic binder in a patient with a complex pelvic ring injury with lateral compression instability. **A,** AP pelvis radiograph shows a multiplanar deformity with cranial displacement of the left hemipelvis. **B,** The reformatted image better identifies the pubic ramus fractures and complex left-sided deformity. **C,** The surface-rendered three-dimensional inlet tilt image reveals the left comminuted iliac-sacroiliac joint fracture dislocation, bilateral ramus fractures, and left hemipelvic internal rotation deformity. The right sacroiliac joint anterior disruption can also be seen on this view. **D,** AP pelvis radiograph shows the deformity corrected by the removal of the pelvic binder and the placement of the patient in 10 lb of left-side distal femoral skeletal traction.

abdominal arterial systems. Inflation of the balloon occludes the pelvic arterial tree to temporarily halt pelvic area bleeding. REBOA is less invasive than resuscitative open aortic cross clamping but is functionally similar. The complications of the technique are related to entry site injury and lower-extremity ischemia from prolonged use. Although early clinical results are promising, especially as surgeon experience improves, REBOA warrants continued assessment[37-40] (**Figure 4**).

Retroperitoneal Packing

Retroperitoneal packing for pelvic area hemorrhage control currently is being investigated. After a surgical incision is made anteriorly, a variety of packing devices may be used to provide internal direct tamponade. Most clinicians believe that retroperitoneal packing is used best in conjunction with overall pelvic volume restoration through closed or open reduction.[21]

Fixation

Skeletal traction is advised for unstable pelvic ring disruptions with associated cranial posterior hemipelvic displacement. Usually, a small-diameter traction wire is placed in the distal femur and tensioned in an appropriately sized bow to fit the patient. No more than 10 to 15 lb of traction is advised for most adult patients. Excessive traction beyond this limit usually indicates the need for open reduction. A plain pelvic radiograph obtained with the patient in traction is helpful to assess the effect of the applied traction. Early traction application for vertically

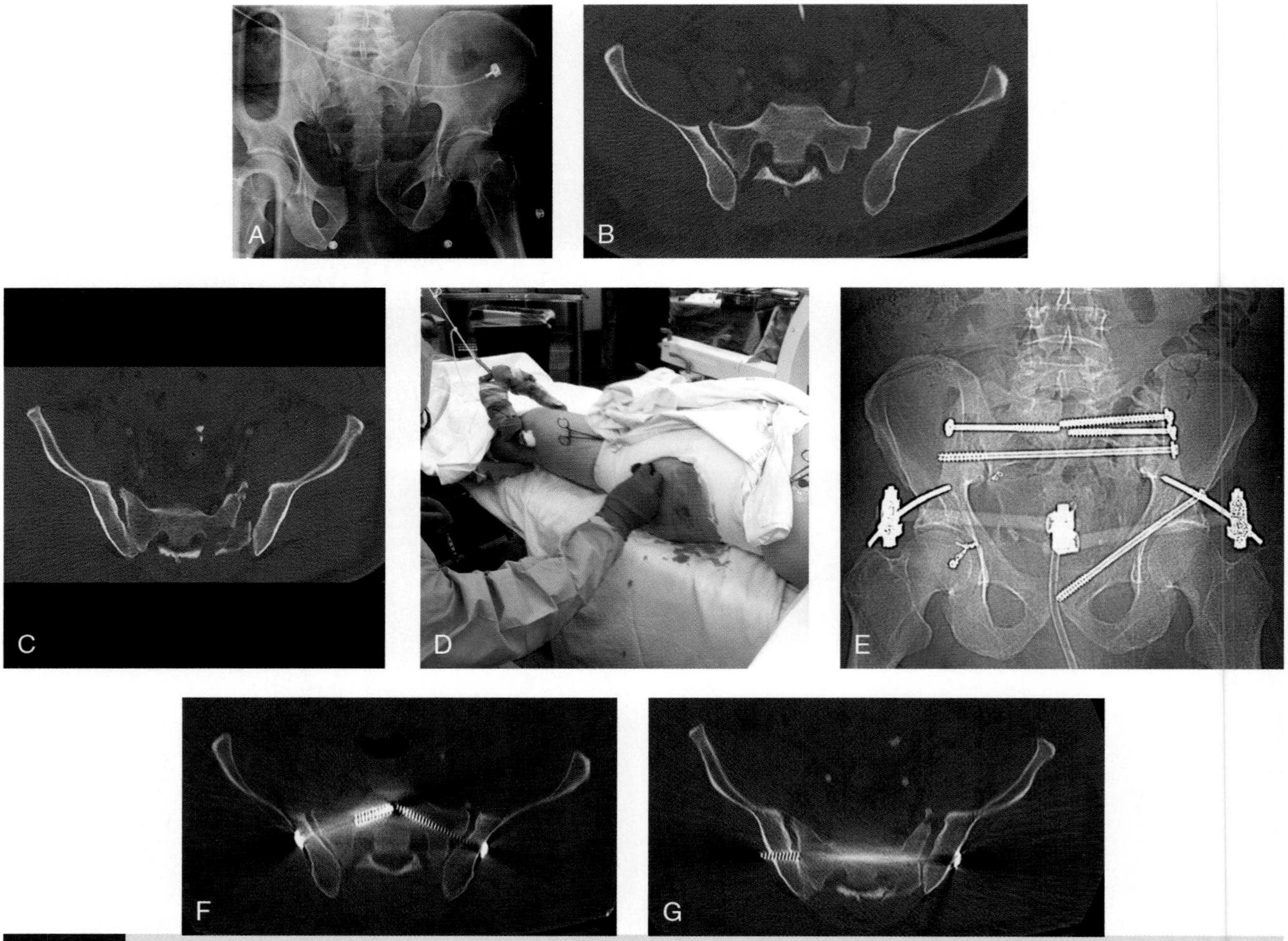

Figure 3 Images depict the use of holes cut in a pelvic circumferential sheet as working portals for the sequential insertion of fluoroscopically guided fixation. **A**, AP pelvis radiograph shows complete symphysis pubis disruption, a left pubic ramus displaced fracture, and bilateral posterior pelvic injuries in a patient who was placed in a pelvic circumferential sheet that resulted in incomplete reductions at the injury sites. **B** The pelvic CT axial image at the upper sacral zone shows the extent of sacroiliac (SI) joint injuries and displacements, as well as the bone available for fixation. C, The axial image at the second sacral level identifies the left-sided SI joint dislocation has an associated displaced dorsal sacral fracture and anterior sacral impaction. **D**, Intraoperative photograph shows holes cut in the sheet and used as working portals for the sequential insertion of fluoroscopically guided iliosacral screws, a medullary ramus screw, and an anterior pelvic external fixation device during urgent percutaneous pelvic fixation. **E**, Iliosacral lag screws were used initially to reduce and compress the posterior pelvic injuries, and then the fully threaded iliosacral screw was subsequently inserted to support the lag screw reduction on the left side. For the anterior ring injuries, the pubic ramus fracture was stabilized with a medullary lag screw and the anterior external fixation frame supported the symphysis injury and the screw fixations. The angiographic embolic coils are also seen on the postoperative film. **F,** On the postoperative CT scan, the upper sacral axial image shows the residual distraction of the right-sided anterior SI joint, and the alar impaction on the left side. **G**, The second sacral level postoperative axial image shows the left dorsal sacral fracture reduction and apparent distraction of the left SI joint due to the anterior alar impaction fracture. The reduction and implant location details are best assessed with a postoperative CT scan.

unstable pelvic ring injuries helps achieve and maintain the reduction so that percutaneous fixation techniques can be considered in the preoperative planning. Traction is not indicated for hemipelvic instability with caudal anterior displacement because the traction will accentuate the deformity and potentially injure the lumbosacral nerve roots and iliac vessels because of stretch.

External Fixation

Anterior pelvic external fixation is used routinely as a resuscitation tool to provide initial pelvic stability and decrease true pelvic volume. Iliac crest and supra-acetabular pin locations are the most commonly used pin sites. A variety of locations and orientations are recommended for supra-acetabular pins. Triplanar fluoroscopy during

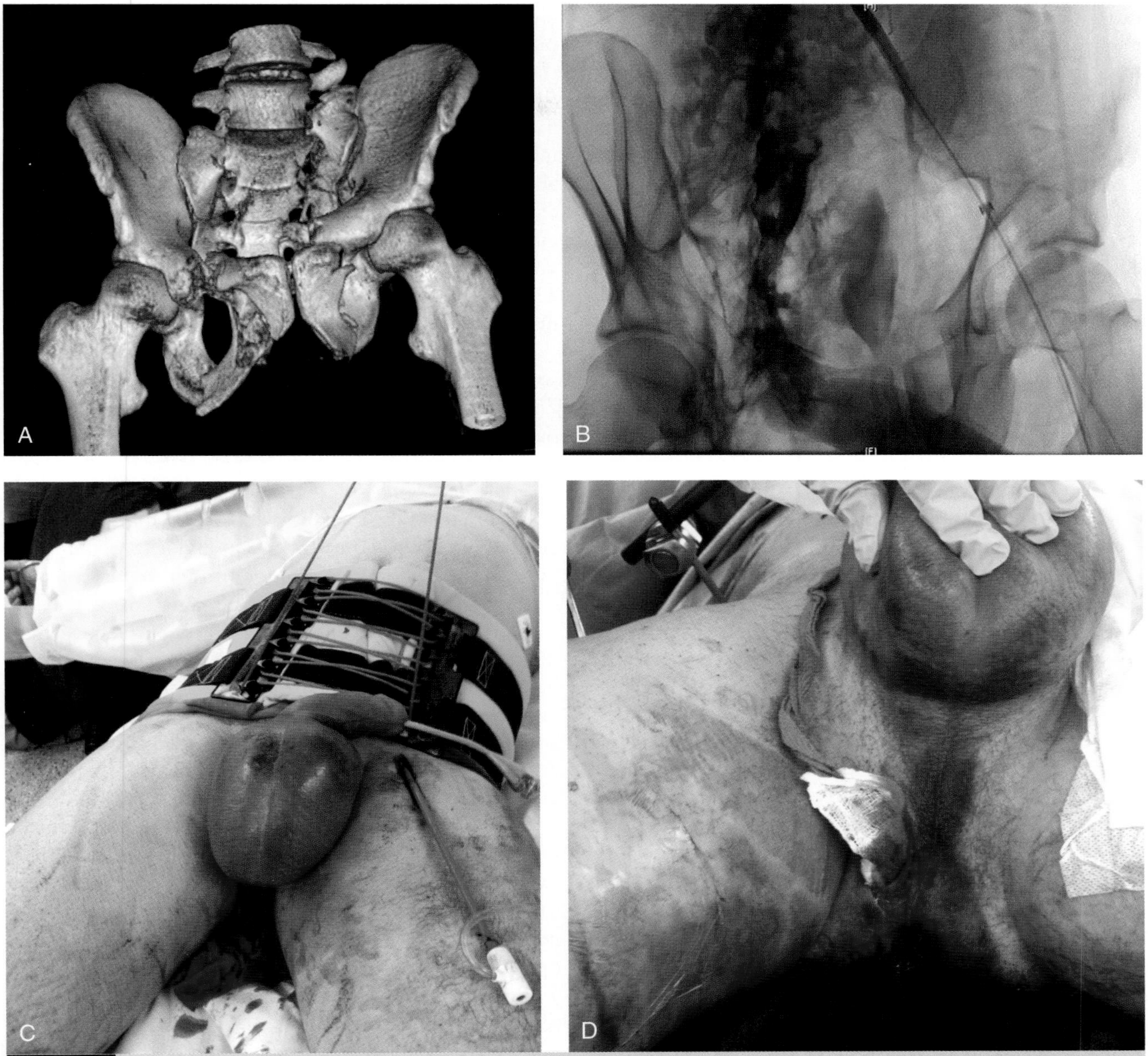

Figure 4 Images demonstrate resuscitative endovascular balloon occlusion of the aorta (REBOA). **A**, Three-dimensional surface-rendered image reveals an unstable and displaced complex pelvic ring injury. The patient had substantial hemorrhaging from a traumatic open perineal wound. **B**, Oblique pelvic angiographic image shows the significant contrast leakage from his arterial injury. **C**, Intraoperative photograph shows REBOA, which was performed to temporarily halt the ongoing pelvic bleeding. The REBOA catheter was inserted in the left femoral artery. **D**, Intraoperative photograph depicts the site after irrigation and packing of the open perineal wound, application of an anterior pelvic external fixation device, and pelvic angiographic embolization.

placement assures that the supra-acetabular pin (1) has an accurate insertion point located at the superior area of the anterior inferior iliac spine well cranial to the hip joint capsule, (2) is aimed properly to allow hip flexion after surgery, (3) is located between the iliac cortical bone surfaces, and (4) is not positioned so deeply that it extrudes through the greater sciatic notch or obstructs subsequent iliosacral screw insertion.[41,42] External pelvic fixation devices are used initially to manipulate a reduction or maintain a manipulative reduction and then to support internal fixation. If noncompliant patient behavior is anticipated, the external bars can be positioned to limit activities. Anterior pelvic external fixation systems with the pins, bars, and clamps located beneath the skin were introduced several years ago, seemed novel, and expectedly were popular. Recent clinical studies have reported important related complications requiring a second surgery to remove these devices. The complications included symptomatic ectopic bone obstructing hip motion that required surgical excision, lateral femoral cutaneous nerve injuries, and even femoral nerve injury.[43-45]

In a recent long-term clinical study, standard anterior pelvic external fixation was advocated because the authors found very few complications and reported the safe removal of the device in the clinic without a second surgery.[46]

Internal Fixation

Internal fixation for pelvic ring disruptions has numerous advantages over external fixation but is much more challenging to apply well. Some surgeons avoid pelvic internal fixation because of (1) unfamiliar surgical exposures, (2) risks of excessive bleeding and of nerve and vascular injuries, (3) unacceptable wound complication rates, and (4) surgeon inexperience. Pelvic internal fixation is biomechanically superior to external fixation. Overall, pelvic ring stability from internal fixation is optimized when the fracture is well reduced and each instability site is stabilized.

Anterior pelvic injuries consist of symphysis pubis disruptions, pubic ramus fractures, and combination injuries. Symphyseal disruptions usually are distracted, but overlapping or locked symphysis also can occur less frequently. Iliac fractures that involve the pelvic ring usually extend from the iliac crest through the greater sciatic notch. Iliac fractures such as anterior superior iliac spine avulsions and comminuted crests spare the overall pelvic ring. Posterior pelvic ring injuries include incomplete SI disruptions, complete SI dislocations, iliac fracture with SI joint disruption, and sacral fractures. Transverse upper-segment sacral fractures include a spectrum of spinopelvic disruptive injuries.

For most adult patients with an unstable symphysis pubis disruption, open reduction and internal fixation (ORIF) with plating remains the standard treatment. A variety of plate designs and lengths have been recommended. The Pfannenstiel or low pubic midline exposure can be used for symphyseal ORIF.[47] One recent study reported reduced fixation failure rates when the symphyseal cartilage was removed at the time of symphyseal ORIF.[48]

Because of their size and comminution, pubic ramus fractures often are treated using external or no anterior fixation. Pubic ramus fracture reductions can be manipulated using (1) remote techniques such as traction and external fixation frames, (2) percutaneous techniques such as blunt elevators or curved retractors, or (3) medullary techniques such as curved wires.[49] For unstable parasymphyseal fractures, plate fixation usually extends across the symphysis pubis to the contralateral side. Midpubic fractures have two available cortical surfaces for plate fixation. If the posterior cortical surface is selected, an intrapelvic exposure is used so the plate can be applied above the acetabulum. If the superior cortical surface is chosen, the fixation plate usually extends to but does not violate the medial acetabulum. Medullary ramus screws are equally effective in stabilizing pubic ramus fractures. These screws are inserted and directed depending on numerous factors.

Pelvic–ring-sparing iliac crest fractures are treated surgically when (1) the fracture is open, (2) considerable displacement is present, causing nerve injury or anticipated healing problems, (3) the fracture causes cosmetic deformity, and (4) closed management fails. These fractures are accessed using the lateral surgical interval of an ilioinguinal exposure, and fixation is accomplished with lag screws between the iliac cortical tables and malleable plates. The abdominal oblique muscle repair must be sound to avoid subsequent hernia formation.

Usually, closed reduction of an incomplete SI joint disruption and of some sacral fractures is accomplished best by accurately reducing the anterior pelvic ring injury. Open reduction of a complete SI dislocation can be accomplished using an anterior iliac exposure or a direct posterior approach. A direct posterior exposure is advocated for open reduction of an unstable sacral fracture.

Iliosacral screws have become the standard and the foundation of posterior pelvic ring stabilization. Clinical experience has matured. Recent series have demonstrated that multiple iliosacral screws of sufficient length within the available pathway at each available sacral level optimize the strength and durability of the construct while diminishing failure rates. To improve iliosacral screw insertion accuracy, the safe pathways for iliosacral screws have been assessed using a variety of radiographic parameters.[50,51]

Unfortunately, the iliosacral screw technique and the understanding of the safe bone pathways continue to be challenging.[52-59] One recent study described alarming rates of screw location error and related nerve root injuries.[60] For the optimally safe use of iliosacral screws, it is imperative for the surgeon to have a complete understanding of the posterior pelvic osteology and its radiology, an accurate reduction, and high-quality intraoperative imaging.

Lumbopelvic fixation supplements iliosacral screw fixation and improves the overall construct strength, especially in the most unstable posterior pelvic injuries.[52-55,61] Like iliosacral screw techniques, lumbopelvic

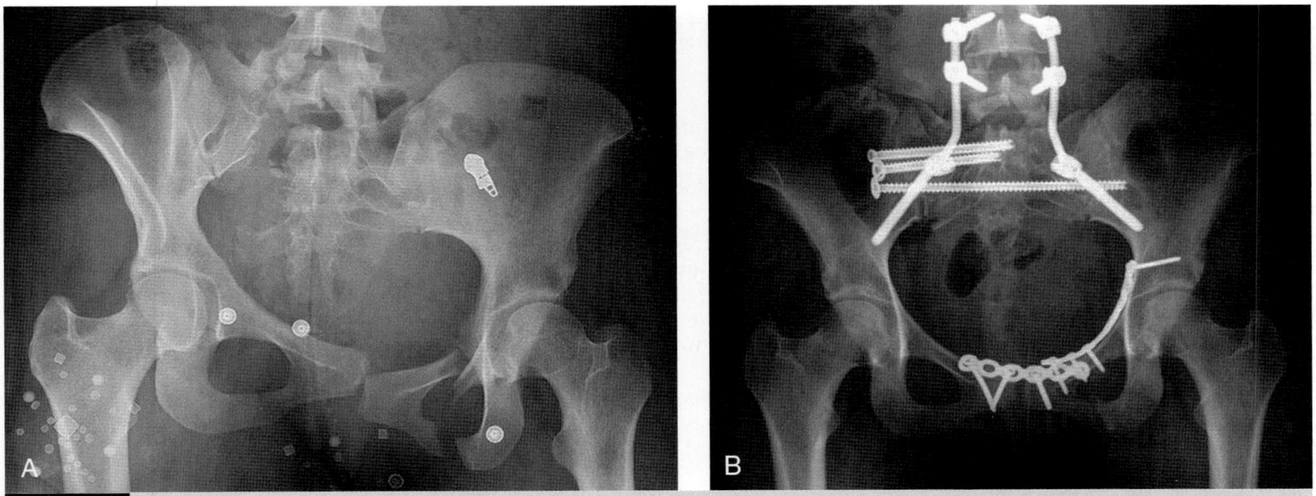

Figure 5 AP pelvis plain radiograph shows a severely displaced right sacral fracture, a complete disruption of the symphysis pubis, and a left-side displaced pubic ramus fracture. **A**, The transforamenal sacral fracture was associated with an S1 facet fracture-dislocation as well as extension of the fracture into the fifth lumbar vertebral body and lamina. **B**, The sacral fracture was treated with open reduction and internal fixation initially with the patient positioned prone. The fracture surfaces allowed for accurate reduction and clamping. Iliosacral screws were first inserted according to her sacral osteology: obliquely at S1, and transiliac transsacral at S2. Fully threaded screws were used to support the clamp compression at the fracture site. The denuded facet was excised and lumbopelvic fixation was used to support the sacral and lumbar fractures. Open reduction and internal fixation of the anterior pelvic injuries was then performed using a low pubic midline exposure.

fixation techniques have evolved to the point that the pedicle and iliac screw placements and the connecting bar attachments routinely are performed percutaneously, using short and focal incisions whenever possible (**Figure 5**). Recessing the iliac screw head and connector beneath the posterior iliac cortical bone diminishes symptoms related to the device.

Summary

Unstable pelvic ring disruptions, whether from high-energy traumatic events or poor bone quality, remain difficult to treat effectively. Recent studies have focused on improved imaging and resuscitation interventions. Pelvic binders and circumferential sheeting have become common and successful modes of early reduction and temporary stabilization. Iliosacral screws remain the foundation of posterior pelvic fixation, but their insertions continue to challenge many surgeons.

Key Study Points

- Pelvic ring instability and related bleeding must be diagnosed and treated early after injury.
- Circumferential pelvic wrapping is useful to initially reduce certain pelvic ring disruptions.
- Contrast-enhanced CT of the pelvis reliably identifies important factors related to unstable pelvic ring injuries.
- Anterior pelvic external fixation devices applied beneath the skin are associated with complications.
- Accurate early pelvic reduction and stable internal fixation are preferred whenever possible.

Annotated References

1. Abrassart S, Stern R, Peter R: Unstable pelvic ring injury with hemodynamic instability: What seems the best procedure choice and sequence in the initial management? *Orthop Traumatol Surg Res* 2013;99(2):175-182.

This study intended to determine the optimal sequence of surgical procedures to restore hemodynamic stability in patients with unstable pelvic ring injuries. The patients were divided into four groups according to the sequence of surgical procedures performed within 24 hours of admission. The authors found that the management of hemorrhagic instability linked to pelvic ring disruption involves a sequence of therapeutic events that is more important than the events themselves. Level of evidence: IV.

2. Clements J, Jeavons R, White C, McMurtry I: The concealment of significant pelvic injuries on computed tomography evaluation by pelvic compression devices. *J Emerg Med* 2015;49(5):675-678.

   This report identified two patients with pelvic ring injuries who had pelvic binders applied before the time of screening evaluations, including pelvic CT. In both cases, CT failed to identify a substantial pelvic injury, which was concealed by the pelvic external compression belt.

3. Bozeman MC, Cannon RM, Trombold JM, et al: Use of computed tomography findings and contrast extravasation in predicting the need for embolization with pelvic fractures. *Am Surg* 2012;78(8):825-830.

   This study attempted to identify the demographic and radiographic findings that predict the need for embolization. The authors found that contrast extravasation was not present in 25% of patients requiring therapeutic transarterial embolization and concluded that the presence of contrast extravasation is associated highly with the need for pelvic embolization in patients with pelvic fractures. Its absence does not exclude the need for pelvic angiography.

4. Matityahu A, Marmor M, Elson JK, et al: Acute complications of patients with pelvic fractures after pelvic angiographic embolization. *Clin Orthop Relat Res* 2013;471(9):2906-2911.

   This study highlighted the complications observed after bilateral or nonselective pelvic arterial embolization. The authors advocate for selective unilateral arterial embolization whenever possible.

5. Schwartz DA, Medina M, Cotton BA, et al: Are we delivering two standards of care for pelvic trauma? Availability of angioembolization after hours and on weekends increases time to therapeutic intervention. *J Trauma Acute Care Surg* 2014;76(1):134-139.

   This study demonstrated that patients admitted at night and on weekends have a statistically significant increase in time to angioembolization compared with those arriving during the daytime and during the week. Multivariate regression noted that after-hours management was associated with an almost 100% increase in mortality. This study suggests that two different standards of care are being delivered for pelvic trauma, depending on the day and time of admission. Level of evidence: II.

6. Tanizaki S, Maeda S, Matano H, Sera M, Nagai H, Ishida H: Time to pelvic embolization for hemodynamically unstable pelvic fractures may affect the survival for delays up to 60 min. *Injury* 2014;45(4):738-741.

   This study found that patients who were embolized within 60 minutes of arrival had a significantly lower mortality rate (16 versus 64%; $P = 0.04$). No embolization-related complications were observed.

7. Hallinan JT, Tan CH, Pua U: Emergency computed tomography for acute pelvic trauma: Where is the bleeder? *Clin Radiol* 2014;69(5):529-537.

   A technique for predicting the location of the bleeding vessel in patients with acute pelvic trauma. This technique is based on knowledge of the cross-sectional anatomical territory of the vessel rather than tracing the vessel's course.

8. Scolaro JA, Wilson DJ, Routt ML: Use of the initial trauma CT scan to aid in diagnosis of open pelvic fractures. *Injury* 2015;46(10):1999-2002.

   In this study of patients with a pelvic disruption, 33% of the open pelvic fractures initially were missed clinically but were subsequently diagnosed because of ectopic air densities identified on the pelvic CT. Pneumothorax, bowel injuries, and open wounds that were previously missed clinically can be identified by these atypical site air densities on routine pelvic CT.

9. Scheyerer MJ, Hüllner M, Pietsch C, Werner CM, Veit-Haibach P: Evaluation of pelvic ring injuries using SPECT/CT. *Skeletal Radiol* 2015;44(2):217-222.

   In this study, single-photon emission computed tomography proved to be helpful in diagnosing occult fractures and instability within the SI joint.

10. Bishop JA, Rao AJ, Pouliot MA, Beaulieu C, Bellino M: Conventional versus virtual radiographs of the injured pelvis and acetabulum. *Skeletal Radiol* 2015;44(9):1303-1308.

    This study showed that virtual radiographs of pelvic and acetabular fractures offer superior image quality, improved comfort, reduced radiation exposure, and a more cost-effective alternative to conventional radiographs.

11. Brun J, Guillot S, Bouzat P, et al: Detecting active pelvic arterial haemorrhage on admission following serious pelvic fracture in multiple trauma patients. *Injury* 2014;45(1):101-106.

    The effectiveness of an institutional algorithm focusing on hemodynamic status on admission and whole-body CT scan in stabilized patients to screen patients in whom transcatheter arterial embolization was required was assessed in a retrospective study of 106 patients.

12. Verbeek DO, Zijlstra IA, van der Leij C, Ponsen KJ, van Delden OM, Goslings JC: Management of pelvic ring fracture patients with a pelvic "blush" on early computed tomography. *J Trauma Acute Care Surg* 2014;76(2):374-379.

    This study found that, in patients with pelvic ring fracture, a pelvic blush on early contrast-enhanced CT is a frequent finding. Many patients with pelvic blushes, particularly those that are isolated, have stable vital signs and can be managed without surgical or radiologic pelvic hemorrhage control. The need for an intervention for a pelvic blush seems to be determined by the presence of clinical signs of ongoing bleeding. Level of evidence: IV.

13. Gabbe BJ, Esser M, Bucknill A, et al: The imaging and classification of severe pelvic ring fractures:

Experiences from two level 1 trauma centres. *Bone Joint J* 2013;95-B(10):1396-1401.

In 187 patients, routine imaging practices of Level 1 trauma centers were described for patients with severe pelvic ring fractures, and the interobserver reliability of the classification systems of these fractures using plain radiographs and three-dimensional (3D) CT reconstructions was assessed.

14. Nüchtern JV, Hartel MJ, Henes FO, et al: Significance of clinical examination, CT and MRI scan in the diagnosis of posterior pelvic ring fractures. *Injury* 2015;46(2):315-319.

This study noted the significance of clinical examination and CT in the detection of fractures in the posterior pelvic ring. MRI examination of the pelvis was found to be superior in detecting undislocated fractures in a cohort of patients with a high incidence of osteoporosis. Using MRI may be beneficial in select cases, especially when reduced bone density is suspected.

15. Pekmezci M, Kandemir U, Toogood P, Morshed S: Are conventional inlet and outlet radiographs obsolete in the evaluation of pelvis fractures? *J Trauma Acute Care Surg* 2013;74(6):1510-1515.

This study showed that virtual inlet and outlet images consistently provided higher rates of adequate radiographs than conventional radiographs. In the evaluation of patients with pelvis fractures, obtaining virtual inlet and outlet views instead of conventional radiographs may provide some advantages, such as reductions in radiation exposure to the patient, overall cost, and repeat radiographs to achieve adequate views. Level of evidence: V.

16. Suzuki T, Morgan SJ, Smith WR, Stahel PF, Flierl MA, Hak DJ: Stress radiograph to detect true extent of symphyseal disruption in presumed anteroposterior compression type I pelvic injuries. *J Trauma* 2010;69(4):880-885.

A stress examination under general anesthesia in patients with acute pelvic injury can help accurately diagnose the extent of injury and select the appropriate treatment.

17. Fu CY, Wang SY, Hsu YP, et al: The diminishing role of pelvic x-rays in the management of patients with major torso injuries. *Am J Emerg Med* 2014;32(1):18-23.

The use of pelvic x-rays is on the decline and is being supplanted by CT. Pelvic x-rays are still obtained for patients in critical condition who are likely to experience retroperitoneal hemorrhage.

18. Bolorunduro OB, Haider AH, Oyetunji TA, et al: Disparities in trauma care: Are fewer diagnostic tests conducted for uninsured patients with pelvic fracture? *Am J Surg* 2013;205(4):365-370.

Using a national database, this study examined the differences in diagnostic and therapeutic procedures administered to patients who underwent trauma with pelvic fractures. The authors found that insurance-based disparities were less evident in level 1 trauma centers, uninsured patients with pelvic fractures get fewer diagnostic procedures than their insured counterparts, and this disparity is much greater for more invasive and resource-intensive tests.

19. Langford JR, Burgess AR, Liporace FA, Haidukewych GJ: Pelvic fractures: Part 1. Evaluation, classification, and resuscitation. *J Am Acad Orthop Surg* 2013;21(8):448-457.

Treatment options and established protocols for open and closed pelvic fractures are discussed.

20. Langford JR, Burgess AR, Liporace FA, Haidukewych GJ: Pelvic fractures: Part 2. Contemporary indications and techniques for definitive surgical management. *J Am Acad Orthop Surg* 2013;21(8):458-468.

The indications for surgical treatment of pelvic fractures is discussed.

21. Mauffrey C, Cuellar DO III, Pieracci F, et al: Strategies for the management of haemorrhage following pelvic fractures and associated trauma-induced coagulopathy. *Bone Joint J* 2014;96-B(9):1143-1154.

This article provides an overview of the classification of pelvic injuries and the current evidence on the best-practice management of high-energy pelvic fractures, including resuscitation, transfusion of blood components, monitoring of coagulopathy, and procedural interventions such as preperitoneal pelvic packing, external fixation, and angiographic embolization.

22. Fitzgerald CA, Morse BC, Dente CJ: Pelvic ring fractures: Has mortality improved following the implementation of damage control resuscitation? *Am J Surg* 2014;208(6):1083-1090, discussion 1089-1090.

This study investigates the outcomes of closed and open pelvic ring fractures at a single institution before and after the formal implementation of damage control resuscitation (DCR) principles. A retrospective chart review was performed in an urban level I trauma center that identified 2,247 patients with pelvic fractures over 10 years. No difference in mortality was observed when comparing DCR and before DCR cohorts for open or closed pelvic fractures.

23. Harvin JA, Peirce CA, Mims MM, et al: The impact of tranexamic acid on mortality in injured patients with hyperfibrinolysis. *J Trauma Acute Care Surg* 2015;78(5):905-909, discussion 909-911.

In this study, tranexamic acid was not associated with a reduction in mortality. Level of evidence: IV.

24. Holcomb JB, Tilley BC, Baraniuk S, et al; PROPPR Study Group: Transfusion of plasma, platelets, and red blood cells in a 1:1:1 vs a 1:1:2 ratio and mortality in patients with severe trauma: The PROPPR randomized clinical trial. *JAMA* 2015;313(5):471-482.

This multicenter study attempted to determine the effectiveness and safety of transfusing patients with severe trauma and major bleeding using plasma, platelets, and red blood cells in a 1:1:1 ratio compared with a 1:1:2 ratio. The authors reported that, among patients with severe trauma and major bleeding, early administration of plasma, platelets, and red blood cells in a 1:1:1 ratio compared with a 1:1:2 ratio did not result in statistically significant differences in mortality at 24 hours or at 30 days.

25. Sagi HC, Coniglione FM, Stanford JH: Examination under anesthetic for occult pelvic ring instability. *J Orthop Trauma* 2011;25(9):529-536.

    Examination under anesthesia is an important diagnostic tool that provides information about pelvic ring instability and helps prevent inadequate treatment of misdiagnosed injuries, which can lead to chronic instability and/or malunion.

26. Morshed S, Knops S, Jurkovich GJ, Wang J, MacKenzie E, Rivara FP: The impact of trauma-center care on mortality and function following pelvic ring and acetabular injuries. *J Bone Joint Surg Am* 2015;97(4):265-272.

    Mortality was reduced for patients with unstable pelvic and severe acetabular injuries when care was provided in a trauma center rather than in a nontrauma center. Moreover, those with severe acetabular fractures experienced improved physical function at 1 year. Patients with these injuries represent a well-defined subset of trauma patients for whom the findings suggest preferential triage or transfer to a level 1 trauma center.

27. Childs BR, Nahm NJ, Dolenc AJ, Vallier HA: Obesity is associated with more complications and longer hospital stays after orthopaedic trauma. *J Orthop Trauma* 2015;29(11):504-509.

    Obesity was noted among 42% of trauma patients in this study. In obese patients, complications occurred more often, and hospital and intensive care unit stays were substantially longer. These increases are likely to be associated with higher hospital costs. Surgeon decisions to delay procedures in medically stable obese patients may have contributed to these findings. Definitive fixation was more likely to be delayed in obese patients.

28. Richards JE, Morris BJ, Guillamondegui OD, et al: The effect of body mass index on posttraumatic transfusion after pelvic trauma. *Am Surg* 2015;81(3):239-244.

    In this study, morbid obesity was a statistically significant risk factor for transfusion. Adjusting by age and fracture patterns less likely to receive transfusion, morbid obesity remained a risk factor for transfusion in isolated pelvic trauma even for fracture patterns less likely to receive transfusion.

29. Cotton BA, Podbielski J, Camp E, et al; Early Whole Blood Investigators: A randomized controlled pilot trial of modified whole blood versus component therapy in severely injured patients requiring large volume transfusions. *Ann Surg* 2013;258(4):527-532, discussion 532-533.

    Modified whole blood reduced transfusion volumes in patients without severe brain injuries but did not reduce transfusion volumes in severely injured patients predicted to receive massive transfusion.

30. Burkhardt M, Kristen A, Culemann U, et al; TraumaRegister DGU; German Pelvic Injury Register: Pelvic fracture in multiple trauma: Are we still up-to-date with massive fluid resuscitation? *Injury* 2014;45(suppl 3):S70-S75.

    Evidence indicates that restrained volume therapy in the preclinical setting may improve trauma outcomes. Hemodilution and concomitant trauma-associated coagulopathy might be reduced with less intravenous fluid administration.

31. Bonner TJ, Eardley WG, Newell N, et al: Accurate placement of a pelvic binder improves reduction of unstable fractures of the pelvic ring. *J Bone Joint Surg Br* 2011;93(11):1524-1528.

    This study assessed the accuracy of placement of pelvic binders and determined whether circumferential compression at the level of the greater trochanters was the best method of reducing a symphyseal diastasis. The authors noted that application of a pelvic binder above the level of the greater trochanters was common but was an inadequate method of reducing pelvic fractures.

32. Prasarn ML, Small J, Conrad B, Horodyski N, Horodyski M, Rechtine GR: Does application position of the T-POD affect stability of pelvic fractures? *J Orthop Trauma* 2013;27(5):262-266.

    This cadaver study found that, in an unstable pelvic injury, placement of a pelvic binder at the level of the greater trochanters provided improved control of the fracture.

33. Prasarn ML, Conrad B, Small J, Horodyski M, Rechtine GR: Comparison of circumferential pelvic sheeting versus the T-POD on unstable pelvic injuries: A cadaveric study of stability. *Injury* 2013;44(12):1756-1759.

    This cadaver study sought to determine whether the trauma pelvic orthotic device (T-POD) pelvic binder would provide more stability to an unstable pelvic injury than circumferential pelvic sheeting. A T-POD or a circumferential sheet was applied in random order for testing. No differences were seen in motion of the injured hemipelvis during application of the T-POD or the circumferential sheet. During the bed transfer, log-rolling, and head of bed elevation, no statistically significant differences in displacements were observed when the pelvis was immobilized with a sheet or the T-POD pelvic binder.

34. Prasarn ML, Horodyski M, Conrad B, et al: Comparison of external fixation versus the trauma pelvic orthotic device on unstable pelvic injuries: A cadaveric study of stability. *J Trauma Acute Care Surg* 2012;72(6):1671-1675.

    This cadaver study assessed whether a pelvic external fixator would provide more stability to an unstable pelvic injury than a commercially available binder. Unstable pelvic injuries classified as Tile C were created surgically in five fresh whole human cadavers. For unstable pelvic injuries, the authors found no statistically significant differences in stability conferred by an external fixator or a T-POD pelvic binder.

35. Fu CY, Wu YT, Liao CH, et al: Pelvic circumferential compression devices benefit patients with pelvic fractures who need transfers. *Am J Emerg Med* 2013;31(10):1432-1436.

This study determined that pelvic circumferential compression devices do benefit patients with pelvic fracture who need to be transferred to trauma centers. Pretransfer placement of the pelvic circumferential compression device appeared to be feasible and safe during the transfer.

36. Pizanis A, Pohlemann T, Burkhardt M, Aghayev E, Holstein JH: Emergency stabilization of the pelvic ring: Clinical comparison between three different techniques. *Injury* 2013;44(12):1760-1764.

The data suggest that emergency stabilization of the pelvic ring by binders and c-clamps is associated with a lower incidence of lethal pelvic bleeding than that provided by sheet wrapping. Level of evidence: III.

37. Brenner ML, Moore LJ, DuBose JJ, et al: A clinical series of resuscitative endovascular balloon occlusion of the aorta for hemorrhage control and resuscitation. *J Trauma Acute Care Surg* 2013;75(3):506-511.

This study found that resuscitative endovascular balloon occlusion of the aorta is a feasible and effective means of proactive aortic control for patients in end-stage shock from blunt and penetrating mechanisms. Level of evidence: V.

38. Saito N, Matsumoto H, Yagi T, et al: Evaluation of the safety and feasibility of resuscitative endovascular balloon occlusion of the aorta. *J Trauma Acute Care Surg* 2015;78(5):897-903, discussion 904.

According to this study, resuscitative endovascular balloon occlusion of the aorta seems to be feasible for trauma resuscitation and may improve survivorship. The serious complication of lower-limb ischemia warrants more research on the safety of the procedure. Level of evidence: V.

39. Morrison JJ, Percival TJ, Markov NP, et al: Aortic balloon occlusion is effective in controlling pelvic hemorrhage. *J Surg Res* 2012;177(2):341-347.

The effectiveness of aortic balloon occlusion to manage noncompressible pelvic hemorrhage was evaluated.

40. Delamare L, Crognier L, Conil JM, Rousseau H, Georges B, Ruiz S: Treatment of intra-abdominal haemorrhagic shock by Resuscitative Endovascular Balloon Occlusion of the Aorta (REBOA). *Anaesth Crit Care Pain Med* 2015;34(1):53-55.

Intra-abdominal hemorrhagic shock was treated by resuscitative endovascular balloon occlusion of the aorta in a 35-year-old man with a ruptured splenic artery aneurysm.

41. Calafi LA, Routt ML: Anterior pelvic external fixation: Is there an optimal placement for the supra-acetabular pin? *Am J Orthop (Belle Mead NJ)* 2013;42(12):E125-E127.

The supra-acetabular bone pin must be placed strategically to provide optimal frame stability, patient comfort, and hip mobility without obstructing subsequent osseous fixation pathways. The technique for the alternative placement of supra-acetabular bone pins is described, and the intraoperative imaging is detailed. The bone pin starting point is located more cranially than described previously, at the anterior inferior iliac spine, and the pin is directed to accommodate better hip motion.

42. Stahel PF, Mauffrey C, Smith WR, et al: External fixation for acute pelvic ring injuries: Decision making and technical options. *J Trauma Acute Care Surg* 2013;75(5):882-887.

43. Hesse D, Kandmir U, Solberg B, et al: Femoral nerve palsy after pelvic fracture treated with INFIX: A case series. *J Orthop Trauma* 2015;29(3):138-143.

This series followed six patients with eight femoral nerve palsies after application of a subcutaneous anterior pelvic fixator (INFIX) device to inform pelvic surgeons using this technique about the potentially devastating complication of femoral nerve palsy. Despite early implant removal after the detection of nerve injury, some patients had residual quadriceps weakness, disturbance of the skin sensation on the thigh, and/or gait disturbance attributable to femoral nerve palsy at the time of early final follow-up. Level of evidence: IV.

44. Cole PA, Gauger EM, Anavian J, Ly TV, Morgan RA, Heddings AA: Anterior pelvic external fixator versus subcutaneous internal fixator in the treatment of anterior ring pelvic fractures. *J Orthop Trauma* 2012;26(5):269-277.

Subcutaneous anterior pelvic fixation was associated with good clinical outcomes (lower wound complication rate and associated morbidity, and fewer surgical site symptoms) in comparison with anterior pelvic external fixation. Level of evidence: III.

45. Schottel PC, Smith CS, Helfet DL: Symptomatic hip impingement due to exostosis associated with supra-acetabular pelvic external fixator pin. *Am J Orthop (Belle Mead NJ)* 2014;43(1):33-36.

A symptomatic exostosis formed at the supra-acetabular pin site, a unique complication in a 35-year-old man with a pelvic fracture. The anterior approach to the hip was used to excise the impinging bone. There was a 40° improvement in the patient's hip flexion range of motion after excision.

46. Mitchell PM, Corrigan CM, Patel NA, et al: 13-Year experience in external fixation of the pelvis: Complications, reduction and removal. *Eur J Trauma Emerg Surg* 2016;42(1):91-96.

Previous data suggest high complication rates in definitive anterior pelvic external fixation. This study, which presents the largest cohort of patients receiving anterior pelvic external fixation and sacroiliac screws, demonstrates a low complication rate while maintaining reduction of the pelvic ring. The study also found that these devices could be removed reliably in a clinic setting.

47. Adams MR, Scolaro JA, Routt ML Jr: The pubic midline exposure for symphyseal open reduction and plate fixation. *J Orthop Traumatol* 2014;15(3):195-199.

5: Axial Skeleton: Pelvis, Acetabulum, and Spine

The authors of this study concluded that pubic midline skin exposure is a reasonable alternative to the Pfannenstiel incision for open reduction and plate fixation of the pubic symphysis. Level of evidence: IV.

48. Lybrand K, Kurylo J, Gross J, Templeman D, Tornetta P III: Does removal of the symphyseal cartilage in symphyseal dislocations have any effect on final alignment and implant failure? *J Orthop Trauma* 2015;29(10):470-474.

    This comparative clinical study suggests that removing the symphyseal cartilage at the time of symphysis pubis open reduction and internal fixation correlates with fewer fixation failures. Level of evidence: III.

49. Scolaro JA, Routt ML: Intraosseous correction of misdirected cannulated screws and fracture malalignment using a bent tip 2.0 mm guidewire: Technique and indications. *Arch Orthop Trauma Surg* 2013;133(7):883-887.

    The authors present a reliable and reproducible technique using a 2.0-mm guidewire that allows for the correction of an initially misdirected drill within the pelvis. This technique also allows for medullary manipulation and the reduction of certain malaligned pelvic fractures before percutaneous cannulated screw placement. The technique is not a substitute for poor surgical technique but can be used to optimize the position of percutaneously placed pelvic screws.

50. Kaiser SP, Gardner MJ, Liu J, Routt ML Jr, Morshed S: Anatomic determinants of sacral dysmorphism and implications for safe iliosacral screw placement. *J Bone Joint Surg Am* 2014;96(14):e120.

    This study attempts to further describe the safe bone pathways available for upper sacral iliosacral screw insertions.

51. Lee JJ, Rosenbaum SL, Martusiewicz A, Holcombe SA, Wang SC, Goulet JA: Transsacral screw safe zone size by sacral segmentation variations. *J Orthop Res* 2015;33(2):277-282.

    Transsacral screw safe zone size is dependent on patient sex and sacral segmentation variations.

52. Tabaie SA, Bledsoe JG, Moed BR: Biomechanical comparison of standard iliosacral screw fixation to transsacral locked screw fixation in a type C zone II pelvic fracture model. *J Orthop Trauma* 2013;27(9):521-526.

    Fixation of unstable zone II sacral fractures using the combination of an iliosacral screw and a locked transsacral screw resists deformation and withstands a greater force to failure than fixation with two standard iliosacral screws. This locked transsacral construct may prove advantageous, especially when a percutaneous technique is used for a type C zone II vertically oriented sacral fracture injury pattern, which can result in residual fracture site separation.

53. Miller AN, Routt ML Jr: Variations in sacral morphology and implications for iliosacral screw fixation. *J Am Acad Orthop Surg* 2012;20(1):8-16.

    The dysmorphic sacrum has many important characteristics, and it is important that the surgeon be knowledgeable about individual patient anatomy, its variations, and related imaging to ensure safe iliosacral screw placement.

54. Bishop JA, Routt ML Jr: Osseous fixation pathways in pelvic and acetabular fracture surgery: Osteology, radiology, and clinical applications. *J Trauma Acute Care Surg* 2012;72(6):1502-1509.

55. Min KS, Zamorano DP, Wahba GM, Garcia I, Bhatia N, Lee TQ: Comparison of two-transsacral-screw fixation versus triangular osteosynthesis for transforaminal sacral fractures. *Orthopedics* 2014;37(9):e754-e760.

    Compared with triangular osteosynthesis fixation, using two transsacral screws provides a comparable biomechanical stability profile in translation and rotation. This newly revised two–transsacral-screw construct offers the traumatologist an alternative method of repair for vertical shear fractures that provides biplanar stability. It also provides the advantage of percutaneous placement with the patient in the prone or supine position.

56. Eastman JG, Routt ML Jr: Correlating preoperative imaging with intraoperative fluoroscopy in iliosacral screw placement. *J Orthop Traumatol* 2015;16(4):309-316.

    Substantial anatomic variation of the posterior pelvic ring exists. The preoperative CT sagittal reconstruction images enable appropriate preoperative planning for anticipated intraoperative fluoroscopic inlet and outlet views within 5°. Knowing the chosen intraoperative views preoperatively prepares the surgeon, aids in efficiently obtaining correct intraoperative views, and contributes to safe iliosacral screw placement.

57. Hopf JC, Krieglstein CF, Müller LP, Koslowsky TC: Percutaneous iliosacral screw fixation after osteoporotic posterior ring fractures of the pelvis reduces pain significantly in elderly patients. *Injury* 2015;46(8):1631-1636.

    Conventional percutaneous iliosacral screw fixation is a successful surgical treatment for elderly patients with persistent low back pain after an unstable posterior ring fracture of the pelvis. Level of evidence: IV.

58. Salazar D, Lannon S, Pasternak O, et al: Investigation of bone quality of the first and second sacral segments amongst trauma patients: Concerns about iliosacral screw fixation. *J Orthop Traumatol* 2015;16(4):301-308.

    The pelvic CT scans of 25 consecutive trauma patients aged 18 to 49 years at a level 1 trauma center were analyzed prospectively. Hounsfield units, a standardized CT attenuation coefficient, were used to measure regional cancellous bone mineral density of the S1 and S2. No change in the clinical protocol or the treatment occurred as a consequence of inclusion in this study. In relatively young otherwise healthy trauma patients, a statically significant difference in bone quality was found when comparing the first and second sacral segment ($P = 0.0001$). Age, sex, and smoking status did not affect bone quality independently.

59. Bishop JA, Behn AW, Castillo TN: The biomechanical significance of washer use with screw fixation. *J Orthop Trauma* 2014;28(2):114-117.

Washers used during screw fixation allow for more compression before intrusion occurs and help salvage compressive force of intruded screws.

60. Tejwani NC, Raskolnikov D, McLaurin T, Takemoto R: The role of computed tomography for postoperative evaluation of percutaneous sacroiliac screw fixation and description of a "safe zone". *Am J Orthop (Belle Mead NJ)* 2014;43(11):513-516.

This clinical study describes an alarming 45% incidence of wayward iliosacral screw locations, with an even more disturbing 22% rate of nerve root injuries from the poorly located screws identified on postoperative pelvic CT scans.

61. Salari P, Moed BR, Bledsoe JG: Supplemental S1 fixation for type C pelvic ring injuries: Biomechanical study of a long iliosacral versus a transsacral screw. *J Orthop Traumatol* 2015;16(4):293-300.

In a comparison of long iliosacral and transsacral screws in providing additional stability to an unstable sacral fracture fixation construct, no biomechanical advantage of one method over the other was found.

In many circumstances, the iliac wing fracture enters the SI joint and results in a partial dislocation. This type of injury is the crescent fracture or fracture-dislocation. The anterior SI joint ligaments are disrupted, but the posterior ilium fragment remains reduced and stabilized to the sacrum by the intact posterior SI joint ligaments (**Figure 3**). Depending on the size and location of the fracture fragment, these fractures can be reduced and stabilized through an anterior or a posterior approach. When the crescent fragment is large and the SI joint involvement is small, the fixation strategy is similar to that used for isolated iliac wing fractures. Lag screws placed between the tables and a pelvic reconstruction plate placed along the iliac crest provide enough stability to allow fracture union. As the fragment becomes smaller, the injury behaves more like an SI joint dislocation, and iliosacral screws with or without an anterior plate may be indicated. Intermediate size displaced fractures, in which the fracture is located at the start site of the iliosacral screws and the intact fragment is too small and posterior to repair from a supine approach, may require an open reduction through a posterior approach and fixation with lag screws and an antiglide plate (**Figure 3**).

Associated Soft Tissues

The soft tissues in the area of the abdomen and pelvis can be severely injured and limit access to the bony anatomy. Along with a search for open wounds, careful inspection for a closed degloving injury, also known as a Morel-Lavallée lesion, is imperative because this soft-tissue injury is reported to be 46% culture positive.[22] Formal surgical débridement with open treatment and vacuum-assisted closure or percutaneous treatment is indicated before open reduction and internal fixation (ORIF).[23] In severe injuries, full-thickness necrosis may result, requiring soft-tissue reconstruction. Sometimes a closed reduction technique is the only option because of the condition of the soft tissues, and an imperfect reduction must be accepted. Without good data, these situations are left to surgeon experience and cautious decision-making in determining how to proceed.

Postoperative Care

Postoperatively, the mobilization of patients with pelvic fracture should begin as soon as the rest of their injuries allow. For complete posterior ring injuries, the patient must not bear weight on the affected extremity for 12 weeks. For complete bilateral injuries, slide board bed-to-chair transfer is necessary. Surgical drains are left in the space of Retzius, internal iliac fossa, and subgluteal space as needed until dry. Aggressive surgical management of wounds that continue to drain is typically necessary to prevent deep infection. Care must be taken to monitor for the return of bowel sounds, and then the diet is advanced slowly as appropriate.

Deep vein thrombosis (DVT) prophylaxis remains a controversial topic in orthopaedics, and limited data is available to guide the clinical care of pelvic and acetabular fracture patients.[24] Without DVT prophylaxis, hospitalized patients who sustain major trauma, including those with pelvic fracture, have a DVT risk that exceeds 50%, and pelvic fracture is an independent predictor.[25] Intermittent pneumatic compression devices have been shown to reduce the incidence of thrombus without the associated bleeding risk inherent with chemical prophylaxis; they should be used on all patients with available extremities. Chemical prophylaxis should be started as soon as bleeding risk allows—typically when the drain output is minimal or 48 hours after open procedures—but must be tailored to individual patient needs. Screening examinations are not indicated for patients having no signs or symptoms concerning for a clot. No data support the thromboprophylactic use of inferior vena cava filters, but they are indicated in patients with proven proximal DVT and a contraindication to full-dose anticoagulation medication or planned major surgery in the near future.[25] Discharge anticoagulation medication should be reviewed and considered in high-risk patients. Aspirin and compression stockings are not considered adequate DVT prophylaxis in trauma patients.[25]

Complications

Treating pelvic fracture patients includes caring for any associated complications. Blood loss, hypotension, open wounds, neurologic injury, or visceral injuries often are present when the patient arrives from the scene. Sometimes, difficulties that result in complications are encountered in the operating theater. Successful management of complications demands early recognition and effective communication among surgeons, anesthesiologists, interventionalists, and intensivists.

The surgical management of pelvic fractures requires a firm understanding of the vascular anatomy. Injury to a vascular structure can happen during the injury or during surgical dissection, fracture reduction, or definitive fixation. Arterial injury and subsequent bleeding can be life threatening. Common sources of bleeding include the superior gluteal artery near the greater sciatic notch, the obturator artery, or the corona mortise, a retropubic anastomosis between the obturator system and the external iliac/inferior epigastric systems. When direct

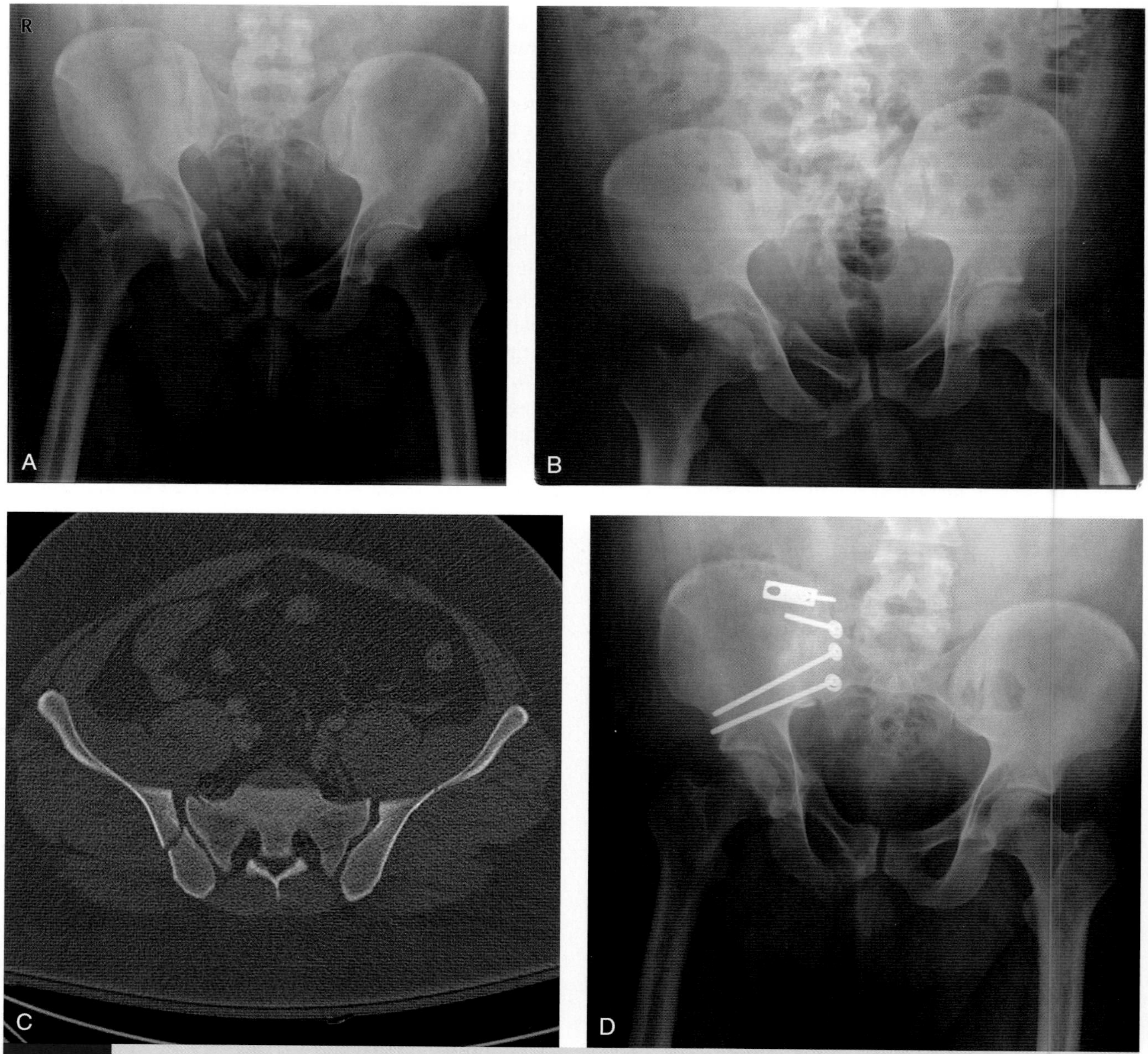

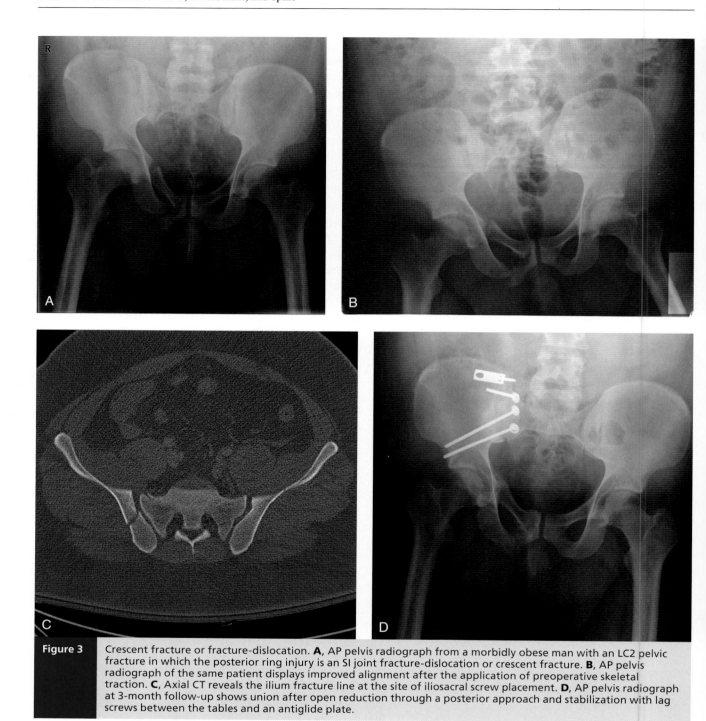

Figure 3 Crescent fracture or fracture-dislocation. **A**, AP pelvis radiograph from a morbidly obese man with an LC2 pelvic fracture in which the posterior ring injury is an SI joint fracture-dislocation or crescent fracture. **B**, AP pelvis radiograph of the same patient displays improved alignment after the application of preoperative skeletal traction. **C**, Axial CT reveals the ilium fracture line at the site of iliosacral screw placement. **D**, AP pelvis radiograph at 3-month follow-up shows union after open reduction through a posterior approach and stabilization with lag screws between the tables and an antiglide plate.

control of these vessels is not possible, the wound should be packed in an attempt to tamponade the bleeding, and the patient should undergo angiography for embolization. In the event of substantial venous bleeding that causes physiologic compromise, the wound should be packed or closed, and the patient should be resuscitated and stabilized in the intensive care unit. The patient can be returned to the operating theater to complete the pelvic fixation after being stabilized.

Following treatment of a pelvic fracture, wound infections require early recognition and aggressive management. Acute infection can be treated with open surgical débridement, intravenous antibiotics that are appropriate to the culture, and retained hardware. Serial débridements may be necessary. Loose hardware needs to be removed and revised, potentially with an intervening period of external fixation and/or traction. Historically, the posterior approach is associated with wound dehiscence and infection rates as high as 25%. A 2012 study reported an infection rate of 3.4% with proper patient selection and surgical technique. No patients needed additional soft-tissue reconstructive procedures other than the surgical débridement.[26] A 2010 study looked at the role obesity played in wound complications in 145 patients treated with any type of open approach and reported an overall wound complication rate of 11% (16 patients). Within that series, the posterior approach to the posterior ring resulted in a deep infection rate of 15% overall and 33% in the group having a body mass index greater than 30 kg/m^2.[27]

Late-presenting infections should be evaluated using the usual laboratory studies, which are helpful over the long term in following a patient's response to treatment. CT with contrast of the abdomen and pelvis also should be obtained to look for an abscess and to evaluate fracture healing. Typically, MRI is not helpful because of metal artifact. If the fractures are healed, the hardware is removed at the time of open débridement. Percutaneous drainage and antibiotics are reserved for patients who are too sick to undergo surgical management.

Conducting a complete and thorough neurologic examination often is challenging or impossible in a preoperative pelvic fracture patient. Subtle deficits may be present preoperatively but may not be detected. It is vital to carefully document the completeness of the examination and its findings. In the case of a new postoperative neurologic injury, CT should be obtained to evaluate for any source of injury. Possible etiologies include fracture manipulation and reduction, misplaced bony fragments, malreduction, or errant hardware. If a motor deficit corresponds to a malpositioned bony fragment or screw, then decompression and/or revision fixation are indicated. Isolated radicular pain or a neurologic deficit without evidence of nerve root impingement can be treated with observation, pain medications, and physical therapy.

The close follow-up of surgical patients is just as important as it is for nonsurgical patients, so that any loss of fixation can be identified and addressed early. For the increasing numbers of patients presenting with poor bone quality and obesity and those with unstable fracture patterns, a delay in diagnosis can lead to pelvic malunion, which can be debilitating. The well-known long-term complications are pelvic obliquity, sitting imbalance, limb-length discrepancy, dyspareunia, and pain. The generally accepted definitions of satisfactory reduction are less than 1 cm of displacement and less than 15° of rotation deformity. A review of the literature reported a 97% incidence of pain in this patient population.[28] Although surgery for nonunion and malunion is reported to relieve posterior pelvic pain in 92.6% of patients and to return 55.9% of patients to preinjury levels of activity, it also is associated with a 15% complication rate, including a 5.3% incidence of neurologic deficit.[28]

Outcomes

The long-term functional outcomes following high-energy pelvic ring fractures are associated with a high incidence of chronic posterior pelvic pain and disability. Outcome studies are difficult to interpret because of the many confounding variables in this population. Radiographic measurements often are used to judge the outcomes, despite the lack of standardization of the measurements.[29] Pelvic surgeons seek anatomic reduction, defined as less than 4 mm of displacement, and rigid stable internal fixation while trying to avoid any associated complications.[30,31] Fractures of the posterior ring often are thought to have a better outcome than purely ligamentous injuries because bony healing provides more stability than scar tissue. One study, however, reported that bony ankylosis of the SI joint had no effect on outcome after complete SI joint dislocation, anatomic reduction, and rigid internal fixation.[30]

The causation of poor outcomes is likely multifactorial, and any substantial urologic, neurologic, or visceral injury affects outcomes.[32-34] For example, male patients report erectile dysfunction, whereas female patients have dyspareunia and child-bearing issues.[35] A 2012 study looked at 31 women with pelvic fractures, including 17 who were treated surgically. Of the total, 16 had 25 vaginal deliveries despite having retained hardware. Cesarean delivery was not related to age, fracture pattern, treatment type, or residual deformity.[36] Data from Musculoskeletal Function Assessment (MFA) questionnaires showed that women with pelvic fractures associated with bladder rupture or lower-extremity injury had worse outcomes than women without those injuries.[37] Additionally, many pelvic fracture patients have depression and anxiety, which complicate their outcomes.[34]

The mortality rate associated with pelvis fractures ranges from 8.6% to 20% and typically is secondary to the other associated life threatening injuries.[38-43] In a recent article reevaluating the predictive ability of the Young-Burgess system, a 2010 study of 1,248 pelvic fracture patients in the same institution as the original article[38] reported a 9.1% mortality rate[41] This rate is unchanged from the 8.6% reported 24 years ago.[38] The lateral compression injuries were associated with more severe chest injuries, but a higher rate of head injuries was not reconfirmed. Additionally, the unstable fractures types (LC3, APC2, APC3) were predictive of higher transfusion requirements and higher rate of abdominal injury.[41]

Summary

The successful definitive care of high-energy pelvic fracture patients requires a multifactorial understanding of the patient's injuries. A thorough understanding of the anatomy, deformity, associated injuries, treatment options, and potential complications is required to care for these patients. The radiographic deformity will direct treatment with most emphasis placed on the displacement of the posterior pelvic ring. Surgical management is dictated by the degree and type of bony and/or ligamentous injury and the surrounding soft tissue envelope. Nonsurgical, percutaneous, or open treatment options can all be used successfully with various challenges and benefits. Long-term outcomes are affected by the associated injuries and often are complicated by posterior pelvic pain.

Key Study Points

- Stable pelvic ring fractures with minimal deformity can be treated nonsurgically with immediate weight bearing, assuming early radiographic follow-up to confirm maintained alignment.
- The most common indication for surgical management of anterior pelvic ring fractures is pubic symphysis instability; most pubic rami fractures are treated nonsurgically as they are inherently more stable due to their periosteal attachments and the intact inguinal ligament.
- Complete posterior pelvic ring injuries are treated surgically with both open and percutaneous techniques depending on the condition of the surrounding soft tissues and the quality of the fracture reduction after closed methods. Iliosacral screws, intra-table lag screws, and/or plate fixation are available stabilization options dictated by fracture pattern.
- Chronic posterior pelvic pain is the most frequent long-term complaint after high-energy pelvic fractures. The poor outcomes are likely multifactorial and are greatly affected by the associated neurologic, urologic, and visceral injuries.
- Mortality rate after pelvic ring fracture ranges from 8.6% to 20% and is typically due to the other associated life-threatening injuries.

Annotated References

1. Kaiser SP, Gardner MJ, Liu J, Routt ML Jr, Morshed S: Anatomic determinants of sacral dysmorphism and implications for safe iliosacral screw placement. *J Bone Joint Surg Am* 2014;96(14):e120.

   The authors evaluated 104 pelvic CT scans of uninjured patients for sacral dysmorphism. The incidence was 41%. The recognition of variations in anatomy is necessary for preoperative planning.

2. McAndrew CM, Merriman DJ, Gardner MJ, Ricci WM: Standardized posterior pelvic imaging: Use of CT inlet and CT outlet for evaluation and management of pelvic ring injuries. *J Orthop Trauma* 2014;28(12):665-673.

   The authors evaluated routine CT scans of pelvic bony anatomy in patients without pelvic fractures and reported that routine imagining does not provide a standardized view of the pelvic bony anatomy. This factor can overestimate and underestimate the size of the safe zone for the placement of iliosacral screws and can affect preoperative planning and, potentially, treatment strategies.

3. Bruce B, Reilly M, Sims S: OTA highlight paper predicting future displacement of nonoperatively managed lateral compression sacral fractures: Can it be done? *J Orthop Trauma* 2011;25(9):523-527.

   Patients with less than 5 mm of displacement on initial radiographs of high-energy sacral fractures were followed to determine which fracture patterns would displace. The authors found that lateral compression pelvic fractures that include complete sacral fractures with bilateral rami fractures are the most likely to displace.

4. Beckmann JT, Presson AP, Curtis SH, et al: Operative agreement on lateral compression-1 pelvis fractures. A survey of 111 OTA members. *J Orthop Trauma* 2014;28(12):681-685.

   Using three plain radiographs and scrollable CT, the authors presented 27 LC1 pelvic fractures of varying types to surgeons at the Orthopaedic Trauma Association annual meeting, along with yes or no questions inquiring whether they would perform surgical stabilization. A total of 111 surgeons participated. Only nine cases resulted in substantial agreement among the surgeons. Surgical case volume, years in practice, and completion of a trauma fellowship did not predict surgical tendency.

5. Gaski GE, Manson TT, Castillo RC, Slobogean GP, O'Toole RV: Nonoperative treatment of intermediate severity lateral compression type 1 pelvic ring injuries with minimally displaced complete sacral fracture. *J Orthop Trauma* 2014;28(12):674-680.

   The authors reviewed 50 lateral compression pelvic fractures that included complete sacral fractures displaced initially less than 1 cm, hypothesizing that these fractures could be managed nonsurgically. Based on the Majeed pelvic score, acceptable functional outcomes were reported. Patients with lower-extremity injuries had lower scores. Radiographic outcomes available on 36 of the patients revealed no fracture displaced more than 1 cm. Level of evidence: IV.

6. Sagi HC, Papp S: Comparative radiographic and clinical outcome of two-hole and multi-hole symphyseal plating. *J Orthop Trauma* 2008;22(6):373-378.

7. Moed BR, Grimshaw CS, Segina DN: Failure of locked design-specific plate fixation of the pubic symphysis: A report of six cases. *J Orthop Trauma* 2012;26(7):e71-e75.

   The authors describe acute clinical fixation failures of specific locking plates designed to stabilize symphyseal disruptions. They observed traditional plating failures with loosening of the hardware at the bone-screw interface and common locked plating failures occurring at the screw-plate junction with pull-out through the bone. The authors concluded that the specific indications for this fixation have yet to be determined. Level of evidence: IV.

8. Lybrand K, Kurylo J, Gross J, Templeman D, Tornetta P III: Does removal of the symphyseal cartilage in symphyseal dislocations have any effect on final alignment and implant failure? *J Orthop Trauma* 2015;29(10):470-474.

   The authors reviewed 96 patients with anterior-posterior compression pelvic fractures treated with 6-hole symphyseal plates. Of the total, 50 patients had the symphyseal cartilage removed, and the remainder kept the cartilage. Fewer revision surgeries and fewer implant failures were seen in the cartilage excision group. Level of evidence: III.

9. Vaidya R, Colen R, Vigdorchik J, Tonnos F, Sethi A: Treatment of unstable pelvic ring injuries with an internal anterior fixator and posterior fixation: Initial clinical series. *J Orthop Trauma* 2012;26(1):1-8.

   The authors presented the initial series of patients treated with supra-acetabular pedicle screws and a subcutaneous bar construct fashioned as a Hannover external fixator but placed completely internally for the management of pelvic fractures. The complications, including lateral femoral cutaneous nerve paresthesia, which resolved, were deemed acceptable. The patients tolerated the devices and could roll in bed, sit, and walk without difficulty. Nursing care was improved. A second surgery is necessary to remove the implant, although some patients have refused it. All fractures healed without a loss of reduction.

10. Merriman DJ, Ricci WM, McAndrew CM, Gardner MJ: Is application of an internal anterior pelvic fixator anatomically feasible? *Clin Orthop Relat Res* 2012;470(8):2111-2115.

    The authors evaluated the pelvic CT scans of 13 patients who had received an internal anterior pelvic fixator for its location and the risk to nearby anatomic structures. There was at least 2 cm between all hardware and the surface of the skin, the neurovascular bundle, the bladder, and the hip joint. With careful adherence to surgical technique, the authors report that the risk of injury to local anatomic structures can be minimized. Level of evidence: IV.

11. Hesse D, Kandmir U, Solberg B, et al: Femoral nerve palsy after pelvic fracture treated with INFIX: A case series. *J Orthop Trauma* 2015;29(3):138-143.

    This case series included six patients with eight femoral nerve palsies attributed to the placement of an anterior internal fixator. The authors hypothesize that insufficient room for the psoas and the femoral nerve was the cause of the palsies. Level of evidence: IV.

12. Lindsay A, Tornetta P III, Diwan A, Templeman D: Is closed reduction and percutaneous fixation of unstable posterior ring injuries as accurate as open reduction and internal fixation? *J Orthop Trauma* 2016;30(1):29-33.

    The authors compared two groups of patients with Bucholz type 3 (OTA type 61-C1) unilateral unstable pelvic ring fractures treated with prone open reduction and internal fixation or supine closed reduction percutaneous fixation with a quadrilateral traction set-up. Closed reduction was found to be as effective as open reduction and internal fixation. Level of evidence: III.

13. Siegel J, Tornetta P: Sacral Fractures, in Wiss D, ed: *Master Techniques in Orthopaedic Surgery: Fractures* ,ed 3Philadelphia, PA, Lippincott Williams & Wilkins, 2013, pp 799-816.

    The authors review sacral fracture classification, radiographic evaluation, and treatment options including surgical tactics. Closed and open reduction techniques are discussed; stabilization options, complications, and outcomes are also reviewed.

14. Matta JM, Yerasimides JG: Table-skeletal fixation as an adjunct to pelvic ring reduction. *J Orthop Trauma* 2007;21(9):647-656.

15. Reilly MC, Bono CM, Litkouhi B, Sirkin M, Behrens FF: The effect of sacral fracture malreduction on the safe placement of iliosacral screws. *J Orthop Trauma* 2003;17(2):88-94.

16. Sagi HC: Technical aspects and recommended treatment algorithms in triangular osteosynthesis and spinopelvic fixation for vertical shear transforaminal sacral fractures. *J Orthop Trauma* 2009;23(5):354-360.

17. Gardner MJ, Routt ML Jr: Transiliac-transsacral screws for posterior pelvic stabilization. *J Orthop Trauma* 2011;25(6):378-384.

    The authors describe the surgical technique and their clinical experience with placement of transiliac-transsacral screws in patients with certain unstable injuries. The authors propose improved holding power and stabilization of a concomitant contralateral posterior pelvic injury as benefits. Osteoporosis, significant posterior instability, patient obesity, noncompliant behavior, and nonunion procedures are offered as indications.

18. Schildhauer TA, Ledoux WR, Chapman JR, Henley MB, Tencer AF, Routt ML Jr: Triangular osteosynthesis and iliosacral screw fixation for unstable sacral fractures: A

cadaveric and biomechanical evaluation under cyclic loads. *J Orthop Trauma* 2003;17(1):22-31.

19. Sagi HC, Militano U, Caron T, Lindvall E: A comprehensive analysis with minimum 1-year follow-up of vertically unstable transforaminal sacral fractures treated with triangular osteosynthesis. *J Orthop Trauma* 2009;23(5):313-319, discussion 319-321.

20. Siebler JC, Hasley BP, Mormino MA: Functional outcomes of Denis zone III sacral fractures treated nonoperatively. *J Orthop Trauma* 2010;24(5):297-302.

    The authors presented the results of their nonsurgical treatment of 11 patients with Denis zone III sacral fractures, including 6 patients with U-type or H-type sacral fractures. They reported neurologic improvement in 10 of 11 patients over the 2-year follow-up period, including 3 patients with an initial loss of bowel and bladder function who recovered completely.

21. Schildhauer TA, Bellabarba C, Nork SE, Barei DP, Routt ML Jr, Chapman JR: Decompression and lumbopelvic fixation for sacral fracture-dislocations with spino-pelvic dissociation. *J Orthop Trauma* 2006;20(7):447-457.

22. Hak DJ, Olson SA, Matta JM: Diagnosis and management of closed internal degloving injuries associated with pelvic and acetabular fractures: The Morel-Lavallée lesion. *J Trauma* 1997;42(6):1046-1051.

23. Tseng S, Tornetta P III: Percutaneous management of Morel-Lavallée lesions. *J Bone Joint Surg Am* 2006;88(1):92-96.

24. Slobogean GP, Lefaivre KA, Nicolaou S, O'Brien PJ: A systematic review of thromboprophylaxis for pelvic and acetabular fractures. *J Orthop Trauma* 2009;23(5):379-384.

25. Geerts WH, Bergqvist D, Pineo GF, et al; American College of Chest Physicians: Prevention of venous thromboembolism: American College of Chest Physicians evidence-based clinical practice guidelines (8th Edition). *Chest* 2008;133(6suppl):381S-453S.

26. Stover MD, Sims S, Matta J: What is the infection rate of the posterior approach to type C pelvic injuries? *Clin Orthop Relat Res* 2012;470(8):2142-2147.

    The authors retrospectively reviewed 236 patients at 6 institutions with OTA type C pelvic ring fractures who underwent open reduction through a posterior approach. They had eight (3.4%) infections, which were treated with surgical débridement, wound closure, and antibiotics. No soft-tissue reconstructions were necessary. The authors concluded that only minimal risk exists for catastrophic wound complication with good patient selection and surgical technique. Level of evidence: IV.

27. Sems SA, Johnson M, Cole PA, Byrd CT, Templeman DC; Minnesota Orthopaedic Trauma Group: Elevated body mass index increases early complications of surgical treatment of pelvic ring injuries. *J Orthop Trauma* 2010;24(5):309-314.

    The authors evaluated 184 consecutive surgically treated pelvic fracture patients to determine the relationship between body mass index (BMI) and early postoperative complications. The 48 patients with a BMI of more than 30 kg/m^2 had more overall complications (54.2% versus 14.9%), including more deep infections (22.9% versus 3.7%) and more loss of reductions (31.3% versus 6%) than those with a lower BMI. Of the obese patients, 16 (33%) had to return to the operating theater for irrigation and débridement or revision fixation, compared with 9.7% of those in the not obese group.

28. Kanakaris NK, Angoules AG, Nikolaou VS, Kontakis G, Giannoudis PV: Treatment and outcomes of pelvic malunions and nonunions: A systematic review. *Clin Orthop Relat Res* 2009;467(8):2112-2124.

29. Lefaivre KA, Slobogean G, Starr AJ, Guy P, O'brien PJ, Macadam SA: Methodology and interpretation of radiographic outcomes in surgically treated pelvic fractures: A systematic review. *J Orthop Trauma* 2012;26(8):474-481.

    The authors performed a systematic review of the methods used to evaluate radiographic outcomes in surgically treated pelvic fracture patients. They found nonstandardized and untested measurement techniques, with inconsistent interpretation, confirming that a reproducible method to evaluate radiographic outcome is needed to allow comparison to functional outcomes.

30. Mullis BH, Sagi HC: Minimum 1-year follow-up for patients with vertical shear sacroiliac joint dislocations treated with iliosacral screws: Does joint ankylosis or anatomic reduction contribute to functional outcome? *J Orthop Trauma* 2008;22(5):293-298.

31. Tornetta P III, Matta JM: Outcome of operatively treated unstable posterior pelvic ring disruptions. *Clin Orthop Relat Res* 1996;329:186-193.

32. Adelved A, Tötterman A, Glott T, Søberg HL, Madsen JE, Røise O: Patient-reported health minimum 8 years after operatively treated displaced sacral fractures: A prospective cohort study. *J Orthop Trauma* 2014;28(12):686-693.

    The authors reported the results of a 10.7-year follow-up of 28 of 31 displaced sacral fracture patients treated surgically. Considerable improvement was observed at 10 years compared with at 1-year, with all patients at 10 years being independent in activities of daily living. Sexual and bowel dysfunction correlated with worse outcomes. The 36-Item Short Form Health Survey scores did not change over time but were statistically significantly lower than the norm-based scores in all domains except mental health. Level of evidence: IV.

33. Holstein JH, Pizanis A, Köhler D, Pohlemann T; Working Group Quality of Life After Pelvic Fractures: What are predictors for patients' quality of life after pelvic ring fractures? *Clin Orthop Relat Res* 2013;471(9):2841-2845.

The authors surveyed 172 patients in the German Pelvic Trauma Registry for predictors of patient quality of life after pelvic fracture using a multivariate linear regression model. The median follow-up was 3 years, and the median age of the follow-up cohort was 47 years. Using the EuroQOL five dimensions questionnaire, the authors concluded that older age, complex trauma, and surgery led to a higher likelihood of reduced quality of life.

34. Kabak S, Halici M, Tuncel M, Avsarogullari L, Baktir A, Basturk M: Functional outcome of open reduction and internal fixation for completely unstable pelvic ring fractures (type C): A report of 40 cases. *J Orthop Trauma* 2003;17(8):555-562.

35. Vallier HA, Cureton BA, Schubeck D: Pelvic ring injury is associated with sexual dysfunction in women. *J Orthop Trauma* 2012;26(5):308-313.

    The authors described the sexual function of 187 women under the age of 55 after pelvic trauma. Of the total, 74 patients had surgical management, and 23 had genitourinary injuries. Dyspareunia is associated with anteroposterior compression and B-type fractures, symphyseal plating, and bladder rupture. Level of evidence: III.

36. Vallier HA, Cureton BA, Schubeck D: Pregnancy outcomes after pelvic ring injury. *J Orthop Trauma* 2012;26(5):302-307.

    The authors evaluated the pregnancy outcomes after pelvic fracture in this retrospective review of 31 women, who had 54 pregnancies. Of the pelvic fractures, 17 were treated surgically. Despite retained hardware, 16 women had 25 vaginal deliveries. Cesarean delivery was not related to age, fracture pattern, treatment type, or residual deformity. The authors recommended developing guidelines for when a trial of labor can be considered. Level of evidence: IV.

37. Vallier HA, Cureton BA, Schubeck D, Wang XF: Functional outcomes in women after high-energy pelvic ring injury. *J Orthop Trauma* 2012;26(5):296-301.

    The authors examined functional outcomes using the Musculoskeletal Function Assessment (MFA) questionnaire in 87 women with an average age of 33.5 years who sustained pelvic trauma. Outcomes were not related to age or injury severity score. Isolated pelvic fracture patients had better MFA scores than patients with multiple injuries (21.2 versus 35.5). Those with other associated lower extremity fractures had worse outcomes (41.7 versus 29.1) than women who did not sustain these other injuries. Bladder rupture portends a poor outcome (mean MFA 50.0). Level of evidence: IV.

38. Burgess AR, Eastridge BJ, Young JW, et al: Pelvic ring disruptions: Effective classification system and treatment protocols. *J Trauma* 1990;30(7):848-856.

39. Dalal SA, Burgess AR, Siegel JH, et al: Pelvic fracture in multiple trauma: Classification by mechanism is key to pattern of organ injury, resuscitative requirements, and outcome. *J Trauma* 1989;29(7):981-1000, discussion 1000-1002.

40. Manson TT, Nascone JW, Sciadini MF, O'Toole RV: Does fracture pattern predict death with lateral compression type 1 pelvic fractures? *J Trauma* 2010;69(4):876-879.

    The authors compared the radiographs and outcome data of 52 patients treated at their institution with LC1 pelvis fractures who died and those with similar fractures who lived. They found no radiographic criteria to indicate that fracture pattern can be used to predict death after sustaining an LC1 pelvis fracture.

41. Manson T, O'Toole RV, Whitney A, Duggan B, Sciadini M, Nascone J: Young-Burgess classification of pelvic ring fractures: Does it predict mortality, transfusion requirements, and non-orthopaedic injuries? *J Orthop Trauma* 2010;24(10):603-609.

    The authors reviewed the data of 1,248 patients with pelvic fractures to determine whether mortality rates in patients with pelvic fractures had changed over time and to evaluate the predictive power of the Young-Burgess classification system. The mortality rate remained consistent at 9.1%. Transfusion requirements were higher in patients with LC2, LC3, APC2, and APC3 fractures. When fractures were grouped into stable and unstable categories, mortality, abdominal injury, and transfusion requirements were predictably higher in the unstable group.

42. O'Sullivan RE, White TO, Keating JF: Major pelvic fractures: Identification of patients at high risk. *J Bone Joint Surg Br* 2005;87(4):530-533.

43. Starr AJ, Griffin DR, Reinert CM, et al: Pelvic ring disruptions: Prediction of associated injuries, transfusion requirement, pelvic arteriography, complications, and mortality. *J Orthop Trauma* 2002;16(8):553-561.

Chapter 32

Evaluation and Management of Acetabular Fractures

Reza Firoozabadi, MD, MA   Conor Kleweno, MD

Abstract

A fracture of the acetabulum is a complex injury best treated by an orthopaedic traumatologist. The injury most often results from a high-energy mechanism in a relatively young patient or from a low-energy mechanism in an older patient. A clear understanding of osseous and soft-tissue anatomy is paramount before treating these injuries. Radiographic classification is useful for determining the specific fracture pattern and the best surgical treatment. Several surgical exposures and fixation constructs are available. Recent outcomes research has focused on decreasing complication rates and assessing the role of acute total hip arthroplasty.

Keywords: acetabular fracture; posterior column fracture; transverse fracture; total hip arthroplasty

Introduction

A clear understanding of acetabular osseous anatomy and the surrounding soft tissue is essential for the evaluation and treatment of an acetabular fracture. These challenging injuries are associated with substantial morbidity and are best treated at a trauma center by an orthopaedic trauma surgeon with specialized training and experience in pelvic and acetabular surgery.[1]

The ischium, ilium, and pubis are the three embryologic elements of the innominate bone; they fuse at skeletal maturity to form the osseous structure of the acetabulum.

Neither of the following authors nor any immediate family member has received anything of value from or has stock or stock options held in a commercial company or institution related directly or indirectly to the subject of this chapter: Dr. Firoozabadi and Dr. Kleweno.

The two-column structural model of the acetabulum includes anterior and posterior columns that join at the sciatic buttress in an inverted-Y shape[2] (**Figure 1**). Like the lamina, pars interarticularis, and pedicle in the vertebral spine, the columns of the acetabulum blend at their borders. In general, however, the anterior column includes the bones of the anterior ilium (the anterosuperior and anteroinferior iliac spine and gluteus medius pillar), anterior wall of the acetabulum, anterior half of the acetabular dome, anterior half of the quadrilateral plate, and superior pubic rami. The posterior column includes the caudal portion of the greater sciatic notch, posterior wall, posterior half of the acetabular dome, posterior half of the quadrilateral plate, and remainder of the ischium including the ischial spine and ischial tuberosity downward toward the inferior ramus of the pubis.

An understanding of the two-column structural model is crucial for fixing acetabular fractures. The general patterns of injury are the consequence of the hip position and force vector applied at the time of impact, and these patterns are described in relation to the columns. Reconstitution of column stability is necessary for a successful outcome.

Respect for the muscular and neurovascular anatomy surrounding the innominate bone is of paramount importance for safe surgical management. Notable neurovascular structures such as the external iliac vessels, gluteal vessels, iliolumbar vessels, obturator vessels, and sciatic nerve must be assessed for a full appreciation of the soft-tissue component of an acetabular fracture.

Radiographic Evaluation

The radiographs necessary for fracture evaluation and preoperative planning include the AP pelvic and oblique (Judet) views. CT with three-dimensional volumetric rendering also is useful for diagnosing an acetabular fracture. The AP pelvis radiograph is critical for identifying injury to the pelvis and acetabulum. This radiograph routinely is

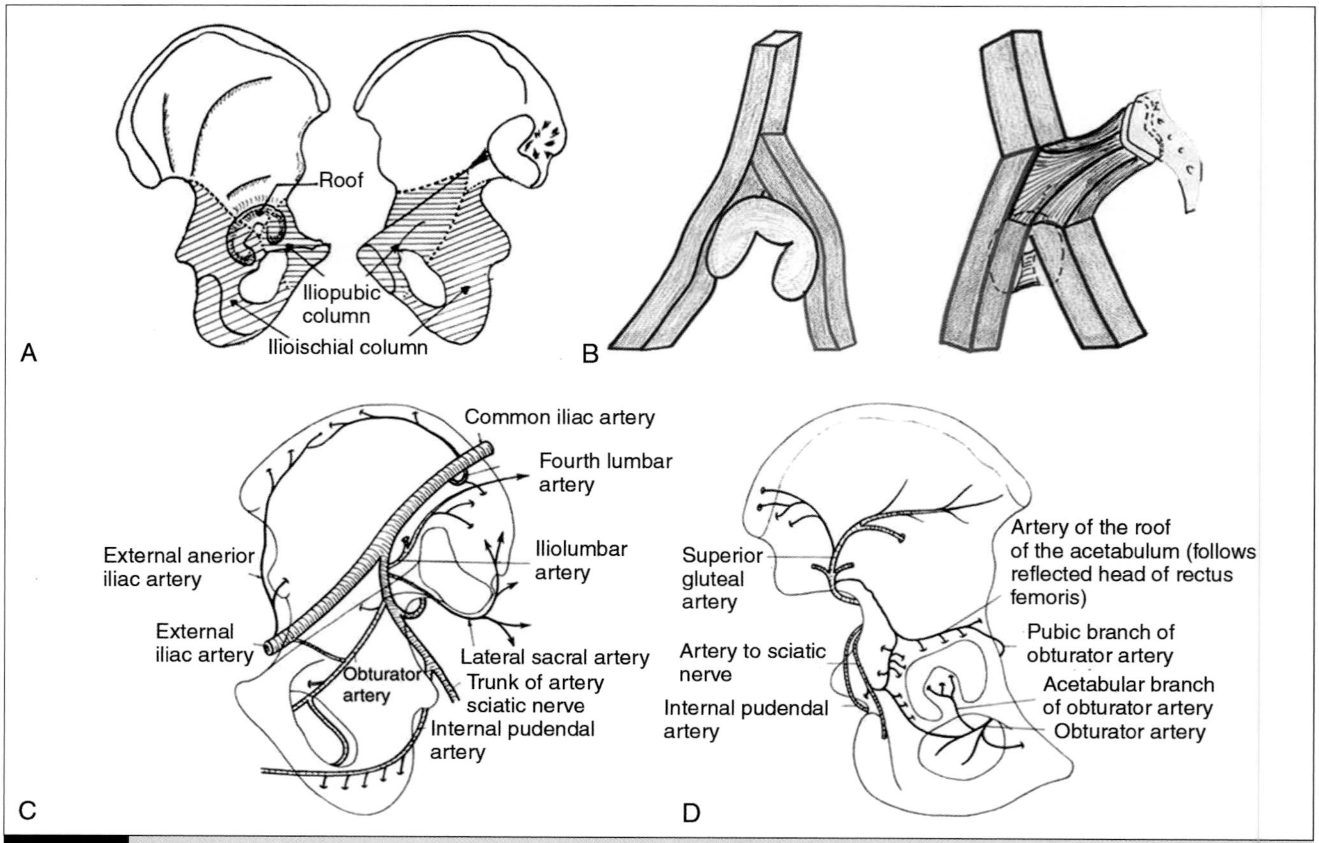

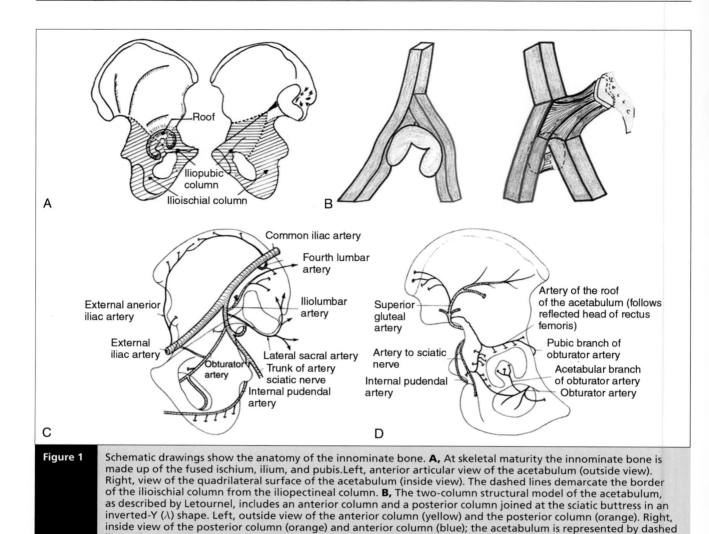

Figure 1 Schematic drawings show the anatomy of the innominate bone. **A,** At skeletal maturity the innominate bone is made up of the fused ischium, ilium, and pubis.Left, anterior articular view of the acetabulum (outside view). Right, view of the quadrilateral surface of the acetabulum (inside view). The dashed lines demarcate the border of the ilioischial column from the iliopectineal column. **B,** The two-column structural model of the acetabulum, as described by Letournel, includes an anterior column and a posterior column joined at the sciatic buttress in an inverted-Y (λ) shape. Left, outside view of the anterior column (yellow) and the posterior column (orange). Right, inside view of the posterior column (orange) and anterior column (blue); the acetabulum is represented by dashed lines. The sciatic buttress (black shading) connects both columns to axial skeleton through the sacroiliac joint. Internal **(C)** and external **(D)** views of the vasculature of the innominate bone. (Reproduced with permission from Letournel E, Judet R: *Fractures of the Acetabulum,* ed 2. New York, NY, Springer-Verlag, 1993, pp 4-21.)

obtained as part of the initial trauma workup but should be reacquired if the initial radiograph was suboptimal. Inlet and outlet views are necessary for every patient with an acetabular fracture to identify associated injuries to the anterior sacroiliac joint and symphysis.

The six cardinal lines on the AP pelvis and their corresponding structures are the ilioischial line (posterior column), iliopectineal line (anterior column), anterior rim (anterior wall), posterior rim (posterior wall), roof (dome of acetabulum), and teardrop (cotyloid fossa, section of the quadrilateral surface, and outer wall of the obturator canal)[3] (**Figure 2**). These cortical densities are secondary to tangential x-ray beams, and they define the structural integrity of acetabulum. Disruption in any of these lines implies fracture, and the location and constellations of disruptions describe the fracture pattern.

In addition to the AP pelvis radiographs, orthogonal 45° obturator oblique and iliac oblique (Judet) views are acquired (**Figure 3**). To obtain these images, each side of the patient's pelvis alternately is raised 45°, and the beam is centered on the acetabulum. The obturator oblique view best shows the integrity of the anterior column and posterior wall, and the iliac oblique view best shows the posterior column and anterior wall. The iliac oblique view also is useful for characterizing the pattern of an anterior column fracture as it exits the iliac crest.

CT is useful for characterizing the fracture (including a nondisplaced fracture that is not apparent on radiographs), identifying free osteochondral fragments, depicting marginal impaction, and identifying the most advantageous position for implant placement. It should be standard practice to obtain reformatted CT of the pelvis,

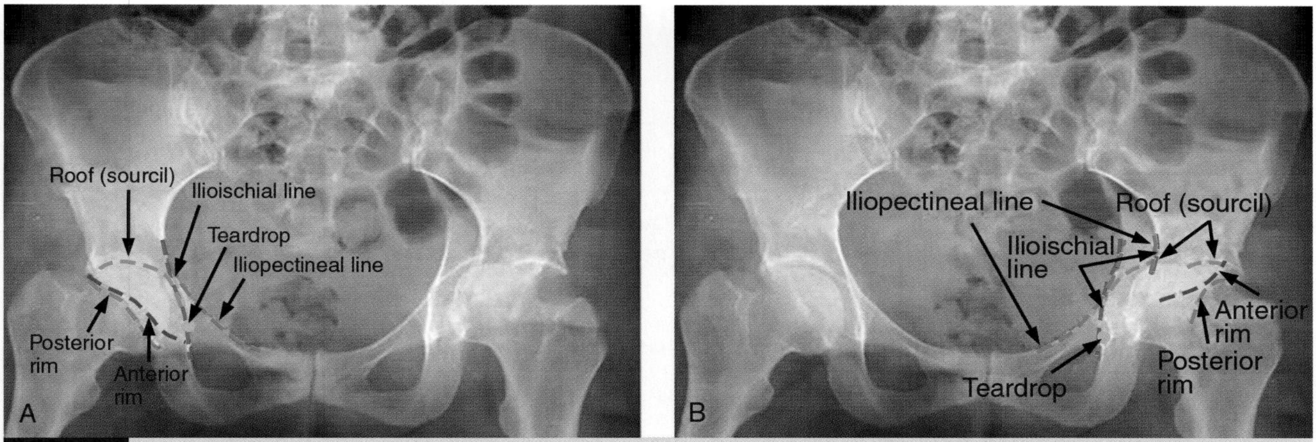

Figure 2 AP pelvis radiographs showing the six cardinal lines (and their corresponding structures) as dashed lines on the uninjured **(A)** and fractured **(B)** sides of the pelvis. Red = ilioischial line (posterior column), dark blue = iliopectineal line (anterior column), purple = anterior rim (anterior wall), orange = posterior rim (posterior wall), green = roof (dome of acetabulum), and circle = teardrop (cotyloid fossa, section of quadrilateral surface and outer wall of obturator canal). (Reproduced from Ahn J, Reilly M, Lorich D, Helfet D: Acetabular fractures: Acute evaluation, in Schmidt A, Teague D: *Orthopaedic Knowledge Update: Trauma 4*. Rosemont, IL, American Academy of Orthopaedic Surgeons, 2010, p 312.)

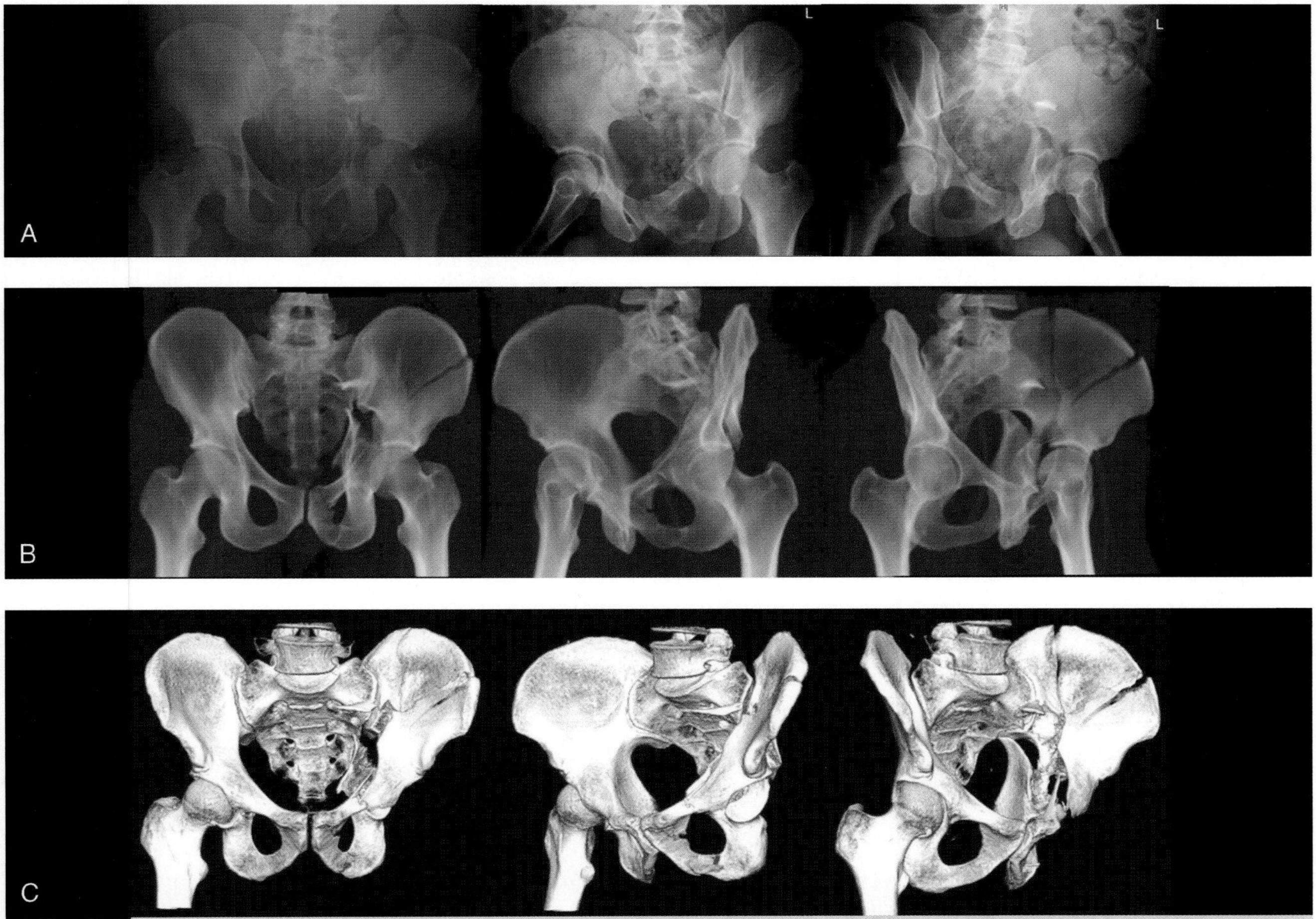

Figure 3 AP (left) and oblique (Judet) radiographs (center, obturator oblique; right, iliac oblique) showing an associated both-column acetabular fracture. **A,** Traditional plain radiographs. **B,** CT-generated AP and Judet images. **C,** CT-generated three-dimensional volumetric surface-rendered images.

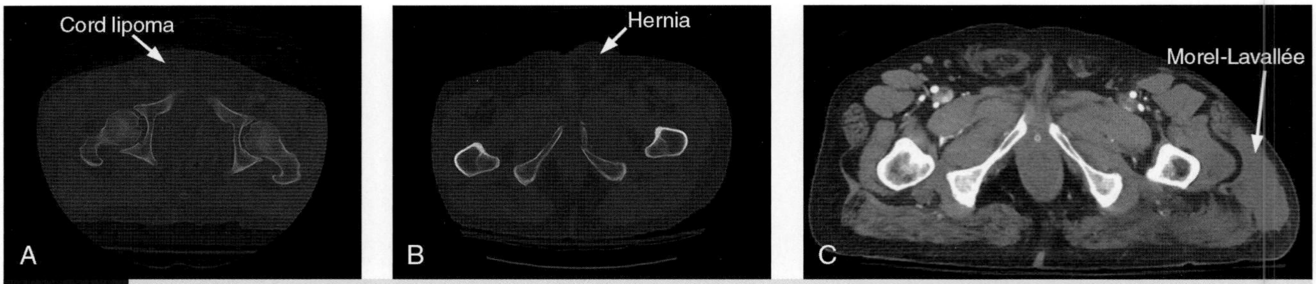

Figure 4 CT identification of soft-tissue abnormalities. **A,** Cord lipoma seen as hypodense and homogenous. **B,** Inguinal hernia seen as a heterogeneous density within the enlarged spermatic cord. **C,** Morel-Lavallée lesion seen on the lateral aspect of the left hemipelvis; hematoma has developed between the subcutaneous tissue and the fascia.

with cuts through the acetabulum of no more than 2 mm. Three-dimensional CT can be used to improve understanding of fracture geometry and diagnostic accuracy. However, nondisplaced and minimally displaced fracture-lines may be volume-averaged and thus difficult to see.[4] A hematoma, Morel-Lavallée lesion, hernia, or soft-tissue abnormality that can influence fracture management can be identified through critical analysis of CT (**Figure 4**).

Plain radiograph-like images, or so-called ghost images, including the Judet view, can be re-created from CT data. These CT-reconstructed Judet radiographs have several potential advantages over traditional Judet radiographs. In traditional radiography, the patient may experience substantial pain when rolled onto the injured side. The quality of the CT-generated ghost images is not affected by large body habitus, bowel gas, or contrast in the bladder, all of which can diminish the quality of plain radiographs. The quality of plain radiographs also can be affected by inaccurate patient placement or inappropriate x-ray penetration, whereas the CT ghost images can be protocoled for reproducible accuracy. With CT re-creation, the amount of radiation exposure is decreased because there is no need to obtain additional oblique radiographs, and avoiding a trip to the radiology department increases the efficiency of care in the emergency department. The quality of CT-reconstructed plain radiographs was reported to be equivalent or superior to that of traditional radiographs.[5,6]

CT-based three-dimensional volumetric imaging of acetabular fractures is useful for fracture classification and surgical planning.[7] AP and Judet images can be created, and the pelvis can be digitally rotated 360° in the horizontal or vertical axis for enhanced evaluation of fracture planes. The posterior iliac oblique view is useful for evaluating complex posterior column and posterior wall fractures but cannot be obtained with traditional Judet view radiography (**Figure 5**). This view is obtained by rotating the three-dimensional CT image approximately 35° from a pure posterior view (with the coccyx approximately bisecting the obturator foramen) to simulate the surgeon's intraoperative perspective. Subtraction of the femoral head allows the articular surface of the acetabulum to be assessed.[8]

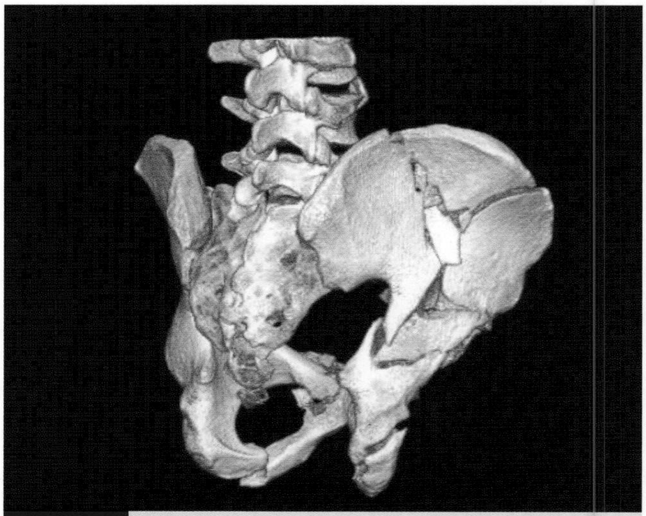

Figure 5 Posterior iliac oblique view from three-dimensional CT demonstrating fracture patterns of the posterior column and posterior wall in this associated both-column acetabular fracture. This image replicates the surgeon's intraoperative perspective of the posterior column.

Increasingly advanced technology appears to be on the horizon to aid in the treatment of acetabular fractures. Computer navigation, including three-dimensional navigation, has been used for improving the accuracy of percutaneous screw placement in acetabular fracture surgery.[9-11] Three-dimensional printing has been proposed as a tool for patient-specific plate contouring before acetabular fracture surgery.[12]

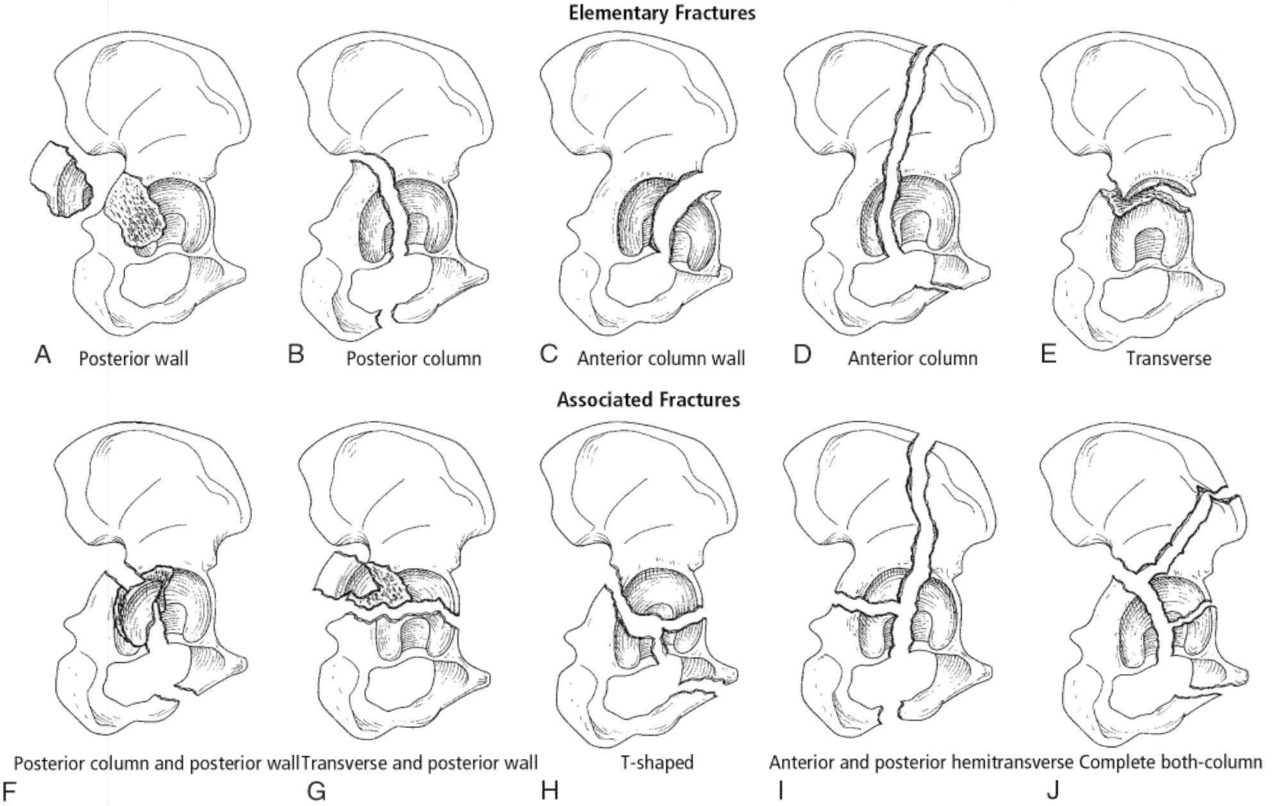

Figure 6 Drawings showing the 10 fractures in the Letournel classification. The elementary fracture patterns are the posterior wall (**A**), posterior column (**B**), anterior wall (**C**), anterior column (**D**), and transverse (**E**). The associated fracture patterns include the posterior column–posterior wall (**F**), transverse–posterior wall (**G**), T-type (**H**), anterior column–posterior hemitransverse (**I**), and associated both-column (**J**). (Reproduced with permission from Alton TB, Gee AO: Classifications in brief: Letournel classification for acetabular fractures. *Clin Orthop Relat Res* 2014; 472:35-38.)

Classification

In 1961 Letournel published the original classification of acetabular fractures based on plain radiographs, and in 1964 the classification was modified to include seven acetabular fracture patterns based on AP pelvic and internal and external 45° oblique (Judet) views.[2,13,14] In 1980 Letournel used radiographic and surgical analysis of 647 acetabular fractures to devise an updated classification of 10 fracture patterns.[15]

There is debate about the usefulness of CT to improve the reliability of the Letournel classification.[16] Some studies found that the addition of three-dimensional CT did not improve the interobserver or intraobserver reliability of the Letournel classification, but other studies found that CT did improve reliability.[17-20] Surgeon experience was found to be correlated with the accuracy of acetabular fracture classification.[19] Algorithms for evaluating pelvic radiographs have improved the accuracy of acetabular fracture classification.[17]

The 10 common acetabular fracture patterns identified by Letournel were divided into two groups of five[3] (**Figure 6**). The so-called elementary fractures, including anterior wall, anterior column, posterior wall, posterior column, and transverse fractures, were described as having a singular fracture plane. The transverse fracture is the only elementary fracture pattern that involves both columns of the acetabulum. The so-called associated fractures, which combine at least two of the elementary patterns, are the anterior column with associated posterior hemitransverse, T-type, posterior column with associated posterior wall, transverse with associated posterior wall, and associated both-column fractures. The posterior column with associated posterior wall fracture is the only associated fracture pattern that does not involve both columns.

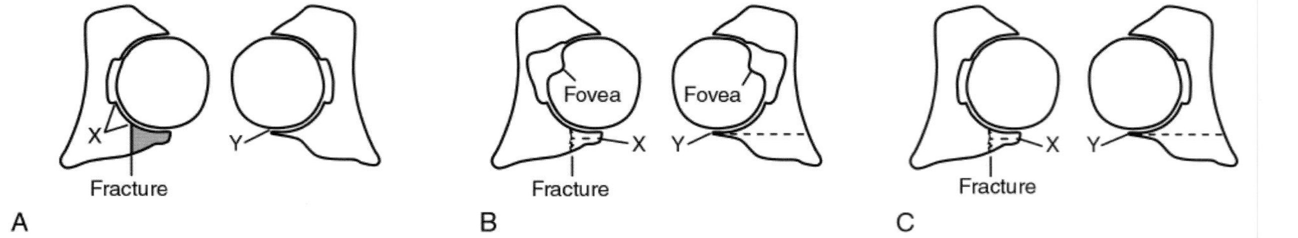

Figure 7 Schematic drawings showing three methods of calculating posterior wall fracture fragment size. **A,** The Calkins et al method is based on measurement of the smallest amount of intact acetabular arc. A straight-line mediolateral measurement is made of the remaining intact articular posterior-wall acetabular segment at the level of the greatest fracture involvement (X), and the length of the posterior acetabular arc is determined from the contralateral uninjured hip at the same level (Y). The index is calculated as X divided by Y and multiplied by 100. **B,** The Keith et al method is based on the wall size at the level of the fovea. The depth of the fracture fragment is measured at the level of the fovea (X), and the percentage of the fragment size is calculated from the ratio of the measured depth of the fracture side to the intact matched contralateral-side acetabular depth (Y). **C,** The Moed et al method is a modification of the Keith et al method in which the level of the largest wall deficit is measured instead of the fovea. (Reproduced with permission from Moed BR, Ajibade DA, Israel H: Computed tomography as a predictor of hip stability status in posterior wall fractures of the acetabulum. *J Orthop Trauma* 2009; 23(1):7-15.)

The Letournel acetabular fracture classification was designed to guide surgeons toward a specific exposure, but it does not guide fracture treatment and is not all-inclusive. Variants of these fracture patterns exist, and the prognosis is not related to the pattern.

Elementary Fracture Patterns

Fracture of the posterior wall of the acetabulum is the most common injury to the hip socket, accounting for 20% to 30% of all acetabular fractures.[3] Nonsurgical management of these injuries is supported if the hip is stable and congruent, as occurs with native anatomy and remaining wall size sufficiently large to maintain the femoral head within the acetabulum.[21-23] The posterior wall fragment size traditionally was used as a predictor of hip stability. In general, a hip with a large wall fragment (larger than 66%, as measured using the Calkins et al technique, larger than 50% using the Moed et al technique, or larger than 40% using the Keith et al technique) is considered unstable and requires open reduction and internal fixation (ORIF)[24-26] (**Figure 7**). A fracture affecting less than 20% of the posterior wall, as measured using the Keith el al or Moed et al technique, is likely to be stable and theoretically can be treated nonsurgically.

A fracture with a size between the large and small categories is considered indeterminate. Experts in acetabular surgery were unable to predict the stability of fractures in this indeterminate group using plain radiographs or CT.[27] The presence of a small posterior wall fragment (less than 20% of the wall) was found to cause the hip to be unstable.[22,28] Therefore, radiographic measurements of wall size have only been marginally successful for predicting instability. Although wall size has been studied extensively and is a critical component of acetabular fracture stability, the complex bony anatomy of the hip joint means that other anatomic factors must be considered. The cranial exit point of the fracture, acetabular version, lateral center edge angle, percentage of femoral head coverage, and history of dislocation are some of the other factors that can be useful for predicting hip stability in patients with a posterior wall acetabular fracture. A cranial exit point within 5 mm of the acetabular dome was found to suggest instability.[29] Examination under anesthesia remains the gold standard for determining hip stability, even in fractures that involve less than 20% of the posterior wall.

Posterior column fractures involve the retroacetabular surface and are less common than posterior wall fractures. The fracture line descends from the greater sciatic notch, migrates through the acetabular dome, and progresses through the obturator foramen. On the AP pelvis radiograph, the ilioischial line is disrupted and the association with the teardrop is lost unless most of the quadrilateral surface remains attached to the posterior column. The iliac oblique view best shows the fracture and is useful for identifying the extent and level of displacement.

Displaced posterior column fractures should be assessed for sciatic and superior gluteal neurovascular bundle injury. The sciatic and superior gluteal neurovascular bundles should be identified in a displaced fracture to make sure they are not entrapped or will not become entrapped during the reduction. If brisk bleeding occurs during the surgery and cannot be packed and identified, prompt closure and angiography should be considered.

Anterior wall fracture is the least common of the 10 acetabular fracture patterns, probably because of the unusual force vector required to cause this injury. An anterior column fracture often is misclassified as an anterior wall fracture, and vice versa. An anterior wall fracture that violates the iliopectineal line is classified as an anterior column fracture because it involves the pelvic brim. If the fracture does not involve the iliopectineal line, it is an anterior wall fracture. The obturator oblique view best shows the relationship of the femoral head to the acetabulum, and the iliac oblique view is useful for showing the extent of anterior wall displacement. In displaced acetabular fractures, as in a posterior column fracture, it is important to assess the neurovascular structures and specifically the femoral nerve and iliac artery and vein.

Anterior column fractures are divided into three groups based on the fracture's iliac exit point. High fractures exit at the crest, intermediate fractures exit at the level of the anterosuperior iliac spine, and low fractures exit at the anteroinferior iliac spine. These fractures are best seen on iliac oblique radiographs; a nondisplaced fracture can be difficult to identify on an AP radiograph. In a displaced fracture, the lateral femoral cutaneous nerve can sustain a traction injury, and, depending on the location and displacement of the superior rami, the obturator neurovascular bundle can be injured.

Transverse acetabular fractures also are divided into three groups, based on dome involvement. Transtectal transverse fractures involve the dome, juxtatectal transverse fractures have a fracture line that is at the junction of the acetabular dome and fossa, and infratectal fractures split the acetabular fossa. In all three types the cranial aspect is the stable portion, and the caudal portion is the mobile displaced portion. The more cranial the fracture line is, the more likely is medial displacement of the caudal portion of the femoral head.

Associated Fracture Patterns

The transverse with associated posterior wall fracture is a common injury that combines a transverse fracture and a posterior wall fracture. The femoral head can follow the posterior wall (as it would in a posterior wall fracture), follow the caudal component of the transverse fracture (as it would in a transverse fracture) and cause a superolateral femoral head impaction injury, or remain under a relatively large, intact dome.

The posterior column with associated posterior wall fracture is rare. A careful assessment of the neurovascular structures in this region is critical. The ilioischial line is seen as disrupted on the AP radiograph. The iliac oblique and obturator oblique views are useful for showing the posterior column component or the posterior wall, respectively.

The anterior column fracture with associated posterior hemitransverse fracture is the most common acetabular injury in elderly patients. Like the anterior column fracture, this associated fracture has three exit points along the ilium, with an accompanying fracture that divides the posterior column through the sciatic notch. Both the iliopectineal and ilioischial lines are seen as disrupted on AP radiographs.

The T-shaped acetabular fracture is complex and is composed of a transverse acetabular fracture with an associated vertical fracture that divides the two unstable caudal segments of the transverse fracture through the quadrilateral surface. Both the caudal segment and the anterior column segment are unstable. Both the iliopectineal and ilioischial lines are disrupted, and CT images should be carefully examined for a nondisplaced fracture through the ischium. A posterior column fracture with an anterior hemitransverse fracture is considered a T-shaped fracture.

The associated both-column fracture separates the entire articular surface of the acetabulum and does not have a connection with the intact hemipelvis. The intact ileum is stable because of its connection with the sacrum. Because the most caudal portion of the intact ileum resembles a rooster's cockspur on the obturator outlet radiograph, the term spur sign is used. The spur sign can be seen only in a displaced fracture in which the unstable segment is medially displaced, and it cannot be seen in a nondisplaced or minimally displaced fracture. It is important to avoid mistaking a displaced posterior wall acetabular fracture for a spur sign. The ilioischial and iliopectineal lines both should be disrupted in an associated both-column acetabular fracture, and they should not be disrupted in a posterior wall acetabular fracture.

Variants that are not specifically identifiable based on the Letournel classification are not uncommon and are called transitional patterns. The surgeon should able to identify a transitional pattern and formulate a treatment plan based on preoperative radiography and CT. It is important to realize that the Letournel classification is useful for deciding on the surgical exposure but not for deciding on the treatment plan or fixation construct.

Treatment

Indications

The goal of surgery is to restore a stable, congruent, anatomic hip while avoiding complications. The complex, decision-making process is based on the patient's medical status rather than the fracture. If the patient's medical condition allows, surgery should be considered for an incongruent, unstable hip joint. The stability of the hip can be difficult to determine, but in general the more intact the acetabular dome, the more stable is the joint. Roof arc angles can be measured to determine the extent of the intact dome, but there is controversy as to the roof arc angles that coincide with hip stability. A large roof arc angle is needed for hip stability, especially during activities of daily living.[30-32] Alternatively, CT cuts from the top of the dome and 1 cm distal on axial images can be used to determine whether the fracture involves the weight-bearing dome.[33] Roof and subchondral arc angles can be used to determine the stability of most acetabular fractures, but these angles do not apply to fractures of the posterior or anterior walls, which occur in a region beyond the plane of measurement. Furthermore, if the femoral head is not centered in the acetabulum, the hip is incongruent and roof arc angles do not need to be measured. Alternative indications for surgery include fracture displacement of 1 to 2 mm through the weight-bearing dome or the presence of substantial loose intra-articular bodies, an open fracture, or decreased sciatic nerve function after closed reduction.[34,35]

Surgical Exposure

Most surgical approaches for the treatment of acetabular fractures are anterior or posterior based. Extended approaches, such as the extended iliofemoral approach, rarely are used because of their high complication rates. The Kocher-Langenbeck and Gibson posterior approaches expose the posterior wall and posterior column and provide clamp access to the quadrilateral surface through the greater sciatic notch. A formal surgical hip dislocation through the posterior approach has been proposed as an alternative for selected acetabular fractures. The advantage of surgical hip dislocation is that it provides the surgeon with a 360° view of the articular surface of the acetabulum.[36]

The traditional ilioinguinal anterior approach with its three windows provides almost full access to the intrapelvic surface of the acetabulum and the pelvic brim including anterior column, anterior wall, and clamp access to the posterior column.[2] The use of the modified Stoppa window has become popular, often in conjunction with the use of the lateral window of the ilioinguinal approach.[37] This approach is similar to the use of the medial and lateral windows of the ilioinguinal approach, except the surgeon crosses the table to the contralateral side to access the medial window. Many surgeons have long used the medial- and lateral-window technique with crossing to the contralateral side of the table. In addition, the lateral window can be extended by opening the inguinal canal without taking down the iliopectineal fascia between the femoral nerve and external iliac vessels or by elevating the soft tissue off of the anterosuperior iliac spine. Alternatively, an osteotomy involving the anterosuperior iliac spine including the inguinal ligament and most of the sartorius origin can be performed. The lateral window thereby is exposed down to the anterior wall, iliopectineal eminence, and even the lateral aspect of the superior ramus. This exposure essentially is a Smith-Peterson approach.

The advantages of the modified Stoppa window are that it allows improved medial-to-lateral reduction maneuvers and fixation as well as access to superior medial dome impaction.[38] However, no definitive difference was found between the standard ilioinguinal and Stoppa approaches, probably because they are similar.[39]

Although the selected surgical approach allows access to the fracture, the quality of the soft-tissue handling and reduction is the most critical factor for obtaining the best outcome. The approach aspects that are best suited to the specific fracture pattern should be used, even in a hybrid fashion.[40]

Fracture Fixation

The design of a fixation construct is based on the principles of fracture fixation. Several different combinations of lag screws and 3.5-mm pelvic reconstruction plates can provide the foundation for the fixation. Buttress plate fixation is used to fix the accessed column, and indirect lag screw fixation is used for the second column. New designs focus on locking and fragment-specific implant options. The use of a reconstruction plate allows overcontouring or undercontouring, which is useful for reducing the fracture or capturing specific fragments, respectively (**Figures 8** and **9**). Locking plates can limit the screw placement trajectory. In osteoporotic bone, 4.0-mm screws can be used to improve fixation if 3.5-mm screws have limited purchase. Some research findings have suggested that a quadrilateral surface implant spanning the anterior and posterior columns is biomechanically comparable to and in some fractures better than a traditional buttress plate.[41] Quadrilateral surface implants have yet to be studied extensively in vivo, however.

Percutaneous Techniques

Percutaneous techniques are best used in a patient who cannot medically tolerate an open procedure; has poor-quality soft tissue; has an unstable, minimally displaced fracture; or, if the patient cannot be followed on a routine basis, has a nondisplaced or minimally displaced fracture. Percutaneous techniques can provide anterior

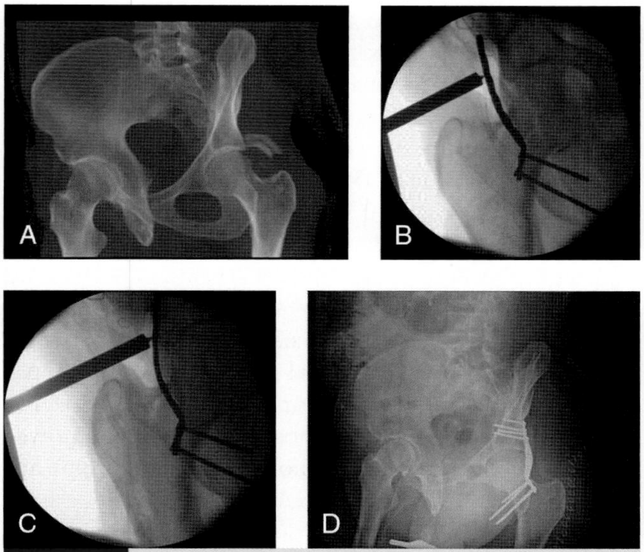

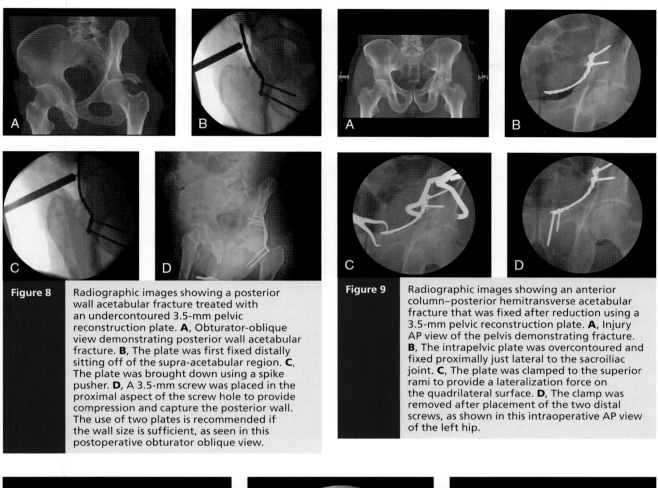

Figure 8 Radiographic images showing a posterior wall acetabular fracture treated with an undercontoured 3.5-mm pelvic reconstruction plate. **A**, Obturator-oblique view demonstrating posterior wall acetabular fracture. **B**, The plate was first fixed distally sitting off of the supra-acetabular region. **C**, The plate was brought down using a spike pusher. **D**, A 3.5-mm screw was placed in the proximal aspect of the screw hole to provide compression and capture the posterior wall. The use of two plates is recommended if the wall size is sufficient, as seen in this postoperative obturator oblique view.

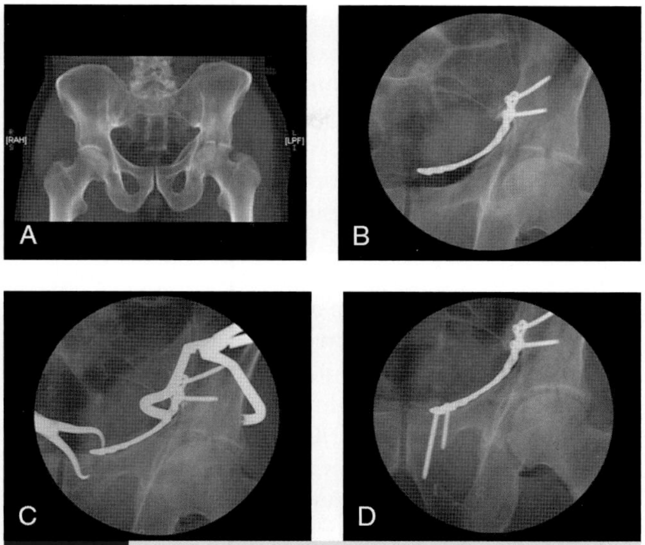

Figure 9 Radiographic images showing an anterior column–posterior hemitransverse acetabular fracture that was fixed after reduction using a 3.5-mm pelvic reconstruction plate. **A**, Injury AP view of the pelvis demonstrating fracture. **B**, The intrapelvic plate was overcontoured and fixed proximally just lateral to the sacroiliac joint. **C**, The plate was clamped to the superior rami to provide a lateralization force on the quadrilateral surface. **D**, The clamp was removed after placement of the two distal screws, as shown in this intraoperative AP view of the left hip.

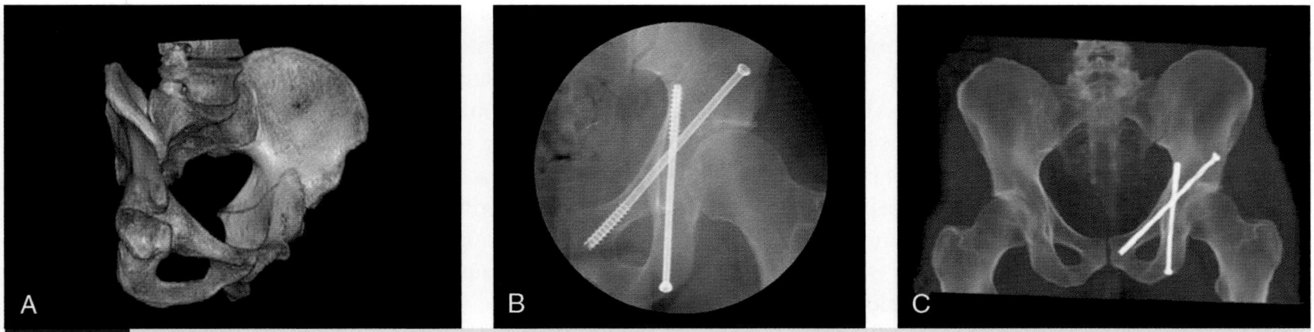

Figure 10 **A,** Three-dimensional CT showing a minimally displaced transverse acetabular fracture before fixation using a percutaneous technique. **B,** Intraoperative view with the patient in the prone position. The anterior and posterior columns were stabilized with 7.0-mm partially threaded cannulated screws. **C,** Postoperative AP pelvis radiograph with definitive fixation.

and posterior column fixation but are not useful for wall fixation (**Figure 10**). It is critical that the surgeon have a keen understanding of the anatomy before attempting percutaneous fixation because neurologic structures such as the sciatic nerve will be located within centimeters of the instrumentation.[42]

Acute Total Hip Arthroplasty

The incidence of acetabular fractures has substantially increased in individuals older than 65 years.[43] The fracture often results from a low-energy fall onto the patient's side, and typically it is classified as a variant of the anterior column–posterior hemitransverse or associated both-column pattern.[44] The common anterior column–posterior hemitransverse variants are characterized by predominant anterior column involvement (with a low exit caudal to the anterosuperior iliac spine), extension into the quadrilateral plate, and medialization of the femoral head. Superomedial dome impaction (the gull sign) and superolateral femoral head damage can occur because of poor bone quality.[45] In a patient with poor bone quality, a fall onto the knee can cause an isolated posterior wall fracture with comminution and impaction.

In some older patients with an acetabular fracture, combined ORIF and acute total hip arthroplasty (THA) should be considered. An almost-30% rate of conversion to THA was reported after ORIF in patients older than 65 years.[46] A fracture involving a comminuted posterior wall, marginal impaction, substantial femoral head cartilage damage, superomedial dome impaction, dislocation, and/or comminution is associated with an increased risk of posttraumatic arthritis.[45,47,48] The quality of reduction also was reported to be the main determinant of a need for conversion to THA.[49]

The primary goal of acute ORIF and THA is the reestablishment of stable columns and/or a stable wall to allow stable acetabular cup placement. The techniques used for this purpose include traditional ORIF with plates and screws, percutaneous reduction and screw placement, and cabling.[48] When a press-fit acetabular component is used, the stability of the cup often depends on an impaction press-fit between the low anterior column and the anterior wall cranially and the ischium caudally, rather than a classic rim fit. However, augmenting initial cup stability with multiple screws is highly recommended and is required if the press-fit is tenuous. Alternatively, a trabecular metal cup-cage construct can be used.[50]

Combined ORIF and THA should be done through a single incision, if possible, to decrease surgical time and the amount of blood loss. The Levine modification of the Smith-Peterson approach can be useful for fracture fixation and direct anterior THA, particularly in the common anterior column–posterior hemitransverse variants.

The combination of acute ORIF and THA in certain acetabular fractures in older patients was reported to lead to excellent functional outcomes.[51,52] The advantages of acute THA include allowing relatively early weight bearing and possibly avoiding the need for additional surgery. THA to relieve posttraumatic arthritis after acetabular fracture was reported to have worse functional outcomes than THA for primary osteoarthritis.[53] THA after ORIF can be challenging because of the presence of hardware from the earlier procedure, difficult dissection because of scarring or heterotopic ossification (HO), and the potential for an indolent infection. The longevity of the acetabular component is of central concern; press-fit components were found to have lower rates of loosening compared with cemented components.[54,55] Further research is needed to identify the patients and specific fracture patterns better suited to combined acute ORIF and THA rather than ORIF alone.

Complications

The complications associated with acetabular fractures have been the focus of recent research. Posttraumatic arthritis is the most important such complication. The most comprehensive long-term follow-up study reported a 79% rate of 20-year hip survivorship after ORIF.[47] Angiographic embolization of pelvic arterial hemorrhage before surgery led to a 58% rate of postoperative deep infection.[56] Determining the extent to which embolization increases the risk of infection requires study of several factors, including the experience of the angiographer and the choice of selective or nonselective embolization as well as the use of an absorbable gelatin compressed sponge or coil embolization. Acute blood loss anemia and the efficacy of intraoperative red blood cell salvage also is a focus of research.[57-59] Red blood cell salvage was found to be cost effective in acetabular surgery, although the rate at which blood was returned to the patient was relatively low. Blood loss in older patients with an associated fracture pattern and in patients requiring an ilioinguinal approach may warrant the use of red blood cell salvage.

Surgical timing is believed to relate to blood loss and anemia. Surgeons in the past believed that intraoperative blood loss could be limited by a so-called cooling-off period before surgery using an open approach. Blood loss and surgical time were not found to be correlated based on whether surgery to treat a variety of acetabular fractures was done within 48 hours of injury or later and whether a posterior- or anterior-based approach was used.[60,61]

Deep vein thrombosis (DVT) is a dreaded complication that causes significant morbidity and mortality. Patients with an acetabular fracture are at high risk for DVT, although the use of anticoagulation medications and mechanical prophylaxis has decreased the rate. In patients with a contraindication to systemic chemoprophylaxis, the use of inferior vena cava (IVC) filters has been promoted to decrease the risk of pulmonary embolism. Retrievable IVC filters provide temporary protection from pulmonary embolism and spare the patient from the long-term complications associated with the use of permanent filters. Unretrieved filters are a risk factor for recurrent DVT, organ penetration, vena cava thrombosis, filter migration, and fracture of the strut.[62,63] The historical reported retrieval rate was 34%, but dedicated protocols and clinics have increased the retrieval rate to 60%.[64,65] It is critical that the orthopaedic surgeon ask patients on a routine basis whether their filters have been removed.

The development of HO can significantly affect outcomes. The risk factors for HO historically were believed to include traumatic brain injury, the use of an extensile surgical approach, and a fracture requiring dual approaches. Additional risk factors continue to be identified. Mechanical ventilation of more than 72 hours' duration was found to be a risk factor for the development of severe HO.[66] The prophylactic use of pharmacologic and radiation therapy is controversial. Early reports supported the use of indomethacin, but subsequent randomized studies did not find significant differences in rates of HO based on administration of indomethacin or placebo.[67,68] A routine 6-week course of indomethacin not only failed to decrease the rate of HO but also was found to increase the risk of nonunion in posterior wall acetabular fractures.[69] Radiation therapy has not been studied as extensively as pharmacologic intervention because of its theoretic risks and high cost. Administering radiation therapy within the first 3 days of surgery was found to be effective.[70] Because the stimuli for HO occur at the time of surgery, it might be assumed that preoperative administration of radiation would be more effective than postoperative administration. However, in a comparison of patients treated with preoperative or postoperative radiation no difference was found.[71]

HO should be discontinued if it limits the patient's range of motion or causes neurologic insult. Although arthroplasty research in general supports removal of HO after it has matured, earlier removal may be preferable after acetabular fracture surgery. A mobile joint is critical for the health of the joint, and neurologic compromise for an extended period of time can lead to permanent deficits. The longer the time from the index surgery to HO removal, the more substantial the scar tissue that must be dissected; resection early but at least 3 months from the index surgery does not increase the risk of recurrence.[72]

Outcomes

Several studies have reported functional outcomes after surgical treatment of acetabular fractures. Conversion to THA was reported in an average 23% of patients (range, 21% to 45%), most often within 2 years of injury.[44,46,73,74] The quality of reduction continues to be the most important predictor of a need for future arthroplasty.[74,75] Patients who did not undergo THA had higher functional scores than those who underwent conversion to THA.[53,73] As a result, some experts recommend initial THA for the treatment of selected acetabular fractures in the elderly.[52]

Summary

Acetabular fractures are complex, and treatment requires the surgeon to have a clear understanding of fracture anatomy and imaging. The treatment is guided by the patient's medical condition and the nature of the bony and soft-tissue injury. The goals of surgical intervention are to obtain and maintain a stable, congruent, and anatomic hip socket and to avoid complications.

Key Study Points

- The goals of surgical intervention are to obtain and maintain a stable, congruent, and anatomic hip socket and to avoid complications.
- Red blood cell salvage is cost-effective and is more likely to be useful in surgery through an anterior approach than through a posterior approach.
- A small posterior wall acetabular fracture can be unstable, especially if it is within 5 mm of the acetabular dome.
- The quality of reduction is the most important predictor of a need for future THA.
- The role of acute THA has not yet been fully determined.

Annotated References

1. Morshed S, Knops S, Jurkovich GJ, Wang J, MacKenzie E, Rivara FP: The impact of trauma-center care on mortality and function following pelvic ring and acetabular injuries. *J Bone Joint Surg Am* 2015;97(4):265-272.

   A study of the effect of trauma center care on outcomes after acetabular and pelvic fractures included 829 patients. The mortality rate was lower in patients treated in a trauma center than in those treated in other centers. Level of evidence: III.

2. Letournel E: Fractures of the cotyloid cavity: Study of a series of 75 cases. *J Chir (Paris)* 1961;82:47-87.

3. Letournel E, Judet R: *Fractures of the Acetabulum, ed* 2. New York, NY, Springer, 1993.

4. O'Toole RV, Cox G, Shanmuganathan K, et al: Evaluation of computed tomography for determining the diagnosis of acetabular fractures. *J Orthop Trauma* 2010;24(5):284-290.

Four orthopaedic traumatologists classified 75 acetabular fractures based on CT or plain radiographs. The accuracy of plain radiographs alone was lower than that of CT.

5. Borrelli J Jr, Peelle M, McFarland E, Evanoff B, Ricci WM: Computer-reconstructed radiographs are as good as plain radiographs for assessment of acetabular fractures. *Am J Orthop (Belle Mead NJ)* 2008;37(9):455-459, discussion 460.

6. Sinatra PM, Moed BR: CT-generated radiographs in obese patients with acetabular fractures: Can they be used in lieu of plain radiographs? *Clin Orthop Relat Res* 2014;472(11):3362-3369.

   Seventeen acetabular fractures in patients with obesity were assessed using CT-generated radiographs, which were found to be as accurate as plain radiographs for classification. Level of evidence: II.

7. Citak M, Gardner MJ, Kendoff D, et al: Virtual 3D planning of acetabular fracture reduction. *J Orthop Res* 2008;26(4):547-552.

8. Scheinfeld MH, Dym AA, Spektor M, Avery LL, Dym RJ, Amanatullah DF: Acetabular fractures: What radiologists should know and how 3D CT can aid classification. *Radiographics* 2015;35(2):555-577.

   Acetabular fracture patterns were reviewed, and the use of CT to classify acetabular fractures was described.

9. Wong JM, Bewsher S, Yew J, Bucknill A, de Steiger R: Fluoroscopically assisted computer navigation enables accurate percutaneous screw placement for pelvic and acetabular fracture fixation. *Injury* 2015;46(6):1064-1068.

   The placement of 162 percutaneous screws using fluoroscopic navigation was found to be accurate. Ten screws perforated cortical bone, however.

10. Schwabe P, Altintas B, Schaser KD, et al: Three-dimensional fluoroscopy-navigated percutaneous screw fixation of acetabular fractures. *J Orthop Trauma* 2014;28(12):700-706, discussion 706.

    Twelve patients with a moderately displaced acetabular fracture underwent three-dimensional fluoroscopically navigated percutaneous screw fixation and reduction. Postoperative CT confirmed anatomic reduction in all patients. Level of evidence: IV.

11. Gras F, Marintschev I, Klos K, Mückley T, Hofmann GO, Kahler DM: Screw placement for acetabular fractures: Which navigation modality (2-dimensional vs. 3-dimensional) should be used? An experimental study. *J Orthop Trauma* 2012;26(8):466-473.

    A comparison of two- and three-dimensional navigation for the placement of percutaneous acetabular screws in a synthetic bone model found that both imaging modalities prevented intra-articular penetration but that three-dimensional navigation was more accurate.

12. Yu AW, Duncan JM, Daurka JS, Lewis A, Cobb J: A feasibility study into the use of three-dimensional printer modelling in acetabular fracture surgery. *Adv Orthop* 2015;2015:617046.

    The feasibility of using three-dimensional printer technology to make models for contouring reconstruction plates was studied.

13. Judet R, Judet J, Letournel E: Fractures of the acetabulum: Classification and surgical approaches for open reduction. Preliminary report. *J Bone Joint Surg Am* 1964;46:1615-1646.

14. Judet R, Judet J, Letournel E: [Fractures of the Acetabulum]. *Acta Orthop Belg* 1964;30:285-293.

15. Letournel E: Acetabulum fractures: Classification and management. *Clin Orthop Relat Res* 1980;151:81-106.

16. Alton TB, Gee AO: Classifications in brief: Letournel classification for acetabular fractures. *Clin Orthop Relat Res* 2014;472(1):35-38.

    The Letournel classification for acetabular fractures is reviewed.

17. Prevezas N, Antypas G, Louverdis D, Konstas A, Papasotiriou A, Sbonias G: Proposed guidelines for increasing the reliability and validity of Letournel classification system. *Injury* 2009;40(10):1098-1103.

18. Hüfner T, Pohlemann T, Gänsslen A, Assassi P, Prokop M, Tscherne H: The value of CT in classification and decision making in acetabulum fractures: A systematic analysis. *Unfallchirurg* 1999;102(2):124-131.

19. Beaulé PE, Dorey FJ, Matta JM: Letournel classification for acetabular fractures: Assessment of interobserver and intraobserver reliability. *J Bone Joint Surg Am* 2003;85(9):1704-1709.

20. Ohashi K, El-Khoury GY, Abu-Zahra KW, Berbaum KS: Interobserver agreement for Letournel acetabular fracture classification with multidetector CT: Are standard Judet radiographs necessary? *Radiology* 2006;241(2):386-391.

21. Moed BR, Spoonamore MJ: *Management of acetabular fractures, in Oxford Textbook of Orthopedics and Trauma* .Oxford, England, Oxford University Press, 2002, pp 2182-2201.

22. Tornetta P III: Non-operative management of acetabular fractures: The use of dynamic stress views. *J Bone Joint Surg Br* 1999;81(1):67-70.

23. Grimshaw CS, Moed BR: Outcomes of posterior wall fractures of the acetabulum treated nonoperatively after diagnostic screening with dynamic stress examination under anesthesia. *J Bone Joint Surg Am* 2010;92(17):2792-2800.

    Twenty-one patients with an acute posterior wall acetabular fracture underwent examination under anesthesia.

Radiographic outcomes were excellent at follow-up, and early clinical outcomes were good to excellent. Level of evidence: IV.

24. Calkins MS, Zych G, Latta L, Borja FJ, Mnaymneh W: Computed tomography evaluation of stability in posterior fracture dislocation of the hip. *Clin Orthop Relat Res* 1988;227(227):152-163.

25. Keith JE Jr, Brashear HR Jr, Guilford WB: Stability of posterior fracture-dislocations of the hip: Quantitative assessment using computed tomography. *J Bone Joint Surg Am* 1988;70(5):711-714.

26. Moed BR, Ajibade DA, Israel H: Computed tomography as a predictor of hip stability status in posterior wall fractures of the acetabulum. *J Orthop Trauma* 2009;23(1):7-15.

27. Davis AT, Moed BR: Can experts in acetabular fracture care determine hip stability after posterior wall fractures using plain radiographs and computed tomography? *J Orthop Trauma* 2013;27(10):587-591.

    Only 53% interobserver reliability was found for stability in posterior wall acetabular fractures involving 20% to 50% of the posterior wall. Orthopaedic traumatologists could not predict stability based on plain radiographs, CT, and history of dislocation.

28. Reagan JM, Moed BR: Can computed tomography predict hip stability in posterior wall acetabular fractures? *Clin Orthop Relat Res* 2011;469(7):2035-2041.

    In a study to determine whether a previously described method for determining stability in posterior wall fractures was reliable, 10 fractures with known outcomes were assessed by three study participant groups. Wall fragment size larger than 50% was the only reliable predictor of stability. A fracture smaller than 50% should be examined under anesthesia.

29. Firoozabadi R, Spitler C, Schlepp C, et al: Determining stability in posterior wall acetabular fractures. *J Orthop Trauma* 2015;29(10):465-469.

    In a retrospective study of prospectively gathered data to determine the risk factors in unstable posterior wall acetabular fractures, fractures that enter the acetabular dome were found to be unstable even with a wall fragment size smaller than 20%. Level of evidence: II.

30. Matityahu A, McDonald E, Buckley JM, Marmor M: Propensity for hip dislocation in gait loading versus sit-to-stand maneuvers: Implications for redefining the dome of the acetabulum needed for stability of the hip during activities of daily living. *J Orthop Trauma* 2012;26(8):e97-e101.

    A cadaver biomechanical study compared the instability of transverse acetabular fractures in relation to single-leg stance loading and sit-to-stand maneuvers. There was significantly more hip instability with sit-to-stand than with single-leg stance loading. Some fractures considered stable may become significantly unstable during activities of daily living. LOE.

31. Matta JM, Merritt PO: Displaced acetabular fractures. *Clin Orthop Relat Res* 1988;230:83-97.

32. Chuckpaiwong B, Suwanwong P, Harnroongroj T: Roof-arc angle and weight-bearing area of the acetabulum. *Injury* 2009;40(10):1064-1066.

33. Olson SA, Matta JM: The computerized tomography subchondral arc: A new method of assessing acetabular articular continuity after fracture. A preliminary report. *J Orthop Trauma* 1993;7(5):402-413.

34. Pascarella R, Maresca A, Reggiani LM, Boriani S: Intra-articular fragments in acetabular fracture-dislocation. *Orthopedics* 2009;32(6):402.

35. Tornetta P III: Displaced acetabular fractures: Indications for operative and nonoperative management. *J Am Acad Orthop Surg* 2001;9(1):18-28.

36. Masse A, Aprato A, Rollero L, Bersano A, Ganz R: Surgical dislocation technique for the treatment of acetabular fractures. *Clin Orthop Relat Res* 2013;471(12):4056-4064.

    A retrospective review of 31 acetabular fractures treated with surgical hip dislocation found anatomic reduction in 65%, imperfect reduction in 16%, and poor reduction in 19%. The mean Merle d'Aubigne score was 15.

37. Cole JD, Bolhofner BR: Acetabular fracture fixation via a modified Stoppa limited intrapelvic approach: Description of operative technique and preliminary treatment results. *Clin Orthop Relat Res* 1994;305:112-123.

38. Shazar N, Eshed I, Ackshota N, Hershkovich O, Khazanov A, Herman A: Comparison of acetabular fracture reduction quality by the ilioinguinal or the anterior intrapelvic (modified Rives-Stoppa) surgical approaches. *J Orthop Trauma* 2014;28(6):313-319.

    A retrospective review of 122 patients treated using an ilioinguinal surgical approach and 103 treated using an anterior intrapelvic approach found anatomic reduction in significantly more patients who had undergone surgery with the anterior intrapelvic approach. The two patient groups had similar fracture types and complications. Level of evidence: III.

39. Elmadağ M, Güzel Y, Acar MA, Uzer G, Arazi M: The Stoppa approach versus the ilioinguinal approach for anterior acetabular fractures: A case control study assessing blood loss complications and function outcomes. *Orthop Traumatol Surg Res* 2014;100(6):675-680.

    The study hypothesis was that the modified Stoppa approach leads to less blood loss than the ilioinguinal approach in the management of anterior column acetabular fractures. No between-group difference was found. Level of evidence: III.

40. Hagen JE, Weatherford BM, Nascone JW, Sciadini MF: Anterior intrapelvic modification to the ilioinguinal approach. *J Orthop Trauma* 2015;29(Suppl 2):S10-S13.

The use of a modification of the medial window of the ilioinguinal approach was found to facilitate intrapelvic visualization.

41. Kistler BJ, Smithson IR, Cooper SA, et al: Are quadrilateral surface buttress plates comparable to traditional forms of transverse acetabular fracture fixation? *Clin Orthop Relat Res* 2014;472(11):3353-3361.

A biomechanical study compared the use of traditional plating and lag-screw techniques to the use of quadrilateral surface buttress plates. Quadrilateral surface buttress plates spanning the posterior and anterior columns were found to be biomechanically comparable or superior.

42. Azzam K, Siebler J, Bergmann K, Daccarett M, Mormino M: Percutaneous retrograde posterior column acetabular fixation: Is the sciatic nerve safe? A cadaveric study. *J Orthop Trauma* 2014;28(1):37-40.

A cadaver study to determine the proximity of neurologic structures to instruments during placement of percutaneous retrograde posterior column screws found that the sciatic nerve was located an average of 58 mm from the screw head.

43. Ferguson TA, Patel R, Bhandari M, Matta JM: Fractures of the acetabulum in patients aged 60 years and older: An epidemiological and radiological study. *J Bone Joint Surg Br* 2010;92(2):250-257.

Epidemiologic changes that have occurred in patients older than 60 years regarding acetabular fracture injury and specific fracture patterns were studied over a 27-year period. The incidence of elderly acetabular fractures has significantly increased (2.4-fold). Fractures involving the anterior column are more common in elderly patients compared with young patients.

44. Daurka JS, Pastides PS, Lewis A, Rickman M, Bircher MD: Acetabular fractures in patients aged > 55 years: A systematic review of the literature. *Bone Joint J* 2014;96(2):157-163.

A systematic review of published studies on the treatment of acetabular fractures in patients older than 55 years included 15 case studies and 415 fractures. The conversion rate to THA was 23%, the nonfatal complication rate was 40%, and the mortality rate was 19%.

45. Anglen JO, Burd TA, Hendricks KJ, Harrison P: The "gull sign": A harbinger of failure for internal fixation of geriatric acetabular fractures. *J Orthop Trauma* 2003;17(9):625-634.

46. O'Toole RV, Hui E, Chandra A, Nascone JW: How often does open reduction and internal fixation of geriatric acetabular fractures lead to hip arthroplasty? *J Orthop Trauma* 2014;28(3):148-153.

A retrospective review of 147 older patients who underwent ORIF for an acetabular fracture found that 28% underwent THA an average 2.5 years after injury. The mortality rate within 1 year was 25%. Level of evidence: III.

47. Tannast M, Najibi S, Matta JM: Two to twenty-year survivorship of the hip in 810 patients with operatively treated acetabular fractures. *J Bone Joint Surg Am* 2012;94(17):1559-1567.

In a study determine survivorship of the hip after ORIF for acetabular fracture, 816 fractures were followed. The authors report a 21% conversion to total hip arthroplasty within 20 years. Level of evidence: II.

48. Mears DC, Velyvis JH: Acute total hip arthroplasty for selected displaced acetabular fractures: Two to twelve-year results. *J Bone Joint Surg Am* 2002;84(1):1-9.

49. Carroll EA, Huber FG, Goldman AT, et al: Treatment of acetabular fractures in an older population. *J Orthop Trauma* 2010;24(10):637-644.

The authors report on outcomes of 93 patients aged 55 years or older who were treated for acetabular fractures. They found an overall rate of total hip replacement of 30% with low complication rates.

50. Chana-Rodríguez F, Villanueva-Martínez M, Rojo-Manaute J, Sanz-Ruíz P, Vaquero-Martín J: Cup-cage construct for acute fractures of the acetabulum: Re-defining indications. *Injury* 2012;43(Suppl 2):S28-S32.

Six acetabular fractures were successfully treated with THA using a cup in a trabecular metal acetabular cage construct.

51. Herscovici D Jr, Lindvall E, Bolhofner B, Scaduto JM: The combined hip procedure: Open reduction internal fixation combined with total hip arthroplasty for the management of acetabular fractures in the elderly. *J Orthop Trauma* 2010;24(5):291-296.

A retrospective study evaluated 22 patients after ORIF and THA done at the same time. At an average 29-month follow-up, four patients had heterotopic ossification, and five had undergone revision surgery for implant loosening or multiple dislocations.

52. Lin C, Caron J, Schmidt AH, Torchia M, Templeman D: Functional outcomes after total hip arthroplasty for the acute management of acetabular fractures: 1- to 14-year follow-up. *J Orthop Trauma* 2015;29(3):151-159.

A retrospective study of 33 patients who underwent ORIF and THA during the index procedure found a 15% complication rate; 93% of patients reported a good to excellent functional outcome, and 94% of hips remained in situ. The functional outcomes were similar to those of patients undergoing primary THA. Level of evidence: IV.

53. Schnaser E, Scarcella NR, Vallier HA: Acetabular fractures converted to total hip arthroplasties in the elderly: How does function compare to primary total hip arthroplasty? *J Orthop Trauma* 2014;28(12):694-699.

In a retrospective review of 171 patients, 17 patients had an acetabular fracture that required THA for posttraumatic arthritis; all other patients underwent primary THA for osteoarthritis. In patients with an acetabular fracture, the average time to conversion to THA was 35 months;

these patients had outcomes scores indicating a lower level of function than the other patients. Level of evidence: III.

54. Weber M, Berry DJ, Harmsen WS: Total hip arthroplasty after operative treatment of an acetabular fracture. *J Bone Joint Surg Am* 1998;80(9):1295-1305.

55. Bellabarba C, Berger RA, Bentley CD, et al: Cementless acetabular reconstruction after acetabular fracture. *J Bone Joint Surg Am* 2001;83(6):868-876.

56. Manson TT, Perdue PW, Pollak AN, O'Toole RV: Embolization of pelvic arterial injury is a risk factor for deep infection after acetabular fracture surgery. *J Orthop Trauma* 2013;27(1):11-15.

    In a study to determine whether embolization of pelvic arteries before ORIF of acetabular fractures was associated with an increase in deep surgical site infections, 7 of 12 patients (58%) who underwent embolization had infections, compared with 14% of patients who had angiography without embolization. Level of evidence: II.

57. Firoozabadi R, Swenson A, Kleweno C, Routt MC: Cell saver use in acetabular surgery: Does approach matter? *J Orthop Trauma* 2015;29(8):349-353.

    In a study to determine whether red blood cell salvage was routinely indicated and whether there was a difference between surgical approaches, 145 consecutive acetabular procedures were retrospectively analyzed. There were significantly more blood loss and salvaged blood return with anterior-based approaches to the acetabulum compared with posterior-based approaches. Level of evidence: II.

58. Scannell BP, Loeffler BJ, Bosse MJ, Kellam JF, Sims SH: Efficacy of intraoperative red blood cell salvage and autotransfusion in the treatment of acetabular fractures. *J Orthop Trauma* 2009;23(5):340-345.

59. Bigsby E, Acharya MR, Ward AJ, Chesser TJ: The use of blood cell salvage in acetabular fracture internal fixation surgery. *J Orthop Trauma* 2013;27(10):e230-e233.

    In a retrospective study of 80 patients, routine use of red blood cell salvage in acetabular ORIF was found to be cost-effective, particularly in associated fracture patterns, and to reduce the need for allogenic blood transfusion. Level of evidence: IV.

60. Dailey SK, Archdeacon MT: Open reduction and internal fixation of acetabulum fractures: Does timing of surgery affect blood loss and OR time? *J Orthop Trauma* 2014;28(9):497-501.

    A retrospective review of 288 consecutive acetabular fractures (176 posterior wall fractures treated through a Kocher-Langenbeck approach and 112 associated both-column and anterior column–posterior hemitransverse fractures treated through an anterior intrapelvic approach) found that estimated blood loss and surgical time were no different based on whether surgery was done less than or more than 48 hours from admission. Level of evidence: III.

61. Furey AJ, Karp J, O'Toole RV: Does early fixation of posterior wall acetabular fractures lead to increased blood loss? *J Orthop Trauma* 2013;27(1):2-5.

    A retrospective review of 49 consecutive posterior wall acetabular fractures over a 1-year period found no difference in estimated blood loss based on whether the fracture was fixed less than 24 hours after injury or later. Level of evidence: II.

62. Sarosiek S, Crowther M, Sloan JM: Indications, complications, and management of inferior vena cava filters: The experience in 952 patients at an academic hospital with a level I trauma center. *JAMA Intern Med* 2013;173(7):513-517.

    A retrospective review of outcomes and complications associated with placement of 679 retrievable IVC filters found that only 58 (8.5%) were successfully removed. Thirteen retrieval attempts were unsuccessful (18% of all removal attempts). A high (7%) rate of venous thrombotic events was observed including 25 (7%), all of which occurred with the IVC filter in place. Approximately 25% of patients were discharged on anticoagulant therapy in addition to the filters. The authors concluded that the use of IVC filters had suboptimal outcomes because of high rates of venous thrombotic events, the low retrieval rate, and inconsistent use of anticoagulant therapy.

63. Nicholson W, Nicholson WJ, Tolerico P, et al: Prevalence of fracture and fragment embolization of Bard retrievable vena cava filters and clinical implications including cardiac perforation and tamponade. *Arch Intern Med* 2010;170(20):1827-1831.

    A retrospective review of 80 first- and second-generation Bard retrievable IVC filters found a high incidence of strut fracture (16%) or embolization, with potentially life-threatening sequelae.

64. Angel LF, Tapson V, Galgon RE, Restrepo MI, Kaufman J: Systematic review of the use of retrievable inferior vena cava filters. *J Vasc Interv Radiol* 2011;22(11):1522-1530.e3.

    A literature review of 37 studies of IVC filters including 6,834 patients found a 1.7% rate of pulmonary embolism after IVC placement, a 34% mean retrieval rate, and multiple complications associated with use for more than 30 days.

65. Minocha J, Idakoji I, Riaz A, et al: Improving inferior vena cava filter retrieval rates: Impact of a dedicated inferior vena cava filter clinic. *J Vasc Interv Radiol* 2010;21(12):1847-1851.

    A retrospective study found that the rate of retrieval of IVC filters improved from 29% before implementation of a dedicated IVC filter clinic to 60% after implementation.

66. Firoozabadi R, O'Mara TJ, Swenson A, Agel J, Beck JD, Routt M: Risk factors for the development of heterotopic ossification after acetabular fracture fixation. *Clin Orthop Relat Res* 2014;472(11):3383-3388.

A retrospective study to evaluate independent risk factors for the development of HO after surgery using a Kocher-Langenbeck approach found severe HO in 38 of 312 patients (12%). Prolonged mechanical ventilation (3 or more days) was the only significant independent risk factor. Level of evidence: IV.

67. Karunakar MA, Sen A, Bosse MJ, Sims SH, Goulet JA, Kellam JF: Indomethacin as prophylaxis for heterotopic ossification after the operative treatment of fractures of the acetabulum. *J Bone Joint Surg Br* 2006;88(12):1613-1617.

68. Matta JM, Siebenrock KA: Does indomethacin reduce heterotopic bone formation after operations for acetabular fractures? A prospective randomised study. *J Bone Joint Surg Br* 1997;79(6):959-963.

69. Sagi HC, Jordan CJ, Barei DP, Serrano-Riera R, Steverson B: Indomethacin prophylaxis for heterotopic ossification after acetabular fracture surgery increases the risk for nonunion of the posterior wall. *J Orthop Trauma* 2014;28(7):377-383.

    A prospective randomized double-blinded study to determine whether indomethacin was efficacious for HO prophylaxis and whether it affected the rate of nonunion found nonunion rates ranging from 19% with placebo to 62% with 6 weeks of treatment. Treatment with 6 weeks of indomethacin did not decrease the rate of HO formation after acetabular fracture surgery and appeared to increase the incidence of nonunion. Level of evidence: II.

70. Blokhuis TJ, Frölke JP: Is radiation superior to indomethacin to prevent heterotopic ossification in acetabular fractures?: A systematic review. *Clin Orthop Relat Res* 2009;467(2):526-530.

71. Archdeacon MT, d'Heurle A, Nemeth N, Budde B: Is preoperative radiation therapy as effective as postoperative radiation therapy for heterotopic ossification prevention in acetabular fractures? *Clin Orthop Relat Res* 2014;472(11):3389-3394.

    A retrospective study found no significant difference in HO rates or severity after radiation therapy was used before or after surgery (22% or 27%, respectively). Level of evidence: III.

72. Wu XB, Yang MH, Zhu SW, et al: Surgical resection of severe heterotopic ossification after open reduction and internal fixation of acetabular fractures: A case series of 18 patients. *Injury* 2014;45(10):1604-1610.

    A retrospective study of 18 patients who underwent HO resection surgery found a 28.6% recurrence rate if the HO resection was done within 6 months of index surgery and a 36.4% rate if the HO resection was done later than 6 months. The complications included one intraoperative femoral neck fracture, one sciatic nerve injury, two incidences of femoral head osteonecrosis, and six mild HO recurrences (33.3%). Early surgical resection of severe HO was found to have satisfactory results, although with a high complication rate.

73. Borg T, Hailer NP: Outcome 5 years after surgical treatment of acetabular fractures: A prospective clinical and radiographic follow-up of 101 patients. *Arch Orthop Trauma Surg* 2015;135(2):227-233.

    A retrospective study of 101 acetabular fractures included conversion to THA or a Girdlestone procedure. The survival rate was 77% 5 years after ORIF. Risk factors for failure included femoral head impaction and age older than 60 years.

74. Briffa N, Pearce R, Hill AM, Bircher M: Outcomes of acetabular fracture fixation with ten years' follow-up. *J Bone Joint Surg Br* 2011;93(2):229-236.

    A retrospective study of 10-year outcomes after 161 acetabular fractures were surgically fixed found that the result was excellent in 47% of patients, good in 25%, fair in 7%, and poor in 20%. The prognostic factors included increasing age, delay to surgery, quality of reduction, and specific fracture patterns.

75. Magu NK, Gogna P, Singh A, et al: Long term results after surgical management of posterior wall acetabular fractures. *J Orthop Traumatol* 2014;15(3):173-179.

    A retrospective analysis of 26 posterior wall acetabular fractures after ORIF found that anatomic reduction was essential for an optimal functional and radiologic outcome. An associated lower limb injury and a body mass index higher than 25 were risk factors for a less than optimal outcome. Level of evidence: IV.

Chapter 33

Management of Traumatic Spinal Cord Injuries

Jay M. Zampini, MD Mitchel B. Harris, MD, FACS

Abstract

Spinal cord injury (SCI) is among the most devastating types of traumatic injury. The lifetime cost of caring for a patient with SCI can reach $5 million, and the global incidence and prevalence of SCI have changed little in past decades. Variations in causation and ethnicity are found between and within regions and countries. The neurologic deficits caused by SCI result from direct trauma to the spinal cord and vasculature, and secondary damage can be caused by inflammatory mediators, free radicals, endogenous opioids, neurotransmitters, neural apoptosis and necrosis, thrombosis, edema, or demyelination. Direct damage is controlled by rapid neural decompression and mechanical stabilization. Each mediator of indirect, secondary damage has been targeted for treatment using specific cellular and pharmacologic agents. Regenerative treatments have focused on the regrowth of both neural and supporting cells. Although the outcome of SCI treatment has not significantly changed in recent decades, considerable advances have been made in the incremental understanding of this complex and challenging condition.

Keywords: cellular regenerative techniques; pharmacologic prevention and treatment of secondary spinal cord damage; spinal cord damage; spinal cord injury epidemiology; spinal cord injury surgery

Dr. Zampini or an immediate family member serves as a paid consultant to or is an employee of Biomet. Dr. Harris or an immediate family member serves as a board member, owner, officer, or committee member of the North American Spine Society.

Introduction

Spinal cord injury (SCI) is one of the most devastating survivable effects of trauma. The medical, social, and economic consequences can dominate almost every aspect of the life of the patient and the patient's family. The ability to function in routine daily activities often is permanently altered, and the risk of compromise to the patient's cardiopulmonary system, skin, coagulation and hemostasis, and metabolism present ongoing medical challenges. It may be difficult or impossible for the patient to find employment. The patient's need for personal assistance often taxes the capacities of the family and friends. The average lifetime cost of medical and other direct personal care of a patient with SCI can reach $5 million; expenditures during the first year alone range from $334,000 to $1,023,000.[1,2]

Although there has been important progress in the management of SCI during the past four decades, the fundamental nature and treatment of the condition have changed little in millennia. Descriptions of axial traction for spinal injury can be found in ancient Egyptian, Hindu, and Greek texts from 4,500 years ago.[3] Galen described a method of neurologic localization in approximately 150 BCE. The concept of laminectomy was first described by Paulus of Aegina during the medieval period. The first documented laminectomy was done in 1564 by Sir Ambrose Pare and was condemned by Charles Bell in the early 19th century as too dangerous to justify. The accelerated pace of scientific discovery that began in the late 19th century has led to a considerably improved understanding of the prevention, stabilization, and rehabilitation of SCI.

Epidemiology

The variable nature of SCI creates difficulty in formulating an accurate estimate of its global prevalence and annual incidence (**Figures 1** and **2**). Recent reports concluded that the global incidence and prevalence of SCI have not appreciably changed during the past two

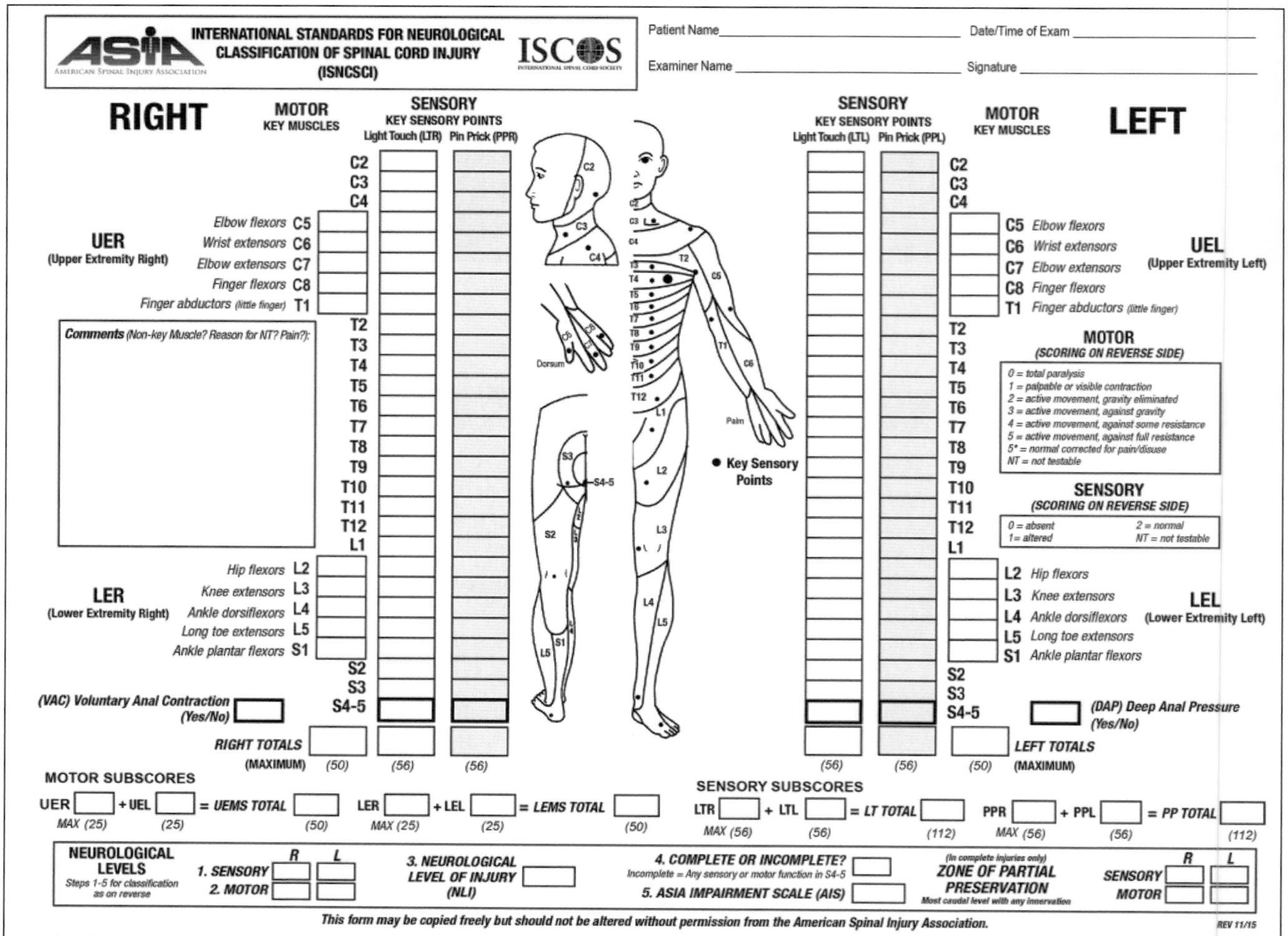

Figure 1 The American Spinal Injury Association Classification of Spinal Cord Injury and Impairment Scale. (Reproduced with permission from the American Spinal Injury Association: Standard Neurological Classification of Spinal Cord Injury. http://www.asia-spinalinjury.org.)

decades.[4] The annual incidence is 23 to 40 per million population, and the number of patients living with SCI is 200 to 1,000 per million.[5,6] The development of the Spinal Cord Injury Model Systems and the National Spinal Cord Injury Statistical Center has led to reports that the United States has the highest incidence and prevalence of SCI. Approximately 12,000 incidences of SCI (40 per million population) occur each year in the United States, and 273,000 patients (906 per million) currently live with SCI.[7] The data notably omit patients who die from SCI before arriving at a hospital. No recent estimates of this number exist, although in the 1970s the prehospital mortality rate after SCI was believed to be 50% to 79%.[8] These percentages are similar to the mortality levels described in 19th-century wartime reports.[9]

Despite considerable regional and national variation, the population of patients with SCI has certain demographic commonalities. The distribution of SCIs is bimodal: patients are injured during the third, fourth, or fifth decade of life by a high-energy mechanism, or they are injured at an age older than 70 years, typically by a fall from a standing position or another low-energy mechanism.[5,6] The average age of a patient when the SCI occurs is 42.6 years.[7] Men are injured two to four times more often than women. Slightly more than half of patients affected by SCI were employed at the time of injury. In the United States, the proportion of patients self-described as African American has increased, and the proportion self-described as Caucasian has decreased. African American patients are more likely than Caucasian or Hispanic patients to be readmitted to a hospital for medical care during the first 10 years after injury.[1] These findings can be explained only by conjecture, but they provide evidence of the need for research

Muscle Function Grading

0 = total paralysis
1 = palpable or visible contraction
2 = active movement, full range of motion (ROM) with gravity eliminated
3 = active movement, full ROM against gravity
4 = active movement, full ROM against gravity and moderate resistance in a muscle specific position
5 = (normal) active movement, full ROM against gravity and full resistance in a functional muscle position expected from an otherwise unimpaired person
5* = (normal) active movement, full ROM against gravity and sufficient resistance to be considered normal if identified inhibiting factors (i.e. pain, disuse) were not present
NT = not testable (i.e. due to immobilization, severe pain such that the patient cannot be graded, amputation of limb, or contracture of > 50% of the normal ROM)

Sensory Grading

0 = Absent
1 = Altered, either decreased/impaired sensation or hypersensitivity
2 = Normal
NT = Not testable

When to Test Non-Key Muscles:

In a patient with an apparent AIS B classification, non-key muscle functions more than 3 levels below the motor level on each side should be tested to most accurately classify the injury (differentiate between AIS B and C).

Movement	Root level
Shoulder: Flexion, extension, abduction, adduction, internal and external rotation **Elbow:** Supination	**C5**
Elbow: Pronation **Wrist:** Flexion	**C6**
Finger: Flexion at proximal joint, extension. **Thumb:** Flexion, extension and abduction in plane of thumb	**C7**
Finger: Flexion at MCP joint **Thumb:** Opposition, adduction and abduction perpendicular to palm	**C8**
Finger: Abduction of the index finger	**T1**
Hip: Adduction	**L2**
Hip: External rotation	**L3**
Hip: Extension, abduction, internal rotation **Knee:** Flexion **Ankle:** Inversion and eversion **Toe:** MP and IP extension	**L4**
Hallux and Toe: DIP and PIP flexion and abduction	**L5**
Hallux: Adduction	**S1**

ASIA Impairment Scale (AIS)

A = Complete. No sensory or motor function is preserved in the sacral segments S4-5.

B = Sensory Incomplete. Sensory but not motor function is preserved below the neurological level and includes the sacral segments S4-5 (light touch or pin prick at S4-5 or deep anal pressure) AND no motor function is preserved more than three levels below the motor level on either side of the body.

C = Motor Incomplete. Motor function is preserved at the most caudal sacral segments for voluntary anal contraction (VAC) OR the patient meets the criteria for sensory incomplete status (sensory function preserved at the most caudal sacral segments (S4-S5) by LT, PP or DAP), and has some sparing of motor function more than three levels below the ipsilateral motor level on either side of the body.
(This includes key or non-key muscle functions to determine motor incomplete status.) For AIS C – less than half of key muscle functions below the single NLI have a muscle grade ≥ 3.

D = Motor Incomplete. Motor incomplete status as defined above, with at least half (half or more) of key muscle functions below the single NLI having a muscle grade ≥ 3.

E = Normal. If sensation and motor function as tested with the ISNCSCI are graded as normal in all segments, and the patient had prior deficits, then the AIS grade is E. Someone without an initial SCI does not receive an AIS grade.

Using ND: To document the sensory, motor and NLI levels, the ASIA Impairment Scale grade, and/or the zone of partial preservation (ZPP) when they are unable to be determined based on the examination results.

AMERICAN SPINAL INJURY ASSOCIATION

INTERNATIONAL STANDARDS FOR NEUROLOGICAL CLASSIFICATION OF SPINAL CORD INJURY

ISCOS
INTERNATIONAL SPINAL CORD SOCIETY

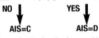

Steps in Classification

The following order is recommended for determining the classification of individuals with SCI.

1. Determine sensory levels for right and left sides.
The sensory level is the most caudal, intact dermatome for both pin prick and light touch sensation.

2. Determine motor levels for right and left sides.
Defined by the lowest key muscle function that has a grade of at least 3 (on supine testing), providing the key muscle functions represented by segments above that level are judged to be intact (graded as a 5).
Note: in regions where there is no myotome to test, the motor level is presumed to be the same as the sensory level, if testable motor function above that level is also normal.

3. Determine the neurological level of injury (NLI)
This refers to the most caudal segment of the cord with intact sensation and antigravity (3 or more) muscle function strength, provided that there is normal (intact) sensory and motor function rostrally respectively.
The NLI is the most cephalad of the sensory and motor levels determined in steps 1 and 2.

4. Determine whether the injury is Complete or Incomplete.
(i.e. absence or presence of sacral sparing)
*If voluntary anal contraction = **No** AND all S4-5 sensory scores = **0** AND deep anal pressure = **No**, then injury is **Complete**.*
*Otherwise, injury is **Incomplete**.*

5. Determine ASIA Impairment Scale (AIS) Grade:

Is injury Complete? **If YES, AIS=A** and can record ZPP (lowest dermatome or myotome on each side with some preservation)

NO ↓

Is injury Motor Complete? **If YES, AIS=B**

NO ↓ (No=voluntary anal contraction OR motor function more than three levels below the motor level on a given side, if the patient has sensory incomplete classification)

Are at least half (half or more) of the key muscles below the neurological level of injury graded 3 or better?

NO ↓ **AIS=C**
YES ↓ **AIS=D**

If sensation and motor function is normal in all segments, AIS=E
Note: AIS E is used in follow-up testing when an individual with a documented SCI has recovered normal function. If at initial testing no deficits are found, the individual is neurologically intact; the ASIA Impairment Scale does not apply.

Figure 1 *(continued)* The American Spinal Injury Association Classification of Spinal Cord Injury and Impairment Scale. (Reproduced with permission from the American Spinal Injury Association: Standard Neurological Classification of Spinal Cord Injury. http://www.asia-spinalinjury.org.)

to further the development of primary and tertiary prevention strategies.

Throughout the developed world, motor vehicle crashes are the most important cause of SCIs (accounting for 36% to 60% of all SCIs), and they are followed in importance by falls (30%), violence (15%), and sports injuries (10%).[5,6] In Alabama and Mississippi, more injuries are caused by violence than by sports.[6] In Canada, the proportion of patients injured in a sport or fall is higher than in the United States, and the proportion attributed to violence is lower. This information has been used to plan primary SCI prevention programs. For example, a retrospective review of 10 years of data from an SCI unit in Spain reported a 54% reduction in motor vehicle crashes as a result of safety improvements in automobiles and on roadways, with a commensurate reduction in the incidence of motor vehicle–related SCIs.[4] Global data have, therefore, supported the belief that improvements in traffic safety measures have led to a reduction in motor vehicle–related SCI in developed countries.

Pathophysiology

Injury to the spinal cord occurs as a result of two distinct mechanisms: the initial direct physical or mechanical injury and the secondary physiologic injury. **Figure 3** summarizes the time course of initial and secondary damage after SCI and outlines the prevention and treatment strategies relevant to each stage. The initial damage is caused by a direct impact to or a mechanical disruption of the neuron cell body, axonal tract, supporting cells, and vasculature, and it occurs at the time of injury.

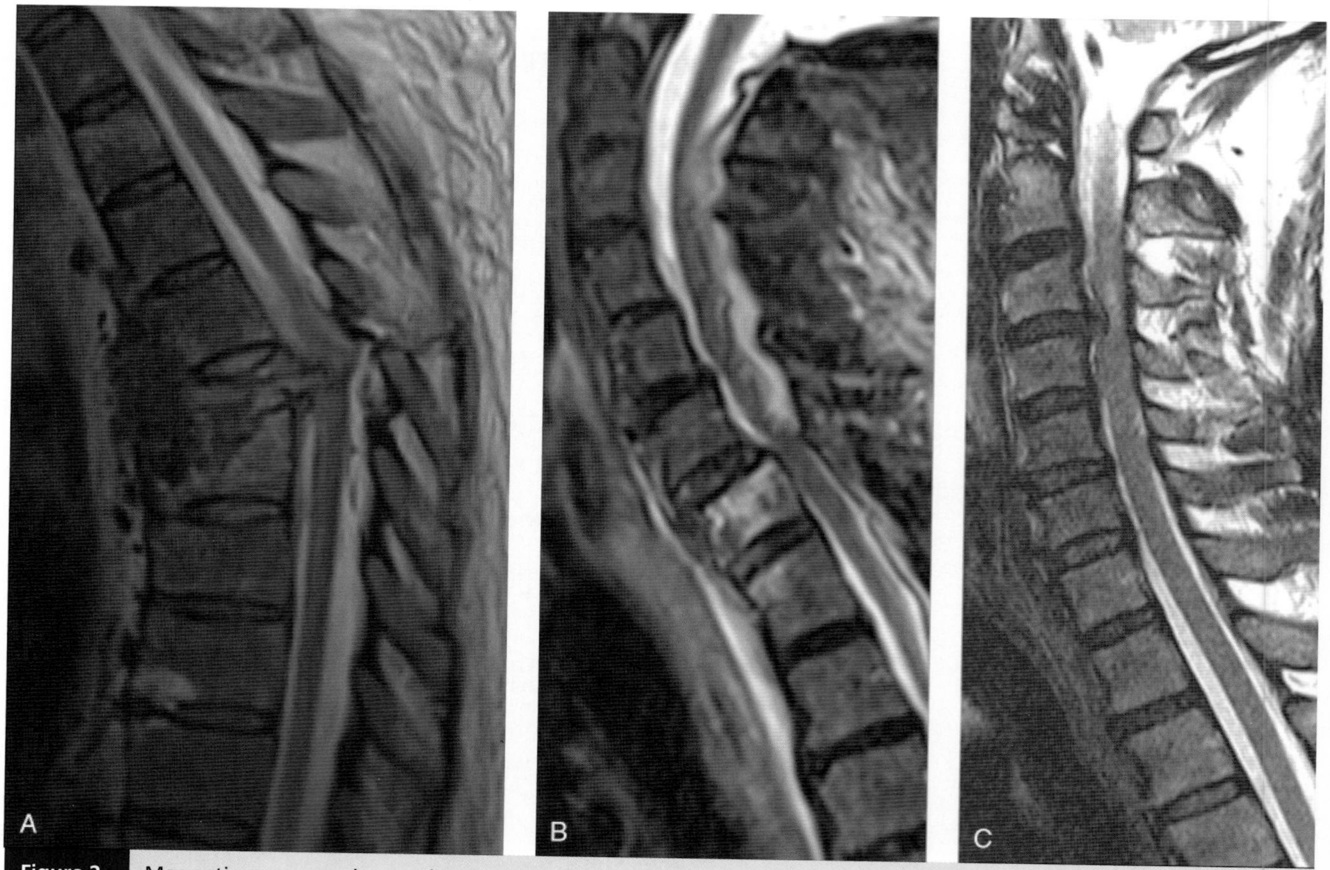

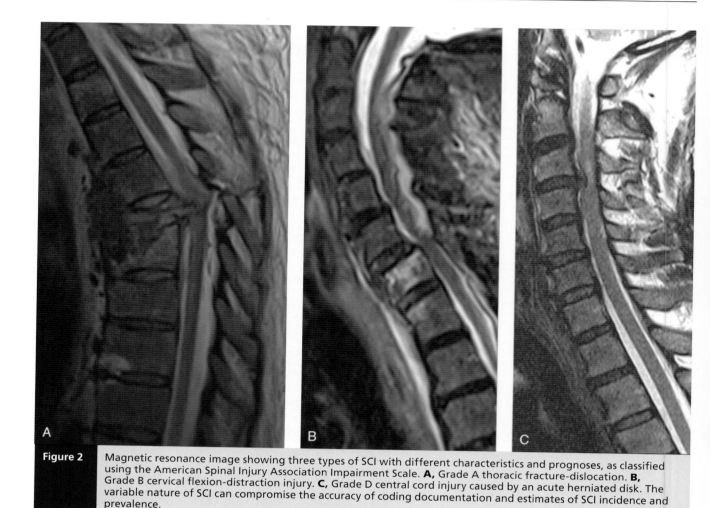

Figure 2 Magnetic resonance image showing three types of SCI with different characteristics and prognoses, as classified using the American Spinal Injury Association Impairment Scale. **A,** Grade A thoracic fracture-dislocation. **B,** Grade B cervical flexion-distraction injury. **C,** Grade D central cord injury caused by an acute herniated disk. The variable nature of SCI can compromise the accuracy of coding documentation and estimates of SCI incidence and prevalence.

Frank transection of the cord is rare. The concept of secondary damage in SCI initially was postulated in 1911 and has been elucidated with increasing sophistication since the 1970s.[10-12] The physiologic response to the initial injury causes secondary damage that involves a complex interaction of several factors: release of inflammatory mediators and endogenous opioids, activation of inflammatory cells, induction of oxidative free radicals, damage to axonal myelin sheaths, increase in vascular permeability and thrombosis, production of excitotoxic neurotransmitters, induction of cellular necrosis and apoptosis, and ingress and differentiation of regenerative cells.[12,13] Some of the most important factors in secondary damage represent a potential target for therapy to limit the extent of injury and promote neurologic recovery. Cellular and pharmacologic agents are currently under investigation for treating the physiologic mediators of damage in SCI.

Initial Evaluation

Since the Advanced Trauma Life Support (ATLS) protocol was developed by the American College of Surgeons in the late 1970s, the initial evaluation of injured patients has become standardized and efficient.[14] All patients who arrive in an emergency department with a high-energy injury or another injury resulting in neurologic impairment should be evaluated using the ATLS protocol. Airway function, breathing, and circulation always are secured first to limit life-threatening risks to the patient. Particular attention should be paid to identifying neurogenic shock, the hallmark of which is hypotension without tachycardia or even with frank bradycardia. (In contrast, the more common hypovolemic shock is marked by hypotension with reflexive tachycardia.) This physiologic response is caused by the loss of autonomic control after SCI and particularly from the loss of sympathetic control.

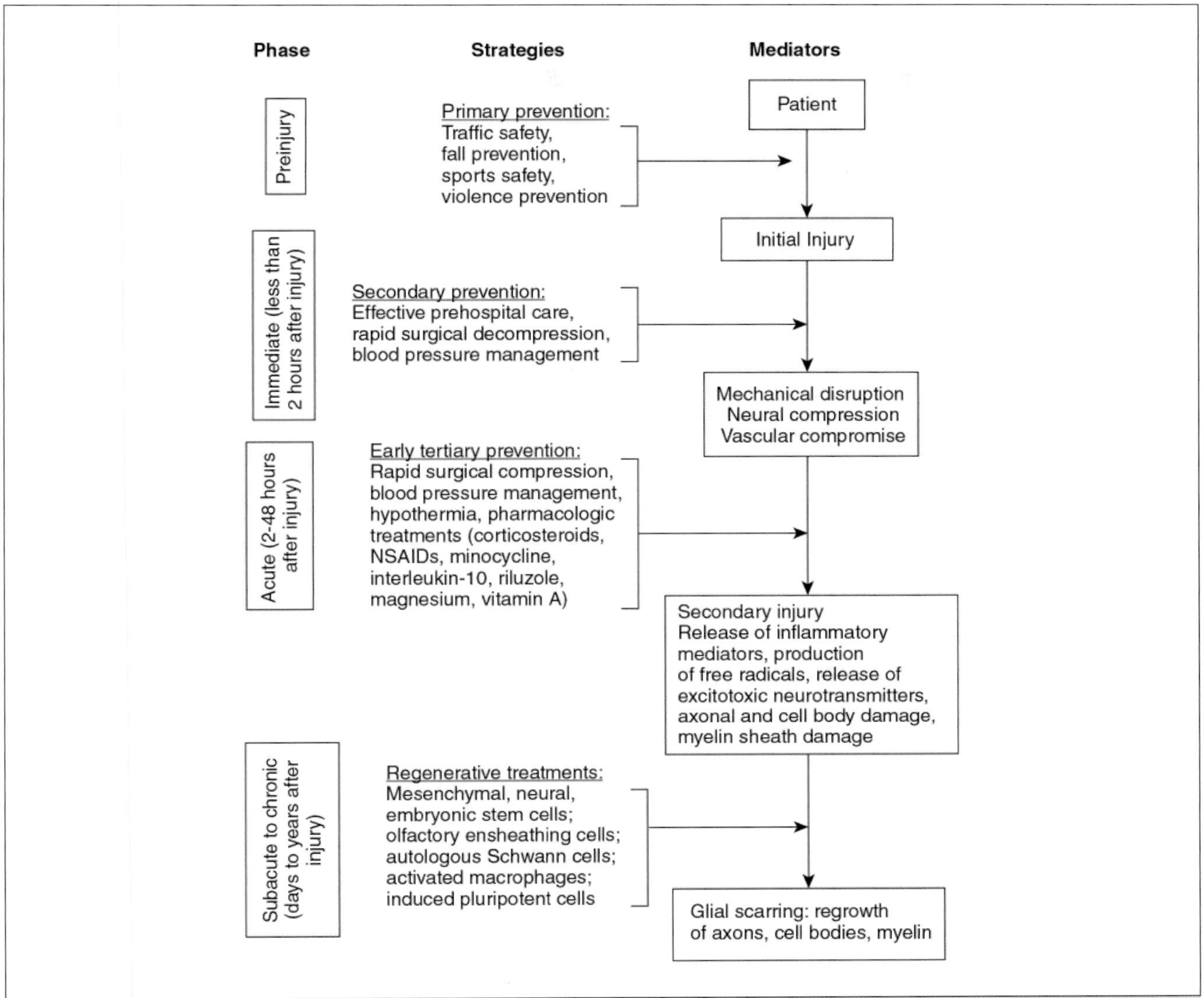

Figure 3 The phases and mediators of initial and secondary SCI, with their targeted prevention and treatment strategies. The factors contributing to impairment after SCI differ based on time from injury.

A mean arterial pressure higher than 85 mm Hg should be maintained to prevent further ischemia of the injured spinal cord.[15] Pressors may be required in addition to fluid resuscitation to maintain spinal cord perfusion.

A thorough neurologic examination (the ATLS disability evaluation) subsequently is done to assess the sensory and motor function of all key innervations of the cervical, thoracic, lumbar, and sacral nerve roots. Lower sacral innervation is evaluated by determining external anal sphincter tone and deep rectal sensation. Assessment of spinal reflex function includes evaluation of the deep tendon reflexes of the extremities, the Hoffman and Babinski signs, ankle clonus, and the bulbocavernosus reflex. The information is used to formulate an accurate neurologic description of the injury. The American Spinal Injury Association (ASIA) Impairment Scale provides an easily used, reproducible method of SCI assessment that can serve as a quantitative tool (as designed) or as a general guideline for SCI understanding and communication (**Figure 1**). Spinal shock, characterized by sensory and motor impairment with areflexia as well as the absence of the bulbocavernosus reflex, is common after SCI and should be specifically documented. Spinal shock can be compared with the loss of consciousness that can occur with head injury: although much of the brain is uninjured, the observable signs of diminished or absent function are more diffuse than is suggested by the actual injury. The return of the bulbocavernosus reflex heralds the resolution of spinal shock by indicating that the inherent function of the spinal cord is returning. The SCI can be fully assessed only after spinal shock has resolved. In a complete SCI, no motor or sensory function remains caudal to the level of the SCI, and sacral root function is absent. If any neural function is preserved caudal to the injury, it is classified as an incomplete SCI. The injury is further categorized into one of several patterns of injury, each of which has a typical propensity for recovery or maintenance of function.

One of the most important aspects of the initial treatment of SCI is prevention of iatrogenic injury to the already-compromised spinal cord. Every suspected spinal injury should be treated as unstable and immobilized until adequate information is available to allow unrestricted spinal motion. This principle is particularly important for the cervical spine, which is involved in approximately 60% of all SCIs.[6] Cervical immobilization is achieved with the use of a cervical collar. If the collar must be temporarily removed or changed, in-line stabilization of the head, neck, and shoulders should be done by one provider while the collar is manipulated by another. Traction should not be applied before the injury pattern is radiographically assessed. An atlanto-occipital dislocation or a C2 pars interarticularis fracture with disk disruption and angular displacement can be exacerbated by the application of traction. The thoracolumbar spine initially is immobilized by positioning the patient on a bed without an elevated head and moving the patient as infrequently as possible. The traditional logroll mobilization method, in which one provider supports the head, neck, and shoulder while two other providers simultaneously turn the trunk, pelvis, and legs, applies torsion to thoracolumbar fractures and can cause further displacement and neural compression.[16] Kinetic treatment beds and mattresses specially designed for transfer should be used whenever possible. Trendelenburg and reverse-Trendelenburg positioning of the bed are allowable as necessary for airway protection and perfusion.

A radiographic evaluation of the spine is the next critical step for understanding SCI. Plain radiography was used in the past for the initial evaluation of the injured spine, but multidetector spiral CT has been established as the optimal imaging study for identification of spinal injuries.[17,18] Axial acquisition images can be rapidly reconstructed in the sagittal and coronal planes to assess alignment as well as fracture and dislocation morphology. CT findings are essential to planning the definitive care of the injury. Particular attention must be paid to the vertebral body and posterior element fracture characteristics, dislocation or translation in the sagittal and coronal planes, and distraction across motion segments. MRI is useful for delineating soft-tissue injury to the disks and ligamentous structures, which is not evident on CT. MRI also allows an accurate assessment of the spinal cord, including differentiation of edema and hemorrhage. MRI is particularly useful for spine care providers who use the Thoracolumbar Injury Classification Score (TLICS) and Subaxial Injury Classification (SLIC) to determine whether surgical treatment is indicated.[19-21] These classification systems consider damage to ligamentous structures as independent factors in surgical planning; the TLICS requires evaluation for damage to the posterior ligamentous complex, and the SLIC requires the diskoligamentous complex to be evaluated.[19,20,21] MRI can reveal these injuries if CT findings are equivocal.

Definitive Treatment

The treatment of SCI has three overarching goals: physical decompression of the spinal cord to minimize the risk of irreversible primary neurologic injury; mechanical stabilization of the osteoligamentous injury to restore anatomic alignment and prevent posttraumatic deformity; and efficient, effective optimization of the local environment in preparation for the reparative or regenerative phase. Each of these three types of treatment should protect the fragile spinal cord and enhance the likelihood of functional recovery. Regaining even a single level of function has important implications for a patient's mobility and independence. For example, improving a patient's neurologic level from C3 to C4 can eliminate dependence on a respirator as diaphragm activity is gained. Improving the neurologic level to C7 can allow a patient to perform independent transfers and even to drive a car with modifications; these activities are impossible at a C6 neurologic level. Improvement from the L2 to the L4 level greatly increases a patient's ability to ambulate by restoring quadriceps, adductor, and anterior tibial muscular function.

Neurologic Stabilization

The neurologic stabilization phase of treatment should begin immediately upon the patient's arrival in the emergency department. The initial injury to the spinal cord disrupts or impairs perfusion of the cord. Mean arterial pressure higher than 85 mm Hg should be ensured to maintain the existing perfusion and prevent further cord ischemia, and aggressive management should continue until the patient can maintain perfusion without assistance.

Several physiologic changes that occur during the early phase of injury have been targeted for treatment to prevent further neurologic injury. An inflammatory response to injury begins rapidly, resulting in the release of early mediators of inflammation and the generation of free radicals. The most thoroughly evaluated molecular treatment of the inflammatory response is the use of corticosteroids, of which methylprednisolone sodium succinate (MPSS) has been the paradigm for SCI. Corticosteroids limit the release of inflammatory mediators, scavenge free radicals, and help maintain vascular integrity to prevent edema.[22] The outcomes of the three iterations of the North American Spinal Cord Injury Studies initially led to enthusiasm for the use of high-dosage MPSS during the early phase after SCI.[23] These studies recommended administration of a bolus of 30 mg/kg of MPSS over 1 hour, with an infusion of 5.4 mg/kg/h for the remainder of the first 24 hours if the infusion was started within 3 hours of injury, or for the remainder of the first 48 hours if the infusion was started 3 to 8 hours after injury. The initial statistical improvement was not found to lead to a dramatic clinical difference, however, and high-dosage MPSS was found to increase the risk of pneumonia, sepsis, pancreatitis, and death. Because the observed risks appear to outweigh any potential benefit of high-dosage MPSS, it has fallen out of favor, and the American Association of Neurologic Surgeons has recommended against its use.[24]

Several other modulators of inflammation have been considered for use during the early phase of SCI, including interleukin-10, minocycline, NSAIDs, and atorvastatin.[25-28] Each of these agents inhibits one or more components of the proinflammatory cascade. Initial preclinical results were positive but were not reproduced, and higher-level SCI model or clinical studies have not been completed. The NSAID dosages found necessary to achieve an effect are several times higher than the safe level for human use.

In addition to inflammation, the initial injury leads to supraphysiologic activation of glutamate receptors, which accentuates the release of sodium and calcium. Overactivation of this pathway, called excitotoxicity, induces neuronal death. The pathway was identified as a target for neuroprotective molecular therapy in SCI. Magnesium and riluzole, a sodium channel blocker approved for use in patients with amyotrophic lateral sclerosis, have received the most attention in this role.[29,30] The initial results of using riluzole and a polyethylene glycol formulation of magnesium in animal models led to the development of clinical studies currently in process.[12]

Mechanical Stabilization

The forces that produce SCI often render the spine mechanically unstable. A mechanically unstable spine cannot withstand physiologic forces without deforming or generating severe pain. Although this definition appears to imply that evaluation under physiologic loading is required to determine the stability of an injured spine, such a test would be unwise if spinal stability is even remotely in question. Radiographic parameters and static neurologic examination are the best methods of assessing spinal stability, and they have been codified into classification schemes that reproducibly predict whether a patient has an unstable spinal injury requiring surgery.[19-21] The TLICS and SLIC systems are used to rate the parameters of spinal stability that typically are considered in surgical planning for a thoracolumbar or cervical injury, respectively. In both systems, a score of 5 or higher implies that surgical stabilization is necessary. The details of the stabilization are left to the discretion of the surgeon, and the choice should be based on biomechanical factors, the fracture or dislocation anatomy including the presence of epidural hematoma or bone in the spinal canal, and the best available evidence to support the choice of technique.

The timing of surgical intervention for mechanical stabilization is controversial because of conflicting reports on the impact of early and late surgical decompression and fusion. In addition, there is a lack of consensus as to what exactly constitutes early surgery. Proponents of early surgery argue that continuing, prolonged pressure on the spinal cord leads to further injury as edema increases and the cord swells in an already-constricted enclosure.[31,32] Others assert that early intervention is unnecessary or even detrimental because of the particular susceptibility of an edematous spinal cord to iatrogenic injury as well as the risk that hypotension during general anesthesia will increase the ischemia of the fragile spinal cord.[33,34] The empirical evidence is contradictory. A 1997 comparison of the neurologic outcomes of patients treated within 72 hours of injury or after 5 days found no between-group difference in ASIA grade, but a meta-analysis of several reports concluded that surgery within 24 hours of injury is feasible and yielded better outcomes than later surgery.[33,35] The best evidence was from the Surgical Timing in Acute Spinal Cord Injury Study, an international, multicenter prospective study that reported that patients treated with surgical decompression and stabilization within 24 hours of injury were more likely than patients treated later to have improvement of two or more points on the ASIA Impairment Scale.[36] The methodology of this study was criticized because of variations in the manner in which patients were assigned to early or late groups (based on time to presentation to the treating surgeon, time to radiographic evaluation, or surgeon discretion). The report discusses the ethical and practical challenges of imposing a scientifically rigorous method such as randomization.

Regenerative Medicine

The final and perhaps most unpredictable aspect of SCI treatment is the establishment of an optimal environment for healing and regeneration of neural tissue. Damage to neural tissue in the central nervous system initiates physiologic and mechanical responses that remove cellular, axonal, and myelin debris. In the wake of debris removal comes a proliferation of reparative glial cells and neurite budding, the intention of which is to restore neural pathway continuity and support. The contradictory effects of molecules that promote or inhibit neural budding or guide or inhibit axonal regeneration creates a poorly coordinated effort that results in a glial scar and lack of meaningful neural regeneration. Several specific mediators of this process have been identified, studied, and proposed as targets of treatment. The best understood is neurite outgrowth inhibitor A (Nogo-A), a myelin-associated membrane protein that binds the neural membrane and arrests growth.[37] The interaction of Nogo-A and its receptor was found to induce the inhibitory effect through the Rho signal transduction pathway.[38] These findings led to the development of an anti–Nogo-A antibody, a Nogo receptor antagonist called NEP1-40 , and a Rho antagonist called BA-210 (Cethrin, BioAxone BioSciences).[39-41] The purpose of each of these agents is to reverse the inhibitory effect of Nogo-A binding and terminate the progress of a regenerating axon. Clinical studies of the anti–Nogo-A antibody are under way. Preclinical results of using NEP1-40 and BA-210 were encouraging but did not lead to significant clinical studies; the initially promising results of NEP1-40 use were not reproduced, and further study of BA-210 was not sufficiently funded. There also is interest in neurotrophic factors capable of inducing growth and guiding the budding axon; among these are brain-derived neurotrophic factor, nerve growth factor, and vascular endothelial growth factor. Several preclinical and clinical studies are under way, but no results are available to guide major changes in clinical practice.[12]

Cellular therapy has been explored for optimization of neural regrowth and support. Cellular therapy includes implantation of cells intended to generate new neural growth, permit and support neural growth, or assist in debris removal and pathway repair.[12] Neural stem cells, mesenchymal stem cells, embryonic stem cells, and induced pluripotent cells have been evaluated for generation of new neural growth.[42-45] Promising studies are under way for the use of each of these cell types. Neural and mesenchymal stem cells must be isolated from the tissue of a patient with SCI and grown in tissue culture before being implanted into the injured spinal cord. The use of embryonic stem cells presents ethical concerns as well as concern that undifferentiated cells might produce teratomas at the site of implantation. The use of induced pluripotent cells requires initial dedifferentiation from their committed cell line back into pluripotent cells. A general drawback of each of these cell types is their failure to naturally differentiate into neural cell lines in vivo. For this reason, many investigators have predifferentiated the pluripotent cells into neural lineages before implanting them at the injury site.

A second method of cellular therapy involves manipulating the environment of the regenerating axon to direct growth toward a target. Two cell lines have been explored for this purpose: Schwann cells produce the supportive myelin of the peripheral nervous system, and olfactory ensheathing cells provide the permissive link between the olfactory receptors of the peripheral nervous system and the olfactory nerve of the central nervous system.[12] Cells of both types are readily harvested from peripheral sites, grown in tissue culture, and reimplanted. Preclinical and clinical studies have had mixed results; the cells often have not had the intended effect of axonal bud guidance. Clinical studies of both Schwann cells and olfactory ensheathing cells are under way.

Activated macrophages represent another cell line that has been used in the treatment of SCI. Appropriately activated macrophages were found to attenuate the negative physiologic effects that follow injury and improve neurologic function in both preclinical and human clinical studies.[12,46] The initial clinical results led to proposals for larger studies that were terminated because of insufficient funding.[12]

Summary

The simplicity and inclusivity of the term spinal cord injury, like the term cancer, belies the complex nature and variability of the condition. A rapid assessment of a patient's objective neurologic deficit and mechanical spinal injury should be done before planning the initial and definitive management of SCI. Early neurologic decompression and mechanical stabilization appear to promote a better environment for neurologic stabilization and improvement than delayed treatment. Several physiologic factors have been identified as contributing to inhibition or promotion of neural regeneration, and they have been targeted for the development of therapeutic interventions. It is clear that a thorough understanding of each factor does not necessarily lead to an understanding of the way in which changes to one variable affect others or improve the overall outcome. Only further study of the nature, timing, control, and interdependence of each variable contributing to SCI can lead to a cure.

Key Study Points

- The United States has the highest known incidence and prevalence of SCI.
- Secondary damage in SCI is caused by several physiologic factors, each of which has been targeted for treatment. Interleukin-10, minocycline, NSAIDs, atorvastatin, riluzole, magnesium, Nogo-A inhibitors, and Rho antagonists have shown promise in preclinical studies.
- Surgical intervention within 24 hours of injury appears to provide the best environment for neural protection and recovery of function.
- Stem cell and pluripotent cell technologies are under evaluation for use in neural and myelin regeneration.

Annotated References

1. Mahmoudi E, Meade MA, Forchheimer MB, Fyffe DC, Krause JS, Tate D: Longitudinal analysis of hospitalization after spinal cord injury: Variation based on race and ethnicity. *Arch Phys Med Rehabil* 2014;95(11):2158-2166.

   The authors utilized the Spinal Cord Injury Model Systems database to follow patients with SCI for 10 years after injury to evaluate the incidence of rehospitalization. Patients identified as African American tended to have the most days of hospitalization and patients identified as Hispanic of having the fewest.

2. Klaas SJ: Avoiding injury. *Nature* 2013;503(7475):S18.

   Current SCI epidemiology is summarized. The author concludes that measures to prevent SCI should include avoidance of cellular phone use while driving and installation of assistance devices in the homes of elderly individuals to help prevent falls.

3. Lifshutz J, Colohan A: A brief history of therapy for traumatic spinal cord injury. *Neurosurg Focus* 2004;16(1):E5.

4. Sebastià-Alcácer V, Alcanyis-Alberola M, Giner-Pascual M, Gomez-Pajares F: Are the characteristics of the patient with a spinal cord injury changing? *Spinal Cord* 2014;52(1):29-33.

   This is a retrospective review of 10 years of data from one SCI unit in Spain. During the time, traffic accidents decreased by 54% as a result of improved traffic safety measures. The incidence of traffic accident related SCI decreased by a commensurate 59%.

5. Lee BB, Cripps RA, Fitzharris M, Wing PC: The global map for traumatic spinal cord injury epidemiology: Update 2011. Global incidence rate. *Spinal Cord* 2014;52(2):110-116.

   The authors report that the incidence of traumatic SCI is highest in North America but is rising in developing countries as a result of increased motor vehicle travel. The incidence by specific cause of SCI is reported for each global region.

6. Singh A, Tetreault L, Kalsi-Ryan S, Nouri A, Fehlings MG: Global prevalence and incidence of traumatic spinal cord injury. *Clin Epidemiol* 2014;6:309-331.

   The incidence and prevalence of SCI have remained nearly unchanged since prior epidemiologic reports. Substantial variation is observed in the cause of SCI between regions of the world and within countries.

7. Spinal cord injury facts and figures at a glance. *J Spinal Cord Med* 2014;37(5):659-660.

   The National Spinal Cord Statistical Center periodically reports statistical observations from the National SCI Database, which represents 13% of all new SCIs in the United States as reported through the SCI Model Systems.

8. Kraus JF, Franti CE, Riggins RS, Richards D, Borhani NO: Incidence of traumatic spinal cord lesions. *J Chronic Dis* 1975;28(9):471-492.

9. Hanigan WC, Shoffer C. Nelson's wound: Treatment of spinal cord injury in the 19th and early 20th century military conflicts. *Neurosurg Focus* 2004;16(1):E4.

10. Allen AR: Surgery of experimental lesions of spinal cord equivalent to crush injury of fracture dislocation of spinal column: A preliminary report. *JAMA* 1911;57:878-880.

11. Tator CH, Fehlings MG: Review of the secondary injury theory of acute spinal cord trauma with emphasis on vascular mechanisms. *J Neurosurg* 1991;75(1):15-26.

12. Silva NA, Sousa N, Reis RL, Salgado AJ: From basics to clinical: A comprehensive review on spinal cord injury. *Prog Neurobiol* 2014;114:25-57.

    The authors provide a thorough review and exhaustive bibliography of the pathophysiology of SCI and all treatment methods currently in practice or under study.

13. Hawryluk GW, Rowland J, Kwon BK, Fehlings MG: Protection and repair of the injured spinal cord: A review of completed, ongoing, and planned clinical trials for acute spinal cord injury. *Neurosurg Focus* 2008;25(5):E14.

14. American College of Surgeons Committee on Trauma: *Advanced trauma life support program for doctors* ,ed 9. Chicago, IL, American College of Surgeons, 2012.

    The American College of Surgeons developed the Advanced Trauma Life Support curriculum to standardize the evaluation and initial treatment of all patients admitted to an emergency department following traumatic injury.

15 Vale FL, Burns J, Jackson AB, Hadley MN: Combined medical and surgical treatment after acute spinal cord injury: Results of a prospective pilot study to assess the

merits of aggressive medical resuscitation and blood pressure management. *J Neurosurg* 1997;87(2):239-246.

16. Conrad BP, Rossi GD, Horodyski MB, Prasarn ML, Alemi Y, Rechtine GR: Eliminating log rolling as a spine trauma order. *Surg Neurol Int* 2012;3(Suppl 3):S188-S197.

    A thorough review of transfer methods for patients with spinal injury describes the inadequacy of the logroll technique. The use of a mattress designed for transfer is a safer technique. The best use of the logroll technique is for an injured patient who is prone in the field and must be transferred to a stretcher in the supine position.

17. Como JJ, Diaz JJ, Dunham CM, et al: Practice management guidelines for identification of cervical spine injuries following trauma: Update from the Eastern Association for the Surgery of Trauma Practice Management guidelines committee. *J Trauma* 2009;67(3):651-659.

18. Brown CV, Antevil JL, Sise MJ, Sack DI: Spiral computed tomography for the diagnosis of cervical, thoracic, and lumbar spine fractures: Its time has come. *J Trauma* 2005;58(5):890-895, discussion 895-896.

19. Vaccaro AR, Hulbert RJ, Patel AA, et al; Spine Trauma Study Group: The subaxial cervical spine injury classification system: A novel approach to recognize the importance of morphology, neurology, and integrity of the disco-ligamentous complex. *Spine (Phila Pa 1976)* 2007;32(21):2365-2374.

20. van Middendorp JJ, Audigé L, Bartels RH, et al: The subaxial cervical spine injury classification system: An external agreement validation study. *Spine J* 2013;13(9):1055-1063.

    The Subaxial Cervical Spine Classification System was developed to assist healthcare providers with decisions to perform surgery for cervical spine injury. Similar to the Thoracolumbar Injury Classification System, the system considers bony injury, neurologic injury, and ligamentous disruption.

21. Harrop JS, Vaccaro AR, Hurlbert RJ, et al; Spine Trauma Study Group: Intrarater and interrater reliability and validity in the assessment of the mechanism of injury and integrity of the posterior ligamentous complex: A novel injury severity scoring system for thoracolumbar injuries. *J Neurosurg Spine* 2006;4(2):118-122.

22. Hall ED, Braughler JM: Effects of intravenous methylprednisolone on spinal cord peroxidation and (Na+ + K+)-ATPase activity: Dose-response analysis during 1st hour after contusion injury in the cat. *J Neurosurg* 1982;57:247-253.

23. Bracken MB, Shepard MJ, Holford TR, et al: Administration of methylprednisolone for 24 or 48 hours or tirilazad mesylate for 48 hours in the treatment of acute spinal cord injury: Results of the Third National Acute Spinal Cord Injury Randomized Controlled Trial. National Acute Spinal Cord Injury Study. *JAMA* 1997;277(20):1597-1604.

24. Hadley MN, Walters BC, Grabb PA, et al: Guidelines for the management of acute cervical spine and spinal cord injuries. *Clin Neurosurg* 2002;49:407-498.

25. Bethea JR, Nagashima H, Acosta MC, et al: Systemically administered interleukin-10 reduces tumor necrosis factor-alpha production and significantly improves functional recovery following traumatic spinal cord injury in rats. *J Neurotrauma* 1999;16(10):851-863.

26. Heo K, Cho YJ, Cho KJ, et al: Minocycline inhibits caspase-dependent and independent cell death pathways and is neuroprotective against hippocampal damage after treatment with kainic acid in mice. *Neurosci Lett* 2006;398(3):195-200.

27. Kwon BK, Okon E, Hillyer J, et al: A systematic review of non-invasive pharmacologic neuroprotective treatments for acute spinal cord injury. *J Neurotrauma* 2011;28(8):1545-1588.

    The authors review pharmacologic agents for which success has been reported in preclinical trials in SCI with an emphasis on agents currently approved for use in unrelated conditions in humans.

28. Mann CM, Lee JH, Hillyer J, Stammers AM, Tetzlaff W, Kwon BK: Lack of robust neurologic benefits with simvastatin or atorvastatin treatment after acute thoracic spinal cord contusion injury. *Exp Neurol* 2010;221(2):285-295.

    The class of pharmacologic agents known as statins has been proposed for neuroprotection in acute SCI treatment. The anti-inflammatory effects seen in initial experiments could not be produced and neuroprotective effects were not observed.

29. Schwartz G, Fehlings MG: Evaluation of the neuroprotective effects of sodium channel blockers after spinal cord injury: Improved behavioral and neuroanatomical recovery with riluzole. *J Neurosurg* 2001;94(2, Suppl):245-256.

30. Wiseman DB, Dailey AT, Lundin D, et al: Magnesium efficacy in a rat spinal cord injury model. *J Neurosurg Spine* 2009;10(4):308-314.

31. Fehlings MG, Perrin RG: The timing of surgical intervention in the treatment of spinal cord injury: A systematic review of recent clinical evidence. *Spine (Phila Pa 1976)* 2006;31(11, Suppl):S28-S35, discussion S36.

32. Papadopoulos SM, Selden NR, Quint DJ, Patel N, Gillespie B, Grube S: Immediate spinal cord decompression for cervical spinal cord injury: Feasibility and outcome. *J Trauma* 2002;52(2):323-332.

33. Vaccaro AR, Daugherty RJ, Sheehan TP, et al: Neurologic outcome of early versus late surgery for cervical spinal cord injury. *Spine (Phila Pa 1976)* 1997;22(22):2609-2613.

34. Kwon BK, Curt A, Belanger LM, et al: Intrathecal pressure monitoring and cerebrospinal fluid drainage in acute

spinal cord injury: A prospective randomized trial. *J Neurosurg Spine* 2009;10(3):181-193.

35. La Rosa G, Conti A, Cardali S, Cacciola F, Tomasello F: Does early decompression improve neurological outcome of spinal cord injured patients? Appraisal of the literature using a meta-analytical approach. *Spinal Cord* 2004;42(9):503-512.

36. Fehlings MG, Vaccaro A, Wilson JR, et al: Early versus delayed decompression for traumatic cervical spinal cord injury: Results of the Surgical Timing in Acute Spinal Cord Injury Study (STASCIS). *PLoS One* 2012;7(2):e32037.

    This study represents the best current evidence that early decompression of spinal cord compression in SCI yields better neurologic function than delayed decompression. A prospective nonrandomized study found a higher likelihood of improving two or more points on the ASIA Impairment Scale when surgery was done within 24 hours of injury.

37. GrandPré T, Nakamura F, Vartanian T, Strittmatter SM: Identification of the Nogo inhibitor of axon regeneration as a Reticulon protein. *Nature* 2000;403(6768):439-444.

38. McKerracher L, Winton MJ: Nogo on the go. *Neuron* 2002;36(3):345-348.

39. Fouad K, Klusman I, Schwab ME: Regenerating corticospinal fibers in the Marmoset (Callitrix jacchus) after spinal cord lesion and treatment with the anti-Nogo-A antibody IN-1. *Eur J Neurosci* 2004;20(9):2479-2482.

40. GrandPré T, Li S, Strittmatter SM: Nogo-66 receptor antagonist peptide promotes axonal regeneration. *Nature* 2002;417(6888):547-551.

41. Fehlings MG, Theodore N, Harrop J, et al: A phase I/IIa clinical trial of a recombinant Rho protein antagonist in acute spinal cord injury. *J Neurotrauma* 2011;28(5):787-796.

    The Rho antagonist, BA-210, has been found to reverse the deleterious effects of Nogo-A on neurite grown in preclinical trials. When treated with 3 mg of BA-210, 66% of patients with cervical SCI converted from ASIA A to ASIA C or D, suggesting that the agent may improve neurologic outcomes of SCI.

42. Lepore AC, Fischer I: Lineage-restricted neural precursors survive, migrate, and differentiate following transplantation into the injured adult spinal cord. *Exp Neurol* 2005;194(1):230-242.

43. Tetzlaff W, Okon EB, Karimi-Abdolrezaee S, et al: A systematic review of cellular transplantation therapies for spinal cord injury. *J Neurotrauma* 2011;28(8):1611-1682.

    Current understanding of cellular treatment for SCI is reviewed, including Schwann cells, olfactory ensheathing cells, stem cells, and bone-marrow stromal cells.

44. Hendricks WA, Pak ES, Owensby JP, et al: Predifferentiated embryonic stem cells prevent chronic pain behaviors and restore sensory function following spinal cord injury in mice. *Mol Med* 2006;12(1-3):34-46.

45. Takahashi K, Yamanaka S: Induction of pluripotent stem cells from mouse embryonic and adult fibroblast cultures by defined factors. *Cell* 2006;126(4):663-676.

46. Knoller N, Aurbach G, Fulga V, et al: Clinical experience using incubated autologous macrophages as a treatment for complete spinal cord injury: Phase I study results. *J Neurosurg* 2005;3(3):173-81.

Chapter 34

Acute Cervical Spine Injuries: Initial Evaluation, Clearance, and Management

Gregory D. Schroeder, MD   Jeffrey A. Rihn, MD

Abstract

All patients who sustain blunt trauma should be treated as if they have an unstable cervical spine until a spine injury is ruled out, because these injuries occur in approximately 2.4% of all blunt trauma patients. Spine precautions, including immobilization in a cervical collar and on a rigid backboard, should be used. After a patient has reached the emergency department, many trauma centers in the United States use CT to evaluate for a cervical spine injury. Expeditiously identifying these injuries is critical, because a missed injury may lead to devastating consequences. Furthermore, high-level evidence shows that early decompression leads to improved long-term neurologic outcomes.

Keywords: cervical spine injury; acute spinal cord injury; subaxial cervical spine fracture; geriatric odontoid fracture

Introduction

Cervical spine injuries are relatively common, occurring in approximately 2.4% of all patients with blunt trauma and in 24% of all fatal motor vehicle accidents. Most commonly, these injuries occur in the subaxial spine (C3-C7), and injuries to this region account for between 66% and 75% of all injuries. They are typically the result of a high-energy mechanism. Upper cervical spine injuries account for 70% of all cervical spine injuries in patients older than 60 years.[1] Unstable cervical spine fractures may develop from relatively minor trauma in patients with spondyloarthropathies such as ankylosing spondylitis or diffuse idiopathic skeletal hyperostosis and in geriatric patients. The early diagnosis and treatment of cervical spine trauma are paramount, because the failure to identify an unstable fracture in a neurologically intact patient can lead to a devastating neurologic injury. Early decompression increases the rate of neurologic recovery in patients with acute spinal cord injuries (SCIs).[2] It is important to identify key principles in the treatment of common cervical spine injuries, including timing of surgery, the treatment of geriatric odontoid fractures, and subaxial fracture classification systems.

Dr. Schroeder or an immediate family member has received nonincome support (such as equipment or services), commercially derived honoraria, or other non–research-related funding (such as paid travel) from Medtronic and AOSpine. Dr. Rihn or an immediate family member serves as a paid consultant of DePuy and is a board member, owner, officer, or committee member of the North American Spine Society.

Initial Management

Evaluation

All patients with a possible cervical spine injury should be treated as if they have an unstable injury until proven otherwise. Spine precautions, including immobilization using a cervical collar and a rigid backboard, should be used. The Advanced Trauma Life Support (ATLS) protocol should be implemented, and a complete neurologic examination should be completed after these patients arrive at the emergency department. If the airway is compromised, a jaw thrust maneuver should be used for intubation rather than extending the neck. Maintaining proper spine precautions throughout the initial examination is critical, because poor immobilization techniques lead to a worsening neurologic deficit in up to 25% of patients with a spinal fracture.[3]

Although vigilance for cervical spine fracture is required, expeditious clearance of the cervical spine of patients who do not have a spinal injury is critical. The ATLS protocol recommends continued cervical immobilization until the patient is stabilized and a complete examination can be performed. Guidelines such as the National Emergency X-Radiography Utilization Study (NEXUS) Low-Risk Criteria (**Table 1**) and the Canadian C-Spine Rule for Radiography in Alert and Stable Trauma Patients have been validated for the safe identification of patients whose cervical spines can be cleared clinically without imaging studies.

A definitive imaging algorithm has yet to be established for patients whose cervical spine cannot be safely cleared clinically. Depending on the resources available, radiography, CT, and MRI all may be used. Although radiography is readily available and is low in cost, up to 20% of traumatic cervical spine injuries may be missed on radiographs alone, because the upper cervical spine and the cervicothoracic junction are difficult to assess with this modality.[4-6] Additionally, the benefit of lateral flexion and extension radiographs in the acute setting is limited, because voluntary guarding due to pain prevents adequate motion. Consequently, many trauma centers routinely use CT as the initial imaging modality in patients whose cervical spine cannot be cleared clinically. The routine use of MRI is controversial. A recently published prospective study on more than 800 awake and alert trauma patients reported that no additional clinically significant injuries were identified from the addition of a cervical MRI in blunt trauma patients.[7] Similarly, a study of more than 14,000 obtunded patients reported that a negative CT had a negative predictive value of 100% (95% CI 0.96-1.00) for detecting unstable cervical spine injuries.[8] Despite the fact that the best evidence available suggests that an MRI is not needed, some authors still believe that routine use of MRI in obtunded patients may reduce the risk of missing a discoligamentous injury. Prompt diagnosis can lead to expedited removal of the rigid cervical orthosis, thus minimizing the risk of collar-related complications, such as pressure ulcers.[9] Additionally, when an unstable fracture is identified, MRI often is needed for surgical planning. If a cervical spine fracture is identified, imaging of the entire spine should be performed, because the overall rate of noncontiguous spine fracture is 17% and has been reported to be as high as 50% in patients with a fracture to the posterior arch of C1.[10]

Acute Spinal Cord Injuries

Prompt recognition and treatment of an acute SCI is critical to the long-term neurologic recovery of the patient. The role of medical therapy in patients with an acute SCI is highly controversial.[11-13] Although the use of different neuroprotective medications is controversial, induced hypertension to ensure spinal cord perfusion commonly is used to decrease the effects of the secondary injury from an acute SCI; however, the literature to support this finding is limited to two case series. No definitive protocol for the exact target blood pressure or treatment duration has been accepted, but the mean arterial pressure routinely is kept above 85 to 90 mm Hg for 5 to 7 days. The only treatment to improve neurologic recovery that is supported by high-level evidence is early decompression of the neural elements.[2]

Table 1

National Emergency X-Radiography Utilization Study, Low-Risk Criteria Patients with suspected cervical spine trauma should undergo radiographic evaluation of the cervical spine unless all of the following five criteria are met.

No posterior midline cervical spine tenderness[a]
No evidence of intoxication[b]
A normal level of alertness[c]
No focal neurologic deficit[d]
No painful distracting injuries[e]

[a] Midline posterior bony cervical spine tenderness is present if the patient reports pain on palpation of the posterior midline neck from the nuchal ridge to the prominence of the first thoracic vertebra, or if the patient evinces pain with direct palpation of any cervical spinous process. [b]Patients should be considered intoxicated if they have either of the following criteria: 1) a recent history of intoxication or intoxicating ingestion provided by the patient or an observer or 2) evidence of intoxication such as an odor of alcohol, slurred speech, ataxia, dysmetria, or other cerebellar findings on physical examination or any behavior consistent with intoxication. Patients also may be considered to be intoxicated if tests of bodily secretions are positive for alcohol or drugs that affect the level of alertness. [c]An altered level of alertness can include any of the following measures: Glasgow Coma Scale score of 14 or less; disorientation to person, place, time, or events; inability to remember 3 objects at 5 minutes; delayed or inappropriate response to external stimuli; or other findings. [d]Defined as any focal neurologic finding on motor or sensory examination [e]No precise definition of a painful distracting injury is possible. The category includes any condition thought by the clinician to be producing pain sufficient to distract the patient from a second neck injury. Such injuries may include, but are not limited to, any long-bone fractures; a visceral injury requiring surgical consultation; a large laceration, degloving injury, or crush injury; large burns; or any other injury causing acute functional impairment. Physicians also may classify any injury as distracting if it is thought to potentially impair the patient's ability to appreciate other injuries.

(Reproduced with permission from Stell IG, Clement CM, McKnight RD, et al: The Canadian C-Spine Rule versus the Nexus Low-Risk Criteria in patients with trauma. *N Engl J Med* 2003;349:2510-2518.)

Upper Cervical Spine Trauma

The upper cervical spine is composed of the occiput to C2 and, unlike the lower cervical spine, the unique morphology of each component precludes a unified classification system. Although a detailed analysis of every possible upper cervical spine injury is beyond the scope of a single chapter, the goal of this section is to highlight the crucial points and new developments in the management of these injuries.

Occipitocervical Dissociation

Atlanto-occipital injuries are rare but devastating injuries that account for less than 1% of all cervical spine injuries. Approximately half of these injuries are fatal, and patients can present with brain stem and cranial nerve lesions as well as spinal cord and cervical root injuries.[14] Because the radiographic findings can be subtle and immediate recognition of this injury is critical, multiple radiographic measurements have been designed to identify this unstable injury. The Wackenheim line is a line drawn along the clivus. When extended, this line should be tangential to the tip of the dens. If it is not, an occipitocervical dissociation may be present. The Powers ratio and the Harris Rule of 12s (**Figure 1**) are two other radiographic methods commonly used to identify occipitocervical dissociations. The C0-C1 articulation should be studied carefully on reformatted CT images to ensure no subluxation of the joint, which may indicate an injury is present. Although multiple classifications of these injuries have been proposed, all injuries resulting in occipitocervical dissociation are unstable. Traction should be avoided, and the patient should undergo urgent surgical stabilization with a posterior occipitocervical fusion. If surgery cannot be performed promptly, the patient should be placed in a halo vest without distraction, and spine precautions should be maintained until surgical stabilization is achieved.

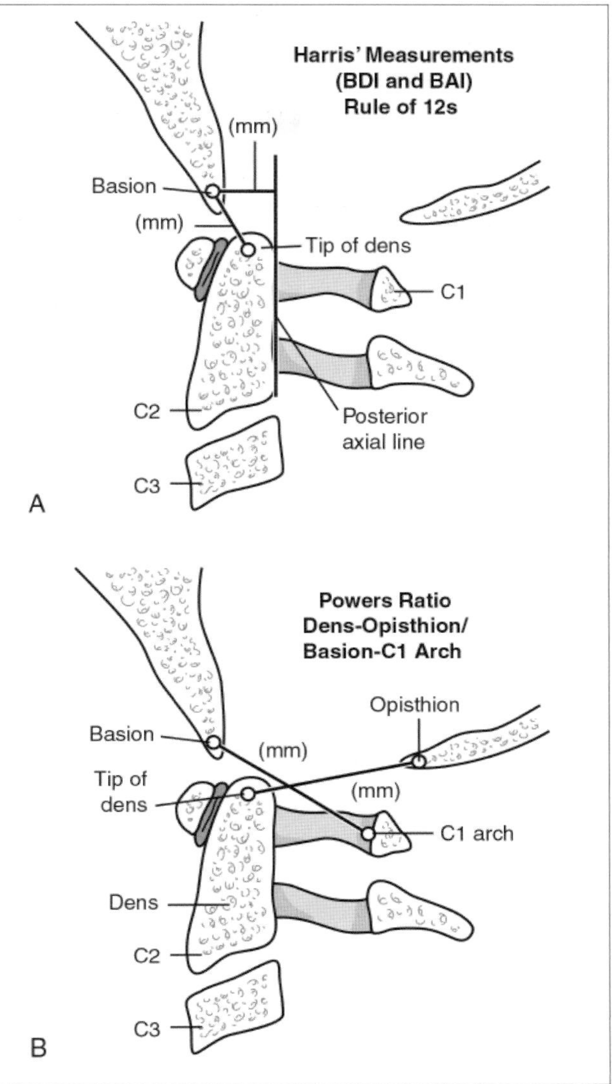

Figure 1 Drawings show two radiographic methods commonly used to identify occipitocervical dissociations. **A**, The measurements for the Harris Rule of 12s are shown. If either measurement is more than 12 mm, an occipitocervical dissociation may be present. **B**, The measurements for the Powers ratio are shown. This ratio represents the distance from the basion to the posterior arch divided by the distance from the anterior arch to the opisthion. If the ratio is greater than 1.0, anterior subluxation may be present. If it is less than 1.0, posterior subluxation may be present.

C1 Fractures

Fractures of the atlas account for approximately 25% of upper cervical fractures and are associated with a concomitant spine fracture in up to 50% of cases.[15-18] Because an injury to C1 usually results in increased space available for the cord, neurologic injury from these fractures is rare. These fractures are categorized into five types: posterior arch fractures, anterior arch fractures, Jefferson (burst) fractures, lateral mass fractures, and transverse process fractures. Stability of the fracture has been determined by the integrity of the transverse ligament. Historically, the combined measured C1 lateral mass overhang on the C2 superior articular process when measured on an open-mouth odontoid radiograph of more than 6.9 mm has been associated with a disrupted transverse ligament, but recent literature has found little correlation between lateral mass overhang and the integrity of the transverse ligament.[19] For this reason, the Dickman classification for transverse ligament disruption, which uses MRI to divide transverse ligament injuries into midsubstance disruptions of the transverse ligament (type 1) or avulsions of the transverse ligament (type 2), commonly is used. This distinction is critical, because patients with a type 1 transverse ligament injury, in which the transverse ligament will not heal, will benefit from early surgery, whereas those with a type 2 lesion, in which the injury often will heal, can be treated in a hard collar, even in cases in which the lateral mass overhang is greater than 6.9 mm. Last, special consideration is needed for patients with a unilateral sagittally oriented C1 fracture lateral to the TAL insertion, because these injuries place the patient at risk for continued displacement and the development of a late cock-robin deformity. For this reason, early surgical intervention also should be considered for patients with this fracture variant.[20]

Odontoid Fractures

Odontoid fractures constitute approximately 9% to 15% of cervical spine fractures in adults, but they are one of the most common types of geriatric spine fractures.[21] A bimodal distribution of odontoid fractures exists. Younger patients tend to sustain an odontoid fracture from a high-energy mechanism, whereas in older patients, a low-energy mechanism is common.

These fractures commonly are classified into one of three types using the Anderson and D'Alonzo classification (**Figure 2**). Type I and III fractures can be treated in a hard cervical orthosis,[21] with the exception of type III fractures having greater than 5 mm of distraction. Such fractures often are vertically unstable and require surgical stabilization.[22]

Comparatively, the treatment algorithm for type II fractures is controversial, requiring different variables to be considered. Because type II fractures in young patients are associated with a high-energy mechanism, this type of fracture often occurs in polytrauma patients. In such cases, the immediate stability afforded by anterior or posterior fixation often is warranted. In younger patients with an isolated type II fracture, the decision to operate commonly is based on risk factors for the development of a nonunion that are fracture specific and patient specific. Fractures with greater than 5 mm of displacement, more than 11° of angulation, or a fracture gap greater than 2 mm have an increased risk for failure to unite. Patients who smoke or are diabetic are also at increased risk for nonunion.

Surgical intervention should be considered for patients with one or more of these risk factors as well as for any patient with neurologic symptoms. Surgical treatment may consist of a posterior C1-C2 fusion or direct osteosynthesis through an anterior approach (**Figure 3**). Because of better bone quality and reduced risk of prolonged dysphagia in young patients, an anterior approach should be considered. The anterior approach can preserve the range of motion at the atlantoaxial joint and can avoid the risk of fracture displacement when positioning the patient prone. This is a technically demanding surgery and is not feasible in patients with barrel chests, comminuted fractures, or reverse oblique fractures in which the fracture is oriented in a way that prevents a screw from being placed perpendicular to the fracture. In young patients without neurologic deficit who have no risk factors for nonunion, treatment should consist of a halo vest or a hard cervical collar. Although the literature devoted specifically to young patients with no risk factors is limited, a systematic review found that the union rate of type II odontoid fractures treated nonsurgically is higher when a halo vest is used (hard collar, 51%; halo, 65%).[21] Given the substantial morbidity associated with a halo, however,

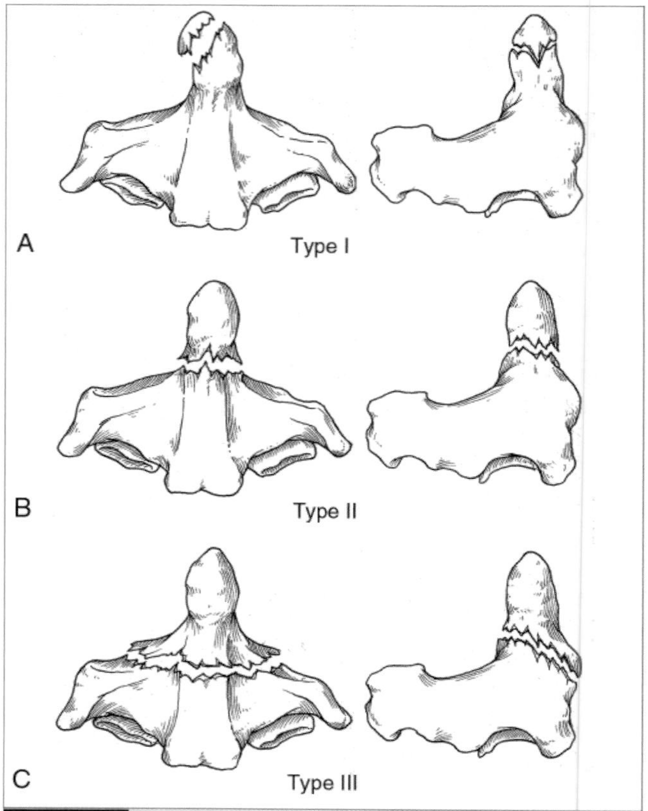

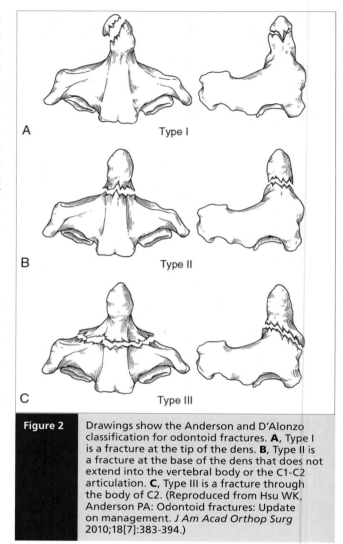

Figure 2 Drawings show the Anderson and D'Alonzo classification for odontoid fractures. **A**, Type I is a fracture at the tip of the dens. **B**, Type II is a fracture at the base of the dens that does not extend into the vertebral body or the C1-C2 articulation. **C**, Type III is a fracture through the body of C2. (Reproduced from Hsu WK, Anderson PA: Odontoid fractures: Update on management. *J Am Acad Orthop Surg* 2010;18[7]:383-394.)

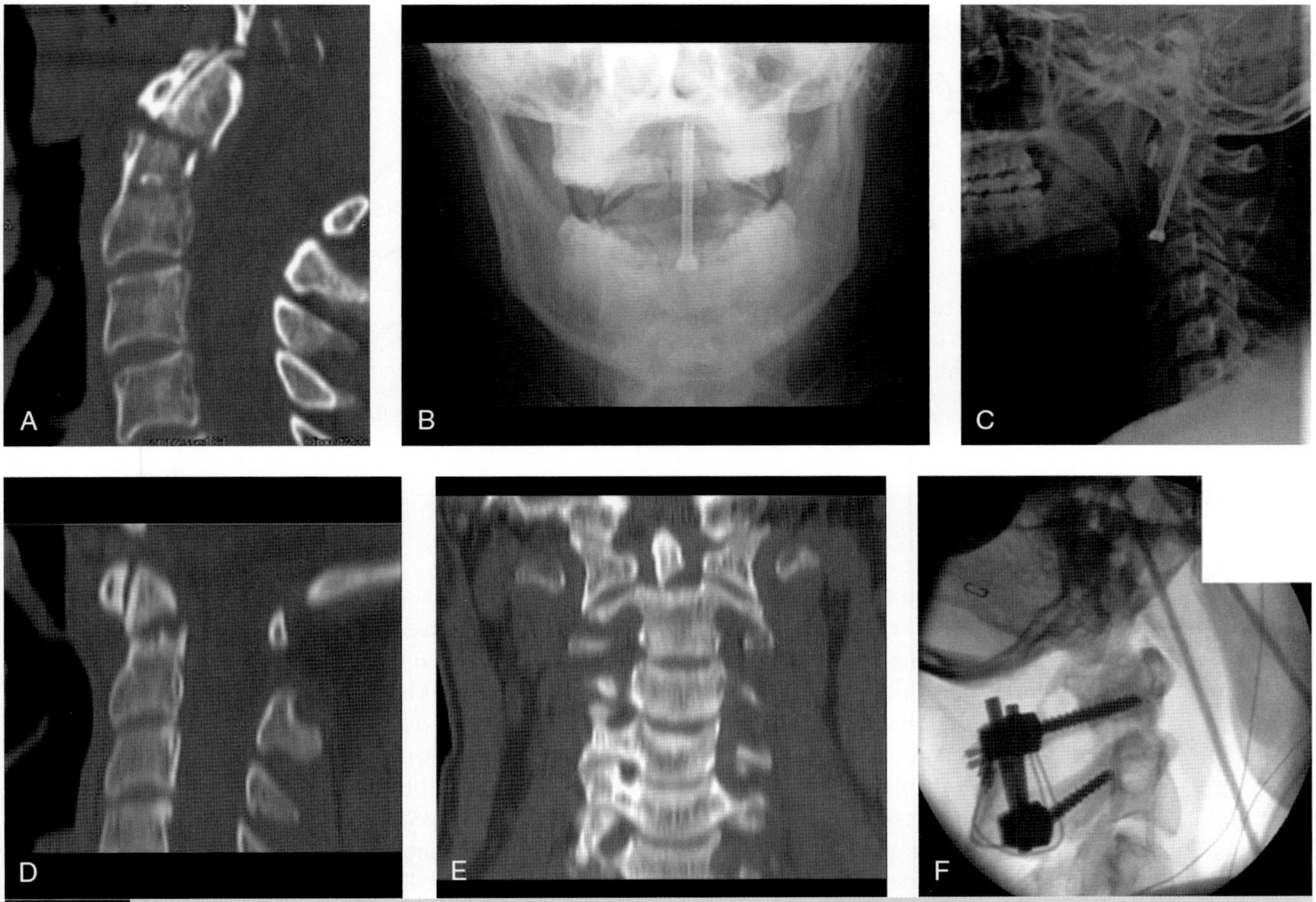

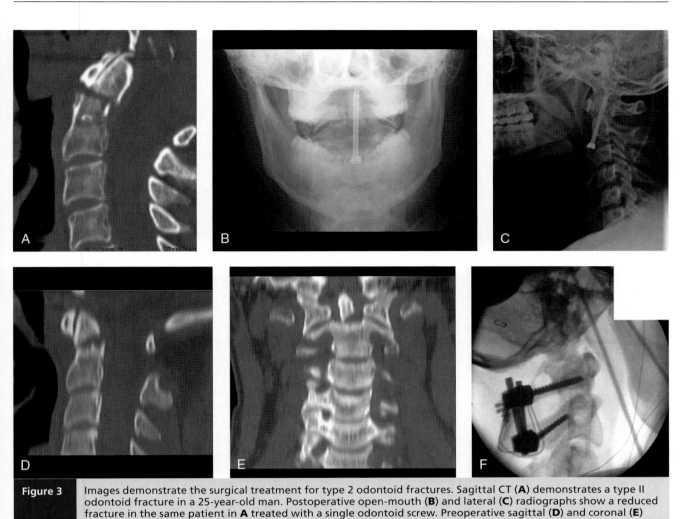

Figure 3 Images demonstrate the surgical treatment for type 2 odontoid fractures. Sagittal CT (**A**) demonstrates a type II odontoid fracture in a 25-year-old man. Postoperative open-mouth (**B**) and lateral (**C**) radiographs show a reduced fracture in the same patient in **A** treated with a single odontoid screw. Preoperative sagittal (**D**) and coronal (**E**) CT views show a type II odontoid fracture in a 70-year-old woman. Postoperative lateral radiograph (**F**) shows the same patient after treatment with a posterior C1-C2 fusion.

the treatment of these injuries often is individualized to the specific patient.

The treatment of type II odontoid fractures in elderly patients is challenging and has been the subject of several recent publications. The risk of nonunion has been reported to increase by as much as 21 times in patients older than 50 years treated nonsurgically. Furthermore, using a halo vest in elderly patients has been shown to increase the risk of complications and mortality. A 2013 retrospective study of type II odontoid fractures in 322 elderly patients demonstrated an increase in 30-day and overall mortality for patients treated nonsurgically.[23] Similarly, a prospective multicenter cohort study of 159 patients older than 65 years with a type II odontoid fracture found that patients who underwent surgery had significantly better scores on the Neck Disability Index and the subscale bodily pain component of the 36-Item Short Form Health Survey compared with the nonsurgical group after 1 year. Furthermore, the annual mortality rate was higher in the nonsurgical group (26% versus 14%, $P = 0.06$).[24]

Traumatic Spondylolisthesis of C2

Traumatic spondylolisthesis of C2, also known as hangman fracture, is commonly the result of a high-energy mechanism and accounts for approximately 4% of all cervical spine fractures. As with C1 fractures, careful scrutiny of the entire spine is required when a hangman fracture is identified, because more than 25% of patients with this injury have a second spine fracture.[25] The Levine and Edwards classification system (**Figure 4**) is commonly used, but an important variant, in which the fracture includes a portion of the C2 posterior vertebral wall, has since been identified. When the fracture fragment includes a portion of the vertebral body, the fragment can compress the spinal cord, leading to an increased rate of neurologic injury, often a Brown-Séquard injury.

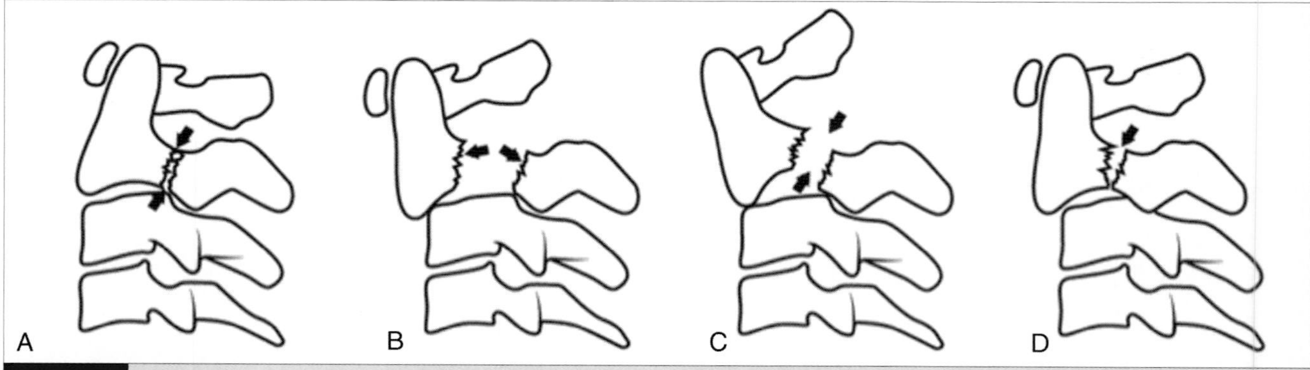

Figure 4 Drawings depict the Levine and Edwards classification system. **A**, Type I fracture is a nondisplaced injury. **B**, Type II involves substantial angulation and more than 3 mm of displacement. **C**, Type IIa involves substantial angulation and less than 3 mm of displacement. **D**, Type III is associated with subluxated or dislocated facets. (Reproduced from Bransford RJ, Alton TB, Patel AR, Bellabarba C: Upper cervical spine trauma. *J Am Acad Orthop Surg* 2014;22[11]:718-729.)

Type I fractures are considered stable and can be treated in a hard cervical collar. Most type II injuries can be treated with closed reduction and a halo vest; however, if substantial angulation, disruption of the C2-3 disk, or an inability to maintain the reduction is present, surgery is recommended. Often the placement of C2 pedicle screws is possible. If this is the case, an isolated C2-3 fusion is preferred. If the placement of C2 pedicle screws is not possible, a C1-3 posterior fusion or a C2-3 anterior cervical discectomy and fusion can be performed. Although traction in type IIa fractures is contraindicated, these fractures often can be reduced and treated with a halo vest. As with type II fractures, if substantial angulation, disruption of the C2-3 disk, or an inability to maintain the reduction is present, surgery is recommended. Finally, all type III fractures are unstable and require a C2-3 or C1-3 fusion.

Subaxial Cervical Spine Injuries

Multiple classifications for the subaxial cervical spine have been proposed with variable amounts of reliability, accuracy, and clinical applicability; however, no current classification system or treatment algorithm has been accepted globally.[26] Commonly used classification systems include the Allen and Ferguson classification, which was the first to classify injuries based on the mechanism that produced the injury; the Magerl system, which was described originally in the thoracolumbar spine but has been extrapolated to the cervical spine, and the Subaxial Cervical Spine Injury Classification System (SLIC). The SLIC was the first system to formally consider the neurologic status of the patient and the integrity of the discoligamentous complex. Furthermore, because it is accompanied by a scoring system, it was the first system to formally guide treatment (**Table 2**). Despite improved reliability compared with previous classifications, global acceptance of the SLIC has been limited by the perception that it promotes the biases of the authors. Therefore, its treatment recommendations are not consistent with worldwide regional treatment algorithms. Furthermore, the SLIC fails to recommend definitive treatment of a neurologically intact patient with a burst fracture and a disrupted posterior ligamentous complex.

Recognizing the limitations of the current classifications, the organization AOSpine published the new AOSpine Subaxial Cervical Spine Injury Classification System in 2015.[27] This classification system combines the benefits of the SLIC and the Magerl systems (**Table 3**). Fractures first are separated into one of three morphologic types: type A, compression injuries; type B, disruption of the tension band; and type C, translational injuries. Additionally, type A fractures are divided into five subtypes, and type B injuries are divided into three subtypes. Next, injuries to the facet joint complex are given a grade of F1 to F4, and the patient's neurologic status is evaluated and assigned a grade. Finally, any patient-specific modifiers that may alter the treatment algorithm are considered. Currently, only the descriptive classification has been published; however, studies are ongoing to validate the classification system and to use the new system to develop a globally applicable treatment algorithm for subaxial cervical spine injuries.

The treatment of individual fracture patterns of the subaxial spine is beyond the scope of this chapter, but a few key principles should be followed. All patients with a cervical spine fracture and an SCI should undergo urgent decompression. In some cases, the decompression may

Table 2

The Subaxial Cervical Spine Injury Classification System

Injuries are assigned points based on the scale below. An injury with a point total of less than 4 typically can be treated nonsurgically, whereas injuries accruing 5 or more points typically require surgical intervention.

Points		
Morphology		
No abnormality	0	
Compression		1
Burst		+1 = 2
Distraction (eg, facet perch, hyperextension)		3
Rotation/translation (eg, facet dislocation, unstable teardrop or advanced staged flexion compression injury)		4
Discoligamentous Complex		
Intact		0
Indeterminate (eg, isolated interspinous widening)		1
Disrupted (eg, widening of disk space, facet perch or dislocation)		2
Neurologic Status		
Intact		0
Root injury		1
Complete cord injury		2
Incomplete cord injury		3
Continuous cord compression in setting of neurodeficit (neuromodifier)		+1

(Reproduced with permission from Vaccaro AR, Hulbert RJ, Patel AA, et al: Spine Trauma Study Group: The subaxial cervical spine injury classification system: A novel approach to recognize the importance of morphology, neurology, and the integrity of the disco-ligamentous complex. *Spine* 2007;32:2365-2374.)

be able to be achieved closed, and surgical stabilization can be delayed. Although in the future the new AOSpine Subaxial Cervical Spine Injury Classification System may be able to help identify specific fractures that are unstable, the treatment algorithm for this classification has yet to be published. Currently, the best available classification

Table 3

The AOSpine Subaxial Injury Classification System

Morphologic Type	
A	**Compression Injury**
A0	Minor injury such as a spinous or transverse process fracture; also may be injury such as central cord syndrome, in which a neurologic injury is present but no fracture
A1	A wedge or compaction fracture
A2	A split or pincer fracture; a fracture through both end plates with an intact posterior wall
A3	A burst fracture involving a single end plate
A4	A burst fracture involving both end plates
B	**Tension Band Injury**
B1	Transosseous disruption (ie, bony chance)
B2	Disruption of the posterior ligamentous tension band
B3	Disruption of the anterior ligamentous tension band
C	**Translation Injury**
Facet	
F1	A nondisplaced fracture in which the fragment is less than 1 cm in height and represents less than 40% of the lateral mass
F2	A displaced fracture or a fracture greater than 1 cm in height or accounting for more than 40% of the lateral mass
F3	A floating lateral mass
F4	Any injury that results in a subluxated, perched, or dislocated facet
BL	Indicates bilateral facet involvement
Neurologic Status	
N0	Neurologically intact
N1	Transient neurologic symptoms
N2	Persistent nerve root symptoms
N3	Incomplete spinal cord injury
N4	Complete spinal cord injury
N+	Any injury with persistent spinal cord compression
Nx	Unable to obtain a neurologic exam

Table 3 *(continued)*

The AOSpine Subaxial Injury Classification System

Morphologic Type	
Patient-Specific Modifiers	
M1	Indeterminate injury to the posterior ligamentous complex
M2	Substantial disk herniation identified
M3	A preexisting stiffening or metabolic bone disease such as diffuse idiopathic skeletal hyperostosis or ankylosing spondylitis
M4	Any injury with a vertebral artery injury

(Reproduced with permission from Vaccaro A, Hulbert R, Patel A, et al: The Spine Trauma Study Group: The subaxial cervical spine injury classification system: A novel approach to recognize the importance of morphology, neurology, and integrity of the disco-ligamentous complex. *Spine* 2007;32:2365-2374.)

system for identifying unstable fractures—and thus, the need for surgical intervention—is the SLIC. Patients with a score of less than 4 points should undergo a trial of nonsurgical care, whereas for patients with a score greater than 4, surgery is recommended.

Special consideration should be given to patients with stiffening bone disease such as diffuse idiopathic skeletal hyperostosis or ankylosing spondylitis. A specialized treatment plan for patients with either of these pathologies is necessary. All individuals should undergo advanced imaging, including CT to rule out any occult fractures, and MRI to evaluate for the presence of an epidural hematoma. Almost all fractures in these patients are unstable and require surgical intervention.

MRI Before Closed Reduction of a Cervical Spine Injury

Because the Surgical Timing in Acute Spinal Cord Injury Study demonstrated a clear long-term improvement in neurologic outcomes with early decompression of the neural elements, most SCI centers now obtain a CT and MRI of the cervical spine for any patient with an SCI and then take the patient directly to the operating room for a surgical decompression. In the case of dislocated cervical facets, however, considerable controversy still exists over the ideal algorithm for the reduction. It may be possible to decompress the neurologic elements rapidly and completely with a closed reduction, thus reducing the time to decompression while allowing for surgical stabilization in a more controlled situation. Controversy remains, however, because acute neurologic deterioration secondary to the displacement of a large herniated disk has been reported in patients who underwent a closed reduction without a preoperative MRI.

It is clear that an MRI scan should be obtained before any type of reduction is performed in a patient who has dislocated cervical facets but is neurologically intact because nothing is to be gained by emergently decompressing the spinal cord. Additionally, a patient with a complete SCI should undergo a closed reduction as soon as the injury is identified because it is highly unlikely that the patient will have any further neurologic deterioration. The need for MRI before reduction in a patient with an incomplete SCI is controversial, however. In a study of nine patients in whom closed reduction of dislocated cervical facets was successful, a prereduction MRI scan demonstrated a herniated disk in two patients, and a postreduction MRI scan demonstrated a herniated disk in five patients.[28] In addition, no patients experienced a worsening of their neurologic status. This led the authors to propose that, if the patient is awake, alert, and cooperative and a dedicated radiology technician is available, closed reduction may be appropriate. Traction should be terminated, however, if a decline in the neurologic status, a lack of reduction progress, or excessive distraction of spinal elements occurs.

Summary

Cervical spine fractures are a diverse group of injuries that can present after a high-energy mechanism or as a geriatric fragility fracture. Important advances in treatment have been made since 2010. During this time, the importance of urgent surgical decompression of patients with an acute SCI has been verified, and the use of high-dose methylprednisolone has declined considerably. An improvement in the mortality rate and the health-related quality of life has been demonstrated in geriatric patients with a type II odontoid fracture who undergo surgery, in contrast to those receiving nonsurgical care. A new classification system for subaxial cervical spine injuries also has been established.

Key Study Points

- In patients with an acute spinal cord injury, early decompression improves the rate of meaningful neurologic recovery.
- The transverse ligament is evaluated best on MRI. C1 fractures rarely require surgery unless a midsubstance disruption of the transverse ligament is present.
- The mortality rate is reduced and the health-related quality of life is improved when geriatric patients with a type II odontoid fracture undergo surgical treatment.
- The bony stability and integrity of the discoligamentous complex and the neurologic status of a patient should be considered in the treatment algorithm for patients with a subaxial cervical spine injury.

Annotated References

1. Spivak JM, Weiss MA, Cotler JM, Call M: Cervical spine injuries in patients 65 and older. *Spine (Phila Pa 1976)* 1994;19(20):2302-2306.

2. Fehlings MG, Vaccaro A, Wilson JR, et al: Early versus delayed decompression for traumatic cervical spinal cord injury: Results of the Surgical Timing in Acute Spinal Cord Injury Study (STASCIS). *PLoS One* 2012;7(2):e32037.

   This prospective observational cohort study of patients with an acute spinal cord injury found that patients treated with early decompression had a statistically significant rate of neurologic improvement. Level of evidence: II.

3. Toscano J: Prevention of neurological deterioration before admission to a spinal cord injury unit. *Paraplegia* 1988;26(3):143-150.

4. Blahd WH Jr, Iserson KV, Bjelland JC: Efficacy of the posttraumatic cross table lateral view of the cervical spine. *J Emerg Med* 1985;2(4):243-249.

5. Antevil JL, Sise MJ, Sack DI, Kidder B, Hopper A, Brown CV: Spiral computed tomography for the initial evaluation of spine trauma: A new standard of care? *J Trauma* 2006;61(2):382-387.

6. Blacksin MF, Lee HJ: Frequency and significance of fractures of the upper cervical spine detected by CT in patients with severe neck trauma. *AJR Am J Roentgenol* 1995;165(5):1201-1204.

7. Resnick S, Inaba K, Karamanos E, et al: Clinical relevance of magnetic resonance imaging in cervical spine clearance: A prospective study. *JAMA Surg* 2014;149(9):934-939.

   In this prospective study of more than 800 patients who underwent blunt trauma, CT was able to identify every clinically significant cervical spine injury. Although MRI did identify additional injuries, none of the injuries that were evident on MRI but not on CT affected the treatment. Level of evidence: II.

8. Panczykowski DM, Tomycz ND, Okonkwo DO: Comparative effectiveness of using computed tomography alone to exclude cervical spine injuries in obtunded or intubated patients: Meta-analysis of 14,327 patients with blunt trauma. *J Neurosurg* 2011;115(3):541-549.

   In this meta-analysis of more than 14,000 patients, the negative predictive value of a normal CT was 100% in patients who were able to be examined reliably. Level of evidence: III.

9. Kaiser ML, Whealon MD, Barrios C, Kong AP, Lekawa ME, Dolich MO: The current role of magnetic resonance imaging for diagnosing cervical spine injury in blunt trauma patients with negative computed tomography scan. *Am Surg* 2012;78(10):1156-1160.

   This article reports the results of a retrospective review of patients who sustained blunt trauma and were not able to be examined reliably. MRI altered the treatment in 7 of 23 patients who underwent an MRI. Level of evidence: IV.

10. Miller CP, Brubacher JW, Biswas D, Lawrence BD, Whang PG, Grauer JN: The incidence of noncontiguous spinal fractures and other traumatic injuries associated with cervical spine fractures: A 10-year experience at an academic medical center. *Spine (Phila Pa 1976)* 2011;36(19):1532-1540.

    This article details a retrospective case series of more than 13,000 trauma patients. Of the total, 492 had an acute fracture to the spinal column. A noncontiguous spinal injury was present in 19% of the cases (93 patients). Level of evidence: IV.

11. Hurlbert RJ, Hadley MN, Walters BC, et al: Pharmacological therapy for acute spinal cord injury. *Neurosurgery* 2013;72(suppl 2):93-105.

    These recommendations from the American Association of Neurological Surgeons/Congress of Neurological Surgeons cover the use of pharmacologic treatment for patients with an acute spinal cord injury (SCI). The authors report a level-1 recommendation against the use of steroids for an acute SCI.

12. Schroeder GD, Kwon BK, Eck JC, Savage JW, Hsu WK, Patel AA: Survey of Cervical Spine Research Society members on the use of high-dose steroids for acute spinal cord injuries. *Spine (Phila Pa 1976)* 2014;39(12):971-977.

    In this survey of members of the Cervical Spine Research Society, the authors reported a substantial reduction in the use of steroids in the last decade.

13. Grossman RG, Fehlings MG, Frankowski RF, et al: A prospective, multicenter, phase I matched-comparison group trial of safety, pharmacokinetics, and preliminary

efficacy of riluzole in patients with traumatic spinal cord injury. *J Neurotrauma* 2014;31(3):239-255.

This phase-1 FDA trial evaluated the safety of using riluzole in patients with an acute SCI. The authors report that, in this small study of only 36 patients, riluzole appeared to be safe. Level of evidence: II.

14. Chaput CD, Torres E, Davis M, Song J, Rahm M: Survival of atlanto-occipital dissociation correlates with atlanto-occipital distraction, injury severity score, and neurologic status. *J Trauma* 2011;71(2):393-395.

    In this retrospective case series of 14 patients with an atlanto-occipital dissociation, the authors reported that this injury is survivable; of the total, 8 patients survived the injury. Mortality was associated with an increased injury severity score, a complete neurologic deficit, and a high basion-dens interval. Level of evidence: IV.

15. Sherk HH, Nicholson JT: Fractures of the atlas. *J Bone Joint Surg Am* 1970;52(5):1017-1024.

16. Levine AM, Edwards CC: Treatment of injuries in the C1-C2 complex. *Orthop Clin North Am* 1986;17(1):31-44.

17. Fowler JL, Sandhu A, Fraser RD: A review of fractures of the atlas vertebra. *J Spinal Disord* 1990;3(1):19-24.

18. Hadley MN, Dickman CA, Browner CM, Sonntag VK: Acute traumatic atlas fractures: Management and long term outcome. *Neurosurgery* 1988;23(1):31-35.

19. Radcliff KE, Sonagli MA, Rodrigues LM, Sidhu GS, Albert TJ, Vaccaro AR: Does C_1 fracture displacement correlate with transverse ligament integrity? *Orthop Surg* 2013;5(2):94-99.

    In this review of 18 patients with a C1 fracture, the authors found that using the lateral mass overhang was not an appropriate way to evaluate the integrity of the transverse acetabularligament. The authors assert that MRI should be used to evaluate the TAL. Level of evidence: IV.

20. Bransford R, Falicov A, Nguyen Q, Chapman J: Unilateral C-1 lateral mass sagittal split fracture: An unstable Jefferson fracture variant. *J Neurosurg Spine* 2009;10(5):466-473.

21. Hsu WK, Anderson PA: Odontoid fractures: Update on management. *J Am Acad Orthop Surg* 2010;18(7):383-394.

    This article details a narrative review of the treatment of odontoid fractures.

22. Jea A, Tatsui C, Farhat H, Vanni S, Levi AD: Vertically unstable type III odontoid fractures: Case report. *Neurosurgery* 2006;58(4):E797, discussion E797.

23. Chapman J, Smith JS, Kopjar B, et al: The AOSpine North America Geriatric Odontoid Fracture Mortality Study: A retrospective review of mortality outcomes for operative versus nonoperative treatment of 322 patients with long-term follow-up. *Spine (Phila Pa 1976)* 2013;38(13):1098-1104.

    The authors of this multicenter retrospective study of geriatric patients with type II odontoid fractures report that nonsurgical treatment leads to an increase in short-term and long-term mortality. Importantly, this study reported an increase in mortality with nonsurgical treatment even when controlling for age, sex, and Charlson comorbidity index. Level of evidence: III.

24. Vaccaro AR, Kepler CK, Kopjar B, et al: Functional and quality-of-life outcomes in geriatric patients with type-II dens fracture. *J Bone Joint Surg Am* 2013;95(8):729-735.

    This prospective observational cohort study of geriatric patients with a type II odontoid fracture found that surgery is associated with improved health-related quality of life metrics and is not associated with an increase in complications. Level of evidence: II.

25. Ryan MD, Henderson JJ: The epidemiology of fractures and fracture-dislocations of the cervical spine. *Injury* 1992;23(1):38-40.

26. van Middendorp JJ, Audigé L, Hanson B, Chapman JR, Hosman AJ: What should an ideal spinal injury classification system consist of? A methodological review and conceptual proposal for future classifications. *Eur Spine J* 2010;19(8):1238-1249.

    This review identifies the benefits of and problems with the existing spine injury classification systems.

27. Vaccaro AR, Koerner JD, Radcliff KE, et al: AOSpine subaxial cervical spine injury classification system. *Eur Spine J* 2015.[Epub ahead of print].

    This article presents the new AOSpine Subaxial Cervical Spine Injury Classification System.

28. Vaccaro AR, Falatyn SP, Flanders AE, Balderston RA, Northrup BE, Cotler JM: Magnetic resonance evaluation of the intervertebral disc, spinal ligaments, and spinal cord before and after closed traction reduction of cervical spine dislocations. *Spine (Phila Pa 1976)* 1999;24(12):1210-1217.

Chapter 35

Diagnosis and Management of Traumatic Thoracic and Lumbar Injuries

Chadi Tannoury, MD Ahmed Yousry Moussa, MD Omar Fawaz Alnori, MD Tony Tannoury, MD

Abstract

Thoracic and lumbar fractures are common injuries associated with substantial morbidities and at times devastating neurologic deficits. Defining clear indications for the surgical and nonsurgical management of such injuries has been the topic of extensive debate and investigations. Many classification schemes have been created, but few have been useful in recommending a surgical decision. Nonsurgical management has shown superiority in patients with stable fractures without neurologic deficits, whereas surgical management has been reserved for patients with selected unstable fractures, fractures with neurologic deficits, and fractures of the ankylosed spine. Morbidities and mortalities have been reported in surgically treated patients. Despite the promising results of trending minimally invasive techniques, high-quality studies still are lacking.

Keywords: spinal trauma; burst fracture; compression fracture; flexion distraction injury; spinal fracture dislocation; Chance fracture; spinal cord injury

Dr. Tony Tannoury or an immediate family member has received royalties from Johnson & Johnson, is a member of a speakers' bureau or has made paid presentations on behalf of Johnson & Johnson, and serves as a paid consultant to Johnson & Johnson. None of the following authors nor any immediate family member has received anything of value from or has stock or stock options held in a commercial company or institution related directly or indirectly to the subject of this chapter: Dr. Chadi Tannoury, Dr. Moussa, and Dr. AlNori.

Introduction

Thoracic and lumbar fractures are common injuries. Most result from blunt trauma and have a male predominance and an incidence of 117 per 100,000 person-years.[1] Management of the injured spine remains a controversial topic, especially for a neurologically intact patient.[2]

As a transitional segment, the thoracolumbar junction (T11-L2) is the most prone to injuries (52%), followed by the thoracic segment (T1-T11), and the lower lumbar spine.[3,4] Depending on the extent of bony and ligamentous involvement, thoracic and lumbar fractures can range from stable compression deformities to devastating osteoligamentous disruptions with neurologic compromise. Despite the lack of mechanical stability in certain burst fractures, neurologic compromise is not encountered frequently.[5-7]

Classification Systems

To better characterize the different injury patterns, numerous classification schemes have been proposed over the past decades. One of the earliest systems is the Denis classification, based on the anatomic extent of the injury as seen on plain radiographs and the integrity of the three columns of the spine[6] (**Figure 1**). If the clinician relies solely on plain radiographs, the presence of ligamentous injuries is underestimated. Therefore, the reliability of the Denis classification to predict spinal column stability is questionable.[8]

Another classification system using CT provided more comprehensive information regarding the integrity of the three spinal columns.[9] The system's limited ability to evaluate soft-tissue injury warranted the later development of other classification systems.[4,10,11] The McCormack classification system took into account the extent of vertebral body fracture, the propagation and displacement of the

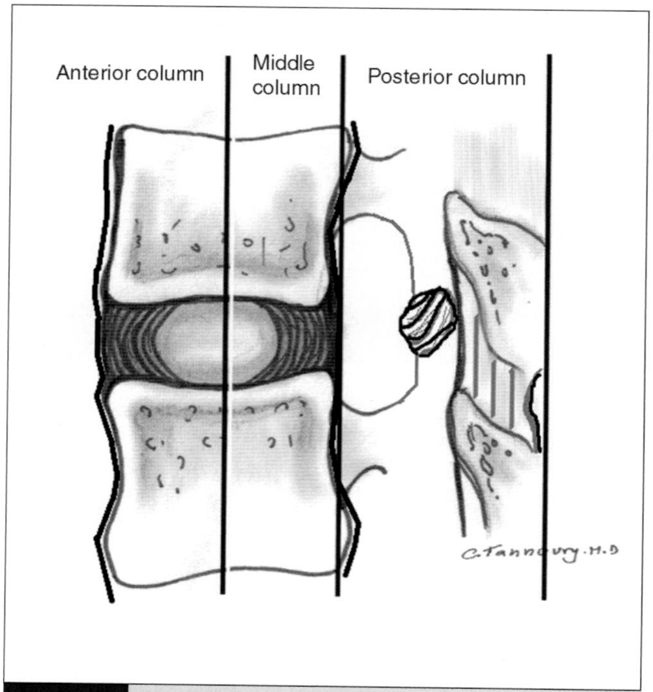

Figure 1 Drawing depicts the three-column Denis classification system. The anterior column includes the anterior longitudinal ligament, the anterior annulus, and the anterior two-thirds of the vertebral body. The middle column includes the posterior longitudinal ligament, the posterior one-third of the vertebral body, and the posterior anulus fibrosus. The posterior column includes the pedicles, facet joints, posterior bony elements, and posterior ligaments.

bony fragments, and the sagittal balance correction[12] (**Table 1**). This "load-sharing" classification gained popularity as being simple to use. However, it overlooked the significance of the patient's neurologic status and the presence of ligamentous injury.[8] The AO-Spine Group also proposed a well detailed and comprehensive classification comprising more than 50 fracture subtypes, but the complexity of this classification system has made its common clinical use unwieldy.[13,14]

The Thoracolumbar Injury Classification and Severity Score (TLICS) is based on the morphology and mechanism of the fracture, the integrity of the posterior ligamentous complex (PLC), and neurologic status. With this classification scheme, a score can be calculated for any given fracture, which leads to a treatment recommendation.[4,8,15]

A recent systematic literature review identified the four most widely used classification schemes: the Denis classification, the AO comprehensive classification, the load-sharing classification, and the TLICS. The authors concluded that TLICS is the best available classification system for its reproducibility and capability of guiding treatment[16] (**Table 2**).

Evaluation

After securing the respiratory and cardiovascular functions, the evaluation of spinal injuries in a polytrauma patient includes detailed history taking, a thorough clinical examination, and radiographic imaging. The initial evaluation may be obscured by the presence of severe distracting injuries, including long bone fractures, pelvic fractures, chest and abdominal trauma, and/or a disturbed level of consciousness (such as from substance intoxication or head injury). The incidence of missed thoracolumbar injuries has been reported to be as high as 24%.[17,18] Therefore, CT with three-dimensional reconstruction and MRI are strongly recommended as adjunct screening tools for vertebral injuries.[4]

In an alert and conscious patient, a comprehensive motor and sensory evaluation should be performed, and a score may be given using the American Spinal Injury Association impairment scale.[17] The log roll maneuver should be performed to inspect the skin for abnormal bruising, evaluate the spine for exaggerated angulations, and feel for abnormal step-offs and point tenderness. Additionally, evaluation of the rectal tone, sphincter control, and the bulbocavernosus reflex are relevant in discerning a spinal cord injury from a spinal shock. Priapism is among the well-noted signs of spinal cord injuries. Its presence indicates acute and complete sensory and motor deficits.[19]

Concomitant cervical and thoracolumbar injuries have been reported in approximately 11% of polytrauma patients. Therefore, an evaluation of the entire spine almost always is warranted after an injury is identified.[20]

Imaging

Although plain radiographs are often used and are easily accessible, they are no longer recommended as the initial screening tool for vertebral injuries in polytrauma patients. The high sensitivity (99%) of high-resolution CT and its superior accuracy in detecting bony injury have promoted this imaging modality as the study of choice for the initial screening.[21] Additionally, CT is being used routinely as a screening tool to evaluate chest, abdomen, and pelvic injuries in multitrauma patients.[22]

The recent recognition of the contribution of the PLC to spine stability has made MRI valuable because of its high specificity and sensitivity for injuries to this structure. The integrity of the PLC and the intervertebral disks plays an important role in surgical decision making. The

Table 1

The McCormack Scoring System

Score	Sagittal Collapse	Displacement	Correction	Total
1 point	30%	1 mm	3°	3 points
2 point	>30%	2 mm	9°	6 points
3 point	60%	>2 mm	10°	9 points

Reproduced with permission from McCormack T, Karaikovic E, Gaines RW. The load sharing classification of spine fractures. *Spine* (Phila Pa 1976) 1994;19(15):1741-1744.

value of MRI as a diagnostic tool has been highlighted in the TLICS algorithm.[10,23,24] Preoperative MRI findings and intraoperative assessments of PLC integrity were prospectively studied and discrepancies were reported, with only a moderate correlation between the two.[24] Therefore, it is recommended that PLC disruption be determined not solely on the MRI findings but rather by collective morphologic criteria using plain radiographs, CT, and MRI.[16]

Table 2

Thoracolumbar Injury Classification and Severity Score Table

Classification Factor	Points
Injury Morphology	
No abnormality	0
Compression	1
Burst	+1 = 2
Translational injury	3
Distraction injury	4
Integrity of Posterior Ligamentous Complex	
Intact	0
Indeterminate (isolated interspinous widening, MRI signal change only)	2
Disrupted (widening of disk space, facet perch, or dislocation)	3
Neurologic Status	
Intact	0
Root injury	1
Complete spinal cord injury	2
Incomplete spinal cord injury	3
Cauda equina injury	3

Reproduced with permission from Vaccaro AR, Lehman RA, Hurlbert RJ, et al: A new classification of thoracolumbar injuries: The importance of injury morphology, the integrity of the posterior ligamentous complex, and neurologic status. *Spine* 2005;30[20]:2325-2333.

Management of Thoracolumbar Fracture

Compression Fractures

Compression fractures typically present without neurologic deficits, involve only one column, and are considered stable injuries (**Figure 2**). Although some studies recommend early ambulation without any external support, others have shown the benefits of braces, including off-the-shelf or well-molded orthoses, and hyperextension casting in preventing flexion load at the fracture site and allowing early mobilization.[25]

Nonsurgically treated patients should be monitored closely with follow-up standing radiographs. Surgical management may be considered for progressive kyphosis of more than 30°, worsening vertebral collapse consisting of more than 50% of vertebral height, an increase in fracture angle of more than 10°, and intractable back pain, despite the nonsurgical management.[26]

Osteoporotic Compression Fractures

According to the World Health Organization, osteoporotic vertebral compression fracture is the most common osteoporotic fracture worldwide.[27] Affected patients, who typically are elderly, commonly present with back pain following a trivial trauma episode (**Figure 3**). Fracture management involves preventing the complications of deconditioning, intractable back pain, depression, adjacent vertebral segment fractures, and a lengthy hospital stay.[28] Nonsurgical management is the first line of treatment and entails bracing, oral pain medicine, and early physical–therapy-assisted mobilization.[29] No additional treatment is required for most osteoporotic fractures without initial kyphosis and with a positive response to nonsurgical management of up to 6 weeks duration. Surgical treatment may be warranted in patients for the indications described previously.

The value of vertebroplasty, the technique involving placement of percutaneous polymethyl methacrylate (PMMA) cement at the fractured vertebra, has been

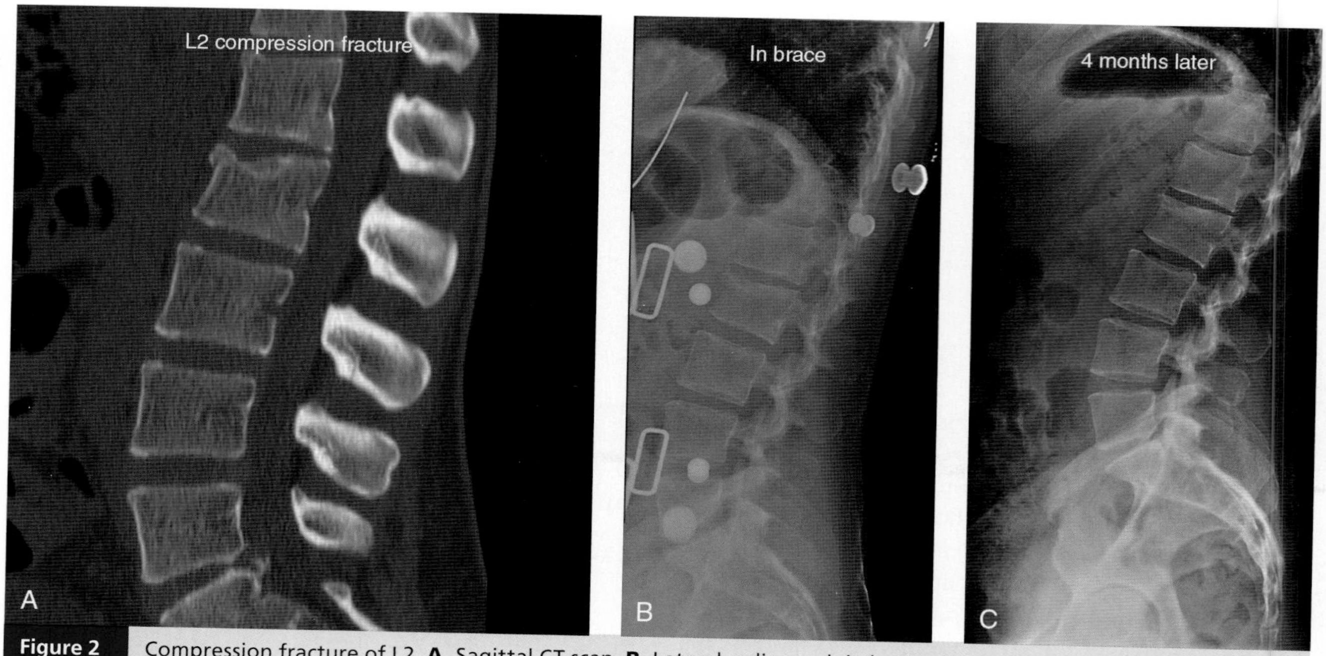

Figure 2 Compression fracture of L2. **A,** Sagittal CT scan, **B,** Lateral radiograph in brace. **C,** Lateral radiograph after successful treatment.

studied.[30] In some patients treated with vertebroplasty, pain relief, improved quality of life, and prevention of pulmonary complications were noted. Similar benefits were nonreproducible in other studies, however.[31-33]

Kyphoplasty is based on the concept of using balloon expansion followed by cement PMMA augmentation to partially correct the kyphosis at the fractured segment. When compared with nonsurgical management, kyphoplasty was found to help restore some of the sagittal alignment and promote a faster recovery and return to function with a lower complication rate.[34,35]

Complications following vertebroplasty and kyphoplasty include cement extravasation, cement embolism, spinal stenosis with cord compression, infection, adjacent vertebrae fractures, and even mortalities.[36] Therefore, vertebroplasty and kyphoplasty are contraindicated in patients with active osteomyelitis, severe coagulopathy, cardiopulmonary disease, PMMA allergy, and a fractured posterior vertebral wall with retropulsed pieces.[37] Based on the evidence, the American Academy of Orthopaedic Surgeons clinical practice guidelines specifically recommend against kyphoplasty and do not support vertebroplasty.[38]

Burst Fractures Without Neurologic Injury

Burst fractures mainly involve the anterior and middle columns of the spine but sometimes involve the posterior column (**Figure 4**). In a neurologically intact patient, the treatment of a burst fracture remains controversial. Management ranges from immobilization with bracing or body casting or temporary bed rest with pain medication to surgical fixation with or without decompression.[25,39-41]

A meta-analysis looked at patients with burst fractures having no neurologic deficits treated with and without surgical intervention. The authors reported equal outcomes as measured by pain, disability scores, and return to work rates. In the surgical group, superior kyphosis correction but higher complication rates and overall costs were noted.[42]

A recent randomized trial with a 16- to 22-year follow-up reported a greater degree of comfort, less pain medication use, and better functional recovery with nonsurgical management than with surgery.[43] Conversely, previous studies highlighted the superiority of surgical management as measured by functional outcomes, pain scores, and early return to work.[7,44] Strong support exists for nonsurgical treatment in a neurologically intact patient with a burst fracture.

Although burst fractures without PLC injury are considered to be inherently stable and suitable for nonsurgical treatment, disruption of the posterior osteoligamentous tension complex and the facet capsules jeopardizes spinal stability.[45] Burst fractures with PLC injuries should be suspected in patients with large vertebral compression of more than 50%, angular deformities greater than 25°, neurologic deficits, and positive MRI findings. Surgical

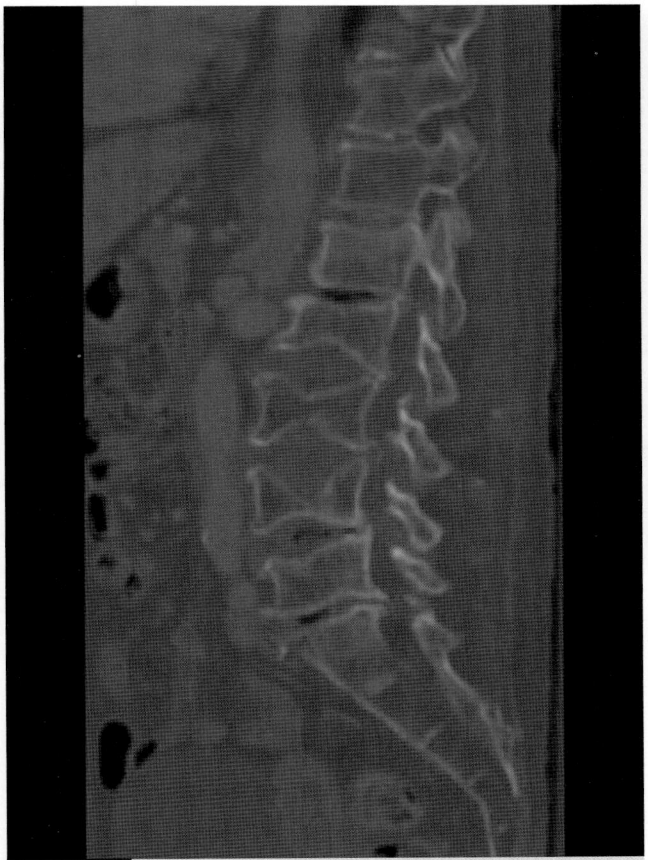

Figure 3 Sagittal CT scan of the lumbar spine shows multiple osteoporotic compression fractures in an elderly woman.

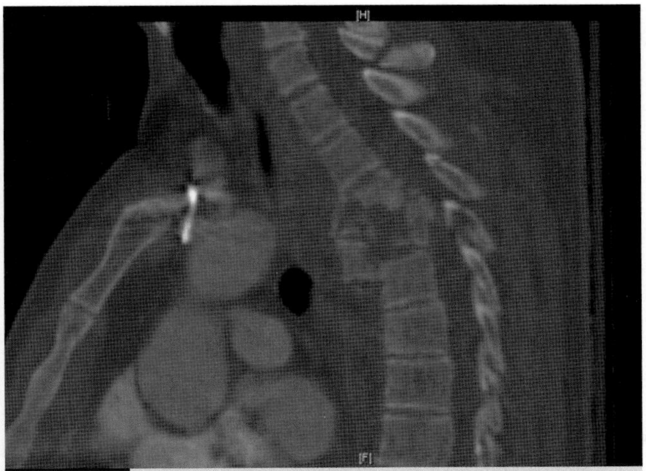

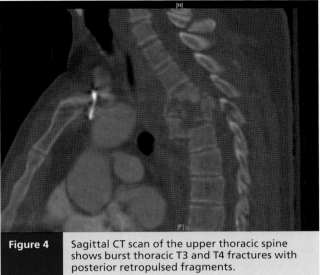

Figure 4 Sagittal CT scan of the upper thoracic spine shows burst thoracic T3 and T4 fractures with posterior retropulsed fragments.

management with direct decompression, kyphosis reduction, and posterior fusion using pedicle screw instrumentation is preferable. Anterior and/or combined anterior-posterior decompression are preferred over posterior decompression alone.[16,24]

Flexion-Distraction Injuries

Flexion-distraction injuries (FDI), also known as a seatbelt injury or Chance fracture, typically are characterized by a disruption to the posterior osteoligamentous complex, in which the middle and posterior columns fail under tension and the anterior column fails under compression.[46] FDI may present as a purely bony variant or an osteoligamentous variant. Both types are associated with a 40% rate of associated intra-abdominal visceral and mesenteric injuries.[47]

Isolated bony Chance fractures can be treated successfully with a hyperextension cast or orthosis for approximately 3 months, followed by rehabilitation.[48] Alternately, FDI in patients who cannot tolerate external immobilization, FDI injuries in polytrauma patients, and ligamentous FDI typically are treated with surgical fixation. The goals of surgical fixation include the correction of the kyphosis, the restoration of sagittal balance, stabilization, and fusion.[49] These goals can be achieved with a posterior compression construct that approximates the fracture gap while avoiding overcompression to prevent the development of neurologic deterioration from displaced disk or bony fragments (**Figure 5**). Studies on the use of anterior short segment fixation for the treatment of FDI reported superior sagittal alignment correction when compared with posterior fixation.[50,51]

More recently, minimally invasive percutaneous fixation has become popular in patients with no neurologic deficits who do not warrant direct decompression. Percutaneous screw fixation is considered as effective in correcting kyphosis as open surgical fixation but with less soft-tissue disruption and surgical blood loss.[52]

Fractures With Incomplete Neurologic Injuries

Surgery generally is recommended for thoracolumbar fractures associated with incomplete neurologic deficits, but the optimal surgical management is still controversial.[53] Many studies have proven the safety, efficiency, and reliability of posterior pedicle screw fixation in providing stabilization and correcting kyphosis[12,43,54,55] (**Figure 6**). Other studies have reported failure of the posterior-only pedicle screw constructs and described the need for anterior column support in fractures with extensive vertebral body damage, substantial kyphosis of 30° or more, and notable fracture displacement of 2 mm or more. The load-sharing classification system predicted the need for anterior column support supplementation to posterior short-segment fixation[12] (**Table 1**). A burst fracture with

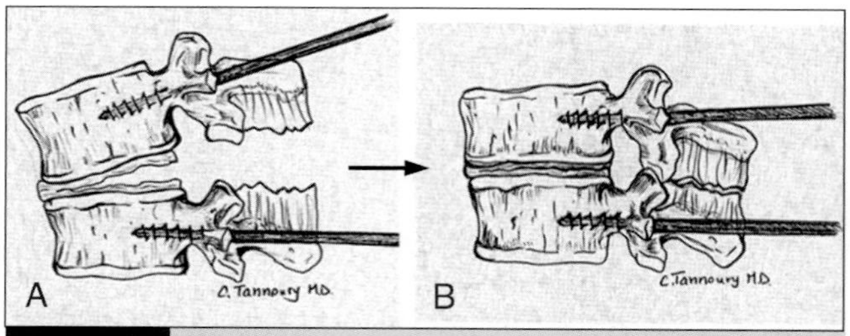

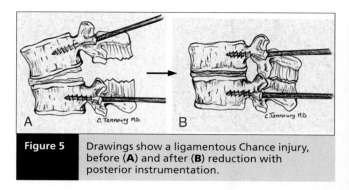

Figure 5 Drawings show a ligamentous Chance injury, before (**A**) and after (**B**) reduction with posterior instrumentation.

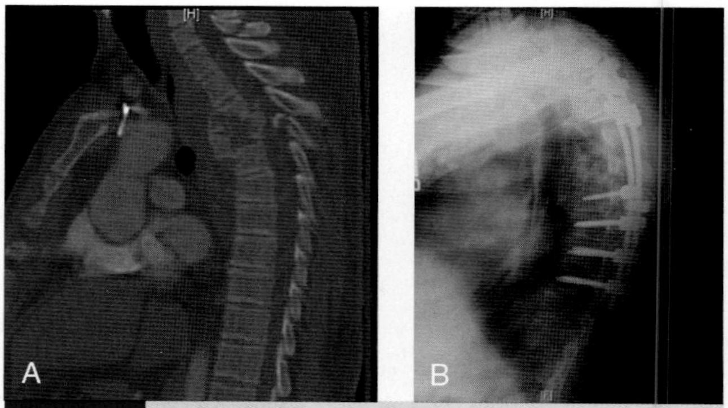

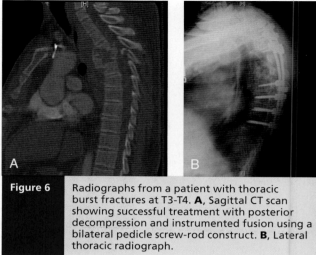

Figure 6 Radiographs from a patient with thoracic burst fractures at T3-T4. **A**, Sagittal CT scan showing successful treatment with posterior decompression and instrumented fusion using a bilateral pedicle screw-rod construct. **B**, Lateral thoracic radiograph.

a load-sharing score less than 6 can be treated with short segment posterior-only fixation. Burst fractures with a load-sharing score higher than 6 warrant long segment posterior fixation and/or combined anterior-posterior approaches.[12]

Many authors strongly advocate the benefits of anterior decompression or corpectomy along with anterior column reconstruction using strut allografts or metallic spacers or cages. This technique enables direct canal decompression and sagittal contour correction and produces fewer complications than posterior-only surgeries[50,56,57] (**Figure 7**). Various surgical options, including anterior decompression and fusion, posterior decompression and fusion, posterior fusion without decompression, combined anterior decompression with posterior fixation, and posterior decompression and stabilization with cement injection at the fractured osteoporotic vertebra, using neurologic recovery and kyphosis correction as the primary and secondary outcomes, were examined in a systematic literature review.[16] The authors noted better kyphosis correction with the combined anterior/posterior approaches when compared with posterior-only techniques. All techniques provided similar outcomes as measured by neurologic recovery and surgical complications, however. Therefore, no single surgical technique is superior or preferred, and the choice of surgical approach should take into account the surgeon's preference, the patient's morbidity factors, and the overall costs.[16,58-60]

Fracture-Dislocations

Fracture-dislocations result from high-energy trauma and are commonly associated with neurologic deficits and other skeletal injuries. The mechanism of injury is a combination of shear with rotation and flexion-extension moments. Patients with incomplete spinal cord injuries benefit from early decompression, fracture reduction, and fusion with instrumentation. Most of these injuries are treated sufficiently with a posterior-only approach without additional anterior column support[61] (**Figure 8**).

The presence of severe vertebral body comminution, large fracture fragments extending into the canal, and ventral cord compression may warrant additional direct anterior decompression of the spinal canal with anterior column support.[50]

Fractures of the Ankylosed Spine

Ankylosing conditions alter the biomechanical behavior of the axial skeleton via progressive ossification of the disks and ligaments. The resultant loss of segmental mobility leads to disuse osteoporosis and increases the risk of catastrophic fractures following minor trauma.[62] Fractures of the ankylosed spine include ankylosing spondylitis and diffuse idiopathic skeletal hyperostosis (DISH).

Ankylosing spondylitis is predominant in men aged 20 to 30 years, with a prevalence of 0.1% to 1.4% of the population. Patients with ankylosing spondylitis (characterized by a wide spectrum of spine radiographic profiles including bony erosive changes, vertebral body squaring, syndesmophytes formation, bamboo spine, and dagger spine with interspinous ligament calcification) have an 11.4 times greater risk of spinal cord injury than the general population.[63]

DISH is associated with flowing osteophytes over at least four consecutive spinal levels, and the injured DISH spine is often misdiagnosed with late or delayed presentation. Therefore, CT and MRI often are warranted.

Following trauma, patients with ankylosing spondylitis are more likely to present with neurologic deficits, whereas DISH patients have an increased risk of mortality.[64,65] Although nonsurgical treatment may be used in a few selected patients with nondisplaced and stable fracture patterns, preinjury hyperkyphosis and the patient's body habitus often make bracing difficult, and

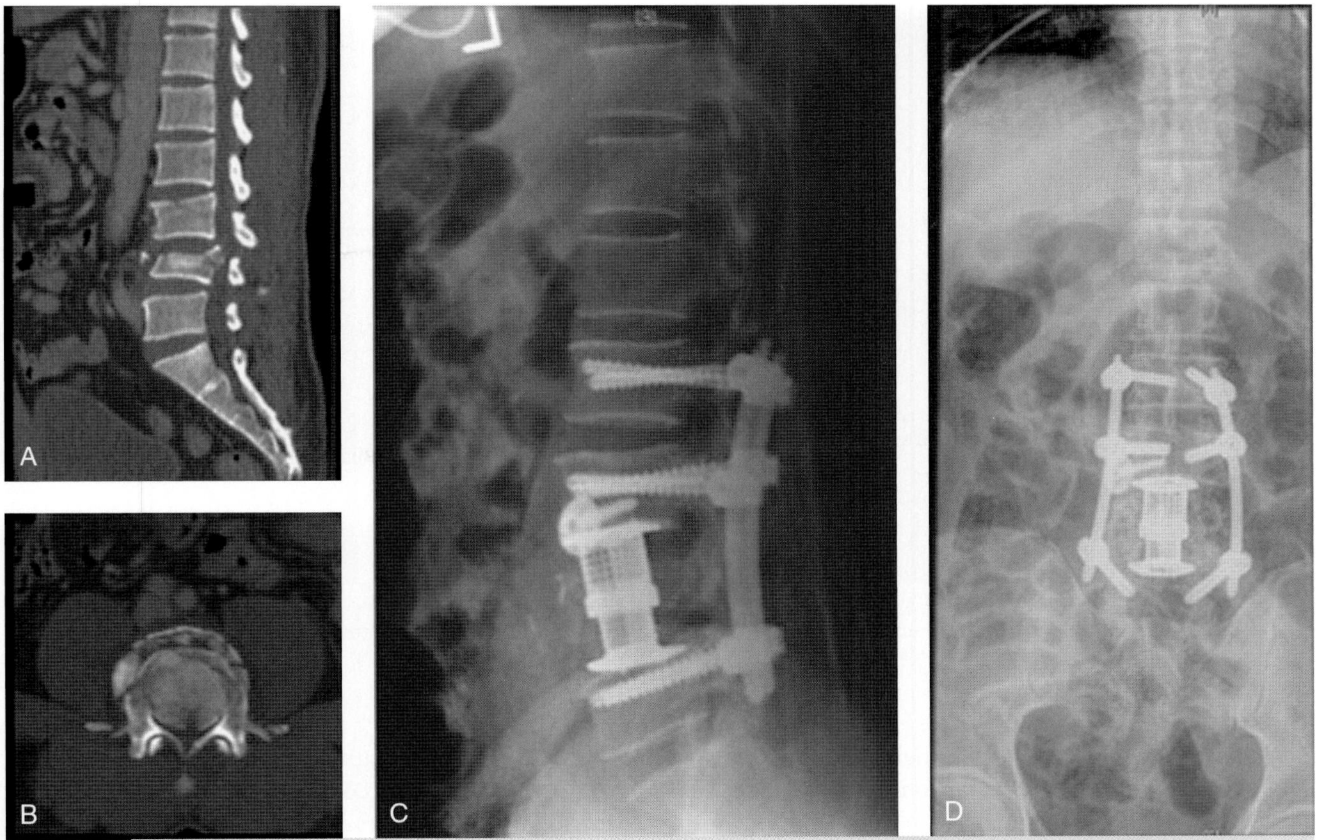

Figure 7 Radiographic images from a patient with thoracolumbar fracture. **A**, Sagittal CT shows L3 and L4 burst fractures with bony fragment retropulsion into the canal, **B**, Axial CT scan at the L4 level shows severe canal compromise. **C**, Lateral lumbar radiographic view. The patient was treated with a minimally invasive psoas sparing anterior L4 corpectomy with direct canal decompression supplemented with posterior percutaneous instrumentation. **D**, AP lumbar radiograph.

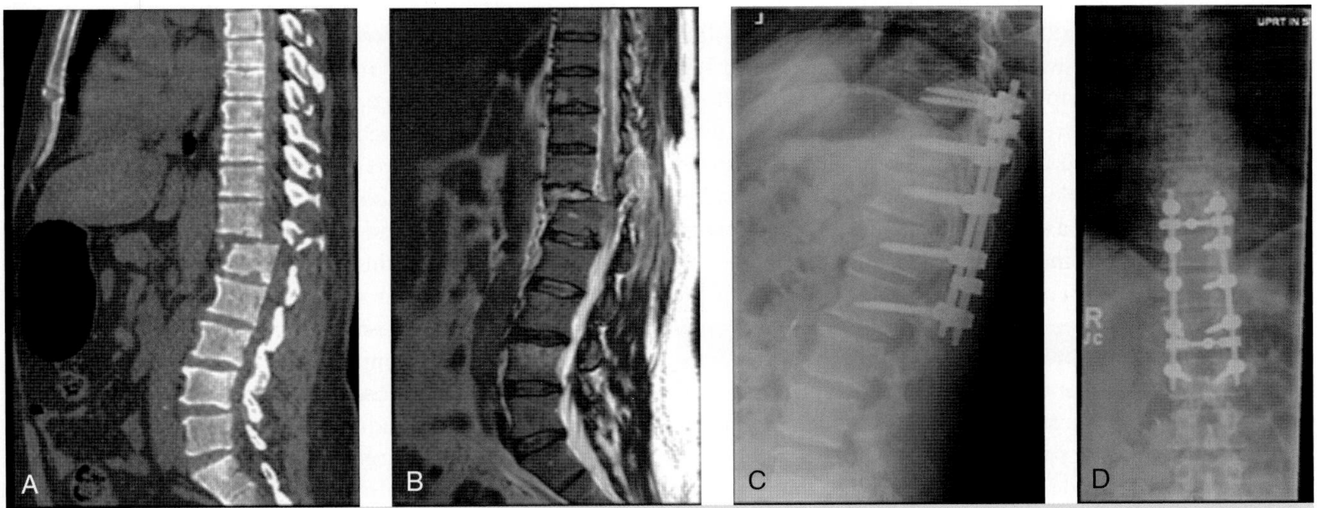

Figure 8 Sagittal CT scan (**A**) and T2-weighted MRI (**B**) show a fracture-dislocation at T12-L1. Posterior reduction, decompression and instrumented fusion using bilateral pedicle screw and rod constructs were performed. **C**, Lateral view. **D**, AP view.

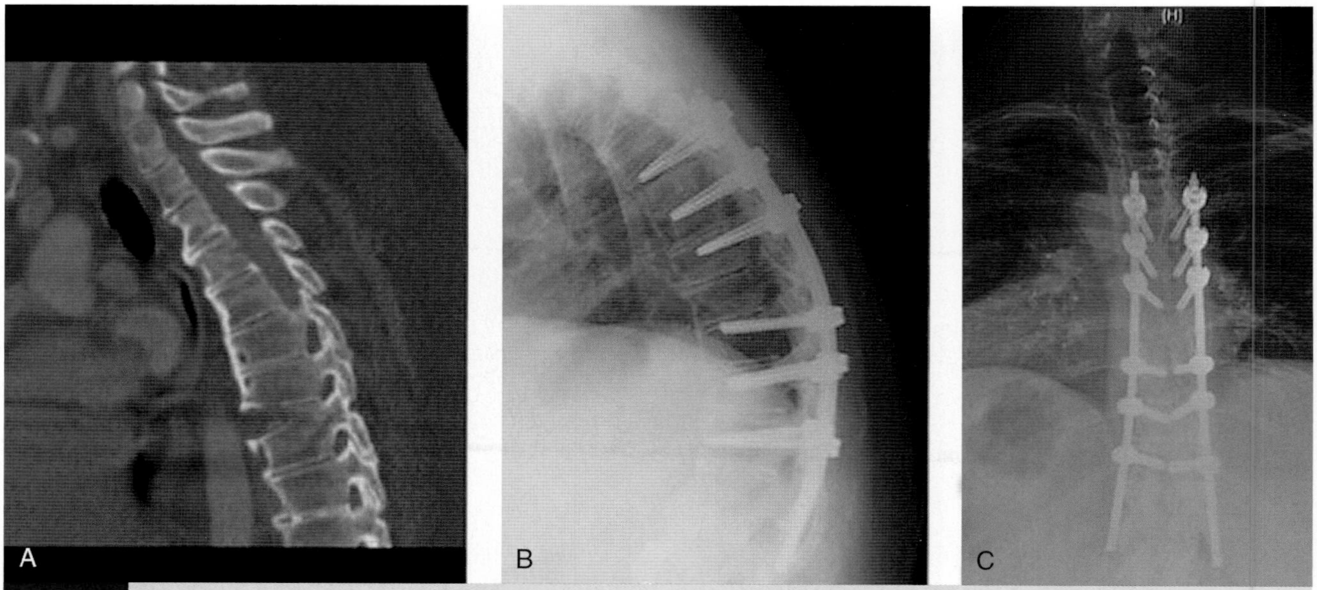

Figure 9 **A**, Sagittal CT scan of the thoracic spine shows a T7-T8 extension distraction injury in a 41-year-old woman with ankylosing spondylitis. **B** and **C**, lateral and AP views, respectively, after closed reduction and long-segment percutaneous pedicle screw and rod fixation from T5-T11.

surgery frequently is needed.[66] Patients with ankylosing conditions often have underlying comorbidities including cardiovascular disorders, diabetes mellitus, obesity, muscular fatty atrophy, and poor tissue healing potentials. Hence, they have an increased risk of mortality, surgical site infection, and pseudarthrosis. These factors should be taken into serious consideration when planning a surgical intervention.[62,67]

In ankylosing spondylitis and DISH, the fractured spine often involves all three columns and behaves like a long bone fracture, which warrants reduction and stabilization using multiple points of fixation of the long segment. Recently, percutaneous fixation has been used with good clinical and functional outcomes as measured by visual analog scale and Oswestry Disability Index scores and has avoided the complications associated with conventional open spinal surgery[68,69] (**Figure 9**).

Adverse Events

Adverse events frequently reported in patients with thoracic and lumbar fractures are urinary tract infections (19.7%), neuropathic pain (12.3%), pneumonia (11.8%), delirium (10.5%), and ileus (6.2%).[70]

Prevention of adverse events helps to improve patient outcomes and limits health care costs. A recent study showed that surgical patients have a higher risk of experiencing an adverse event (56%, with an average of 1.4 adverse events per patient) than nonsurgical patients (13%, with an average of 0.2 adverse events per patient).[3] Additionally, patients with complete neurologic injury were noted to have a 3.4 times higher risk of experiencing an adverse event than were patients who were neurologically intact (75% versus 25%, respectively). Finally, the complications found to most substantially affect a patient's length of stay are delirium and pneumonia.[3]

Minimally Invasive Spine Surgery

The goals of minimally invasive spine surgery are to minimize soft-tissue damage, limit the morbidities associated with open exposures such as blood loss and surgical time, reduce postoperative pain, and allow an earlier return to activities.[71-75] Endoscopic thoracic decompression (including diskectomy and corpectomy) and stabilization techniques have been described and show successful fusion rates of 90%, very low conversion rates to open surgery (1.4%), and substantial reductions in postoperative pain.[72,75] When compared with patients having open surgery, the duration of analgesic medication required by patients undergoing endoscopic thoracic decompression was reduced by 31%, and the overall dosage intake was reduced by 42%.[72,75] However, complications related to thoracoscopic techniques reportedly range between 1.3% and 20% and include pleural effusions, intercostal and sympathetic neuralgias, pneumothorax, portal infections, vascular injuries, neurologic deterioration, and implant loosening, making these techniques less appealing.[72,73]

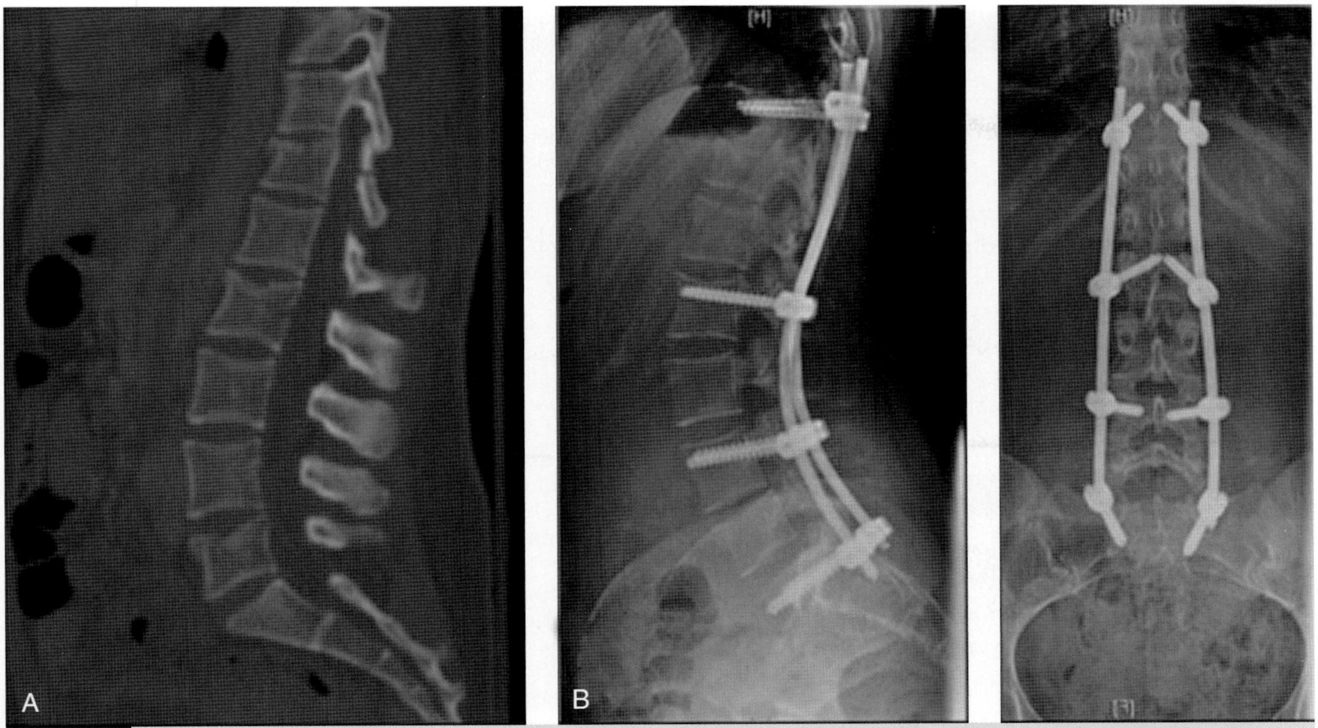

Figure 10 Images demonstrate T12, L2, and L5 burst fractures in a 29-year-old patient with associated abdominal visceral injuries precluding the use of external bracing. **A**, Sagittal CT scan of the lumbar spine shows the fractures at T12, L2, and L5. Lateral (**B**) and AP (**C**) radiographs show the spine after treatment with a percutaneous spanning internal fixator using pedicle screws and rods in place for approximately 6 months, followed by hardware removal after successful fracture healing was achieved.

The direct lateral transpsoas approach is gaining popularity because it allows mini-open access to the spine using special retractors. In combination with neuromonitoring, the approach improves the safety of the lumbar plexus as it travels within the psoas muscle. When safely performed, this technique affords a surgical corridor for canal decompression (diskectomy or corpectomy) and anterolateral instrumentation.[76]

Percutaneous stabilization with pedicle screws and rods is increasing in popularity for treatment of spinal fractures. Percutaneous stabilization with pedicle screws and rods primarily is indicated in patients with no neurologic compromise who are not good candidates for nonsurgical bracing or cast immobilization. Such patients include those with polytrauma, morbid obesity, and restrictive pulmonary disease[77-79] (**Figures 9** and **10**). Prospective and retrospective series have demonstrated equal outcomes when comparing open approaches with percutaneous procedures with and without fusion.[78,80] Because arthrodesis cannot be achieved with stand-alone percutaneous stabilization with pedicle screws and rods, the authors of a 2011 study recommended its application in neurologically stable patients with intact intervertebral disks having no major structural loss of the anterior column. The recommended indication is a fracture with a comminution not exceeding 30% of the vertebral body, height loss of 25% or less, and a kyphosis not exceeding 15°.[81] Although percutaneous short-segment stabilization has been used as a stand-alone construct, it also may be used as additional fixation complementing anterior minimally invasive spine surgery decompression and reconstruction techniques.[82] Minimally invasive anterior column decompression with partial or total corpectomy allows greater and direct canal decompression. Corpectomy is preferred in fractures with severe comminution, canal obliteration of 70% or more, and kyphosis greater than 30° at the fracture site[83] (**Figure 7**).

More recently, the percutaneous placement of PMMA or calcium phosphate at the fracture site combined with percutaneous stabilization with pedicle screws and rods have shown promising results as measured by pain relief, sagittal contour correction, and neurologic improvement in patients with thoracolumbar burst fractures.[84,85]

Despite the encouraging results with minimally invasive spine surgery, high-quality studies comparing the practice with traditional open surgery are still lacking.

Summary

Thoracolumbar injuries are not uncommon, and the management of these injuries should consider the neural, bony, and ligamentous involvements. Nonsurgical management is recommended for compression fractures and stable burst fractures without neurologic involvement. Surgical management, including traditional surgery and minimally invasive surgery, is indicated in posttraumatic deformities, fractures with spinal column instability, and spinal injuries with neurologic compromise. Surgical treatment should aim at relieving the neurologic compression, correcting spinal alignment, and providing appropriate stability.

Key Study Points

- An understanding of the available thoracolumbar injury classifications systems will guide treatment decisions. A full evaluation in the setting of polytrauma patients is important to avoid overlooking associated spinal injuries.
- The integrity of the posterior ligamentous complex injury has an important role in surgical decision making.

Annotated References

1. Cooper C, Atkinson EJ, O'Fallon WM, Melton LJ III: Incidence of clinically diagnosed vertebral fractures: A population-based study in Rochester, Minnesota, 1985-1989. *J Bone Miner Res* 1992;7(2):221-227.

2. Ghobrial GM, Maulucci CM, Maltenfort M, et al: Operative and nonoperative adverse events in the management of traumatic fractures of the thoracolumbar spine: A systematic review. *Neurosurg Focus* 2014;37(1):E8.

   This systematic review looked at the complication rates associated with the surgical and nonsurgical treatment of thoracolumbar fractures. The surgical group was noted to have higher overall complications and infection rates. Level of evidence: I.

3. Glennie RA, Ailon T, Yang K, et al: Incidence, impact, and risk factors of adverse events in thoracic and lumbar spine fractures: An ambispective cohort analysis of 390 patients. *Spine J* 2015;15(4):629-637.

   This ambispective cohort study examined the adverse events encountered in patients with thoracolumbar fractures. More adverse events were noted in patients with neurologic deficit and in those treated surgically. Level of evidence: III.

4. Wood KB, Li W, Lebl DR, Ploumis A: Management of thoracolumbar spine fractures. *Spine J* 2014;14(1):145-164.

   This study is a comprehensive literature review of the management of thoracolumbar spine fractures. Classifications, fracture types, and available surgical and nonsurgical managements were presented thoroughly. Level of evidence: III.

5. Limb D, Shaw DL, Dickson RA: Neurological injury in thoracolumbar burst fractures. *J Bone Joint Surg Br* 1995;77(5):774-777.

6. Denis F: The three column spine and its significance in the classification of acute thoracolumbar spinal injuries. *Spine (Phila Pa 1976)* 1983;8(8):817-831.

7. Denis F, Armstrong GW, Searls K, Matta L: Acute thoracolumbar burst fractures in the absence of neurologic deficit. A comparison between operative and nonoperative treatment. *Clin Orthop Relat Res* 1984;189:142-149.

8. Sethi MK, Schoenfeld AJ, Bono CM, Harris MB: The evolution of thoracolumbar injury classification systems. *Spine J* 2009;9(9):780-788.

9. McAfee PC, Yuan HA, Fredrickson BE, Lubicky JP: The value of computed tomography in thoracolumbar fractures. An analysis of one hundred consecutive cases and a new classification. *J Bone Joint Surg Am* 1983;65(4):461-473.

10. Whang PG, Vaccaro AR, Poelstra KA, et al: The influence of fracture mechanism and morphology on the reliability and validity of two novel thoracolumbar injury classification systems. *Spine (Phila Pa 1976)* 2007;32(7):791-795.

11. Aebi M: Classification of thoracolumbar fractures and dislocations. *Eur Spine J* 2010;19(suppl 1):S2-S7.

    This comprehensive review of the existent thoracolumbar fractures classification systems placed a special focus on the AO-Spine Group classification system. Level of evidence: III.

12. McCormack T, Karaikovic E, Gaines RW: The load sharing classification of spine fractures. *Spine (Phila Pa 1976)* 1994;19(15):1741-1744.

13. Chhabra HS, Kaul R, Kanagaraju V: Do we have an ideal classification system for thoracolumbar and subaxial cervical spine injuries: What is the expert's perspective? *Spinal Cord* 2015;53(1):42-48.

    Data collected from online questionnaire surveys were used to review the experts' opinions on the availability of practical and useful classification systems for the different types of spine injuries. Level of evidence: V.

14. Magerl F, Aebi M, Gertzbein SD, Harms J, Nazarian S: A comprehensive classification of thoracic and lumbar injuries. *Eur Spine J* 1994;3(4):184-201.

15. Vaccaro AR, Lehman RA Jr, Hurlbert RJ, et al: A new classification of thoracolumbar injuries: The importance of injury morphology, the integrity of the posterior ligamentous complex, and neurologic status. *Spine (Phila Pa 1976)* 2005;30(20):2325-2333.

16. Oner FC, Wood KB, Smith JS, Shaffrey CI: Therapeutic decision making in thoracolumbar spine trauma. *Spine (Phila Pa 1976)* 2010;35(21suppl):S235-S244.

    A comprehensive search was conducted of the published systematic reviews in English. Standardized grading systems were used to assess the level of evidence and the quality of articles affecting decision making in thoracolumbar spine trauma. Level of evidence: I.

17. Maynard FM Jr, Bracken MB, Creasey G, et al; American Spinal Injury Association: International Standards for Neurological and Functional Classification of Spinal Cord Injury. *Spinal Cord* 1997;35(5):266-274.

18. Anderson S, Biros MH, Reardon RF: Delayed diagnosis of thoracolumbar fractures in multiple-trauma patients. *Acad Emerg Med* 1996;3(9):832-839.

19. Todd NV: Priapism in acute spinal cord injury. *Spinal Cord* 2011;49(10):1033-1035.

    This prospective literature review examined the presence of priapism in complete motor and sensory spinal cord injuries. Level of evidence: III.

20. Terregino CA, Ross SE, Lipinski MF, Foreman J, Hughes R: Selective indications for thoracic and lumbar radiography in blunt trauma. *Ann Emerg Med* 1995;26(2):126-129.

21. Hauser CJ, Visvikis G, Hinrichs C, et al: Prospective validation of computed tomographic screening of the thoracolumbar spine in trauma. *J Trauma* 2003;55(2):228-234, discussion 234-235.

22. Chang CH, Holmes JF, Mower WR, Panacek EA: Distracting injuries in patients with vertebral injuries. *J Emerg Med* 2005;28(2):147-152.

23. Schweitzer KM, Vaccaro AR, Harrop JS, et al: Interrater reliability of identifying indicators of posterior ligamentous complex disruption when plain films are indeterminate in thoracolumbar injuries. *J Orthop Sci* 2007;12(5):437-442.

24. Vaccaro AR, Rihn JA, Saravanja D, et al: Injury of the posterior ligamentous complex of the thoracolumbar spine: A prospective evaluation of the diagnostic accuracy of magnetic resonance imaging. *Spine (Phila Pa 1976)* 2009;34(23):E841-E847.

25. Wood K, Buttermann G, Mehbod A, Garvey T, Jhanjee R, Sechriest V: Operative compared with nonoperative treatment of a thoracolumbar burst fracture without neurological deficit. A prospective, randomized study. *J Bone Joint Surg Am* 2003;85-A(5):773-781.

26. Mehta JS, Reed MR, McVie JL, Sanderson PL: Weight-bearing radiographs in thoracolumbar fractures: Do they influence management? *Spine (Phila Pa 1976)* 2004;29(5):564-567.

27. Genant HK, Cooper C, Poor G, et al: Interim report and recommendations of the World Health Organization Task-Force for Osteoporosis. *Osteoporos Int* 1999;10(4):259-264.

28. Schwab F, Lafage V, Patel A, Farcy JP: Sagittal plane considerations and the pelvis in the adult patient. *Spine (Phila Pa 1976)* 2009;34(17):1828-1833.

29. Kim HJ, Yi JM, Cho HG, et al: Comparative study of the treatment outcomes of osteoporotic compression fractures without neurologic injury using a rigid brace, a soft brace, and no brace: A prospective randomized controlled non-inferiority trial. *J Bone Joint Surg Am* 2014;96(23):1959-1966.

    This study reported equal benefits of different nonsurgical managements of osteoporotic compression fractures, with and without the use of bracing. Level of evidence: I.

30. McGraw JK, Cardella J, Barr JD, et al; Society of Interventional Radiology Standards of Practice Committee: Society of Interventional Radiology quality improvement guidelines for percutaneous vertebroplasty. *J Vasc Interv Radiol* 2003;14(9 Pt 2):S311-S315.

31. Lee JS, Kim KW, Ha KY: The effect of vertebroplasty on pulmonary function in patients with osteoporotic compression fractures of the thoracic spine. *J Spinal Disord Tech* 2011;24(2):E11-E15.

    This prospective study looked at the effect of vertebroplasty in treating osteoporotic fractures and reported improvement in pulmonary functions and back pain scores. Level of evidence: III.

32. Buchbinder R, Osborne RH, Ebeling PR, et al: A randomized trial of vertebroplasty for painful osteoporotic vertebral fractures. *N Engl J Med* 2009;361(6):557-568.

33. Kallmes DF, Comstock BA, Heagerty PJ, et al: A randomized trial of vertebroplasty for osteoporotic spinal fractures. *N Engl J Med* 2009;361(6):569-579.

34. Luo J, Bertram W, Sangar D, Adams MA, Annesley-Williams DJ, Dolan P: Is kyphoplasty better than vertebroplasty in restoring normal mechanical function to an injured spine? *Bone* 2010;46(4):1050-1057.

    This cadaver study showed an equal effectiveness of vertebroplasty and kyphoplasty in restoring mechanical function of the injured spine. It also reported the superiority of kyphoplasty in vertebral wedging correction. Level of evidence: V.

35. Wardlaw D, Cummings SR, Van Meirhaeghe J, et al: Efficacy and safety of balloon kyphoplasty compared with non-surgical care for vertebral compression

fracture (FREE): A randomised controlled trial. *Lancet* 2009;373(9668):1016-1024.

36. Lee MJ, Dumonski M, Cahill P, Stanley T, Park D, Singh K: Percutaneous treatment of vertebral compression fractures: A meta-analysis of complications. *Spine (Phila Pa 1976)* 2009;34(11):1228-1232.

37. Robinson Y, Heyde CE, Försth P, Olerud C: Kyphoplasty in osteoporotic vertebral compression fractures—guidelines and technical considerations. *J Orthop Surg Res* 2011;6:43.

    The indications, limitations, and technical considerations of kyphoplasty in the treatment of vertebral compression fractures are discussed in detail. Level of evidence: V.

38. American Academy of Orthopaedic Surgeons: The Treatment of Symptomatic Osteoporotic Spinal Compression Fractures – Guideline and Evidence Report. Rosemont, IL, American Academy of Orthopaedic Surgeons September 2010. http://www.aaos.org/research/guidelines/SCFguideline.pdf.

39. Mumford J, Weinstein JN, Spratt KF, Goel VK: Thoracolumbar burst fractures. The clinical efficacy and outcome of nonoperative management. *Spine (Phila Pa 1976)* 1993;18(8):955-970.

40. Cantor JB, Lebwohl NH, Garvey T, Eismont FJ: Nonoperative management of stable thoracolumbar burst fractures with early ambulation and bracing. *Spine (Phila Pa 1976)* 1993;18(8):971-976.

41. Shen WJ, Shen YS: Nonsurgical treatment of three-column thoracolumbar junction burst fractures without neurologic deficit. *Spine (Phila Pa 1976)* 1999;24(4):412-415.

42. Gnanenthiran SR, Adie S, Harris IA: Nonoperative versus operative treatment for thoracolumbar burst fractures without neurologic deficit: A meta-analysis. *Clin Orthop Relat Res* 2012;470(2):567-577.

    This meta-analysis compared the clinical, functional, and radiographic outcomes as well as the complication rates and health costs of the surgical and nonsurgical management of thoracolumbar burst fractures. Level of evidence: II.

43. Wood KB, Buttermann GR, Phukan R, et al: Operative compared with nonoperative treatment of a thoracolumbar burst fracture without neurological deficit: A prospective randomized study with follow-up at sixteen to twenty-two years. *J Bone Joint Surg Am* 2015;97(1):3-9.

    This long-term follow-up study highlights the superiority of nonsurgical treatment as measured by pain and functional improvement in patients with stable burst fractures. Level of evidence: I.

44. Siebenga J, Leferink VJ, Segers MJ, et al: Treatment of traumatic thoracolumbar spine fractures: A multicenter prospective randomized study of operative versus nonsurgical treatment. *Spine (Phila Pa 1976)* 2006;31(25):2881-2890.

45. Bailey CS, Dvorak MF, Thomas KC, et al: Comparison of thoracolumbosacral orthosis and no orthosis for the treatment of thoracolumbar burst fractures: Interim analysis of a multicenter randomized clinical equivalence trial. *J Neurosurg Spine* 2009;11(3):295-303.

46. Ivancic PC: Biomechanics of thoracolumbar burst and Chance-type fractures during fall from height. *Global Spine J* 2014;4(3):161-168.

    This article reports the results of an in vitro investigation of the biomechanics of thoracolumbar burst and Chance-type fractures following a fall from a height. Level of evidence: V.

47. Hasankhani EG, Omidi-Kashani F: Posterior tension band wiring and instrumentation for thoracolumbar flexion-distraction injuries. *J Orthop Surg (Hong Kong)* 2014;22(1):88-91.

    This study reports good outcomes in patients with flexion distraction injuries treated with tension band wiring followed by posterior spinal fusion with instrumentation. Level of evidence: IV.

48. Rajasekaran S: Thoracolumbar burst fractures without neurological deficit: The role for treatment. *Eur Spine J* 2010;19(suppl 1):S40-S47.

    This article reports the results of a literature review highlighting the outcomes of the nonsurgical management of thoracolumbar burst fractures. Level of evidence: V.

49. Karargyris O, Morassi L, Zafeiris C, Evangelopoulos D, Pneumaticos S: The unusual chance fracture: Case report & literature review. *Open Orthop J* 2013;7:301-303.

    This case report discusses an unrestrained driver who sustained a Chance-type injury to the thoracolumbar spine. Level of evidence: V.

50. Sasso RC, Renkens K, Hanson D, Reilly T, McGuire RA Jr, Best NM: Unstable thoracolumbar burst fractures: Anterior-only versus short-segment posterior fixation. *J Spinal Disord Tech* 2006;19(4):242-248.

51. Alanay A, Acaroglu E, Yazici M, Oznur A, Surat A: Short-segment pedicle instrumentation of thoracolumbar burst fractures: Does transpedicular intracorporeal grafting prevent early failure? *Spine (Phila Pa 1976)* 2001;26(2):213-217.

52. Grossbach AJ, Dahdaleh NS, Abel TJ, Woods GD, Dlouhy BJ, Hitchon PW: Flexion-distraction injuries of the thoracolumbar spine: Open fusion versus percutaneous pedicle screw fixation. *Neurosurg Focus* 2013;35(2):E2.

    This prospective study compared percutaneous fixation with open techniques in treating flexion distraction injuries. It reported equivalent American Spinal Injury Association scores and kyphosis correction for both techniques, along with trends toward shorter surgical times with less blood loss using percutaneous fixation. Level of evidence: III.

53. Vaccaro AR, Lim MR, Hurlbert RJ, et al; Spine Trauma Study Group: Surgical decision making for unstable thoracolumbar spine injuries: Results of a consensus panel review by the Spine Trauma Study Group. *J Spinal Disord Tech* 2006;19(1):1-10.

54. Verlaan JJ, Diekerhof CH, Buskens E, et al: Surgical treatment of traumatic fractures of the thoracic and lumbar spine: A systematic review of the literature on techniques, complications, and outcome. *Spine (Phila Pa 1976)* 2004;29(7):803-814.

55. Acosta FL Jr, Aryan HE, Taylor WR, Ames CP: Kyphoplasty-augmented short-segment pedicle screw fixation of traumatic lumbar burst fractures: Initial clinical experience and literature review. *Neurosurg Focus* 2005;18(3):e9.

56. Wood KB, Bohn D, Mehbod A: Anterior versus posterior treatment of stable thoracolumbar burst fractures without neurologic deficit: A prospective, randomized study. *J Spinal Disord Tech* 2005;(18 suppl):S15-S23.

57. Korovessis P, Baikousis A, Zacharatos S, Petsinis G, Koureas G, Iliopoulos P: Combined anterior plus posterior stabilization versus posterior short-segment instrumentation and fusion for mid-lumbar (L2-L4) burst fractures. *Spine (Phila Pa 1976)* 2006;31(8):859-868.

58. Blondel B, Fuentes S, Metellus P, Adetchessi T, Pech-Gourg G, Dufour H: Severe thoracolumbar osteoporotic burst fractures: Treatment combining open kyphoplasty and short-segment fixation. *Orthop Traumatol Surg Res* 2009;95(5):359-364.

59. Toyone T, Tanaka T, Kato D, Kaneyama R, Otsuka M: The treatment of acute thoracolumbar burst fractures with transpedicular intracorporeal hydroxyapatite grafting following indirect reduction and pedicle screw fixation: A prospective study. *Spine (Phila Pa 1976)* 2006;31(7):E208-E214.

60. Sasani M, Ozer AF: Single-stage posterior corpectomy and expandable cage placement for treatment of thoracic or lumbar burst fractures. *Spine (Phila Pa 1976)* 2009;34(1):E33-E40.

61. Fehlings MG, Perrin RG: The timing of surgical intervention in the treatment of spinal cord injury: A systematic review of recent clinical evidence. *Spine (Phila Pa 1976)* 2006;31(11suppl):S28-S35, discussion S36.

62. Westerveld LA, Verlaan JJ, Oner FC: Spinal fractures in patients with ankylosing spinal disorders: A systematic review of the literature on treatment, neurological status and complications. *Eur Spine J* 2009;18(2):145-156.

63. Mathews M, Bolesta MJ: Treatment of spinal fractures in ankylosing spondylitis. *Orthopedics* 2013;36(9):e1203-e1208.

This article discussed a case series of 11 patients with ankylosing spondylitis treated for spinal fractures. Clinical data, treatment modalities, and outcomes were reviewed. Level of evidence: IV.

64. Whang PG, Goldberg G, Lawrence JP, et al: The management of spinal injuries in patients with ankylosing spondylitis or diffuse idiopathic skeletal hyperostosis: A comparison of treatment methods and clinical outcomes. *J Spinal Disord Tech* 2009;22(2):77-85.

65. Westerveld LA, van Bemmel JC, Dhert WJ, Oner FC, Verlaan JJ: Clinical outcome after traumatic spinal fractures in patients with ankylosing spinal disorders compared with control patients. *Spine J* 2014;14(5):729-740.

This retrospective cohort study compared the neurologic deficits, morbidities, and mortalities following spinal injuries in patients having an ankylosed spine with those of a control group. Level of evidence: III.

66. Chaudhary SB, Hullinger H, Vives MJ: Management of acute spinal fractures in ankylosing spondylitis. *ISRN Rheumatol* 2011;2011:150484.

This article reports the results of a review study highlighting the mechanism of injury, treatment considerations, and surgical management of spine fractures in ankylosing spondylitis. Level of evidence: V.

67. Kiltz U, Sieper J, Braun J: Development of morbidity and mortality in patients with spondyloarthritis. *Z Rheumatol* 2011;70(6):473-479.

This paper reviewed the course of illness in patients with ankylosing spondylitis and associated morbidities including cardiovascular disease and spine fragility. Level of evidence: V.

68. Yeoh D, Moffatt T, Karmani S: Good outcomes of percutaneous fixation of spinal fractures in ankylosing spinal disorders. *Injury* 2014;45(10):1534-1538.

This article reports the results of a retrospective review of 10 patients with an ankylosed injured spine who were treated with percutaneous fixation with good outcomes. Level of evidence: IV.

69. Krüger A, Frink M, Oberkircher L, El-Zayat BF, Ruchholtz S, Lechler P: Percutaneous dorsal instrumentation for thoracolumbar extension-distraction fractures in patients with ankylosing spinal disorders: A case series. *Spine J* 2014;14(12):2897-2904.

This paper examines a case series of 10 patients with an ankylosed spine who were treated with percutaneous fixation for spinal extension distraction fractures with good outcomes. Level of evidence: IV.

70. Street JT, Noonan VK, Cheung A, Fisher CG, Dvorak MF: Incidence of acute care adverse events and long-term health-related quality of life in patients with TSCI. *Spine J* 2015;15(5):923-932.

This prospective cohort study of patients with traumatic spinal cord injury highlighted the associated adverse events and their effects on the duration of the hospital stay and the health-related quality of life. Level of evidence: II.

71. Rampersaud YR, Annand N, Dekutoski MB: Use of minimally invasive surgical techniques in the management of thoracolumbar trauma: Current concepts. *Spine (Phila Pa 1976)* 2006;31(11suppl):S96-S102, discussion S104.

72. Kim DH, Jahng TA, Balabhadra RS, Potulski M, Beisse R: Thoracoscopic transdiaphragmatic approach to thoracolumbar junction fractures. *Spine J* 2004;4(3):317-328.

73. Khoo LT, Beisse R, Potulski M: Thoracoscopic-assisted treatment of thoracic and lumbar fractures: A series of 371 consecutive cases. *Neurosurgery* 2002;51(5suppl):S104-S117.

74. Oh T, Scheer JK, Fakurnejad S, Dahdaleh NS, Smith ZA: Minimally invasive spinal surgery for the treatment of traumatic thoracolumbar burst fractures. *J Clin Neurosci* 2015;22(1):42-47.

    This systematic review suggests a low level of evidence for minimally invasive surgery in the treatment of thoracolumbar fractures. Level of evidence: II.

75. Lee MC, Coert, B.A., Kim, S.H., Kim, D.H.: Endoscopic techniques for stabilization of the thoracic spine, in Vaccaro AR, Bono CM, eds: *Minimally Invasive Spine Surgery* .Boca Raton, FL; CRC Press, 2007, pp 189-202.

76. Gandhoke GS, Tempel ZJ, Bonfield CM, Madhok R, Okonkwo DO, Kanter AS: Technical nuances of the minimally invasive extreme lateral approach to treat thoracolumbar burst fractures. *Eur Spine J* 2015;24(suppl 3):353-360.

    The authors report their experience, emphasizing the value of the extreme lateral approach as an effective surgical option for the management of thoracolumbar burst fractures. Level of evidence: V.

77. Palmisani M, Gasbarrini A, Brodano GB, et al: Minimally invasive percutaneous fixation in the treatment of thoracic and lumbar spine fractures. *Eur Spine J* 2009;18(suppl 1):71-74.

78. Wild MH, Glees M, Plieschnegger C, Wenda K: Five-year follow-up examination after purely minimally invasive posterior stabilization of thoracolumbar fractures: A comparison of minimally invasive percutaneously and conventionally open treated patients. *Arch Orthop Trauma Surg* 2007;127(5):335-343.

79. Logroscino CA, Proietti L, Tamburrelli FC: Minimally invasive spine stabilisation with long implants. *Eur Spine J* 2009;18(suppl 1):75-81.

80. Wang ST, Ma HL, Liu CL, Yu WK, Chang MC, Chen TH: Is fusion necessary for surgically treated burst fractures of the thoracolumbar and lumbar spine?: A prospective, randomized study. *Spine (Phila Pa 1976)* 2006;31(23):2646-2652, discussion 2653.

81. Blondel B, Fuentes S, Pech-Gourg G, Adetchessi T, Tropiano P, Dufour H: Percutaneous management of thoracolumbar burst fractures: Evolution of techniques and strategy. *Orthop Traumatol Surg Res* 2011;97(5):527-532.

    This retrospective study of 29 patients treated with balloon kyphoplasty and percutaneous fixation with good outcomes supports the value of minimally invasive techniques in treating spinal injuries without neurologic deficit. Level of evidence: IV.

82. Assaker R: Minimal access spinal technologies: State-of-the-art, indications, and techniques. *Joint Bone Spine* 2004;71(6):459-469.

83. Kirkpatrick JS: Thoracolumbar fracture management: Anterior approach. *J Am Acad Orthop Surg* 2003;11(5):355-363.

84. Marco RA, Meyer BC, Kushwaha VP: Thoracolumbar burst fractures treated with posterior decompression and pedicle screw instrumentation supplemented with balloon-assisted vertebroplasty and calcium phosphate reconstruction. Surgical technique. *J Bone Joint Surg Am* 2010;92(suppl 1 Pt 1):67-76.

    This study looked at a series of 38 patients with unstable burst fractures treated with decompression, pedicle screw fixation, and kyphoplasty with good overall outcomes. Level of evidence: IV.

85. Oner FC, Verlaan JJ, Verbout AJ, Dhert WJ: Cement augmentation techniques in traumatic thoracolumbar spine fractures. *Spine (Phila Pa 1976)* 2006;31(11suppl):S89-S95, discussion S104.

Section 6

Lower Extremity

SECTION EDITOR

Kyle J. Jeray, MD

Chapter 36

Hip Dislocations and Femoral Head Fractures

Brian Mullis, MD Christopher A. DeFalco, MD

Abstract

Hip dislocations not associated with a fracture can be managed routinely by closed reduction if a concentric reduction can be achieved. Associated fractures such as femoral head fractures can complicate the management and the outcomes. If a concentric reduction can be achieved, Pipkin type I femoral head fractures typically are treated by closed means, but Pipkin type II femoral head fractures usually require surgical intervention. Percutaneous or arthroscopic removal of loose bodies is a good alternative to the standard approaches. Although percutaneous and arthroscopic fixation of femoral head fractures have been described, more reliable reduction and fixation can be achieved through a standard anterior or posterior approach to the hip, especially if a trochanteric flip osteotomy is used with a posterior approach.

Keywords: hip dislocation; femoral head fracture; Pipkin; loose bodies; trochanteric flip osteotomy; osteonecrosis

Introduction

Traumatic hip dislocations are relatively high-energy injuries that often are associated with other injuries. Simple hip dislocation refers to an isolated hip dislocation without an associated fracture such as a fracture of the acetabulum, femoral head, or femoral neck. Although these fractures can be treated by closed reduction, an incongruent reduction is an absolute indication for surgical intervention. This type of surgery routinely is done through an anterior or posterior approach to the hip, but recent evidence shows that percutaneous[1] or arthroscopic[2-4] intervention may play a role in removing loose bodies and even in fixing associated femoral head fractures.[5,6] Complex hip dislocation refers to a hip dislocation having an associated fracture, which usually is a fracture of the acetabulum, but also can be a femoral neck or femoral head fracture.

Femoral head fractures are associated with hip dislocations in 10% to 15% of cases.[7,8] The most common classification system used to describe femoral head fractures is the Pipkin classification, which helps inform treatment decisions, but does not predict the prognosis[9] (**Figure 1**). Pipkin type I fractures typically are treated by closed reduction alone if a congruent joint can be restored, but surgical intervention for these injuries might be considered even in the setting of a congruent reduction.[3,10] Pipkin type II fractures usually are fixed through an anterior or posterior approach using bioabsorbable or standard screws. A trochanteric flip osteotomy should be considered with a posterior approach, because such an approach allows a better exposure and reduction and may reduce operating room time and blood loss.[11] If fixation cannot be achieved, mosaicplasty with fragment excision may be considered as an alternative.[12]

Hip Dislocations

Traumatic hip dislocations are high-energy injuries and are associated with other musculoskeletal and systemic injuries in up to 75% of cases.[13] These injuries typically occur in young patients and pose a high risk for post-traumatic arthritis. This risk can be as high as 26% for

Dr. Mullis or an immediate family member is a member of a speakers' bureau or has made paid presentations on behalf of Biomet, serves as a paid consultant to Biomet, and serves as a board member, owner, officer, or committee member of the Orthopaedic Trauma Association. Neither Dr. DeFalco nor any immediate family member has received anything of value from or has stock or stock options held in a commercial company or institution related directly or indirectly to the subject of this chapter.

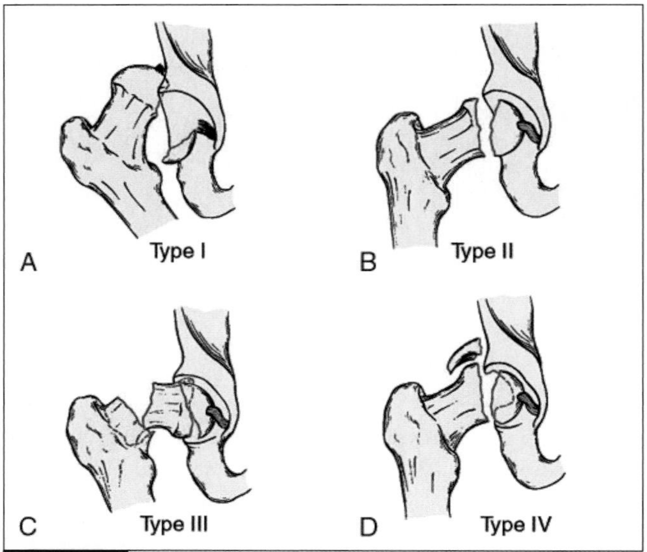

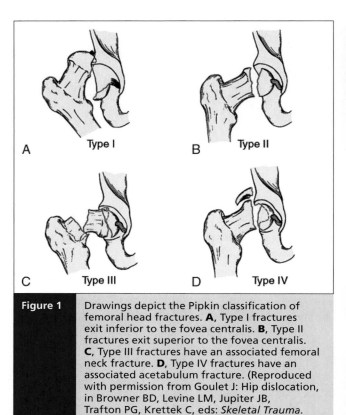

Figure 1 Drawings depict the Pipkin classification of femoral head fractures. **A**, Type I fractures exit inferior to the fovea centralis. **B**, Type II fractures exit superior to the fovea centralis. **C**, Type III fractures have an associated femoral neck fracture. **D**, Type IV fractures have an associated acetabulum fracture. (Reproduced with permission from Goulet J: Hip dislocation, in Browner BD, Levine LM, Jupiter JB, Trafton PG, Krettek C, eds: *Skeletal Trauma*. Philadelphia, PA, WB Saunders, 1994, pp 1575-1596.)

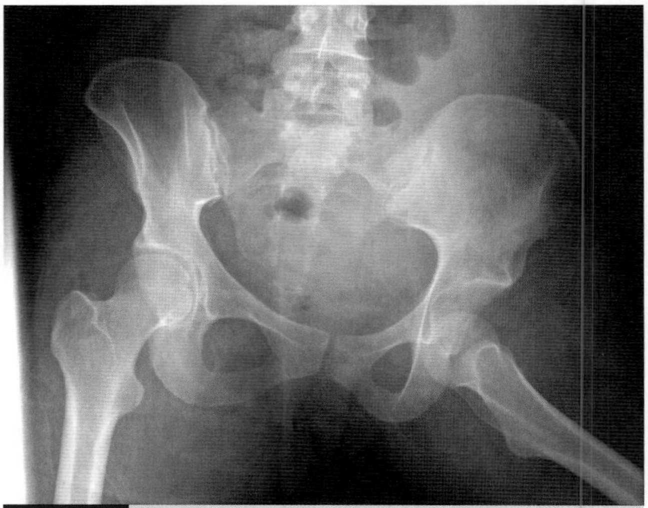

Figure 2 AP pelvis radiograph shows an anterior hip dislocation. Note the typical abducted and externally rotated position, with the obvious deformity of the left hip.

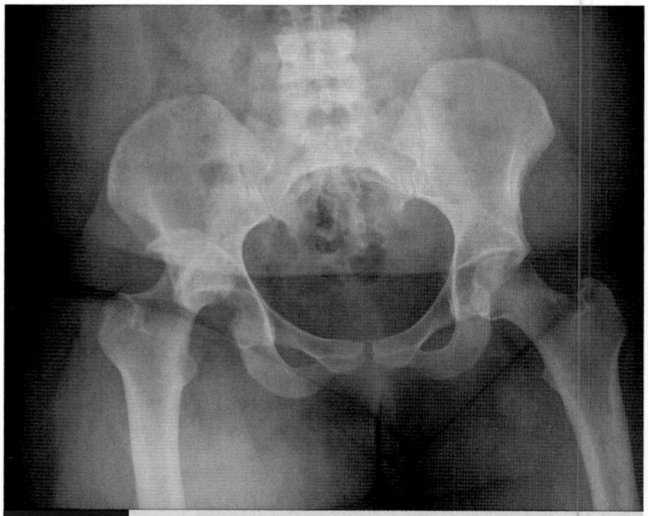

Figure 3 AP pelvis radiograph shows a posterior hip dislocation with an associated posterior wall acetabulum fracture. Note the typical adducted and shortened radiographic appearance that corresponds with the clinical presentation.

simple dislocations and can rise up to 90% for complex fracture-dislocations.[14] The most common description of hip dislocations divides them into anterior or posterior dislocations. Anterior dislocations are less common, with an incidence of approximately 10%, and can be further subclassified as obturator, pubic, or iliac dislocations, depending on where the femoral head is positioned when seen on an AP pelvis radiograph[15,16] (**Figure 2**).

An anterior hip dislocation typically occurs as an abduction and external rotation injury, which is more common in motorcycle or industrial injuries. The mechanism of action for posterior hip dislocations is typically an axial load through a flexed hip and knee, commonly known as a dashboard injury (**Figure 3**).

A hip dislocation is a surgical emergency, because the blood supply to the femoral head is placed at risk. It is believed that the longer the hip is dislocated, the higher the risk for osteonecrosis, although this assumption has been difficult to quantify or prove.[17] Most surgeons still would attempt an urgent reduction in the emergency department with the patient under deep sedation; however, some authors advocate that reduction should not be attempted unless complete paralysis has been achieved, which may require a delay in reduction while awaiting operating room availability.

After reduction has been achieved, an AP pelvis radiograph should be obtained to evaluate for a concentric reduction. Because it is more sensitive than plain radiographs, CT should be obtained to evaluate for loose bodies; however, loose bodies still can be missed even by CT, although this omission may be more common in complex fracture-dislocations.[3] In a series of 117 patients with simple dislocations, a 2011 study found that 12 patients

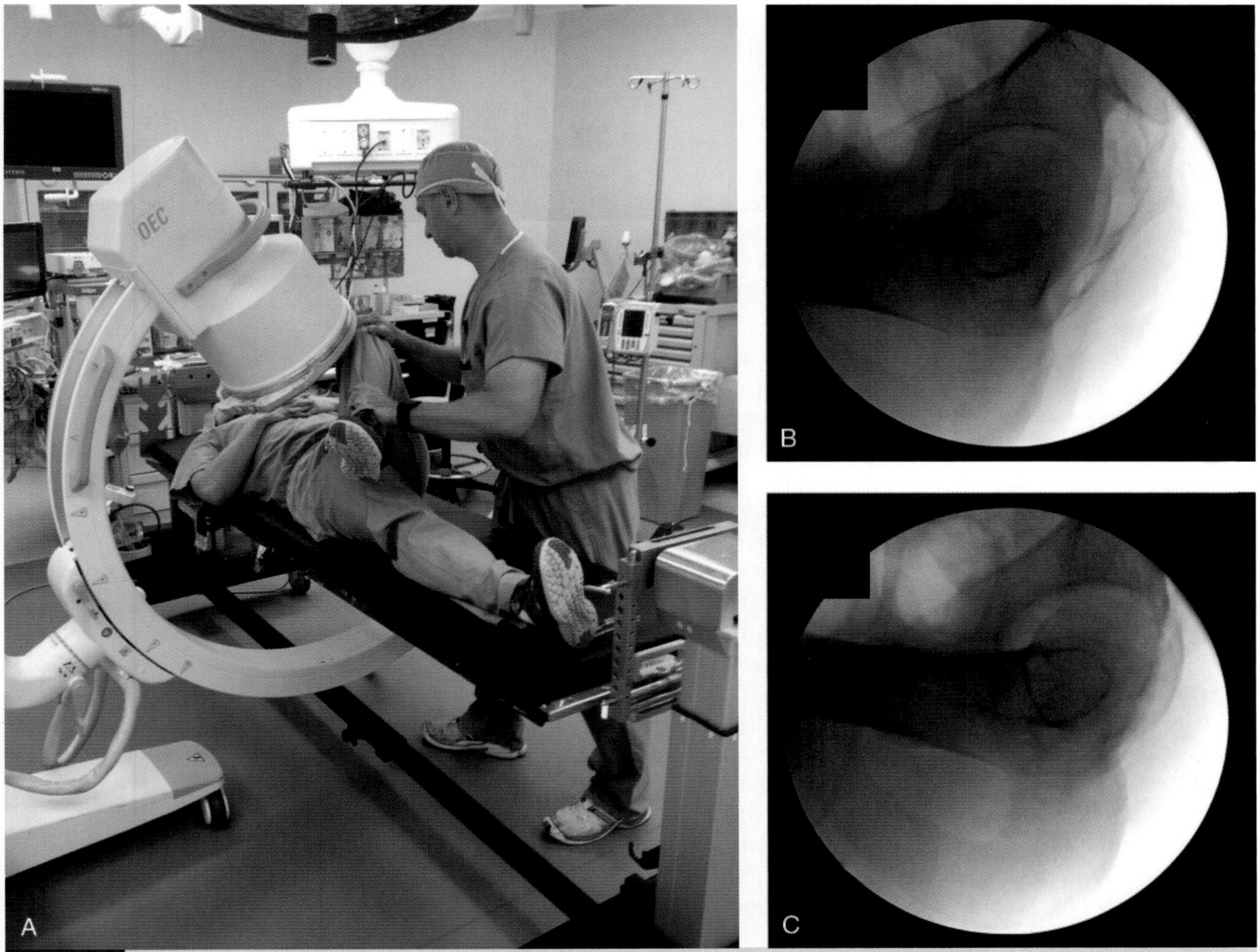

Figure 4 Images show stability testing with stress views for a complex dislocation typically associated with a posterior wall fracture. Clinical photograph (**A**) demonstrates the positioning of the surgeon, the patient, the fluoroscope, and the adducted, flexed, internally rotated, and axially loaded hip. Fluoroscopic stress views show a concentric reduction (**B**) and a nonconcentric reduction (**C**).

(10%) had loose bodies present.[18] In addition to plain radiographs and CT, the authors recommended performing a dynamic study under fluoroscopy to help determine incongruency. If loose bodies are present, percutaneous or arthroscopic removal may be an option. The authors of a 2014 study described a percutaneous technique in which the joint is "swept" under fluoroscopic guidance to remove loose bodies.[1] Early hip arthroscopy also has been described but may not be familiar to most orthopaedic trauma surgeons.[3] Delayed hip arthroscopy is indicated for patients with mechanical symptoms following closed reduction, because the cause typically is found to be loose bodies and labral tears, which may improve following arthroscopic treatment.[4]

For simple dislocations, stability testing with stress views typically is not indicated. For complex dislocations usually associated with posterior wall fractures, stress testing can be helpful in determining whether surgery is indicated to fix the posterior wall. Generally, posterior wall fractures greater than 40% require surgery, wall fractures between 20% and 40% may benefit from stress testing to determine if surgery is indicated, and wall fractures less than 20% typically are stable; although some authors still would advocate for routine stress testing to rule out instability. Stress testing is performed with the patient supine under a general anesthetic, with flexion, internal rotation, adduction, and axial load of the hip. In general, it is easier to use an obturator oblique fluoroscopic view during this test to clear the knee from the fluoroscopy machine while performing the test (**Figure 4**).

It remains difficult to predict which patients have the highest risk for osteonecrosis following hip dislocation.

Studies evaluating single-photon emission CT and MRI following hip dislocation were unable to correlate findings with the risk for osteonecrosis.[17,19] It appears that a posterior hip approach with a trochanteric osteotomy, often referred to as a surgical hip dislocation, is safe to perform in adolescents who require an open approach. A 2015 study of 11 patients with an average age of 12 years and an average follow-up of 2 years found that osteonecrosis had developed in none of the patients following surgical hip dislocations for traumatic hip dislocations requiring surgery.[20]

Osteonecrosis rates for posterior dislocations are reported to be less than 6% in those with no fracture or associated with a simple posterior wall. In patients sustaining posterior dislocations with more complex acetabular fractures, osteonecrosis rates up to 50% were noted.[21,22] Osteonecrosis has been observed to occur as long as 5 years from the initial injury; however, it usually is seen within 2 years.[23] Thus, it is important to follow these patients with continued imaging. The time that elapses between injury and reduction has a considerable effect on the outcome. Femoral head necrosis was seen at a rate of 18% when reduced within 12 hours of the injury but was observed at a rate of 57% when reduced after 12 hours postinjury.[23] Anterior dislocations with femoral head fractures have been found to have a better long-term prognosis when compared with posterior dislocations with femoral head fractures.[24-26] In one study, only 25% of the anterior dislocations had fair results, compared with more than 50% of those in the posterior group.

Posttraumatic arthritis of the hip joint is a fairly common complication that is usually evident within 5 years of the index injury.[24,27,28] The incidence of posttraumatic osteoarthritis increases from 16% to 88% if the dislocation is associated with severe concomitant fractures of the femoral head or the acetabulum.[28]

Sciatic nerve injury is another complication associated with posterior hip dislocations. The cumulative incidence of injury reported in the literature is 10%. In 60% to 70% of these patients, at least partial recovery of nerve function occurs.[29] The likelihood of a major motor deficit is higher in delayed reductions, however.[30] Recurrent dislocations following an anterior or posterior dislocation are rare. In 264 traumatic dislocations, only 4 cases of redislocation were reported.[23] In an early review of the literature, only 11 cases with recurrent dislocations were found.[31]

After ensuring that concentric reduction has been achieved, it is important to begin early mobilization and passive range of motion of the hip to prevent intra-articular adhesions and arthritis. Extremes of motion should be delayed for 4 to 6 weeks to allow capsular and soft-tissue healing.[32] Controversy still exists over weight-bearing status following reduction. Many surgeons allow immediate weight bearing as tolerated. If the patient is at increased risk for osteonecrosis because of a delay to reduction of greater than 6 hours, however, some surgeons recommend waiting 8 to 12 weeks before permitting weight bearing. The rationale behind this is that the amount of collapse may be diminished in those in whom osteonecrosis does develop.[33]

Femoral Head Fractures

Approximately 10% to 15% of hip dislocations are associated with femoral head fractures.[8,34] Pipkin type II fractures appear to occur two to three times more frequently than Pipkin type I fractures[11,34] and usually require surgery, because the fracture line in Pipkin type II fractures extends superior to the fovea centralis. In Pipkin type III injuries, the femoral head fracture is associated with a fracture of the femoral neck. A type IV injury is associated with a fracture of the acetabulum.

The initial treatment is the same as isolated hip dislocations, with emergent reduction of the dislocation being a priority. Some would advocate Pipkin III injuries should always be reduced in the surgical suite under a general anesthetic to prevent further displacement of the femoral neck fracture, but this should be weighed against any delay needed to perform in the surgical suite versus immediately in the emergency department. Plain films and CT should be performed following the reduction just as with simple hip dislocations.

A 2011 study randomized 16 patients in China with Pipkin type I fractures to open treatment with fragment excision or closed reduction and skeletal traction for 6 weeks. This small series showed better outcomes with surgery, but it is difficult to draw conclusions from the study given the prolonged traction that typically would not be done in North American centers.[10] This group also conducted a small randomized study of 24 patients with Pipkin type II fractures that compared surgical treatment using an anterior approach with closed reduction and skeletal traction for 6 weeks. The authors found that surgical reduction yielded better outcomes, but the prolonged traction again makes it difficult to extrapolate these findings to North American centers.[8] In a retrospective review of 110 patients with mixed femoral head fracture types I through IV treated by surgery (78 patients) or closed reduction alone (32 patients), the authors could not determine whether surgery was of benefit. The study was notable, however, because 20 patients (in 5 patients this was the primary treatment, 15 patients had secondary surgery within 6 months) required total hip arthroplasty within 6 months of injury.[35] A prospective randomized study compared emergent open surgical reduction and internal fixation with emergent closed reduction followed by delayed open reduction and internal fixation (ORIF). Of all Pipkin type I femoral head fractures involving more than 25% of the femoral head, the authors found a shorter hospital stay in the emergent ORIF group and a higher complication and osteonecrosis rate in the delayed ORIF group.[36] In a retrospective review of 21 patients with a mix of Pipkin type I, II, and IV fractures, 95% (20 patients) had posttraumatic arthritis demonstrated radiographically at an average of 4 years following surgery. Many of these patients still had good to excellent outcomes. ORIF appeared to provide better outcomes than excision of the fragments.[37]

The most common surgical approaches for femoral head fractures are the anterior and posterior approaches, although a medial approach and arthroscopic treatment have been described.[35] The trochanteric flip osteotomy is used routinely with the posterior approach to aid exposure. In one retrospective review comparing the trochanteric flip osteotomy with a standard posterior approach, less operating room time and less blood loss were found with the trochanteric flip osteotomy, but no significant difference was seen in outcomes.[11] Another retrospective review of 23 patients with Pipkin type I and II fractures all treated with trochanteric flip osteotomies showed a low complication rate, with 77% (17 patients) obtaining good to excellent results.[34] Arthroscopic fixation has been described, but few cases were reported, likely because of the difficulty in achieving an anatomic reduction and fixation with an arthroscopic approach and because of the technique's lack of familiarity to most orthopaedic trauma surgeons.[5,6,35]

Although previous studies had advocated against using the anterior approach, because it was believed that any residual blood supply would be damaged, the recent literature has refuted this assertion. A 2009 meta-analysis did show a statistically significant difference in the likelihood of osteonecrosis that was 3.7 times higher when a posterior approach was used when compared to a trochanteric flip osteotomy. A difference was also noted in the estimated incidence of posttraumatic arthritis when comparing the anterior or posterior approaches to the trochanteric flip osteotomy. A 20.3 and 30.6 times higher incidence of posttraumatic arthritis, respectively, was found.[38] For surgical fixation of Pipkin type I and II fractures, a Smith-Petersen approach to the hip allows better visualization of the head, a shorter surgical time, and less blood loss compared with a Kocher-Langenbeck approach.[39] Historically, Pipkin type IV fractures have been fixed through the Kocher-Langenbeck approach; however, a trochanteric flip digastric osteotomy has been used with promising results.[40,41]

Fixation of the small femoral head fragments can be quite difficult. Although 3.5-mm small fragment screws typically can be used and countersunk, even smaller mini-fragment screws, headless screws, or bioabsorbable screws often are needed.[42] Mosaicplasty also has been described as an alternative if ORIF cannot be achieved.[12]

Summary

Treatment of hip dislocations and associated femoral head fractures can be challenging. If a concentric reduction is achieved, many surgeons would advocate for closed treatment of simple hip dislocations and Pipkin type I fractures. Most would agree that ORIF is indicated for Pipkin type II fractures, even in the setting of a concentric reduction, to allow early ambulation and range of motion. Arthroscopic and percutaneous techniques can be employed to definitively treat nonconcentric reductions. A posterior approach with a trochanteric flip osteotomy likely affords the best exposure to facilitate ORIF of femoral head fractures, but other approaches can be considered.

Key Study Points

- A trochanteric flip osteotomy commonly is used for femoral head fractures and may give the best exposure.
- An absolute indication for surgery following the reduction of a simple hip dislocation is a nonconcentric reduction.
- The benefit of performing ORIF for a Pipkin type II femoral head fracture is that it allows early ambulation and range of motion and may reduce the risk of posttraumatic arthritis.

Acknowledgments

The authors would like to thank Dr. Charles Maloy for his assistance in completing this chapter.

Annotated References

1. Marecek GS, Routt ML Jr: Percutaneous manipulation of intra-articular debris after fracture-dislocation of the femoral head or acetabulum. *Orthopedics* 2014;37(9):603-606.

The authors describe a technique for patients with a nonconcentric reduction of the hip secondary to interposed debris between the acetabular dome and femoral head, using fluoroscopy to percutaneously sweep away debris with a right-angled instrument. They present a case series of three patients who underwent the percutaneous manipulation with successful removal of debris with no wound infections or other early complications. Level of evidence: IV.

2. Khanna V, Harris A, Farrokhyar F, Choudur HN, Wong IH: Hip arthroscopy: Prevalence of intra-articular pathologic findings after traumatic injury of the hip. *Arthroscopy* 2014;30(3):299-304.

   Using hip arthroscopy, the authors viewed intra-articular pathologic disorders in 29 patients with posttraumatic hip injuries. Seventeen hips had loose bodies, 11 had intra-articular step deformities, 14 had osteochondral lesions, and 27 had a labral tear. Correlation with plain radiographs and CT for identification of loose bodies and step deformities showed low sensitivity with these tests, whereas MRI/magnetic resonance angiography was noted to be an accurate tool for labral tears (91% of tears on arthroscopy were also identified by MRI/magnetic resonance angiography). MRI/magnetic resonance angiography failed to identify osteochondral lesions identified by arthroscopy in four hips. Level of evidence: IV.

3. Mullis BH, Dahners LE: Hip arthroscopy to remove loose bodies after traumatic dislocation. *J Orthop Trauma* 2006;20(1):22-26.

4. Ilizaliturri VM Jr, Gonzalez-Gutierrez B, Gonzalez-Ugalde H, Camacho-Galindo J: Hip arthroscopy after traumatic hip dislocation. *Am J Sports Med* 2011;39(suppl):50S-57S.

   The authors found that arthroscopy was indicated when loose fragments were present inside the joint and in patients with mechanical hip symptoms. Level of evidence: IV.

5. Park MS, Yoon SJ, Choi SM: Arthroscopic reduction and internal fixation of femoral head fractures. *J Orthop Trauma* 2014;28(7):e164-e168.

   A case series of three patients with displaced large-fragment femoral head fractures (OTA 31-C1.3) using arthroscopic reduction and internal fixation (anterolateral viewing portal, an anterior portal, and an accessory distal anterior working portal) was presented. By 3 months postoperatively all three patients had returned to full function. Level of evidence: IV.

6. Lansford T, Munns SW: Arthroscopic treatment of Pipkin type I femoral head fractures: A report of 2 cases. *J Orthop Trauma* 2012;26(7):e94-e96.

   The authors present two cases of displaced Pipkin type I fractures secondary to posterior hip dislocations treated with arthroscopic excision of the fragment. One patient returned to work and full activity whereas the other returned to work and light activities without pain but has been unable to return to running. Level of evidence: IV.

7. Mullis BH, Anglen JO: Hip Trauma, in Flynn JM, ed: *Orthopaedic Knowledge Update 10* .Rosemont, IL, American Academy of Orthopaedic Surgeons, 2011, pp 49-58.

8. Feng Y, Wang S, Jin D, et al: Free vascularised fibular grafting with OsteoSet®2 demineralised bone matrix versus autograft for large osteonecrotic lesions of the femoral head. *Int Orthop* 2011;35(4):475-481.

   Twenty-four patients (30 hips) with large osteonecrotic lesions of the femoral head (stage IIC in 6 hips, stage IIIC in 14, and stage IVC in 10) underwent free vascularized fibular grafting with OsteoSet2 DMB. This group was retrospectively matched to 24 patients (30 hips) who underwent free vascularized fibular grafting with autologous cancellous bone. After a mean follow-up duration of 26 months, no statistically significant differences between the two groups in overall clinical outcome or radiographic assessment were noted. Also, no adverse events were related to the use of OsteoSet2 DBM. Level of evidence: III.

9. Pipkin G: Treatment of grade IV fracture-dislocation of the hip. *J Bone Joint Surg Am* 1957;39-A(5):1027-1042, passim.

10. Chen ZW, Lin B, Zhai WL, et al: Conservative versus surgical management of Pipkin type I fractures associated with posterior dislocation of the hip: A randomised controlled trial. *Int Orthop* 2011;35(7):1077-1081.

    Sixteen patients with Pipkin type I fractures following posterior hip dislocation (8 treated with closed reduction and surgical excision of fragment, 8 with closed reduction alone) were followed with assessment of functional outcomes using the Thompson and Epstein score and the Merle d'Aubigne and Postel score. Follow-up between 25 to 52 months (39.3 +/- 8.91 months) in the conservative group and 28 to 60 months (39.5 +/- 12.82 months) noted a statistically significant difference with the surgical group reporting better outcomes. Level of evidence: I.

11. Mostafa MF, El-Adl W, El-Sayed MA: Operative treatment of displaced Pipkin type I and II femoral head fractures. *Arch Orthop Trauma Surg* 2014;134(5):637-644.

    A retrospective review of 23 patients with Pipkin I and II fractures treated surgically with Kocher-Langenbeck approach (11 patients) and Ganz trochanteric flip osteotomy (12) with modified Merle d'Aubigne and Postel and Thompson and Epstein scores showing no statistically significant difference in outcome scores. The digastric osteotomy group was associated with less surgical time and less blood loss when compared with the Kocher-Langenbeck group. Level of evidence: III.

12. Gagała J, Tarczyńska M, Gawęda K: Fixation of femoral head fractures with autologous osteochondral transfer (mosaicplasty). *J Orthop Trauma* 2014;28(9):e226-e230.

    A case review is presented of three patients with 31-C1 femoral head fractures treated with trochanteric flip osteotomy followed by osteochondral autologous transfer from the lateral femoral condyle of the ipsilateral knee. Follow-ups of 80 months, 62 months, and 24 months revealed good Harris hip score and Oxford hip scores and

6: Lower Extremity

imaging revealed no evidence of osteonecrosis of the femoral head or heterotopic ossification. Level of evidence: IV.

13. Epstein HC: Traumatic dislocations of the hip. *Clin Orthop Relat Res* 1973;92:116-142.

14. Upadhyay SS, Moulton A: The long-term results of traumatic posterior dislocation of the hip. *J Bone Joint Surg Br* 1981;63B(4):548-551.

15. Foulk DM, Mullis BH: Hip dislocation: Evaluation and management. *J Am Acad Orthop Surg* 2010;18(4):199-209.

    A dislocated hip should be treated with surgery when nonconcentric reduction, associated proximal femur fracture (including hip, femoral neck, and femoral head), and associated acetabular fracture producing instability are present.

16. Bastian JD, Turina M, Siebenrock KA, Keel MJ: Long-term outcome after traumatic anterior dislocation of the hip. *Arch Orthop Trauma Surg* 2011;131(9):1273-1278.

    A retrospective review of anterior traumatic hip dislocations (10 out of 100 hip dislocations) was performed. Four cases had impaction fractures of femoral head and three had fractures of the anterior acetabular wall. Four cases yielded fair Thompson and Epstein clinical outcomes.

17. Yue JJ, Sontich JK, Miron SD, et al: Blood flow changes to the femoral head after acetabular fracture or dislocation in the acute injury and perioperative periods. *J Orthop Trauma* 2001;15(3):170-176.

18. Karthik K, Sundararajan SR, Dheenadhayalan J, Rajasekaran S: Incongruent reduction following post-traumatic hip dislocations as an indicator of intra-articular loose bodies: A prospective study of 117 dislocations. *Indian J Orthop* 2011;45(1):33-38.

    The authors found 12 of 117 reduced hip dislocations to have nonconcentric reduction on radiographs and/or passive range of motion fluoroscopy. Of these 12, 11 were found to have intra-articular loose bodies and 1 had an inverted posterior labrum.

19. Tannast M, Pleus F, Bonel H, Galloway H, Siebenrock KA, Anderson SE: Magnetic resonance imaging in traumatic posterior hip dislocation. *J Orthop Trauma* 2010;24(12):723-731.

    MRI was obtained acutely in 19 traumatic posterior hip dislocations immediately after closed reduction to evaluate integrity of the obturator externus tendon. All 19 were found to have intact tendons and subsequent osteonecrosis of the femoral head had not developed at 3-year follow-up. It was concluded that integrity of the obturator externus implies integrity of the medial femoral circumflex artery.

20. Podeszwa DA, De La Rocha A, Larson AN, Sucato DJ: Surgical hip dislocation is safe and effective following acute traumatic hip instability in the adolescent. *J Pediatr Orthop* 2015;35(5):435-442.

    A retrospective review is presented of 11 patients with nonconcentric reductions following posterior traumatic hip dislocations. Treatment was with transtrochanteric surgical hip dislocations and fixation of osteochondral fractures and/or removal of loose bodies. At follow-up no osteonecrosis was noted and the mean Harris hip score was excellent (95.8 with range of 84.7 to 100). Level of evidence: IV.

21. Hougaard K, Thomsen PB: Coxarthrosis following traumatic posterior dislocation of the hip. *J Bone Joint Surg Am* 1987;69(5):679-683.

22. Dwyer AJ, John B, Singh SA, Mam MK: Complications after posterior dislocation of the hip. *Int Orthop* 2006;30(4):224-227.

23. Brav E: Traumatic dislocation of the hip: Army experience and results over a 12 year period. *J Bone Joint Surg Am* 1962;44(6):1115-1134.

24. Dreinhöfer KE, Schwarzkopf SR, Haas NP, Tscherne H: Isolated traumatic dislocation of the hip. Long-term results in 50 patients. *J Bone Joint Surg Br* 1994;76(1):6-12.

25. DeLee JC, Evans JA, Thomas J: Anterior dislocation of the hip and associated femoral-head fractures. *J Bone Joint Surg Am* 1980;62(6):960-964.

26. Amihood S: Anterior dislocation of the hip. *Injury* 1975;7(2):107-110.

27. Hougaard K, Thomsen PB: Traumatic posterior dislocation of the hip—prognostic factors influencing the incidence of avascular necrosis of the femoral head. *Arch Orthop Trauma Surg* 1986;106(1):32-35.

28. Upadhyay SS, Moulton A, Srikrishnamurthy K: An analysis of the late effects of traumatic posterior dislocation of the hip without fractures. *J Bone Joint Surg Br* 1983;65(2):150-152.

29. Cornwall R, Radomisli TE: Nerve injury in traumatic dislocation of the hip. *Clin Orthop Relat Res* 2000;377:84-91.

30. Hillyard RF, Fox J: Sciatic nerve injuries associated with traumatic posterior hip dislocations. *Am J Emerg Med* 2003;21(7):545-548.

31. Liebenberg F, Dommisse GF: Recurrent post-traumatic dislocation of the hip. *J Bone Joint Surg Br* 1969;51(4):632-637.

32. Tornetta P III, Mostafavi HR: Hip dislocation: Current treatment regimens. *J Am Acad Orthop Surg* 1997;5(1):27-36.

33. Stuck WG, Thompson MS: Treatment of fractures of the forearm with intramedullary pins. *Am J Surg* 1949;77(1):12-18.

34. Lin S, Tian Q, Liu Y, Shao Z, Yang S: Mid- and long-term clinical effects of trochanteric flip osteotomy for treatment of Pipkin I and II femoral head fractures. *Nan Fang Yi Ke Da Xue Xue Bao* 2013;33(9):1260-1264.

In a retrospective review of 23 patients with femoral head fractures and posterior hip dislocation, trochanteric flip osteotomy was found to be an effective and reliable treatment option. Level of evidence: IV.

35. Tonetti J, Ruatti S, Lafontan V, et al: Is femoral head fracture-dislocation management improvable: A retrospective study in 110 cases. *Orthop Traumatol Surg Res* 2010;96(6):623-631.

In a retrospective review of 102 posterior and 8 anterior traumatic hip dislocations, the authors found Chiron grade 3 and femoral neck fractures were significantly predictive for a total hip arthroplasty, whereas the Pipkin classification at the time of injury was not prognostic. Level of evidence: IV.

36. Lin D, Lian K, Chen Z, Wang L, Hao J, Zhang H: Emergent surgical reduction and fixation for Pipkin type I femoral fractures. *Orthopedics* 2013;36(6):778-782.

The authors found that in patients with Pipkin type I fractures with fragments greater than one-fourth of the femoral head, complications and osteonecrosis rates were higher in those treated with secondary surgical fixation after emergent closed reduction versus those treated with emergent surgical reduction and fixation. No differences were noted with blood loss or surgical time; however, the emergent surgical reduction and fixation group had a shorter hospital stay in comparison to the secondary surgical fixation group.

37. Oransky M, Martinelli N, Sanzarello I, Papapietro N: Fractures of the femoral head: A long-term follow-up study. *Musculoskelet Surg* 2012;96(2):95-99.

The authors present a retrospective review of 21 patients with femoral head fractures (four Pipkin type I, nine Pipkin type II, eight Pipkin type IV) and found that 95.2% of patients had radiographic criteria of posttraumatic hip arthritis at average follow-up of 81.19 +/- 37.4 months. Open reduction and internal fixation of fragments provided better functional outcome results according to Thompson-Epstein and Merle d'Aubigne-Postel scores when compared with the excision group. Level of evidence: IV.

38. Giannoudis PV, Kontakis G, Christoforakis Z, Akula M, Tosounidis T, Koutras C: Management, complications and clinical results of femoral head fractures. *Injury* 2009;40(12):1245-1251.

39. Stannard JP, Harris HW, Volgas DA, Alonso JE: Functional outcome of patients with femoral head fractures associated with hip dislocations. *Clin Orthop Relat Res* 2000;377:44-56.

40. Henle P, Kloen P, Siebenrock KA: Femoral head injuries: Which treatment strategy can be recommended? *Injury* 2007;38(4):478-488.

41. Solberg BD, Moon CN, Franco DP: Use of a trochanteric flip osteotomy improves outcomes in Pipkin IV fractures. *Clin Orthop Relat Res* 2009;467(4):929-933.

42. Bassuener SR, Mullis BH, Harrison RK, Sanders R: Use of bioabsorbable pins in surgical fixation of comminuted periarticular fractures. *J Orthop Trauma* 2012;26(10):607-610.

In treating highly comminuted periarticular fractures (OTA C2 and 3), the authors used bioabsorbable pins instead of Kirschner wires or other buried implants to maintain reduction of articular fragments. Two patients were lost to follow-up; however, none of the remaining 78 fractures were found to have a loss of reduction at the articular surface on images obtained 6 weeks after surgery. Seventy-two of 73 fractures with records available at 3 months postoperatively showed stable unchanged articular surfaces (one was treated with a below-knee amputation for worsening infection from Gustilo-Anderson type 3B open pilon fracture. Level of evidence: IV.

Chapter 37

Femoral Neck Fractures in the Younger Patient

Cory Collinge, MD   Hassan Mir, MD, MBA, FACS

Abstract

Displaced femoral neck fractures in healthy young adults are difficult to treat and typically result from high-energy mechanisms causing a vertically oriented fracture through the femoral neck. Complications associated with femoral neck fractures in young patients are frequent and often catastrophic, and include nonunion (often associated with failed fixation), osteonecrosis, and malunion. Several ongoing controversies exist regarding these injuries, including open versus closed reduction, surgical approach, optimal fixation construct, and where the line should be drawn between surgical repair versus replacement.

Keywords: femoral neck; young adult; vertical; Pauwels; Pauwels III; fracture; younger; young patient

Dr. Collinge or an immediate family member has received royalties from Biomet, Smith & Nephew, Advanced Orthopedic Solutions, and Synthes, serves as a paid consultant to Biomet, Stryker, and Smith & Nephew, and serves as a board member, owner, officer, or committee member of the Foundation for Orthopedic Trauma. Dr. Mir or an immediate family member serves as a paid consultant to Acumed and Smith & Nephew, has stock or stock options held in Core Orthopaedics, and serves as a board member, owner, officer, or committee member of the American Academy of Orthopaedic Surgeons Council on Advocacy, the American Academy of Orthopaedic Surgeons Diversity Advisory Board, the FOT Nominating and Membership Committees, and the Orthopaedic Trauma Association PR Committee.

Introduction

The treatment of displaced femoral neck fractures in healthy young adults remains an unsolved challenge in orthopaedic surgery. These injuries typically result from high-energy mechanisms causing a vertically oriented fracture through the femoral neck. Pauwels described this injury and classified these fractures according to the verticality of the fracture, with respect to the injury pattern. The type I Pauwels angle injury is less than 30°, the type II angle is 30° to 50°, and the type III angle greater than 50°[1] (**Figure 1**). These factors contribute to the difficulty of obtaining alignment and construct stability to resist vertical shear forces around the hip, and the risk of complications increases as the fracture's angle of inclination increases, despite several fixation strategies. Complications associated with femoral neck fractures in young patients are frequent (20% to 60%) and often catastrophic, including nonunion (often associated with failed fixation) (**Figure 2**), osteonecrosis, and malunion[2-5] (**Figure 3**). Open versus closed reduction, surgical approach, optimal fixation construct, and where the line should be drawn between surgical repair versus replacement are controversial factors.

Injury Pattern

Pauwels characterized the vertical femoral neck fracture pattern in the young adult more than 80 years ago, and until very recently little had been added to the biomechanical understanding of the injury.[1] The advent of high-quality CT has allowed for a more complete morphologic description (**Figure 1**). A 2014 radiographic study reported further details of fracture orientation and comminution of femoral neck fractures in adults younger than 50 years.[6] The coronal (vertical) fracture angled 60° and the axial fracture plane obliquity averaged 24° with relative deficiency of the posterior neck. Major femoral neck comminution (>1.5 cm) was identified in 96% of cases, with most located in the inferior (94%)

and posterior (84%) neck regions. Nondisplaced fractures and those associated with femur and acetabular injury were excluded because those injuries may present with different morphology. Fracture displacement and deformity in these injuries seem intuitive but do not appear to be discussed at length in the literature. The degree of displacement would seem to be an obvious predictor of complications, but nondisplaced fractures also can lead to similar complications.[7,8] Displacement has ranged significantly in series from 70% to 96%, and seems to depend on patient age, mechanism of injury, and presence of associated femur injury. Average deformity in an isolated, displaced fracture population was described as external rotation of 44° and cranial femoral shortening as 18 mm.[6] Based on this definition of deformity, an internal rotation traction view was suggested as an effective imaging study of the femoral neck fracture.

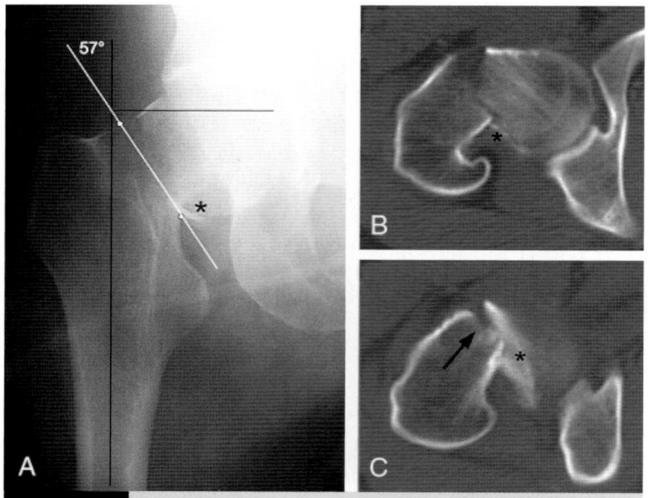

Figure 1 Imaging studies from a 49-year-old man who was thrown from a horse and sustained vertical femoral neck fracture. **A**, AP radiograph of the hip demonstrates Pauwels III vertical fracture. **B** and **C**, Axial CT images show typical fracture morphology. The cannulated screws are of questionable functionality because of the comminution (asterisk) and apical defect seen at the femoral calcar (black arrow).

Assessment

In the aforementioned 2014 radiographic study from three trauma centers including 120 patients younger than 50 years with femoral neck fracture,[6] 90% of patients had AP radiographs of the pelvis, 85% had two views of the hip, 52% had a CT of the pelvis (all but two screening trauma scans), and only two patients had a traction (dynamic) view radiograph. A good AP pelvis radiograph is helpful for preoperative planning and intraoperative reference with regard to restoring the anatomic neck-shaft axis to match the contralateral uninjured limb as well as an internal rotation traction view. Similarly, a CT scan allows the surgeon to judge fracture deformity and comminution (**Figure 1**) and plan for reduction maneuvers and implant configuration to maximize the chances for an anatomically aligned reconstruction with a stable construct.

Timing of Surgery

For many years, displaced femoral neck fractures were managed on an emergent basis with the goal of preserving blood flow to the femoral head. Early studies indicated that early fixation may decrease osteonecrosis and increase functional outcome.[3] In the fractured femoral neck of an adult, the interosseous blood flow is lost, so that the ascending cervical branches (mostly posterior) of the medial femoral circumflex artery provide the main blood supply to the head. Theoretically, fracture reduction was thought to unkink these vessels or restore some of the intraosseous blood supply. However, subsequent studies specifically evaluating outcomes have found little or no

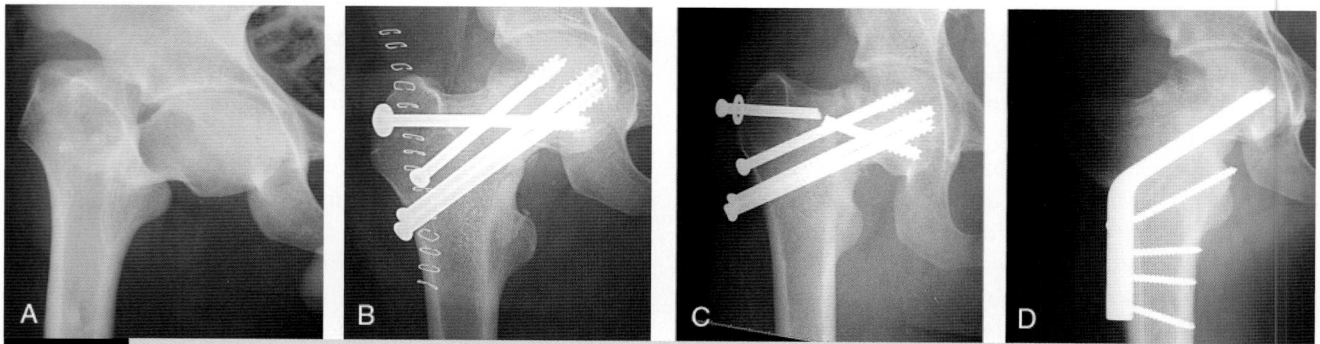

Figure 2 Imaging studies from a 17-year-old boy injured in a motorcycle crash. AP radiographs show the injury (**A**), fracture repair (**B**), loss of fixation and nonunion at 4 months (**C**), and results of a proximal femoral osteotomy 1 year after the revision surgery (**D**).

6: Lower Extremity

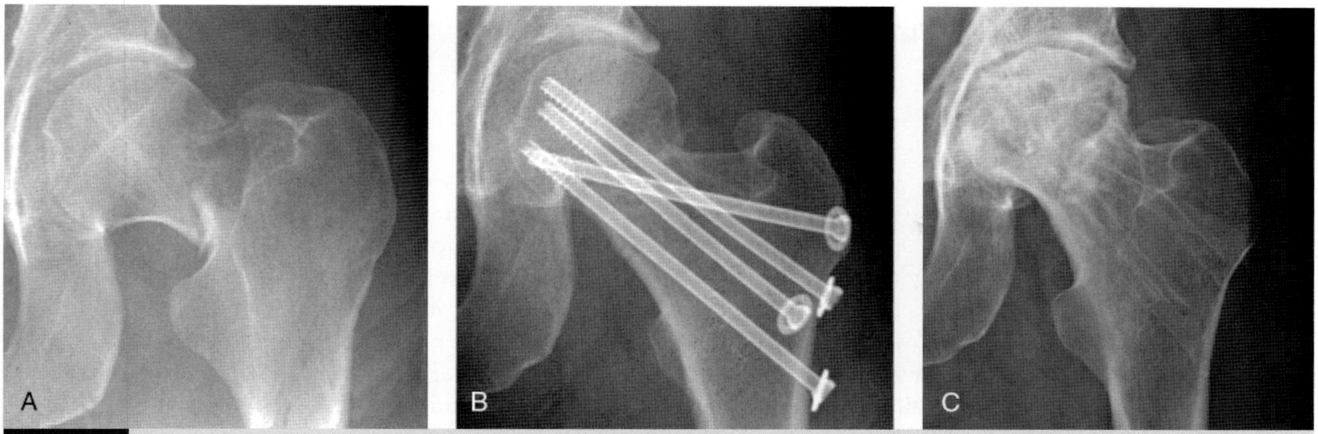

Figure 3 Imaging studies from a 42-year-old man who fell 12 feet from a ladder and injured his left hip. AP radiographs show displaced vertical neck fracture (**A**), fracture repair (**B**), and profound osteonecrosis of the head with hip arthritis (**C**). A hip arthroplasty is planned.

difference in osteonecrosis rates or clinical results between early and delayed time to fixation.[9-11] A 2012 retrospective study reported on 92 patients with femoral neck fractures and no difference was found in osteonecrosis rates comparing treatment within 6 hours postinjury and delayed treatment at 48 hours postinjury.[11] Given the evidence regarding outcomes of emergent versus "early" surgery for this injury, most experts currently recommend treating displaced femoral neck fractures on an early basis, when the patient is stable and appropriate resources are mobilized to allow for a quality surgical experience.[12,13]

Reduction

Amid modifiable factors, the quality of fracture reduction has been shown to be among the most consistent predictors of successful treatment.[4,5,13] The use of closed versus open reduction techniques remains a topic of debate. Some surgeons have been reluctant in the past to perform open reduction of femoral neck fractures for several reasons, including difficulty in assessing intraoperative quality of reduction, lack of familiarity of open approaches, and further disruption of femoral head blood supply. Several strategies and methods are currently recommended for femoral neck fractures in young adults. A cornerstone of treatment is anatomic reduction of the fracture, whether using open or closed (indirect) means. Anatomic reduction of the fracture, in addition to restoring the normal anatomy, should allow for maximal stability of the fixation construct. Open approaches during repair of a femoral neck fracture may provide the best opportunity for achieving anatomic reduction, as the fracture can be inspected and manipulated under direct visualization.[14] For example, many of these fractures have an apical fracture spike that, if anatomically reduced, may dramatically increase the stability of the repair construct. An open approach to the hip also allows the surgeon to apply supplemental fixation into the neck area that may be desirable in some cases.[15] In addition, an open approach provides decompression of the intracapsular hematoma (if it is not already decompressed by the injury), which if left untreated may increase the risk for osteonecrosis from increased intracapsular pressure and prevent adequate blood flow to the femoral head.[3]

Open surgical fixation of a femoral neck fracture may be performed on either a flat radiolucent table or a fracture table. A flat radiolucent table allows for greater freedom to manipulate the limb, which may aid with exposure and reduction. A disadvantage may be the need for a surgical assistant to provide traction, which may be inconsistent. A fracture table provides consistent traction on the injured limb. Some disadvantages of a fracture table include limited ability to manipulate the limb, as well as some challenges with draping and exposure due to the presence of the perineal post.

There are two commonly used surgical approaches to the femoral neck, a direct anterior approach as described by Smith-Petersen (or Heuter) and an anterolateral approach as described by Watson-Jones.[16] The modified Smith-Petersen approach allows for excellent direct visualization of the anterior femoral neck; the vertical fracture line typically exits in the anteroinferior region of the femoral neck to the level of the lesser trochanter[14] (**Figure 4**). The fracture can be reduced with a combination of manipulation of the femur, joystick Kirschner wires in the femoral head or neck, and the use of modified fracture reduction clamps and provisional Kirschner wires. Restoring bony stability through a quality reduction with

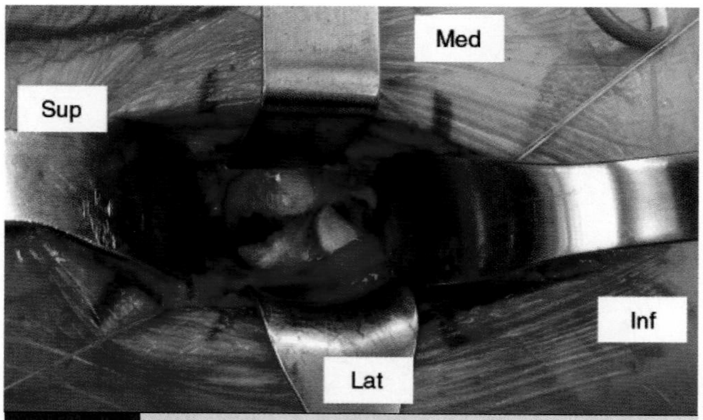

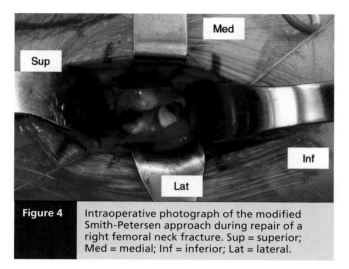

Figure 4 Intraoperative photograph of the modified Smith-Petersen approach during repair of a right femoral neck fracture. Sup = superior; Med = medial; Inf = inferior; Lat = lateral.

bony apposition is helpful, and can be achieved in these cases by re-approximating the fracture apex at the calcar. The disadvantage of the Smith-Petersen approach is that traditional implants must still be applied through a lateral incision; thus, a second incision is necessary for fixation. Through the Watson-Jones approach, the entire surgical procedure can be performed through the anterolateral window, although access for reduction and instrumentation of the neck is limited, especially in muscular or obese patients.

Fixation

Shortening with resultant malunion or loss of fixation and nonunion have been common problems. For optimal treatment of vertical femoral neck fractures, fixation must be able to resist the high shear forces across the fracture with hip motion, weight bearing, and muscle tone. Several fracture fixation constructs have been recommended for vertical femoral neck fractures; however, none of these constructs have been found to optimally resist the shearing forces across the hip with this fracture pattern. Three parallel, cannulated lag screws placed along the axis of the femoral neck have been frequently described.[3,15] These screws, however, while optimally applied perpendicular to most femoral neck fractures (for example, Pauwels type I), are applied obliquely in relation to more vertically oriented factures (for example, Pauwels type II and III). Thus, instability, especially the ability to resist shearing forces across the fracture, is possible. Also, the mechanical advantage of placing a screw along the shaft-neck's inferior cortex or calcar, as in repairing a typical osteoporotic neck fracture, is lost, as this part of the fracture is attached to the head fragment in the vertical fracture pattern[6] (**Figure 1**). Shearing deformity may be exacerbated further with tightening of typical parallel lag screws due to the mismatch of the implant forces and the vertical fracture obliquity. In contrast, subcapital fracture patterns with intact cortical calcar bone prevent the screw from collapsing inferiorly, resisting failure into varus. Clinical failure rates using parallel screws appear greater than the sliding hip screw (SHS) in several studies[4,17,18] and have been shown to have the worst performance compared with other methods in mechanical testing using a younger fracture model, with a more vertically oriented fracture.[19-21] Other studies have recommended a nonparallel screw configuration, where two of the three screws are placed in typical orientation, but the third screw is modified to be placed more horizontally into the head or neck and more perpendicular to the vertical fracture line. This allows for a true lag effect, compressing the major fragments across the vertical fracture to gain stability and possibly control shearing better than an all-parallel screw construct. Although never proven in a comparative clinical series, the nonparallel screw configuration has performed significantly better in several mechanical testing studies using a vertical neck fracture model.[20,21]

The SHS, which has been used with success for typical hip fractures, is a fixed angle device that provides increased resistance to varus collapse compared with parallel screws while also allowing compression along the axis of the femoral neck; for most femoral neck fractures the SHS is approximately parallel to the femoral neck axis, and perpendicular to the fracture pattern. However, in the more vertically oriented fracture pattern, the SHS will induce shearing forces with axial compression. This implant has shown improved mechanical testing strength compared with three parallel screws in a vertical fracture model, similar to the nonparallel screw construct described previously. Some clinicians have added a long parallel screw superior to the SHS lag screw for antirotation and intramedullary buttress effect, which seems to have decreased failure rates. However, some amount of varus collapse still occurred in 10% of cases.[22] The dynamic compression screw (DCS) is similar in design to the SHS, only with a 95° angle. This device appears to have had limited use for femoral neck fractures, but theoretically allows for dynamic compression in the desired axis for fixation of vertical fractures. This device, like the SHS, has minimal rotational control when used alone.

Less frequently used implants have been proposed as improvements to traditional methods. Reconstruction nails, which are intramedullary femoral nails with dual points of cephalomedullary fixation, have been proposed for femoral neck fractures to allow for rotational control of the head and may provide resistance to shaft medialization and varus collapse. Nonetheless, problems with the Z-effect (screw displacement) and violation of the abductors have dampened enthusiasm for the use of reconstruction nails. A recent mechanical study showed that in a Pauwels III fracture model with posterior comminution, cephalomedullary fixation failed at 40% higher failure load and 41% lower loaded construct displacement compared to a SHS.[23] Only one study has evaluated the clinical results of femoral neck fractures treated with cephalomedullary nails; a high proportion of failures (38%) were reported in patients with osteoporotic subcapital femoral neck fractures.[24] Interestingly, this same study reported that five of six patients with Pauwels III femoral neck fractures in their series healed well, with the only failure in an 88-year-old man injured from a ground-level fall.

Proximal femoral locking plates are relatively new implants whereby the use of nonlocking screws for fracture compression at 95° can be followed by locking screws for fixed angle support in the 120° to 125° range. One study showed high failure rates after using static fixed angled plates on a variety of femoral neck fracture types, such as locking proximal femur plates, even after compression has been applied.[25] Several cohort studies using small fixed-angle locking plates that combine multiple points for head and neck fixation along the head-neck axis have shown promising results in femoral neck fractures in the "younger" elderly (age 60–70 years).[26-29] A comparative cohort study of patients with femoral neck fractures treated with three parallel cannulated screws (47 patients) or a small fixed-angle locking lateral hip plate (31 patients) with cancellous femoral neck screws was performed.[29] The mean Pauwels angle was 59° and mean age was 59 years. Revision surgery was required in 34% of those treated with screws only and 13% of those treated with the plate construct ($P < 0.04$).

Orthopaedic surgeons frequently apply the concept of buttress (or antiglide) plate fixation to other fractures that require resistance to shear forces. Buttress plates are applied over the apex of fractures and act by resisting shear forces and converting them into compressive forces. The Smith-Petersen anterior approach provides excellent visualization of the femoral neck fracture as it is anatomically reduced along the anteroinferior aspect of the femoral neck[14,15] (**Figure 5**). The apical fracture spike for most of these injuries is oriented along the femoral neck axis or anteriorly, where after provisional clamping and pinning gentle external rotation and flexion of the hip allows for easy access for plating of the femoral neck. A Weber clamp or modified small-pointed clamp is helpful at obtaining reduction. A short third-tubular plate, 2.7 mm reconstruction or dynamic compression plate, or spider washer is placed over the apex of the fracture spike with a bicortical screw just inferior to the spike's tip.[15] Fracture compression can still be accomplished using laterally based implants, but the ability to resist shear forces across a vertical fracture is enhanced by the interdigitation of the fracture's interstices and by the buttress effect of the plate. A 2015 study evaluated the use of a medial 2.7-mm buttress plate in a vertical femoral neck model repaired with three parallel screws or a SHS.[30] Failure loads were increased by an average of 83%, energy absorbed to failure by 183%, and stiffness by 35%.

Complications and Outcomes

Complications, some of which are devastating, are common after femoral neck fractures in the young adult population. A meta-analysis of patients younger than 60 years was recently performed to assess complication risks after a femoral neck fracture.[13] Forty-one studies with 1,558 patients were reviewed and osteonecrosis was found in 14.7% and nonunion in 10% of patients with displaced fractures; reoperation was necessary in 18% of these patients.

Malunion

Malunion occurs in most cases, according to careful measurements and strict definitions. Moderate (5 mm to 10 mm) to severe (>10 mm) shortening of 66% and >5° of varus was found in 39% of 70 patients with a femoral neck fracture in a multicenter cohort study.[31] Patients with either moderate or severe shortening of the femoral neck had dramatically poorer Medical Outcomes Study Short Form-36 and EuroQol questionnaire function scores versus those with none or mild shortening (<5 mm). Authors of a 2015 study reported shortening greater than 5 mm in 54% of patients younger than 60 years with femoral neck fracture treated with repair, including 32% of patients with shortening greater than 10 mm.[32] Ninety-three percent of patients had Pauwels II or III fractures. Initially displaced fractures shortened more than nondisplaced fractures. Patients treated with a SHS and antirotation screw had shortening of 2.2 mm more than those treated with screws alone, although the authors assert that this finding was likely the result of selection bias (use of SHS in more difficult fractures). Treatment of symptomatic femoral neck malunion may include observation, a shoe lift, corrective osteotomy, or arthroplasty depending on the patient's symptoms, physiology, and age.

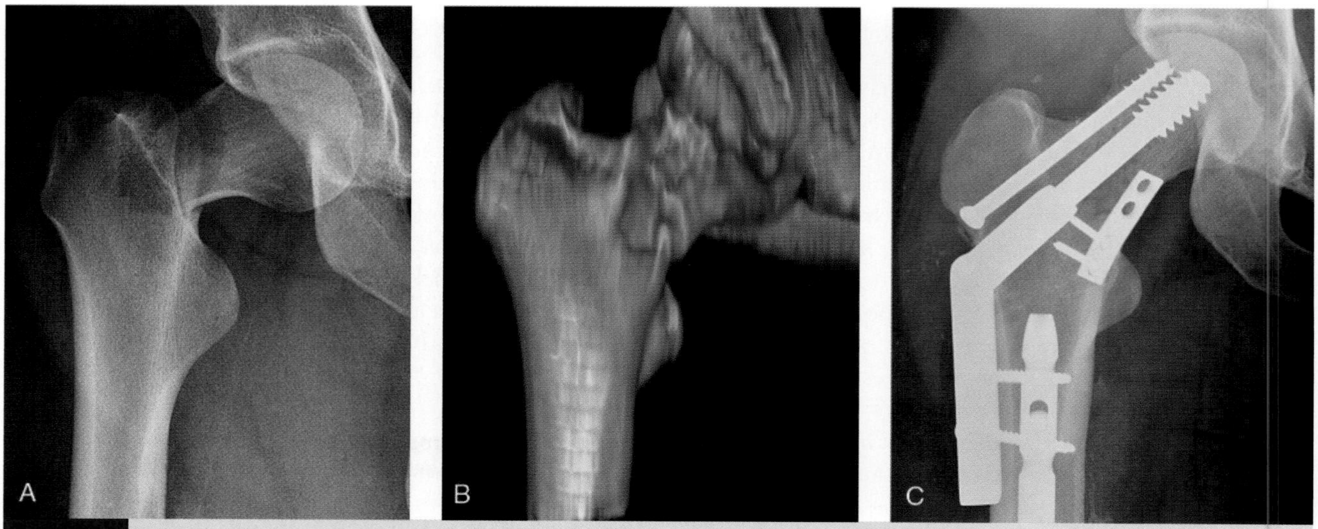

Figure 5 Imaging studies from a 22-year-old woman with a vertical femoral neck fracture. **A**, Radiograph showing the injury. **B**, CT showing the injury. Reconstruction was performed with open reduction and internal fixation using a sliding hip screw, antirotation screw, and medial buttress plate (**C**).

Nonunion

Nonunion appears closely related to a loss of mechanical stability in young adult patients with a femoral neck fracture. Initial fracture displacement, quality of reduction, fixation construct, and increasing patient age has correlated with an increased risk of nonunion.[6,33,34] It is accepted that mechanical factors (as opposed to biologic factors) are more central to the occurrence of nonunion in vertical fractures in young patients compared with typical femoral neck fractures in older patients. Nonunion rates for displaced femoral neck fractures in young adults are reportedly 10% to 33%.[34] Treatment of femoral neck nonunion may include a valgus intertrochanteric osteotomy or arthroplasty depending on the viability of the femoral head and the physiology and age of the patient.

Osteonecrosis

Osteonecrosis of the hip is found in 2% to 24% of patients treated in modern series. The incidence of osteonecrosis for isolated fractures is reportedly 14.3%.[8] Fracture displacement was the only contributing factor identified for osteonecrosis (14.7% versus 6.4%). Direct arterial injury and/or local pressure increases (such as compartment syndrome) may be additional contributing factors. Treatment of femoral head osteonecrosis may include observation, medication, osteotomy, a vascularized fibular strut, or arthroplasty depending on the stage of osteonecrosis and the physiology and age of the patient.[16,35,36]

Summary

Fracture treatment has evolved in recent years to improve implant mechanics and biology. Although several characteristics of femoral neck fractures in the young adult have been identified, few biomechanical methods have been developed that appear to have improved outcomes. It does appear that several new implants and ideas on implant application are imminent but only time will tell if these efforts are successful. Both clinical and laboratory studies of this injury are lacking. Only recently have substantial efforts been made to improve mechanical testing models to better reflect in vivo findings or assemble large, multicenter clinical studies to evaluate patient treatment and outcomes.

Key Study Points

- The characteristic differences between femoral neck fractures in young adult patients and typical osteoporotic femoral neck fractures contribute to a specific set of clinical problems.
- Several complications frequently occur after femoral neck fractures; the physician should be aware of how these complications may affect patients and how they might be avoided.

Annotated References

1. Pauwels F: *Biomechanics of the Normal and Diseased Hip: Theoretical Foundation, Technique, and Results of Treatment: An Atlas* .Berlin, Springer-Verlag, 1976.

   The classic: this book from the "father of biomechanics" describes his discoveries and thoughts about the hip, mostly from early in his career.

2. Protzman RR, Burkhalter WE: Femoral-neck fractures in young adults. *J Bone Joint Surg Am* 1976;58(5):689-695.

3. Swiontkowski MF, Winquist RA, Hansen ST Jr: Fractures of the femoral neck in patients between the ages of twelve and forty-nine years. *J Bone Joint Surg Am* 1984;66(6):837-846.

4. Haidukewych GJ, Rothwell WS, Jacofsky DJ, Torchia ME, Berry DJ: Operative treatment of femoral neck fractures in patients between the ages of fifteen and fifty years. *J Bone Joint Surg Am* 2004;86-A(8):1711-1716.

5. Liporace F, Gaines R, Collinge C, Haidukewych GJ: Results of internal fixation of Pauwels type-3 vertical femoral neck fractures. *J Bone Joint Surg Am* 2008;90(8):1654-1659.

6. Collinge CA, Mir H, Reddix R: Fracture morphology of high shear angle "vertical" femoral neck fractures in young adult patients. *J Orthop Trauma* 2014;28(5):270-275.

   This CT-based radiographic study described other morphologic elements of isolated displaced Pauwels III femoral neck fractures in adults younger than 50 years with a high-energy mechanism. In addition to the vertical (coronal) fracture, there was axial fracture obliquity (mean 24°) with relative deficiency of the posterior neck on the head–neck fragment, and >1.5 cm comminution in 96% of cases (typically posterior-inferior).

7. Damany DS, Parker MJ, Chojnowski A: Complications after intracapsular hip fractures in young adults. A meta-analysis of 18 published studies involving 564 fractures. *Injury* 2005;36(1):131-141.

8. Slobogean GP, Sprague SA, Scott T, Bhandari M: Complications following young femoral neck fractures. *Injury* 2015;46(3):484-491.

   This 17-item survey of North American fracture surgeons was developed to assess treatment preferences for femoral neck fractures in young patients. Five hundred forty surgeons completed the survey, with a similar proportion of respondents from academic and community hospitals. Most surgeons treat fewer than five young adult femoral neck fractures per year. There was a lack of surgeon consensus for closed versus open reduction, fixation with multiple screws versus SHS, and other treatment decisions. Level of evidence: V.

9. Upadhyay A, Jain P, Mishra P, Maini L, Gautum VK, Dhaon BK: Delayed internal fixation of fractures of the neck of the femur in young adults. A prospective, randomised study comparing closed and open reduction. *J Bone Joint Surg Br* 2004;86(7):1035-1040.

10. Karaeminogullari O, Demirors H, Atabek M, Tuncay C, Tandogan R, Ozalay M: Avascular necrosis and nonunion after osteosynthesis of femoral neck fractures: Effect of fracture displacement and time to surgery. *Adv Ther* 2004;21(5):335-342.

11. Razik F, Alexopoulos AS, El-Osta B, et al: Time to internal fixation of femoral neck fractures in patients under sixty years—does this matter in the development of osteonecrosis of femoral head? *Int Orthop* 2012;36(10):2127-2132.

    A retrospective study of 92 patients younger than 60 years with a surgically treated femoral neck fracture was performed to assess effects of time delay and fixation method on the development of osteonecrosis. Osteonecrosis of the femoral head developed in 13 patients (14.1%), the highest incidence being in the cannulated screw fixation group (24%). Time to surgery for internal fixation was not a predictor in the development of osteonecrosis.

12. Pauyo T, Drager J, Albers A, Harvey EJ: Management of femoral neck fractures in the young patient: A critical analysis review. *World J Orthop* 2014;5(3):204-217.

    Modern treatments and remaining controversies for young patients with femoral neck fractures are reviewed.

13. Slobogean GP, Sprague SA, Scott T, McKee M, Bhandari M: Management of young femoral neck fractures: Is there a consensus? *Injury* 2015;46(3):435-440.

    A pooled review of the literature is presented. Level of evidence: IV.

14. Blair JA, Stinner DJ, Kirby JM, Gerlinger TL, Hsu JR; Skeletal Trauma Research Consortium (STReC): Quantification of femoral neck exposure through a minimally invasive Smith-Petersen approach. *J Orthop Trauma* 2010;24(6):355-358.

    This anatomic study demonstrates wide exposure of the femoral neck accessible via the modified Smith-Petersen approach to the hip.

15. Mir H, Collinge C: Application of a medial buttress plate may prevent many treatment failures seen after fixation of vertical femoral neck fractures in young adults. *Med Hypotheses* 2015;84(5):429-433.

    The authors present a technical guide and rationale for the use of a medial buttress plate for adjunctive repair of vertical femoral neck fractures.

16. Ly TV, Swiontkowski MF: Treatment of femoral neck fractures in young adults. *J Bone Joint Surg Am* 2008;90(10):2254-2266.

17. Gardner S, Weaver MJ, Jerabek S, Rodriguez E, Vrahas M, Harris M: Predictors of early failure in young patients with displaced femoral neck fractures. *J Orthop* 2015;12(2):75-80.

This study compared early failure rates of SHS and cannulated screw constructs in young patients. One patient (3%) with SHS fixation and 6 patients (21%) with CS fixation experienced implant failure within 6 months. Regression analysis demonstrated type of fixation and reduction quality are independent predictors of early failure. Level of evidence: III.

18. Hoshino CM, O'Toole RV: Fixed angle devices versus multiple cancellous screws: What does the evidence tell us? *Injury* 2015;46(3):474-477.

    The authors present a review of the literature and opinion piece regarding cancellous screws versus a sliding hip screw for femoral neck fractures.

19. Kauffman JI, Simon JA, Kummer FJ, Pearlman CJ, Zuckerman JD, Koval KJ: Internal fixation of femoral neck fractures with posterior comminution: A biomechanical study. *J Orthop Trauma* 1999;13(3):155-159.

20. Sirkin M, Grossman MG, Renard RL, Behrens, FF: A biomechanical analysis of fixation constructs in high angle femoral neck fractures. *J Orthop Trauma* 2000;14(2):131.

21. Aminian A, Gao F, Fedoriw WW, Zhang LQ, Kalainov DM, Merk BR: Vertically oriented femoral neck fractures: Mechanical analysis of four fixation techniques. *J Orthop Trauma* 2007;21(8):544-548.

22. Boraiah S, Paul O, Hammoud S, Gardner MJ, Helfet DL, Lorich DG: Predictable healing of femoral neck fractures treated with intraoperative compression and length-stable implants. *J Trauma* 2010;69(1):142-147.

23. Rupprecht M, Grossterlinden L, Sellenschloh K, et al: Internal fixation of femoral neck fractures with posterior comminution: A biomechanical comparison of DHS® and Intertan nail®. *Int Orthop* 2011;35(11):1695-1701.

    A cadaver mechanical testing study of Pauwels III femoral neck fractures was performed with and without comminution using a cephalomedullary nail (with integrated antirotation) versus a sliding hip screw. The cephalomedullary nail outperformed the SHS in stiffness and construct displacement with cyclic loading, and load to failure in comminuted and noncomminuted models.

24. Mir HR, Edwards P, Sanders R, Haidukewych G: Results of cephallomedullary nail fixation for displaced intracapsular femoral neck fractures. *J Orthop Trauma* 2011;25(12):714-720.

    In a case series of patients with femoral neck fractures treated with cephalomedullary nailing, the overall failure rate was 38%, but a small subset of young patients with vertical fractures notably healed well.

25. Berkes MB, Little MT, Lazaro LE, Cymerman RM, Helfet DL, Lorich DG: Catastrophic failure after open reduction internal fixation of femoral neck fractures with a novel locking plate implant. *J Orthop Trauma* 2012;26(10):e170-e176.

    Open reduction and internal fixation using a locking plate construct yielded a 37% rate of failed fixation in 18 patients with a femoral neck fracture (mean age 72 years).

26. Lin D, Lian K, Ding Z, Zhai W, Hong J: Proximal femoral locking plate with cannulated screws for the treatment of femoral neck fractures. *Orthopedics* 2012;35(1):e1-e5.

    The safety and effectiveness of the proximal femoral locking plate with cannulated screws for the treatment of femoral neck fractures was evaluted. Fewer complications were noted.

27. Osarumwense D, Tissingh E, Wartenberg K, et al: The Targon FN system for the management of intracapsular neck of femur fractures: Minimum 2-year experience and outcome in an independent hospital. *Clin Orthop Surg* 2015;7(1):22-28.

    In a case series of mostly nondisplaced femoral neck fractures treated with a multiple sliding screw and side plate construct, clinical results were successful.

28. Eschler A, Brandt S, Gierer P, Mittlmeier T, Gradl G: Angular stable multiple screw fixation (Targon FN) versus standard SHS for the fixation of femoral neck fractures. *Injury* 2014;45(suppl 1):S76-S80.

    This comparative cohort study revealed less subsidence of the head fragment, lower cutout rate, and lower rate of conversion to hemiarthroplasty after multiple sliding screw and side plate fixation compared with a standard SHS fixation in a small number of patients with hip fractures.

29. Thein R, Herman A, Kedem P, Chechik A, Shazar N: Osteosynthesis of unstable intracapsular femoral neck fracture by dynamic locking plate or screw fixation: Early results. *J Orthop Trauma* 2014;28(2):70-76.

    In a comparative case series of displaced femoral neck fractures treated with internal fixation by a multiple sliding screw and side plate device or cannulated screws, nonunion rates and revision rates were decreased in the dynamic plated group.

30. Kunapuli SC, Schramski MJ, Lee AS, et al: Biomechanical analysis of augmented plate fixation for the treatment of vertical shear femoral neck fractures. *J Orthop Trauma* 2015;29(3):144-150.

    Repairs of a vertical femoral neck osteotomy using cannulated screws or a sliding hip screw augmented with medially applied 2.7-mm locking plates were evaluated in a mechanical study. Medial plating increased failure loads on average by 83%, energy absorbed to failure by 183%, and constructs' stiffness by 35%.

31. Zlowodzki M, Brink O, Switzer J, et al: The effect of shortening and varus collapse of the femoral neck on function after fixation of intracapsular fracture of the hip: A multi-centre cohort study. *J Bone Joint Surg Br* 2008;90(11):1487-1494.

32. Stockton DJ, Lefaivre KA, Deakin DE, et al: Incidence, magnitude, and predictors of shortening in young femoral neck fractures. *J Orthop Trauma* 2015;29(9):e293-e298.

The authors reviewed radiographs from 65 patients averaging 51 years old treated with repair of femoral neck fractures. Shortening "likely to interfere with gait" (>1 cm) was seen in 32% of patients.

33. Yang JJ, Lin LC, Chao KH, et al: Risk factors for nonunion in patients with intracapsular femoral neck fractures treated with three cannulated screws placed in either a triangle or an inverted triangle configuration. *J Bone Joint Surg Am* 2013;95(1):61-69.

In a clinical series of 202 patients treated with cannulated screws for an intracapsular hip fracture, risk factors for nonunion were identified, including a noninverted triangle configuration (one proximal, two distal) screws, a displaced fracture, and poor reduction.

34. Parker MJ, Raghavan R, Gurusamy K: Incidence of fracture-healing complications after femoral neck fractures. *Clin Orthop Relat Res* 2007;458(458):175-179.

35. Tidermark J, Ponzer S, Svensson O, Söderqvist A, Törnkvist H: Internal fixation compared with total hip replacement for displaced femoral neck fractures in the elderly. A randomised, controlled trial. *J Bone Joint Surg Br* 2003;85(3):380-388.

36. Heetveld MJ, Rogmark C, Frihagen F, Keating J: Internal fixation versus arthroplasty for displaced femoral neck fractures: What is the evidence? *J Orthop Trauma* 2009;23(6):395-402.

Chapter 38

Subtrochanteric Femoral Fractures

William D. Lack, MD Madhav A. Karunakar, MD

Abstract

The unique surgical challenges of subtrochanteric femoral fractures are related to the local biomechanical environment of the proximal femur and the anatomic transition from metaphyseal to diaphyseal bone. Reduction requires counteracting the strong deforming muscular forces acting on the proximal femur and is further complicated by the anatomic features of the proximal femur. The intramedullary canal widens as it approaches the proximal metaphysis, and this factor must be considered if an intramedullary implant is to be used for a midshaft fracture. The risk of malunion or construct failure is greater in these fractures than in more distal diaphyseal fractures. Reduction requires manipulation of both the proximal and distal segments of the fracture. The use of an intramedullary or cephalomedullary implant or a fixed-angle plate is appropriate for fixation. The implant is selected based on the fracture characteristics (the proximal extent of the fracture and trochanter involvement), patient age, and surgeon preference. Subtrochanteric femoral fractures are vulnerable to loss of reduction during implant insertion, and avoiding malunion requires an accurate intraoperative reduction and starting point as well as careful attention to the orientation of the fixation construct as related to the fracture segments.

Keywords: proximal femur fracture; subtrochanteric femur fracture

Dr. Karunakar or an immediate family member serves as a board member, owner, officer, or committee member of the American Academy of Orthopaedic Surgeons and the Orthopaedic Trauma Association. Neither Dr. Lack nor any immediate family member has received anything of value from or has stock or stock options held in a commercial company or institution related directly or indirectly to the subject of this chapter.

Introduction

The subtrochanteric region of the femur extends from the inferior aspect of the lesser trochanter to the junction of the proximal and middle thirds of the femoral shaft. The distal border is more specifically described as a point 5 cm distal to the inferior border of the lesser trochanter. A subtrochanteric femoral fracture may extend outside this zone, but significant involvement of the subtrochanteric region requires consideration of specific treatment issues. These fractures have a bimodal distribution of incidence, and the patient's age can affect the treatment.[1-5] High-energy fractures typically occur in younger patients. Low-energy fractures occur in older patients and are associated with dementia and obesity.[6] The incidence of subtrochanteric femoral fractures among older patients is increasing, as is the incidence of atypical subtrochanteric femoral fractures secondary to long-term diphosphonate use.[7]

The treatment of subtrochanteric femoral fractures presents unique challenges. Strong deforming muscular forces act on the proximal femur, affecting the alignment of both fracture segments. The proximal segment is flexed by the pull of the iliopsoas, abducted by the gluteus medius and minimus, and externally rotated by the short external rotators. The distal segment is shortened and medialized by the pull of the adductors (**Figure 1**). The anatomic features of the proximal femur further complicate treatment. The widening of the intramedullary canal as it approaches the proximal metaphysis must be considered when using an intramedullary implant. Reduction requires manipulating both the proximal and distal segments of the fracture and precisely aligning the fixation construct with both fracture segments. These fractures involve cortical bone that heals more slowly than the adjacent metaphyseal bone of the intertrochanteric region. Furthermore, compressive stresses in the proximal femur peak at the medial cortex 1 to 2 inches distal to the lesser trochanter. Compressive stresses in the femur are greatest in the medial cortex of the subtrochanteric region below the lesser trochanter, where they can exceed 1,200 lb per square inch.[8] These factors increase the risk of malunion and

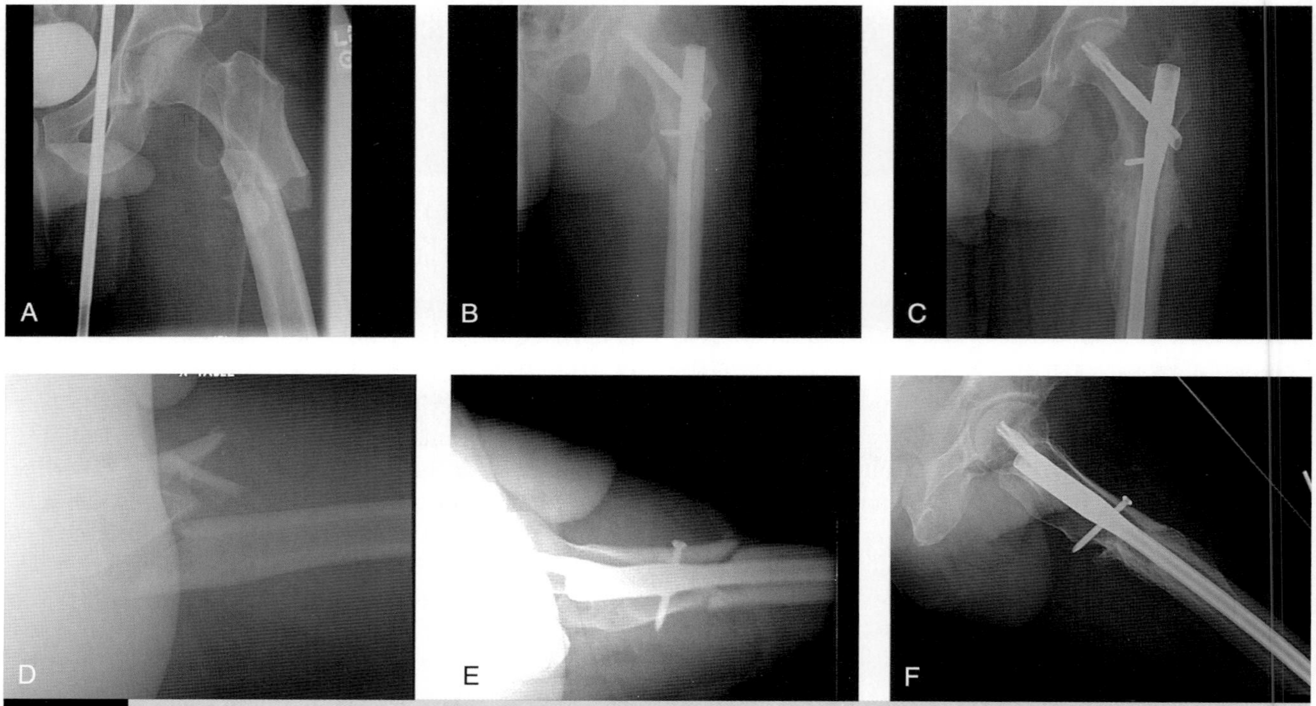

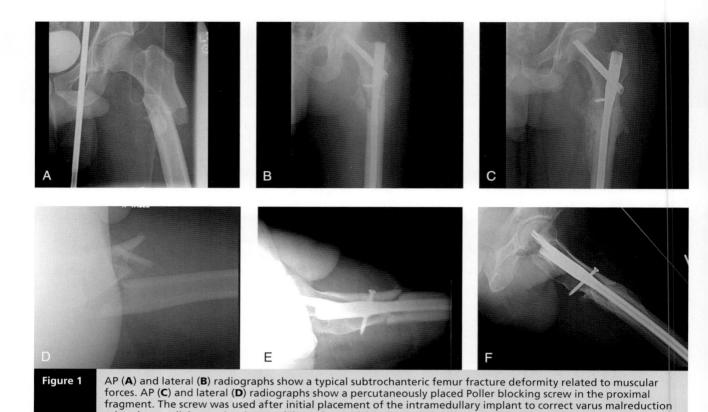

Figure 1 AP (**A**) and lateral (**B**) radiographs show a typical subtrochanteric femur fracture deformity related to muscular forces. AP (**C**) and lateral (**D**) radiographs show a percutaneously placed Poller blocking screw in the proximal fragment. The screw was used after initial placement of the intramedullary implant to correct varus malreduction related to medial comminution. AP (**E**) and lateral (**F**) radiographs show the healed fracture.

construct failure in subtrochanteric fractures compared with more distal diaphyseal fractures.

The appropriate fixation constructs include intramedullary or cephalomedullary devices as well as fixed-angle plate constructs. The choice of implant depends on the characteristics of the fracture, including comminution and proximal extension, the patient's age, and the surgeon's preference. Avoiding malunion requires accurate intraoperative reduction. Because subtrochanteric femoral fractures are vulnerable to loss of reduction during implant insertion, careful attention is required during the reaming process to orient the fixation construct relative to the fracture segments.

Classification

Fifteen classification systems have been developed for subtrochanteric femoral fractures.[9] The Russell-Taylor classification is most common in clinical practice and is useful for implant selection. The presence or absence of posteromedial buttress involvement is emphasized, as is the presence or absence of extension into the greater trochanter and piriformis fossa.[2] A group I fracture does not extend into the piriformis fossa or the greater trochanter and is considered amenable to the use of an intramedullary device with a standard piriformis or trochanteric starting point. A group IA fracture does not involve the posteromedial buttress and is amenable to the use of standard locking nails. A group IB fracture involves the posteromedial buttress, so the use of standard locking nails is inadvisable. A group IIA fracture extends into the greater trochanter and the piriformis fossa, so the use of a trochanteric nail or a 95° fixed-angle implant is preferable to a piriformis nail. A group IIB fracture, unlike a group IIA fracture, has posteromedial buttress involvement, which increases the risk of implant failure.

Atypical subtrochanteric femoral fractures are not included in the classification. These injuries occur in patients with osteoporosis in the setting of diphosphonate use. The risk of an atypical femur fracture appears to increase with prolonged diphosphonate use.[10] These fractures are associated with a characteristic lateral beaking (**Figure 2**). Consultation with an endocrinologist should be considered because implicit bone turnover deficit occurs in these injuries. The endocrinologist can advise on lessening the risk of future fractures and treating delayed union if necessary. Treatment with teriparatide was found to promote union in atypical subtrochanteric femur fractures with delayed union.[11,12]

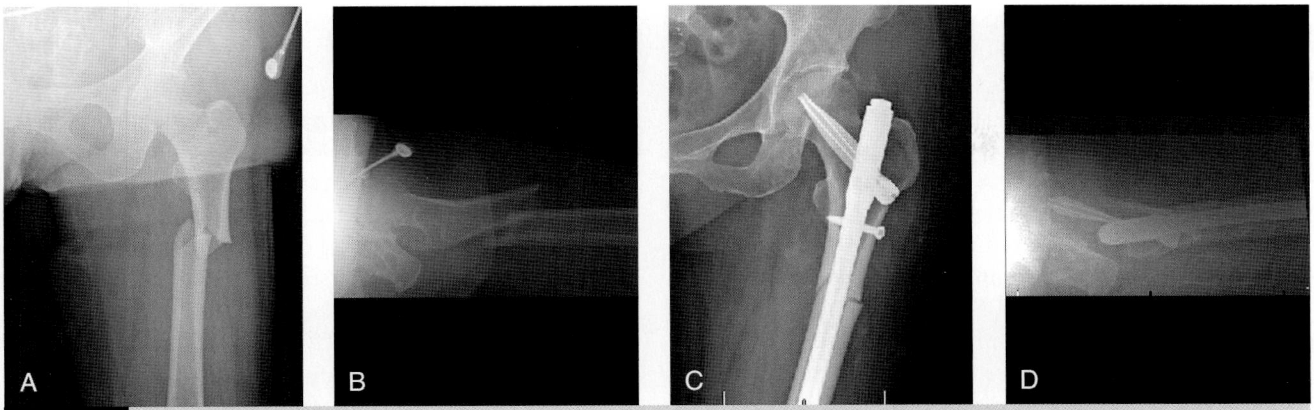

Figure 2 AP (**A**) and lateral (**B**) radiographs show an atypical subtrochanteric femur fracture associated with diphosphonate use. AP (**C**) and lateral (**D**) radiographs show fracture reduction and intramedullary fixation.

Treatment

Nonsurgical treatment of subtrochanteric femoral fractures in adult patients is associated with significant morbidity and mortality as well as nonunion, malunion, and local soft-tissue complications.[13,14] As a result, nonsurgical management is used only for patients who are nonambulatory, have minimal pain, and have significant surgical risk factors. Surgery also is recommended for treating nondisplaced atypical subtrochanteric femoral fractures. A retrospective study of 11 patients with 14 nonsurgically treated nondisplaced atypical subtrochanteric femoral fractures found a 36% risk of late displacement and a 36% risk of intractable pain that required surgery. All patients who did not undergo surgery had persistent pain at a minimum 12-month follow-up.[15]

Surgical Options

The options for surgical fixation include using an intramedullary implant or an extramedullary plate implant. Several fixed-angle plate constructs are available, including a 95° fixed-angle device (condylar blade plate and dynamic condylar screw), a proximal femoral locking plate, and a 135° sliding hip screw. The use of sliding hip screws to treat subtrochanteric femoral fractures has a relatively high complication rate and should be avoided for these fractures.[16,17] The intramedullary device options include piriformis or trochanteric nails as well as standard locking or cephalomedullary locking nails. These devices offer increased resistance to implant failure because of their intramedullary location. Intramedullary implants are unforgiving, however, in that an inaccurate starting point and a proximal reaming path can lead to displacement when the nail is inserted. Care must be taken to avoid varus and apex anterior angulation (flexion of the proximal fragment), which is associated with intramedullary nailing of these fractures.

Surgical Considerations

The rotation and length of the contralateral femur are assessed with fluoroscopy before the patient is positioned. Supine or lateral positioning can be used with any implant, depending on the surgeon's preference, the patient's body habitus, and associated injuries. Lateral positioning is useful for exposing the proximal femur in an open approach (particularly if the patient is obese), aids in the correction of deformity, avoids varus malalignment, improves access to the proximal femoral starting point for intramedullary nail insertion, and frees the surgeon's hands and equipment from interference by the adjacent operating table surface.[18,19] Internal rotation of the distal fragment is necessary in the lateral position to avoid an external rotation deformity. Many surgeons prefer a compromise between the supine and lateral positions, in which a radiolucent bump is used beneath the ipsilateral pelvis and thorax to position the patient at an approximately 45° angle relative to the table surface.

All techniques used for the available implants require an acceptable reduction that includes femoral length, rotation, and alignment. Percutaneous reduction can be accomplished by using a plate or intramedullary construct. Because of the possibility of a simultaneous asymptomatic contralateral fracture, preoperative imaging of the contralateral limb should be obtained in a patient with an atypical subtrochanteric femur fracture.[20]

The fracture can be generally aligned with limb positioning and traction. The proximal fragment may be reducible with a ball-spike pusher or a similar instrument placed through an anterolateral percutaneous incision while flexion and abduction of the proximal segment are resisted. Reduction of the distal segment may require percutaneous use of a bone hook over the anterior shaft to resist medialization of the distal segment. The proximal and distal segments must be simultaneously manipulated to achieve the reduction. Schanz pins can be used to allow more direct control of the fracture segments. Clamps can be placed percutaneously if the fracture geometry permits their use.[21] An adequate reduction must be maintained throughout reaming. If reaming is inaccurate, nail passage will result in malalignment. Nail removal and reorientation of the reaming path are required to salvage the reduction while continuing to use the intramedullary device. The use of a Poller blocking screw may be necessary to correct the nail path (**Figure 1**).

It is possible to fix a fixed-angle plate to the proximal fragment and subsequently reduce the proximal construct to the distal segment. This powerful technique facilitates the reduction through application of the construct itself. However, if the initial relationship of the plate to the proximal segment is inaccurate, the resulting deformity can be corrected only by revising the proximal fixation. Simple fractures treated with plate fixation can be compressed with an articulated tensioning device. In general, the outcomes of plate fixation are improved by using a technique that preserves the vascular supply to the fracture and surrounding bone.[22] However, significant failure rates continue to be reported, as in proximal femoral locking-plate fixation.[23]

In using an intramedullary device, the starting point and the trajectory of reaming in the proximal segment are crucial to final fracture alignment. With a trochanteric starting point for a subtrochanteric fracture, great care must be taken to avoid reaming from lateral to medial, which can lead to varus malalignment with implant insertion. The ideal starting point for a subtrochanteric fracture varies based on individual patient anatomy, but most commonly, it is just medial to the tip of the greater trochanter. Medializing the starting point on the AP fluoroscopic view can aid in avoiding varus deformity during implant insertion.[24,25]

Open reduction and internal fixation sometimes is necessary (**Figure 3**). Regardless of whether a percutaneous or open surgical technique is used, vascularity to the fracture site should be preserved by avoiding aggressive retraction and stripping of soft tissue from the surrounding bone. It is preferable to avoid the use of cerclage wire implants, although they can be successfully inserted while the surrounding soft tissue is protected.[26,27] At the conclusion of the procedure, all instrumentation and implants should be kept sterile while the drapes are removed, and the length and rotation of the limb should be examined while the patient remains under anesthesia in a completely supine position. Any errors can be corrected after repreparation and draping.

Postoperative Management

The patient's weight-bearing status depends on the nature of the injury and the construct used. Patients who have a simple fracture with cortical opposition that was treated with an intramedullary construct without extension into the piriformis fossa or greater trochanter can be allowed to bear weight as tolerated, with the use of an assistive device. Patients with a comminuted fracture, a fracture extending into the piriformis fossa and greater trochanter, or a fracture treated with a plate construct are restricted from touchdown weight bearing for 6 to 8 weeks until callus formation is seen on radiographs.

Outcomes

Complications, including nonunion, implant failure, and infection, are relatively common after the treatment of subtrochanteric femoral fractures. The risk of such complications has decreased, however, with the increasing use of biomechanically superior constructs as well as approaches that preserve the vascular supply to the fracture site. Intramedullary implants increasingly are used to treat these fractures.

Subtrochanteric femoral fractures that involve only diaphyseal bone and are treated with a standard locking intramedullary nail have outcomes similar to those of diaphyseal femoral shaft fractures.[28-31] Cephalomedullary nails have been used with success in fractures with involvement of the posteromedial buttress; union rates have been high, and malunion rates have been low.[2,32-35] The likelihood of functional recovery appears to be best predicted by patient age; patients younger than 60 years are most likely to regain their prefracture level of activity.[33]

The development of trochanteric-entry cephalomedullary nails has expanded the use of intramedullary implants to include subtrochanteric fractures with extension into the piriformis fossa and involvement of the lesser trochanteric region. The use of such devices for the treatment of subtrochanteric femmoral fractures has led to high union and low complication rates.[1,4,36-38] At 1-year follow-up of 211 low-energy subtrochanteric femoral fractures treated with trochanteric long cephalomedullary nails, the union rate was 98%, and the reoperation rate was 8.9%. The 1-year mortality and functional status recovery rates were similar to those of similar patients who sustained femoral neck fractures; the mortality rate was 24%, and approximately one-half of the patients could not return to their home or preinjury functional status.[38]

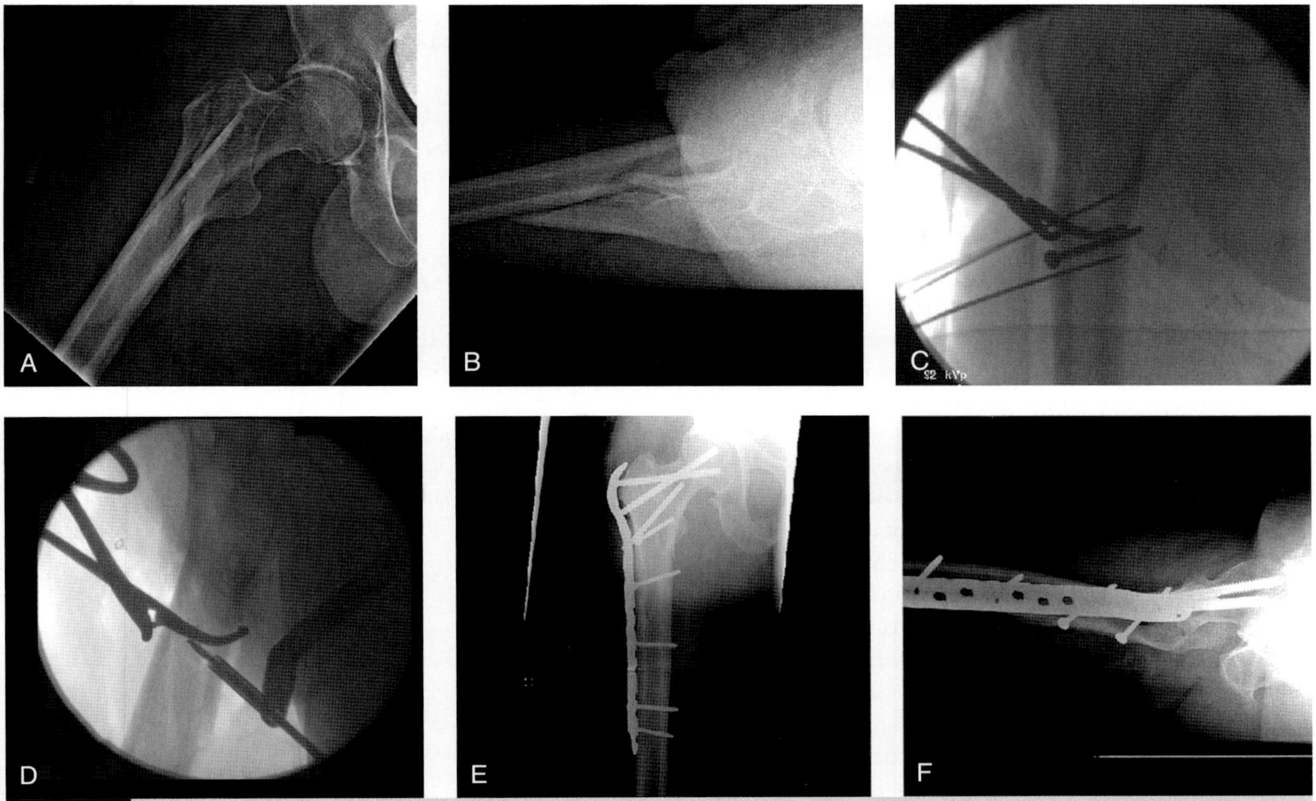

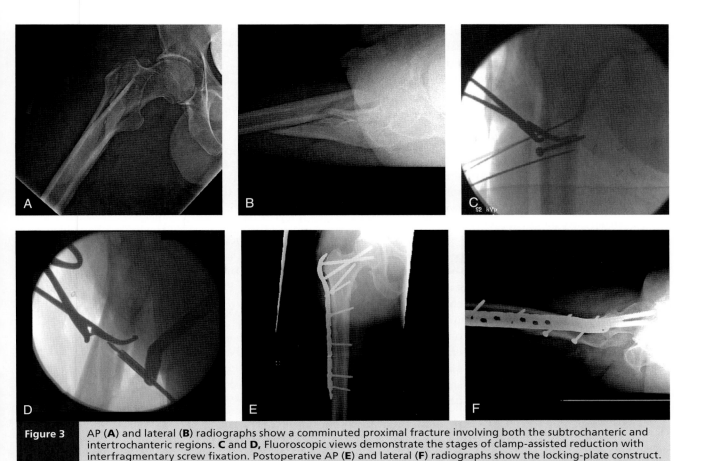

Figure 3 AP (**A**) and lateral (**B**) radiographs show a comminuted proximal fracture involving both the subtrochanteric and intertrochanteric regions. **C** and **D,** Fluoroscopic views demonstrate the stages of clamp-assisted reduction with interfragmentary screw fixation. Postoperative AP (**E**) and lateral (**F**) radiographs show the locking-plate construct.

Because of the usefulness of trochanteric cephalomedullary implants in treating fractures involving both the posteromedial buttress and the piriformis fossa as well as their perceived ease of insertion, some surgeons recommend that this implant be used to treat almost all complex proximal femur fractures. Trochanteric cephalomedullary implants have several disadvantages, however. They generally require the removal of a relatively large volume of bone from the proximal femur as well as a large footprint for the abductor insertion. Other concerns include insertion site pain, abductor weakness, and limited reconstruction options. No clinical evidence exists, however, that these factors lead to poor patient outcomes, but they remain a topic of discussion. The surgeon must understand the risk of varus malreduction of a subtrochanteric femoral fracture when using the relatively lateral starting point of a trochanteric nail.

A 95° fixed-angle plate construct also has been suggested as being suitable for the treatment of almost all subtrochanteric femoral fractures. Initial reports on these implants found high rates of nonunion (16% to 20%) and infection (20%).[3,5,39] However, as discussed previously, less invasive reduction and implant insertion techniques also can be used with plate constructs. Later reports of the use of 95° fixed-angle plate constructs generally found nonunion rates of 0% to 7% and low infection rates, likely related to use of improved technique.[4,17,22,40-46]

Complications

The likelihood of complications during the treatment of a patient with a subtrochanteric femoral fracture is affected by both modifiable and nonmodifiable factors. The modifiable factors include the adequacy of reduction, the surgical approach, soft-tissue stripping, and the choice of fixation construct. The nonmodifiable factors include the fracture pattern and the patient's age and comorbidities. The bimodal distribution of subtrochanteric femoral fractures requires the surgeon to consider the individual patient's bone quality, ability to maintain weight-bearing precautions, and overall surgical risk factors. An increased rate of complications, including nonunion and implant failure, was found in atypical subtrochanteric femoral fractures.[47]

The extent to which the fracture reduction is achieved and maintained throughout the surgical procedure is the single factor that most affects the outcome and is under the surgeon's control, regardless of implant selection. More than 10° of malreduction in any plane increases the risk of delayed union or nonunion of a subtrochanteric femoral fracture.[48] An understanding of the available reduction techniques and implant options can be useful for minimizing the risk of complications with a specific fracture pattern. Given the complexity of treating subtrochanteric femoral injuries, checking the clinical length and rotation of the limb before the patient is awakened from anesthesia avoids having technical errors become clinical complications. If nonunion occurs, revision fixation and bone grafting have a high success rate.[49-51]

Summary

Obtaining and maintaining an acceptable reduction of a subtrochanteric femoral fracture is a challenging surgical task, which can be accomplished through a variety of reduction techniques and fixation constructs. The unifying concepts in successful treatment are a thorough understanding of the fracture pattern and the deforming forces acting on the proximal and distal segments of the fracture. The treating surgeon should be well versed in the challenges posed by the specific fracture pattern and the relative benefits and limitations of the available fixation constructs.

Key Study Points

- Reduction of a subtrochanteric femoral fracture requires simultaneous manipulation of both fracture segments. The proximal segment is flexed, abducted, and externally rotated, whereas the distal segment is shortened and medialized.
- During intramedullary nailing of a subtrochanteric femoral fracture, the starting point and the vector used for reaming the proximal metaphysis must be accurate. Inaccuracy in reaming the proximal segment leads to malalignment after implant insertion.
- For plate fixation of a subtrochanteric femoral fracture, the use of a fixed-angle implant and a biologic surgical approach leads to a high rate of union and few complications.

Annotated References

1. Cheng MT, Chiu FY, Chuang TY, Chen CM, Chen TH, Lee PC: Treatment of complex subtrochanteric fracture with the long gamma AP locking nail: A prospective evaluation of 64 cases. *J Trauma* 2005;58(2):304-311.

2. Russell TA, Taylor JC: Subtrochanteric fractures of the femur, in Browner BD, Jupiter JB, Levine AM, Trafton PG, eds: *Skeletal Trauma: Fractures, Dislocations, Ligamentous Injuries* . Philadelphia, PA, Saunders, 1992, pp 1485-1525.

3. Sanders R, Regazzoni P: Treatment of subtrochanteric femur fractures using the dynamic condylar screw. *J Orthop Trauma* 1989;3(3):206-213.

4. Vanderschot P, Vanderspeeten K, Verheyen L, Broos P: A review on 161 subtrochanteric fractures: Risk factors influencing outcome. Age, fracture pattern and fracture level. *Unfallchirurg* 1995;98(5):265-271.

5. Waddell JP: Subtrochanteric fractures of the femur: A review of 130 patients. *J Trauma* 1979;19(8):582-592.

6. Maravic M, Ostertag A, Cohen-Solal M: Subtrochanteric/femoral shaft versus hip fractures: Incidences and identification of risk factors. *J Bone Miner Res* 2012;27(1):130-137.

   The incidence of subtrochanteric and femoral shaft fractures increased from 2002 to 2009. Compared with hip fractures, obesity and dementia were identified as risk factors for these fractures. Level of evidence: III.

7. Shane E, Burr D, Abrahamsen B, et al: Atypical subtrochanteric and diaphyseal femoral fractures: Second report of a task force of the American Society for Bone and Mineral Research. *J Bone Miner Res* 201429(1):1-23.

   Atypical femoral fractures are associated with diphosphonate use, and the risk increases with long-term use. The risk may decline when diphosphonate use ends. Inconsistent evidence indicates that teriparatide may advance the healing of an atypical femoral fracture. Level of evidence: III.

8. Koch JC: The laws of bone architecture. *Am J Anat* 1917;21(2):177-298.

9. Loizou CL, McNamara I, Ahmed K, Pryor GA, Parker MJ: Classification of subtrochanteric femoral fractures. *Injury* 2010;41(7):739-745.

   The subtrochanteric zone was defined as the area of bone extending 5 cm below the lower border of the lesser trochanter. Level of evidence: III.

10. Park-Wyllie LY, Mamdani MM, Juurlink DN, et al: Bisphosphonate use and the risk of subtrochanteric or femoral shaft fractures in older women. *JAMA* 2011;305(8):783-789.

    Women at least age 68 years who were treated with a diphosphonate for more than 5 years had an increased risk of a subtrochanteric or femoral shaft fracture, although the absolute risk of such a fracture remained low. Level of evidence: III.

11. Chiang CY, Zebaze RM, Ghasem-Zadeh A, Iuliano-Burns S, Hardidge A, Seeman E: Teriparatide improves bone quality and healing of atypical femoral fractures associated with bisphosphonate therapy. *Bone* 2013;52(1):360-365.

    Improvement in fracture healing was found in atypical femoral fractures treated with teriparatide. Level of evidence: Level IV.

12. Fukuda F, Kurinomaru N, Hijioka A: Weekly teriparatide for delayed unions of atypical subtrochanteric femur fractures. *Biol Ther* 2014;4(1-2):73-79.

    A case report described successful teriparatide treatment of a delayed union of an atypical subtrochanteric femoral fracture. Level of evidence: IV.

13. Hibbs RA: The management of the tendency of the upper fragment to tilt forward in fractures of the upper third of the femur. *NY Med J* 1902;75:177-179.

14. Johnson KD, Johnston DW, Parker B: Comminuted femoral-shaft fractures: Treatment by roller traction, cerclage wires and an intramedullary nail, or an interlocking intramedullary nail. *J Bone Joint Surg Am* 1984;66(8):1222-1235.

15. Ha YC, Cho MR, Park KH, Kim SY, Koo KH: Is surgery necessary for femoral insufficiency fractures after long-term bisphosphonate therapy? *Clin Orthop Relat Res* 2010;468(12):3393-3398.

    Nonsurgical treatment of femoral insufficiency fractures in the setting of prolonged diphosphonate therapy often is unsuccessful, and surgery is required for fracture displacement or intractable pain. Level of evidence: IV.

16. Haidukewych GJ, Israel TA, Berry DJ: Reverse obliquity fractures of the intertrochanteric region of the femur. *J Bone Joint Surg Am* 2001;83(5):643-650.

17. Wile PB, Panjabi MM, Southwick WO: Treatment of subtrochanteric fractures with a high-angle compression hip screw. *Clin Orthop Relat Res* 1983;175:72-78.

18. Bishop JA, Rodriguez EK: Closed intramedullary nailing of the femur in the lateral decubitus position. *J Trauma* 2010;68(1):231-235.

    The safety and effectiveness of intramedullary femoral nailing were described for patients in the lateral decubitus position. Level of evidence: III.

19. Connelly CL, Archdeacon MT: The lateral decubitus approach for complex proximal femur fractures: Anatomic reduction and locking plate neutralization. A technical trick. *J Orthop Trauma* 2012;26(4):252-257.

    A case study supported the use of the lateral decubitus position for locking-plate fixation of proximal femur fractures. Level of evidence: IV.

20. Capeci CM, Tejwani NC: Bilateral low-energy simultaneous or sequential femoral fractures in patients on long-term alendronate therapy. *J Bone Joint Surg Am* 2009;91(11):2556-2561.

21. Afsari A, Liporace F, Lindvall E, Infante A Jr, Sagi HC, Haidukewych GJ: Clamp-assisted reduction of high subtrochanteric fractures of the femur: Surgical technique. *J Bone Joint Surg Am* 2010;92(suppl 1, pt 2):217-225.

    Clamp-assisted reduction was found to be successful for the treatment of subtrochanteric femoral fractures with careful preservation of the surrounding soft-tissue attachment to bone. Level of evidence: IV.

22. Kinast C, Bolhofner BR, Mast JW, Ganz R: Subtrochanteric fractures of the femur: Results of treatment with the 95 degrees condylar blade-plate. *Clin Orthop Relat Res* 1989;238:122-130.

23. Glassner PJ, Tejwani NC: Failure of proximal femoral locking compression plate: A case series. *J Orthop Trauma* 2011;25(2):76-83.

    Proximal femoral locking compression plates had a high failure rate even after surgery by experienced and fellowship-trained traumatologists. Level of evidence: IV.

24. Ostrum RF, Marcantonio A, Marburger R: A critical analysis of the eccentric starting point for trochanteric intramedullary femoral nailing. *J Orthop Trauma* 2005;19(10):681-686.

25. Streubel PN, Wong AH, Ricci WM, Gardner MJ: Is there a standard trochanteric entry site for nailing of subtrochanteric femur fractures? *J Orthop Trauma* 2011;25(4):202-207.

    Preoperative templating using the contralateral femur helped determine the appropriate starting point for a trochanteric entry nail on a patient-specific basis. Level of evidence: IV.

26. Tomás J, Teixidor J, Batalla L, Pacha D, Cortina J: Subtrochanteric fractures: Treatment with cerclage wire and long intramedullary nail. *J Orthop Trauma* 2013;27(7):e157-e160.

    A cerclage wire was used through a minimally invasive approach to maintain reduction in certain subtrochanteric fracture patterns. Level of evidence: IV.

27. Kennedy MT, Mitra A, Hierlihy TG, Harty JA, Reidy D, Dolan M: Subtrochanteric hip fractures treated with cerclage cables and long cephalomedullary nails: A review of 17 consecutive cases over 2 years. *Injury* 2011;42(11):1317-1321.

    Cerclage wiring was used in the treatment of subtrochanteric femoral fractures without a deleterious effect on healing. The number of wires should be minimized. Level of evidence: IV.

28. Brumback RJ, Uwagie-Ero S, Lakatos RP, Poka A, Bathon GH, Burgess AR: Intramedullary nailing of femoral shaft fractures: Part II. Fracture-healing with static interlocking fixation. *J Bone Joint Surg Am* 1988;70(10):1453-1462.

29. Thoresen BO, Alho A, Ekeland A, Strømsøe K, Folleräs G, Haukebø A: Interlocking intramedullary nailing in femoral shaft fractures: A report of forty-eight cases. *J Bone Joint Surg Am* 1985;67(9):1313-1320.

30. Wiss DA, Brien WW, Stetson WB: Interlocked nailing for treatment of segmental fractures of the femur. *J Bone Joint Surg Am* 1990;72(5):724-728.

31. Wiss DA, Fleming CH, Matta JM, Clark D: Comminuted and rotationally unstable fractures of the femur treated with an interlocking nail. *Clin Orthop Relat Res* 1986;212:35-47.

32. Bose WJ, Corces A, Anderson LD: A preliminary experience with the Russell-Taylor reconstruction nail for complex femoral fractures. *J Trauma* 1992;32(1):71-76.

33. Garnavos C, Peterman A, Howard PW: The treatment of difficult proximal femoral fractures with the Russell-Taylor reconstruction nail. *Injury* 1999;30(6):407-415.

34. Kang S, McAndrew MP, Johnson KD: The reconstruction locked nail for complex fractures of the proximal femur. *J Orthop Trauma* 1995;9(6):453-463.

35. Smith JT, Goodman SB, Tischenko G: Treatment of comminuted femoral subtrochanteric fractures using the Russell-Taylor reconstruction intramedullary nail. *Orthopedics* 1991;14(2):125-129.

36. Borens O, Wettstein M, Kombot C, Chevalley F, Mouhsine E, Garofalo R: Long gamma nail in the treatment of subtrochanteric fractures. *Arch Orthop Trauma Surg* 2004;124(7):443-447.

37. Pakuts AJ: Unstable subtrochanteric fractures—gamma nail versus dynamic condylar screw. *Int Orthop* 2004;28(1):21-24.

38. Robinson CM, Houshian S, Khan LA: Trochanteric-entry long cephalomedullary nailing of subtrochanteric fractures caused by low-energy trauma. *J Bone Joint Surg Am* 2005;87(10):2217-2226.

39. Nungu KS, Olerud C, Rehnberg L: Treatment of subtrochanteric fractures with the AO dynamic condylar screw. *Injury* 1993;24(2):90-92.

40. Kulkarni SS, Moran CG: Results of dynamic condylar screw for subtrochanteric fractures. *Injury* 2003;34(2):117-122.

41. Neher C, Ostrum RF: Treatment of subtrochanteric femur fractures using a submuscular fixed low-angle plate. *Am J Orthop (Belle Mead NJ)* 2003;32(9, suppl):29-33.

42. Siebenrock KA, Müller U, Ganz R: Indirect reduction with a condylar blade plate for osteosynthesis of subtrochanteric femoral fractures. *Injury* 1998;29(suppl 3):C7-C15.

43. Vaidya SV, Dholakia DB, Chatterjee A: The use of a dynamic condylar screw and biological reduction techniques for subtrochanteric femur fracture. *Injury* 2003;34(2):123-128.

44. Tornetta P III: Subtrochanteric femur fracture. *J Orthop Trauma* 2002;16(4):280-283.

45. Saini P, Kumar R, Shekhawat V, Joshi N, Bansal M, Kumar S: Biological fixation of comminuted subtrochanteric fractures with proximal femur locking compression plate. *Injury* 2013;44(2):226-231.

Proximal femoral locking-plate fixation of subtrochanteric femur fractures achieved a high union rate with a low complication rate. Level of evidence: IV.

46. Hu SJ, Zhang SM, Yu GR: Treatment of femoral subtrochanteric fractures with proximal lateral femur locking plates. *Acta Ortop Bras* 2012;20(6):329-333.

A case study supported the use of lateral femoral locking-plate fixation. A high union rate and a low complication rate were observed. Level of evidence: IV.

47. Teo BJ, Koh JS, Goh SK, Png MA, Chua DT, Howe TS: Post-operative outcomes of atypical femoral subtrochanteric fracture in patients on bisphosphonate therapy. *Bone Joint J* 2014;96-B(5):658-664.

Atypical subtrochanteric femur fractures were associated with slow healing and prolonged postoperative immobility. Level of evidence: IV.

48. Riehl JT, Koval KJ, Langford JR, Munro MW, Kupiszewski SJ, Haidukewych GJ: Intramedullary nailing of subtrochanteric femur fractures: Does malreduction matter? *Bull Hosp Jt Dis* 2014;72(2):159-63.

In subtrochanteric femoral fractures treated with an intramedullary device, malreduction of more than 10° in any plane was associated with a significantly increased rate of delayed union and/or nonunion. Level of evidence: IV.

49. Barquet A, Mayora G, Fregeiro J, López L, Rienzi D, Francescoli L: The treatment of subtrochanteric nonunions with the long gamma nail: Twenty-six patients with a minimum 2-year follow-up. *J Orthop Trauma* 2004;18(6):346-353.

50. Haidukewych GJ, Berry DJ: Nonunion of fractures of the subtrochanteric region of the femur. *Clin Orthop Relat Res* 2004;419:185-188.

51. Pascarella R, Maresca A, Palumbi P, Boriani S: Subtrochanteric nonunion of the femur. *Chir Organi Mov* 2004;89(1):1-6.

Chapter 39

Femoral Shaft Fractures

Toni M. McLaurin, MD Charisse Y. Sparks, MD

Abstract

Femur fractures in adults are usually the result of high-energy trauma and can have a substantial effect on the overall physiology of the trauma patient. Understanding the importance of this injury and the most appropriate management are critical to ensuring an optimal outcome.

Keywords: femoral shaft fracture; diaphyseal; intramedullary nail; temporary external fixation; reaming

Introduction

Along with unstable pelvis and spine fractures, femoral shaft fractures are one of the orthopaedic injuries that can substantially affect the overall physiology of the trauma patient. Understanding the importance of this injury and the most appropriate management are critical to ensuring an optimal outcome, whereas not recognizing the physiologic effect or potential complications of a femur fracture can have a deleterious effect on the patient.

Initial Evaluation and Management

Femur fractures in adults are usually the result of high-energy trauma, and a standard Advanced Trauma Life Support protocol should be used at initial presentation. After the airway is secured, the primary survey is completed, and appropriate resuscitation is underway, attention can be turned to the evaluation of the femur fracture. Patients may present with an obvious deformity but often are brought in by emergency medical services with a traction splint already applied. Historically, after the patient was hemodynamically stabilized, skeletal traction was applied, using either a distal femoral or proximal tibial traction pin. Although the use of skeletal traction has more recently been abandoned by some in favor of long leg splinting or skin (cutaneous) traction, distal femoral traction has been shown to result in less pain during and after immobilization than long leg splinting, with no subsequent knee dysfunction.[1] However, cutaneous traction shows the same reduction in pretraction and posttraction pain using visual analog scale scores, no difference in pain medication requirements or time to reduction intraoperatively, and a significant reduction in time of application compared with skeletal traction,[2] so cutaneous traction can be considered a viable alternative to skeletal traction. After the femur is placed in traction, the overall status of the patient can be more definitively evaluated, and additional studies such as CT can be performed as needed.

Physical Examination

A thorough motor and sensory examination must be performed to rule out any vascular or neurologic injury. Diminished or absent pulses may be noted on initial presentation but often return to normal after the angular and rotational deformities of the femur are corrected using splinting or traction. If pulses remain diminished, asymmetric, or not palpable, the ankle-brachial index should be measured and further evaluation pursued if the ankle-brachial index is less than 0.9. Although rare with femoral shaft fractures, any neurologic injury must be carefully documented. The secondary survey can then be used to rule out any additional injuries associated with high-energy trauma such as those involving the pelvis, spine, or other extremities.

Although the details of resuscitation and management of the trauma patient are not discussed in this chapter, it is important to realize and understand the physiologic effect of a femoral shaft fracture. Estimated blood loss from a closed femoral shaft fracture can range from

Dr. McLaurin or an immediate family member serves as a board member, owner, officer, or committee member of the Orthopaedic Trauma Association. Dr. Sparks or an immediate family member is a member of a speakers' bureau or has made paid presentations on behalf of DePuy and Synthes; and has stock or stock options held in Synthes.

6: Lower Extremity

500 to 1,000 mL; this number increases with an open fracture.[3] Therefore, the potential for hypovolemic shock must be recognized and the appropriate resuscitation initiated. The patient's physiologic status must be continually monitored throughout the initial workup and early stages of treatment to confirm successful ongoing resuscitation efforts.

Imaging

Plain radiographs are obtained after the patient and the fracture have been initially stabilized, and should include AP and lateral femur radiographs, as well as AP and lateral hip and knee views. In addition, an AP pelvis view is often obtained according to the Advanced Trauma Life Support protocol. Most polytrauma patients and many of those with only isolated femur fractures will have had an abdomen/pelvis CT scan obtained, allowing evaluation for the presence of an ipsilateral femoral neck fracture, which can be missed on the AP pelvic view. This injury pattern is associated with high-energy femur fractures in the young patient, and although it occurs in only approximately 1% to 9% of femoral shaft fractures,[4] missing this injury can have devastating consequences for the patient. Historically, 20% to 50% of these injuries were missed on initial presentation, but this can be improved with the combined use of axial and sagittal CT cuts through the femoral neck, an internal rotation AP view of the hip preoperatively (which can be difficult to obtain in the setting of a fractured femur), fluoroscopic examination intraoperatively, and postoperative AP and lateral hip radiographs.[5,6] Many centers have now established protocols for appropriately evaluating the femoral neck. Although initially a 91% reduction in the incidence of missed femoral neck fractures was found when CT was added to radiographic evaluation of the femoral neck,[6] more recently it has been shown that both CT scans and plain radiographs alone have similar high rates of false-negative results, with poor sensitivity of 64% and 56%, respectively, but a low rate of false-positive results, with specificity of 96% and 94%, respectively.[5] This change may be a result of increased vigilance in looking for ipsilateral femoral neck fractures, resulting in less of a difference between the findings of CT and plain radiography. However, combining multiple imaging modalities resulted in a low rate (3%) of missed femoral neck fractures.

Classification

Historically, femoral shaft fractures have been classified based on the amount of comminution and cortical contact present (Winquist classification),[7] but with the routine use of statically locked intramedullary nails and immediate postoperative weight bearing as tolerated for diaphyseal fractures, this type of classification scheme becomes less important because it no longer determines either treatment or postoperative management and it has no prognostic importance. The Orthopaedic Trauma Association classification[8] is useful for descriptive and comparative purposes for research, but is also not widely used in practice.

Treatment

Timing

Although the first prospective study on the reduction and stabilization of acute femoral shaft fractures that resulted in decreased pulmonary complications, days in the hospital, days in the intensive care unit, mortality, and the cost of hospital care was published in 1989,[9] the controversy over the timing and technique for definitive management remains ongoing. Retrospective and prospective studies,[10,11] as well as systematic reviews,[12] have reported disparate results when examining the previously mentioned parameters and comparing early with delayed definitive fixation. However, despite weak supporting evidence, there is a consensus that early definitive treatment (less than 24 hours after injury) of femoral shaft fractures is safe and beneficial for most trauma patients, including those with head injury, when appropriate intraoperative intracranial pressure monitoring is used.[12] Resuscitation with correction of systemic inflammatory markers such as lactate, base deficit, and pH levels can help determine the optimum time for definitive treatment. Earlier literature supported delaying definitive treatment in patients with thoracic trauma and advocated acute damage control orthopaedics for these borderline patients,[10,11] but this approach has not been supported in more recent literature, which shows patients with thoracic trauma to have better outcomes following early instead of delayed definitive treatment.[13]

Treatment Options

The gold standard for definitive treatment of femoral shaft fractures remains reamed, statically locked intramedullary nailing, but there are options regarding the direction of nailing (antegrade versus retrograde) and location of starting point with antegrade nails (piriformis versus trochanteric). The question of reamed versus unreamed nailing remains controversial but has largely been answered because the concerns about negative pulmonary effects with reaming have not been proved,[14,15] and reamed nails have higher union rates, shorter time to union, and lower perioperative complication rates (including implant failure) than unreamed nails, with no difference in mortality or rates of adult respiratory distress syndrome (ARDS).[14,16,17] Another issue for surgeons who do not frequently perform intramedullary nailing is the freehand placement of either the distal interlocking screws in antegrade nailing or the proximal interlocking screws in retrograde nailing. Multiple-insertion jig extensions have been tried without success, but more recently, an electromagnetic targeting device has been shown to result in substantially decreased exposure to ionizing radiation and a potential decrease in surgical time, with similar accuracy compared with freehand interlocking screw placement.[18-20]

Provisional Stabilization

Skeletal Traction

Although external fixation has become the mainstay of damage control orthopaedics, evidence exists that the outcomes of temporary stabilization using skeletal traction during the acute phase are no different than those of external fixation with respect to rates of ARDS, multiple organ failure, pulmonary embolism, deep vein thrombosis, pneumonia, mechanical ventilation days, intensive care unit length of stay, or death in the severely injured patient.[21] Because external fixation offers no advantage over skeletal traction in the critically injured patient, temporary skeletal traction is a simple, inexpensive option that avoids an additional trip to the operating room for those patients who do not require general anesthesia for some other lifesaving procedures.

External Fixation

External fixation is well established as the method of stabilization most often used acutely in the unstable polytrauma patient. External fixation is fast, with low morbidity and a limited complication profile. However, it is not without risks:[22] if conversion to intramedullary nailing is planned, it should be completed in less than 2 weeks to avoid an increased risk of infection.[23,24] Immediate external fixation with early conversion to closed nailing is a safe practice, with an infection rate reported from 1.7% to 3.6% and a union rate of 97%.[23,25,26]

Unreamed Retrograde Nailing

Unreamed retrograde nailing has been described for rapid provisional stabilization of femur fractures, but this is an extremely technique-intensive option that is probably not feasible for most surgeons. Although this technique has advantages over temporary external fixation, including the elimination of concern for pin tract infections and contamination of a future surgical site, the disadvantages include the need for a secondary procedure and that the technique is not well established or particularly rapid. However, the surgical procedure still involves anesthesia, blood loss, and the possibility of fat embolism, even with unreamed intramedullary nails.

Any of the previously mentioned techniques can be used to stabilize the femur acutely until the patient's physiologic status has improved enough to allow definitive treatment. In addition, if the patient remains unfit for any additional surgery, either external fixation or the unreamed nail can act as definitive fixation. To avoid exacerbation of the "second hit" phenomenon, definitive stabilization should not be performed when the patient is in a proinflammatory state, and should be delayed until the effect of the "second hit" on the patient's overall physiologic status is diminished, usually not until about the fifth day.[27]

Antegrade Intramedullary Nailing

Trochanteric Versus Piriformis Fossa Entry Portals

The starting point of an antegrade intramedullary nail has two options: the piriformis fossa and trochanteric entry. Because the piriformis fossa is in line with the femoral canal, using a piriformis start nail is cited as better than a trochanteric entry point. However, this issue was more pronounced with straight nails that have no proximal lateral bend and were not specifically designed for trochanteric entry; placing a straight nail through a trochanteric entry point can result in fracture comminution, eccentric reaming of the medial cortex, and varus deformity.[7,28] Current nail designs with a 4° to 5° proximal lateral bend have effectively eliminated these problems.[29] Selecting the appropriate location for the trochanteric starting point, which is just medial to the tip of the greater trochanter (**Figure 1**) and in line with the femoral shaft in the sagittal plane, also helps minimize these intraoperative complications. Concerns also exist about increased damage to the abductor muscles caused by a trochanteric entry point. However, cadaver, electromyographic, MRI, and functional outcome evaluations have all shown nailing through a piriformis entry portal can result in more damage to the abductor and external rotator muscles, and even the superior gluteal nerve, resulting in a positive Trendelenburg sign.[30,31] The medial femoral circumflex artery is also at greater risk with a piriformis fossa starting point.[30] With current nail designs, either no functional difference[28,32] or even improved functional outcomes[31] have been shown when a trochanteric starting point instead of the piriformis fossa is used for antegrade intramedullary nailing. Additionally, a trochanteric starting point can result in decreased surgical time, smaller incisions, and decreased fluoroscopy time, with these differences increased in obese patients. With proper nail insertion technique and nails designed for a specific entry

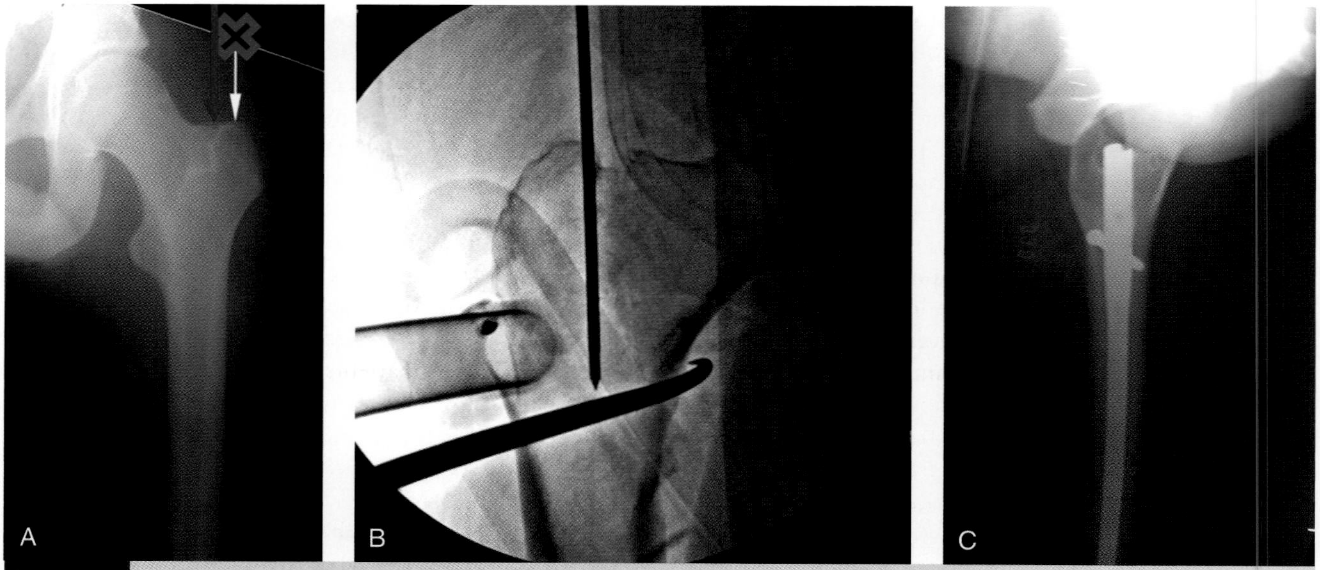

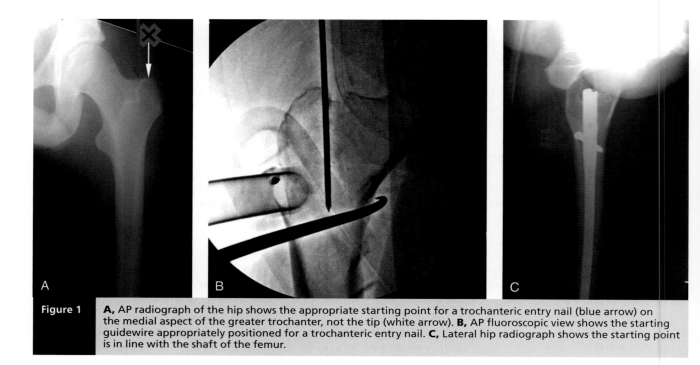

Figure 1 **A,** AP radiograph of the hip shows the appropriate starting point for a trochanteric entry nail (blue arrow) on the medial aspect of the greater trochanter, not the tip (white arrow). **B,** AP fluoroscopic view shows the starting guidewire appropriately positioned for a trochanteric entry nail. **C,** Lateral hip radiograph shows the starting point is in line with the shaft of the femur.

portal, no difference exists in malalignment.[28,32] It is not the nail starting point but technical errors that result in malreduction and malalignment.

Retrograde Nailing

In addition to provisional stabilization, reamed retrograde nails are frequently used for definitive treatment of femoral shaft fractures. The advantages of retrograde nailing are well known and include a starting point that is easier to find, easier nail placement in obese patients, and the capability to position the patient supine and allow other surgical services simultaneous access to the patient, which is particularly important in the polytrauma patient. Relative indications are obesity; pregnancy; ipsilateral fractures of the tibia, femoral neck, pelvis, acetabulum, and/or patella; traumatic knee lacerations; distal femoral fractures; bilateral femoral shaft fractures; spine fractures; polytrauma; and the presence of other extremity injuries that could be treated simultaneously with the patient in a supine position, avoiding the need for a change in patient positioning.[33] Despite the use of an intercondylar starting point, no long-term effects on knee cartilage have been reported due to this intra-articular insertion, with union rates equal to antegrade nailing when reamed nails were used.[34] Knee sepsis after retrograde nailing through a traumatic knee arthrotomy or retrograde nailing of open fractures has always been of concern and has been anecdotally reported in the past, but retrospective reviews have shown no increased rate of knee sepsis in either scenario.[33,35]

Plating

The role of plating is limited in the treatment of femoral shaft fractures. Plating has long been shown not to confer any benefits over reamed nailing with respect to ARDS, pneumonia, pulmonary embolism, failure of multiple organs, or death.[36] Percutaneous plating is a viable alternative in adults with small femoral canal diameters for which even the smallest-diameter nail could be difficult to place, but is a technique more often reserved for the pediatric population with axially unstable fractures. Open plating is indicated for periprosthetic fractures and also can be used for cases in which the fracture has been exposed during repair of a vascular injury, and a plate can be applied to the medial femur via the same incision. One disadvantage of plating, especially in the polytrauma population, is that patients must limit weight bearing after femoral plating.

Special Considerations

Ipsilateral Femoral Neck and Shaft Fractures

The reported incidence of this injury is approximately 1% to 9%, but failure to diagnose it can be devastating. After diagnosis, multiple treatment options are available, but it must be determined which injury takes precedence, especially in an unstable patient for whom it can become impossible to definitively treat all injuries acutely. Multiple small, underpowered retrospective series have examined treatment options, but little prospective or randomized data are available to guide treatment.[4]

Although delay in treatment of the femoral shaft has a more immediate effect on the patient's physiology, delay in treatment of the femoral neck can result in more long-term problems such as osteonecrosis, posttraumatic arthrosis, or nonunion, and most centers advocate anatomic reduction and fixation of the femoral neck before focusing on the femoral shaft. Numerous fixation constructs have been proposed; the two most frequently used are fixation of both fractures with a single implant (a reconstruction nail), or the use of two separate implants. Using two implants involves anatomic fixation of the femoral neck fracture either with multiple cannulated screws or with a sliding hip screw plus antirotation screw, and fixation of the femoral shaft with a retrograde nail. There is an increased risk of femoral neck nonunion, malreduction, and loss of reduction with the use of reconstruction nailing, and most authors now think that this implant is not appropriate for use in this fracture pattern.[4,37-39] Although a sliding hip screw with antirotation screw has been shown to be a more biomechanically sound construct than multiple cannulated screws for isolated Pauwels III femoral neck fractures, in ipsilateral femoral neck and shaft fractures, no difference is noted between the two constructs in femoral neck union rates or malreduction when combined with a reamed retrograde intramedullary nail.[40] For cases in which the patient is unable to tolerate intramedullary nailing after the femoral neck has been treated, temporary external fixation can be used and the femur treated definitively whenever the patient is stable.[4]

Bilateral Femur Fractures

Bilateral femur fractures are a marker of severe injury and have been associated with increased mortality as well as increased incidence of fat embolism syndrome, respiratory failure, and other associated injuries.[41] This increase in morbidity and mortality persists even after early fracture fixation.[42] In addition, multiple intramedullary procedures, which would be necessary for this injury, are an independent risk factor (along with thoracic injury) for respiratory failure. Intramedullary nailing triggers an inflammatory response, and the associated increased soft-tissue injury with bilateral femur fractures also contributes to this inflammatory response, exacerbating the problem.[43] Improvements in reamer head and shaft design, improved surgical technique, and the use of smaller-diameter nails, along with overall improved trauma care, have helped to decrease the incidence of these complications.

An overall decrease in mortality from both bilateral and unilateral femur fractures has occurred over the past 2 decades, but bilateral femur fractures still have a higher mortality rate (6% to 10% versus approximately 2%), with more associated injuries than unilateral femur fractures.[42,44-46] The increased number of associated injuries occurring with bilateral femur fractures appears to play as much, if not more, of a role in the mortality rate than the femoral injuries themselves, as is shown by a substantially increased mortality rate seen in bilateral femur fractures with associated injuries compared with isolated bilateral femur fractures (31.6% versus 9.8%).[46] Other than multiple intramedullary procedures known to be an independent risk factor, literature is sparse on whether bilateral femur fractures should be nailed in a single procedure, staged, or if bilateral nailing should be avoided in more critically ill patients.

Open Femur Fractures

Because of the substantial soft-tissue disruption and periosteal stripping necessary for a femur fracture to break through such a robust soft-tissue envelope, almost all open femur fractures should be considered and treated as type IIIA open fractures, irrespective of wound size, with the exception of an outside-in type of open injury. Open femur fractures have an increased rate of infection, time to union, and rate of nonunion compared with closed femur fractures, and these rates are unaffected by the choice of implant.[47,48] The infection rate for open femur fractures following intramedullary nailing ranges from 3% to 5%; type IIIB open fractures have a higher risk of infection than lower grade fractures.[47] However, as long as the principles of open fracture management are followed, including enlargement of the wound, meticulous débridement and irrigation, and stable fixation, any appropriate method of stabilization can be used.[33]

Fat Embolism Syndrome

The pathophysiology of fat embolism syndrome (FES) is not fully understood, and is generally thought to be mediated by two main processes: mechanical obstruction and biochemical injury.[49] It is important to differentiate the clinical signs and symptoms of FES from the subclinical phenomenon of fat embolization that occurs frequently with long bone and pelvic fractures. Pulmonary fat embolism has been found in up to 82% of trauma patients at autopsy,[50] but the incidence of FES in patients with long bone fractures is 0.5% to 11.0%.[51] Diagnosis can be difficult because no standard diagnostic criteria exist, but the classic triad of the clinical presentation is hypoxemia, neurologic abnormalities, and petechiae in nondependent regions (conjunctiva, head, neck, anterior thorax, or axilla), all of which occur after an asymptomatic latent period of 24 to 48 hours postinjury. Radiographic and laboratory findings also can be nonspecific. Despite some evidence that corticosteroids can play a role in reducing the incidence of FES,[52] supportive care of the respiratory failure and hypovolemia, along with frequent monitoring of neurologic status, still remains the only current treatment. Early surgical fixation can help decrease the risk of FES.[9] The mortality rate of FES has decreased to less than 10%, and the outcome for survivors is usually favorable, with the pulmonary, neurologic, and dermatologic manifestations generally completely resolving.[49]

Postoperative Treatment

Patients with diaphyseal femur fractures treated with statically-locked intramedullary nails can begin immediate weight bearing as tolerated, irrespective of degree of comminution, as long as interlocking screws are at least 5.0 mm in diameter.[53] Union rates are reported at 97% to 99%. Even with this high union rate, functional deficits can still be seen 2 years or longer after injury, including abductor and external rotator muscle dysfunction, decreased leg endurance, gait disturbance, and decreased functional outcome scores compared with baseline.[29,31,54,55] No differences in functional outcomes with respect to knee function have been found for antegrade versus retrograde intramedullary nailing.[56] In addition, reamed intramedullary nailing has been shown to be a moderate risk factor for the development of cognitive impairment 12 months after injury, even in the absence of any known brain injury at the time of initial presentation with the femur fracture.[57] Femoral shaft fractures are a substantial physical and physiologic insult that require multidisciplinary long-term rehabilitation for optimal recovery.

Summary

Fractures of the femoral diaphysis are typically the result of high-energy trauma, can have a substantial effect on the overall physiology of the polytrauma patient, and have a high association with injuries to other body systems as well other extremities, especially when the injury is bilateral. The gold standard for treatment remains reamed, statically locked, intramedullary nailing, but the direction of nailing and the starting point can be left up to the surgeon because union rates and rates of malreduction are similar with any modern nailing system used. Decision making should account for the patient's other injuries and/or comorbidities, fracture characteristics, and surgeon preference as well as experience. Although early stabilization of femur fractures results in decreased morbidity and mortality, in an unstable patient, provisional fixation such as an external fixator can be used in the acute setting, and definitive fixation with an intramedullary nail delayed until the patient is more stable. Early postoperative weight bearing, improved overall management of trauma patients, high union rates, and low rates of malreduction and malunion have resulted in most patients with femoral shaft fractures returning to their preinjury level of function, but it is important to recognize the risk of prolonged functional and cognitive deficits.

Key Study Points

- The gold standard for the treatment of diaphyseal femoral shaft fractures is reamed, statically locked, intramedullary nailing.
- Early stabilization of femur fractures (within 24 hours after injury) results in decreased pulmonary complications, days in the hospital, days in the intensive care unit, mortality, and cost of hospital care, but the type of stabilization needs to be tailored to the patient's physiologic status.
- Temporary external fixation of the femoral shaft can be performed acutely in the unstable patient and safely converted to definitive fixation with an intramedullary nail within 2 weeks.
- Secondary definitive nailing should be delayed until the patient is out of the proinflammatory phase (approximately days 2 through 4) to minimize the pulmonary and organ effects of a new physiologic insult.
- Piriformis fossa and trochanteric starting points can both be used with appropriately designed antegrade nails, with no differences in malreduction or malalignment and potentially less soft-tissue disturbance and neurovascular risk with a trochanteric starting point.

Annotated References

1. Bumpass DB, Ricci WM, McAndrew CM, Gardner MJ: A prospective study of pain reduction and knee dysfunction comparing femoral skeletal traction and splinting in adult trauma patients. *J Orthop Trauma* 2015;29(2):112-118.

The authors compared patients with femoral shaft fractures placed either into distal femoral traction (85 patients) or a long-leg splint (35 patients) with respect to preinjury and postinjury knee pain and function, as well as pain before, during, and immediately after fracture immobilization. During and after application of immobilization, visual analog scale pain scores were significantly lower in the traction group ($P < 0.01$). Although the entire cohort showed a slight decrease in Lysholm knee survey scores from baseline to 6 months postinjury, there was no significant difference between the two groups, showing no detectable knee dysfunction resulting from distal femoral traction. Level of evidence: II.

2. Even JL, Richards JE, Crosby CG, et al: Preoperative skeletal versus cutaneous traction for femoral shaft fractures treated within 24 hours. *J Orthop Trauma* 2012;26(10):e177-e182.

   The authors compared the use of cutaneous traction versus skeletal traction in 65 patients with 66 femoral shaft fractures treated within 24 hours. There was a significant reduction in time of application for cutaneous traction ($P \leq 0.001$), but no significant differences in posttraction visual analog scale pain scores, pain medication requirements, or time of reduction in the operating room. Level of evidence: II.

3. Gulli B, Ciatolla JA, Barnes L, American Academy of Orthopaedic Surgeons. *Emergency Care and Transportation of the Sick and Injured*. 10th ed.Sudbury, MA: Jones and Bartlett; 2011, pp 672-673.

   In this classic textbook that has now become the gold standard training program for Emergency Medical Services (EMS) education, Chapter 29: Orthopaedic Injuries provides an overview of the anatomy and physiology of the musculoskeletal system. This includes the proper assessment for suspected and obvious injuries and details the emergency treatment of orthopaedic injuries.

4. Boulton CL, Pollak AN: Special topic: Ipsilateral femoral neck and shaft fractures—does evidence give us the answer? *Injury* 2015;46(3):478-483.

   The authors review the incidence, mechanism of injury, diagnosis, and treatment options for ipsilateral femoral neck and shaft fractures and present their preferred method of treatment: anatomic open reduction and internal fixation of the femoral neck followed by retrograde nailing to treat the femoral shaft fracture. Functional outcomes for treatment of this injury are generally reported as good (63% to 94%), but few studies use validated outcome instruments and most are underpowered, indicating the need for prospective, randomized trials.

5. O'Toole RV, Dancy L, Dietz AR, et al: Diagnosis of femoral neck fracture associated with femoral shaft fracture: Blinded comparison of computed tomography and plain radiography. *J Orthop Trauma* 2013;27(6):325-330.

   The authors hypothesized that axial CT of the pelvis is superior to plain AP pelvic radiography at detecting ipsilateral femoral neck fractures, but found in a blinded, randomized, retrospective review of image sets that axial CT and AP pelvic radiographs had similar high rates of missed femoral neck fractures, with poor sensitivity of 64% and 56%, respectively.

6. Tornetta P III, Kain MS, Creevy WR: Diagnosis of femoral neck fractures in patients with a femoral shaft fracture. Improvement with a standard protocol. *J Bone Joint Surg Am* 2007;89(1):39-43.

7. Winquist RA, Hansen ST Jr, Clawson DK: Closed intramedullary nailing of femoral fractures. A report of five hundred and twenty cases. *J Bone Joint Surg Am* 1984;66(4):529-539.

8. Marsh JL, Slongo TF, Agel J, et al: Fracture and dislocation classification compendium - 2007: Orthopaedic Trauma Association classification, database and outcomes committee. *J Orthop Trauma* 2007;21(10suppl):S1-S133.

9. Bone LB, Johnson KD, Weigelt J, Scheinberg R: Early versus delayed stabilization of femoral fractures. A prospective randomized study. *J Bone Joint Surg Am* 1989;71(3):336-340.

10. Pape HC, Grimme K, Van Griensven M, et al; EPOFF Study Group: Impact of intramedullary instrumentation versus damage control for femoral fractures on immunoinflammatory parameters: Prospective randomized analysis by the EPOFF Study Group. *J Trauma* 2003;55(1):7-13.

11. Pape HC, Rixen D, Morley J, et al; EPOFF Study Group: Impact of the method of initial stabilization for femoral shaft fractures in patients with multiple injuries at risk for complications (borderline patients). *Ann Surg* 2007;246(3):491-499, discussion 499-501.

12. Nahm NJ, Vallier HA: Timing of definitive treatment of femoral shaft fractures in patients with multiple injuries: A systematic review of randomized and nonrandomized trials. *J Trauma Acute Care Surg* 2012;73(5):1046-1063.

    This systematic review of randomized and nonrandomized studies compared early and delayed treatment or early treatment and damage control orthopaedics and was performed to determine the effect of timing of definitive treatment of femoral shaft fractures on the incidence of ARDS, mortality rate, and length of stay in patients with multiple injuries. The authors concluded early definitive treatment may be safe in most multiplyinjured patients. Level of evidence: III.

13. Gandhi RR, Overton TL, Haut ER, et al: Optimal timing of femur fracture stabilization in polytrauma patients: A practice management guideline from the Eastern Association for the Surgery of Trauma. *J Trauma Acute Care Surg* 2014;77(5):787-795.

    Based on a systematic review and meta-analysis, The Practice Management Guideline Committee of EAST suggests early (less than 24 hours) definitive fixation of femoral shaft fractures. Although the strength of the evidence is low, early stabilization shows a trend toward lower risk of infection, mortality, and venous thromboembolism.

14. Canadian Orthopaedic Trauma Society: Reamed versus unreamed intramedullary nailing of the femur: Comparison of the rate of ARDS in multiple injured patients. *J Orthop Trauma* 2006;20(6):384-387.

15. Giannoudis PV, Tzioupis C, Pape H-C: Fat embolism: The reaming controversy. *Injury* 2006;37(4suppl 4):S50-S58.

16. Duan X, Li T, Mohammed AQ, Xiang Z: Reamed intramedullary nailing versus unreamed intramedullary nailing for shaft fracture of femur: A systematic literature review. *Arch Orthop Trauma Surg* 2011;131(10):1445-1452.

This systematic literature review compared reamed with unreamed nailing among 7trials with 952 patients and found reamed nailing had a substantially lower reoperation rate, lower nonunion rate, and lower delayed union rate, with no substantial differences in implant failure rates, mortality or ARDS.

17. Canadian Orthopaedic Trauma Society: Nonunion following intramedullary nailing of the femur with and without reaming. Results of a multicenter randomized clinical trial. *J Bone Joint Surg Am* 2003;85-A(11):2093-2096.

18. Langfitt MK, Halvorson JJ, Scott AT, et al: Distal locking using an electromagnetic field-guided computer-based real-time system for orthopaedic trauma patients. *J Orthop Trauma* 2013;27(7):367-372.

The authors compared distal interlocking screw placement in 24 femoral and 24 tibial nails using either a freehand technique or an electromagnetic field real-time system (EFRTS). EFRTS was significantly faster ($P < 0.0001$) regardless of training level, and there were fewer screw misses with EFRTS. Level of evidence: II.

19. Maqungo S, Horn A, Bernstein B, Keel M, Roche S: Distal interlocking screw placement in the femur: Free-hand versus electromagnetic assisted technique (sureshot). *J Orthop Trauma* 2014;28(12):e281-e283.

The authors compared distal interlocking screw placement using either a freehand technique or an EM targeting system in a prospectively randomized group of 100 consecutive femoral shaft fractures in 99 patients requiring intramedullary nailing with respect to operating time, radiation dose, and accuracy of screw placement. There was a significant reduction in radiation exposure ($P < 0.0001$) but no differences in operating time or accuracy of drill bit placement. Level of evidence: II.

20. Somerson JS, Rowley D, Kennedy C, Buttacavoli F, Agarwal A: Electromagnetic navigation reduces surgical time and radiation exposure for proximal interlocking in retrograde femoral nailing. *J Orthop Trauma* 2014;28(7):417-421.

In a cadaver model, the authors showed that proximal femur interlocking screw insertion using an EM navigation system was significantly faster ($P = 0.002$) than the standard fluoroscopic freehand method, with the potential to prevent ionizing radiation exposure.

21. Scannell BP, Waldrop NE, Sasser HC, Sing RF, Bosse MJ: Skeletal traction versus external fixation in the initial temporization of femoral shaft fractures in severely injured patients. *J Trauma* 2010;68(3):633-640.

The major physiologic clinical outcomes of provisional skeletal traction (ST) versus damage control external fixation of femoral shaft fractures in severely injured patients with an Injury Severity Score of 17 or higher were evaluated in this retrospective review. The authors concluded that external fixation of femur fractures in severely injured patients offers no significant advantage in clinical outcomes compared with ST, and recommend the continued use of ST as a temporization method, reserving external fixation only for those patients already undergoing anesthesia for another procedure.

22. Beltran MJ, Collinge CA, Patzkowski JC, Masini BD, Blease RE, Hsu JR; Skeletal Trauma Research Consortium (STReC): The safe zone for external fixator pins in the femur. *J Orthop Trauma* 2012;26(11):643-647.

This cadaver study determined that the safe zone for anterior external fixator pin placement in the femur is distal to the last crossing branch of the femoral nerve and proximal to the superior reflection of the suprapatellar pouch, is, on average, 20 cm in length, and can be as narrow as 12 cm.

23. Bhandari M, Zlowodzki M, Tornetta P III, Schmidt A, Templeman DC: Intramedullary nailing following external fixation in femoral and tibial shaft fractures. *J Orthop Trauma* 2005;19(2):140-144.

24. Harwood PJ, Giannoudis PV, Probst C, Krettek C, Pape HC: The risk of local infective complications after damage control procedures for femoral shaft fracture. *J Orthop Trauma* 2006;20(3):181-189.

25. Della Rocca GJ, Crist BD: External fixation versus conversion to intramedullary nailing for definitive management of closed fractures of the femoral and tibial shaft. *J Am Acad Orthop Surg* 2006;14(10 Spec No.):S131-S135.

26. Nowotarski PJ, Turen CH, Brumback RJ, Scarboro JM: Conversion of external fixation to intramedullary nailing for fractures of the shaft of the femur in multiply injured patients. *J Bone Joint Surg Am* 2000;82(6):781-788.

27. Pape HC, van Griensven M, Rice J, et al: Major secondary surgery in blunt trauma patients and perioperative cytokine liberation: Determination of the clinical relevance of biochemical markers. *J Trauma* 2001;50(6):989-1000.

28. Stannard JP, Bankston L, Futch LA, McGwin G, Volgas DA: Functional outcome following intramedullary nailing of the femur: A prospective randomized comparison of piriformis fossa and greater trochanteric entry portals. *J Bone Joint Surg Am* 2011;93(15):1385-1391.

This prospective, randomized trial reported no difference in functional outcome postoperatively at 1-year follow-up between patients treated with trochanteric nailing and those treated with nailing through the piriformis fossa. Intraoperatively, trochanteric nailing resulted in shorter surgical time, fluoroscopy time, and incision length. Level of evidence: I.

29. Ricci WM, Devinney S, Haidukewych G, Herscovici D, Sanders R: Trochanteric nail insertion for the treatment of femoral shaft fractures. *J Orthop Trauma* 2005;19(8):511-517.

30. Dora C, Leunig M, Beck M, Rothenfluh D, Ganz R: Entry point soft tissue damage in antegrade femoral nailing: A cadaver study. *J Orthop Trauma* 2001;15(7):488-493.

31. Ansari Moein C, ten Duis H-J, Oey L, et al: Functional outcome after antegrade femoral nailing: A comparison of trochanteric fossa versus tip of greater trochanter entry point. *J Orthop Trauma* 2011;25(4):196-201.

    In this small, retrospective series, five of nine patients with nails placed through the piriformis fossa had a positive Trendelenburg sign compared with no patients in the trochanteric entry group; four of these five had electromyographic evidence of recovering superior gluteal nerve injury. The piriformis entry group also had substantially diminished abduction and external rotator function on isokinetic testing.

32. Ricci WM, Schwappach J, Tucker M, et al: Trochanteric versus piriformis entry portal for the treatment of femoral shaft fractures. *J Orthop Trauma* 2006;20(10):663-667.

33. O'Toole RV, Riche K, Cannada LK, et al: Analysis of postoperative knee sepsis after retrograde nail insertion of open femoral shaft fractures. *J Orthop Trauma* 2010;24(11):677-682.

    This retrospective review of prospective trauma registries and fracture databases reported on 93 open femoral fractures treated with retrograde intramedullary nailing from 2003 through 2007. A 1.1% rate of knee sepsis (1 patient with a severe degloving injury) was noted, a rate comparable with elective knee arthroscopy (1.8%) and primary total knee arthroplasty (range, 1% to 2%).

34. Ricci WM, Bellabarba C, Evanoff B, Herscovici D, DiPasquale T, Sanders R: Retrograde versus antegrade nailing of femoral shaft fractures. *J Orthop Trauma* 2001;15(3):161-169.

35. Bible JE, Kadakia RJ, Choxi AA, Bauer JM, Mir HR: Analysis of retrograde femoral intramedullary nail placement through traumatic knee arthrotomies. *J Orthop Trauma* 2013;27(4):217-220.

    This report analyzed the rate of postoperative infection after retrograde femoral nail placement in the setting of traumatic knee arthrotomy over a 10-year time span. Thirty-four retrograde nails placed through a traumatic knee arthrotomy were compared with a control group of 23 antegrade nails with a traumatic knee arthrotomy. No infections of the knee or fractures in the retrograde group were reported; one infection was reported in the antegrade group. Level of evidence: III.

36. Bosse MJ, MacKenzie EJ, Riemer BL, et al: Adult respiratory distress syndrome, pneumonia, and mortality following thoracic injury and a femoral fracture treated either with intramedullary nailing with reaming or with a plate. A comparative study. *J Bone Joint Surg Am* 1997;79(6):799-809.

37. Watson JT, Moed BR: Ipsilateral femoral neck and shaft fractures: Complications and their treatment. *Clin Orthop Relat Res* 2002;399:78-86.

38. Singh R, Rohilla R, Magu NK, Siwach R, Kadian V, Sangwan SS: Ipsilateral femoral neck and shaft fractures: A retrospective analysis of two treatment methods. *J Orthop Traumatol* 2008;9(3):141-147.

39. Bedi A, Karunakar MA, Caron T, Sanders RW, Haidukewych GJ: Accuracy of reduction of ipsilateral femoral neck and shaft fractures—an analysis of various internal fixation strategies. *J Orthop Trauma* 2009;23(4):249-253.

40. Ostrum RF, Tornetta P III, Watson JT, Christiano A, Vafek E: Ipsilateral proximal femur and shaft fractures treated with hip screws and a reamed retrograde intramedullary nail. *Clin Orthop Relat Res* 2014;472(9):2751-2758.

    Of 95 ipsilateral proximal femur and shaft fractures treated over 9 years with either cannulated screws or a sliding hip screw and a reamed retrograde nail, 92 were reviewed. A low risk of proximal malunions (5%) was reported, with no difference in femoral neck union or alignment comparing cannulated screws to a sliding hip screw. The union rate was 98% for femoral neck fractures and 91.3% for femoral shaft fractures. Level of evidence: IV.

41. Copeland CE, Mitchell KA, Brumback RJ, Gens DR, Burgess AR: Mortality in patients with bilateral femoral fractures. *J Orthop Trauma* 1998;12(5):315-319.

42. Nork SE, Agel J, Russell GV, Mills WJ, Holt S, Routt ML Jr: Mortality after reamed intramedullary nailing of bilateral femur fractures. *Clin Orthop Relat Res* 2003;415:272-278.

43. Kobbe P, Vodovotz Y, Kaczorowski DJ, Billiar TR, Pape H-C: The role of fracture-associated soft tissue injury in the induction of systemic inflammation and remote organ dysfunction after bilateral femur fracture. *J Orthop Trauma* 2008;22(6):385-390.

44. Stavlas P, Giannoudis PV: Bilateral femoral fractures: Does intramedullary nailing increase systemic complications and mortality rates? *Injury* 2009;40(11):1125-1128.

45. O'Toole RV, Lindbloom BJ, Hui E, et al: Are bilateral femoral fractures no longer a marker for death? *J Orthop Trauma* 2014;28(2):77-82.

    The authors compared the mortality rate of 54 patients with bilateral femur fractures from 2000 to 2006 with those of historical control patients from the same institution 15 years prior, and also to current and historical unilateral control patients. Although mortality rates were still substantially higher for bilateral (7%) than for unilateral (2%) fractures, both rates had decreased over time from 26% and 12%, respectively. Level of evidence: III.

46. Willett K, Al-Khateeb H, Kotnis R, Bouamra O, Lecky F: Risk of mortality: The relationship with associated injuries and fracture treatment methods in patients with unilateral or bilateral femoral shaft fractures. *J Trauma* 2010;69(2):405-410.

    In this observational cohort study of the prospectively recorded England and Wales Trauma Registry data from 1989 to 2003, the authors identified unilateral and

6: Lower Extremity

bilateral femoral fracture patients with or without injuries to other body regions. Bilateral femur fracture patients had an 80% likelihood of substantial associated injuries in other body systems and those with associated injuries had a 31.6% mortality rate compared with 9.8% in patients with isolated bilateral femur fractures.

47. Brumback RJ, Ellison PS Jr, Poka A, Lakatos R, Bathon GH, Burgess AR: Intramedullary nailing of open fractures of the femoral shaft. *J Bone Joint Surg Am* 1989;71(9):1324-1331.

48. O'Brien PJ, Meek RN, Powell JN, Blachut PA: Primary intramedullary nailing of open femoral shaft fractures. *J Trauma* 1991;31(1):113-116.

49. Kosova E, Bergmark B, Piazza G: Fat embolism syndrome. *Circulation* 2015;131(3):317-320.

    This case presentation of a 49-year-old man,with a history of metastatic prostate cancer, who sustained a pathologic left femur fracture and in whom the classis signs and symptoms of fat embolism syndrome developed provides an overview of FES including pathophysiology, clinical presentation, diagnosis, management, prevention, and prognosis.

50. Eriksson EA, Pellegrini DC, Vanderkolk WE, Minshall CT, Fakhry SM, Cohle SD: Incidence of pulmonary fat embolism at autopsy: An undiagnosed epidemic. *J Trauma* 2011;71(2):312-315.

    Prospectively, 50 consecutive patients presenting for autopsy were evaluated for evidence of pulmonary and brain fat embolism. Of these, 68% were trauma patients, 88% of whom had died within 1 hour of injury. Pulmonary fat embolism was present in 82% of all trauma patients, and 80% of those who died within the "golden hour." Knowledge of how acutely pulmonary fat embolism occurs can assist in early management of trauma patients.

51. Akoh CC, Schick C, Otero J, Karam M: Fat embolism syndrome after femur fracture fixation: A case report. *Iowa Orthop J* 2014;34:55-62.

    This case report discusses a healthy 24-year old man who sustained a left olecranon fracture and closed bilateral midshaft femur fractures in a head-on motor vehicle collision and in whom cerebral fat embolism syndrome developed 12 hours after immediate bilateral intramedullary nail fixation. The signs and symptoms of cerebral fat embolism syndrome are reviewed along with the history, incidence, pathophysiology, presentation, diagnosis, and management.

52. Bederman SS, Bhandari M, McKee MD, Schemitsch EH: Do corticosteroids reduce the risk of fat embolism syndrome in patients with long-bone fractures? A meta-analysis. *Can J Surg* 2009;52(5):386-393.

53. Brumback RJ, Toal TR Jr, Murphy-Zane MS, Novak VP, Belkoff SM: Immediate weight-bearing after treatment of a comminuted fracture of the femoral shaft with a statically locked intramedullary nail. *J Bone Joint Surg Am* 1999;81(11):1538-1544.

54. Archdeacon M, Ford KR, Wyrick J, et al: A prospective functional outcome and motion analysis evaluation of the hip abductors after femur fracture and antegrade nailing. *J Orthop Trauma* 2008;22(1):3-9.

55. Helmy N, Jando VT, Lu T, Chan H, O'Brien PJ: Muscle function and functional outcome following standard antegrade reamed intramedullary nailing of isolated femoral shaft fractures. *J Orthop Trauma* 2008;22(1):10-15.

56. Daglar B, Gungor E, Delialioglu OM, et al: Comparison of knee function after antegrade and retrograde intramedullary nailing for diaphyseal femoral fractures: Results of isokinetic evaluation. *J Orthop Trauma* 2009;23(9):640-644.

57. Richards JE, Guillamondegui OD, Archer KR, Jackson JC, Ely EW, Obremskey WT: The association of reamed intramedullary nailing and long-term cognitive impairment. *J Orthop Trauma* 2011;25(12):707-713.

    In this prospective observational cohort study, 108 trauma intensive care unit survivors presenting over a 1-year span underwent a comprehensive battery of neuropsychologic tests 12 months after injury. Of these, 18 had received a reamed intramedullary nail and 14 of these (78%) had cognitive deficit at follow-up. Reamed intramedullary nail was found to be a moderate risk factor for the development of cognitive impairment.

Chapter 40

Fractures of the Distal Femur

Frank R. Avilucea, MD   Michael T. Archdeacon, MD, MSE

Abstract

Fractures of the distal femur are well suited to treatment with a precontoured lateral locking plate or an intramedullary nail. Knowledge of relevant anatomy and appropriate clinical and radiographic evaluation, in addition to long-term outcomes and complications, is important for management of these injuries, which focuses on surgical technique.

Keywords: distal femur; fracture; plate fixation; retrograde intramedullary nail

Introduction

The primary goals in the surgical treatment of distal femur fractures include restoring anatomic congruity of the articular surface; obtaining correct limb alignment, length, and rotation; and simultaneously applying stable fixation to enable early knee motion. These surgical goals should be completed to create a biologically favorable environment that enables osseous union.

Demographically, distal femur fractures have a bimodal distribution: high-energy injuries occur in a younger, often male population, and lower energy fractures occur in the elderly, typically in females. Higher energy injuries of the distal femur often involve metaphyseal comminution. Moreover, in the setting of intercondylar fracture extension, coronal plane fractures of the condyles (Hoffa fractures) are often present, injuries that can be radiographically occult.[1] To better delineate these fractures, CT is required to localize the presence of this injury pattern.

Neither of the following authors nor any immediate family member has received anything of value from or has stock or stock options held in a commercial company or institution related directly or indirectly to the subject of this chapter: Dr. Avilucea and Dr. Archdeacon.

Unique Anatomy of the Distal Femur

Knowledge of distal femur anatomy is particularly important when applying anatomically based plating systems to avoid malalignment and implant-related complications.

Osseous Anatomy

The femoral shaft is essentially a cylinder that flares distally into lateral and medial condyles separated by a large intercondylar fossa. The large medial flare provides a broad condylar weight-bearing surface for the knee. The medial and lateral condyles coalesce anteriorly to form the trochlea, which articulates with the patella. Immediately posterior to the trochlea is the intercondylar notch, which houses the cruciate ligaments. Medially, the maximal point of flare is formed by the adductor tubercle. From a radiographic standpoint, the lateral fluoroscopic view will show the subchondral arc of the trochlea and the limits of the intercondylar notch, which is represented by the Blumensaat line (**Figure 1**). Axially, the condyles of the distal femur represent a trapezoid such that the inclination of the lateral and medial surfaces is approximately 10° and 25°, respectively (**Figure 2**). On the sagittal view, the shaft of the femur is aligned with the anterior half of the condyles; the posterior half lies posterior to the femoral shaft axis.

The anatomic axis of the femoral shaft differs from that of the weight-bearing (mechanical) axis in that the weight-bearing axis passes from the center of the femoral head through the center of the knee. The anatomic axis is an average 6° from vertical; the mechanical axis subtends an average angle of 3°. The articulation of the knee is typically parallel to the floor, which results in an anatomic lateral distal femoral angle of 81° (**Figure 3**). The surgical reconstruction of a distal femur fracture aims to restore the correct valgus angulation (anatomic axis), enabling the articulation of the knee to remain parallel to the ground. Two reports discuss the importance of understanding the aforementioned anatomic description to achieve proper fracture reduction, correct alignment, and minimize excessive articular wear resulting in arthritis.[2,3]

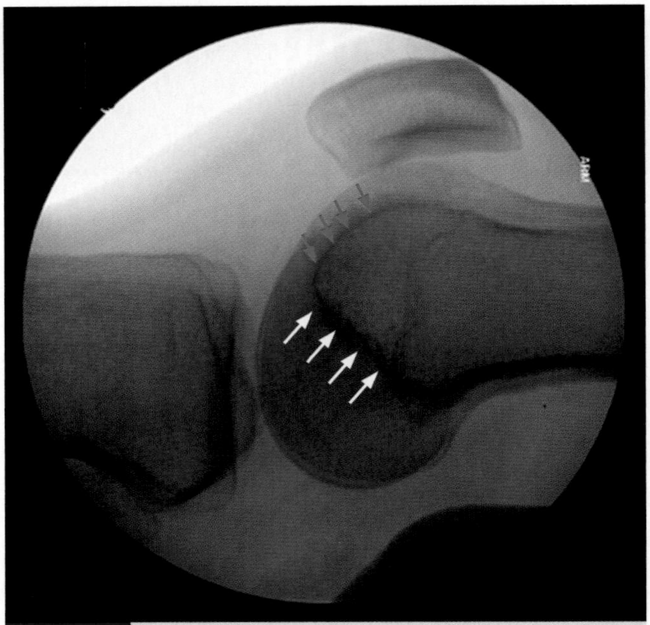

Figure 1 Lateral fluoroscopic image shows the Blumensaat line (white arrows) and the subchondral surface (red arrows) of the trochlea. Implants placed in the distal femur should remain within these lines to avoid chondral injury and intra-articular hardware placement.

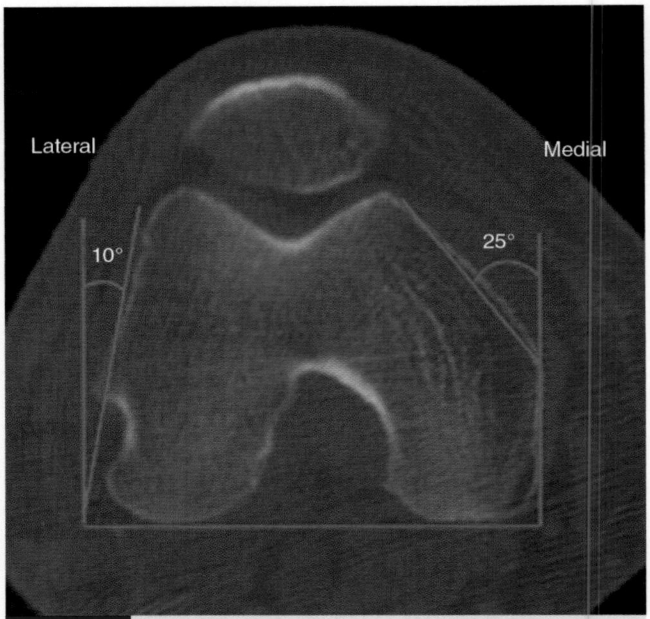

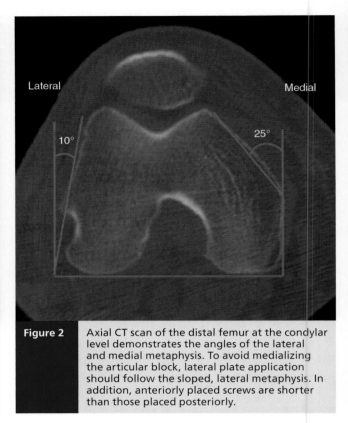

Figure 2 Axial CT scan of the distal femur at the condylar level demonstrates the angles of the lateral and medial metaphysis. To avoid medializing the articular block, lateral plate application should follow the sloped, lateral metaphysis. In addition, anteriorly placed screws are shorter than those placed posteriorly.

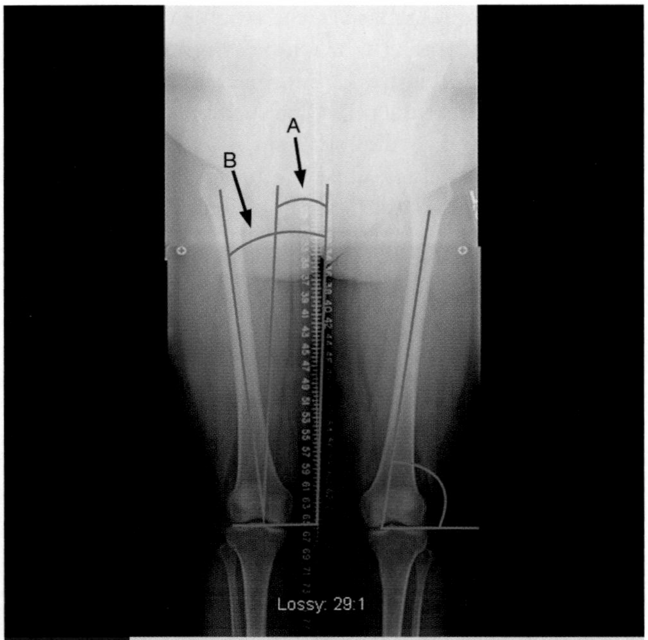

Figure 3 Long-standing radiograph depicting the anatomic and mechanical axis and the respective angle relative to a vertical line. The lateral distal femoral anatomic axis is also shown.

Soft-Tissue Anatomy

The anterior or extensor compartment of the thigh is composed of the quadriceps femoris superficially, and the vastus lateralis, vastus intermedius, and vastus medialis in the deeper layer. The lateral and medial intermuscular septum are important partitions and landmarks for surgical approaches to either the medial or lateral aspect of the distal femur and knee. Medially, the superficial femoral artery traverses the thigh between the extensor and adductor compartments and enters the popliteal space approximately 10 cm proximal to the knee joint by passing through the adductor magnus. In the setting of fracture, displacement is secondary to the deforming forces, including the powerful pull of the extensor mechanism and hamstrings, which result in shortening of the femur. The contraction of the gastrocnemius produces posterior translation and angulation of the distal segment. In the setting of an intercondylar split, resultant rotational malalignment is also seen because of the unrestrained gastrocnemius pull and overriding anterior femoral shaft.

Initial Evaluation

Distal femur fractures are often one of several injuries in the setting of high-energy trauma. A multidisciplinary team approach is used for thorough patient assessment and to rule out associated injuries. Typically, fractures of the distal femur are the result of direct trauma to a flexed knee, as often occurs when the knee strikes the dashboard of a rapidly decelerating vehicle. The presence of concomitant fractures of the patella, femoral shaft, femoral neck, and acetabular fractures, as well as hip dislocation, must be determined. Substantial soft-tissue injury, particularly involving ligaments, can also be associated with fracture. By virtue of the fracture, such ligamentous disruptions of the knee are difficult to diagnose with clinical examination and stress radiographs until the femur is stabilized. Tethering the popliteal artery at the adductor hiatus in the medial distal thigh and at the soleus arch distal to the knee makes the vessel susceptible to stretch, tear, or intimal damage. Therefore, heightened suspicion for injury to this vessel is necessary because displacement of the fracture was likely much greater at the time of injury than what the static radiographs demonstrate as fragments return to their original position due to soft-tissue recoil.

Routine AP and lateral radiographs of the supracondylar region, as well as traction views in the setting of deformity and shortening, are customary. To evaluate for associated fractures, AP pelvis as well as AP and lateral femoral views are indicated. In addition to analysis of the soft tissues for evidence of an open fracture, a thorough vascular examination must be completed to assess for a palpable pulse difference between the distal lower extremities. So that an occult vascular injury is not missed, an ankle-brachial index of the injured extremity should be obtained; a value less than 0.9 has been reported to have 100% sensitivity, specificity, and positive predictive value for a substantial arterial lesion.[4] If intra-articular involvement is suspected, CT should be performed to delineate the fracture pattern as well as the presence of any osteochondral lesions or impaction fractures. CT is particularly helpful in identifying any associated Hoffa fragment, a coronal plane condylar fracture with a reported incidence of 38% in high-energy supracondylar-intercondylar distal femur fractures, because it is often missed on radiographs.[5]

Classification

A relatively simple classification scheme of supracondylar and intercondylar femoral fractures has been described that divides intercondylar fractures into those with minimal displacement, displacement of the condyles, and fractures with supracondylar and shaft patterns.[6] Subsequently, other classification systems have been described, all of which delineate extra-articular, intra-articular, and condylar patterns. Currently, no universal classification system exists; however, the Orthopaedic Trauma Association (OTA) scheme provides adequate documentation of the injury and permits the surgeon to develop a basic surgical treatment plan for a particular pattern.[7] The classification systems are limited in that not every fracture fits nicely in any one system. In addition, data are limited on clinical outcome for many patterns; thus, providing prognostic information to patients is difficult.

Indications for Fixation

The targeted goals for surgical intervention include restoring and stabilizing the articular surface; reducing the articular block to the shaft of the femur aiming to correct length, alignment, and rotation; preserving microvascular blood supply to metaphyseal comminution; and applying stable fixation to enable early knee range of motion. The patient's overall health and functional capacity must be assessed to determine whether surgical intervention is appropriate. Important factors to consider include patient age, level of activity (community ambulatory versus wheelchair dependent), medical condition, hemodynamic status, associated injuries, and presence of previous implants (such as previous total knee arthroplasty). Equally important is the surgeon's expertise with this injury and his or her fundamental understanding of the pathomechanics and morphology of the fracture. If the surgeon is not experienced with this injury, if the appropriate implant is unavailable, or a skilled surgical team is lacking, the patient should be transferred to the appropriate health care facility to avoid complications related to poor surgical intervention and prolonged immobilization. A reasonable interim step before patient transfer would be the application of a temporizing spanning knee external fixator. This minimally invasive procedure provides stability during transfer, decreasing patient pain and maintaining provisional alignment.

Role of Temporizing External Fixation

External fixation is an excellent option to provide provisional stability in the setting of extensive soft-tissue injury or open fracture, an injury with comminution and resultant shortening not amenable to stabilization with a splint or knee immobilizer, limb ischemia, or systemic injury precluding the ability to safely proceed with definitive fixation. Given the complexity and difficulty of reconstructing the distal femur, many surgeons opt for provisional stabilization with spanning knee external fixation in most distal femur fractures, irrespective of other factors. Such an intervention enables soft-tissue and bony stabilization and permits patient mobilization, pain

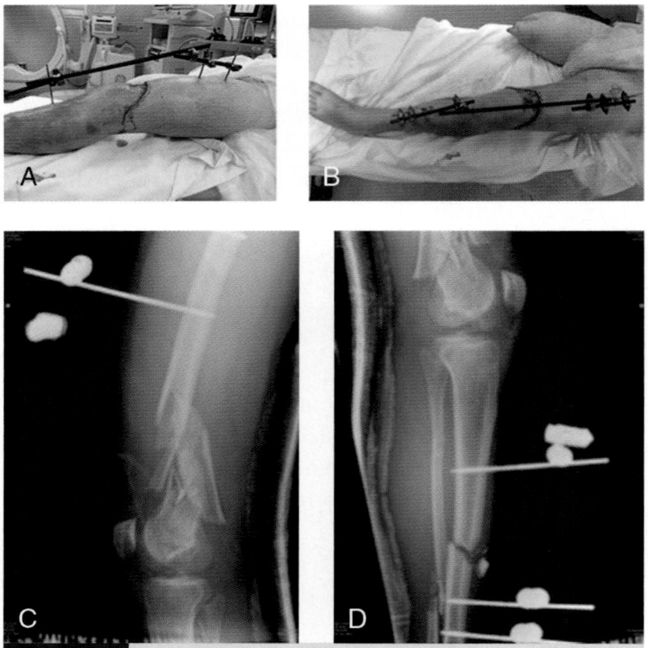

Figure 4 **A** and **B**, Photographs demonstrate a temporary external fixator used for a patient with polytrauma, including traumatic amputation of the contralateral limb. Radiographs demonstrate a comminuted distal femur fracture (**C**) and an ipsilateral tibia fracture (**D**).

relief, nursing care, and local wound care until definitive stabilization can be performed.

When an external fixator is applied, not only should the zone of injury be accounted for, but future definitive fixation should also be anticipated so that, if possible, the pin tracts remain outside the zone of the definitive implant used. Although no current evidence exists regarding optimal pin placement to minimize injury to the quadriceps muscle, two pins are typically placed in the mid to proximal aspect of the femur and two pins in the tibia to permit axial, rotational, and angular control of the fracture site[8] (**Figure 4**). Moreover, it is necessary to establish appropriate length because prolonged use of an external fixator with a shortened extremity results in difficulty with reestablishing correct length at the time of definitive fixation. After the patient has been appropriately resuscitated and is deemed stable to undergo an extended procedure, a single-stage conversion procedure can be performed with minimal complications expected because of previous pin tracts. One of the largest series reported on a series of 59 fractures of the femoral shaft initially treated with external fixation for a short duration (less than 2 weeks), followed by planned conversion to intramedullary fixation with a one-stage procedure in the absence of systemic or pin site infection.[9] Of 58 fractures that were followed until union, 97% healed within 6 months, with an infection rate of 1.7%. The methodology is a safe treatment strategy in patients who cannot undergo definitive fixation at the index procedure.

Principles of Surgical Approaches

The OTA classification scheme is a helpful tool to determine which surgical approach can be used, particularly because fractures are categorized based on the complexity of the fracture pattern and the degree of articular surface injury. In general, extra-articular fractures do not require visualization of the articular surface; therefore, exposure is based on whether direct anatomic reduction and compression of the fracture site is required (as in a simple extra-articular pattern) or if exposure of only the lateral femoral condyle is needed in the setting of bridge plating across metaphyseal comminution. However, the presence of an articular fracture warrants a direct, anatomic articular reconstruction, particularly in a young patient. Articular injuries with displacement thus require formal arthrotomy; the degree of exposure is predicated on the extent of the articular injury.

Open treatment of distal femur fractures has evolved from large surgical exposures to what is now considered a biologic approach. Initially described in 1979, the concept of maintaining soft-tissue attachments and preserving the vascularity of cortical bone fragments was demonstrated in 1996 as an effective method to achieve union of supracondylar femur fractures.[10-12] Since then, not only are indirect reduction techniques used but the length of the incision is minimized to avoid microvascular injury to metadiaphyseal portions of the fracture. Currently, the aforementioned goals can be accomplished with the use of submuscular plating or retrograde intramedullary nailing.

Surgical Approaches

Preoperative Considerations

Preoperative planning is essential to understand the fracture pattern and help improve the clinical outcome. Identification of an articular fracture, such as a Hoffa fragment, and the degree of the metaphyseal comminution, will help determine the surgical approach used and the amount of articular exposure required. Simple metaphyseal patterns benefit from direct compression via formal open reduction. When substantial metaphyseal comminution is present, a minimally invasive approach is often used to preserve the vasculature along the zone of comminution. In such circumstances, a submuscular tunnel along the lateral femur should be considered for plate fixation or a transtendinous or parapatellar arthrotomy for insertion of a retrograde intramedullary nail.

Exposure of the Lateral Femur

The traditional open exposure of the lateral distal femur is centered over the lateral epicondyle. A longitudinal incision on the skin is extended to allow gentle soft-tissue retraction. The fibers of the iliotibial band are visualized and the tendon is incised and split in a single line, enabling visualization of the vastus lateralis, which is reflected anteriorly off the intermuscular septum. Perforator vessels are identified and carefully ligated or coagulated. To avoid osseous devascularization, dissection on the medial aspect is avoided and the periosteum is kept intact. Depending on the amount of articular visualization needed, the incision can be extended distally toward the lateral edge of the patellar tendon to permit increased medial subluxation of the extensor mechanism and greater visualization of the intercondylar notch and medial femoral condyle.

After the advent of submuscular plating, a limited incision is required. The dissection proceeds as described for the lateral approach, but is limited to the length of the lateral femoral condyle. Visualization of the anterior half of the lateral femoral condyle is necessary, particularly of the vermillion border of the chondral/cortical interface, which defines the boundary for both peripheral screw and plate placement. Because of limited exposure of the distal femur and fracture site with this approach, fracture reduction and correct plate application relies on indirect methods that require excellent AP and lateral fluoroscopic images to avoid fracture malreduction and plate malposition.[13]

Modifications of the lateral approach have been described, including the swashbuckler and mini-swashbuckler approaches to the distal femur. The swashbuckler involves a lateral parapatellar approach that extends into an S-shaped incision enabling complete exposure of the articular block while sparing the extensor mechanism.[14] The mini-swashbuckler involves a lateral parapatellar incision extending from the tibial tubercle to the superolateral corner of the patella followed by retinacular dissection and excision of the retropatellar fat pad to enable complete exposure of the articular surface of the distal femur.[15] Unique to these methods is the ability to optimize the articular exposure (without a tibial tubercle osteotomy) by placing the incision at the lateral parapatellar border to optimize medial subluxation of the patella and gaining exposure of the entire articular surface.[14,15]

Access for Retrograde Intramedullary Nail Insertion

In the setting of an articular segment that is reduced and fixed with screws and the nail is used to bridge the metadiaphyseal comminution, retrograde intramedullary nailing can be completed through a 3- to 4-cm incision either directly on the midline or medial border of the patellar tendon or through a formal arthrotomy (**Figure 5**). For the transtendinous approach, the skin is incised directly on the midline over the tendon, the paratenon is split longitudinally and elevated, and a single split of the central portion of the tendon is completed to gain access to the joint. With a medial parapatellar tendon approach, the skin is incised at the medial border of the tendon and intra-articular access is gained by dissecting sharply and in a single flap through the retinaculum and capsule.

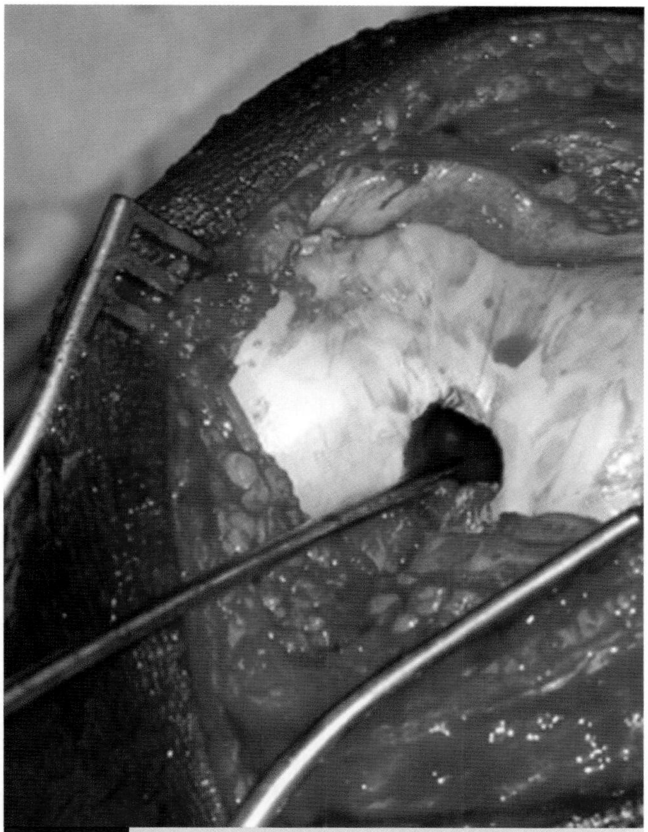

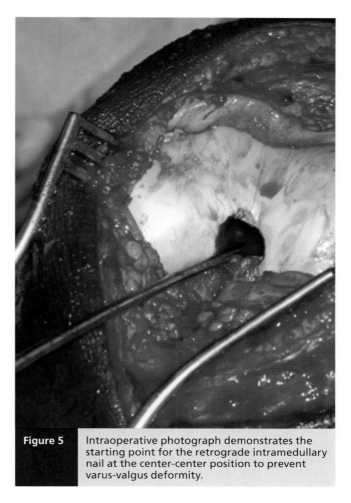

Figure 5 Intraoperative photograph demonstrates the starting point for the retrograde intramedullary nail at the center-center position to prevent varus-valgus deformity.

Plating

The locked plate is an important advance in distal femur fracture fixation. The use of angular stable screws (secured to the plate using threaded holes) enables numerous fixed-angle points of fixation in the distal articular block, which is critical in the setting of a comminuted fracture with multiplanar articular involvement, a short distal femoral block, or presence of limited bone stock.[16] In 1994,

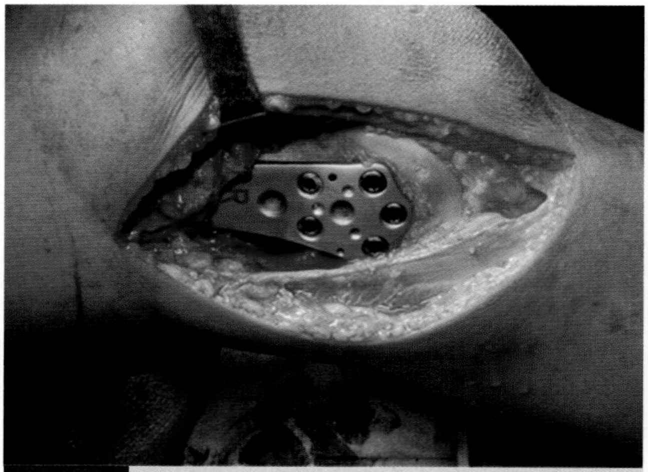

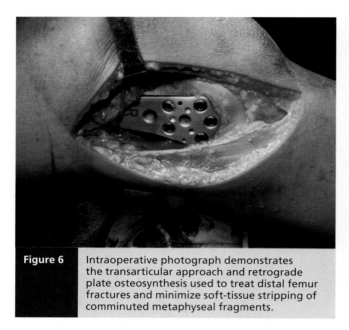

Figure 6 Intraoperative photograph demonstrates the transarticular approach and retrograde plate osteosynthesis used to treat distal femur fractures and minimize soft-tissue stripping of comminuted metaphyseal fragments.

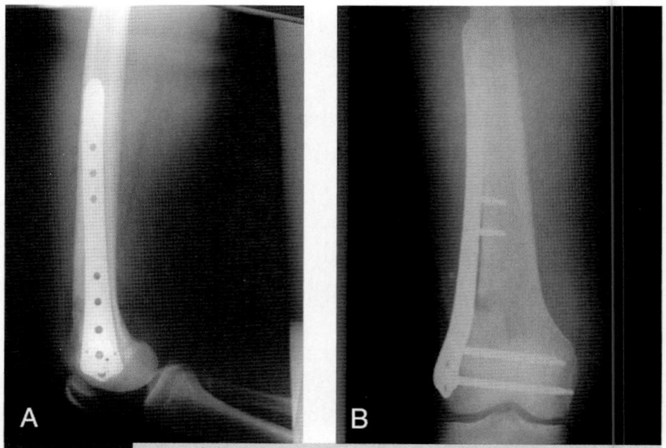

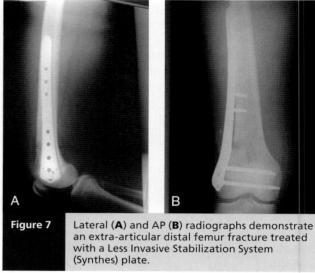

Figure 7 Lateral (**A**) and AP (**B**) radiographs demonstrate an extra-articular distal femur fracture treated with a Less Invasive Stabilization System (Synthes) plate.

the first locked plate was developed for this purpose, and several series describe its use and effective short- and midterm results[17-20] (**Figures 6** and **7**). The plate not only featured locking technology, but also incorporated submuscular insertion technique. Several locked plating systems have been developed as the construct and technique have become the favored approach to the surgical treatment of many distal femur fractures.

Current Plating Techniques

Modern plates are contoured and have various screw fixation options including conventional cortical screws, cannulated locking and nonlocking screws, solid locking screws, and the necessary guide attachments that can be used for percutaneous fixation. Additionally, some plates also allow variable-angle screw trajectories that permit screws to be angled away from the articular surface in a native knee or the implant in the setting of total knee arthroplasty. In general, plates should be used for OTA A- and C-type fracture patterns only. B-type patterns (partial articular) require absolute stability and should be treated using interfragmentary compression of the articular surface and supported with buttress plate fixation (**Figure 8**). Although many fracture patterns are amenable to either plate or nail fixation, the specific indications for using a plate include a condylar segment too short to allow nailing, a periprosthetic fracture about a total knee implant with a closed box design, a preexisting total hip arthroplasty, or an existing intramedullary implant.

In the setting of metaphysis comminution, a biologic-preserving approach combined with submuscular plate application is recommended (**Figure 9**). Following open reduction and internal fixation of the condylar block, attention is focused on intraoperative assessment of femoral length and rotation (as with nailing). Techniques that facilitate plate application include chemical paralysis, longitudinal traction with either a femoral distractor or skeletal traction, carefully placed clamps and Kirschner wires to facilitate preliminary application of the plate, a rolled towel placed beneath the condylar segment to help correct sagittal plane deformity, and using the plate and cortical screws to facilitate correcting coronal plane alignment.

Serious consideration must be given to the length of the plate and the number and placement of screws. A plate allows the surgeon to control how stiff a construct to build based on the fracture pattern. This so-called stress modulation provides stable fixation to support physiologic loading until union is achieved and concomitantly provides the necessary flexibility to allow micromotion and result in callus formation.[21] Much attention has been given to this topic given that delayed healing and nonunion is a substantial complication that occurs at a higher rate than previously believed.[22]

Based on recent findings, recommendations for modulating construct stiffness include using a longer plate (more than eight holes) when possible with a balanced spread of screws in the proximal segment[22] (**Figure 10**). In the setting of bridge plating, no more than 50% of the available holes in the proximal segment should be filled. The working length and stiffness of the construct is determined by the distalmost screw in the diaphyseal segment. Although decreased working length is theorized as an independent factor contributing to nonunion, this

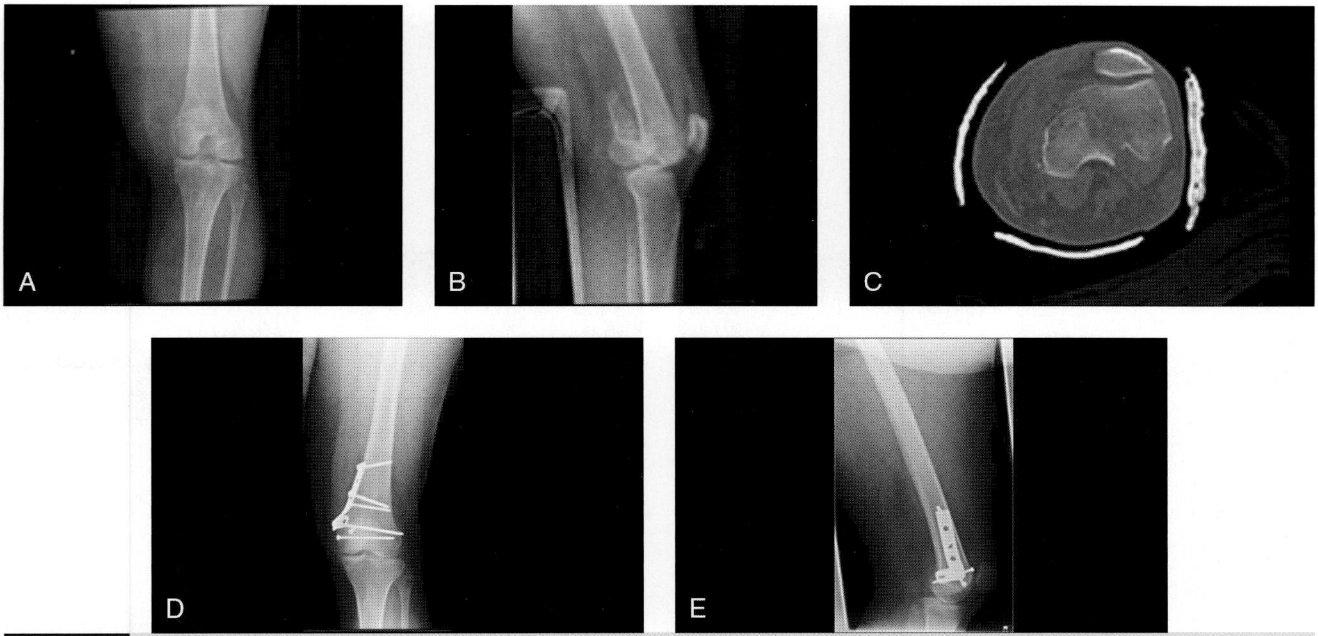

Figure 8 AP (**A**) and lateral (**B**) radiographs and axial CT scan (**C**) demonstrate a partial articular (B-type) distal femur fracture of the medial femoral condyle. AP (**D**) and lateral (**E**) radiographs obtained following treatment with direct compression of the articular surface and buttress plate fixation. Medial condylar fractures should undergo fixation using a medially based subvastus surgical approach.

remains to be determined.[23] Moreover, increased stiffness has been suggested as a contributor to asymmetric callus formation.[23,24] Therefore, the use of far cortical locking implants or near-cortical slotting techniques has been recommended to decrease stiffness, resulting in increased near-cortex callus formation because of increased stiffness and a higher nonunion rate when locking screws near the fracture site are used.[24,25] These constructs have been assessed clinically, with nonunion rates of 3.0% and 11.1%.[26,27] Future studies will be needed to directly compare similar fracture patterns and plate/screws constructs using the aforementioned technology or techniques to confirm these early results.

Retrograde Intramedullary Nailing

Recent Advances

In the late 1980s, retrograde intramedullary nailing was used for indirect reduction that theoretically provides less interference with fracture healing because of limited soft-tissue exposure. Limitations of the technique include the need to proceed with an open approach in the setting of articular fracture, awareness that a nail will not restore anatomic alignment in the setting of metaphyseal comminution, and the current lack of long-term data regarding articular problems that remain a concern. For carefully selected OTA type A and C fractures, however, retrograde intramedullary nailing is a valuable tool, particularly in the setting of severe soft-tissue disruption, obese habitus, a floating knee, a patient with multiple injuries, and appropriate periprosthetic fractures.[28-30]

As with plating systems, the design of retrograde intramedullary nails has also evolved with improved implant design and instrumentation. Recent biomechanical studies demonstrate that the strength of a nail depends substantially on the number and orientation of the distal locking screws, as well as the quality of distal screw purchase. In an osteoporotic synthetic bone model, the presence of four multiplanar distal locking screws optimizes torsional and axial stability compared with not only other screw configurations, but also with a lateral locked plate.[31] Consequently, many implants now offer the capability of locking several interlocking screws to create fixed-angle devices, which help stabilize fractures with short condylar segments and/or osteoporotic bone.

Insertion Technique

During the preoperative planning phase, it is necessary to assess the length of the condylar segment, including the anticipated insertion depth of the nail and how many locking screws from the nail's distal end will be available to obtain condylar fixation.

The presence of an articular fracture requires direct fixation so that lag screws are placed to prevent interference with either the nail or the traversing interlocking

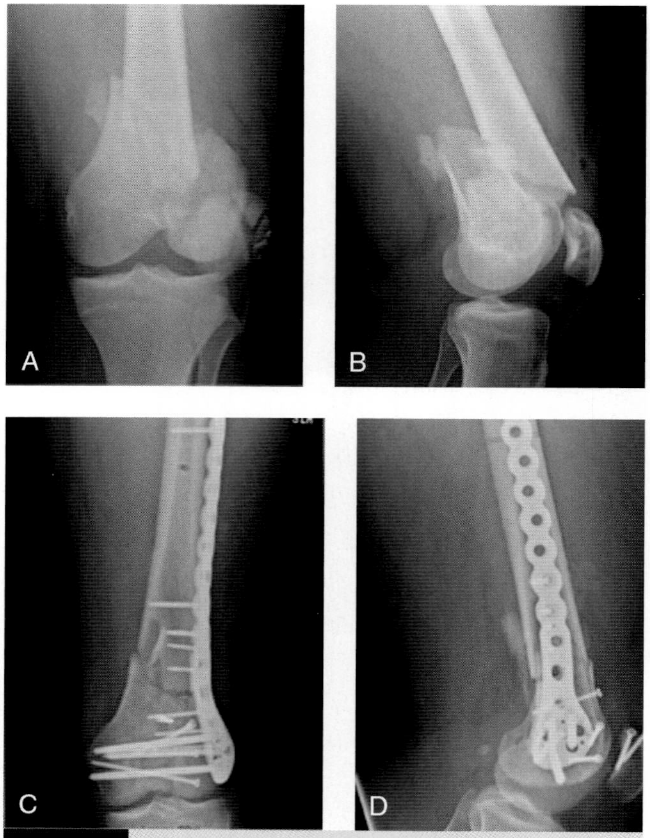

Figure 9 AP (**A**) and lateral (**B**) radiographs demonstrate a distal femur fracture with articular involvement. Postoperative AP (**C**) and lateral (**D**) radiographs. The condylar block was repaired first, followed by plate application.

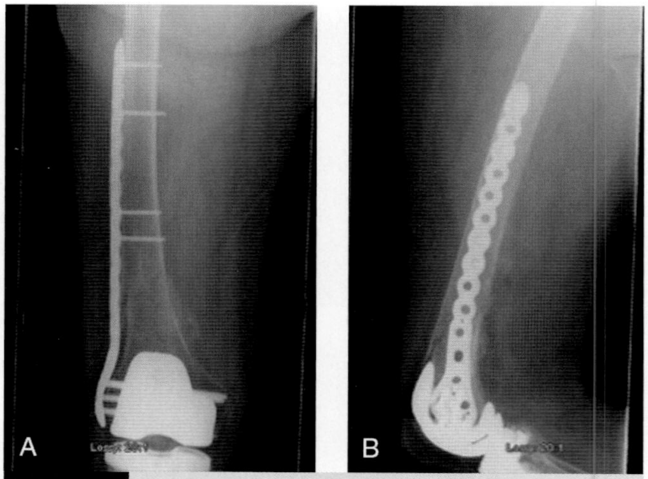

Figure 10 AP (**A**) and lateral (**B**) radiographs demonstrate a distal femur fracture superior to a total knee arthroplasty treated with plate fixation. The construct demonstrates the concept of stress modulation given the length of the plate to balance the length of the fracture, and screw placement positioned to control the degree of micromotion at the fracture site.

screws. Intraoperative techniques for intramedullary nail insertion are similar to those for plate application to obtain anatomic metaphyseal reduction: skeletal paralysis, traction or use of a distractor, sagittal plane correction with a bump or Schanz pins, use of percutaneous clamps or blocking screws to treat coronal plane deformity, and comparison with the lesser trochanter profile or femoral neck anteversion of the contralateral side to correct rotation.

The entry portal for nail insertion is located immediately anterior to the femoral origin of the posterior cruciate ligament. Radiographically, this portal is located just anterior to the distal extent of the Blumensaat line (**Figure 11**). Typically, a threaded tip guidewire is placed at this position with its trajectory parallel to the anterior femoral cortex and in line with the anatomic axis of the femoral shaft. A cannulated drill is used to create the entry portal, with care taken to protect the surrounding tissues and chondral surface of the patella. A guidewire is passed into the proximal segment at the level of the lesser trochanter under fluoroscopic guidance. To avoid creating a deformity, AP and lateral fluoroscopic images of the fracture reduced should be obtained to ensure the guidewire is located center-center on each image. Similarly, during reaming and nail passage, it is essential that the fracture is reduced. Prior to placing the interlocking bolts, the nail must be inserted past the Blumensaat line and deep to the subchondral bone visualized on the lateral fluoroscopic view to avoid chondral damage to the patellofemoral articulation. After the final position of the nail has been determined fluoroscopically, distal locking bolts are placed through cannulated guides and proximally using the perfect circle freehand technique (**Figure 12**). If comminution of the metaphysis is present following distal locking of the nail, the IM nail can be backslapped to restore femoral length. The joint should be copiously irrigated to prevent mechanical issues or heterotopic bone formation.

Postoperative Management

As with all periarticular fractures, early active motion is encouraged to facilitate articular motion and function. Gentle active motion is initiated in a conscious patient; continuous passive motion may be better in an obtunded or intubated patient. If the patient is not limited by other substantial injuries, early gait training is also initiated. The amount of weight bearing is typically predicated on the amount of intraoperative stability achieved. If stable

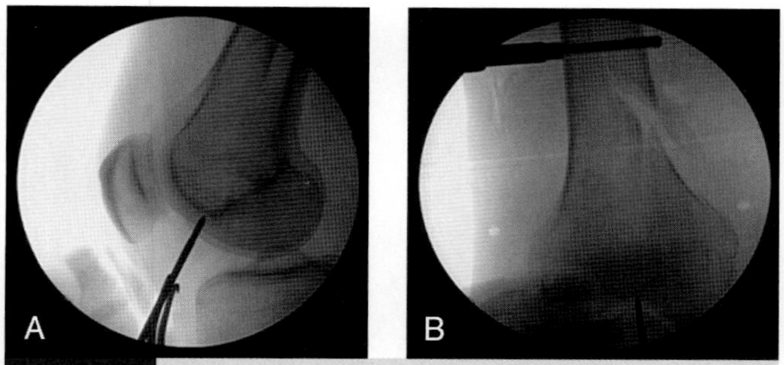

Figure 11 Fluoroscopic images demonstrate the starting point for retrograde intramedullary nail insertion localized just anterior to the Blumensaat line on the lateral view (**A**) and slightly medial within the trochlear groove as seen on the AP view (**B**).

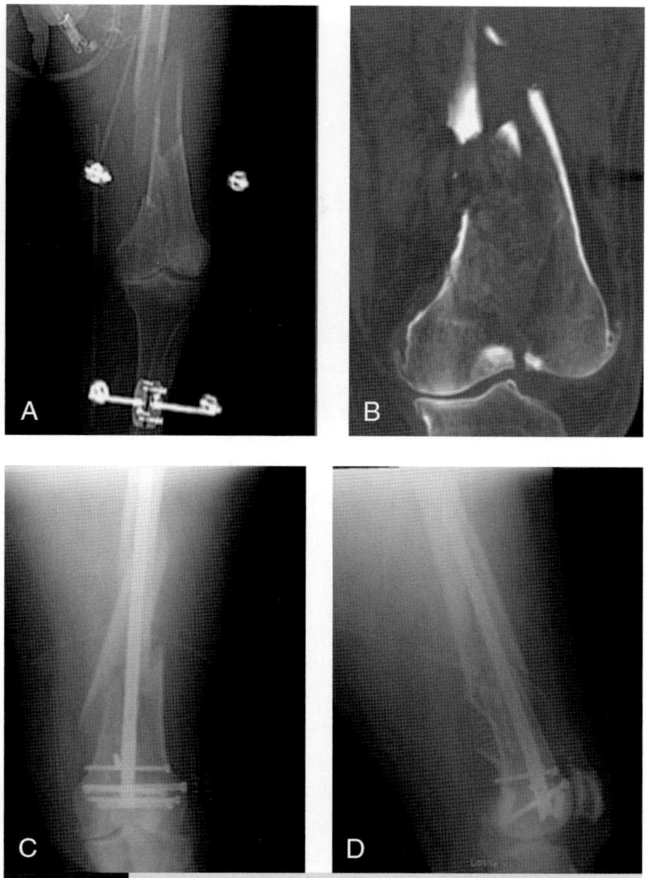

Figure 12 AP radiograph (**A**) and coronal CT (**B**) images demonstrate an intra-articular distal femur fracture. AP (**C**) and lateral (**D**) radiographs obtained following open reduction and internal fixation of the articular block followed by retrograde intramedullary nailing.

fixation is obtained, most surgeons recommend no weight bearing or touchdown weight bearing for 10 to 12 weeks in the setting of an articular fracture and partial weight bearing with progression over 4 to 12 weeks for an extra-articular fracture. At the conclusion of 12 weeks, most patients should be able to tolerate substantial weight, although use of an assistive ambulatory device is common.

Complications

Malalignment/Malunion

Following open reduction and internal fixation, distal femur fixation has a tendency to fail and collapse into varus in the presence of substantial metaphyseal comminution[32] (**Figure 13**). More commonly, the iatrogenic deformity results from using a fixed-angle device from the lateral side. Valgus malalignment is typically created when condylar fragment malreduction occurs to the plate (**Figure 14**). To prevent this complication, normal alignment is determined from the contralateral side and precise plate placement is attained using intraoperative fluoroscopic images.[2,3]

Nonunion

Even with biologic-preserving techniques, nonunion remains a substantial complication related to locked-plate fixation of distal femur fractures, with an incidence ranging from 15% to 20%.[22,33] Additional investigations have identified independent risk factors for surgical intervention to promote healing, including open fracture, obesity, the use of stainless steel instruments, infection, diabetes, and shorter plate length.[22,34] The treatment of nonunion is difficult, particularly if the complication is long-standing and much of the motion occurs through the pseudarthrosis, resulting in a stiff knee. Successful management requires not only stable fixation but also restoration of knee motion, both of which can be treated in a single stage. In the setting of an osseous defect, bone grafting is necessary. Aseptic nonunion is often best treated with bone grafting alone; hypertrophic nonunion requires increased stability, which can be gained with a 95° condylar blade plate.

Infection

Factors predisposing to infection include high-energy injuries with resultant bony devascularization, open fractures, extensive surgical dissection, and inadequate fixation. In the literature of the 1960s, postoperative infection was noted at a rate of approximately 20%.[6,35] More recent studies document infection rates ranging from 3% to 16%[20,36,37] in closed injuries and up to 25% in open fractures.[38] The presence of a deep infection mandates aggressive management, including a thorough irrigation and débridement, and the possibility of either

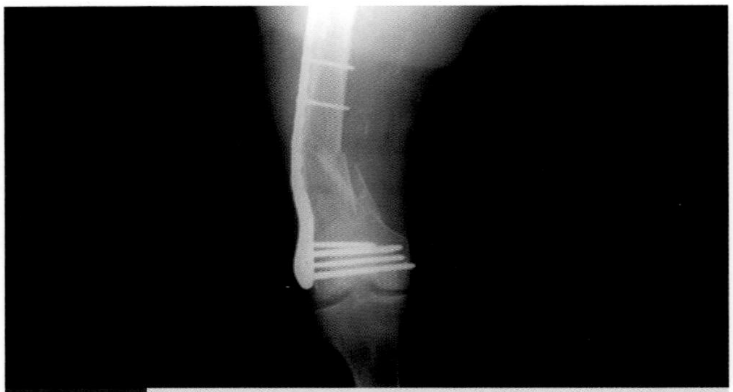

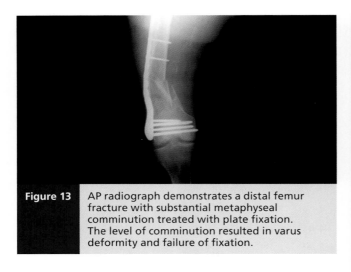

Figure 13 AP radiograph demonstrates a distal femur fracture with substantial metaphyseal comminution treated with plate fixation. The level of comminution resulted in varus deformity and failure of fixation.

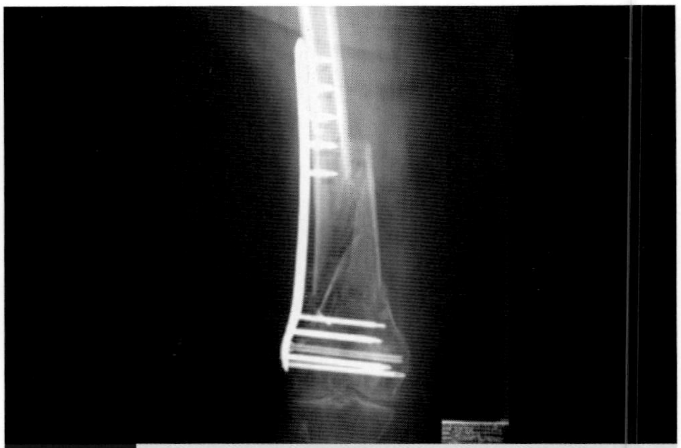

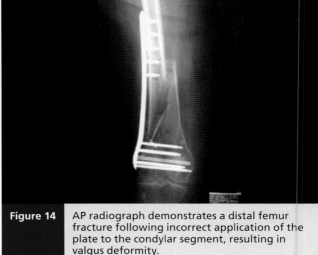

Figure 14 AP radiograph demonstrates a distal femur fracture following incorrect application of the plate to the condylar segment, resulting in valgus deformity.

negative-pressure dressing or an antibiotic bead pouch followed by serial washouts until the wound appears clean and soft tissues are without gross evidence of necrosis or infectious changes. Cultures should direct intravenous antibiotic treatment, which is typically administered for 3 to 12 consecutive weeks. Implants are typically left in place when no evidence of loosening exists. However, in the setting of loose hardware, implants should be removed and the fracture is temporarily stabilized using a spanning external fixator.

Knee Stiffness

It is common for some loss of motion to occur following surgical treatment of a distal femur fracture. However, a functional range of motion (full extension to 110° of flexion) is necessary. Following stable fixation along with meticulous soft-tissue handling, early motion of the knee should commence soon after surgery, particularly in the setting of an articular fracture. If motion is not regained approximately 1 month after surgery, aggressive physical therapy should be initiated. If this measure fails, manipulation under anesthesia may be necessary along with surgical releases including lysis of adhesions, capsular release and, in persistent cases, quadricepsplasty as a late surgical intervention.

Outcomes

Although numerous implants have previously been used in the treatment of distal femur fractures, many of these implants are not particularly relevant currently because implant design, material, and surgical technique have drastically improved. In the past decade, reports demonstrate a favorable trend toward the use of titanium intramedullary devices. Similarly, lateral locking plates remain a well-supported intervention despite recent evidence questioning efficacy. To date, no published randomized studies have compared plating with retrograde nailing. Smaller series have demonstrated relatively good outcomes with either technique: one study reported an increased rate of revision surgery for patients treated with a nail,[39] another report demonstrated increased rates of malunion and the need for bone grafting in the setting of plate fixation.[40] Overall, the physical function portion of the Medical Outcomes Study 36-Item Short Form was decreased in both groups by approximately 2 SD.

Summary

Substantial improvements in implant design and understanding the determinants of achieving a good clinical outcome have been achieved in the treatment of distal femur fractures. The evaluation and treatment of these injuries requires an understanding of the injury mechanism, the potential associated injuries, and the radiographic and clinical goals. Surgical treatment requires a clear understanding of the unique anatomy of the distal femur as well as a comprehensive knowledge of the implant and how it can be used in a biologic preserving manner to achieve an anatomic reduction and enable fracture healing.

Key Study Points

- It is necessary to understand the unique anatomy of the distal femur so that an anatomic reduction may be achieved as well as successful maintenance of reduction using modern implants.
- Clinical and radiographic assessment of both soft-tissue and osseous injury to the distal femur helps define surgical treatment options.
- An understanding of expected outcomes and potential postoperative complications related to the surgical treatment of these injuries is important for optimal results.

Annotated References

1. Baker BJ, Escobedo EM, Nork SE, Henley MB: Hoffa fracture: A common association with high-energy supracondylar fractures of the distal femur. *AJR Am J Roentgenol* 2002;178(4):994.

2. Karunakar MA, Kellam JF: Avoiding malunion with 95degrees fixed-angle distal femoral implants. *J Orthop Trauma* 2004;18(7):443-445.

3. Collinge CA, Gardner MJ, Crist BD: Pitfalls in the application of distal femur plates for fractures. *J Orthop Trauma* 2011;25(11):695-706.

   This review article discusses common errors with the use of a lateral locking plate resulting in malunion.

4. Mills WJ, Barei DP, McNair P: The value of the ankle-brachial index for diagnosing arterial injury after knee dislocation: A prospective study. *J Trauma* 2004;56(6):1261-1265.

5. Nork SE, Segina DN, Aflatoon K, et al: The association between supracondylar-intercondylar distal femoral fractures and coronal plane fractures. *J Bone Joint Surg Am* 2005;87(3):564-569.

6. Neer CS II, Grantham SA, Shelton ML: Supracondylar fracture of the adult femur. A study of one hundred and ten cases. *J Bone Joint Surg Am* 1967;49(4):591-613.

7. Marsh JL: OTA fracture classification. *J Orthop Trauma* 2009;23(8):551.

8. Haidukewych GJ: Temporary external fixation for the management of complex intra- and periarticular fractures of the lower extremity. *J Orthop Trauma* 2002;16(9):678-685.

9. Nowotarski PJ, Turen CH, Brumback RJ, Scarboro JM: Conversion of external fixation to intramedullary nailing for fractures of the shaft of the femur in multiply injured patients. *J Bone Joint Surg Am* 2000;82(6):781-788.

10. Mast JW, Jakob R, Ganz R: *Planning and Reduction Technique in Fracture Surgery* .New York, Springer-Verlag, 1979.

11. Gerber C, Mast JW, Ganz R: Biological internal fixation of fractures. *Arch Orthop Trauma Surg* 1990;109(6):295-303.

12. Bolhofner BR, Carmen B, Clifford P: The results of open reduction and internal fixation of distal femur fractures using a biologic (indirect) reduction technique. *J Orthop Trauma* 1996;10(6):372-377.

13. Kregor PJ: Distal femur fractures with complex articular involvement: Management by articular exposure and submuscular fixation. *Orthop Clin North Am* 2002;33(1):153-175, ix.

14. Starr AJ, Jones AL, Reinert CM: The "swashbuckler": A modified anterior approach for fractures of the distal femur. *J Orthop Trauma* 1999;13(2):138-140.

15. Beltran MJ, Blair JA, Huh J, Kirby JM, Hsu JR; Skeletal Trauma Research Consortium(STReC): Articular exposure with the swashbuckler versus a "Mini-swashbuckler" approach. *Injury* 2013;44(2):189-193.

    This anatomic study assessed the exposure gained through the mini-swashbuckler approach. The authors report sufficient exposure of the distal femur articular surface, enabling anatomic reduction.

16. Higgins TF, Pittman G, Hines J, Bachus KN: Biomechanical analysis of distal femur fracture fixation: Fixed-angle screw-plate construct versus condylar blade plate. *J Orthop Trauma* 2007;21(1):43-46.

17. Schütz M, Müller M, Regazzoni P, et al: Use of the less invasive stabilization system (LISS) in patients with distal femoral (AO33) fractures: A prospective multicenter study. *Arch Orthop Trauma Surg* 2005;125(2):102-108.

18. Weight M, Collinge C: Early results of the less invasive stabilization system for mechanically unstable fractures of the distal femur (AO/OTA types A2, A3, C2, and C3). *J Orthop Trauma* 2004;18(8):503-508.

19. Ricci AR, Yue JJ, Taffet R, Catalano JB, DeFalco RA, Wilkens KJ: Less Invasive Stabilization System for treatment of distal femur fractures. *Am J Orthop (Belle Mead NJ)* 2004;33(5):250-255.

20. Kregor PJ, Stannard JA, Zlowodzki M, Cole PA: Treatment of distal femur fractures using the less invasive stabilization system: Surgical experience and early clinical results in 103 fractures. *J Orthop Trauma* 2004;18(8):509-520.

21. Perren SM: Evolution of the internal fixation of long bone fractures. The scientific basis of biological internal fixation: Choosing a new balance between stability and biology. *J Bone Joint Surg Br* 2002;84(8):1093-1110.

22. Ricci WM, Streubel PN, Morshed S, Collinge CA, Nork SE, Gardner MJ: Risk factors for failure of locked plate fixation of distal femur fractures: An analysis of 335 cases. *J Orthop Trauma* 2014;28(2):83-89.

In this retrospective review, 326 patients with 335 distal femur fractures were treated with lateral locking plates. A nonunion rate of 19% (64 patients) was identified. Identifiable risk factors include diabetes, smoking, open fracture, and short overall plate length (eight holes or less). Level of evidence: III.

23. Lujan TJ, Henderson CE, Madey SM, Fitzpatrick DC, Marsh JL, Bottlang M: Locked plating of distal femur fractures leads to inconsistent and asymmetric callus formation. *J Orthop Trauma* 2010;24(3):156-162.

This retrospective cohort study assessed the rate of callus formation in distal femur fractures treated with lateral locking plate fixation. Using a titanium plate enhances callus formation compared with stainless steel implants. Level of evidence: III.

24. Bottlang M, Lesser M, Koerber J, et al: Far cortical locking can improve healing of fractures stabilized with locking plates. *J Bone Joint Surg Am* 2010;92(7):1652-1660.

An established ovine tibial osteotomy model is used to assess the rate of callus formation in fractures treated with either a lateral locking plate or far cortical locking implant. At 9 weeks, far cortical locking specimens had 36% greater callus volume and 44% greater bone mineral content than those in the locked plating group.

25. Linn MS, McAndrew CM, Prusaczyk B, Brimmo O, Ricci WM, Gardner MJ: Dynamic locked plating of distal femur fractures. *J Orthop Trauma* 2015;29(10):447-450.

This prospective study of 34 patients assessed the efficacy of dynamic plating (overdrilling the near cortex) versus standard locking plating technique. The dynamic plating group had significantly greater callus formation than the control group. All patients were followed until union or the development of nonunion (mean, 10 months). Level of evidence: II.

26. Bottlang M, Fitzpatrick DC, Sheerin D, et al: Dynamic fixation of distal femur fractures using far cortical locking screws: A prospective observational study. *J Orthop Trauma* 2014;28(4):181-188.

In this observational cohort study, 31 consecutive patients were treated with far cortical locking. Patients were followed for a minimum of 1 year: 30 of 31 fractures (96.7%) healed at an average of 15.6 weeks. All diaphyseal screws maintained fixation. Level of evidence: II.

27. Ries Z, Hansen K, Bottlang M, Madey S, Fitzpatrick D, Marsh JL: Healing results of periprosthetic distal femur fractures treated with far cortical locking technology: A preliminary retrospective study. *Iowa Orthop J* 2013;33:7-11.

Retrospective review of 20 patients who underwent open reduction internal fixation of a distal femur periprosthetic femur fracture treated with far cortical locking constructs. Complete clinical and radiographic data was available on 18 patients. Sixteen of 18 patients (88.9%) healed by 24 weeks, the remaining two underwent revision surgery. Level of evidence: III.

28. Gliatis J, Megas P, Panagiotopoulos E, Lambiris E: Midterm results of treatment with a retrograde nail for supracondylar periprosthetic fractures of the femur following total knee arthroplasty. *J Orthop Trauma* 2005;19(3):164-170.

29. Patel K, Kapoor A, Daveshwar R, Golwala P: Percutaneous intramedullary supracondylar nailing for fractures of distal femur. *Med J Malaysia* 2004;59(Suppl Bsuppl B):206-207.

30. Markmiller M, Konrad G, Südkamp N: Femur-LISS and distal femoral nail for fixation of distal femoral fractures: Are there differences in outcome and complications? *Clin Orthop Relat Res* 2004;426:252-257.

31. Wähnert D, Hoffmeier KL, von Oldenburg G, Fröber R, Hofmann GO, Mückley T: Internal fixation of type-C distal femoral fractures in osteoporotic bone. *J Bone Joint Surg Am* 2010;92(6):1442-1452.

This biomechanics study assessed three different screw configurations for intramedullary fixation compared with a lateral locking plate. For intramedullary nails, the interlocking pattern affects stabilization such that four-screw distal locking provides the highest axial stability and almost comparable torsional stability to that of an angular stable plate.

32. Sanders R, Swiontkowski M, Rosen H, Helfet D: Double-plating of comminuted, unstable fractures of the distal part of the femur. *J Bone Joint Surg Am* 1991;73(3):341-346.

33. Vallier HA, Hennessey TA, Sontich JK, Patterson BM: Failure of LCP condylar plate fixation in the distal part of the femur. A report of six cases. *J Bone Joint Surg Am* 2006;88(4):846-853.

34. Rodriguez EK, Boulton C, Weaver MJ, et al: Predictive factors of distal femoral fracture nonunion after lateral locked plating: A retrospective multicenter case-control study of 283 fractures. *Injury* 2014;45(3):554-559.

This retrospective review of 283 fractures identified patient comorbidities, injury, and construct characteristics that are independent predictors of nonunion requiring a secondary procedure. Body mass index > 30 kg/m^2, open fracture, infection, and use of a stainless steel plate were predictive of nonunion. Level of evidence: III.

35. Stewart MJ, Sisk TD, Wallace SL: Fractures of the distal third of the femur: A comparison of methods of treatment. *J Bone Joint Surg Am* 1966;48(4):784-807.

36. Henderson CE, Lujan TJ, Kuhl LL, Bottlang M, Fitzpatrick DC, Marsh JL: 2010 mid-America Orthopaedic Association Physician in Training Award: Healing complications

are common after locked plating for distal femur fractures. *Clin Orthop Relat Res* 2011;469(6):1757-1765.

In this retrospective review, distal femur fractures were treated with a lateral locking plate aiming to assess healing rates, degree of callus formation, and complications associated with the procedure. Notable findings include a nonunion rate of 20%; infection was identified in 13%. Level of evidence: III.

37. Parekh AA, Smith WR, Silva S, et al: Treatment of distal femur and proximal tibia fractures with external fixation followed by planned conversion to internal fixation. *J Trauma* 2008;64(3):736-739.

38. Ricci WM, Collinge C, Streubel PN, McAndrew CM, Gardner MJ: A comparison of more and less aggressive bone debridement protocols for the treatment of open supracondylar femur fractures. *J Orthop Trauma* 2013;27(12):722-725.

This retrospective review compared the degree of bony fragment removal in open distal femur fractures treated with lateral locked plating. Infection ranged from 18% to 25% between the two groups with a trend toward increased healing with less aggressive bony excision. Level of evidence: III.

39. Hartin NL, Harris I, Hazratwala K: Retrograde nailing versus fixed-angle blade plating for supracondylar femoral fractures: A randomized controlled trial. *ANZ J Surg* 2006;76(5):290-294.

40. Thomson AB, Driver R, Kregor PJ, Obremskey WT: Long-term functional outcomes after intra-articular distal femur fractures: ORIF versus retrograde intramedullary nailing. *Orthopedics* 2008;31(8):748-750.

Chapter 41

Patella Fractures and Extensor Mechanism Injuries

Thomas Jones, MD   Michael C. Tucker, MD

Abstract

The extensor mechanism of the knee is composed of the quadriceps tendon, the patella, the patellar tendon, and the extensor retinaculum. The integrity of these structures is necessary for active knee extension and normal gait. A common mechanism of injury is eccentric loading of the quadriceps muscle with knee flexion, although a direct blow to the knee also can disrupt the extensor mechanism. After a disruption of the extensor mechanism is diagnosed, surgery typically is required. The surgical management of patella fractures usually involves open reduction and internal fixation, but partial patellectomy may be performed in highly comminuted fractures. Acute repair of the quadriceps and patellar tendons is typically performed using nonabsorbable suture passed through transpatellar bone tunnels, often augmented with cerclage of some type. The goals of surgery for displaced patella fractures and disruptions of the quadriceps and patellar tendons are restoration of the integrity of the extensor mechanism, stable fixation, and early protected range of motion.

Keywords: extensor mechanism; patella fracture; quadriceps tendon rupture; patellar tendon rupture

Introduction

The quadriceps tendon, the patella, the patellar tendon, and the extensor retinaculum are key components of the extensor mechanism of the knee. Disruption of any of these structures can compromise physiologic function of the knee. Thus, surgery to repair these structures usually is indicated to restore active extensor mechanism function.

Neither of the following authors nor any immediate family member has received anything of value from or has stock or stock options held in a commercial company or institution related directly or indirectly to the subject of this chapter: Dr. Jones and Dr. Tucker.

Patella Fractures

Fractures of the patella represent 1% of all fractures.[1] The patella is the largest human sesamoid bone and functions as a key component of the knee extensor mechanism, along with the quadriceps tendon, the patellar ligament, and the extensor retinaculum. Biomechanically, the patella transmits tensile forces of the quadriceps muscle to the patellar ligament and increases the moment arm of the extensor mechanism by displacing it anterior to the axis of knee rotation.

Most patella fractures result from a combination of direct and indirect trauma. Because the patella is a relatively subcutaneous bone, it is subject to injury from a direct blow, as when a flexed knee strikes a dashboard in a motor vehicle collision or strikes the ground in a fall. These fractures are typically more comminuted and may be associated with substantial chondral damage. Indirect trauma also may lead to a fracture. The patella is loaded in tension with quadriceps contraction and is subject to three-point bending during knee flexion. This combination of forces, as during eccentric quadriceps contraction in the course of a fall, can generate enough strain within the patella to cause a fracture. Because these fractures result from tension failure, they are often simple and transverse in nature, and the chondral surfaces may be relatively uninjured.[2]

Clinical Evaluation

Patient evaluation should begin with a detailed history. The mechanism of injury may suggest the extent of injury. A low-energy mechanism such as a ground-level fall with eccentric loading of the quadriceps should raise suspicion for a patella fracture or rupture of the quadriceps or patellar tendons. A higher-energy mechanism such as a direct blow from a dashboard should alert the surgeon to a possible extensor mechanism injury and other associated ipsilateral injuries such as proximal tibia fractures, knee ligamentous injuries, distal, midshaft, and proximal femur fractures, acetabular fractures, and/or hip dislocations.

The physical examination should start with inspection of the soft tissues. Lacerations and abrasions alert the physician to a possible open fracture or traumatic arthrotomy. In cases that are equivocal, a saline load test (SLT) can detect the presence of a traumatic arthrotomy found with an open fracture of the patella. A 2013 study reviewed a series of 50 patients with a suspected traumatic arthrotomy who underwent an SLT with an average of 75 mL of fluid injected. The study revealed a sensitivity of 94% and a specificity of 91% of the SLT.[3] Another study yielded a much lower sensitivity rate with larger volumes, and the addition of methylene blue to the SLT was not shown to improve its sensitivity.[4]

Other physical examination findings can include anterior ecchymosis, knee effusion, pain with palpation of the patella, and occasionally a palpable gap (**Figure 1**). If the injury is thought to be isolated, the extensor mechanism can be tested with a straight leg raise examination. If pain prevents an accurate examination, aspiration of the joint hematoma and intra-articular anesthetic injection may provide enough relief to perform the test.

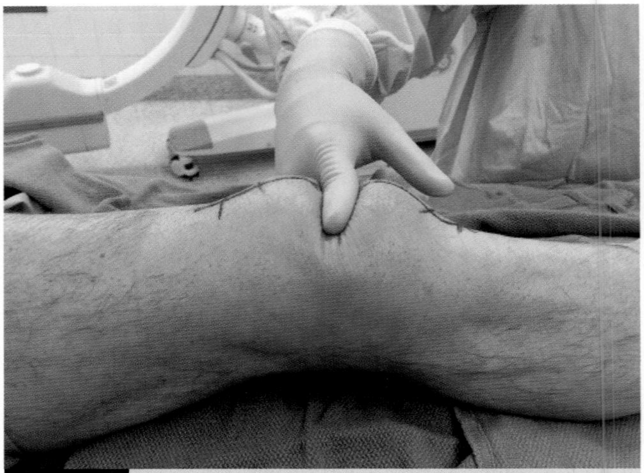

Figure 1 Clinical photograph demonstrates a palpable gap noted on physical examination of a patient with a patella fracture.

Radiographic Evaluation

Radiographic examination should begin with AP and lateral radiographs of the affected knee. Because the patella is superimposed on the distal femur on the AP view, interpretation may be difficult. The lateral view is most helpful for fractures in the axial or transverse plane. Vertically oriented patellar fractures may be best seen on an axial (Merchant or sunrise) view. Radiographs are often inadequate to evaluate the extent of comminution of patella fractures, especially those of the inferior pole. CT may improve the delineation of fracture patterns and facilitate preoperative planning.[5] CT also can help diagnose open patella fractures by demonstrating intra-articular air, which is associated with a traumatic arthrotomy. One series of 63 patients demonstrated a sensitivity and specificity of 100%.[6]

Treatment

Nonsurgical Treatment

Indications for nonsurgical treatment include an intact extensor mechanism with minimal fracture displacement, typically less than 2 mm of articular incongruity or fracture gap, although no standard measurement defines displacement. Management includes extension casting or bracing for 4 to 6 weeks, weight bearing as tolerated, and physical therapy for range of motion (ROM) and strengthening. In these cases, nonsurgical treatment has been shown to yield good to excellent results with minimal residual pain and full ROM in most cases.[7,8] Nonsurgical treatment can be considered in patients with substantial medical comorbidities that might preclude surgery or in patients who are minimal ambulators or nonambulators. One study of nonsurgical treatment of displaced patella fractures greater than 1 cm demonstrated substantial extensor lag in all patients, but none had severe pain. Minimal to moderate activity restrictions were seen in 75% of patients.[9]

Surgical Treatment

The relative surgical indications for displaced patella fractures include disruption of the extensor mechanism, substantial fracture displacement or articular incongruity, the presence of an open fracture, or free-floating intra-articular osteochondral fragments. As stated previously, no standard measurement defines displacement, but 2 mm of articular incongruity or a fracture gap on a lateral radiograph has been suggested as a reasonable threshold of displacement for surgical management.[10,11] As with any displaced articular fracture, the surgical goals remain the anatomic reduction of the articular surface, if possible, followed by stable fixation that restores extensor mechanism integrity and allows early ROM.

The surgical exposure of the patella typically involves an anterior, midline incision centered over the patella. The incision should be adequate enough to evaluate the entire extensor mechanism. As with any fracture exposure, appropriate soft-tissue handling and meticulous surgical technique are paramount. Full-thickness flaps should be elevated as a single layer medially and laterally. Fracture exposure should be limited to the identification and visualization of fragments necessary for anatomic reduction without excessive soft-tissue stripping. The surgeon then proceeds with reduction and temporary fixation. For most simple transverse and multifragmentary fractures with large, reconstructible fragments, this step often is achieved by positioning the knee in extension and using reduction forceps and temporary Kirschner wires (K-wires). Larger individual fragments sometimes can be secured to the intact patella using mini-fragment screws before the placement of definitive fixation. Reduction can be assessed with direct visualization of the dorsal cortex of the patella in conjunction with orthogonal intraoperative fluoroscopic views. These methods may not identify a malreduction at the articular surface, however. The articular reduction is confirmed best by placing a palpating finger on the articular surface or by directly visualizing it through an existing retinacular tear or a limited arthrotomy[12] (**Figure 2**).

Multiple techniques have been described for the definitive fixation of simple transverse patella fractures, including cerclage wiring, screw fixation, tension band wiring, and several modifications of the tension band technique. Simple cerclage wiring and traditional tension band techniques have been shown to be inferior to a modified anterior tension band with K-wires.[13] In addition, it has been shown that retinacular repair contributed to the stability of the overall patellar fracture treatment construct; therefore, it is recommended.[13] The technique was refined further to include a stainless steel wire woven in a figure-of-8 pattern around two parallel K-wires and over the anterior cortex of the patella with two wire twists.[14]

Tension band techniques work by converting tension forces into compression forces when they are applied to a fracture that is loaded eccentrically. In a transverse fracture of the patella, the tensioned wires are thought to convert the distracting force of the quadriceps across the anterior cortex of the patella to a compressive force at the articular surface.[10]

For simple transverse patella fractures, a typical modified tension band construct involves placing two parallel K-wires perpendicular to the fracture. A stainless steel wire is passed posterior to the K-wires at the proximal and distal poles of the patella and crossed over the anterior cortex in a figure-of-8 pattern. After tensioning, the wire twists and the proximal and distal ends of the K-wires are clipped, bent, and buried in the soft tissue (**Figure 3**). The

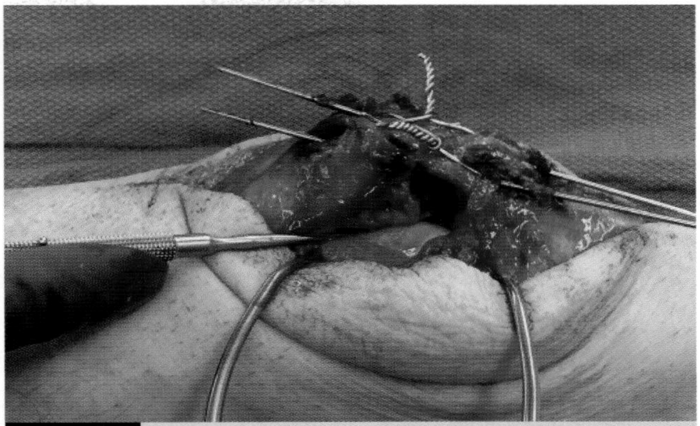

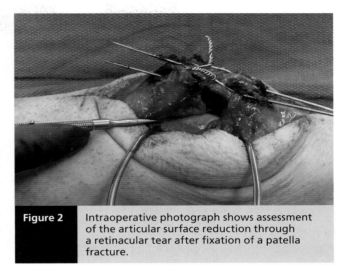

Figure 2 Intraoperative photograph shows assessment of the articular surface reduction through a retinacular tear after fixation of a patella fracture.

bending of the proximal and distal ends of the K-wires is associated with a reduced risk of wire migration.[15]

When anatomic reduction and stable fixation are achieved, tension band wire constructs can be associated with high union rates and a good functional result.[16] One series of patients treated with a tension band wire construct showed a 100% union rate and satisfactory functional outcomes in all patients.[17] Other series have not reproduced these results. In a series of 51 surgically treated displaced patella fractures, fracture displacement before healing was noted in 11 patients (22%). This displacement was attributed to technical errors and patient noncompliance. Soft-tissue irritation requiring hardware removal in 18% of patients also was observed.[18] The issue of symptomatic hardware also has been seen in other studies. A 2013 series of 315 patients with displaced patella fractures treated with tension band and K-wire constructs showed that 116 patients (37%) elected to have their implants removed secondary to soft-tissue irritation.[19]

One possible reason for such soft-tissue irritation is the inability to cut the wires short enough without causing substantial dissection of the quadriceps and patellar tendons.[10] A second reason might be the ability to impact the wires adjacent to only one pole of the patella, leaving the other ends protruding from the opposite pole. A 2010 study described a modification to the tension band wire technique that used four wires: two placed from the proximal pole and two placed from the distal pole. Each wire crossed the fracture but was not advanced through the opposite cortex. A figure-of-8 wire was tensioned around the ends of the four wires. The ends of the wires then were cut, bent 180°, and impacted into the cortices of the proximal and distal poles. The authors reported that hardware removal was required less frequently when using this technique.[20]

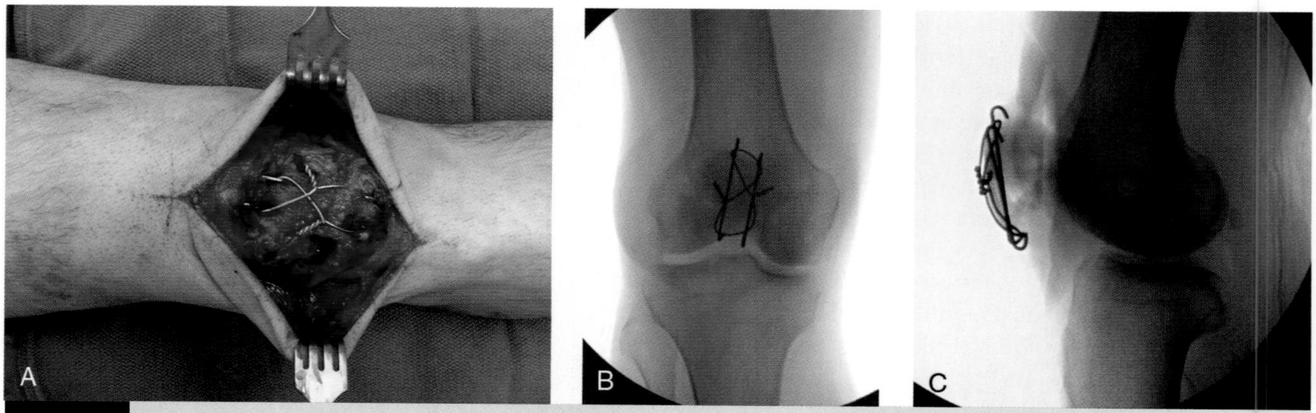

Figure 3 Intraoperative images show a typical modified tension band wire construct used to treat a simple transverse patella fracture. **A**, Photograph shows the tension band wire construct with two parallel Kirschner wires and a figure-of-8 wire with two twists. **B**, AP fluoroscopic view. **C**, Lateral fluoroscopic view.

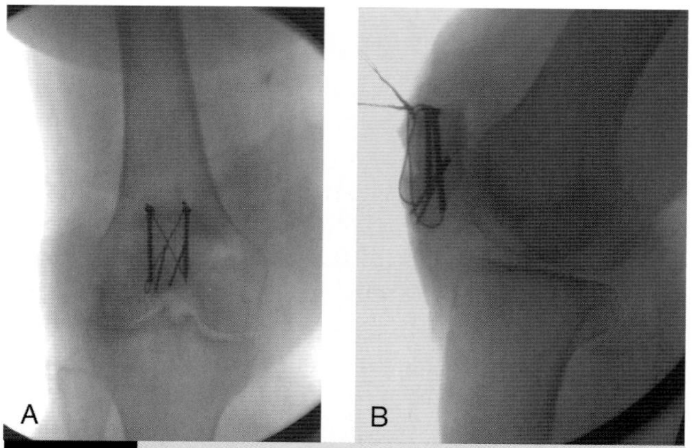

Figure 4 Intraoperative fluoroscopic AP (**A**) and lateral (**B**) images show a tension band construct using two cannulated screws with a tensioned wire passing through the cannulae of the screws. Note the intraosseous mini-fragment screws used to treat a separate inferior fragment. These screws were placed initially, thus creating a simple transverse fracture pattern amenable to tension band fixation.

Another modification to the tension band technique involves using cannulated, partially threaded screws in lag fashion with a tensioned wire passed through the cannulae of the screws (**Figure 4**). This technique has been demonstrated to be superior to the modified tension band wire construct in biomechanical testing.[21] In a clinical series of 10 displaced patella fractures treated with this technique, union was noted in all cases and good to excellent clinical results observed in 7 patients, which was comparable to previously published reports.[22] A 2012 review of 173 patella fractures studied factors predicting the failure of fixation in surgically treated patella fractures. Using a tension band wire construct reportedly was a predictor of failure, whereas using screws or other fixation was not.[23]

A 2013 study also examined fixation failure in surgically treated patella fractures, comparing a tension band used with wires with a tension band used with screws.[19] Of 448 patella fractures, a trend toward increased failure when using screws was noted, but this trend was not statistically significant. Patients with a tension band wire construct were twice as likely to undergo implant removal for symptomatic hardware.

Because of some of the technical difficulties and symptomatic hardware issues associated with traditional tension band constructs, alternative fixation techniques have been suggested. Using heavy, nonabsorbable suture as a tensioning device has been studied biomechanically and described clinically for patella fractures. In biomechanical testing, heavy, braided suture as a tension band was shown to result in less fracture gap and superior fixation strength compared with traditional tension band techniques using stainless steel wire.[24,25] In a 2013 clinical study, a cohort of 25 patients with displaced patella fractures treated with a tension band technique using transosseous suture were matched with a historical control group that underwent modified tension band wire fixation. No difference in union rate or time to union was noted, but shorter hospital stays, less soft-tissue irritation, and lower reoperation rates were noted for the transosseous suture cohort; all of these factors were statistically significant.[26]

As patella fractures become more complex, a tension band construct in isolation no longer may be acceptable. When reconstructible, major fragments can be reduced anatomically and fixed with interfragmentary compression using mini-fragment implants. With lesser degrees of comminution, these fractures sometimes can be converted

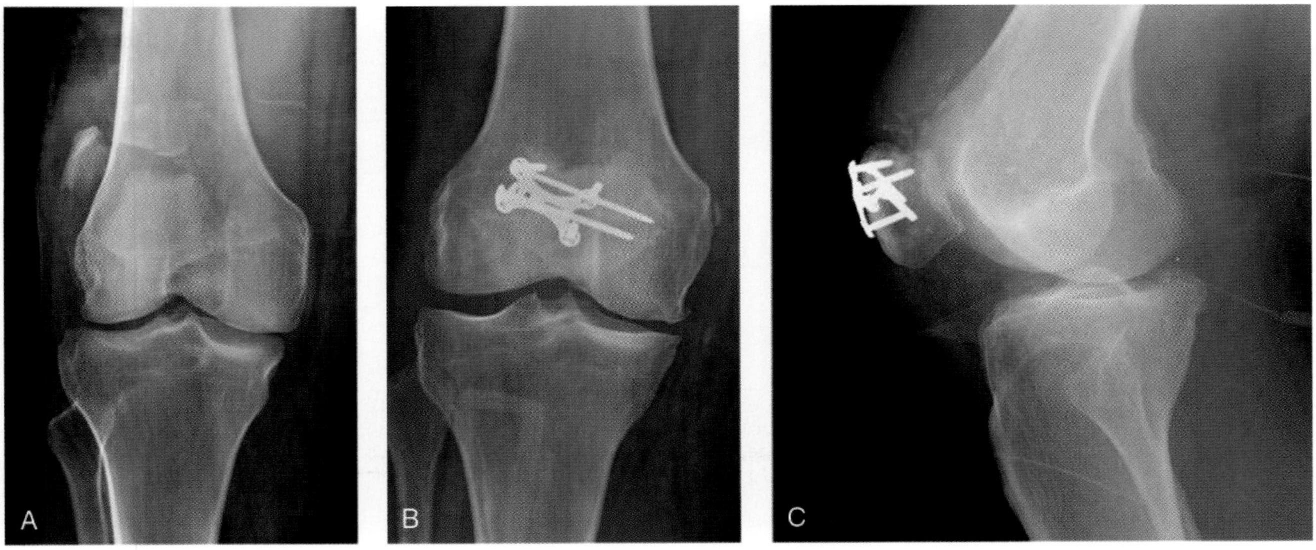

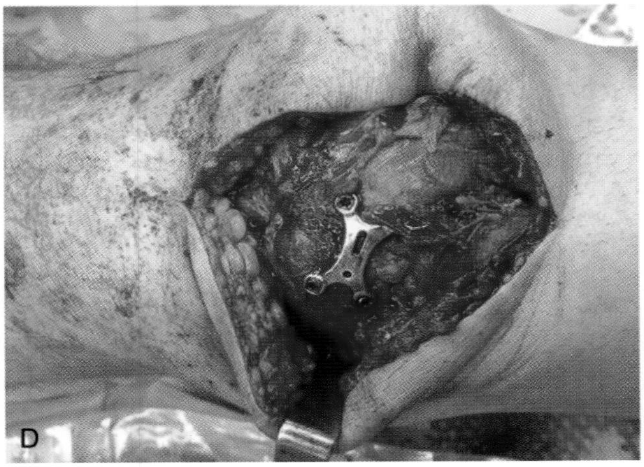

Figure 5 Images demonstrate open reduction and internal fixation using a plating technique of a comminuted patella fracture with relatively large fragments. **A**, Preoperative AP radiograph. **B** and **C**, AP and lateral radiographs of the fixation construct. Note the independent lag screws placed prior to neutralization with the locked plate. **D**, Photograph demonstrates the locked plate and screw construct. (Reproduced with permission from Taylor BC, Mehta S, Castaneda J, French BG, Blanchard C: Plating of patella fractures: Techniques and outcomes. *J Orthop Trauma* 2014;28[9]:231-235.)

to a simple transverse pattern and subsequently fixed using a tension band technique. In more comminuted cases, traditional fixation techniques can be augmented with cerclage wiring of the patella. In cadaver testing, this technique has been shown to improve the fixation stability of a tension band-wire construct.[27]

Fixed-angle plating of patella fractures has been studied in cadaver testing. These constructs have been shown to be substantially stronger than tension band constructs with K-wires or screws.[28] In a 2014 clinical series of eight patients, the technique of fixed angle plating of displaced patella fractures was described. With simple fractures, lag screw fixation was attempted if possible, then the screws neutralized with a mini-fragment fixed-angle plate placed on the anterior surface of the patella (**Figure 5**). For highly comminuted fractures, plating portions of the patella amenable to fixation and performing limited excision of the fragments that were not amenable to associated soft-tissue repair were described.[29] All patients went on to union, and none required hardware removal.

Fractures of the proximal and distal poles of the patella provide a surgical treatment challenge. Often, the fragments are very small and highly comminuted and make anatomic reduction and stable fixation more difficult. The ideal strategy for these fractures has been debated. Some surgeons advocate osteosynthesis, whereas others recommend partial patellectomy (PP) with excision of the comminuted fragments and advancement and fixation of the adjacent tendon into the fracture bed of the remaining patella with heavy, nonabsorbable suture. For the remaining patella to which the tendon is repaired, anterior and posterior attachment sites have been described. Because these reconstructions are not anatomic, alterations in patellofemoral biomechanics are to be expected.[10] This expectation was demonstrated in a biomechanical study that compared the patellofemoral contact pressures in a

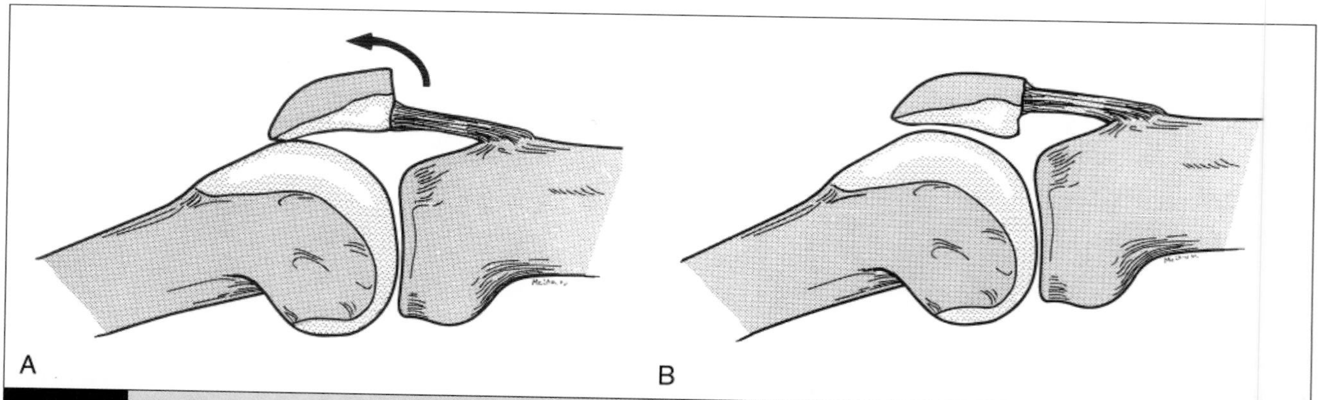

Figure 6 Illustration shows the possible reattachment locations for the patellar tendon after partial patellectomy. A posterior attachment site (**A**) tilts the distal aspect of the patella anteriorly (arrow) and shifts the contact area more proximally. An anterior attachment (**B**) minimizes this effect. (Reproduced with permission from Marder RA, Swanson TV, Sharkey NA, Duwelius PJ: Plating of patella fractures: Techniques and outcomes. *J Bone Joint Surg Am* 1993;75[1]:35-45.)

group of cadaver knees that had undergone PP with a group that had intact patellae.[30] An anterior attachment point produced contact areas most similar to the unaltered specimens; a posterior attachment point was associated with the greatest decrease in contact area (**Figure 6**).

Good clinical results have been achieved for patella fractures treated with PP. In a series of 40 patients treated with PP and tendon advancement to a posterior articular location, excellent results were seen in 20 patients and good results were noted in 11.[31] Mean active ROM of 94% and quadriceps strength of 85% of the surgical extremity were reported in comparison with the contralateral extremity. Worse clinical outcomes were found in patients sustaining comminuted fractures.[31]

Advocates of osteosynthesis for these types of fractures believe the technique preserves patellar bone—and thus, patellar height—and may allow earlier ROM and weight bearing. One osteosynthesis technique using a basket plate has been described in two clinical studies, which compared it with PP. A study of 24 inferior pole patella fractures described a technique of suturing the inferior pole fragments into a bundle and then capturing them using a curved plate with hooks.[32] The plate is then fixed to the main patellar fragment using cancellous screws, thus capturing the inferior pole. Improved patellofemoral scores, improved ROM, increased work intensity, and reduced pain were noted in the group that underwent osteosynthesis, compared with those undergoing pole resection. A retrospective study noted similar results when comparing the two techniques.[33] In both groups, patella baja was associated with poor functional outcomes.

In extreme cases of soft-tissue and bony compromise for which stable fixation is impossible, total patellectomy may be indicated. This technique is associated with cosmetic and functional compromises. Total patellectomy effectively shortens the moment arm of the extensor mechanism, thus decreasing its overall efficiency. Episodes of instability may result, because the knee remains loaded and in a flexed position at full extension. In patients having undergone total patellectomy, one study reported mean quadriceps strength to be 60% of the normal side.[34] The study also found that, when walking, patients experienced a feeling of instability, which occurred more frequently as quadriceps strength diminished. In these extreme cases of highly comminuted patella fractures, the retention of substantial patellar fragments may preserve some of the biomechanical advantage of the extensor mechanism. Such retention should remain a surgical goal, if possible.

Outcomes

Historically, reported healing rates have been high, and complication rates have been low for surgically treated patella fractures, whereas clinical outcomes have been mixed. A 2012 meta-analysis of 24 studies involving 737 patellae found the nonunion, infection, and reoperation rates to be 1.9%, 3.2%, and 33.6%, respectively.[35] These rates were consistent with reported rates in the literature. The study did not address patient-centered outcomes such as ROM, satisfaction, or return to function, because these metrics often were not reported or were reported in a nonuniform fashion.

Recently, studies examining functional outcomes after the surgical treatment of patella fractures demonstrate consistently poor results with surgical treatment. A 2012 series of 40 patients with a median follow-up time of 6.5 years found that, overall, long-term outcomes after patella fractures were not good.[36] The patients in the study group showed considerably poorer outcome scores than normalized population values. Objective measurements of quadriceps strength and knee ROM on the affected side showed substantial deficits compared with the contralateral side.

A similar 2013 study prospectively obtained outcome scores from 30 patients with isolated unilateral patella fractures treated with surgery.[37] All fractures healed with minimal complications. Residual deficits in muscle performance and functional ability were found that persisted 12 months after surgical intervention, with 24 patients (80%) reporting anterior knee pain. More than one-third of all patients elected to undergo hardware removal. In more than one-half of these patients, patella baja developed, which has been shown to be a risk factor for poor functional outcomes.

More recently, a 2015 study prospectively compared the functional outcomes of 52 displaced patella fractures treated with open reduction and internal fixation or PP.[38] No difference in union rates, complication rates, ROM, or outcome measures were noted between the two groups. Irrespective of treatment, functional outcomes after patella fracture are inferior to those of population norms.

Extensor Mechanism Injuries

Knee extensor mechanism injuries occur infrequently but occur predominantly in males and African Americans.[39-42] Quadriceps tendon ruptures generally occur in patients older than 40 years[39] and often exhibit degenerative changes within the tendon.[41,43] Patellar tendon ruptures demonstrate a bimodal age distribution, with younger patients often injured during sports participation.[39,40,42,44] High-risk patient populations have been identified. Systemic comorbidities, including chronic renal failure, rheumatoid arthritis, diabetes, systemic steroid use, hyperparathyroidism, gout, connective tissue disorders, obesity, and fluoroquinolone use, often are noted and are associated with quadriceps tendon ruptures in particular.[41,45-47] Generally, healthy tendons do not rupture and can tolerate substantial tensile forces without injury. As a result, many knee extensor mechanism injuries manifest as tendon-bone interface avulsions, with quadriceps ruptures occurring at the superior patellar pole[48] and patellar tendon ruptures occurring at the inferior patellar pole as opposed to the tibial tubercle.[43]

Anatomy and Biomechanics

Four separate muscles—the rectus femoris, vastus lateralis, vastus intermedius, and vastus medialis—converge for insertion primarily as the single quadriceps tendon on the proximal pole of the patella. The patellar tendon, or ligament, is the concluding distal component of the knee extensor complex, originating from the lower pole of the patella and inserting at the tibial tubercle. The quadriceps tendon is generally thicker than the patellar tendon, which also transitions from being wider and thinner proximally to being more narrow and thicker distally. The femoral nerve supplies all four quadriceps muscles. Vascularly, the quadriceps tendon is supplied by the descending branches of the lateral femoral circumflex, descending geniculate along with the medial and lateral superior geniculate arteries. A somewhat avascular area exists in the deeper portions of the quadriceps tendon, located 1 to 2 cm from the proximal pole of the patella. The patellar tendon has contrastingly less vascular supply and is supplied primarily by the infrapatellar fat pad along with the inferior medial and lateral geniculate arteries.

The knee extension mechanism serves as the force-transmitting connector from the quadriceps muscle group to the proximal tibia. The patella is the largest sesamoid bone in the body and possesses the thickest articular cartilage, thereby offering protection against the considerable pressures routinely generated, particularly during eccentric contractions of the quadriceps. Overall, the thickness of the patella provides substantial mechanical advantage to the quadriceps by increasing the moment arm relative to the knee center of rotation. The greatest intratendinous extensor mechanism forces are generated in a position of flexion and during eccentric contraction, and these positions are consistent with the occurrence of several injuries.

Physical Examination

Extensor mechanism soft-tissue disruption typically presents with a history of a sudden forceful knee flexion, subsequent severe pain, and an inability to extend the knee or bear weight without knee flexion collapse. Often, quadriceps or patellar tendon ruptures also demonstrate a clearly palpable soft-tissue defect at the respective patellar poles. Vigilance must be maintained, because this seemingly straightforward presentation continues to result in a 10% to 50% rate of missed diagnoses.[49] Diagnostic hindrances include the typical tense knee effusion, making palpation more difficult. Knee aspiration followed by intra-articular anesthetic injection may result in improved patient participation. Findings range from the absence of active knee extension to the inability to maintain the passively extended knee, often associated with complete tendon and retinacular tears, or perhaps weak knee extension and terminal active extension lag, indicating a less extensive injury.

Diagnostic Imaging

Initial AP and lateral radiographs may reveal patella alta, likely representing patellar tendon rupture with associated retinacular tears, or may appear relatively normal in a scenario of quadriceps tendon rupture. Findings on traditional radiographs are often more helpful in cases of patella fracture. Ultrasonography has proven to be a helpful diagnostic tool in experienced hands, is relatively inexpensive, and can be available quickly in the emergency department setting.[50] Ultrasonography does require caution, however, because reports of overdiagnosis and underdiagnosis have been published. In particular, differentiating between partial and complete tears has proven more unpredictable with ultrasonography alone, likely affecting treatment decisions.[51,52] Although more expensive and time consuming, MRI has proven highly sensitive and accurate and therefore should be used to confirm any equivocal ultrasonographic findings.[52] High rates of false-positive ultrasonographic findings resulting in unnecessary surgical intervention have led to a recommendation to abandon ultrasonography and pursue MRI in cases of clinical ambiguity.[51] Also, although uncommonly associated with knee extensor mechanism ruptures, additional knee injuries are more accurately diagnosed using MRI than ultrasonography.[53]

Treatment

Quadriceps Tendon Rupture

The type of treatment (nonsurgical or surgical) depends on whether the tear is incomplete or complete. Historically, incomplete tears without a functional deficit have responded satisfactorily to nonsurgical management, which includes immobilization in full extension for 6 weeks followed by a course of physical therapy designed to regain motion and strength. Controversial aspects of nonsurgical treatment, including initial joint aspiration for pain control, early anti-inflammatory medication, and more aggressive early ROM, remain unresolved.

Surgical treatment is indicated for incomplete tears with functional deficits and for all complete tears. Acute repair is preferred, because delays in treatment generally result in less satisfactory outcomes,[54] although isolated cases of successful chronic tear treatment have been reported.[55] The location of the rupture determines surgical treatment, because midsubstance tears with adequate proximal and distal tendon portions allow primary end-to-end repair. A recent literature review reveals this location to be more common than is perceived by many surgeons—between 1 and 2 cm from the superior pole of the patella.[54] Most commonly, primary end-to-end repair uses heavy No. 2 to No. 5 nonabsorbable suture material placed in a running locked Krackow stitch. The optimal number of suture strands or "bites" per strand remains undetermined and is left to the discretion of the surgeon. Ruptures occurring at or near the tendon-bone interface, which account for approximately one-third of quadriceps tears,[54] are not candidates for end-to-end repair techniques. Most commonly, a heavy nonabsorbable continuous locking-stitch technique combined with vertical patellar drill tunnels is used (**Figure 7**). The superior pole of the patella may be decorticated, which may facilitate healing. Sutures then are pulled through the patellar tunnels with a suture passer or long straight needle assistance and tied at the inferior pole of the patella, with care taken to minimize the soft tissue captured under the suture knot location. A 2012 study revealed use of the patellar drill hole technique in 50% of cases, although rupture location at the tendon insertion occurred only one-third of the time.[54]

Alternative methods of distal quadriceps tendon rupture repair using suture anchors continue to be reported, although in small series. Biomechanical studies have demonstrated equivalent or even superior results when using suture anchors versus the traditional patellar drill hole technique.[56] Proponents of the suture anchor technique stress its simplicity, smaller incisions, shorter surgical times, and stronger repair. Less appealing aspects include the cost and the difficulty of hardware removal if necessary.[57]

Augmentation techniques may be used in addition to the patellar drill tunnel or suture anchor methods of primary repair. Various historically reported options include using wire, Mersilene tape (Ethicon), available soft tissue in the partial quadriceps turn-down or Scuderi technique, or the fascia lata.

Chronic or neglected quadriceps tendon ruptures continue to present a much more difficult treatment dilemma, because substantial tendon retraction and scarring typically are present. Extensive mobilization of the quadriceps tendon, including release from the femur along with medial and lateral release, may still leave a tendon gap. Successful reports of late reconstruction have been published.[55] For a persistent tendon gap, some form of tendon lengthening or a major augmentation procedure, such as a V-Y plasty, is necessary.

Patellar Tendon Rupture

Like a quadriceps tendon rupture, an incomplete patellar tendon rupture with an intact extensor mechanism may be managed successfully with 2 to 4 weeks of immobilization in extension followed by progressive ROM and strengthening exercises beginning at 6 weeks after injury. Surgery is reserved for incomplete tears with a functional deficit or complete tears.

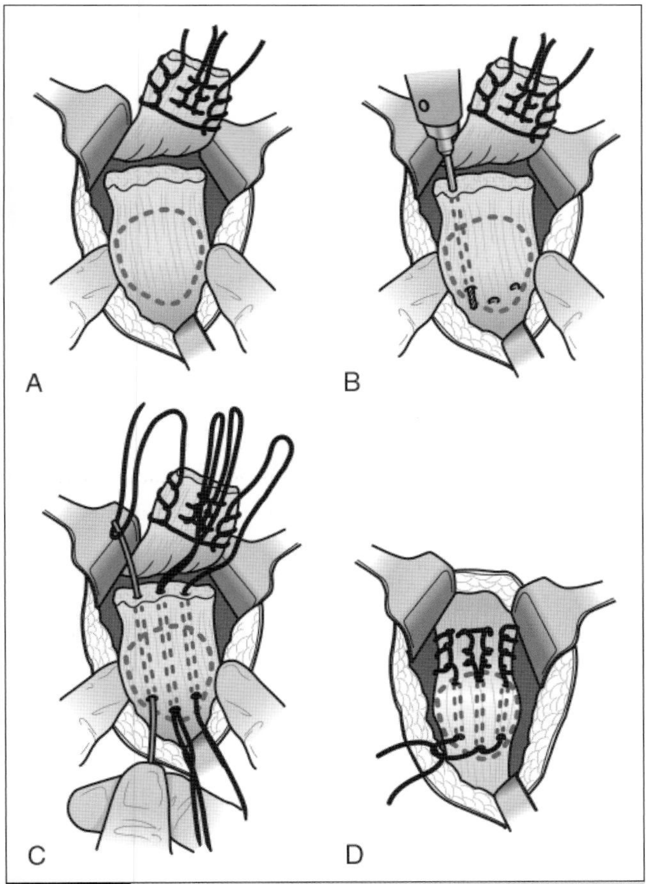

Figure 7 Illustrations demonstrate the suture technique for a typical quadriceps tendon repair. **A,** Krackow-style stitch is placed in the proximal quadriceps tendon stump. **B,** Drill holes (three) are placed vertically through patella. **C,** Previously placed sutures are passed through patellar drill holes. **D,** Final construct as sutures are tied securely at the inferior pole of the patella.

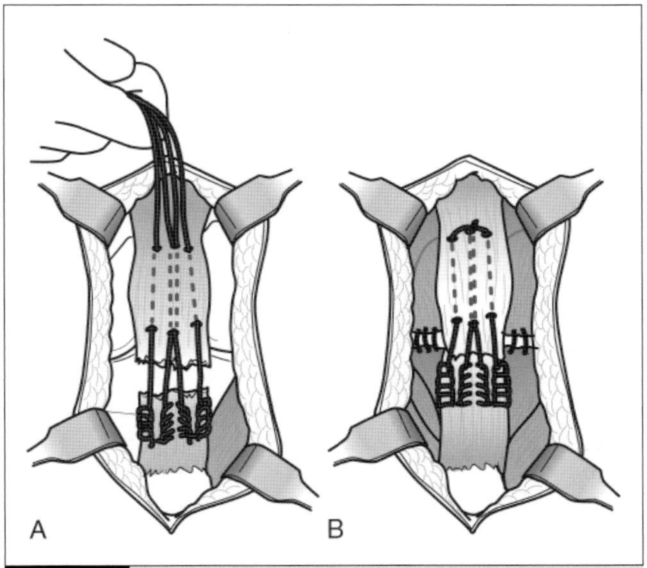

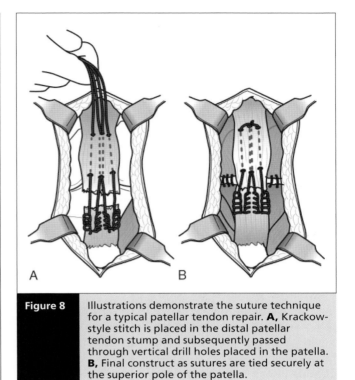

Figure 8 Illustrations demonstrate the suture technique for a typical patellar tendon repair. **A,** Krackow-style stitch is placed in the distal patellar tendon stump and subsequently passed through vertical drill holes placed in the patella. **B,** Final construct as sutures are tied securely at the superior pole of the patella.

Acute repair is preferred, and several techniques have been described, including intraoperative decision making regarding possible augmentation of the repair.[58] The surgical technique is guided largely by the location of the rupture. Unlike quadriceps tendon rupture, the location of a patellar tendon injury is predominantly at the bone-tendon interface, not intrasubstance. Injury typically occurs at the inferior pole of the patella, not at the tibial tubercle.[42,58] Given this location, the most common repair technique uses two rows of locking, heavy-gauge, nonabsorbable suture to capture the patellar tendon, pass it proximally through the vertical patellar bone tunnels, and tie it over the superior patellar pole with a minimum of underlying soft tissue. The inferior patellar pole bone surface often is débrided to create a fresh and exposed surface, which is thought to enhance healing potential and the strength of repair. Any associated retinacular tears also are repaired now. The knee is held in extension during this portion of the procedure.

Although less common, midsubstance tears can be repaired successfully using continuous heavy-gauge locking suture, culminating in end-to-end tendon apposition. Should either tendon portion be a concern in terms of length and adequate purchase, drill holes may be incorporated through the patella or, if appropriate, the tibial tubercle (**Figure 8**).

Using suture anchors in cases of bone-tendon interface disruption is also an option and has demonstrated superior results in a recent biomechanical cadaveric study.[59] Clinical results using suture anchor repair have been reported infrequently and demonstrate relatively high failure rates of up to 21% along with increased implant costs.[60]

Historically, patellar tendon repair augmentation has been a popular technique. A 2015 study reported a 66% overall augmentation rate with primary repairs in an extensive review of the published literature.[58] Augmentation has been described using wire, cables, additional heavy-gauge suture, or Mersilene tape. The additional implant typically is placed in a cerclage fashion through a tibial tubercle drill hole, then passed medial and lateral along the patella, with final completion of the loop over the superior patellar pole. This technique is designed to further protect or offload the actual tendon repair. Few publications have addressed augmented versus nonaugmented acute repair of patellar tendon ruptures specifically. Findings vary, with a possible trend toward more infrequent use of augmentation, because good results have been demonstrated in younger, seemingly healthy patients when using nonaugmented primary repair.[61] A 2015 study recommended the continued use of augmentation, because this review demonstrated only a 2% failure rate in augmented repairs versus a 5% failure rate in nonaugmented repairs.[58] Additional augmentation techniques have been described using autogenous tissue derived from semitendinosus, gracilis, quadriceps, or gastrocnemius tendons, but they are used almost exclusively for the repair of chronic and neglected patellar tendon ruptures or for those associated with total knee arthroplasty.[58]

Postoperative Rehabilitation

Similar rehabilitation and physical therapy regimens are recommended for quadriceps tendon rupture and patellar tendon repair patients. Early guarded motion is indicated for most acute repairs except in cases of exceptionally poor tissue or a concerning soft-tissue envelope. Improved results have been demonstrated with a hinged knee brace that can be locked in extension for weight bearing during ambulation but can be released for early initiation of graduated active flexion and passive only extension for 6 weeks.[61] Higher complication rates and failure rates were noted in acute repairs after longer periods of immobilization in a recent review.[58]

Summary

Traditional fixation techniques for patella fractures usually involve some variation of a tension band construct, although, more recently, alternative fixation strategies, such as screw fixation with plating and suturing, have been described. For highly comminuted patella fractures, PP may be performed; however, some authors advocate preserving patellar bone stock and have moved toward fixation of these comminuted fractures if possible. Fixation of patella fractures is associated with high union rates and low infection rates, but symptomatic hardware and persistent functional deficits can remain a problem postoperatively. Specifically, patella baja is associated with poor functional outcomes. For the repair of quadriceps and patellar tendon ruptures occurring adjacent to the patellar poles, fixation usually consists of nonabsorbable sutures passed through the patella. For midsubstance ruptures, the sutures may be tied together for an end-to-end tendon repair. Often, repair of the patellar tendon is augmented with cerclage. The acute repair of quadriceps and patellar tendon ruptures is associated with low rerupture rates and good to excellent functional results, although few studies include validated outcome measures. In all cases, the surgical goals remain the restoration of extensor mechanism integrity, stable fixation, and early ROM.

Key Study Points

- The integrity of the extensor mechanism is necessary for active knee extension and normal gait.
- Two common mechanisms of injury are eccentric loading of the quadriceps with knee flexion and a direct blow to the anterior aspect of the knee.
- The straight leg raise is an important physical examination tool for assessing the integrity of the extensor mechanism.
- The goals of surgery include the repair of the extensor mechanism with stable fixation to allow early ROM.

Annotated References

1. Harris RM: Fractures of the patella and injuries to the extensor mechanism, in Bucholz RW, Heckman JD, Court-Brown CC, eds: *Rockwood and Green's Fractures in Adults,* ed 6. Philadelphia, PA, Lippincott Williams & Wilkins, 2006, p 1974, vol 2.

2. Carpenter JE, Kasman R, Matthews LS: Fractures of the patella. *Instr Course Lect* 1994;43:97-108.

3. Konda SR, Howard D, Davidovitch RI, Egol KA: The saline load test of the knee redefined: A test to detect traumatic arthrotomies and rule out periarticular wounds not requiring surgical intervention. *J Orthop Trauma* 2013;27(9):491-497.

   This is a retrospective review of 50 consecutive patients who underwent an SLT for a suspected traumatic knee arthrotomy. The mean wound size was 3.9 cm, and the mean saline load volume was 74.9 mL. The sensitivity and specificity of the SLT were 94% and 91%, respectively. The authors noted that knees with small periarticular wounds, a negative SLT, and no other evidence of a traumatic arthrotomy have an infection rate of 0% with nonsurgical management. Level of evidence: III.

4. Metzger P, Carney J, Kuhn K, Booher K, Mazurek M: Sensitivity of the saline load test with and without methylene blue dye in the diagnosis of artificial traumatic knee arthrotomies. *J Orthop Trauma* 2012;26(6):347-349.

   This is a randomized, prospective study of 58 patients scheduled to undergo elective arthroscopy. During the course of surgery, an inferior, lateral arthrotomy was made, and normal saline or methylene blue solution was injected. The authors noted an overall false-negative rate of 67% (39 patients). In patients with a positive test, the mean volume injected at observed fluid outflow was 105 mL in the methylene blue group and 95 mL in the normal saline group. The authors conclude that the sensitivity of the SLT is unacceptably low and that the addition of methylene blue does not improve the diagnostic value. Level of evidence: I.

5. Lazaro LE, Wellman DS, Pardee NC, et al: Effect of computerized tomography on classification and treatment plan for patellar fractures. *J Orthop Trauma* 2013;27(6):336-344.

This is a prospective study designed to evaluate the effect of CT on the fracture classification and surgical planning of patellar fractures. Radiographs of 41 patellar fractures were reviewed, each fracture was classified, and a treatment plan was developed. The process was repeated with CT. The entire process was repeated 12 months later, and interobserver reliability and intraobserver reproducibility were assessed. After the addition of CT, the reviewers modified the classification in 66% of cases, or an average of 27 fractures, and modified the treatment plan in 49% of cases, or an average of 20 fractures. In 88% of cases, or 36 fractures, CT identified a distinctive, comminuted inferior pole fracture, which was unappreciated on plain radiographs in 44%, or 16 fractures. Level of evidence: II.

6. Konda SR, Davidovitch RI, Egol KA: Computed tomography scan to detect traumatic arthrotomies and identify periarticular wounds not requiring surgical intervention: An improvement over the saline load test. *J Orthop Trauma* 2013;27(9):498-504.

This retrospective review was designed to report the authors' experience with CT in detecting traumatic arthrotomies of the knee (TAK) based on the presence of intra-articular air. In all, 63 knees with wounds suspicious for TAK underwent CT. A subgroup of 37 patients also underwent the SLT. The authors found that the sensitivity and specificity of CT for diagnosing TAK were 100%. In the subgroup of 37 patients who underwent both CT and SLT, the sensitivity and specificity of CT were 100%, versus 92% for the SLT. Level of evidence: III.

7. Boström A: Fracture of the patella. A study of 422 patellar fractures. *Acta Orthop Scand Suppl* 1972;143:1-80.

8. Braun W, Wiedemann M, Rüter A, Kundel K, Kolbinger S: Indications and results of nonoperative treatment of patellar fractures. *Clin Orthop Relat Res* 1993;289:197-201.

9. Pritchett JW: Nonoperative treatment of widely displaced patella fractures. *Am J Knee Surg* 1997;10(3):145-147, discussion 147-148.

10. Della Rocca GJ: Displaced patella fractures. *J Knee Surg* 2013;26(5):293-299.

This review article discusses displaced patella fractures and evaluation of the patient via history, physical examination, and imaging techniques. The author identifies some surgical indications and discusses multiple techniques for surgical treatment, including open reduction and internal fixation as well as partial patellectomy.

11. Melvin JS, Mehta S: Patellar fractures in adults. *J Am Acad Orthop Surg* 2011;19(4):198-207.

A comprehensive review of patellar anatomy, biomechanics, and the typical mechanisms of injury is presented, along with a discussion of clinical and radiographic assessment of the patient and classification of patella fractures, surgical indications and surgical techniques, recommended postoperative management protocols, and reported complications.

12. Gardner MJ, Griffith MH, Lawrence BD, Lorich DG: Complete exposure of the articular surface for fixation of patellar fractures. *J Orthop Trauma* 2005;19(2):118-123.

13. Weber MJ, Janecki CJ, McLeod P, Nelson CL, Thompson JA: Efficacy of various forms of fixation of transverse fractures of the patella. *J Bone Joint Surg Am* 1980;62(2):215-220.

14. Müller ME, Allgöwer M, Schneider R, Willeneger H: *Manual of Internal Fixation: Techniques Recommended by the AO Group*. Berlin, Germany, Springer, 1979, pp 248-253.

15. Eggink KM, Jaarsma RL: Mid-term (2-8 years) follow-up of open reduction and internal fixation of patella fractures: Does the surgical technique influence the outcome? *Arch Orthop Trauma Surg* 2011;131(3):399-404.

This retrospective study of 60 patients evaluates the clinical and radiographic results of tension band wiring techniques for patella fractures, comparing proximally bent only and proximally and distally bent K-wires. The authors noted three failures due to the migration of the K-wires, all of which occurred in the proximally bent only group. No migrations occurred in the proximal and distal bend group. The authors recommend proximally and distally bending K-wires to prevent migration. Level of evidence: III.

16. Levack B, Flannagan JP, Hobbs S: Results of surgical treatment of patellar fractures. *J Bone Joint Surg Br* 1985;67(3):416-419.

17. Wu CC, Tai CL, Chen WJ: Patellar tension band wiring: A revised technique. *Arch Orthop Trauma Surg* 2001;121(1-2):12-16.

18. Smith ST, Cramer KE, Karges DE, Watson JT, Moed BR: Early complications in the operative treatment of patella fractures. *J Orthop Trauma* 1997;11(3):183-187.

19. Hoshino CM, Tran W, Tiberi JV, et al: Complications following tension-band fixation of patellar fractures with cannulated screws compared with Kirschner wires. *J Bone Joint Surg Am* 2013;95(7):653-659.

This retrospective study of 448 patella fractures treated with a tension band construct compared the incidence of complications observed in techniques using K-wires with complications in those using cannulated screws. The authors noted no difference in fixation failure or infection rates. Patients treated with K-wires were twice as likely to undergo implant removal compared with those treated with screws. Level of evidence: III.

20. Lefaivre KA, O'Brien PJ, Broekhuyse HM, Guy P, Blachut PA: Modified tension band technique for patella fractures. *Orthop Traumatol Surg Res* 2010;96(5):579-582.

    In this case series, the authors describe their modification to the tension band technique for the surgical treatment of patella fractures. The technique of using four individual K-wires, which allows each wire to be bent and impacted into the patella, was an effective alternative to the traditional tension band wire technique. In their experience, hardware removal is required less frequently with this technique. Level of evidence: IV.

21. Carpenter JE, Kasman RA, Patel N, Lee ML, Goldstein SA: Biomechanical evaluation of current patella fracture fixation techniques. *J Orthop Trauma* 1997;11(5):351-356.

22. Berg EE: Open reduction internal fixation of displaced transverse patella fractures with figure-eight wiring through parallel cannulated compression screws. *J Orthop Trauma* 1997;11(8):573-576.

23. Miller MA, Liu W, Zurakowski D, Smith RM, Harris MB, Vrahas MS: Factors predicting failure of patella fixation. *J Trauma Acute Care Surg* 2012;72(4):1051-1055.

    This retrospective study of 109 surgically treated patella fractures compares fixation techniques and evaluates the etiology of fixation failure. Failure was defined as hardware breakage, loss of reduction resulting in nonunion, or displacement from the initial reduction on immediate postoperative radiographs. Twelve factors were examined independently for their predictive value using univariate and multivariate analysis; 12% (13 fractures) were found to have failed. Increasing patient age and using K-wires with or without tension band wires were important predictors of failure. A longer follow-up period was the only noteworthy predictor of reoperation and hardware removal. Level of evidence: III.

24. Hughes SC, Stott PM, Hearnden AJ, Ripley LG: A new and effective tension-band braided polyester suture technique for transverse patellar fracture fixation. *Injury* 2007;38(2):212-222.

25. Wright PB, Kosmopoulos V, Coté RE, Tayag TJ, Nana AD: FiberWire is superior in strength to stainless steel wire for tension band fixation of transverse patellar fractures. *Injury* 2009;40(11):1200-1203.

26. Chen CH, Huang HY, Wu T, Lin J: Transosseous suturing of patellar fractures with braided polyester — a prospective cohort with a matched historical control study. *Injury* 2013;44(10):1309-1313.

    In this study, the authors describe their technique of transosseous suture fixation. They identified 25 patients treated with this technique and prospectively followed them for an average of 11 months. This cohort was compared with a matched historical cohort that had undergone fixation with a traditional AO-modified tension band wiring technique. Union time and surgical time did not differ between the two groups. The mean hospitalization days, number of procedures, and frequency of complications were substantially lower in the transosseous suture group, however. Level of evidence: III.

27. Fortis AP, Milis Z, Kostopoulos V, et al: Experimental investigation of the tension band in fractures of the patella. *Injury* 2002;33(6):489-493.

28. Thelen S, Schneppendahl J, Jopen E, et al: Biomechanical cadaver testing of a fixed-angle plate in comparison to tension wiring and screw fixation in transverse patella fractures. *Injury* 2012;43(8):1290-1295.

    In a cadaver test, the authors divided patients into three groups to compare using a 2.7-mm fixed-angle plate designed for the treatment of patella fractures against modified anterior tension wiring or cannulated lag screws with anterior tension wiring. In their model of 100 cycles of nondestructive loads simulating knee motion, both tension band constructs showed considerable fracture displacement. In contrast, the patellae stabilized with fixed-angle plates showed no fracture displacement, and the authors noted this finding to be statistically significant. Level of evidence: V.

29. Taylor BC, Mehta S, Castaneda J, French BG, Blanchard C: Plating of patella fractures: Techniques and outcomes. *J Orthop Trauma* 2014;28(9):e231-e235.

    In this case series, the authors describe their technique of plating displaced patella fractures and patella nonunions and provide early clinical and radiographic results. They assert that their technique can be used in simple transverse fractures as well as comminuted fractures. In this series of 8 patients, all went on to successful union at a mean of 3.2 months. At a mean follow-up of 13.6 months, no implant prominence requiring removal was seen. The authors note that their technique is an off-label use of these devices. Level of evidence: IV.

30. Marder RA, Swanson TV, Sharkey NA, Duwelius PJ: Effects of partial patellectomy and reattachment of the patellar tendon on patellofemoral contact areas and pressures. *J Bone Joint Surg Am* 1993;75(1):35-45.

31. Saltzman CL, Goulet JA, McClellan RT, Schneider LA, Matthews LS: Results of treatment of displaced patellar fractures by partial patellectomy. *J Bone Joint Surg Am* 1990;72(9):1279-1285.

32. Kastelec M, Veselko M: Inferior patellar pole avulsion fractures: Osteosynthesis compared with pole resection. *J Bone Joint Surg Am* 2004;86-A(4):696-701.

33. Matejčić A, Puljiz Z, Elabjer E, Bekavac-Beslin M, Ledinsky M: Multifragment fracture of the patellar apex: Basket plate osteosynthesis compared with partial patellectomy. *Arch Orthop Trauma Surg* 2008;128(4):403-408.

34. Lennox IA, Cobb AG, Knowles J, Bentley G: Knee function after patellectomy. A 12- to 48-year follow-up. *J Bone Joint Surg Br* 1994;76(3):485-487.

35. Dy CJ, Little MT, Berkes MB, et al: Meta-analysis of re-operation, nonunion, and infection after open reduction and internal fixation of patella fractures. *J Trauma Acute Care Surg* 2012;73(4):928-932.

    The rates of reoperation, nonunion, and infection after open reduction and internal fixation of the patella were studied to pinpoint the factors that contribute to these events. The authors identified 24 studies with a total of 737 patella fractures; 20 contained Level IV evidence. The reoperation rate was 33.6% in 24 studies; the infection rate was 3.2% in 18 studies, and the frequency of nonunion was 1.3% among 15 studies. The authors found no significant predictors for reoperation, nonunion, or infection in any regression analyses. Level of evidence: III.

36. LeBrun CT, Langford JR, Sagi HC: Functional outcomes after operatively treated patella fractures. *J Orthop Trauma* 2012;26(7):422-426.

    In their study of isolated, unilateral, surgically treated patella fractures, the authors enrolled 40 patients with a minimum of 1-year follow-up. The patients were evaluated with the Short Form-36 Health Survey Questionnaire, the Knee Injury and Osteoarthritis Outcome Score, an injury-specific questionnaire, and asked to self-report symptomatic hardware. Patients also underwent physical examinations and quadriceps strength testing. The patients' validated outcomes measures were significantly different from reference population norms. It was concluded that, at a mean of 6.5 years, many symptoms and functional deficits persist.

37. Lazaro LE, Wellman DS, Sauro G, et al: Outcomes after operative fixation of complete articular patellar fractures: Assessment of functional impairment. *J Bone Joint Surg Am* 2013;95(14):e96, 1-8.

    In this study, outcomes data on 30 patients with an isolated unilateral patellar fracture were obtained prospectively. Of the 30 patients, 37%, or 11 patients, underwent removal of symptomatic implants. Patella baja was seen in more than one-half of the patients. Functional impairment of the injured extensor mechanism persisted at 12 months, measured in terms of strength, power, and endurance when compared with the uninjured side. The authors conclude that patients should be counseled regarding potential outcomes, specifically ongoing patellofemoral symptoms. Level of evidence: IV.

38. Bonnaig NS, Casstevens C, Archdeacon MT, et al: Fix it or discard it? A retrospective analysis of functional outcomes after surgically treated patella fractures comparing ORIF with partial patellectomy. *J Orthop Trauma* 2015;29(2):80-84.

    In this study, outcomes data were prospectively obtained on 52 patients with isolated displaced patella fractures treated surgically with a minimum of 1-year follow-up. Patients were evaluated with outcomes questionnaires and physical examinations. A group of 26 patients who underwent PP was compared with another group of 26 who underwent open reduction and internal fixation. No significant differences were seen in any of the outcomes scores between the two groups, but the scores of both were lower than normal population values. The authors conclude that functional impairment persists after the surgical treatment of patella fractures and that, in spite of its purported benefits, open reduction and internal fixation does not result in superior outcomes compared with PP. Level of evidence: III.

39. Clayton RA, Court-Brown CM: The epidemiology of musculoskeletal tendinous and ligamentous injuries. *Injury* 2008;39(12):1338-1344.

40. White DW, Wenke JC, Mosely DS, Mountcastle SB, Basamania CJ: Incidence of major tendon ruptures and anterior cruciate ligament tears in US Army soldiers. *Am J Sports Med* 2007;35(8):1308-1314.

41. Boudissa M, Roudet A, Rubens-Duval B, Chaussard C, Saragaglia D: Acute quadriceps tendon ruptures: A series of 50 knees with an average follow-up of more than 6 years. *Orthop Traumatol Surg Res* 2014;100(2):217-220.

    The long-term results of quadriceps tendon repair in a series of 50 knees are presented. Most patients were male, and the mean age was 55 years. Most cases (75%; 38 knees) were repaired with the suture-and-drill tunnel technique, although suture anchors were added in 8 knees. All repairs occurred acutely. The results included a low complication rate of 4% (2 of 50 knees), excellent mean flexion of 125°, and high reported patient satisfaction. Level of evidence: IV.

42. Roudet A, Boudissa M, Chaussard C, Rubens-Duval B, Saragaglia D: Acute traumatic patellar tendon rupture: Early and late results of surgical treatment of 38 cases. *Orthop Traumatol Surg Res* 2015;101(3):307-311.

    In this retrospective study of acute patellar tendon rupture in 38 knees, 34 knees were of male patients. Augmentation of the repair was used in 95% of cases (36 knees). Short-term 7-month and long-term 9-year results are presented. Overall, patients were satisfied or very satisfied in 96% of cases, or 35 of 37 patients. All patients returned to previous employment, and most returned to some form of sports activity. Level of evidence: IV.

43. Kannus P, Józsa L: Histopathological changes preceding spontaneous rupture of a tendon. A controlled study of 891 patients. *J Bone Joint Surg Am* 1991;73(10):1507-1525.

44. Siwek CW, Rao JP: Ruptures of the extensor mechanism of the knee joint. *J Bone Joint Surg Am* 1981;63(6):932-937.

45. Loehr J, Welsh RP: Spontaneous rupture of the quadriceps tendon and patellar ligament during treatment for chronic renal failure. *Can Med Assoc J* 1983;129(3):254-256.

46. Lombardi LJ, Cleri DJ, Epstein E: Bilateral spontaneous quadriceps tendon rupture in a patient with renal failure. *Orthopedics* 1995;18(2):187-191.

47. Stinner DJ, Orr JD, Hsu JR: Fluoroquinolone-associated bilateral patellar tendon rupture: A case report and review of the literature. *Mil Med* 2010;175(6):457-459.

This case report links knee extensor mechanism rupture occurring as a result of minimal trauma with some form of systemic predisposing factor, in this case, precedent fluoroquinolone use.

48. Evans EJ, Benjamin M, Pemberton DJ: Variations in the amount of calcified tissue at the attachments of the quadriceps tendon and patellar ligament in man. *J Anat* 1991;174:145-151.

49. Rauh M, Parker R: Patellar and quadriceps tendinopathies and ruptures, in DeLee JC, ed: *DeLee and Drez's Orthopaedic Sports Medicine* .Philadelphia, PA, Saunders, 2009, pp 1513-1577.

50. Phillips K, Costantino TG: Diagnosis of patellar tendon rupture by emergency ultrasound. *J Emerg Med* 2014;47(2):204-206.

This case report describes the successful use of ultrasonography in the emergency department for the diagnostic confirmation of patellar tendon rupture. It specifically cites the advantages of dynamic ultrasonography and recommends it as a diagnostic aid in the hands of experienced users while the patient is in the emergency department. Using ultrasonography also avoids the higher cost of MRI.

51. Swamy GN, Nanjayan SK, Yallappa S, Bishnoi A, Pickering SA: Is ultrasound diagnosis reliable in acute extensor tendon injuries of the knee? *Acta Orthop Belg* 2012;78(6):764-770.

This retrospective review describes 51 consecutive patients who underwent surgery for patellar rupture or quadriceps tendon rupture. Diagnosis was reached by clinical examination and plain radiographs alone in 13 patients. Ultrasonography was added in 24 patients, and MRI was added in 14 patients. False-positive results based on intraoperative findings were reported in 33% (8 patients) of the ultrasonography group, whereas MRI was 100% accurate. Level of evidence: III.

52. Perfitt JS, Petrie MJ, Blundell CM, Davies MB: Acute quadriceps tendon rupture: A pragmatic approach to diagnostic imaging. *Eur J Orthop Surg Traumatol* 2014;24(7):1237-1241.

In this study assessing the diagnostic accuracy of ultrasonography versus MRI, patients initially were evaluated with ultrasonography, resulting in a 9% rate of inaccurate diagnoses. In the second group of patients MRI was used much more frequently (42% versus 4%), and the misdiagnosis rate dropped to 5%. The authors recommend more aggressive use of MRI versus ultrasonography. Level of evidence: III.

53. McKinney B, Cherney S, Penna J: Intra-articular knee injuries in patients with knee extensor mechanism ruptures. *Knee Surg Sports Traumatol Arthrosc* 2008;16(7):633-638.

54. Ciriello V, Gudipati S, Tosounidis T, Soucacos PN, Giannoudis PV: Clinical outcomes after repair of quadriceps tendon rupture: A systematic review. *Injury* 2012;43(11):1931-1938.

This article reports on the published literature on quadriceps tendon rupture repair over a 25-year period. Of the 474 studies initially identified, only 12 (319 patients) met the methodological requirements for inclusion. The mean age was 57 years, and the most common site of the tear was 1 to 2 cm from the superior pole of the patella. The patellar drill hole technique was used most commonly. The type of repair did not appear to influence the clinical results, and the overall rerupture rate was only 2%. Level of evidence: III.

55. Pocock CA, Trikha SP, Bell JS: Delayed reconstruction of a quadriceps tendon. *Clin Orthop Relat Res* 2008;466(1):221-224.

56. Petri M, Dratzidis A, Brand S, et al: Suture anchor repair yields better biomechanical properties than transosseous sutures in ruptured quadriceps tendons. *Knee Surg Sports Traumatol Arthrosc* 2015;23(4):1039-1045.

This cadaver biomechanical study compares quadriceps tendon repair performed with transosseous sutures and repair with suture anchors. The suture anchor technique demonstrated less gap formation during cyclic loading and higher ultimate failure loads. Further clinical study is recommended. Level of evidence: V.

57. Bushnell BD, Whitener GB, Rubright JH, Creighton RA, Logel KJ, Wood ML: The use of suture anchors to repair the ruptured quadriceps tendon. *J Orthop Trauma* 2007;21(6):407-413.

58. Gilmore JH, Clayton-Smith ZJ, Aguilar M, Pneumaticos SG, Giannoudis PV: Reconstruction techniques and clinical results of patellar tendon ruptures: Evidence today. *Knee* 2015;22(3):148-55.

In this detailed review of the literature published since 1947, 41 manuscripts representing 503 patients were evaluated. Of these 503 patients, 383 underwent primary repair. Augmentation of repair was used in 254 of 383 cases. Acute repair with augmentation produced the best outcome. Immediate postoperative mobilization is recommended. Level of evidence: III.

59. Ettinger M, Dratzidis A, Hurschler C, et al: Biomechanical properties of suture anchor repair compared with transosseous sutures in patellar tendon ruptures: A cadaveric study. *Am J Sports Med* 2013;41(11):2540-2544.

This cadaver biomechanical study compares patellar tendon repair using transpatellar suture tunnels with patellar tendon repair using suture anchor repair. The suture anchor technique resulted in less gap formation during cyclic loading and higher ultimate failure loads. Future clinical studies are needed to further verify the technique. Level of evidence: V.

60. Bushnell BD, Tennant JN, Rubright JH, Creighton RA: Repair of patellar tendon rupture using suture anchors. *J Knee Surg* 2008;21(2):122-129.

61. Marder RA, Timmerman LA: Primary repair of patellar tendon rupture without augmentation. *Am J Sports Med* 1999;27(3):304-307.

Chapter 42

Knee Dislocations

James P. Stannard, MD John D. Adams, MD

Abstract

The assumption that knee dislocations and multiligament knee injuries exist only in the realm of sports medicine is false. Although knee dislocations occasionally occur from low-energy mechanisms such as athletic injuries, most injuries occur as the result of a high-energy trauma such as a motor vehicle accident or fall. Orthopaedic trauma management of knee dislocations is a complex, multifactorial treatment dilemma for surgeons. Although a high risk of complications is associated with these injuries, surgeons are improving outcomes through earlier recognition and treatment, especially surgical treatment within 4 weeks after injury.

Keywords: knee dislocations; anterior cruciate ligament; posterior cruciate ligament; posteromedial corner; posterolateral corner

Introduction

Knee dislocations or multiligament knee injuries are commonly thought of as sports medicine injuries, but they rarely occur as a result of an athletic injury. Commonly, the mechanism of injury is high energy and motor vehicle related. Knee dislocations are being recognized more frequently, most likely because of an increase in survival following motor vehicle trauma as a result of airbags and safety devices, combined with better recognition that many dislocations present after spontaneous reduction. These injuries can result in knee stiffness, chronic instability, arthritis, and poor functional outcomes. Therefore, orthopaedic management of knee dislocations represents a multifactorial treatment challenge.

Anatomy

The anterior cruciate ligament (ACL) is composed of the anteromedial and posterolateral bundles, which run from the posterior aspect of the lateral part of the femoral notch and attach to the anterior aspect of the tibia. The posterior cruciate ligament (PCL) also is composed of two bundles, anterolateral and posteromedial, which run from the anterior aspect of the medial part of the femoral notch to the posterior aspect of the tibia. The anterolateral bundle of the PCL and the anteromedial bundle of the ACL are both the larger bundles. The posterolateral corner (PLC) is composed of dynamic and static stabilizers. PLC reconstruction re-creates the fibular collateral ligament (FCL) (or lateral collateral ligament), the popliteofibular ligament, and the popliteus. The anatomy and details of the posteromedial corner (PMC) have been the subject of increased recent research. The PMC is composed of the superficial and deep medial collateral ligament (MCL) and the posterior oblique ligament, all of which are re-created in PMC reconstruction.[1]

The other important anatomic structures involved in knee dislocations are neurovascular structures. Because of its proximity to the posterior aspect of the tibia, the popliteal artery is at high risk for damage at the time of the injury. Both the tibial and peroneal divisions of the sciatic nerve can be injured in a knee dislocation, with the common peroneal nerve having the highest risk for palsy. The identification, location, and protection of the peroneal nerve are also important in the approach for PLC reconstruction. This nerve emerges from the posterior aspect of the thigh as it runs beneath the biceps tendon and becomes more superficial as it wraps around the neck of the fibula.

Dr. Stannard or an immediate family member serves as a paid consultant to DePuy, Ellipse Technologies, Regeneration Technologies, and Smith & Nephew, has received research or institutional support from Arthrex, DePuy, and Synthes, and serves as a board member, owner, officer, or committee member of the AO Board of Trustees, the AO Research Review Commission, and the Orthopaedic Trauma Association. Neither Dr. Adams nor any immediate family member has received anything of value from or has stock or stock options held in a commercial company or institution related directly or indirectly to the subject of this chapter.

Initial Evaluation

Because of the high-energy mechanisms associated with knee dislocations, every patient should be evaluated as a trauma patient. Therefore, the Advanced Trauma Life Support protocols developed by the American College of Surgeons should be instituted. After life-threatening injuries have been treated and the patient has been stabilized, a secondary survey is completed. Beginning with inspection, the soft-tissue envelope around the knee should be evaluated. If knee dislocation is diagnosed, closed reduction should be attempted as soon as possible. If closed reduction is unsuccessful, open reduction should be performed. After the knee is reduced clinically, a postreduction radiograph should be obtained to ensure knee joint congruency. If congruency can be maintained in an external brace (knee immobilizer or hinged knee brace), external fixation is not needed, but if the knee remains subluxated, a spanning external fixator is warranted. As with open fractures, dislocations that are open injuries should be treated with antibiotics, tetanus prophylaxis, and surgical débridement with irrigation. In most cases of open dislocation, spanning external fixators are used because of severe knee instability and to help with soft-tissue management after reduction. At least two-thirds of all knee dislocations present after spontaneous reduction before evaluation. A high percentage of patients present with the knee spontaneously reduced.[2]

The popliteal artery is intimate to the posterior aspect of the tibia and is at risk during a dislocation event. The incidence of vascular injury as a result of dislocation has been reported to range from 1.6% to 18.0%.[3-6] Therefore, these limb-threatening injuries need to be diagnosed and treated expeditiously.

Controversy exists regarding the best method to evaluate the popliteal artery for injury. Options for evaluation include physical examination, ankle-brachial index (ABI), or routine imaging modalities. Recently, it has been shown that clinical examination alone is adequate to detect substantial vascular injuries.[7] A thorough vascular examination should be conducted both before and after reduction. If bilateral lower extremities have symmetric blood flow, the patient can be followed with serial examinations during the first 48 hours. If any uncertainty exists regarding clinical examination results, the ABI should be obtained. The ABI is calculated by the ratio of the systolic blood pressure obtained from just superior to the ankle to the systolic blood pressure of the upper arm. A 100% sensitivity and specificity for substantial vascular injury with ABI values less than 0.9 has been reported.[8] When ABI is less than 0.9, additional diagnostic studies are warranted. Although ultrasonography has high sensitivity and specificity, it is technician dependent. Conventional angiography has been the gold standard for years, but has a false-positive rate of approximately 5%.[7] CT angiography has been shown to have high specificity and sensitivity for arterial injuries, and only exposes the patient to 25% of the radiation dose from conventional angiography.[9] Although magnetic resonance angiography is a good option to detect arterial injury, its role in traumatic knee dislocation with vascular compromise is not yet determined.

Nerve injury following knee dislocation occurs frequently, with an overall rate of 25%.[5] The most common nerve-sustaining injury is the peroneal nerve. A tibial nerve injury is seen less frequently than peroneal nerve injury. The incidence of tibial nerve injury is approximately 7% to 10%,[10,11] and can present as a complete or partial palsy. Of patients with palsy of the peroneal nerve, 83% with partial palsies regained active ankle dorsiflexion; 38% of those with complete palsies saw the same improvement.[12]

Because knee dislocations are almost completely a ligamentous injury, they are associated with substantial skin and other soft-tissue injuries. Prior to any intervention, a thorough examination of the soft tissues should be undertaken in addition to a ligamentous examination. It is not uncommon for patients to have substantial edema, fracture blisters, and even Morel-Lavallée lesions after knee dislocation.

Following the neurovascular examination, a detailed ligamentous knee examination is performed. When available, it always helps to compare the injured extremity with the contralateral healthy knee. The ACL is usually tested using the Lachman test at 30° of knee flexion and the pivot shift test. The PCL is tested using the posterior drawer test. In these multiligament injuries, it is important to remember that the knee may not be in its normal "station," so what may seem to be substantial anterior translation on the Lachman test can in fact be because the PCL is injured and the tibia is resting more posteriorly than normal. The PLC is tested using a combination of the varus stress test and the dial test. The physical examination helps delineate an isolated MCL injury from an injury involving the entire PMC. Laxity at 30° of flexion with valgus stress is indicative of an MCL injury but does not differentiate between MCL and PMC injuries. Patients with a PMC injury will demonstrate anteromedial rotatory instability, which can be diagnosed using the anterior drawer test with the foot in external rotation. Patients with anteromedial rotatory instability will show an increased amount of anterior translation on the anterior drawer test when the tibia is placed in 10° to 15° of external rotation compared with neutral rotation.[2]

Diagnostic imaging usually includes a combination of radiographs, stress radiographs, and MRIs for further delineation of the injury. Fluoroscopic views obtained under anesthesia can also be helpful. Stress radiographs were examined to help diagnose PLC injuries.[13] In patients with isolated FCL injuries, a 2.7-mm side-to-side difference could be shown on varus stress radiographs; patients with complete PLC injuries showed at least a 4.0-mm difference. After radiography, MRI is the preferred modality. MRI shows the extent of the injury and helps with preoperative planning. Many knee dislocations are associated with tibial plateau fractures. In these cases, MRI should be obtained before definitive fixation of the plateau fracture because metal artifact compromises MRI sensitivity. For complex tibial plateau fractures, CT and MRI may be warranted for bony and soft-tissue detail, respectively. In most cases, MRI can provide enough bony detail to preoperatively plan for surgical fixation of the tibial plateau. A combined CT scan and MRI is a good strategy for a complex articular injury.

Treatment

Surgical Versus Nonsurgical Treatment

A systematic review in 2009 identified four articles that addressed surgical versus nonsurgical treatment:[14] In total, 227 surgically treated patients were compared with 107 nonsurgically treated patients. Patients in the surgical group consistently showed higher outcome scores: three studies showed a higher percentage of excellent/good International Knee Documentation Committee (IKDC) scores for patients in the surgical group compared with patients in the nonsurgical group. Patients who were treated surgically also demonstrated an earlier return to work and athletic activities.[14,15] Most experts in the field of multiligament knee injuries agree that surgery is the treatment of choice; however, indications for nonsurgical management persist. Patients with severe polytrauma, head injury, substantial comorbidities, soft-tissue compromise, and those who are elderly can all be considered for nonsurgical management.[16] Patients who are morbidly obese can be challenging to treat. Even minor traumas such as falls from standing height can result in knee dislocation. These patients should not be ignored; many could benefit from surgery, but the complication rate has been shown to increase by 9.2% for every increase in body mass index of 1 kg/m^2.[17] Coordinated care is extremely important in these patients.

Surgical Strategy

The goal of surgery for knee dislocation is to provide the patient a stable, functional knee. The decision to reconstruct certain ligaments is based on the physical examination findings of the individual ligaments. Typically, if the only ligaments involved are the ACL and MCL, and there is no history of dislocation, the MCL is treated nonsurgically. However, given that dislocations are normally associated with a more complex ligamentous injury compared with those associated with athletic activities, a low threshold exists to reconstruct everything that has positive physical examination findings that correlate with MRI findings.

External Fixation

One of the earliest treatment decisions to make is whether the patient would benefit from external fixation. In patients who present with a dislocated knee, emergency reduction is necessary. If postreduction radiographs demonstrate concentric reduction, external fixation is not needed. In these cases, an external brace in the form of a knee immobilizer, posterior splint, or hinged knee brace can be applied. Repeat radiographs should be obtained in a few days to confirm that reduction has been maintained, because patients with knees that were concentrically reduced in the emergency department sometimes present to the clinic days or weeks later with the knee dislocated. If subluxation is seen on postreduction radiographs, external fixation is indicated. The other indications are open dislocation and vascular injury. Usually, only a simple uniplanar spanning external fixator is warranted until definitive reconstruction.

Early Versus Late Reconstruction

The timing of reconstruction is debatable: most studies that examined early versus late reconstruction were retrospective and had inherent selection biases that added controversy. In most circumstances, early reconstruction was defined as within 3 to 4 weeks of injury. Although somewhat arbitrary, 4 weeks is usually considered the maximum amount of time in which the tissue planes are still identifiable and the tissue integrity facilitates repair with suture placement. In general, early surgical treatment has been shown to result in higher Lysholm scores and a higher percentage of excellent/good IKDC scores. Higher sports activity scores are also associated with early surgery.[14] Although most studies favor early surgery, other studies have not demonstrated a difference in functional outcomes or range of motion. Further prospective randomized studies are needed to truly address the issue of timing.

Repair Versus Reconstruction

One study compared three different treatment options for ACL/PCL injuries[18]: ACL reconstruction with PCL repair, ACL/PCL repair, and ACL/PCL reconstruction. The groups had similar final Lysholm scores and percentages of good/excellent IKDC scores, but the groups that underwent repair reported lower rates of return to preinjury level and a higher incidence of PCL instability. The data on isolated ACL reconstruction also seem to support reconstruction instead of repair of both cruciate ligaments.

Historically, regarding the PLC, it was generally thought that repair alone yielded good results. A 2005 prospective study of 57 patients directly compared repair with reconstruction.[19] Although a functional difference was not demonstrated between groups, the difference in failure rate was significant: The rate of repair was 37% for failure and 9% for reconstruction. This resulted in the preference of PLC reconstruction over repair. A similar study in 2010 reported on 18 PLC reconstructions compared with 10 PLC repairs: 40% of repairs failed, but only 6% of reconstructions failed.[20] The study results favored PLC reconstruction over repair in the setting of multiligament knee injuries.[20]

A 2012 study reported on reconstruction versus repair for 73 PMC tears: 25 patients underwent repair, and 48 underwent reconstruction.[21] Reconstruction had better results; the failure rate for reconstruction was 4% compared with 20% in the repair group.

Fracture-Dislocations

Ligament injuries with concomitant tibial plateau fractures are common, with an incidence up to approximately 75%.[22,23] The precise management of these injuries and their effect on outcomes has not been determined. One protocol for fracture-dislocations is that the fracture is usually treated first using open reduction and internal fixation. If severe coronal plane instability exists after internal fixation, acute reconstruction of the medial or lateral ligaments may be warranted. Because of the techniques involved in ACL and PCL reconstructions, some of the tibial plateau implants may need to be removed. Therefore, ACL and PCL reconstructions are usually performed in a staged fashion after adequate bony healing has occurred and signs or symptoms of instability have persisted.

Surgical Reconstructions

Grafts

As with any ligamentous reconstruction, autograft or allograft can be used. In the patient with multiligament knee injury, allograft can be used. Because of the sheer number of tendons needed for these reconstructions, autograft could potentially be associated with significant morbidity. Also, harvesting autograft would add more time to an already lengthy surgical case. Regarding allograft, tremendous variety exists in allograft use based on the techniques for certain reconstructions.[1,2,9,19,20] Achilles tendon allograft can be used for the PCL, and either semitendinosus or tibialis anterior allograft for the other reconstructions.

Anterior Cruciate Ligament

Patients with ACL tears with concomitant PCL and corner injuries can undergo staged reconstruction. The initial reconstruction of the PCL and the injured corner(s) is performed around 4 weeks postinjury. If the ACL also requires reconstruction, it is performed 6 weeks after the initial reconstruction.

Waiting 6 weeks to perform the ACL reconstruction can have several benefits. First, many patients are stiff at 6 weeks following reconstruction of the other ligaments and benefit from manipulation under anesthesia that can be performed in conjunction with the ACL reconstruction. Also, delaying the ACL reconstruction shortens the first surgical stage a little bit, which likely benefits both the patient and the surgeon. Finally, rehabilitation of the ACL and PCL are slightly different. Separating them allows the therapist to concentrate on the PCL during the initial phase of rehabilitation.

Several ACL reconstruction options exist, and the debate concerning the best technique remains controversial. One method is to use a FlipCutter (Arthrex) to produce an independent femoral socket using an outside-in method and a tibial socket at the anatomic footprint of the ACL. Suspensory fixation of the allograft or autograft has the added benefit of removing bone quality as a potential concern and is currently our preferred method.

Posterior Cruciate Ligament

PCL reconstruction techniques are continually evolving; currently, three distinct approaches are used. The transtibial reconstruction fixes the PCL graft proximally in a femoral tunnel and distally in the proximal tibia. Transtibial reconstructions have typically been associated with residual laxity. This is thought to be a result of "the killer turn" created by the acute angle that the graft must take around the posterior lip of the tibia. This turn is thought to gradually abrade the graft, resulting in laxity. Another reconstruction option to prevent "the killer turn" is the tibial inlay approach, which secures the distal tibial fixation by placing a bone plug into a trough positioned at the anatomic footprint of the PCL. Both of the techniques described produce a single-bundle reconstruction of the PCL. The third option is a two-tailed femoral technique

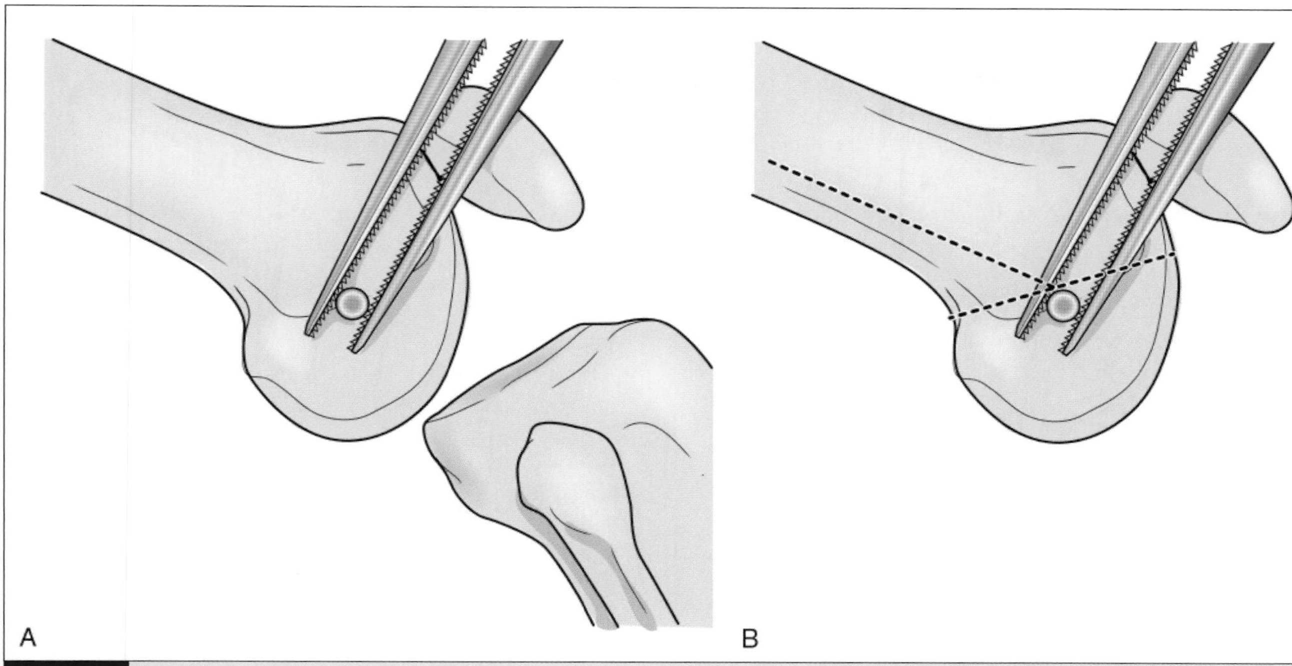

Figure 1 **A** and **B**, illustrations demonstrate the isometric point of the knee, determined by the intersection of a line drawn from the anterior aspect of the posterior femoral cortex and the Blumensaat line.

combined with the tibial inlay to produce an anatomic double-bundle PCL reconstruction.

An open approach to the posterior tibia to produce a double-bundle PCL via the tibia inlay technique has been used; a double-bundle PCL reconstruction has also been performed. A FlipCutter is used for both femoral sockets and the tibial socket. With an arthroscope placed in the posteromedial portal, the tibial socket is intentionally drilled at the distal aspect of the PCL insertion. Placing the tunnel more distally helps prevent "the killer turn." The anterolateral bundle is tensioned at approximately 80° of flexion; the posteromedial bundle is tensioned at 10° of flexion. In most cases, allograft is used.[2]

Posterolateral Corner

The goal of any PLC reconstruction is to reproduce the FCL, the popliteus, and the popliteofibular ligament. A detailed understanding of the anatomy is needed. The popliteus originates along the posteromedial tibia and inserts on the lateral distal femur just anterior and distal to the FCL. The FCL originates off the isometric point of the femur and inserts on the anterolateral aspect of the fibular head. The popliteofibular ligament extends from the popliteus to the posteromedial aspect of the fibula.

Determining the isometric point is paramount to the success of this type of reconstruction. Two techniques are used to determine the isometric point: an anatomic and a radiographic technique. The anatomic technique uses the patient's anatomy to determine the exact origin of the FCL on the femur. One disadvantage of this technique is that in most cases, the soft tissues have been injured and the exact origin may not be recognizable. The radiographic method uses a perfect lateral radiograph of the distal femur. The isometric point is located at the intersection of a line drawn down the anterior aspect of the posterior femoral cortex to the Blumensaat line (**Figure 1**). Recent studies have compared the radiographic method with the anatomic method at identification of the isometric point.[24,25] The radiographic method produced more reliable placement at the true isometric point.[24,25] Reproducing the isometric point is thought to result in less stretching of the grafts and ultimately a lower incidence of failure.

Two separate grafts for anatomic PLC reconstruction can be used. In almost all cases, allograft is used. The popliteus is reconstructed using an anterior-to-posterior tibial tunnel and a femoral tunnel placed slightly distal and anterior to the isometric point. The graft is passed under the FCL when secured to the femur. The FCL and the popliteofibular ligament are reconstructed using another graft. The FCL is secured to the femur at the isometric point and passed through a fibular tunnel from anterolateral to posteromedial. The popliteofibular ligament is passed from the posteromedial aspect of the fibula under the FCL and secured with the popliteus to the femur (**Figure 2**). Graft tensioning is performed with

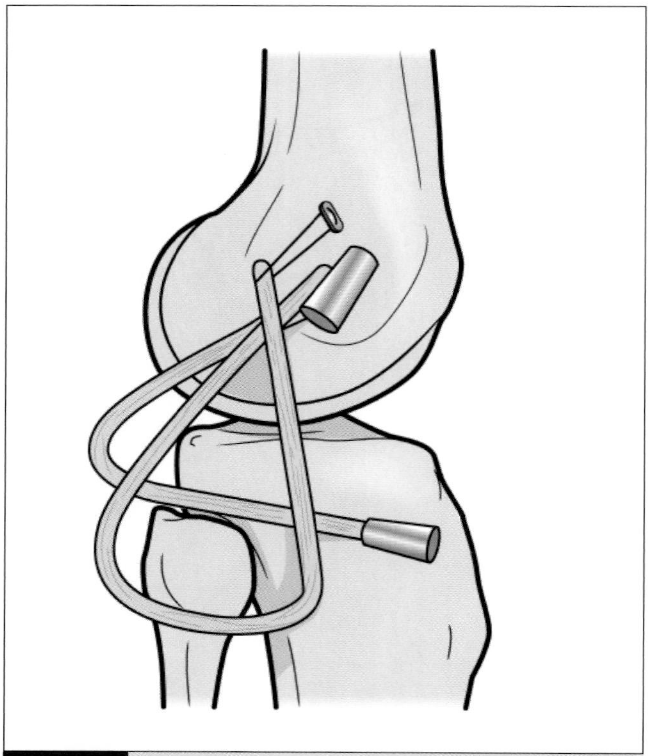

Figure 2 Illustration demonstrates anatomic posterolateral corner reconstruction with suspensory fixation for the popliteus, popliteofibular ligament, and fibular collateral ligament.

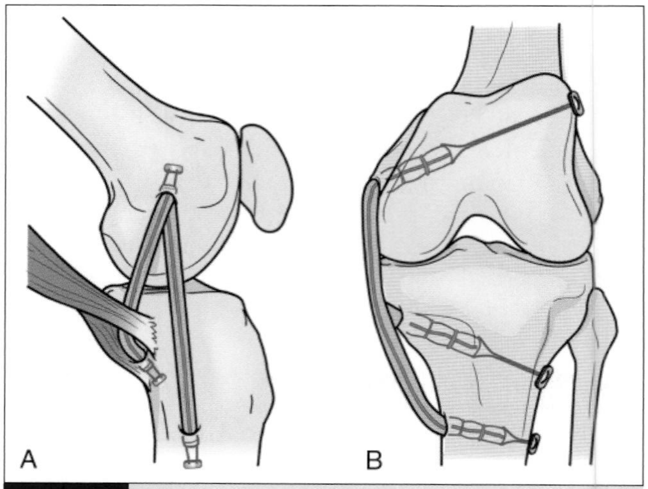

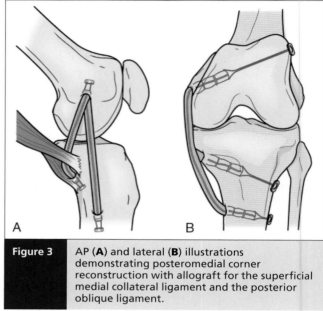

Figure 3 AP (**A**) and lateral (**B**) illustrations demonstrating posteromedial corner reconstruction with allograft for the superficial medial collateral ligament and the posterior oblique ligament.

the knee in 20° to 30° of flexion, neutral rotation, and a valgus stress.[19]

Posteromedial Corner

The goal of PMC reconstruction is to prevent anteromedial rotatory instability as well as valgus stress instability, and is accomplished with reconstruction of the MCL and the posterior oblique ligament. A posteromedial approach to the proximal tibia and distal femur is used for exposure. The exposure should provide access to the medial femoral condyle down to the pes anserinus tendons.[26] As with the PLC, the isometric point of the femur is identified using fluoroscopic imaging. To reconstruct the posterior oblique ligament, the direct head of the semimembranosus muscle is identified. Allograft is routinely used with a two-tailed configuration and secured to the femur at the isometric point. The posterior oblique ligament portion of graft is routed under the semimembranosus and rejoins the MCL graft at the insertion point on the tibia (**Figure 3**). The graft can either be sutured to the semitendinosus with a strong nonabsorbable suture or secured in a tunnel with an interference screw in the tibia. The graft is tensioned in 30° of flexion with slight varus stress.[2,21,27,28]

Hinged External Fixation

In the setting of a four-ligament reconstruction or a remarkably unstable three-ligament reconstruction, a hinged external fixator can be used to protect the reconstruction for 6 weeks. A prospective, randomized study published in 2014 reported that a hinged external fixator protected the reconstructions more efficiently than a hinged knee brace: 21% of reconstructed grafts failed in the brace group and only 7% failed in the external fixator group, a substantial difference.[29] This resulted in the recommendation to use hinged external fixation in patients with highly unstable knee dislocation after reconstruction of three or more ligaments. Another indication for the use of a hinged external fixator is the patient with polytrauma and concomitant extremity injuries. Although anecdotal, the external fixator can help the patient ambulate while protecting the reconstruction.

Rehabilitation

Stiffness and contractures are relatively common after a multiligament knee injury. The treatment of these injuries does not stop after surgical reconstruction; rehabilitation is an important part of treatment. The surgeon should be comfortable with the rehabilitation techniques that will help reproduce functional range of motion. A systematic review in 2009 reported that immobilization after reconstruction resulted in increased laxity posteriorly and that early mobilization is warranted.[30] Immobilization resulted in an increased incidence of flexion and extension loss. Functional rehabilitation (flexion allowed at least to 60° postoperatively) has also been shown to improve outcome scores.[31] A detailed description of the rehabilitation protocol is outside the scope of this chapter because the protocols are determined by which ligaments are reconstructed. In general, the rehabilitation protocol used was first described in 2007; knee motion is begun immediately following surgery.[32]

Complications and Outcomes

Adverse outcomes and complications are common following knee dislocations. In addition to injuries that occur at the accident, pain, loss of motion, and recurrent instability occur frequently. Complications have two major categories: those related to the injury and those that are a result of the treatment. The most common complications related to the injury are neurovascular complications. A careful neurovascular examination is warranted on initial evaluation and a multidisciplinary approach is used in the setting of vascular compromise.

Infection, heterotopic ossification, posttraumatic osteoarthritis, and arthrofibrosis are common complications associated with the treatment of knee dislocation. Infections have a reported rate of 12.5% and can be problematic.[33] Infections can result in multiple débridements, and if fistulas form, soft-tissue flap coverage may be required. The reported incidence of heterotopic ossification is approximately 25% and is more frequently found medially and posteriorly.[34] PCL reconstruction is one independent risk factor for the development of heterotopic ossification.[35] In one retrospective long-term follow-up study of 44 multiligament reconstructions, the incidence of posttraumatic arthritis was 23%.[36] Although current surgical reconstructions and rehabilitation protocols have improved final knee range of motion, it has been shown that a mean of 38% of patients (range, 5% to 71%) require surgical treatment of arthrofibrosis.[37]

Because of anatomic distortion and substantial scarring after a knee dislocation, surgical dissection is challenging. Because of this, iatrogenic neurovascular injury is a concern. Although no specific publications address the incidence of iatrogenic injuries, the patient should be counseled on the risk of injury during surgery. Recurrent instability and pain after reconstruction is common. Several outcome studies have reported recurrent instability with a mean incidence of approximately 40%.[38-40] It is more common for patients to report anterior-posterior instability rather than medial-lateral instability. Pain after knee dislocation can be a result of various etiologies. Factors contributing to pain can include chronic instability, posttraumatic arthritis, and arthrofibrosis. The incidence of pain following these injuries has been reported from 25% to 68%.[37]

Although knee dislocation is associated with a relatively high rate of complications and adverse outcomes, patients can return to work and recreational activity. Nine outcome studies demonstrated that most patients can return to work (93%), but many return to light duty or a less demanding job (31%).[37] Patients who underwent surgical reconstruction after dislocation had a higher incidence of returning to athletic activity compared with nonsurgical treatment (56% versus 17%).[31]

Summary

Knee dislocation is commonly associated with high-energy trauma and represents a complex injury that requires a multidisciplinary approach. Optimal care results from a thorough initial evaluation, a detailed understanding of the anatomy, and diligent reconstruction of the injured ligamentous structures. Although nonsurgical management can be considered in certain high-risk patients, surgical reconstruction within the first 4 weeks produces better outcomes. In general, reconstruction is preferred over acute repair. Various techniques can be used for reconstruction, but generally, anatomic reconstruction is recommended. Although surgical intervention is associated with a high risk of complications and adverse outcomes, most patients can expect to return to work and many can return to athletic activities.

Key Study Points

- Outcomes are generally more favorable following surgical reconstruction than with nonsurgical treatment.
- Some data suggest that treatment within the acute period (the first 4 weeks) yields better results than treatment during the chronic period.
- More than one-fourth of patients require surgical intervention to improve range of motion following ligament reconstruction.
- Although knee dislocation is associated with a relatively high rate of complications and adverse outcomes, patients can expect to return to work and recreational activity.

Annotated References

1. Jacobson KE, Chi FS: Evaluation and treatment of medial collateral ligament and medial-sided injuries of the knee. *Sports Med Arthrosc* 2006;14(2):58-66.

2. Stannard JP, Bauer KL: Current concepts in knee dislocations: PCL, ACL, and medial sided injuries. *J Knee Surg* 2012;25(4):287-294.

   This article describes the senior author's preferred management of injuries involving the ACL, PCL, and PMC. Management strategies include surgical technique, timing for surgery, and rehabilitation.

3. Sillanpää PJ, Kannus P, Niemi ST, Rolf C, Felländer-Tsai L, Mattila VM: Incidence of knee dislocation and concomitant vascular injury requiring surgery: A nationwide study. *J Trauma Acute Care Surg* 2014;76(3):715-719.

   In this retrospective study from 1998 to 2011, patients with acute knee dislocations and concomitant vascular injuries underwent surgical treatment. Young men had the highest incidence, and the rate of popliteal injury requiring surgery was 1.6%. Level of evidence: I.

4. Laprade RF, Wijdicks CA: The management of injuries to the medial side of the knee. *J Orthop Sports Phys Ther* 2012;42(3):221-233.

   This review article describes the anatomy, physical examination, and treatment strategies regarding the management of injuries to the medial side of the knee.

5. Medina O, Arom GA, Yeranosian MG, Petrigliano FA, McAllister DR: Vascular and nerve injury after knee dislocation: A systematic review. *Clin Orthop Relat Res* 2014;472(9):2621-2629.

   In this retrospective review of 862 knee dislocations, 18% had vascular injury and 25% had associated nerve injury. Of the patients with vascular injury, 12% underwent amputation.

6. Natsuhara KM, Yeranosian MG, Cohen JR, Wang JC, McAllister DR, Petrigliano FA: What is the frequency of vascular injury after knee dislocation? *Clin Orthop Relat Res* 2014;472(9):2615-2620.

   This population-based study evaluated diagnostic codes of 11 million orthopaedic patients. The overall frequency of vascular injury was 3.3%; men age 20 to 39 years had the highest incidence; 13% of patients with vascular injury required surgical intervention. Level of evidence: IV.

7. Stannard JP, Sheils TM, Lopez-Ben RR, McGwin G Jr, Robinson JT, Volgas DA: Vascular injuries in knee dislocations: The role of physical examination in determining the need for arteriography. *J Bone Joint Surg Am* 2004;86-A(5):910-915.

8. Mills WJ, Barei DP, McNair P: The value of the ankle-brachial index for diagnosing arterial injury after knee dislocation: A prospective study. *J Trauma* 2004;56(6):1261-1265.

9. Fanelli GC, Stannard JP, Stuart MJ, et al: Management of complex knee ligament injuries. *Instr Course Lect* 2011;60:523-535.

   This instructional course lecture reviewed the management of complex knee ligament injuries. Topics include initial management, vascular and neurologic assessment, treatment options, reconstruction techniques, and rehabilitation.

10. Wascher DC, Dvirnak PC, DeCoster TA: Knee dislocation: Initial assessment and implications for treatment. *J Orthop Trauma* 1997;11(7):525-529.

11. Becker EH, Watson JD, Dreese JC: Investigation of multiligamentous knee injury patterns with associated injuries presenting at a level I trauma center. *J Orthop Trauma* 2013;27(4):226-231.

    In this retrospective study of 102 patients (106 knees), almost one-half of multiligamentous knee injuries involved the ACL, PCL, and PLC; one-fourth had associated ipsilateral tibial plateau fractures. The incidence of peroneal nerve injury (25%) was higher than previously reported (20%); the incidence of arterial injury (21%) was comparable with previous reports (19%). Level of evidence: III.

12. Krych AJ, Giuseffi SA, Kuzma SA, Stuart MJ, Levy BA: Is peroneal nerve injury associated with worse function after knee dislocation? *Clin Orthop Relat Res* 2014;472(9):2630-2636.

    In this retrospective review of prospective data, patients with peroneal nerve injury also had associated knee dislocation. This study compared recovery between patients with partial and complete palsies: 69% regained ankle dorsiflexion to gravity and partial palsy resulted in a higher incidence of recovery. Level of evidence: III.

13. LaPrade RF, Heikes C, Bakker AJ, Jakobsen RB: The reproducibility and repeatability of varus stress radiographs in the assessment of isolated fibular collateral ligament and grade-III posterolateral knee injuries. An in vitro biomechanical study. *J Bone Joint Surg Am* 2008;90(10):2069-2076.

14. Levy BA, Dajani KA, Whelan DB, et al: Decision making in the multiligament-injured knee: An evidence-based systematic review. *Arthroscopy* 2009;25(4):430-438.

    Systematic review of the treatment of multiligament knee injuries regarding nonsurgical versus surgical treatment, repair versus reconstruction, and early versus late surgery. They found that early surgical treatment and reconstruction rather than repair yields better results.

15. Peskun CJ, Whelan DB: Outcomes of operative and nonoperative treatment of multiligament knee injuries: An evidence-based review. *Sports Med Arthrosc* 2011;19(2):167-173.

This meta-analysis compared nonsurgical and surgical treatment strategies for multiligament knee injuries. Surgical treatment had better results in functional outcome, instability, contracture, and return to activity. Surgically treated patients returned to work and sport quicker.

16. Dwyer T, Marx RG, Whelan D: Outcomes of treatment of multiple ligament knee injuries. *J Knee Surg* 2012;25(4):317-326.

    This review article summarized outcomes associated with surgical versus nonsurgical management, early versus delayed surgery, repair versus reconstruction, autograft versus allograft, and rehabilitation.

17. Ridley TJ, Cook S, Bollier M, et al: Effect of body mass index on patients with multiligamentous knee injuries. *Arthroscopy* 2014;30(11):1447-1452.

    This 10-year study evaluate 126 multiligament knee injuries: 87 occurred in nonobese patients and 39 occurred in obese patients. Patients in the obese group were most likely to have a multiligament knee injury from low-energy mechanisms, disregarding sports-related injuries (51.28%, $P = 0.02$). Using a logistic model and body mass index as a continuous variable, researchers found that an increase in body mass index of 1 kg/m^2 increased the odds ratio of complications by 9.2%, with significance ($P = 0.0174$). Level of evidence: III.

18. Mariani PP, Santoriello P, Iannone S, Condello V, Adriani E: Comparison of surgical treatments for knee dislocation. *Am J Knee Surg* 1999;12(4):214-221.

19. Stannard JP, Brown SL, Farris RC, McGwin G Jr, Volgas DA: The posterolateral corner of the knee: Repair versus reconstruction. *Am J Sports Med* 2005;33(6):881-888.

20. Levy BA, Dajani KA, Morgan JA, Shah JP, Dahm DL, Stuart MJ: Repair versus reconstruction of the fibular collateral ligament and posterolateral corner in the multiligament-injured knee. *Am J Sports Med* 2010;38(4):804-809.

    This retrospective review of a prospective database compared PLC repair with reconstruction: 4 of 10 repairs (40%) failed; 1 of 18 reconstructions (6%) failed. Level of evidence: III.

21. Stannard JP, Black BS, Azbell C, Volgas DA: Posteromedial corner injury in knee dislocations. *J Knee Surg* 2012;25(5):429-434.

    This study compared the outcomes of repair versus reconstruction for 73 PMC tears: 25 patients underwent repair, with 5 failures; 48 patients underwent reconstruction, which had a failure rate of 4%.

22. Stannard JP, Lopez R, Volgas D: Soft tissue injury of the knee after tibial plateau fractures. *J Knee Surg* 2010;23(4):187-192.

    This paper is a prospective case series of 73 consecutive high energy tibial plateau fractures evaluated with MRI scanning. 71% sustained at least one torn ligament, with 53% having multiple ligament injuries. There were also 35 lateral meniscus tears and 25 medial meniscus tears in these patients.

23. Gardner MJ, Yacoubian S, Geller D, et al: The incidence of soft tissue injury in operative tibial plateau fractures: A magnetic resonance imaging analysis of 103 patients. *J Orthop Trauma* 2005;19(2):79-84.

24. Leiter JR, Levy BA, Stannard JP, et al: Accuracy and reliability of determining the isometric point of the knee for multiligament knee reconstruction. *Knee Surg Sports Traumatol Arthrosc* 2014;22(9):2187-2193.

    This cadaver study of four specimens compared the accuracy and reliability of the anatomic and radiographic techniques to determine the isometric point of the knee. On the medial side, no difference was found; on the lateral side, surgeons had more accurate results with the anatomic method.

25. Stannard JP, Hammond A, Tunmire D, Clayton M, Johnson C, Moura C: Determining the isometric point of the knee. *J Knee Surg* 2012;25(1):71-74.

    This cadaver study of 20 specimens compared anatomic and radiographic landmarks to determine the isometric point of the knee. Although the medial side showed no difference, the lateral isometric point was more accurately determined using radiographic landmarks.

26. Bauer KL, Stannard JP: Surgical approach to the posteromedial corner: Indications, technique, outcomes. *Curr Rev Musculoskelet Med* 2013;6(2):124-131.

    This review article focused on the anatomy, biomechanics, diagnosis, and treatment of PMC injuries.

27. Lind M, Jakobsen BW, Lund B, Hansen MS, Abdallah O, Christiansen SE: Anatomical reconstruction of the medial collateral ligament and posteromedial corner of the knee in patients with chronic medial collateral ligament instability. *Am J Sports Med* 2009;37(6):1116-1122.

    In this case series, 61 patients with grade 3 or 4 medial instability were treated with MCL reconstruction: 98% had normal to near-normal results and 91% were satisfied or very satisfied. Level of evidence: IV.

28. Laprade RF, Wijdicks CA: Surgical technique: Development of an anatomic medial knee reconstruction. *Clin Orthop Relat Res* 2012;470(3):806-814.

    This article described anatomic reconstruction of the medial knee. The prospective results of 28 patients showed improved valgus instability and overall patient function.

29. Stannard JP, Nuelle CW, McGwin G, Volgas DA: Hinged external fixation in the treatment of knee dislocations: A prospective randomized study. *J Bone Joint Surg Am* 2014;96(3):184-191.

    This prospective, randomized study compared a hinged external fixator with a hinged knee brace in patients undergoing multiligament knee reconstruction. The hinged external fixator group had more favorable results (7% compared with 21%). Level of evidence: I.

30. Mook WR, Miller MD, Diduch DR, Hertel J, Boachie-Adjei Y, Hart JM: Multiple-ligament knee injuries: A systematic review of the timing of operative intervention and postoperative rehabilitation. *J Bone Joint Surg Am* 2009;91(12):2946-2957.

31. Richter M, Bosch U, Wippermann B, Hofmann A, Krettek C: Comparison of surgical repair or reconstruction of the cruciate ligaments versus nonsurgical treatment in patients with traumatic knee dislocations. *Am J Sports Med* 2002;30(5):718-727.

32. Medvecky MJ, Zazulak BT, Hewett TE: A multidisciplinary approach to the evaluation, reconstruction and rehabilitation of the multi-ligament injured athlete. *Sports Med* 2007;37(2):169-187.

33. Fanelli GC: *Complications of Multiple Ligamentous Injuries*. Rosemont, IL, American Academy of Orthopaedic Surgeons, 2002.

34. Stannard JP, Wilson TC, Sheils TM, McGwin G Jr, Volgas DA, Alonso JE: Heterotopic ossification associated with knee dislocation. *Arthroscopy* 2002;18(8):835-839.

35. Whelan DB, Dold AP, Trajkovski T, Chahal J: Risk factors for the development of heterotopic ossification after knee dislocation. *Clin Orthop Relat Res* 2014;472(9):2698-2704.

    In this retrospective study of patients undergoing multiligament reconstruction, risk factors for the development of heterotopic ossification were identified. PCL reconstruction was the only independent predictor of heterotopic ossification. Level of evidence: III.

36. Fanelli GC, Sousa PL, Edson CJ: Long-term follow-up of surgically treated knee dislocations: Stability restored, but arthritis is common. *Clin Orthop Relat Res* 2014;472(9):2712-2717.

    In this retrospective study, 127 multiligament reconstructions performed by a single surgeon were assessed for stability, function, and the development of arthritis at 10-year follow-up. Almost 25% will develop arthritis at 10 years. Level of evidence: IV.

37. Stannard JP: *Surgical Treatment of Orthopaedic Trauma* .New York, NY, Thieme, 2007.

38. Aglietti P, Buzzi R, De Biase P, Giron F: Surgical treatment of recurrent dislocation of the patella. *Clin Orthop Relat Res* 1994;308:8-17.

39. Mehta VM, Inoue M, Nomura E, Fithian DC: An algorithm guiding the evaluation and treatment of acute primary patellar dislocations. *Sports Med Arthrosc* 2007;15(2):78-81.

40. Kohn LM, Meidinger G, Beitzel K, et al: Isolated and combined medial patellofemoral ligament reconstruction in revision surgery for patellofemoral instability: A prospective study. *Am J Sports Med* 2013;41(9):2128-2135.

    This study followed 42 patients (median age, 22 years; range, 13 to 46 years) who underwent revision surgery for persistent patellofemoral instability between January 2007 and December 2009. At 24-month follow-up, 87% of patients were satisfied or very satisfied with the treatment. No apprehension or redislocation was reported at follow-up, and pain was significantly decreased during daily activities. Significant improvements ($P < 0.001$) were noted in IKDC scores (from 50 to 80), Kujala scores (from 51 to 85), and Tegner scores (from 2.4 to 4.9). Level of evidence: IV.

Chapter 43

Fractures of the Tibial Plateau

Robert Zura, MD   Mani Kahn, MD

Abstract

The proper treatment of tibial plateau fractures necessitates an understanding of the injury mechanism. The Schatzker and AO/Orthopaedic Trauma Association classification systems can be supplemented with the three-column classification. Treatment goals should focus on restoring the articular congruity and axial alignment while minimizing complications and carefully monitoring the soft-tissue envelope. Treatment usually can yield satisfactory results for patients. Several treatment modalities have been proposed, but the mainstay of treatment remains open reduction and internal fixation. Staged treatment plays an important role in reducing complications in high-energy injuries. Other treatment options include thin wire fixation and arthroscopy. Although several recent advancements have contributed to improvements in fracture care, further exploration is warranted in several areas.

Keywords: tibial plateau fractures; knee dislocation; Schatzker classification; buttress plate; dual plating; articular reconstruction; bone graft substitutes; thin wire fixation

Dr. Zura or an immediate family member is a member of a speakers' bureau or has made paid presentations on behalf of Bioventus and Cardinal Health, serves as a paid consultant to Cardinal Health, Smith & Nephew, and Bioventus, has received research or institutional support from Synthes, and has received nonincome support (such as equipment or services), commercially derived honoraria, or other non–research-related funding (such as paid travel) from a Synthes fellowship. Neither Dr. Kahn nor any immediate family member has received anything of value from or has stock or stock options held in a commercial company or institution related directly or indirectly to the subject of this chapter.

Introduction

Tibial plateau fractures are fractures of the articular portion of the proximal tibia. This group of injuries results from a combination of indirect coronal and direct axial compressive loads to the knee joint of varying magnitude. They represent 1% of all adult fractures, with an increased incidence of 8% of all fractures in the elderly.[1] Injury severity correlates to the tibial anatomy and the amount of energy delivered. Fractures of the tibial plateau have been found to represent a broad category of high-energy and low-energy injuries.[2] Early encouraging results set the trend of surgical fixation for these injuries.[3]

Plateau fractures affect a large weight-bearing joint, imposing functional deficits that can be mitigated best by properly recognizing the severity of the bony and soft-tissue injuries. Research over the past decade has identified several injury factors and treatment factors that determine the prognosis of these injuries. Although several surgical techniques have been used in the treatment of tibial plateau fractures, a treatment algorithm that properly addresses joint articular reconstruction and mechanical axis restoration and respects the concomitant soft-tissue insult is imperative to maximize functional recovery. At the heart of this algorithm lies the goal of restoring stability for the early resumption of motion to maximize functional recovery and minimize long-term complications.

Pathoanatomy

Several factors determine the injury characteristics of tibial plateau fractures. The knee is aligned with an average anatomic axis of 6° of valgus. The proximal tibia is in 3° of varus, with the lateral plateau sitting slightly higher than the medial plateau. The lateral plateau is smaller and has a convex shape, whereas the larger, concave medial plateau accommodates 60% of the weight distributed through the knee. According to the Wolff law, this distribution of weight results in increased bone density of the medial plateau. The combination of the valgus knee anatomy, the denser medial plateau, and the typical

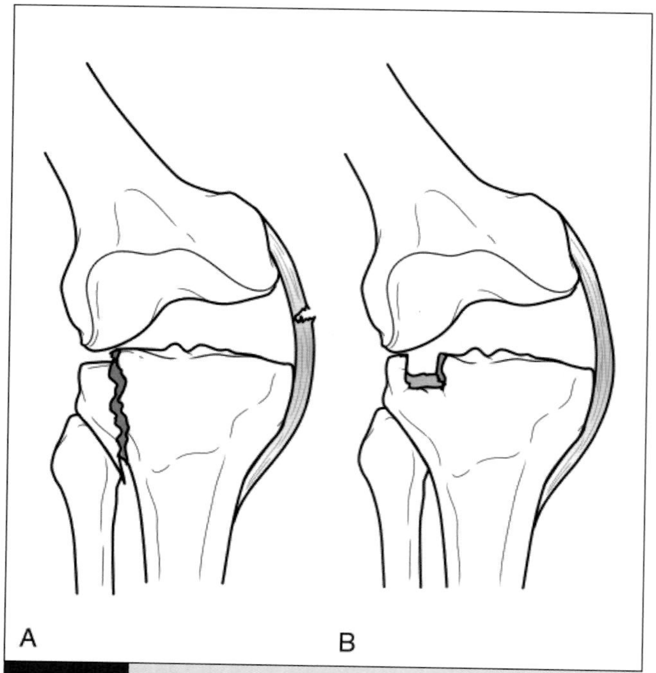

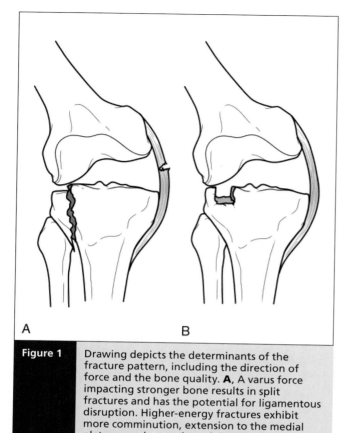

Figure 1 Drawing depicts the determinants of the fracture pattern, including the direction of force and the bone quality. **A**, A varus force impacting stronger bone results in split fractures and has the potential for ligamentous disruption. Higher-energy fractures exhibit more comminution, extension to the medial plateau, and metaphyseal dissociation. **B**, In patients with poorer bone quality, articular depression is more common.

mechanism of lateral-to-medial forces on the knee leads to a higher proportion of lateral plateau injuries.[4] The lateral plateau is affected exclusively in 55% to 70% of fractures. By comparison, medial plateau unicondylar fractures occur 10% to 23% of the time, and bicondylar fractures occur 10% to 30% of the time.[3]

Other determinants of the fracture pattern include the age and bone quality of the patient and the mechanism of injury, specifically, the force vector applied and the position of the knee during energy transfer[5] (**Figure 1**). In younger patients with more robust bone quality, the plateau is broken into various fragments after high-energy trauma. These fractures are typified by more comminution and less joint line depression. Trademarks of higher-energy fractures include involvement of the medial plateau and the tibial spine and complete dissociation of the proximal tibial metaphysis.[4] In the elderly, however, low-energy mechanisms result in lateral plateau fractures with articular depression.[5]

Concomitant injury to the soft tissues also should be considered because the associated soft-tissue damage can have a considerable negative effect on outcome and functional recovery. The combination of shearing and compressive loads imparts a high risk of injury to the menisci, ligaments, peroneal nerve, and popliteal vessels, not to mention the risk of skin damage. Over the past decade, the ubiquity and severity of soft-tissue damage related to these fractures have become more apparent and have affected the way these fractures are managed, particularly in terms of surgical timing and the role of staged fixation.[6]

Classification

The classification systems of Schatzker and the Orthopaedic Trauma Association (OTA) are the most widely accepted and used. The Schatzker classification accounts for the mechanism of injury, the amount of energy delivered, and the location of the deformity, categorizing fractures as low energy (types I through III) and high energy (types IV through VI).[2] The AO/OTA classification distinguishes articular, periarticular, and nonarticular fractures, which then are subclassified further by the amount of comminution present (**Figure 2**). This classification has been shown to have higher interobserver reliability than the Schatzker classification, but both have equal intraobserver reliability. When CT is added as a diagnostic adjunct, it has been shown that the interobserver and intraobserver agreement between these classifications are the same.[7]

Both classifications have been criticized for failing to account for the spectrum of knee dislocations and for ignoring the sagittal deformity of the tibial plateau, although the Schatzker classification continues to be favored in North America because of its simplicity.[4] One proposal that addresses these inconsistencies is the three-column classification, which uses the axial view of a diagnostic CT of the knee to divide the proximal tibia into the medial, lateral, and posterior columns[1] (**Figure 3**).

When describing fractures using the Schatzker classification, the number of fractures and the locations of the planned reduction and fixation are designated. For example, a "zero-column" fracture is a pure depression Schatzker type III fracture. A simple lateral split or lateral split depression Schatzker type I or II fracture is termed a one-column lateral fracture. When an anterolateral fracture and a distinct posterolateral depression are present, the fracture is considered a two-column lateral and posterior fracture. The isolated posterior column articular fracture is termed a one-column posterior fracture. This designation takes into account isolated posterior column fractures that are otherwise outside of the Schatzker classification system. An anteromedial fracture combined with a distinct posteromedial fracture

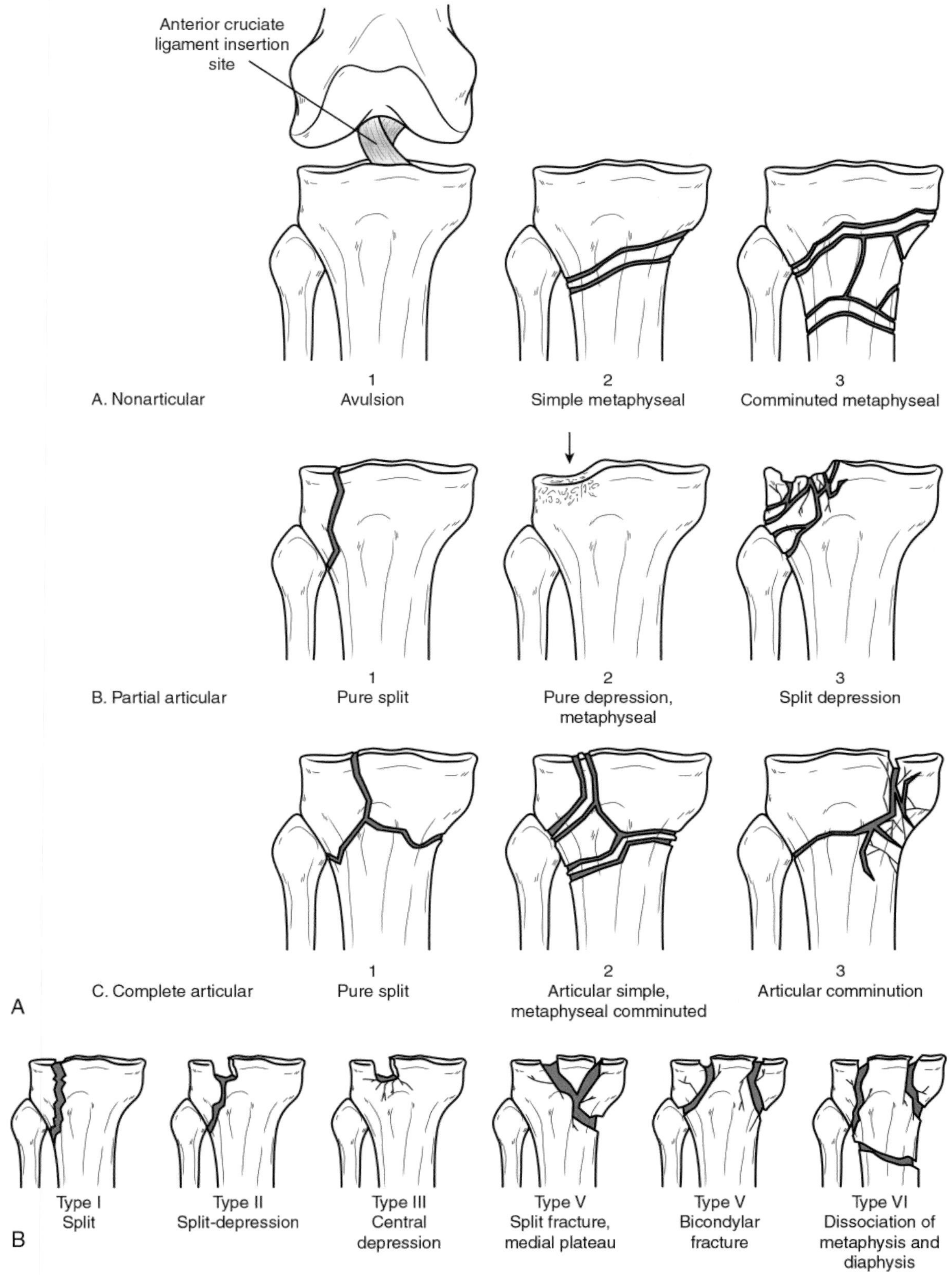

Figure 2 Chart demonstrates the two classifications systems that categorize fractures of the tibial plateau, the AO/Orthopaedic Trauma Association classification (**A**) and the Schatzker classification (**B**).

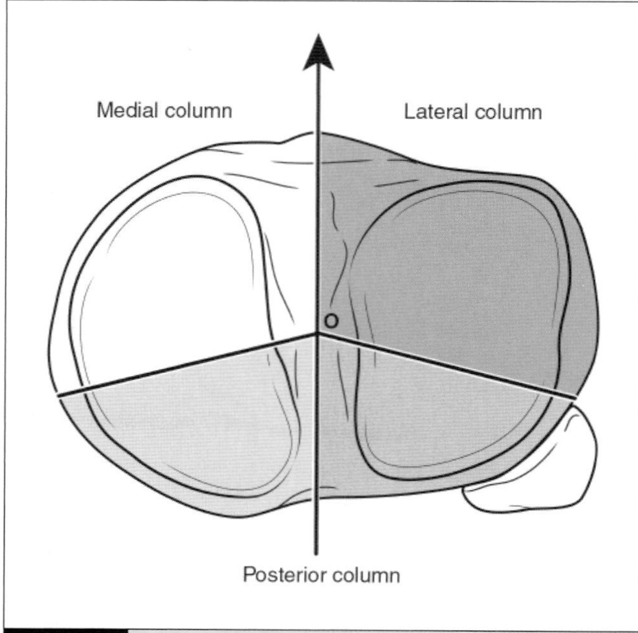

Figure 3 Drawing depicts the three-column classification, which uses the axial CT view of the knee to compartmentalize fractures in the medial, lateral, and posterior columns.

is the other common type of two-column medial and posterior fracture, which is a type of Schatzker type IV fracture that cannot be distinguished from more simple fracture patterns. The three-column fracture, which is composed of distinct fracture fragments in each column, correlates to Schatzker types V and VI fractures that have a separate posterolateral articular fragment.[1] When evaluated for reliability, the three-column classification system exhibited an interobserver reliability superior to that of the Schatzker and OTA/AO classifications.[8] The three-column system can influence how the surgeon approaches fracture fixation by addressing each column independently.

Patient Assessment

As with every trauma patient, it is imperative to begin with Advanced Trauma Life Support protocols and abide by the treatment principles consistent with damage control orthopaedics when necessary. When examining the affected extremity, evaluation of the soft-tissue envelope should include careful assessment for the presence of edema, effusion of the knee, abrasions, contusions, and blisters. Often, subtle findings may be indicative of severe injury, and a higher-energy fracture mechanism should heighten the suspicion for soft-tissue injury. The surfaces known to be susceptible to open injury, such as the subcutaneous location of the anteromedial surface of the proximal tibia, should be checked routinely. Early definitive management in a high-energy injury with unforeseen soft-tissue damage may lead to devastating complications in wound healing.

The neurovascular status of the limb should be assessed. The tethering of the trifurcation of the popliteal artery at the interosseous membrane can lead to vascular injury when fracture fragments of the proximal tibia are displaced. A normal pulse examination can be misleading because pulses may be normal despite vascular injury in up to 15% of cases.[9] Any asymmetry in pulses mandates an assessment of the ankle-brachial index; if less than 0.9, further work-up with conventional angiography, CT angiography, or duplex ultrasonography is warranted. Failure to recognize a vascular injury promptly is associated with a lower-extremity amputation rate as high as 86%.[9] Collaboration between the vascular, trauma, and orthopaedic surgical teams is essential to address combined injuries appropriately.

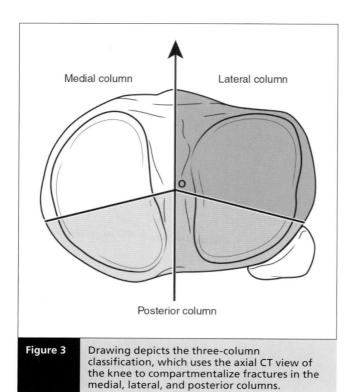

In high-energy fractures, the possibility of acute compartment syndrome (ACS) exists. Serial evaluation of the compartments in the awake patient and the judicious use of intracompartmental pressure monitoring in the obtunded patient are essential to avoid missing the diagnosis of compartment syndrome. In one series, the rate of ACS in high-energy tibial plateau fractures requiring staged treatment was as high as 27% and disproportionately affected patients with medial plateau fracture-dislocations, with an incidence of 53%.[10] When concomitant vascular injury is present, even more vigilance in the diagnosis should be maintained as reported in another series, which showed a 59% incidence of ACS in patients with blunt trauma and vascular injuries.[11]

Also important to consider is the potential for intracapsular soft-tissue injury, which has been postulated to be more common in younger patients with denser bone.[5] The ligamentous injury pattern can correlate with fracture type. For example, higher-energy medial tibial plateau fractures commonly are accompanied by lateral collateral ligament and anterior cruciate ligament injuries, which can result in a combined fracture-dislocation of the knee. Fractures of the tibial spine correlate to cruciate ligament dysfunction.[4] One series using MRI evaluation of surgical tibial plateau fractures found that the incidence of intracapsular soft-tissue injuries was almost universal. Of the 103 patients evaluated, only 1 lacked an identifiable meniscal or ligamentous injury. A lateral meniscus injury was found in 91% of fractures (94 patients), medial meniscus injury in 44% of fractures (45 patients), and ligamentous injury in 77% of fractures (79 patients).[6] Intraoperative correlation has shown that only 30% of fractures

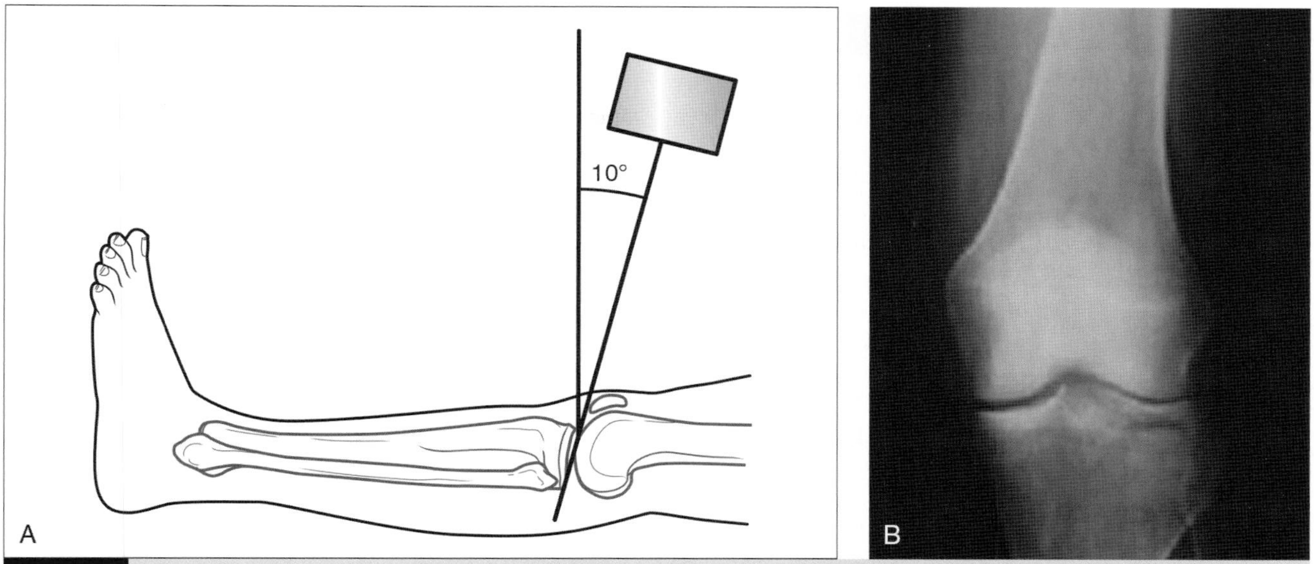

Figure 4 Drawing (**A**) shows the assessment of a proximal tibial articular surface using an AP radiograph of the knee (**B**) tilted 10° caudal to match the posterior slope of the proximal tibia.

have lateral meniscus tears that actually require surgical repair.[12]

Imaging

Plain radiographs provide a substantial amount of information and enable a rapid assessment that can help differentiate high-energy and low-energy mechanisms of injury. The AP knee radiograph should be tilted 10° caudal to attempt to match the posterior slope of the proximal tibia and accurately assess the articular surface (**Figure 4**). The lateral view assesses for coronal fracture planes; oblique views also can be insightful. CT with coronal and sagittal reconstructions typically is obtained for preoperative assessment; it may be delayed in cases of staged treatment of substantial comminution so that imaging may be conducted under ligamentotaxis after application of an external fixator. Three-dimensional (3D) reconstructions can help in surgical planning for more complex cases, and substantial improvements in interobserver and intraobserver reliability have been shown in determining the AO/OTA and Schatzker classifications when compared with two-dimensional (2D) CT.[13] Although helpful in diagnosing the intra-articular soft-tissue injuries that often accompany tibial plateau fractures,[6] MRI is not obtained routinely at most centers. Advocates suggest its use can improve the early diagnosis of accompanying ligamentous and meniscal injuries and can enhance interobserver reliability when compared with 2D CT.[14]

Goals of Treatment

The overall goal of treatment is to promote fracture healing in a manner that allows the return of knee function with good motion while eliminating residual pain or instability. Historically, the management of fractures of the tibial plateau focused on achieving anatomic reduction through open approaches using rigid internal fixation. Outcome studies have reported soft-tissue complications as high 50% and unacceptable nonunion rates when soft-tissue rest and bone vascularity are not emphasized.[15] Modern techniques aim to avoid the osteosynthesis of devascularized bony fragments (avoiding the so-called "dead bone sandwich") and emphasize the prevention of soft-tissue complications.

Articular reduction remains the guiding principle for surgical indications and surgical approaches, because tibial plateau articular defects have been shown to affect the biomechanics of the knee joint.[16] Similarly, studies continue to correlate functional outcomes with articular reduction.[17] The tibial plateau can tolerate some articular incongruity, however, which is believed to be related to the thickness of the cartilage in this region.[18] Although postulated to contribute to posttraumatic arthritis, the degree of articular step-off that can be tolerated continues to be an area of exploration, and no consensus exists. Joint stability and axial alignment have been established as important prognostic indicators.[19] Factors such as sagittal and coronal plane alignment and meniscus retention and repair also have been identified as determinants of functional outcome.[18]

Nonsurgical Treatment and Surgical Indications

Several large series with long-term follow-up support the continued role of nonsurgical treatment in certain fracture patterns. In one early outcomes study of 260 patients, treatment was directed exclusively by one factor: instability on examination to varus/valgus stress in extension. When reevaluated 20 years later, 90% (92 patients) available for follow-up achieved good or excellent results, whereas the 10% (10 patients) with poor results correlated with persistent instability or greater than 10 mm of articular depression.[19] In another large series, 131 tibial plateau fractures with up to 5 mm of condylar widening, 3 mm of articular incongruity, and 5° valgus healed with minimal short-term and long-term complications. Of knees with moderate to severe instability, 70% underwent deteriorated clinical function. Minimally displaced medial and bicondylar fractures were functionally unacceptable, and any amount of varus also was tolerated poorly.[20] These findings have defined the currently accepted parameters for treatment, in which instability and unacceptable articular displacement form the basis of surgical decision making.

It is widely accepted that nonsurgical treatment be reserved for low-energy fractures with a stable knee joint or for patients with unacceptable surgical risks. Although no universal protocol exists, a treatment protocol should stress early immobilization with transition to a hinged knee brace that allows knee motion as early as possible. Knee aspiration may precede casting or the placement of a rigid knee brace to relieve pain and reduce the inflammatory burden, although scant support for this practice exists in the literature. Immobilization should be implemented for 4 to 6 weeks, followed by progressive range of motion exercises over another 4 to 6 weeks. Progressive advancement from no weight bearing to gradual full weight bearing between 8 and 12 weeks should take place to parallel the early signs of healing visualized on the radiographs. In the rare cases in which open reduction and internal fixation (ORIF) of unstable, displaced, or comminuted fractures is not possible, traction or external fixation for ligamentotaxis can be implemented as definitive treatment. In these cases and with radiographs as a guide, range of motion exercises should be initiated between 6 and 12 weeks in a hinged brace, with weight bearing restricted for a total of 12 weeks.

Timing of Surgery and Staged Management

Certain circumstances warrant immediate intervention to address open fractures, compartment syndrome, and vascular injuries. Early extensile approaches through swollen tissue for the internal fixation of tibial plateau fractures are associated with an unacceptable complication rate, however.[15] In the absence of emergent conditions, delaying fixation based on the soft-tissue status, the medical condition, and adherence to damage control principles has reduced the incidence of soft–tissue-related complications.[21]

For high-energy injury patterns in which substantial soft-tissue swelling is possible, staged external fixation has been used. This treatment principle also has applications for low-energy injuries in patients who already have poor soft-tissue quality. Both applications involve the early placement of external fixation and close monitoring of the soft tissues until definitive fixation can be pursued (**Figure 5**). By aligning the fracture fragments during a period of rest before surgical fixation, the staged approach facilitates improved imaging for surgical planning as well as a reduction in soft-tissue complications. Reported infection rates have declined from a high of 50% to less than 8% when multiple surgical approaches are used in conjunction with the staged approach for bicondylar fractures. An increased incidence of complications related to knee stiffness has been reported when using the staged approach.[15,17,22]

The timing of definitive fixation in the context of ACS treated with fasciotomies remains controversial. In a retrospective review, 81 tibial plateau fractures complicated with compartment syndrome were treated using four compartment fasciotomies with variations in the timing of definitive fixation. Infection developed in 7 of 30 fractures (23%) treated with fixation before fasciotomy closure. Infection developed in 3 of 26 fractures (12%) treated with fixation at the time of fasciotomy closure. Infection also developed in 4 of 25 fractures (16%) treated with fixation after fasciotomy closure. No statistical significance was noted in these differences.[23] Another retrospective review of bicondylar plateau fractures treated with dual plating found that fasciotomy closure before definitive fixation was associated with substantially fewer deep infections than internal fixation with open fasciotomy wounds (11.8% versus 50.0%).[24]

Surgical Planning

Beginning with the initial decision for staged treatment, the preoperative plan requires careful evaluation of the injury radiographs and CT with or without 3D reconstruction; 3D reconstruction is deferred until after external fixation when using a staged treatment protocol. ORIF with plate-and-screw constructs and hybrid external fixation with limited open treatment of the joint help provide optimal surgical and functional results. Adjunct

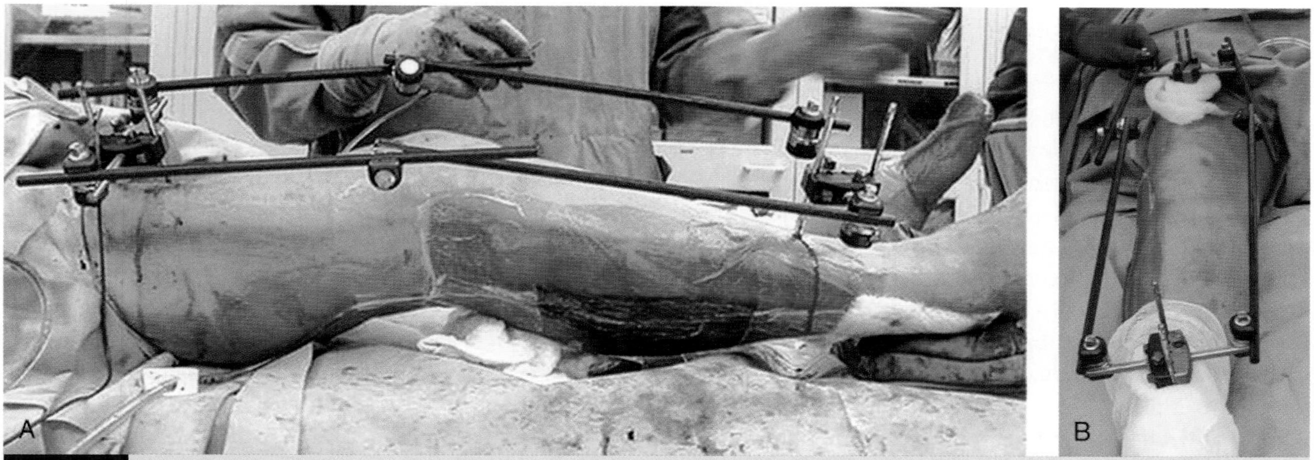

Figure 5 Intraoperative photographs of the lower extremity demonstrate a knee-spanning external fixation frame used to stabilize a bicondylar tibial plateau fracture with associated lower leg compartment syndrome in profile (**A**) and on fos (**B**). (Reproduced from Tejwani N, Polonet D, Wolinsky PR: External fixation of tibial fractures. *J Am Acad Orthop Surg* 2015;23[2]:126-130.)

techniques such as a femoral distractor, arthroscopy, or bone substitutes aid in fracture reduction. The surgical algorithm should involve consideration of the method of reduction, the need for one or multiple surgical approaches, the instrumentation and plating techniques to be used, and the need for adjunct techniques. The method of fixation selected should be tailored to the injury characteristics, obtain adequate articular reduction and stability, and maintain metaphyseal alignment.

Surgical Approaches

Anterior Approach

The traditional midline approach uses the same incision as a total knee arthroplasty (TKA) (**Figure 6**) and permits simultaneous exposure of both tibial condyles and facilitates possible eventual salvage arthroplasty. Its use for extensive exposure has fallen out of favor because of complications related to bony devascularization and the inability to address posterior fragments. A medial or lateral parapatellar arthrotomy with a unilateral full-thickness flap that addresses only one condyle is favorable because of its simplicity, familiarity, good visualization, ease of reduction in certain fracture patterns, and scar location for any future procedures.[25]

Anterolateral Approach

The anterolateral approach for isolated lateral condyle fractures is used in conjunction with other incisions for the treatment of bicondylar plateau injuries. It can allow for soft-tissue sparing, and can be useful for minimally invasive submuscular plating. An anterolateral straight,

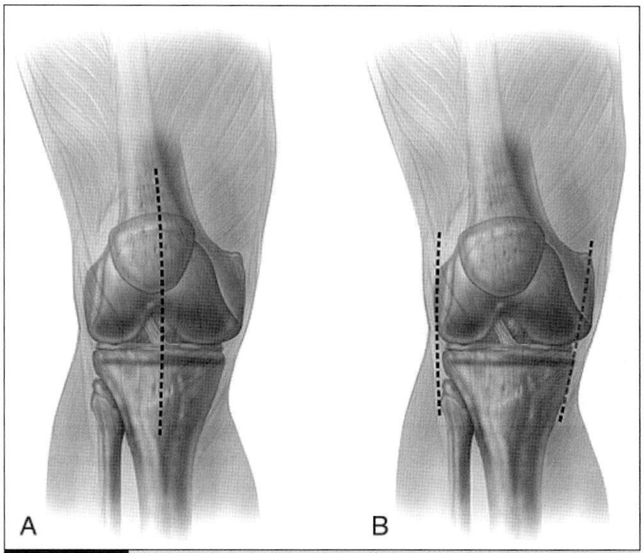

Figure 6 Drawings depict the alternative approaches to the tibial plateau. The traditional midline approach (**A**) uses the same incision as a total knee arthroplasty. Dual incisions (**B**) allow the fragments of bicondylar fractures to be addressed individually. Commonly, an anterolateral approach is combined with a posteromedial approach to approach the apex of the fractures properly and allow for an adequate skin bridge. (Reproduced with permission from Hall JA, Beuerlein MJ, McKee MD, Canadian Orthopaedic Trauma Society: Open reduction and internal fixation compared with circular fixator application for biocondylar tibial plateau fractures: Surgical technique. *J Bone Joint Surg Am* 2009[suppl 2 Pt 1];91:74-88.)

hockey-stick, or lazy S incision is made just lateral to the tibial tubercle. It is extended proximally and posteriorly toward the Gerdy tubercle, then proximally to the level of the distal thigh (**Figure 6**). The iliotibial band is exposed and can be divided in line with fibers or with the skin incision. The anterior compartment fascia is exposed, and the tibialis anterior is elevated off the proximal tibial metaphysis, taking care to preserve soft-tissue and periosteal attachments when possible. A horizontal capsulotomy is used to expose the meniscus, and the submeniscal coronary ligament is incised to elevate the meniscus off the plateau. Joint visualization can be aided with sutures placed in the meniscus for its manipulation, flexion and varus maneuvers of the knee, and the use of a distractor or external fixator. One of the limitations of the anterolateral approach is difficulty with visualization of the posterolateral plateau.

Posteromedial Approach

The posteromedial approach can be used alone for Schatzker type IV fractures or in conjunction with a second incision to address the lateral plateau in Schatzker type V and VI fractures. The posteromedial fracture fragment is present in 31% to 59% of bicondylar fractures and it involves an average of 25% of the joint surface. In 55% of cases, it involves more than 5 mm of displacement.[26] Failure to address this fragment or indirect attempts to address it using laterally placed hardware have been associated with poor results.[27]

The posteromedial tibia is approached with an incision just posterior to the posteromedial border of the tibia, extending proximally over the hamstring. Care is taken to provide an adequate skin bridge of 7 to 8 cm[28] for any planned lateral incisions in bicondylar plateau fractures. The fascia is exposed and incised between the medial gastrocnemius and the pes anserinus anteriorly. The semimembranosus insertion may be detached to improve posterior visualization if necessary. The popliteus muscle is elevated directly off the bone. In the absence of comminution, an indirect reduction can be achieved without arthrotomy. Otherwise, a submeniscal arthrotomy is performed next for articular visualization, although this procedure is more difficult on the medial side secondary to the medial collateral ligament attachment to the medial meniscus. A femoral distractor or external fixator can be used on the medial side for traction. A recent retrospective review of 27 patients treated with this approach alone or in conjunction with a second approach, with an average of 3.5 year follow-up, found no wound complications, good functional scores, and reduction that was maintained in 75% of cases.[28]

Posterior Approach

The Lobenhoffer approach facilitates increased visualization of posterior fragments for reduction and stabilization. The direct approach is advocated for highly unstable posteromedial fracture-dislocations because it provides direct access of shear fragments for buttress plating. A 6- to 8-cm incision is made in the popliteal fossa along the medial border of the gastrocnemius muscle. The medial gastrocnemius is dissected bluntly and retracted laterally, whereas the semimembranosus muscles are dissected bluntly and retracted medially. The partial subperiosteal detachment of the popliteus allows direct access to the posterior plateau. The tibial insertion of the semimembranosus on the medial side can be incised if needed. Visualization extends from the posteromedial border of the tibia to the fibula, also providing access to the medial meniscus and posterior cruciate ligament.[29,30]

Internal Fixation

Advances in plating technology and a gained appreciation for soft-tissue management have defined the evolution of internal fixation for tibial plateau fractures. When necessary, multiple approaches are combined to address separate fracture fragments. Careful incision planning should allow for an adequate skin bridge of 7 to 8 cm.[28] The external fixator placed for staged management may be left in place for distraction and reduction. It often is recommended to avoid pin site incorporation into definitive incisions to reduce the risk of infection. A recent retrospective review of bicondylar tibial plateau fractures reported a statistically significant increased rate of deep infection in patients who had pin site overlap (24%) compared with those whose pin sites had been separated from the incision sites (10%).[31]

Unicondylar fractures in healthy bone generally should be treated with nonlocked buttress fixation. To preserve mechanical alignment, the metaphyseal-diaphyseal relationship should be reestablished, which often is done using a combination of traction, reduction tool placement, and indirect plate reduction. Sometimes it is necessary to address articular reconstruction first. Fracture fragments can be spread apart using the open-door technique. Impacted fragments should be elevated with an osteotome or bone tamp. Isolated depression fragments require an osteotomy. After the joint is reestablished and pinned into place with Kirschner wires, the articular reconstruction can be supported using the rafting screw concept. By spreading screws across the subchondral region, hardware can assist in preventing articular subsidence. This step can be performed by placing the screws through a precontoured periarticular lateral buttress plate, with a

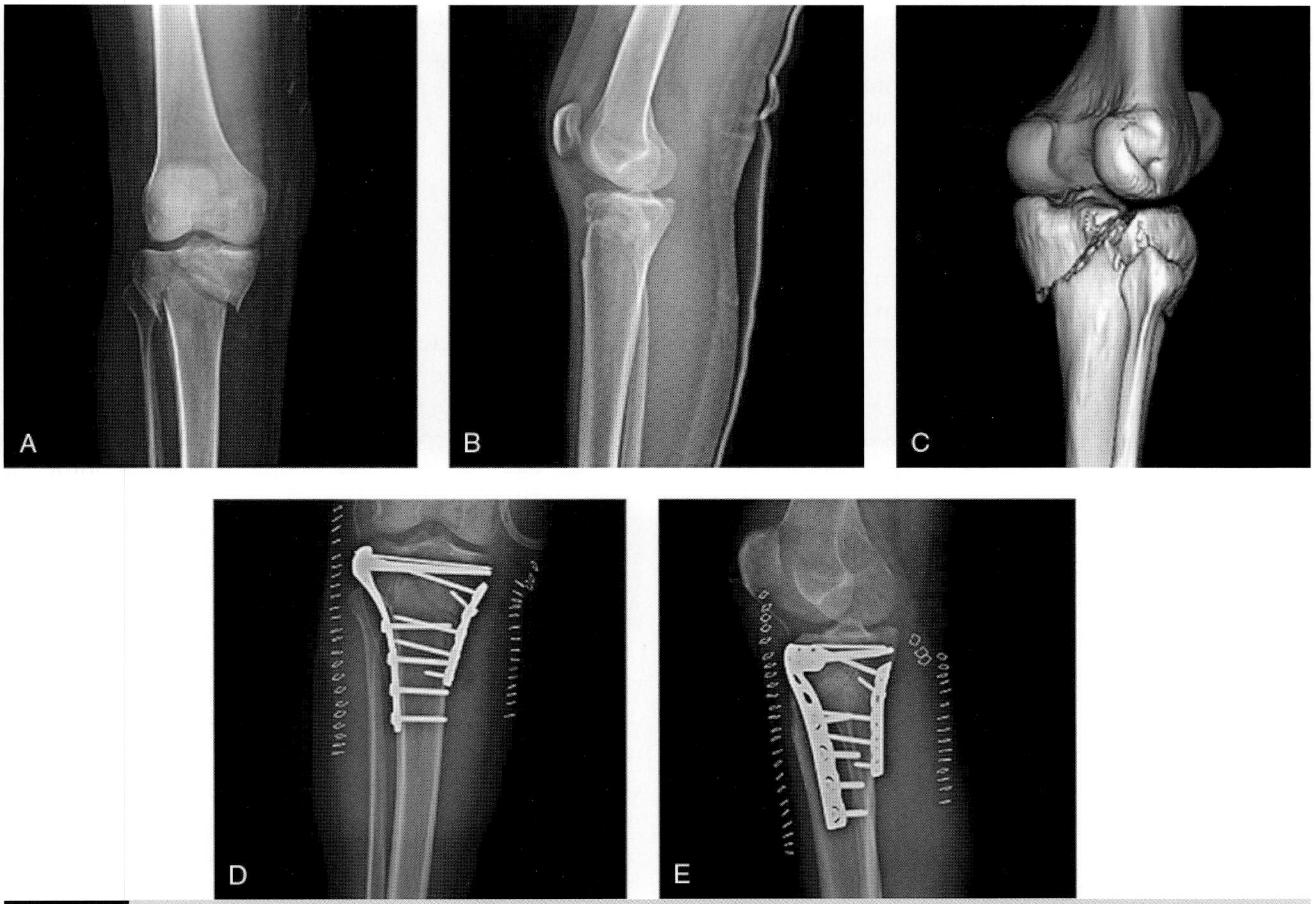

Figure 7 Images depict dual plating for a bicondylar tibial plateau fracture in a 26-year-old man following a motor vehicle accident. Preoperative AP (**A**) and lateral (**B**) radiographs and a CT reconstruction (**C**) show a bicondylar tibial plateau fracture. Postoperative AP (**D**) and lateral (**E**) radiographs show dual plating with a fixed angle construct applied laterally and a posteromedial antiglide plate. (Reproduced from Berkson EM, Virkus WW: High-energy tibial plateau fractures. *J Am Acad Orthop Surg* 2006;14[1]:20-31.)

separate short rafting plate placed parallel to the joint surface or using screws independent of a plate.

The widespread adoption of locked plating has introduced a debate over whether a laterally based locking plate could address medial side fracture fragments. The isolated lateral-based fixation strategy has the advantage of minimizing surgical time, blood loss, and soft-tissue disruption.[32] A recent biomechanical study found that, for bicondylar fractures involving a posteromedial fragment, combining a lateral nonlocked plate with a posteromedial buttress plate was superior to the lateral locking plate (**Figure 7**) with a higher load to failure.[33] Additionally, multiple clinical comparisons have reported that lateral locked plating for medial fractures is related to varus failure and articular subsidence.[27,34] The order of fixation is debated, although performing posteromedial fixation first to provide a stable medial column to which the lateral plateau can be reduced and fixed is advocated in one study.[28] Using both incisions simultaneously also can aid visualization in certain situations.

Defect Augmentation

In unstable fractures with bone graft or graft substitutes, defect augmentation is aimed at preventing articular collapse. Calcium phosphate cement commonly is used, as supported by several studies favorably comparing it to bone graft and other substitutes. In a prospective, multicenter randomized trial of 120 acute tibial plateau fractures treated with ORIF, 82 tibial plateau fractures had subarticular support provided by calcium phosphate cement, whereas iliac crest autograft was used in 38 fractures. Patients were followed clinically and radiographically for up to 1 year. The authors found a statistically significant increase in articular subsidence of 30% in the autograft group, compared with 9% in the calcium phosphate cement group.[35] A recent biomechanical study compared the augmentation of plate fixation using calcium phosphate with autograft in split plateau fractures created in eight matched pairs of tibias in fresh frozen cadavers. The group treated with calcium cement had a reduced subsidence, increased stiffness during fatigue loading, and an increased load to failure.[36]

Meniscal Repair

MRI studies report high rates of meniscus pathology in tibial plateau fractures, citing rates as high as 91% laterally and 44% medially.[6] The proper identification and management of meniscal injuries can improve outcomes and prevent postoperative arthrosis.[37] At the time of submeniscal arthrotomy, the meniscus should be evaluated thoroughly. Sutures are placed into the periphery of the meniscus for its mobilization. Identified bucket-handle and peripheral longitudinal tears should be repaired, and radial tears with flaps should be excised partially. A recent retrospective review of 602 tibial plateau fractures found that 179 patients (30%) had lateral meniscus tears, which occurred more frequently in males, that required repair. The authors further subdivided the cases by fracture type and found a 12% incidence in Schatzker type I fractures, 18% in type II fractures, 45% in type III fractures, 22% in type V fractures, and 26% in type VI fractures. Schatzker type III fractures commonly had peripheral rim tears, whereas other fracture types had a mix of peripheral and radial tears.[12]

Locked and Minimally Invasive Plating

Locking technology increases construct rigidity and has been advocated for complex fractures of the proximal tibia. Most precontoured plate designs now have locking screw options, with or without variable angle features. Locking screws can be useful in severely osteoporotic bone, extensive metaphyseal-diaphyseal comminution, and short-segment articular and periarticular fragments.[38]

Percutaneous plating techniques with precontoured plates have gained popularity. A small arthrotomy is used for articular visualization if a reduction of the articular surface is required. The plate then is passed submuscularly through the same incision, and percutaneous screws are placed through the plate with the help of fluoroscopy in the tibial shaft (**Figure 8**). Caution is recommended if the plate length accommodates more than 11 holes to avoid damage to the peroneal nerve, and screws placed in its territory should be done so with a larger incision to identify and protect it.[38]

A prospective study of 34 Schatzker type V or VI fractures treated with a minimally invasive approach and followed for a minimum of 1 year found that all fractures were united at a mean of 15.6 weeks, with a mean knee

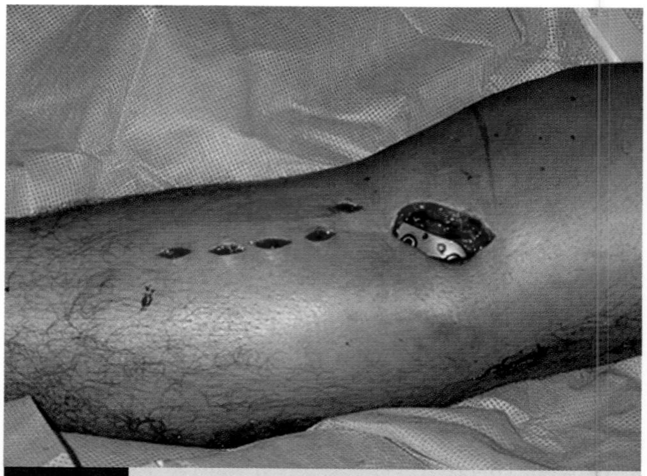

Figure 8 Intraoperative photograph shows the extremity of a patient treated with minimally invasive plate osteosynthesis. (Reproduced from Lowe JA, Tejwani N, Yoo BJ, Wolinsky PR: Surgical techniques for complex proximal tibial fractures. *Instr Course Lect* 2012;61:39-51.)

range of motion (ROM) of from 1° of extension (range, 0° to 10°) to 127° of flexion (range, 90° to 145°). The overall incidence of infection was 5.9%. Plate removal was needed in 10 of 34 patients (29%).[39] Varying rates of complications have been reported using this technique. In one review of high-energy proximal tibia fractures, deep infection was reported in 22% of patients and loss of alignment in 8%.[27] A multicenter review of open plateau fractures treated with percutaneous plating with a mean follow-up of 16.8 months found that deep infection developed in only 6.3% of tibial plateau fractures. The authors propose minimally invasive techniques as a way of reducing infection rates in open and high-energy injuries.[40]

Geriatric Patients

To achieve the goals of treatment in the geriatric population, the quality of the bone, the patient's functional abilities, and any comorbidities must be considered. Older age at the time of injury and poor bone quality have been correlated with overall higher rates of fixation failure and poorer functional outcomes.[17,41] The authors of a review of fracture care in the elderly asserted that, when substantial osteoporosis is present, surgeons should use lateral locked plates instead of separate nonlocked rafting plates and should use medial locking plates to support posteromedial buttress plates when substantial metaphyseal-diaphyseal comminution is present. They also suggested that bridging external fixation can be added to protect fixation constructs for a period of 6 to 8 weeks, with immediate resumption of knee ROM exercises after removal. Weight bearing should be delayed for a full 12 weeks.[42]

Postoperative Management

Swelling and vascular status should be assessed frequently in the immediate postoperative period. Regional anesthesia and continuous nerve blocks preclude this assessment and should be avoided for this reason. In general, the knee should be placed in a soft dressing. Some surgeons may place a hinged knee brace for support. Early mobilization and passive ROM are essential for optimizing outcomes. If the construct is deemed stable, passive ROM exercises should begin immediately. The use of continuous passive motion (CPM) remains controversial. A 2014 prospective randomized study of intra-articular knee fractures treated with ORIF found a statistically significant increase in knee ROM of 66.6 in the CPM group and an increase of 33.5 in the control group at 48 hours. No difference was found during further follow-up up after 6 months postoperatively, however.[43] The initiation of active ROM exercises and weight bearing can be variable, and decisions should be made based on the fracture type and the stability of the construct. Most surgeons recommend at least 6 to 8 weeks of restricted weight bearing, using radiographs to assist the decision making based on healing.

Functional Outcomes

A direct comparison between surgical and nonsurgical treatment is lacking, but the literature includes studies of tibial plateau fractures treated with ORIF that have high union rates and postoperative function. These outcomes sometimes are juxtaposed with high short-term and long-term complication rates. Early studies show 80% to 96% acceptable results in unicondylar and bicondylar injuries treated with ORIF using plating with and without bone grafting.[2,44] A more recent retrospective review of 71 patients treated with ORIF who were followed at an average of 6.1 years using the Knee Injury and Osteoarthritis Score questionnaire found fair to good results in symptoms, pain, and daily function. The authors found poorer functional results in the sports and recreational activity scores. Age and the development of postoperative arthrosis on radiographs had no impact on functional results.[45]

Several studies evaluated high-energy fracture patterns in isolation. One study evaluated the functional results of 41 bicondylar tibial plateau fractures treated with ORIF using a dual approach and followed for 4.9 years; 31 fractures had postoperative radiographs. Using the Musculoskeletal Function Assessment Questionnaire, the authors found lower functional scores in the 45% of patients with articular step-off greater than 2 mm, as well as in older and polytrauma patients.[17] A recent retrospective review of 69 bicondylar fractures treated with dual buttress plating followed for a mean of 27 months found that 81.2% (56 of 69) of patients had good or excellent functional results using the Rasmussen Anatomic and Functional System Score. The authors found no correlation between functional score and age, sex, mechanism of injury, or open fracture, but reported that worse functional scores were correlated with a lower quality of reduction and increased fracture complexity.[46]

A 2010 prospective cohort study followed patients with three-column fractures treated with fixation of all three fractures individually using dual anterolateral and posterior incisions. Patients were followed clinically and radiographically for an average of 27.3 months. All but one case had satisfactory reduction, no cases of secondary articular depression were reported, and no revision surgeries were performed, although angular deformity was present in two patients. Short Form-36 Health Survey and Hospital for Special Surgery knee scores were 89 and 90, respectively. Average ROM at 2 years was 2.7° to 123.4°. The authors concluded that this classification scheme and technique promote satisfactory fixation in these difficult fracture patterns.[1]

Complications

Early complications relate predominantly to the soft tissues. Violating soft tissues with early wide-open approaches has been associated with rates of infections as high 80% in higher-energy injuries.[15] Modern techniques that minimize soft-tissue disruption are associated with much lower infection rates. A recent review of 519 tibial plateau fractures of all types in the American College of Surgeons National Surgical Quality Improvement Program database found infections in only 4% of patients. They were associated with male sex, increased American Society of Anesthesiologists classification, smoking, and bicondylar fractures. A higher American Society of Anesthesiologists classification was associated with severe adverse events, extended length of stay, and readmission within 30 days.[47] In a 2013 retrospective review of surgically treated tibial plateau fractures, 24 of 309 fractures were complicated by infection (7.8% infection rate). Risk factors for infection included open fracture, compartment syndrome treated with fasciotomies, and increased surgical time. No relationship to infection was found for smoking, diabetes, bicondylar fractures, or dual incisions.[48] Recent retrospective reviews of bicondylar injuries treated with dual plating report infection rates of 14.2% to 23.6%, which is higher than the rates reported in studies that include all fracture subtypes.[24,49]

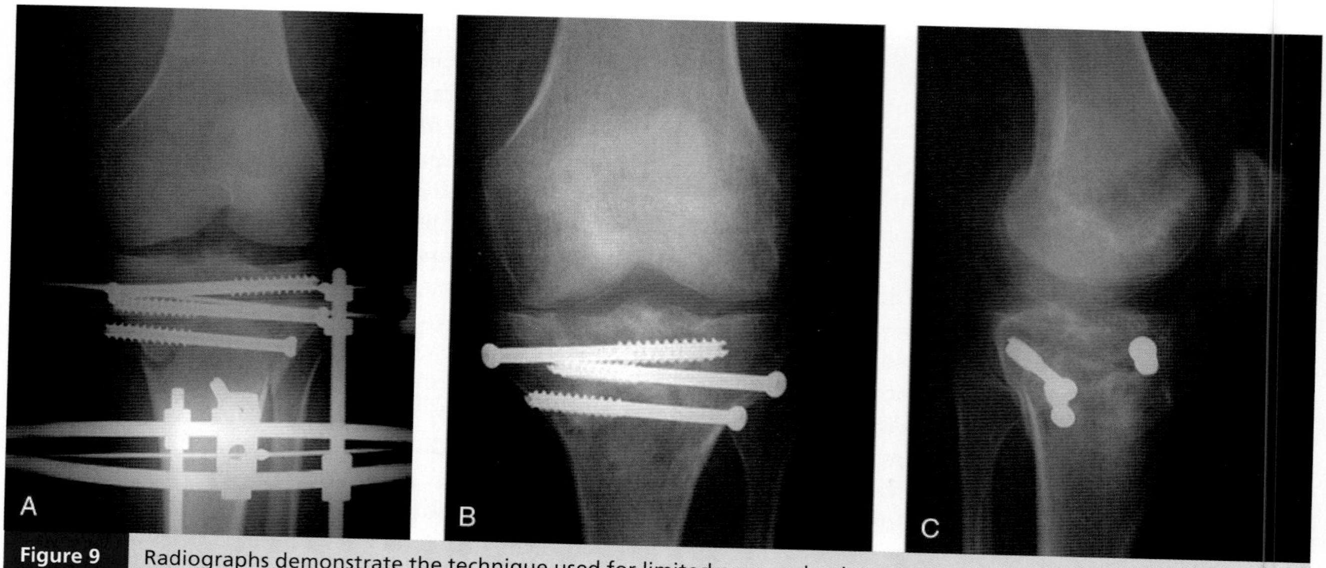

Figure 9 Radiographs demonstrate the technique used for limited open reduction percutaneous screw fixation combined with a circular fixator in a bicondylar tibial plateau fracture. AP radiograph (**A**) shows the fixation immediately postoperatively. AP (**B**) and lateral (**C**) radiographs depict the fixation 2 years postoperatively. (Reproduced with permission from Hall JA, Beuerlein MJ, McKee MD: Open reduction and internal fixation compared with circular fixator application for bicondylar tibial plateau fractures. *J Bone Joint Surg Am* 2009;91[suppl 2 Pt 1]:74-88.)

Other early complications include pyarthrosis, skin necrosis, compartment syndrome, and deep vein thrombosis.[50] A recent study assessed the radiographic factors predictive of compartment syndrome and found a higher Schatzker classification, increased tibial width, and femoral displacement to correlate positively.[51] Vancomycin and negative-pressure wound therapy may hold promise in preventing soft-tissue complications, but more research in these areas is needed.[52,53]

Late complications predominantly relate to mechanical and biologic issues. When fixation strategies address individual fracture fragments and stable fixation is achieved, low rates of articular and condylar subsidence are reported.[34] Loss of fixation is higher in the geriatric population and may be minimized using supplemental spanning external fixation and locking plates.[17,41,54] Nonunion is uncommon, but disruption of the metadiaphysis, as seen in high-energy Schatzker type VI injuries, is a risk factor. It can be limited by avoiding distraction or using bone grafting.[4] Malunion requiring secondary intervention is also uncommon, but often involves a valgus deformity with intra-articular depression. Intra-articular osteotomy has been proposed to delay salvage arthroplasty and prevent posttraumatic arthritis.[55]

Posttraumatic arthritis has been reported with a high frequency of 30% to 40% in long-term follow-up. Risk factors for posttraumatic arthritis include advanced age, meniscal resection, and residual deformity. Articular incongruity has not been well established as a risk factor for posttraumatic arthritis, but this relationship remains controversial.[17,19,37] Arthrodesis and arthroplasty are surgical options for substantial degenerative changes. Following tibial plateau fracture ORIF, TKA was required 7.3% of the time (616 patients) at 10-year follow-up in a retrospective review of 8,426 patients.[56] In this subset of patients, TKA is more challenging technically and has less reliable results.[57]

Alternative Techniques

Thin Wire Fixation

In certain situations, thin wire fixation can be the ideal method of treatment. Some surgeons prefer this technique, and its advantages should not be overlooked in cases of bicondylar injuries with considerable diaphyseal extension or substantial persistent soft-tissue compromise. Ring fixators can be combined with percutaneous lag screw fixation (**Figure 9**). Thin wire fixation enables deformity correction in multiple planes, allows early joint motion, and can permit the treatment of ipsilateral distal tibia fractures with the same device, all while minimizing soft-tissue disruption. Obtaining accurate articular reduction with small incisions can be challenging. Intra-articular pin placement should be avoided, using 15 mm from the joint line as a rough guideline, because it has been associated with septic arthritis. Care also should be taken to avoid the articulation between the proximal tibia and the fibula.[58]

Biomechanically, thin wire frame constructs have stability and strength comparable to plate fixation when compared on sawbones models.[59] Early clinical studies support using this technique in high-energy injuries, with 16 of 23 patients having good to excellent results.[60] A more recent retrospective study reviewed the long-term results of combined thin wire circular frame fixation with limited internal fixation performed in 129 fractures. At 5-year follow-up, 38 of 129 fractures (29%) had excellent results, 63 of 129 (49%) had good results, 18 of 129 (14%) had fair results, and 10 of 129 (8%) had poor results based on responses to a patient questionnaire. A statistically significant correlation was recorded between the magnitude of the articular step-off and the radiologic result. An interesting finding in this study was the worsening of the radiologic results between the 3- and 5-year follow-up. This change in radiographic arthritis also correlated with loss of knee motion.[61]

A multicenter randomized controlled trial evaluated circular external fixation and dual plating in bicondylar tibial plateau fractures. Patients treated with fixators had a shorter hospital stay, a marginally faster return of function, a reduced infection rate (17.5% versus 2.3%), and a lower rate of reoperation. A similar quality of reduction and similar clinical outcomes were noted, however. At 2-year follow-up, the authors reported similar function as measured by Hospital for Special Surgery knee scores, Western Ontario and McMaster Universities Osteoarthritis Index scores, return to preinjury activity, and knee ROM.[62]

Arthroscopy

Arthroscopically assisted ORIF can serve as a useful adjunct technique that offers the advantage of direct visualization of the articular surface without an open approach, and can be used in the treatment of unicondylar and bicondylar injuries.[63] Advantages of arthroscopically assisted ORIF include the benefit of intra-articular lavage, easier retrieval of intra-articular loose bodies, the ability to perform a complete diagnostic ligamentous examination, the ability to repair torn menisci, and direct visualization of the intra-articular reduction. Concerns with the technique include the development of compartment syndrome, a prolonged surgical time, and a potentially steep learning curve for the surgeon.[64]

Summary

The evaluation and treatment of tibial plateau fractures must include an understanding of whether the injury mechanism is high energy or low energy, along with an understanding of associated soft-tissue injuries, the patient's age and physical demands, and radiographic and clinical goals.

If surgical treatment is indicated, the goals should focus on restoring articular congruity and axial alignment, treating the soft-tissue envelope, and minimizing further complications. Careful treatment may yield satisfactory results for patients. Several controversies still remain, but the potential exists to improve the overall functional outcomes of patients with these fractures.

Key Study Points

- Fractures should be differentiated, based on mechanism, into high-energy and low-energy types. Fracture classifications can be used to stratify the risk of complications.
- Radiographic features, patient characteristics, and an understanding of the pathoanatomy should be used to guide the treatment algorithm.
- The advantages and disadvantages of treatment strategies should be comprehended. The soft tissues should guide surgical management, and staged management should be incorporated when necessary.
- Lateral locked plating, dual plating, arthroscopic assistance, and thin wire fixation all have advantages and disadvantages of which the surgeon should be aware.

Annotated References

1. Hohl M: Fractures of the proximal tibia and fibula, in: Rockwood C, Green D, Bucholz R, eds: *Fractures in Adults*, 3rd ed. Philadelphia, JB Lippincott, 1991, pp 1725-1761.

2. Schatzker J, McBroom R, Bruce D: The tibial plateau fracture. The Toronto experience 1968-1975. *Clin Orthop Relat Res* 1979;138:94-104.

3. Luo CF, Sun H, Zhang B, Zeng BF: Three-column fixation for complex tibial plateau fractures. *J Orthop Trauma* 2010;24(11):683-692.

   The authors present a prospective study of 29 complex tibial plateau fractures classified as three-column fractures treated with a combined approach addressing each column. All but one case had had satisfactory reduction. Follow-up at 2 years showed good functional results.

4. Berkson EM, Virkus WW: High-energy tibial plateau fractures. *J Am Acad Orthop Surg* 2006;14(1):20-31.

5. Koval KJ, Helfet DL: Tibial Plateau Fractures: Evaluation and Treatment. *J Am Acad Orthop Surg* 1995;3(2):86-94.

6. Gardner MJ, Yacoubian S, Geller D, et al: The incidence of soft tissue injury in operative tibial plateau fractures: A magnetic resonance imaging analysis of 103 patients. *J Orthop Trauma* 2005;19(2):79-84.

7. Brunner A, Horisberger M, Ulmar B, Hoffmann A, Babst R: Classification systems for tibial plateau fractures; does computed tomography scanning improve their reliability? *Injury* 2010;41(2):173-178.

   Four independent reviewers classified 45 consecutive fractures of the tibial plateau using the OTA/AO classification, Schatzker classification, and the Hohl classification. Moderate interobserver reliability and good and moderate intraobserver reliability were obtained with radiographs in all classifications. CT improved interobserver and intraobserver reliability in all classifications.

8. Zhu Y, Hu CF, Yang G, Cheng D, Luo CF: Inter-observer reliability assessment of the Schatzker, AO/OTA and three-column classification of tibial plateau fractures. *J Trauma Manag Outcomes* 2013;7(1):7.

   Radiographs and CT images from 50 tibial plateau fractures were classified by four observers using the three-column classification, Schatzker classification, and the AO/OTA classification. Substantial agreement in the assessment of interobserver reliability was found, and was higher than the conventional Schatzker and AO/OTA classifications.

9. Halvorson JJ, Anz A, Langfitt M, et al: Vascular injury associated with extremity trauma: Initial diagnosis and management. *J Am Acad Orthop Surg* 2011;19(8):495-504.

   This review article highlights important considerations for the workup and treatment of tibial plateau fractures with concomittant vascular injuries. Physical examination, ankle-brachial index testing, CT, and ultrasonography all can help diagnose vascular injuries. The authors underscore that results are dependent on early detection of vascular injury followed by immediate treatment.

10. Stark E, Stucken C, Trainer G, Tornetta P III: Compartment syndrome in Schatzker type VI plateau fractures and medial condylar fracture-dislocations treated with temporary external fixation. *J Orthop Trauma* 2009;23(7):502-506.

11. Rozycki GS, Tremblay LN, Feliciano DV, McClelland WB: Blunt vascular trauma in the extremity: Diagnosis, management, and outcome. *J Trauma* 2003;55(5):814-824.

12. Stahl D, Serrano-Riera R, Collin K, Griffing R, Defenbaugh B, Sagi HC: Operatively treated meniscal tears associated with tibial plateau fractures: A report on 661 patients. *J Orthop Trauma* 2015;29(7):322-324.

    This retrospective review of 602 surgically treated tibial plateau fractures shows that 179 (30%) had lateral meniscus tears requiring surgical repair. Tear type correlated with fracture type. Level of evidence: IV.

13. Hu YL, Ye FG, Ji AY, Qiao GX, Liu HF: Three-dimensional computed tomography imaging increases the reliability of classification systems for tibial plateau fractures. *Injury* 2009;40(12):1282-1285.

14. Yacoubian SV, Nevins RT, Sallis JG, Potter HG, Lorich DG: Impact of MRI on treatment plan and fracture classification of tibial plateau fractures. *J Orthop Trauma* 2002;16(9):632-637.

15. Young MJ, Barrack RL: Complications of internal fixation of tibial plateau fractures. *Orthop Rev* 1994;23(2):149-154.

16. McKinley TO, Bay BK: Trabecular bone strain changes associated with cartilage defects in the proximal and distal tibia. *J Orthop Res* 2001;19(5):906-913.

17. Barei DP, Nork SE, Mills WJ, Coles CP, Henley MB, Benirschke SK: Functional outcomes of severe bicondylar tibial plateau fractures treated with dual incisions and medial and lateral plates. *J Bone Joint Surg Am* 2006;88(8):1713-1721.

18. Schenker ML, Mauck RL, Ahn J, Mehta S: Pathogenesis and prevention of posttraumatic osteoarthritis after intra-articular fracture. *J Am Acad Orthop Surg* 2014;22(1):20-28.

    This review article discusses epidemiology, risk stratification, multifactorial pathogenesis, and proposed treatment algorithms.

19. Lansinger O, Bergman B, Körner L, Andersson GB: Tibial condylar fractures. A twenty-year follow-up. *J Bone Joint Surg Am* 1986;68(1):13-19.

20. Honkonen SE: Indications for surgical treatment of tibial condyle fractures. *Clin Orthop Relat Res* 1994;302:199-205.

21. Crist BD, Ferguson T, Murtha YM, Lee MA: Surgical timing of treating injured extremities. *J Bone Joint Surg Am* 2012;94(16):1514-1524.

    The many injuries in orthopaedics requiring emergent and urgent treatment are reviewed. Evidence and trends are weighed to provide insight in the decision-making process.

22. Egol KA, Tejwani NC, Capla EL, Wolinsky PL, Koval KJ: Staged management of high-energy proximal tibia fractures (OTA types 41): The results of a prospective, standardized protocol. *J Orthop Trauma* 2005;19(7):448-455, discussion 456.

23. Zura RD, Adams SB Jr, Jeray KJ, Obremskey WT, Stinnett SS, Olson SA; Southeastern Fracture Consortium Foundation: Timing of definitive fixation of severe tibial plateau fractures with compartment syndrome does not have an effect on the rate of infection. *J Trauma* 2010;69(6):1523-1526.

    This retrospective review of 81 patients with tibial plateau fractures and four compartment fasciotomies could not establish a difference in infection rate among those who underwent osteosynthesis before, during, or after definitive fasciotomy closure.

24. Ruffolo MR, Gettys FK, Montijo HE, Seymour RB, Karunakar MA: Complications of high-energy bicondylar tibial plateau fractures treated with dual plating through 2 incisions. *J Orthop Trauma* 2015;29(2):85-90.

    The authors present a retrospective review of complications associated with 140 bicondylar tibial plateau fractures treated with ORIF using dual plating through two incisions. Complications occurred at a rate of 27.9%, including deep infection and nonunion. Level of evidence: IV.

25. Espinoza-Ervin CZ, Starr AJ, Reinert CM, Nakatani TQ, Jones AL: Use of a midline anterior incision for isolated medial tibial plateau fractures. *J Orthop Trauma* 2009;23(2):148-153.

26. Higgins TF, Kemper D, Klatt J: Incidence and morphology of the posteromedial fragment in bicondylar tibial plateau fractures. *J Orthop Trauma* 2009;23(1):45-51.

27. Phisitkul P, McKinley TO, Nepola JV, Marsh JL: Complications of locking plate fixation in complex proximal tibia injuries. *J Orthop Trauma* 2007;21(2):83-91.

28. Weil YA, Gardner MJ, Boraiah S, Helfet DL, Lorich DG: Posteromedial supine approach for reduction and fixation of medial and bicondylar tibial plateau fractures. *J Orthop Trauma* 2008;22(5):357-362.

29. Galla M, Lobenhoffer P: [The direct, dorsal approach to the treatment of unstable tibial posteromedial fracture-dislocations]. *Unfallchirurg* 2003;106(3):241-247.

30. Fakler JK, Ryzewicz M, Hartshorn C, Morgan SJ, Stahel PF, Smith WR: Optimizing the management of Moore type I postero-medial split fracture dislocations of the tibial head: Description of the Lobenhoffer approach. *J Orthop Trauma* 2007;21(5):330-336.

31. Shah CM, Babb PE, McAndrew CM, et al: Definitive plates overlapping provisional external fixator pin sites: Is the infection risk increased? *J Orthop Trauma* 2014;28(9):518-522.

    In a retrospective review, 85 OTA 41C plateau fractures and 97 OTA 43C pilon fractures treated with staged internal fixation were stratified by pin site and incisional overlap and evaluated for development of infection. Twenty-five wound infections developed, with a statistically significant increase in rate of wound infection when pin sites overlapped (24% versus 10%). Level of evidence: III.

32. Partenheimer A, Gösling T, Müller M, et al: Management of bicondylar fractures of the tibial plateau with unilateral fixed-angle plate fixation. *Unfallchirurg* 2007;110(8):675-683.

33. Yoo BJ, Beingessner DM, Barei DP: Stabilization of the posteromedial fragment in bicondylar tibial plateau fractures: A mechanical comparison of locking and nonlocking single and dual plating methods. *J Trauma* 2010;69(1):148-155.

    A biomechanical study of 30 bicondylar tibial plateau models treated with 6 constructs is presented. Posteromedial fragment tolerated higher loads with 3.5 conventional plate and 1/3 tubular plate.

34. Weaver MJ, Harris MB, Strom AC, et al: Fracture pattern and fixation type related to loss of reduction in bicondylar tibial plateau fractures. *Injury* 2012;43(6):864-869.

    One hundred forty patients with bicondylar tibial plateau fractures treated with lateral locking plate or dual plating were retrospectively reviewed. Patients with coronal fracture lines treated with dual plating had substantially less loss of reduction than those treated with lateral locked plating. Level of evidence: III.

35. Russell TA, Leighton RK, Alpha-BSM Tibial Plateau Fracture Study Group: Comparison of autogenous bone graft and endothermic calcium phosphate cement for defect augmentation in tibial plateau fractures. A multicenter, prospective, randomized study. *J Bone Joint Surg Am* 2008;90(10):2057-2061.

36. McDonald E, Chu T, Tufaga M, et al: Tibial plateau fracture repairs augmented with calcium phosphate cement have higher in situ fatigue strength than those with autograft. *J Orthop Trauma* 2011;25(2):90-95.

    Biomechanical evaluation of fatigue strength of calcium phosphate augmented repairs versus autogenous bone graft in lateral tibial plateau fractures was assessed using eight matched pairs of tibias harvested from fresh frozen cadavers. Calcium phosphate repairs have significantly higher fatigue strength and ultimate load than autograft.

37. Honkonen SE: Degenerative arthritis after tibial plateau fractures. *J Orthop Trauma* 1995;9(4):273-277.

38. Lowe JA, Tejwani N, Yoo B, Wolinsky P: Surgical techniques for complex proximal tibial fractures. *J Bone Joint Surg Am* 2011;93(16):1548-1559.

    The authors review strategies to approach surgical treatment of complex proximal tibial fractures.

39. Stannard JP, Wilson TC, Volgas DA, Alonso JE: The less invasive stabilization system in the treatment of complex fractures of the tibial plateau: Short-term results. *J Orthop Trauma* 2004;18(8):552-558.

40. Stannard JP, Finkemeier CG, Lee J, Kregor PJ: Utilization of the less-invasive stabilization system internal fixator for open fractures of the proximal tibia: A multi-center evaluation. *Indian J Orthop* 2008;42(4):426-430.

41. Ali AM, El-Shafie M, Willett KM: Failure of fixation of tibial plateau fractures. *J Orthop Trauma* 2002;16(5):323-329.

42. Horwitz DS, Kubiak EN: Surgical treatment of osteoporotic fractures about the knee. *J Bone Joint Surg Am* 2009;91(12):2970-2982.

43. Hill AD, Palmer MJ, Tanner SL, Snider RG, Broderick JS, Jeray KJ: Use of continuous passive motion in the postoperative treatment of intra-articular knee fractures.2014;96(14):e118.

A prospective randomized controlled trial of 40 patients with tibial plateau or distal femur fractures compared continuous passive motion and traditional therapy for effect on knee range of motion at interval periods between 48 hours and 6 months. No difference in knee range of motion for all time points except at 48 hours, where knee flexion was greater in the continuous passive motion group. Level of evidence: II.

44. Savoie FH, Vander Griend RA, Ward EF, Hughes JL: Tibial plateau fractures. A review of operative treatment using AO technique. *Orthopedics* 1987;10(5):745-750.

45. van Dreumel RL, van Wunnik BP, Janssen L, Simons PC, Janzing HM: Mid-to long-term functional outcome after open reduction and internal fixation of tibial plateau fractures. *Injury* 2015;46(8):1608-1612.

The authors retrospectively reviewed mid- to long-term functional outcome after ORIF for all types of tibial plateau fractures using Knee Injury and Osteoarthritis Outcome Score questionnaire. Lower functional outcomes in the mid- to longterm did not correlate with radiographic osteoarthritis.

46. Yao Y, Lv H, Zan J, Li J, Zhu N, Jing J: Functional outcomes of bicondylar tibial plateau fractures treated with dual buttress plates and risk factors: A case series. *Injury* 2014;45(12):1980-1984.

The authors retrospectively reviewed 74 bicondylar tibial plateau fractures treated with dual buttress plates using dual incisions. Anatomic and functional scores were good to excellent. Fracture reduction quality and AO fracture type were independent risk factors for clinical function.

47. Basques BA, Webb ML, Bohl DD, Golinvaux NS, Grauer JN: Adverse events, length of stay, and readmission after surgery for tibial plateau fractures. *J Orthop Trauma* 2015;29(3):e121-e126.

A retrospective review of National Surgical Quality Improvement Program database identified patient characteristics in relation to adverse events. Increased American Society of Anesthesiologists class and pulmonary disease correlated with adverse events. Level of evidence: II.

48. Colman M, Wright A, Gruen G, Siska P, Pape HC, Tarkin I: Prolonged operative time increases infection rate in tibial plateau fractures. *Injury* 2013;44(2):249-252.

In a retrospective review of 309 tibial plateau fractures treated with ORIF, surgical times approaching 3 hours and open fractures correlated to an increased overall risk for infection. Dual plating did not increase infection risk.

49. Morris BJ, Unger RZ, Archer KR, Mathis SL, Perdue AM, Obremskey WT: Risk factors of infection after ORIF of bicondylar tibial plateau fractures. *J Orthop Trauma* 2013;27(9):e196-e200.

In a retrospective review of 302 bicondylar tibial plateau fractures treated with ORIF, smoking, open fracture, and compartment syndrome and dual incisions increased risk of infection. Level of evidence: II.

50. Barei DP, Nork SE, Mills WJ, Henley MB, Benirschke SK: Complications associated with internal fixation of high-energy bicondylar tibial plateau fractures utilizing a two-incision technique. *J Orthop Trauma* 2004;18(10):649-657.

51. Ziran BH, Becher SJ: Radiographic predictors of compartment syndrome in tibial plateau fractures. *J Orthop Trauma* 2013;27(11):612-615.

In a retrospective case-control study, 162 tibial plateau fractures were evaluated. Radiographic parameters predictive of compartment syndrome were identified. Level of evidence: II.

52. Stannard JP, Volgas DA, McGwin G III, et al: Incisional negative pressure wound therapy after high-risk lower extremity fractures. *J Orthop Trauma* 2012;26(1):37-42.

The authors performed a prospective randomized multicenter clinical trial on the use of incisional negative pressure wound therapy for closed surgical incisions after treatment of fractures of the tibial plateau, pilon, or calcaneus. Decreased incidence of wound dehiscence and infections after high-risk fractures was noted with the use of negative pressure wound therapy.

53. Singh K, Bauer JM, LaChaud GY, Bible JE, Mir HR: Surgical site infection in high-energy peri-articular tibia fractures with intra-wound vancomycin powder: A retrospective pilot study. *J Orthop Traumatol* 2015;16(4):287-291.

In a retrospecive review of tibial plateau and pilon fractures treated with vancomycin powder into the surgical wound, no statistically significant difference in surgical site infection was found.

54. Stevens DG, Beharry R, McKee MD, Waddell JP, Schemitsch EH: The long-term functional outcome of operatively treated tibial plateau fractures. *J Orthop Trauma* 2001;15(5):312-320.

55. Kerkhoffs GM, Rademakers MV, Altena M, Marti RK: Combined intra-articular and varus opening wedge osteotomy for lateral depression and valgus malunion of the proximal part of the tibia. Surgical technique. *J Bone Joint Surg Am* 2009;91(suppl 2 Pt 1):101-115.

56. Wasserstein D, Henry P, Paterson JM, Kreder HJ, Jenkinson R: Risk of total knee arthroplasty after operatively treated tibial plateau fracture: A matched-population-based cohort study. *J Bone Joint Surg Am* 2014;96(2):144-150.

The authors performed a retrospective review of 8,426 tibial plateau fracture patients matched to 33,698 control patients. The rates of total knee arthroplasty at 10 years significantly increased in those treated for tibial plateau fractures.

57. Saleh KJ, Sherman P, Katkin P, et al: Total knee arthroplasty after open reduction and internal fixation of fractures of the tibial plateau: A minimum five-year follow-up study. *J Bone Joint Surg Am* 2001;83-A(8):1144-1148.

58. Weiner LS, Kelley M, Yang E, et al: The use of combination internal fixation and hybrid external fixation in severe proximal tibia fractures. *J Orthop Trauma* 1995;9(3):244-250.

59. Ali AM, Saleh M, Bolongaro S, Yang L: The strength of different fixation techniques for bicondylar tibial plateau fractures—a biomechanical study. *Clin Biomech (Bristol, Avon)* 2003;18(9):864-870.

60. Stamer DT, Schenk R, Staggers B, Aurori K, Aurori B, Behrens FF: Bicondylar tibial plateau fractures treated with a hybrid ring external fixator: A preliminary study. *J Orthop Trauma* 1994;8(6):455-461.

61. Katsenis D, Dendrinos G, Kouris A, Savas N, Schoinochoritis N, Pogiatzis K: Combination of fine wire fixation and limited internal fixation for high-energy tibial plateau fractures: Functional results at minimum 5-year follow-up. *J Orthop Trauma* 2009;23(7):493-501.

62. Canadian Orthopaedic Trauma Society: Open reduction and internal fixation compared with circular fixator application for bicondylar tibial plateau fractures. Results of a multicenter, prospective, randomized clinical trial. *J Bone Joint Surg Am* 2006;88(12):2613-2623.

63. Hartigan DE, McCarthy MA, Krych AJ, Levy BA: Arthroscopic-assisted reduction and percutaneous fixation of tibial plateau fractures. *Arthrosc Tech* 2015;4(1):e51-e55.

    The technique for the arthroscopic-assisted fixation of lateral tibial plateau fractures is described.

64. Chen XZ, Liu CG, Chen Y, Wang LQ, Zhu QZ, Lin P: Arthroscopy-assisted surgery for tibial plateau fractures. *Arthroscopy* 2015;31(1):143-153.

    In a meta-analysis of arthroscopic-assisted fixation of tibial plateau fractures, a total of 609 patients with mean follow-up of 52.5 months found this technique to be reliable, effective, and safe. Level of evidence: IV.

6: Lower Extremity

Chapter 44

Tibial Shaft Fractures

Jennifer L. Bruggers, MD

Abstract

Tibial shaft fracture is the most common type of long bone fracture. The treatment modalities include casting as well as plate, intramedullary nail, and ring fixation. Recent modifications to intramedullary nails allow for stable fixation of proximal and distal fractures. Research continues to elucidate the best care of open fractures. Complications including compartment syndrome, nonunion, and infection remain issues in managing tibial shaft fractures.

Keywords: diaphyseal fracture; open fracture; tibia fracture

Introduction

Tibial shaft fracture is the most common type of long bone fracture. A low- or high-energy mechanism may be responsible for the injury. No specific classification scheme is consistently used. Instead, tibial shaft fractures typically are described by their location (proximal, middle, or distal third) and orientation (transverse, oblique, spiral, segmental, or comminuted).

Nonsurgical Treatment

Nonsurgical treatment of a tibial shaft fracture is indicated if the fracture alignment meets certain criteria: varus or valgus angulation of less than 5° to 10°, procurvatum or recurvatum of less than 10° to 15°, rotation of less than 10°, shortening of less than 1 cm, and displacement of less than 25%.[1] A tibial shaft fracture that does not meet these criteria sometimes can be treated nonsurgically if both tibial length and alignment are maintained and the fibula is intact. Varus alignment in particular can be an issue if the fibula is intact. If all criteria for nonsurgical treatment are met, the patient can be initially treated with protected weight bearing and a long leg splint. At 2 to 4 weeks, the use of a patellar tendon-bearing short leg cast or a fracture brace is begun, and as the fracture heals weight bearing is advanced as tolerated.[2] For a distal-third tibial shaft fracture, the initial use of a long leg splint may not be necessary. Cast use can be discontinued in favor of a boot when bridging callus begins to form, typically at 8 to 12 weeks. The average healing time for a nonsurgically managed tibial shaft fracture is 4 to 5 months.

Open Fractures

The treatment of open fractures of the tibia continues to be a source of controversy. The Gustilo-Anderson classification system traditionally is used after surgical débridement, which determines the extent of the soft-tissue injury.[3] The Orthopaedic Trauma Association classification system delineates the components of an open fracture that may require treatment.[4]

The timing of definitive irrigation and débridement after open fracture has been investigated.[5-9] Each hour of delay after injury was found to lead to a linear increase in the rate of infection.[6] The time from injury to arrival in the definitive care center was the most important risk factor for infection, rather than the time to surgical débridement.[7] Patients who had bone loss of more than 2 cm and/or a Gustilo type III-C open fracture had an increased rate of major infection. The timing of antibiotic therapy was found to be more important for decreasing the risk of infection after an open fracture than the time to débridement, and it was recommended that antibiotics initially be administered within 1 hour of injury.[8] Another study found that the rate of infection was higher in tibia fractures than in upper extremity fractures and in Gustilo type III fractures over type I, but the timing of antibiotics or surgical débridement were not considered significant factors.[9]

Irrigation and thorough débridement are mainstays of treatment for an open fracture. The risk of infection may

Neither Dr. Bruggers nor any immediate family member has received anything of value from or has stock or stock options held in a commercial company or institution related directly or indirectly to the subject of this chapter.

be affected by the method of irrigation and the use of additives. The use of an antibiotic solution was not found to provide any benefit over the use of a soap solution, and it may impede wound healing.[10] Although a pilot study found that low-pressure lavage led to better outcomes than high-pressure irrigation, the final study found no such difference in outcomes.[11] The use of a supplement such as benzalkonium, bacitracin, cefazolin, or castile soap in the irrigation fluid was not found to lead to a smaller bacterial load than plain saline and might increase the infection risk.[12]

Wound closure is an essential part of treating an open fracture. The timing of wound closure depends on variables including the amount of soft-tissue injury, the presence of wound contamination, and the anticipated type of closure. To decrease the risk of infection, repeat débridement is recommended until healthy tissue is obtained. The risk of infection is significantly increased if the patient has a comorbidity such as diabetes mellitus or a body mass index greater than or equal to 25 kg/m^2. Closing an open wound before negative cultures were obtained was found to have no effect on the infection rate.[13] Compared with the use of standard dressings, the use of negative pressure wound therapy to provide a clean environment before soft-tissue coverage was found to decrease the risk of infection by 80%.[14,15] It is recommended that an open wound be closed or covered as soon as possible. Recent studies found that closure or coverage within 3 to 5 days of an open fracture decreased the risk of infection.[8,16] Negative pressure wound dressings have been used on closed incisions to decrease swelling and deep hematoma, promote wound healing, and decrease the risk of infection.[17,18]

The use of bone morphogenetic protein–2 (BMP-2) during definitive stabilization of open fractures with unreamed nails was found to decrease the risk of fracture nonunion.[19] However, there was no significant difference in time to union when open fractures were treated using reamed nails, with or without BMP-2.[20] An increased rate of adverse events was found after reamed nailing in open fractures compared with unreamed nailing.[21]

Surgical Treatment

The optimal timing for surgical treatment of an isolated tibial shaft fracture can be difficult to determine. In an evaluation of the timing of intramedullary nailing, procedures done outside of normal operating room hours were more likely to lead to reoperation compared with procedures done during the normal workday.[22] In addition, after-hours surgery is significantly more costly than surgery done during the normal workday if the facility does not have 24-hour operating room staff and must call in a surgical team.[23]

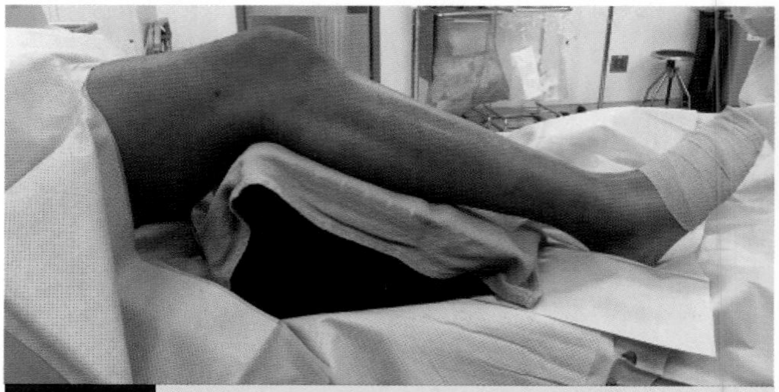

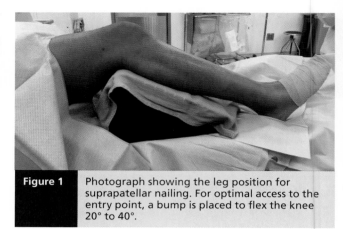

Figure 1 Photograph showing the leg position for suprapatellar nailing. For optimal access to the entry point, a bump is placed to flex the knee 20° to 40°.

Intramedullary Nailing

The indications for intramedullary nailing in tibial shaft fractures are expanding because the nail design allows improved control of very proximal or very distal fracture fragments. In addition, semiextended and suprapatellar nailing with specialized instruments has become popular as a technique for decreasing the risk of malreduction in proximal-third fractures treated with intramedullary nailing.

Surgical Approach

Incisions for intramedullary nail insertion are made anteriorly along the midline of the knee. The incision for a traditional nail insertion is made from the inferior border of the patella to the tibial tubercle, with the knee hyperflexed. A deep incision then can be made in the center of the patellar tendon, in line with the tendon fibers, or parapatellar on the medial or lateral side of the tendon. For a parapatellar incision, the approximate starting point for the guidewire on the proximal tibia should be evaluated under fluoroscopy to determine whether a medial or a lateral approach should be used.

Semiextended or suprapatellar nailing originally was done through a proximal anterior midline incision; a medial parapatellar arthrotomy at the superior aspect of the patella allows for subluxation of the patella and exposure of the starting point with the knee flexed only 20° to 40°[24] (**Figure 1**). In a more minimally invasive approach for use with this nailing technique, a smaller quadriceps tendon-splitting incision is made just cephalad to the proximal pole of the patella. Modified instrumentation has been developed for this approach. A protective guideis placed through the patellofemoral joint and onto

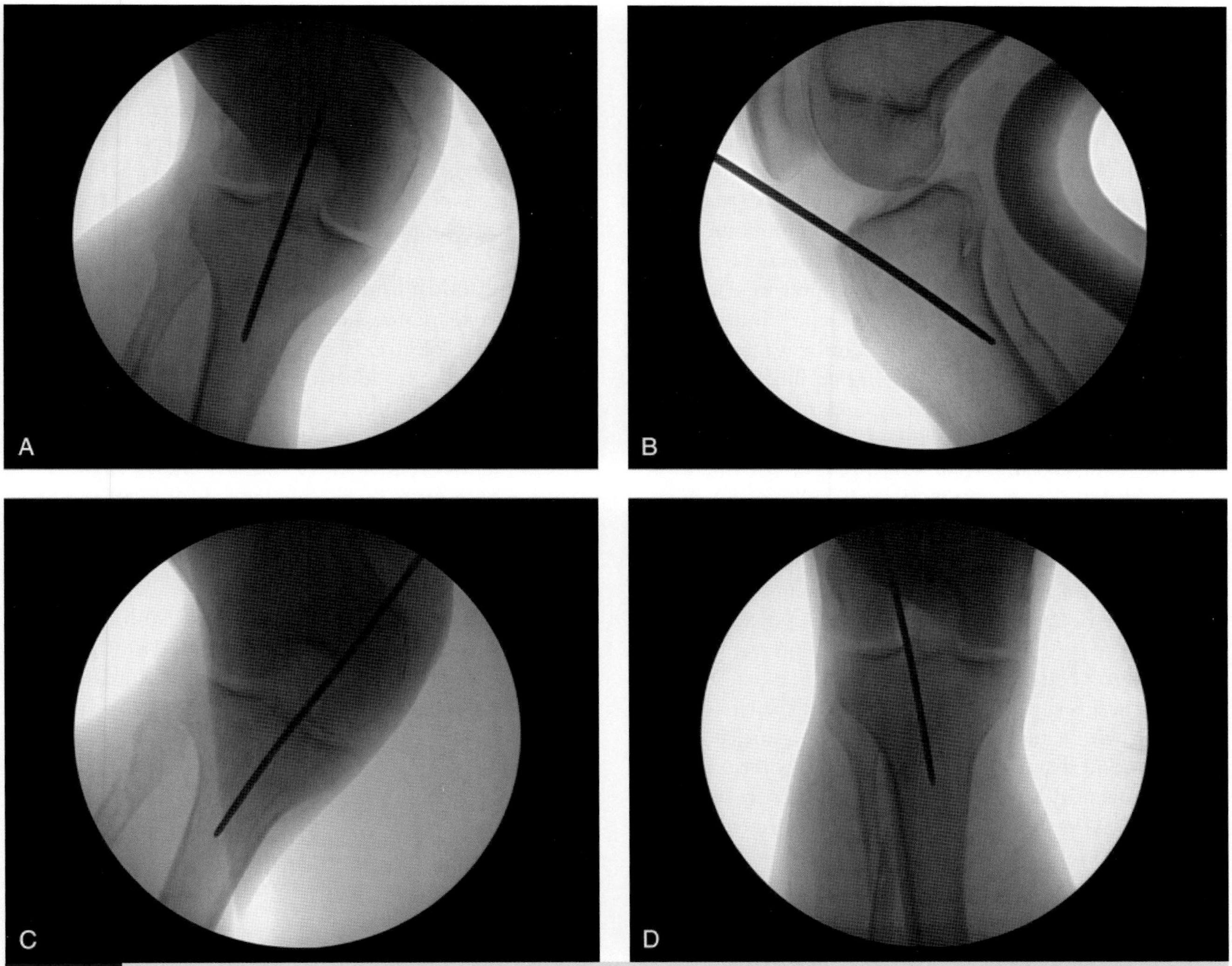

Figure 2 AP **(A)** and lateral **(B)** intraoperative fluoroscopic images showing the correct position of the starting guidewire for intramedullary nailing of a tibial shaft fracture. In **(A)**, the lateral plateau can be seen to bisect the fibular head. Rotation of the leg internally **(C)** or externally **(D)** appears to show the correct wire position as being incorrect.

the anterior proximal tibia, through which the guidewire and nail are inserted. Optimal guidewire positioning is achieved at approximately 50° of knee flexion.[25] In an extra-articular approach, the patella is mobilized and the plane between the patellar tendon and synovium is developed; tissue over the trochlea is retained to minimize contamination of the joint with reamings.[26]

Nail Starting Point

The position of the tibial nail starting point is aligned with the medial border of the lateral tibial spine (on AP fluoroscopy) and the anterior border of the tibial plateau (on lateral fluoroscopy). This starting point places the entry hole for the nail in alignment with the medullary canal of the tibia, where there is little risk of damage to surrounding intra-articular structures.

Actual and apparent guidewire positions can differ greatly, as revealed by rotation of the leg under fluoroscopy during guidewire insertion. For placement of the guidewire in the optimal position, a fluoroscopic AP image of the knee should be obtained in which the lateral border of the tibial plateau bisects the proximal fibula.[27] If the leg is internally or externally rotated, the fibula will not be seen as bisected by the plateau, and the actual guidewire entry position will appear far more medial or lateral than desired. The result could be nail insertion in an incorrect location, which can lead to malreduction[28] (**Figure 2**).

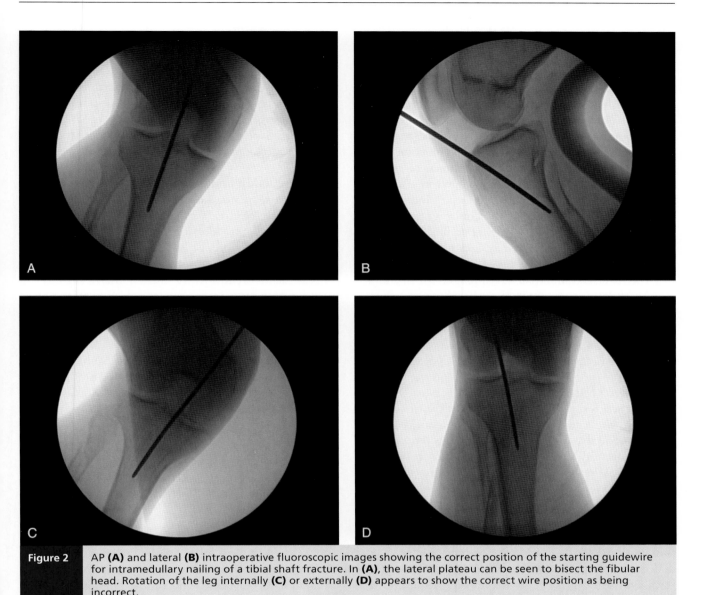

Suprapatellar Versus Infrapatellar Nailing

The suprapatellar and infrapatellar entry points for intramedullary nailing have individual benefits and costs related to reduction, ease of use, and potential damage to surrounding structures. Several studies evaluated each of these techniques with regard to the proximity of the entry point to intra-articular structures. The parapatellar approach was associated with greater bone loss in the proximal tibia and more damage to intra-articular structures, particularly the anterior intermeniscal ligament, than the suprapatellar approach.[29] Injury to the intermeniscal ligament also may occur in as many as 80% of patients treated with suprapatellar nailing.[29,30] Optimal positioning of the entry point may help minimize this risk.

Damage to patellar cartilage often is cited as a reason to avoid using the suprapatellar approach for tibial nailing. An alternative approach can be used to minimize the risk of this damage.[25,27] Although patellofemoral contact pressures are greater during suprapatellar nailing than infrapatellar nailing, the pressures remain below experimental thresholds for inducing chondrocyte apoptosis.[31]

Nail-Screw Constructs

Simple fractures in the mid-diaphysis of the tibia can be stabilized with a nail and a single static interlocking screw proximal and distal to the fracture site. Additional fixation may be needed for a more complex fracture or a proximal or distal metaphyseal fracture. In a proximal-third fracture, a biomechanical study found that increasing the number of proximal interlocking screws increased the load to failure.[32] The correlation with uneventful fracture healing is not known, however. Angular-stable screws can be used for patients with poor bone quality. These screws initially increased resistance against torsional deformation, but this effect did not appear to alter the time to ultimate failure compared with regular screws.[33] In a distal-third fracture treated with intramedullary nailing, adding a third interlocking screw to a construct with two distal interlocking screws increased the construct stiffness and decreased motion at the fracture site.[34]

Reduction Techniques

Multiple tools are available to help with reduction of a tibial shaft fracture during intramedullary nail placement. A universal distractor or external fixator can be applied proximally and distally near the level of the physeal scars to realign the fracture and hold it in position during nailing. Care must be taken to place the pins outside the intended nail trajectory. In addition, unicortical plates can be applied across the fracture to hold the reduction during nail placement. In a proximal-third fracture, this technique is particularly useful to prevent the procurvatum deformity when the knee is flexed for infrapatellar nail preparation and insertion. Blocking screws can be applied on the concave side of the deformity to provide correction when the nail is inserted; practice in determining the optimal placement is required. Percutaneous clamps can be applied, regardless of whether a nail or plate construct is being used, to help reduce and hold the fracture fragments in proper alignment.

Open Reduction and Internal Fixation

If an external fixator is used for temporary fixation before definitive treatment, there may be concern that the plate will overlap the location of the external fixator pins. Available data conflict on whether plate overlap of pin sites increases the risk of infection.[35] One study found a nonsignificant trend toward slightly increased rates of infection correlated with a longer delay to conversion to internal fixation.[36]

Nail Versus Plate Fixation

Outcome studies that compared intramedullary nailing with plating of tibial shaft fractures found no significant differences in the incidence of nonunion. In distal tibial shaft fractures treated with intramedullary nailing, a trend toward an increased rate of fracture nonunion was found when an associated distal fibula fracture also was fixed.[37] Intramedullary nailing was associated with a higher rate of malalignment than with plate fixation. Plate fixation of distal or proximal tibial shaft fractures was associated with a higher rate of implant removal than intramedullary nailing.[37,38]

Patients with multiple traumatic injuries who underwent reamed intramedullary nailing of a long bone fracture were found to have more cognitive dysfunction 1 year after injury than those who did not undergo reamed nailing.[39] Knee pain also is a potential complication of intramedullary nailing, but the pain was found to steadily decrease as the fracture healed to the 20-week mark.[40] After 20 weeks, there appeared to be no correlation between the pain level and progress toward union.

Distal tibial shaft fractures can extend into the articular surface of the plafond or occur with a posterior malleolus fracture. Articular injuries were found in 46% of distal tibial shaft fractures, but only about half of them were detectable on plain radiographs.[41] CT of the ankle is recommended before surgical management if such an injury is identified or suspected on initial radiographs. If an articular fracture is identified, it should be stabilized before intramedullary nailing using screws or a plate-screw construct placed very distal at the level of the epiphyseal scar and outside the intended path of the intramedullary nail.

Fibula fractures commonly occur in conjunction with tibial shaft fractures. Fractures at the fibular head and shaft rarely are fixed. Fibula fixation may be helpful for achieving stability, however, if there is proximal tibiofibular joint disruption or severe tibial comminution. However, distal fibula fractures may require reduction and fixation for ankle stability, particularly if the fracture is at or below the level of the syndesmosis.

Complications

Compartment Syndrome

Compartment syndrome can develop after a fracture of the tibial shaft.[42] The reported incidence varies widely but is higher after a diaphyseal fracture than a proximal or a distal fracture.[43] The exception is fracture caused by a gunshot wound, in which a significantly higher rate of compartment syndrome was found after proximal tibia or proximal fibula fractures than after diaphyseal fractures.[44] Relatively young patients are at increased risk for compartment syndrome, and it is important to note that the presence of an open fracture does not eliminate this risk. Medial condyle fracture dislocation (a Schatzker type IV tibial plateau fracture) appeared to be most likely to lead to compartment syndrome, especially if large portions of the condyle were involved.[45] High-risk fractures often are provisionally stabilized with external fixation for 7 to 14 days before definitive treatment. A high index of suspicion for compartment syndrome must be maintained immediately after external fixation.

Compartment syndrome classically is identified by the presence of paresthesias, paralysis, pulselessness, poikilothermia, pain with passive motion, and pallor (the so-called six Ps). Many of these signs are not present until irreversible muscle and nerve damage have occurred, and therefore they should not be used clinically. Perhaps the only early and reliable signs of compartment syndrome are paresthesias and pain out of proportion to that expected from the injury during passive motion of the ankle or foot. These signs imply compression of the small blood vessels in the limb and resulting early, reversible ischemia, and their presence should prompt emergency fasciotomy to prevent irreversible damage. Manual palpation of compartment firmness has low sensitivity for detection of compartment syndrome and should not be used in isolation.[46]

A patient with a high-energy injury often is closely monitored for compartment syndrome, but compartment syndrome also has been documented after a lower energy fracture sustained during an athletic event. Soccer and football players with a low-energy tibial shaft fracture were found to have five to ten times the risk of compartment syndrome as other patients with a similar fracture.[47] These patients should be monitored for compartment syndrome, and overnight observation may be warranted.

The diagnosis of acute compartment syndrome can be made clinically if the patient is alert. If the patient is obtunded or intubated, commercially available pressure measurement devices can be used to obtain serial or continuous measurements. Accurate pressure measurements can be obtained using bevel tip needles, slit catheters, or an arterial line setup.[48] Careful attention to technique is required, because errors can lead to incorrect measurements. Even with correct technique, as many as 40% of readings were reported to have variability in measurement.[49] Noninvasive methods of identifying compartment syndrome, in particular by detecting a lack of normal hyperemia after trauma in compartments with elevated tissue pressure, are under investigation but not in routine use.[50]

Fasciotomies can be performed using a single- or double-incision technique. In single-incision fasciotomy (also called perifibular fasciotomy), a laterally based incision is made, and all four compartments are released. Care must be taken to expose and release the deep posterior compartment. The benefits of single-incision fasciotomy include a relatively low risk of wound complications and exposure of a relatively small amount of muscle that might require skin graft coverage. Two-incision fasciotomy involves the release of the anterior and lateral compartments through a laterally based incision and release of the superficial posterior and deep posterior compartments through a medially based incision. If the medial incision is too far proximal, the soleus must be taken down for release of the posterior compartment. Both fasciotomy techniques are effective if done in a meticulous and thorough fashion. One study found that single-incision fasciotomy led to slightly a higher rate of fracture nonunion, but there was no difference in infection rates between the two techniques.[51]

Nonunion

Nonunion classically was defined as a failure of fracture healing within 6 months, with no progression of callus formation on three consecutive radiographs. To avoid unnecessary surgical intervention, waiting 6 months after initial fixation was recommended before surgical treatment for nonunion.[52] The patient-associated risk factors for fracture nonunion include tobacco use, diabetes mellitus, segmental bone loss, and infection. Undertaking a smoking cessation program immediately after acute fracture was found to decrease the risk of complications related to healing and infection.[53]

A thorough workup is required to evaluate the cause of a nonunion and plan treatment. The workup should include an evaluation for infection as the possible cause of nonunion. Significant predictors of infection include an elevated erythrocyte sedimentation rate, C-reactive protein level, and intraoperative white blood cell count per high-power field. The positive predictive value of these tests for infection increases with the number of positive results and is as high as 100% if all three tests are positive. There was a greater than 75% probability that infection could be excluded if two or more tests were negative.[54]

Adjuvant treatments including ultrasound and electromagnetic field stimulation have been used to stimulate additional bone formation in concert with or in place of nonunion surgery. These treatments were not found to decrease the incidence of nonunion or delayed union in acute fractures.[55]

Iliac crest autograft commonly is used for bone grafting in the treatment of nonunion. The Reamer/Irrigator/Aspirator system (Synthes) allows more bone for grafting to be harvested from the medullary canals of long bones than can be obtained from the iliac crest. A histologic and genetic comparison of the two types of graft harvest found similar quantities of genetic expression for many of the factors believed to be important for early fracture healing, but expression of BMPs and vascular endothelial growth factor was greater in patients treated with the Reamer/Irrigator/Aspirator system.[56] Percutaneous injection of bone marrow from the iliac crest was found to improve healing in patients treated for nonunion and delayed union without additional surgery.[57]

Infection

Infection remains a concern after fracture stabilization using implants. Seventy-one percent of fractures with an acute postoperative infection went on to union after débridement without chronic infection and with retention of implants and antibiotic suppression. The rates of chronic infection are highest in patients who have an open fracture, are tobacco smokers, undergo intramedullary nail fixation, or have an initial *Pseudomonas* infection.[58] Stress-induced hyperglycemia can occur after trauma, regardless of whether the patient has diabetes. The risk of infection is increased as much as sevenfold in patients with hyperglycemia, even if the average blood glucose level is only 140 mg/dL.[59,60]

Venous Thromboembolism

No evidence supports thromboprophylaxis in patients with an isolated below-the-knee fracture.[61] Patients thought to be at high risk for venous thromboembolism based on the presence of comorbidities or associated injuries should be evaluated for thromboprophylaxis on an individual basis.

Summary

Tibial shaft fractures most often are surgically treated, but in certain patients with acceptable fracture alignment the fracture can be treated nonsurgically using a cast or functional brace. Intramedullary nailing has improved the fixation of more proximal and distal fractures with modified surgical approaches and nails that allow interlocking screw fixation to provide a stable construct. Open fracture treatment continues to evolve, although the optimal timing of antibiotic administration and surgical débridement has not been determined. Tibial shaft fractures carry a high risk for infection, nonunion, and compartment syndrome. Diligent care is required to minimize the risk of these complications.

Key Study Points

- Both nonsurgical and surgical treatment options for tibial shaft fractures have been successful.
- The treatment of open fractures is controversial; the timing of antibiotics, surgical débridement, and wound closure are important factors.
- The likelihood of complications related to the treatment of tibial shaft fractures is high.

Annotated References

1. Trafton P. Tibia Shaft Fractures. In: Browner B, Jupiter J, Levine A, Trafton P, Krettek C, eds. *Skeletal Trauma*, 4th ed. Philadelphia, Saunders, 2009, pp 2319-2451.

2. Sarmiento A: A functional below-the-knee brace for tibial fractures: A report on its use in one hundred thirty-five cases. *J Bone Joint Surg Am* 1970;52(2):295-311.

3. Gustilo RB, Mendoza RM, Williams DN: Problems in the management of type III (severe) open fractures: A new classification of type III open fractures. *J Trauma* 1984;24(8):742-746.

4. Orthopaedic Trauma Association Open Fracture Study Group: A new classification scheme for open fractures. *J Orthop Trauma* 2010;24(8):457-464.

   A review of open fracture classification systems led to a proposed new classification to improve the description of the characteristics of an open fracture, including injury to the skin, muscle, bone, and arteries as well as the level of wound contamination.

5. Schenker ML, Yannascoli S, Baldwin KD, Ahn J, Mehta S: Does timing to operative debridement affect infectious complications in open long-bone fractures? A systematic review. *J Bone Joint Surg Am* 2012;94(12):1057-1064.

In a meta-analysis of time to surgical débridement as a risk factor for infection and other complications, no significant association was found, nor was the site of open fracture significant. Level of evidence: III.

6. Hull PD, Johnson SC, Stephen DJ, Kreder HJ, Jenkinson RJ: Delayed debridement of severe open fractures is associated with a higher rate of deep infection. *Bone Joint J* 2014;96-B(3):379-384.

The risk of deep infection was increased in type II and III fractures by 3% with each hour of delay. Severity of fracture, gross contamination, and tibia fracture were significant additional factors. Level of evidence: IV.

7. Pollak AN, Jones AL, Castillo RC, Bosse MJ, MacKenzie EJ; LEAP Study Group: The relationship between time to surgical debridement and incidence of infection after open high-energy lower extremity trauma. *J Bone Joint Surg Am* 2010;92(1):7-15.

A subanalysis of the LEAP study evaluated the risk of infection in major open lower extremity fractures. Increased time from injury to arrival at the treating facility was a statistically significant predictor of infection. Time from injury to surgical débridement was not a significant predictor. Level of evidence: II.

8. Lack WD, Karunakar MA, Angerame MR, et al: Type III open tibia fractures: Immediate antibiotic prophylaxis minimizes infection. *J Orthop Trauma* 2015;29(1):1-6.

A retrospective study evaluated risk factors for deep infection in open type III tibia fractures. Significant risk factors included initial antibiotic administration more than 66 minutes after injury and wound coverage more than 5 days from injury. Level of evidence: II.

9. Weber D, Dulai SK, Bergman J, Buckley R, Beaupre LA: Time to initial operative treatment following open fracture does not impact development of deep infection: A prospective cohort study of 736 subjects. *J Orthop Trauma* 2014;28(11):613-619.

A study of three trauma centers found that time to antibiotic administration and time to initial surgery were not risk factors for infection after open fracture, but severity of type of open fracture was significant.

10. Anglen JO: Comparison of soap and antibiotic solutions for irrigation of lower-limb open fracture wounds: A prospective, randomized study. *J Bone Joint Surg Am* 2005;87(7):1415-1422.

11. Petrisor B, Sun X, Bhandari M, et al; FLOW Investigators: Fluid lavage of open wounds (FLOW): A multicenter, blinded, factorial pilot trial comparing alternative irrigating solutions and pressures in patients with open fractures. *J Trauma* 2011;71(3):596-606.

Comparison of low- or high-pressure lavage and normal saline or castile soap irrigation for open fractures found no significant difference in infection rates or nonunions. There was a trend toward improved outcomes with low-pressure irrigation. Level of evidence: I.

12. Bhandari M, Jeray KJ, Petrisor BA, et al; FLOW Investigators: A trial of wound irrigation in the initial management of open fracture wounds. *N Engl J Med* 2015;373(27):2629-2641.

A randomized study of open fractures found no significant difference in reoperation rate based on irrigation pressure. The use of soap solution led to a higher rate of reoperation than the use of plain saline irrigation.

13. Lenarz CJ, Watson JT, Moed BR, Israel H, Mullen JD, Macdonald JB: Timing of wound closure in open fractures based on cultures obtained after debridement. *J Bone Joint Surg Am* 2010;92(10):1921-1926.

A retrospective analysis of an open fracture protocol involving repeat débridement every 2 days after a positive culture until cultures were negative found that diabetes and high body mass index had a significant effect on infection rate. Level of evidence: IV.

14. Stannard JP, Volgas DA, Stewart R, McGwin G Jr, Alonso JE: Negative pressure wound therapy after severe open fractures: A prospective randomized study. *J Orthop Trauma* 2009;23(8):552-557.

15. Blum ML, Esser M, Richardson M, Paul E, Rosenfeldt FL: Negative pressure wound therapy reduces deep infection rate in open tibial fractures. *J Orthop Trauma* 2012;26(9):499-505.

A retrospective cohort study of 211 tibial fractures treated with conventional dressings or negative pressure wound therapy found a 78% reduction in the infection rate in fractures treated with negative pressure wound therapy. Level of evidence: III.

16. Wood T, Sameem M, Avram R, Bhandari M, Petrisor B: A systematic review of early versus delayed wound closure in patients with open fractures requiring flap coverage. *J Trauma Acute Care Surg* 2012;72(4):1078-1085.

A systematic review of the literature found that flap coverage within 72 hours was associated with a decreased infection risk and a nonsignificant trend toward lower complication rates. Level of evidence: I.

17. Meeker J, Weinhold P, Dahners L: Negative pressure therapy on primarily closed wounds improves wound healing parameters at 3 days in a porcine model. *J Orthop Trauma* 2011;25(12):756-761.

An animal study compared incisional negative pressure dressings with conventional pressure dressings. After 3 days, negative pressure–treated wounds had a statistically higher load and energy to failure and less hematoma compared with conventionally dressed wounds.

18. Stannard JP, Volgas DA, McGwin G III, et al: Incisional negative pressure wound therapy after high-risk lower extremity fractures. *J Orthop Trauma* 2012;26(1):37-42.

A multicenter prospective randomized controlled study compared wound complications with the use of standard dressings with negative pressure wound therapy in patients with high-energy lower leg fractures. The incidence of infection and wound dehiscence was significantly lower in patients with negative pressure therapy. Level of evidence: I.

19. Govender S, Csimma C, Genant HK, Valentin-Opran A, Amit Y, Arbel R,Aro H, et al; BMP-2 Evaluation in Surgery for Tibial Trauma (BESTT) Study Group: Recombinant human bone morphogenic protein-2 for treatment of open tibia fractures: A prospective, controlled, randomized study for four hundred and fifty patients. *J Bone Joint Surg Am* 2002;84(12):2123-2134.

20. Aro HT, Govender S, Patel AD, et al: Recombinant human bone morphogenetic protein-2: A randomized trial in open tibial fractures treated with reamed nail fixation. *J Bone Joint Surg Am* 2011;93(9):801-808.

A randomized blinded study of open tibia fractures treated with reamed intramedullary nailing with or without the addition of rhBMP-2 at the fracture site found no significant difference with regard to time to union, infection rate, or need for additional procedures. Level of evidence: I.

21. Schemitsch EH, Bhandari M, Guyatt G, et al; Study to Prospectively Evaluate Reamed Intramedullary Nails in Patients with Tibial Fractures (SPRINT) Investigators: Prognostic factors for predicting outcomes after intramedullary nailing of the tibia. *J Bone Joint Surg Am* 2012;94(19):1786-1793.

Multivariate analysis of risk factors for negative outcomes after intramedullary nailing found greater risk in open fractures treated with reamed nailing compared with those treated with unreamed nailing. Level of evidence: II.

22. Ricci WM, Gallagher B, Brandt A, Schwappach J, Tucker M, Leighton R: Is after-hours orthopaedic surgery associated with adverse outcomes? A prospective comparative study. *J Bone Joint Surg Am* 2009;91(9):2067-2072.

23. Schenker ML, Ahn J, Donegan D, Mehta S, Baldwin KD: The cost of after-hours operative debridement of open tibia fractures. *J Orthop Trauma* 2014;28(11):626-631.

The cost of after-hours surgical débridement was higher in facilities that used on-call staff requiring overtime pay compared with facilities having in-house staff.

24. Tornetta P III, Collins E: Semiextended position of intramedullary nailing of the proximal tibia. *Clin Orthop Relat Res* 1996;328:185-189.

25. Eastman J, Tseng S, Lo E, Li CS, Yoo B, Lee M: Retropatellar technique for intramedullary nailing of proximal tibia fractures: A cadaveric assessment. *J Orthop Trauma* 2010;24(11):672-676.

In a technique for suprapatellar nailing through a small longitudinal split in the quadriceps tendon, optimal positioning of the guidewire was achieved with increasing flexion of the knee more than 20°, with the highest rate of correct positioning at 50°.

26. Kubiak EN, Widmer BJ, Horwitz DS: Extra-articular technique for semiextended tibial nailing. *J Orthop Trauma* 2010;24(11):704-708.

In a technique for semiextended nailing that avoids violating the joint surface, the patella is mobilized and an incision is made deep to the tendon and superficial to the synovium to prevent articular contamination from reaming.

27. Walker RM, Zdero R, McKee MD, Waddell JP, Schemitsch EH: Ideal tibial intramedullary nail insertion point varies with tibial rotation. *J Orthop Trauma* 2011;25(12):726-730.

A cadaver study evaluated the effect of tibial rotation on the appearance of the correct entry point for nails under fluoroscopy. An AP image with the fibular head bisected by the lateral tibial plateau provided the most accurate view.

28. Buehler KC, Green J, Woll TS, Duwelius PJ: A technique for intramedullary nailing of proximal third tibia fractures. *J Orthop Trauma* 1997;11(3):218-223.

29. Bible JE, Choxi AA, Dhulipala S, Evans JM, Mir HR: Quantification of anterior cortical bone removal and intermeniscal ligament damage at the tibial nail entry zone using parapatellar and retropatellar approaches. *J Orthop Trauma* 2013;27(8):437-441.

A cadaver study examined damage from the opening reamer in infrapatellar and suprapatellar approaches. The parapatellar approach caused more bone loss and more damage to intra-articular structures, most commonly the anterior intermeniscal ligament.

30. Eastman JG, Tseng SS, Lee MA, Yoo BJ: The retropatellar portal as an alternative site for tibial nail insertion: A cadaveric study. *J Orthop Trauma* 2010;24(11):659-664.

A cadaver study determined the entry position for a suprapatellar nail and the proximity of this position to intra-articular structures about the knee. The intermeniscal ligament was at highest risk of damage in 80% of specimens.

31. Gelbke MK, Coombs D, Powell S, DiPasquale TG: Suprapatellar versus infra-patellar intramedullary nail insertion of the tibia: A cadaveric model for comparison of patellofemoral contact pressures and forces. *J Orthop Trauma* 2010;24(11):665-671.

A cadaver study measured contact pressures on articular cartilage with infrapatellar and suprapatellar nailing. Suprapatellar nailing caused approximately twice the mean peak contact pressures of infrapatellar nailing but remained far below the threshold for inducing chondrocyte apoptosis.

32. Freeman AL, Craig MR, Schmidt AH: Biomechanical comparison of tibial nail stability in a proximal third fracture: Do screw quantity and locked, interlocking screws make a difference? *J Orthop Trauma* 2011;25(6):333-339.

In a biomechanical evaluation of tibial nail locking constructs, several different nails had screw interlocks placed proximally. An osteotomy simulated a fracture with bone loss. A nail with four proximal screws that locked into the nail had the greatest resistance to failure.

33. Gueorguiev B, Ockert B, Schwieger K, et al: Angular stability potentially permits fewer locking screws compared with conventional locking in intramedullary nailed distal tibia fractures: A biomechanical study. *J Orthop Trauma* 2011;25(6):340-346.

A biomechanical study compared stiffness and failure of tibial nail constructs. Constructs with angular stable interlocking screws had lower torsional deformation than constructs with conventional screws for the first 1,000 cycles. The number of cycles to failure was similar in the two constructs.

34. Chan DS, Nayak AN, Blaisdell G, et al: Effect of distal interlocking screw number and position after intramedullary nailing of distal tibial fractures: A biomechanical study simulating immediate weight-bearing. *J Orthop Trauma* 2015;29(2):98-104.

An evaluation of distal locking constructs found that those with three interlocking screws had greater stiffness and less fracture motion than those with two distal interlocking screws, with or without a blocking screw

35. Shah CM, Babb PE, McAndrew CM, et al: Definitive plates overlapping provisional external fixator pin sites: Is the infection risk increased? *J Orthop Trauma* 2014;28(9):518-522.

A retrospective comparison study compared infection rates in patients who had or did not have a definitive implant that crossed external fixator pin sites. Infection rates were increased if the plate crossed the pin sites. Level of evidence: III.

36. Laible C, Earl-Royal E, Davidovitch R, Walsh M, Egol KA: Infection after spanning external fixation for high-energy tibial plateau fractures: Is pin site-plate overlap a problem? *J Orthop Trauma* 2012;26(2):92-97.

A retrospective review of a trauma database that compared patients with or without definitive constructs that overlapped external fixator pin sites found no increase in the infection rate with pin site overlap. Level of evidence: III.

37. Vallier HA, Cureton BA, Patterson BM: Randomized, prospective comparison of plate versus intramedullary nail fixation for distal tibia shaft fractures. *J Orthop Trauma* 2011;25(12):736-741.

A prospective randomized study compared distal tibia intramedullary nailing to plating. A higher rate of nonunion was found with open fractures, and a higher incidence of malalignment was found with nailing. No significant between-group difference in nonunion rate was found. Level of evidence: I.

38. Lindvall E, Sanders R, Dipasquale T, Herscovici D, Haidukewych G, Sagi C: Intramedullary nailing versus percutaneous locked plating of extra-articular proximal tibial fractures: Comparison of 56 cases. *J Orthop Trauma* 2009;23(7):485-492.

39. Richards JE, Guillamondegui OD, Archer KR, Jackson JC, Ely EW, Obremskey WT: The association of reamed intramedullary nailing and long-term cognitive impairment. *J Orthop Trauma* 2011;25(12):707-713.

In a prospective study of long-term neurologic outcomes in patients with multiple trauma, patients who underwent reamed intramedullary nailing of a long bone fracture had a greater cognitive dysfunction than other patients. Level of evidence: II.

40. Ryan SP, Tornetta P III, Dielwart C, Kaye-Krall E: Knee pain correlates with union after tibial nailing. *J Orthop Trauma* 2011;25(12):731-735.

A retrospective study of knee pain in tibial fractures treated with intramedullary nailing found that knee pain diminished to the 20-week point as the fracture healed. Beyond 20 weeks, there was no correlation between knee pain and progress toward union. Level of evidence: IV.

41. Purnell GJ, Glass ER, Altman DT, Sciulli RL, Muffly MT, Altman GT: Results of a computed tomography protocol evaluating distal third tibial shaft fractures to assess noncontiguous malleolar fractures. *J Trauma* 2011;71(1):163-168.

A prospective CT study found an associated intra-articular malleolar fracture in 43% of distal tibial shaft fractures. Fixation of the articular fracture was required in 56% for instability or a fragment larger than 25% of the articular surface. Level of evidence: II.

42. McQueen MM, Gaston P, Court-Brown CM: Acute compartment syndrome: Who is at risk? *J Bone Joint Surg Br* 2000;82(2):200-203.

43. Park S, Ahn J, Gee AO, Kuntz AF, Esterhai JL: Compartment syndrome in tibial fractures. *J Orthop Trauma* 2009;23(7):514-518.

44. Meskey T, Hardcastle J, O'Toole RV: Are certain fractures at increased risk for compartment syndrome after civilian ballistic injury? *J Trauma* 2011;71(5):1385-1389.

A retrospective review of fractures after ballistic injury found that compartment syndrome occurred in 3.5% and only tibia and fibula fractures had significantly higher rates (11.4% and 11.6%, respectively). Proximal fractures and associated arterial injury were most likely to lead to compartment syndrome. Level of evidence: IV.

45. Stark E, Stucken C, Trainer G, Tornetta P III: Compartment syndrome in Schatzker type VI plateau fractures and medial condylar fracture-dislocations treated

with temporary external fixation. *J Orthop Trauma* 2009;23(7):502-506.

46. Shuler FD, Dietz MJ: Physicians' ability to manually detect isolated elevations in leg intracompartmental pressure. *J Bone Joint Surg Am* 2010;92(2):361-367.

A cadaver study found that the ability of orthopaedic residents and faculty members to detect elevated pressure in one of four compartments of the leg was poor using manual palpation.

47. Wind TC, Saunders SM, Barfield WR, Mooney JF III, Hartsock LA: Compartment syndrome after low-energy tibia fractures sustained during athletic competition. *J Orthop Trauma* 2012;26(1):33-36.

A retrospective review of tibia fractures found a 5.4% rate of compartment syndrome. Patients who sustained a fracture playing soccer or football had a significantly greater rate of compartment syndrome (55.4% or 27.3%, respectively) than other patients. Level of evidence: III.

48. Hammerberg EM, Whitesides TE Jr, Seiler JG III: The reliability of measurement of tissue pressure in compartment syndrome. *J Orthop Trauma* 2012;26(1):24-31, discussion 32.

A laboratory study compared pressure measurements obtained using different types of needles for measurement of compartment syndrome in a standardized model. With the use of a digital transducer, there was no statistically significant variation in measurements regardless of type of needle or catheter used.

49. Large TM, Agel J, Holtzman DJ, Benirschke SK, Krieg JC: Interobserver variability in the measurement of lower leg compartment pressures. *J Orthop Trauma* 2015;29(7):316-321.

A cadaver study with known compartment pressures evaluated variation in pressure readings when a standard pressure monitor system was used. Only 60% of measurements obtained using proper technique were within 5 mm Hg of actual pressure.

50. Shuler MS, Reisman WM, Kinsey TL, et al: Correlation between muscle oxygenation and compartment pressures in acute compartment syndrome of the leg. *J Bone Joint Surg Am* 2010;92(4):863-870.

A prospective study correlated the ability to diagnose compartment syndrome on clinical examination with intracompartmental monitoring using near-infrared spectroscopy. There was a lack of hyperemia in compartments with elevated pressure in the injured leg. Level of evidence: II.

51. Bible JE, McClure DJ, Mir HR: Analysis of single-incision versus dual-incision fasciotomy for tibial fractures with acute compartment syndrome. *J Orthop Trauma* 2013;27(11):607-611.

In a retrospective evaluation of nonunion and infection in patients undergoing single- or double-incision fasciotomy for acute compartment syndrome after tibia fracture, those with a single-incision procedure had a nonsignificantly higher incidence of nonunion. Level of evidence: III.

52. Study to Prospectively Evaluate Reamed Intramedullary Nails in Patients with Tibial Fractures Investigators;Bhandari M, Guyatt G, Tornetta P III, et al: Randomized trial of reamed and unreamed intramedullary nailing of tibial shaft fractures. *J Bone Joint Surg Am* 2008;90(12):2567-2578.

53. Nåsell H, Adami J, Samnegård E, Tønnesen H, Ponzer S: Effect of smoking cessation intervention on results of acute fracture surgery: A randomized controlled trial. *J Bone Joint Surg Am* 2010;92(6):1335-1342.

In a randomized blinded study of complication rates in patients with acute fracture, patients assigned to a smoking cessation program had a higher rate of abstinence from smoking than other patients at 2-week follow-up and were at less risk for one or more complications. Level of evidence: I.

54. Stucken C, Olszewski DC, Creevy WR, Murakami AM, Tornetta P III: Preoperative diagnosis of infection in patients with nonunions. *J Bone Joint Surg Am* 2013;95(15):1409-1412.

In an evaluation of a preoperative laboratory protocol for nonunion, erythrocyte sedimentation rate and C-reactive protein level were significant predictors of nonunion. Combining positive tests improved the positive predictive value for infection. The presence of more than two negative test results had a negative predictive value higher than 75%. Level of evidence: III.

55. Adie S, Harris IA, Naylor JM, et al: Pulsed electromagnetic field stimulation for acute tibial shaft fractures: A multicenter, double-blind, randomized trial. *J Bone Joint Surg Am* 2011;93(17):1569-1576.

A prospective randomized study compared the use of pulsed electromagnetic fields and placebo in acute tibial shaft fractures. There was no significant improvement in the incidence of nonunion or delayed union or patient satisfaction with early use of electromagnetic stimulation. Level of evidence: I.

56. Sagi HC, Young ML, Gerstenfeld L, Einhorn TA, Tornetta P: Qualitative and quantitative differences between bone graft obtained from the medullary canal (with a Reamer/Irrigator/Aspirator) and the iliac crest of the same patient. *J Bone Joint Surg Am* 2012;94(23):2128-2135.

Cancellous graft was harvested from the iliac crest and the femur or tibia on the same patient and compared histologically and genetically. The Reamer/Irrigator/Aspirator graft had overexpression of BMP and vascular endothelial growth factor compared with iliac crest.

57. Braly HL, O'Connor DP, Brinker MR: Percutaneous autologous bone marrow injection in the treatment of distal meta-diaphyseal tibial nonunions and delayed unions. *J Orthop Trauma* 2013;27(9):527-533.

In a case study of patients with tibial metadiaphyseal nonunion who underwent percutaneous injection of posterior iliac crest bone marrow at the nonunion site, 82% of patients healed without any need for a change in implants or additional débridement at the nonunion site. Level of evidence: IV.

58. Berkes M, Obremskey WT, Scannell B, Ellington JK, Hymes RA, Bosse M; Southeast Fracture Consortium: Maintenance of hardware after early postoperative infection following fracture internal fixation. *J Bone Joint Surg Am* 2010;92(4):823-828.

    In a retrospective study of osseous union and chronic infection after acute postoperative infection, 71% of patients had union with retained hardware. Relatively high rates of chronic infection were found in patients who were tobacco smokers or had an open fracture, an intramedullary nail, a *Pseudomonas* infection, or a lower extremity fracture. Level of evidence: IV.

59. Karunakar MA, Staples KS: Does stress-induced hyperglycemia increase the risk of perioperative infectious complications in orthopaedic trauma patients? *J Orthop Trauma* 2010;24(12):752-756.

    A retrospective analysis of trauma patients found a seven times higher risk of perioperative infection in patients with a hyperglycemic index higher than 3.0 (an average blood glucose level higher than 220 mg/dL) than in patients with a lower hyperglycemic index. Level of evidence: IV.

60. Richards JE, Kauffmann RM, Obremskey WT, May AK: Stress-induced hyperglycemia as a risk factor for surgical-site infection in nondiabetic orthopedic trauma patients admitted to the intensive care unit. *J Orthop Trauma* 2013;27(1):16-21.

    A retrospective study evaluated the effect of hyperglycemia on the risk of surgical site infection in orthopaedic trauma patients without a known history of diabetes. An elevated hyperglycemic index (correlated with an average blood glucose level higher than 139 mg/dL [odds ratio, 1.8]) was a significant risk factor. Level of evidence: IV.

61. Goel DP, Buckley R, deVries G, Abelseth G, Ni A, Gray R: Prophylaxis of deep-vein thrombosis in fractures below the knee: A prospective randomised controlled trial. *J Bone Joint Surg Br* 2009;91(3):388-394.

Chapter 45

Ankle Fractures

Patrick M. Osborn, MD, Lt Col, USAF, MC

Abstract

Ankle fractures remain among the most commonly encountered injuries. An abundance of new research has been conducted on the radiographic evaluation of ankle fractures, particularly in syndesmotic injuries. Small fragment constructs continue to be used with good results. The significance of posterior malleolus fractures to ankle stability has been noted and has increased the use of the posterior approach for fixation. Anatomic reduction remains the goal of treatment. To attain this goal, substantial research has been performed to identify intraoperative malreductions. Geriatric fractures are seen in increasing numbers and may require novel fixation constructs because of the poor bone quality in the aged population.

Keywords: malleolar ankle fractures; syndesmosis injury; outcomes of ankle fractures

Introduction

Ankle fractures remain one of the most commonly treated types of fractures in the United States. Injuries range from low-energy rotational injuries that may be treated nonsurgically to severe fracture-dislocations with soft-tissue compromise requiring surgical treatment and often leading to substantial postinjury morbidity. Although these injuries are common, management can be difficult, and multiple treatment pitfalls exist that can negatively affect patient outcomes.

Ankle Anatomy

The ankle joint is composed of the talus, which sits in the mortise created by the tibial plafond and the more posterolateral fibula. The stability of the ankle is conferred partly by the bony anatomy of the talus seated in the mortise. The lateral and medial malleoli provide bony restraints to lateral and medial translation, respectively. The posterior curvature of the plafond is referred to as the posterior malleolus and provides a constraint to posterior translation of the talus and a ligamentous anchor of the syndesmosis. The talus is shaped like a trapezoid that is wider in the anterior body than in the posterior body. Therefore, dorsiflexion of the ankle widens the mortise as the fibula migrates proximally and externally rotates through the syndesmosis. Medial ligamentous support of the tibiotalar joint is provided primarily by the deep deltoid ligament, which limits lateral translation and external rotation of the talus in the mortise. Disruption of the deep deltoid in association with a lateral injury creates an unstable ankle joint that may require surgical fixation.

The fibula sits posterior to the anterior colliculus of the lateral tibia and is supported by the anterior-inferior tibiofibular ligament, the posterior-inferior tibiofibular ligament (PITFL), the interosseous ligament, and the interosseous membrane. The PITFL provides most of the ligamentous support. Vigilance for a greater degree of ankle and syndesmosis instability must be maintained even in the absence of a posterior malleolus fracture.

Radiographic Analysis

Understanding the normal anatomy of the ankle is critical to the radiographic analysis of ankle fractures. The medial clear space should measure less than 5 mm on AP and mortise radiographic views. The tibiofibular clear space should be no more than 6 mm on the AP and mortise views. In most patients, at least a 1-mm overlap of the fibula on the tibial incisura should be seen on the mortise view. A recent study noted a population with less than 1 mm of overlap on the mortise view as being a normal variant. In this case, further evaluation of syndesmosis instability with comparison to the uninjured ankle's radiographs may be warranted.[1] On a good talar lateral radiograph, the posterior edge of the fibula should align with the edge of the posterior subchondral bone of the tibia. This relationship between the tibia and fibula is

Neither Dr. Osborn nor any immediate family member has received anything of value from or has stock or stock options held in a commercial company or institution related directly or indirectly to the subject of this chapter.

especially helpful in the operating room to assess syndesmotic reduction.[2]

Incompetence of the deltoid can be determined radiographically by several means. Gravity and external rotation stress tests are both reliable tests to detect injury to the deep deltoid. Ultrasound is sensitive and specific and provides a more pain-free method of evaluating an unstable ankle fracture.[3] MRI was compared with external rotation stress views in a 2014 study of supination-external rotation (SER) injuries. The authors found that all patients demonstrated deltoid injury when a stress view was used for evaluation, regardless of medial clear space widening. The use of MRI for surgical decision making was not recommended.[4]

CT provides excellent detail in evaluating the syndesmosis, especially in comparison with the contralateral side.[5] Although variations in the larger population are found, very little difference in syndesmosis alignment exists between ankles in individuals. In one series, 24% of patients experienced a change in the surgical plan based on CT findings. Plans were altered most often for patients with trimalleolar ankle fractures, dislocations, suprasyndesmotic fractures, and fractures obscured by plaster.[6] Many of these findings likely are defined by critically reviewing available radiographs.

The initial assessment of ankle fractures includes an evaluation of the soft-tissue envelope and the neurovascular status. A carefully documented motor and sensory examination also should be performed. In the absence of abnormal neurologic or vascular signs, radiographs of the ankle before reduction may allow better characterization of the fracture characteristics and more appropriate initial treatment than postreduction films that can be obscured by splint material.[7] Unlike pilon fractures, most ankle fractures are amenable to early fixation. A series of closed ankle fractures found that early fixation resulted in better patient outcomes and fewer complications.[8] A series of open ankle fractures also showed reasonable complication rates with immediate surgical fixation.[9]

The AO/Orthopaedic Trauma Association (OTA), Danis-Weber, and Lauge-Hansen classification systems of ankle fractures often are used and may aid in directing treatment. The latter system demonstrates typical fractures that may be dependent on the position of the foot and the direction of forces at the time of injury. The OTA and Danis-Weber classifications are based on the location of the fibula fracture and the elements of the ankle joint that are fractured. Depending on the fracture type, the treating surgeon may plan a fixation strategy or anticipate syndesmosis instability. A pilon variant has been recognized in some posterior malleolus fractures[10] (**Figure 1**). In a review of posterior malleolus fractures, this posteromedial variant comprised 40% of all posterior malleolus fractures.[10] It was seen more commonly in older patients, females, and patients with diabetes mellitus. It was surmised that this variant represents a different mechanism than a purely rotational injury. This variant should be suspected in cases in which a double density sign is seen on the posteromedial aspect of the medial malleolus. Another study recognized this type as a hyperplantar flexion injury and termed the pathognomonic posteromedial radiographic finding the spur sign, which was found in 79% of these injuries.[11] In both studies, this fracture pattern was noted to be more common in SER type IV injuries. The latter study noted a high occurrence of ankle fracture-dislocations associated with this variant.

Treatment

Bimalleolar ankle fractures or an equivalent fracture such as the lateral malleolus fracture with deep deltoid injury are considered unstable and often require open anatomic reduction and internal fixation. Instability can be observed on injury radiographs in many cases; in other cases, external rotation or gravity stress tests should be performed after local or general anesthesia is administered to determine instability. Anatomic reduction of the talus under the mortise is required, because minimal displacements of the talus can lead to greatly increased joint contact pressures. For stable Danis-Weber type A and B ankle fractures without talar subluxation, however, one study found that good functional and pain results were obtained when the mortise remained reduced despite late displacement of the fibula.[12]

Multiple options for fixation are available, so fixation can be tailored to the fracture characteristics. Lag screw fixation with a lateral neutralization plate has been a common construct. Lag screw-only constructs also have had success, depending on the length of the fracture. Locking plate technology gives additional options for fractures with comminution or in osteoporotic bone; however, no specific benefits of locked plates have been shown over unlocked plates. Percutaneous methods of fixation may be beneficial to protect soft-tissue injuries. A recent review of intramedullary fixation of the fibula showed excellent results using a nail or intramedullary screws; however, no superiority over more standard techniques was noted.[13] A recent review of 111 medial malleolus fractures of multiple configurations showed good results for most constructs except Kirschner wires. Small fractures below the talar shoulder were treated effectively with lag screws or tension band constructs, but the tension band group required fewer revisions and encountered fewer complications at 6-month follow-up.[14] An additional option for smaller medial malleolus fractures not amenable to screw fixation may be a new hook plate type of device designed to capture the distal tip of the medial malleolus. This construct was shown to be equivalent in torsion and load to failure when compared to lag screws in a biomechanical study.[15] In a 2013 randomized trial, it was suggested that fixation may not be required for minimally displaced medial malleoli in unstable ankle fractures. Similar outcomes and a similar incidence of arthritis were noted in the no fixation group when the medial malleolus had residual displacement of 2 mm or less after fixation of the fibula.[16]

The presence of a posterior malleolus fracture resulted in poorer pain outcomes and functional outcomes at 1-year follow-up than when no posterior malleolus fracture was present. These differences were less prominent at the 2-year follow-up, suggesting that these fractures are more severe injuries, and patients may take longer to recover function.[17] Fragment size is typically the guide used in making the decision to specifically address the posterior malleolus, although precise recommendations have varied. A retrospective review of 131 isolated ankle fractures with associated posterior malleolus fractures noted a greater incidence of radiographic posttraumatic arthritis (PTA) in fragments involving more than 5% of the joint surface. An increased risk of PTA also was observed when the postoperative reduction showed a step-off greater than 1 mm. At a mean of 6.9 years, no difference in function was observed despite the size of the fragment.[18] The PITFL attachment to the posterior malleolus fragment plays a critical role in ankle stability. For larger fragments, the ligamentous attachments of the syndesmosis are likely intact, and anatomic reduction and rigid fixation of the posterior malleolus should restore the normal alignment and stability of the distal tibiofibular joint. Syndesmosis stability still must be confirmed in all cases, however. Stable fixation can be achieved with screws or a buttress plate. A 2014 study compared posterior buttress plating with screw fixation through an open posterolateral approach. No distinct advantage of either construct was shown.[19] Another study compared percutaneous reduction and anterior to posterior screw fixation with open reduction and fixation through a posterolateral approach. The latter group was noted to have more improved function over the screw-only group. Postoperative reductions were similar between groups, but the authors suggested that directly treating the posterior malleolus fracture may have a positive effect.[20]

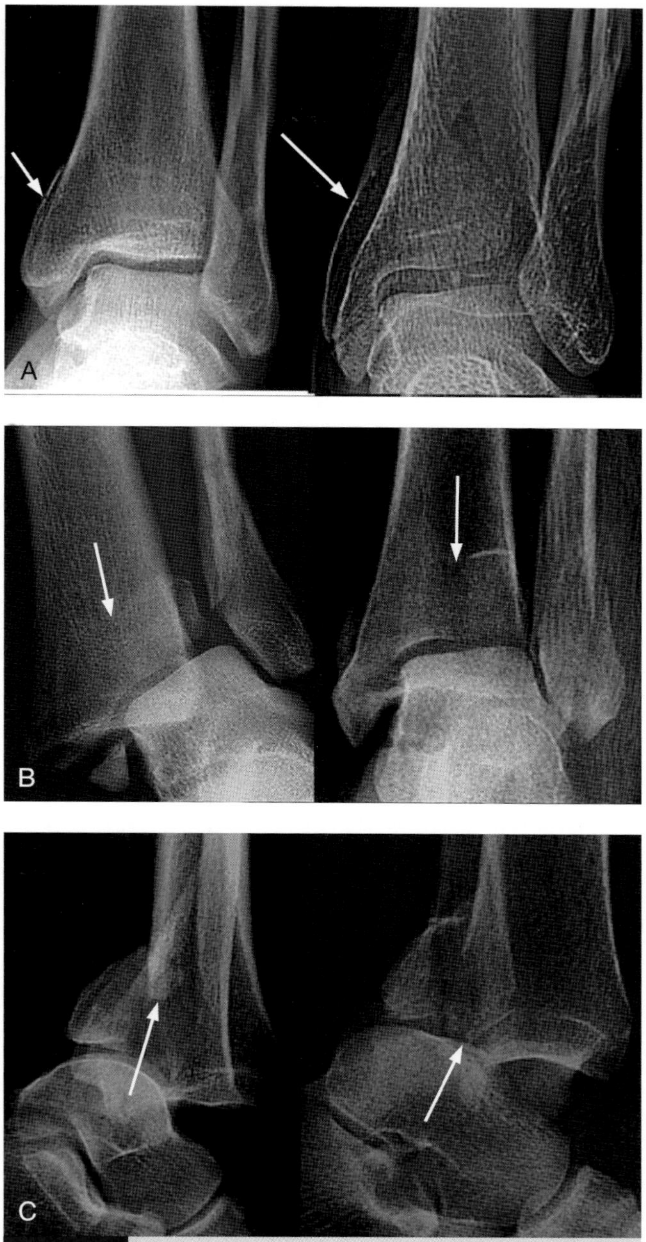

Figure 1 Radiographs show the posterior pilon variant fracture pattern. Arrows on the AP radiograph (**A**) highlight the medial malleolus double contour sign. The ankle on the right shows greater displacement of the medial fragment, with resulting posterior subluxation of the talus. Mortise view (**B**) of both ankles shows the additional sagittal split of the posterior malleolus (arrows). Lateral radiographs (**C**) demonstrate displacement of the posterior malleolus, with the arrows showing the coronal fracture in the posterior malleolus and an articular impaction piece in both images. (Reproduced with permission from Switaj PJ, Weatherford B, Fuchs D, et al: Evaluation of posterior malleolar fractures and the posterior pilon variant in operatively treated ankle fractures. *Foot Ankle Int* 2014:35[9]:886-895.)

Syndesmosis Injury

For any ankle fracture, it is imperative that the syndesmosis be evaluated for instability and that appropriate reduction and stabilization be performed if needed. Radiographs and advanced imaging can indicate syndesmotic instability, as described previously. After fixation of the other fractures involved, the syndesmosis can be evaluated under fluoroscopy with lateral traction on the fibula using a bone hook or a pointed reduction tenaculum, or with external rotation stress. Gapping of the syndesmosis or widening of the medial clear space indicates syndesmosis instability in either test. Studies comparing the Cotton test with external rotation stress show somewhat conflicting results. One study showed that both of these tests were highly specific in detecting a syndesmosis injury in SER fractures but that their sensitivity was questionable.[21] Another study demonstrated significantly greater medial clear space widening with manual stress external rotation.[22] Predicting syndesmosis injury based on fracture type or on the site of the fibula fracture is difficult. To date, no clinical evidence shows improved patient outcomes using a particular test to evaluate the syndesmosis.

Malreduction of the syndesmosis, particularly rotational malalignment, appears to be more common than previously appreciated. Determining rotational malalignment, especially external rotation malalignment, is difficult to gauge with fluoroscopy.[23] A CT study of normal ankles showed that, in most patients, the fibula sits anterior or central in the syndesmosis. The authors concluded that posterior translation of the fibula may indicate a malreduction. Alignment of the fibula in each ankle of individual patients was consistent.[24] Therefore, on a bilateral ankle CT, any displacement of the fibula on the injured ankle not seen on the uninjured side may indicate a syndesmosis injury. Such an evaluation may be beneficial if a syndesmosis injury is suspected but not evident on plain radiographs. In one study, malreductions requiring immediate revision of fixation occurred in 32% of patients after evaluation with intraoperative three-dimensional (3D) imaging. Anterior displacement and internal rotation of the syndesmosis were the most common malreductions.[25] The radiographic results of surgeries performed with intraoperative 3D imaging have been compared with those using intraoperative fluoroscopy, and no particular advantage was noted after comparison on postoperative CT.[26] No functional assessment of the advantages of advanced intraoperative imaging has been undertaken. Intraoperative CT-quality images are not universally available, but methods have been described for assessing the reduction of the syndesmosis using fluoroscopy. Comparing the final reduction of the injury to the patient's contralateral uninjured side appears to be beneficial. When using fibular length on the mortise view and the intersection of the anterior and posterior fibula with the plafond on the lateral view, excellent reductions were obtained as confirmed with intraoperative CT.[27] The utility of the contralateral ankle was further suggested in a cadaver study. Overall, malreductions were easier to identify than appropriate reductions. Anterior displacement and greater amounts of translation of the fibula were identified reliably in most cases.[2]

Debate exists over the best method of obtaining an accurate syndesmosis reduction. Previous findings of poor outcomes with malreduction have been reproduced, and some authors recommend direct visualization to minimize this risk. In a study of 68 syndesmosis injuries, one series found that 44% of closed reductions and 15% of open reductions were malreduced on postoperative CT. These findings did not reach significance, however.[28] Clamp reduction is a common reduction method, but care should be taken during application of the clamp. A cadaver study revealed overcompression of the joint and greater sagittal malreductions when the clamp was placed off-axis.[29] Another study showed similar overcompression and noted that all variations in clamp placement angulation led to malreduction. This study also noted that screw trajectory influenced the eventual reduction.[30] Both studies used periarticular reduction forceps and cautioned against using smaller clamps that may not allow appropriate clamping. An additional method of suggested reduction uses a suspensory fixation device such as TightRope (Arthrex) to guide the fibula into an appropriate reduction rather than forcing a potential malreduction with a clamp and screw.[31,32] Functional outcomes correlate with the accuracy of reductions, but the particular fixation type did not influence outcomes in the presence of an appropriately reduced syndesmosis.

Small and large fragment screws engaging three or four cortices are accepted methods of fixation. Bioabsorbable screws demonstrated similar outcomes and improved sagittal motion but have considerably more complications, particularly foreign body reactions, than metallic implants.[33] Screw removal continues to show no advantage over leaving the screws in place,[34] and removal may lead to an increased rate of complications, including superficial and deep infection, screw breakage during removal, and recurrent diastasis. In patients with recurrent diastasis, the mean time to screw removal was 6.7 weeks, whereas in those without diastasis, the screws remained in place for 3 additional weeks.[35]

Concerns about transsyndesmotic fixation have prompted efforts to find more anatomic and physiologic methods of syndesmosis repair. Direct repair of the PITFL with a soft-tissue washer, coupled with deltoid repair when persistent medial clear space widening is noted, recently showed results similar to those of transsyndesmotic screw fixation and reduced the need for hardware removal. No differences in functional outcomes were observed and, unexpectedly, the transsyndesmotic fixation group showed better ankle dorsiflexion.[36] Suture button devices have been suggested to allow more physiologic motion of the syndesmosis and because of their potential advantage in not requiring removal. Reports of the performance of such devices conflict with studies showing good reduction and functional outcomes.[37,38] Complications have been reported after using the devices, and their use does not obviate the need for further surgical intervention such as implant removal. Additional concern exists for increasing syndesmosis diastasis at early follow-up, but the functional consequence of this process is not known.[39] Regardless of the fixation method, clinical outcomes appear to be similar for a well-reduced mortise.

Postoperative Rehabilitation

The postoperative care of ankle fractures commonly involves a period of no weight bearing. More aggressive early weight bearing has been advocated by some authors, and no additional complications involving the loss of fixation, malunion, or nonunion were noted in one meta-analysis. Early motion and weight bearing appeared to allow patients more rapid return to work.[40] A Cochrane Database Review showed no benefit to early range of motion and noted that no convincing available evidence advocates early range of motion or weight bearing.[41] A recent study suggested that routine postoperative radiographs may not be needed during the follow-up period. Complications were found at similar rates when postoperative radiographs were taken during early postoperative visits and at later times.[42] Debate also continues over the need for thromboembolic prophylaxis after ankle fracture. One large study noted a low rate of venous thromboembolic events and observed no difference between the small group of patients who received prophylaxis and those who did not.[43]

Complications

The treatment of ankle fractures is subject to the typical complications of treating any fracture. PTA is common, and treatment options include activity modification, bracing, distraction arthroplasty, ankle arthrodesis, and ankle arthroplasty. Treatment should be tailored to the severity of the symptoms and to patient needs and characteristics. Smoking has been implicated in an increased risk of overall complications and of deep infection in particular.[44] In one series, wound complications were more common in patients with diabetes mellitus, peripheral neuropathy, open fractures, and older age. The use of medications that can impair wound healing and noncompliance with a postoperative protocol of no weight bearing for 6 weeks also were associated with a higher incidence of wound healing complications.[45] Patients with end-organ damage due to complicated diabetes exhibit an even higher risk of postsurgical noninfectious complications and the need for revision surgery. Open ankle fractures in the complicated diabetes group had a higher number of postsurgical complications and infections.[46] Other factors implicated in the development of deep infections after surgical treatment of ankle fractures include more severe soft-tissue injuries, fracture-dislocations, and alcohol abuse. Surgeon-controlled factors implicated in the development of deep infections included late antibiotic administration, a surgical time longer than 90 minutes, poor reductions, and wound complications.[47]

Patients with diabetes mellitus need to be counseled about the risks of infection and Charcot neuroarthropathy. A greater consideration for soft-tissue injury, glucose control, and the presence of end-organ damage may guide treatment plans. For severe soft-tissue damage, external fixation for temporization or definitive treatment may be prudent. Minimally invasive techniques such as percutaneous pinning or tibiotalocalcaneal (TTC) nailing also can be considered. Prolonged non-weight bearing commonly is employed, regardless of the fixation technique.

Outcomes

A 21-year follow-up in two separate studies—one of SER type injuries and one of pronation-eversion-external rotation type injuries—conducted by the same authors shows good or excellent results in more than 90% of all patients in both studies.[48,49] Ankle fractures appear to cause most cases of PTA. An imprecise reduction greater than 2 mm of gap or step-off in SER type IV fractures has been found to contribute to more arthritic symptoms, increased pain, and difficulty with daily and sports activities at an average of 21 months.[50] A review of Maisonneuve injuries showed good or excellent results in 92% of patients. Although radiographic findings of PTA were identified in almost half the patients, patient-reported pain was found to be more important in determining the outcome.[51] Arthroscopically identified cartilage lesions of the anterolateral talus and the medial malleolus resulted in worse radiographic and clinical outcomes.[52] Early patient satisfaction and activity may be achieved through patient education. Patients receiving enhanced information, including basic information on ankle fractures and a simple rehabilitation protocol had greater satisfaction and greater improvement in activity at 6 weeks. At 3 months,

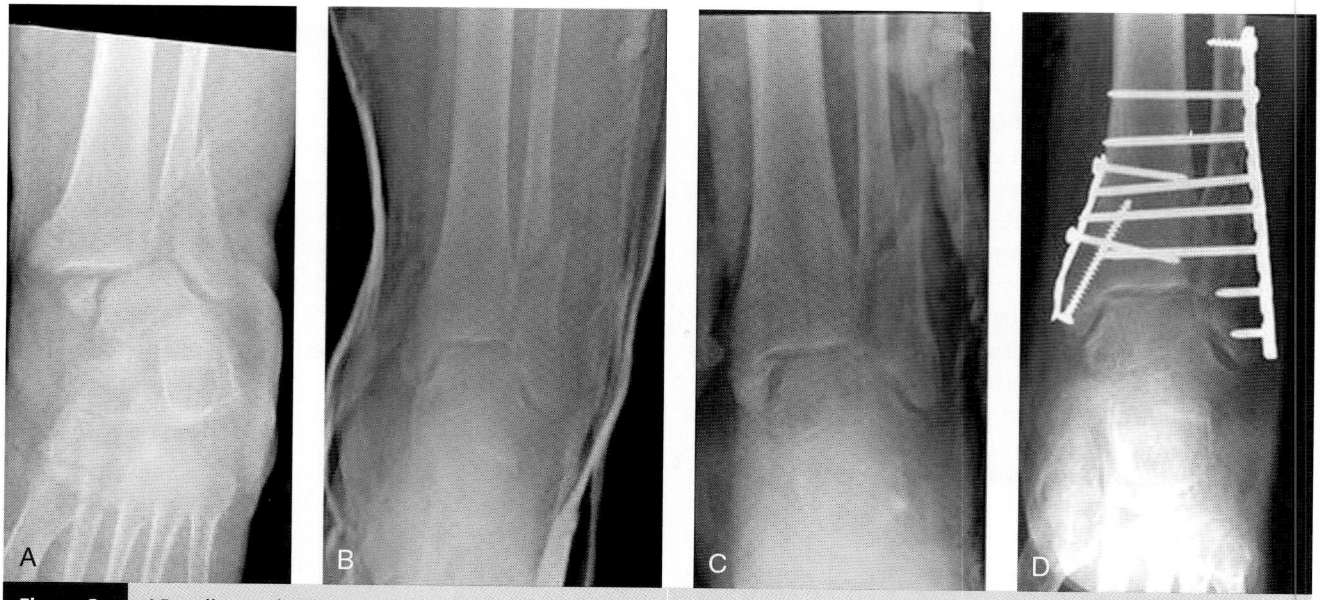

Figure 2 AP radiographs depict the comb technique, which uses multiple quadricortical screws to potentially improve construct strength in the treatment of geriatric ankle fractures. Radiograph of the injury (**A**) shows unreduced bimalleolar ankle fracture that was initially managed nonsurgically in a non–weight-bearing cast (**B**). Subsequently, the patient had a loss of reduction (**C**). The final construct after ORIF is shown (**D**). (Reproduced with permission from Olsen JR, Hunter J, Baumhauer JF: Osteoporotic ankle fractures. *Orthop Clin North Am* 2013;44[2]:225-241.)

the differences in the ability to perform work and other activity were no longer noted.[53]

Geriatric Fractures

Ankle fractures are increasing in incidence in the geriatric population and pose particular difficulties because of the poor bone and soft-tissue quality, medical comorbidities, and poor functional reserve in these individuals. Outcomes can be favorable, however. In a study examining 92 patients older than 80 years with surgically treated fractures, Weber type B injuries occurred most commonly. The 30-day mortality rate was 5.4% (5 patients). Diabetes mellitus, dementia, and peripheral vascular disease were noted as risk factors for wound complications.[54] A direct comparison of the surgical outcomes of geriatric and nongeriatric populations with SER type IV fractures showed similar outcomes between the two groups, however.[55]

Geriatric patients sometimes may have difficulty maintaining protected weight bearing, and strict non–weight-bearing precautions may put patients at an additional risk of falls. Alternative or augmented fixation methods may be considered necessary and beneficial to protect patients who cannot comply fully with restrictions. In a 2011 study, augmentation of a construct used to treat AO/OTA type 44-B fractures with an intramedullary wire and cement allowed immediate weight bearing with no cases of nonunion.[56] TTC nailing has been used with good results, allowing early weight bearing. In one series, 29 of 31 patients returned to their original level of mobility without complication.[57] In another patient cohort in which a femoral nail was used, TTC nailing returned 90% of patients to their preinjury functional level. This study did note a higher (35%) mortality rate; however, the complication rate was low.[58] Other authors have suggested multiple transfibular-transtibial screw fixation depending on the patient's bone quality (**Figure 2**). Placing multiple quadricortical screws proximally may provide maximal fixation to improve construct strength. Fully threaded cancellous screw fixation or bicortical fixation of the medial malleolus also were recommended as biomechanically sound options. No published outcomes are available for this technique to date.[59]

Summary

Ankle fractures remain common, but patients often experience good function after surgical and nonsurgical treatment. Multiple pitfalls in the diagnosis and treatment of these injuries remain. Syndesmotic injury in particular must be recognized, reduced anatomically, and stabilized appropriately. Although multiple new methods of fixation are available, including locking plates and suture buttons, small fragment fixation with syndesmosis screw fixation continues to show consistently good results. Patients should be counseled on the risk factors for complications, including the development of PTA. Patients with diabetes mellitus and other comorbidities should be advised of additional risks. Patients with diabetes mellitus in particular should warrant additional consideration to methods of fixation, prolonging weightbearing restrictions, total contact casting, and the risk of the development of Charcot arthropathy. Surgeons should be prepared to deal with an increasing number of geriatric ankle fractures and should strive to use appropriate treatment methods to return affected patients to their original level of function as soon as practicable.

Key Study Points

- The difficulty in diagnosing syndesmosis instability and the contribution of the posterior malleolus to ankle stability should be recognized, and methods to ensure appropriate reduction should be understood.
- Several methods are available for evaluating an appropriate reduction of the ankle joint intraoperatively.
- The complications of ankle fracture treatment and the factors that contribute to patient outcomes need to be recognized.

Annotated References

1. Shah AS, Kadakia AR, Tan GJ, Karadsheh MS, Wolter TD, Sabb B: Radiographic evaluation of the normal distal tibiofibular syndesmosis. *Foot Ankle Int* 2012;33(10):870-876.

   The lack of a tibia-fibula overlap on the mortise view can be normal. The mortise view was thought to be most accurate when it was compared to that of the contralateral ankle.

2. Koenig SJ, Tornetta P III, Merlin G, et al: Can We Tell if the Syndesmosis Is Reduced Using Fluoroscopy? *J Orthop Trauma* 2015;29(9):e326-e330.

   Anterior-posterior displacement of 2.5 or 5 mm was induced. The 5-mm displacement and anterior displacement were noted reliably. Posterior translation of less than 5 mm was difficult to identify. Reliability was improved by comparing these relationships to the uninjured ankle.

3. Chen P-Y, Wang T-G, Wang CL: Ultrasonographic examination of the deltoid ligament in bimalleolar equivalent fractures. *Foot Ankle Int* 2008;29(9):883-886.

4. Nortunen S, Lepojärvi S, Savola O, et al: Stability assessment of the ankle mortise in supination-external rotation-type ankle fractures: Lack of additional diagnostic value of MRI. *J Bone Joint Surg Am* 2014;96(22):1855-1862.

   In this study, 61 SER fractures were evaluated with MRI. Whether stable or unstable with external rotation stress, all ankles had deep deltoid injuries. The authors do not recommend MRI for further evaluation to guide treatment decisions. Level of evidence: II.

5. Dikos GD, Heisler J, Choplin RH, Weber TG: Normal tibiofibular relationships at the syndesmosis on axial CT imaging. *J Orthop Trauma* 2012;26(7):433-438.

   In this study, 30 uninjured patients (60 ankles) underwent CT. Despite wide variations between patients, comparisons between ankles in individual patients showed that intervals and rotational angles do not vary by more than 2.3 mm or 6.5°, respectively.

6. Black EM, Antoci V, Lee JT, et al: Role of preoperative computed tomography scans in operative planning for malleolar ankle fractures. *Foot Ankle Int* 2013;34(5):697-704.

   CT findings most commonly resulted in changes to the plan for medial and/or posterior malleolus fracture fixation. Of all patients, 9% had findings that prompted the authors to address an anterior plafond fracture. The authors concluded that CT may have considerable value in certain fracture types. Level of evidence: III.

7. Hastie GR, Divecha H, Javed S, Zubairy A: Ankle injury manipulation before or after X-ray—does it influence success? *Injury* 2014;45(3):583-585.

   In 90 ankles, radiographs were obtained before reduction. When these ankles were compared with 31 ankles that were reduced before obtaining radiographs, no difference was seen in the need for surgery or in time to surgery. The latter group had more repeat manipulations. The authors proposed that early radiographs provide good information and reduce the need for repeat reduction in neurovascularly normal injuries.

8. Schepers T, De Vries MR, Van Lieshout EM, Van der Elst M: The timing of ankle fracture surgery and the effect on infectious complications; a case series and systematic review of the literature. *Int Orthop* 2013;37(3):489-494.

   In this study, 145 consecutive ankle fractures were reviewed. Those undergoing surgery within 1 day had no wound complications. Similar findings were observed when comparing patients having surgery within 1 week and those having surgery after 7 days. These findings were corroborated by the authors' review of the literature.

9. Hong-Chuan W, Shi-Lian K, Heng-Sheng S, Gui-Gen P, Ya-Fei Z: Immediate internal fixation of open ankle fractures. *Foot Ankle Int* 2010;31(11):959-964.

   The authors surmised that appropriate antibiotic administration and early irrigation and débridement of these open fractures led to their good results. Of 92 patients, two had a superficial infection, and one diabetic patient had a deep infection. Most injuries were classified as type II and IIIA.

10. Switaj PJ, Weatherford B, Fuchs D, Rosenthal B, Pang E, Kadakia AR: Evaluation of posterior malleolar fractures and the posterior pilon variant in operatively treated ankle fractures. *Foot Ankle Int* 2014;35(9):886-895.

    Of 270 fractures in this series, 50% had posterior malleolus fractures. The pilon variant was seen in 20% of the cohort. Axial load of the ankle was suspected as the cause of this variant. Level of evidence: III.

11. Hinds RM, Garner MR, Lazaro LE, et al: Ankle fracture spur sign is pathognomonic for a variant ankle fracture. *Foot Ankle Int* 2015;36(2):159-164.

    The incidence of the pilon variant was 43 of 640 ankles. The spur sign was found to be 100% specific and was not seen in any nonvariant fractures. Level of evidence: III.

12. Pakarinen HJ, Flinkkil TE, Ohtonen PP, Ristiniemi JY: Stability criteria for nonoperative ankle fracture management. *Foot Ankle Int* 2011;32(2):141-147.

    In this study, 130 patients were followed for 2 years. Stable ankle fractures were treated nonsurgically, and patients showed better pain and functional scores than those in the surgical group. Stability largely was defined as the noting of no talar shift on initial radiographs. Level of evidence: III.

13. Jain S, Haughton BA, Brew C: Intramedullary fixation of distal fibular fractures: A systematic review of clinical and functional outcomes. *J Orthop Traumatol* 2014;15(4):245-254.

    This review identified 17 studies that included 1,008 patients with fibula fractures treated with intramedullary fixation. The union rate was 98.5%, with good or excellent functional outcomes in 91% of patients. Locked and unlocked nails performed similarly. Level of evidence: IV.

14. Ebraheim NA, Ludwig T, Weston JT, Carroll T, Liu J: Comparison of surgical techniques of 111 medial malleolar fractures classified by fracture geometry. *Foot Ankle Int* 2014;35(5):471-477.

    In this study, 111 medial malleolus fractures were reviewed. For transverse fractures below the shoulder of the talus, tension bands had fewer nonunions (15) and complications (37) than other methods. Complications included displacement, infection, wound problems, and hardware failure. Level of evidence: III.

15. Patel T, Owen JR, Byrd WA, et al: Biomechanical performance of a new device for medial malleolar fractures. *Foot Ankle Int* 2013;34(3):426-433.

    In this cadaver study, the sled device required a greater load to cause fracture gapping. Solid screws and the sled device had similar strength in torsion and load to failure.

16. Hoelsbrekken SE, Kaul-Jensen K, Mørch T, et al: Nonoperative treatment of the medial malleolus in bimalleolar and trimalleolar ankle fractures: A randomized controlled trial. *J Orthop Trauma* 2013;27(11):633-637.

    After fibula and syndesmosis fixation, the residual displacement of the medial malleolus was observed intraoperatively, and patients were randomized if displacement was more than 2 mm. Functional scores and incidence of radiographic arthritis were similar. The nonsurgical group had four nonunions, but none were symptomatic. Level of evidence: II.

17. Tejwani NC, Pahk B, Egol KA: Effect of posterior malleolus fracture on outcome after unstable ankle fracture. *J Trauma* 2010;69(3):666-669.

    In this study, 54 posterior malleolus fractures from a larger group of 309 were examined retrospectively. American Orthopaedic Foot and Ankle Society total scores and pain scores and Short Form-36 Health Survey scores were worse for posterior malleolus fractures. When 41 patients had 2-year follow-up, these differences no longer were noted. The authors proposed that posterior malleolus fractures may be higher-energy injuries leading to more short-term dysfunction.

18. Drijfhout van Hooff CC, Verhage SM, Hoogendoorn JM: Influence of fragment size and postoperative joint congruency on long-term outcome of posterior malleolar fractures. *Foot Ankle Int* 2015;36(6):673-678.

    In 42% of posterior malleolus fractures that had been fixed, a step-off greater than 1 mm remained. This percentage was not significantly less than those without fixation. PTA did not appear to correlate with function in this study. Fixation of larger fragments also did not appear to affect function. Level of evidence: IV.

19. Erdem MN, Erken HY, Burc H, Saka G, Korkmaz MF, Aydogan M: Comparison of lag screw versus buttress plate fixation of posterior malleolar fractures. *Foot Ankle Int* 2014;35(10):1022-1030.

    This study was a review of 40 patients alternatively treated with lag screws or a buttress plate. American Orthopaedic Foot and Ankle Society scores and reduction quality were similar at approximately 3 years' follow-up. Level of evidence: II.

20. O'Connor TJ, Mueller B, Ly TV, Jacobson AR, Nelson ER, Cole PA: "A to p" screw versus posterolateral plate for posterior malleolus fixation in trimalleolar ankle fractures. *J Orthop Trauma* 2015;29(4):e151-e156.

    This small study of 27 patients showed improved Short Musculoskeletal Function Assessment bother index scores and trends to better scores for the buttress plate group. Although no differences in radiographic reduction were apparent, a direct approach and reduction of the fracture may translate to improved function and allow more stable fixation. Level of evidence: III.

21. Pakarinen H, Flinkkilä T, Ohtonen P, et al: Intraoperative assessment of the stability of the distal tibiofibular joint in supination-external rotation injuries of the ankle: Sensitivity, specificity, and reliability of two clinical tests. *J Bone Joint Surg Am* 2011;93(22):2057-2061.

In this study, 140 SER fractures were tested with the hook test or external rotation stress using a special tool. Both tests were very specific for syndesmosis injury. External rotation stress was more sensitive but still was considered lacking. Combining the two tests did not improve the results. Level of evidence: I.

22. Matuszewski PE, Dombroski D, Lawrence JT, Esterhai JL Jr, Mehta S: Prospective intraoperative syndesmotic evaluation during ankle fracture fixation: Stress external rotation versus lateral fibular stress. *J Orthop Trauma* 2015;29(4):e157-e160.

    Lateral and manual external rotation stress was placed on 20 consecutive fractures. No special tool was used. External rotation stress showed an additional 1 to 2 mm of medial clear space widening. No functional correlation was made. Level of evidence: IV.

23. Marmor M, Hansen E, Han HK, Buckley J, Matityahu A: Limitations of standard fluoroscopy in detecting rotational malreduction of the syndesmosis in an ankle fracture model. *Foot Ankle Int* 2011;32(6):616-622.

    This cadaveric study showed that up to 30° of external malrotation of the fibula may be unrecognized on fluoroscopic examination. Excessive internal rotation of as little as 10° was identified. The views evaluated were the AP and mortise tibiofibular clear space and overlap views.

24. Lepojärvi S, Pakarinen H, Savola O, Haapea M, Sequeiros RB, Niinimäki J: Posterior translation of the fibula may indicate malreduction: CT study of normal variation in uninjured ankles. *J Orthop Trauma* 2014;28(4):205-209.

    In 97% of normal ankles, the fibula sits anterior or central in the incisura. The width of the posterior aspect of the syndesmosis is wider than that of the anterior aspect, and the center of the fibula is anterior to the center of the incisura. Posterior translation may indicate malalignment of the fibula.

25. Franke J, von Recum J, Suda AJ, Grützner PA, Wendl K: Intraoperative three-dimensional imaging in the treatment of acute unstable syndesmotic injuries. *J Bone Joint Surg Am* 2012;94(15):1386-1390.

    Iso-C three-dimensional fluoroscopy and standard fluoroscopy were compared. Syndesmosis alignment was revised in 25.5% of cases. Only 5.2% of cases required revision of the fracture fragments. Level of evidence: III.

26. Davidovitch RI, Weil Y, Karia R, et al: Intraoperative syndesmotic reduction: Three-dimensional versus standard fluoroscopic imaging. *J Bone Joint Surg Am* 2013;95(20):1838-1843.

    Postoperative CT evaluated the reductions of syndesmosis injuries intraoperatively evaluated with standard fluoroscopy or Iso-C three-dimensional fluoroscopy. Both groups showed similar numbers of malreductions. More rotational malreductions occurred when using standard fluoroscopy, but the authors suggested that this finding resulted from the reduction technique instead of the radiographic technique. Level of evidence: II.

27. Summers HD, Sinclair MK, Stover MD: A reliable method for intraoperative evaluation of syndesmotic reduction. *J Orthop Trauma* 2013;27(4):196-200.

    Reduction of the fractures was performed to re-create a profile similar to the mortise and lateral views noted on the uninjured ankle in the same patient. After intraoperative CT, only 1 of 18 ankles required immediate revision.

28. Sagi HC, Shah AR, Sanders RW: The functional consequence of syndesmotic joint malreduction at a minimum 2-year follow-up. *J Orthop Trauma* 2012;26(7):439-443.

    Clinical and CT evaluations of syndesmosis injuries showed that more malreductions occurred with closed reduction (44%) than with open reduction (15%). Functional scores were lower in the closed reduction group. Level of evidence: II.

29. Phisitkul P, Ebinger T, Goetz J, Vaseenon T, Marsh JL: Forceps reduction of the syndesmosis in rotational ankle fractures: A cadaveric study. *J Bone Joint Surg Am* 2012;94(24):2256-2261.

    Off-axis clamp placement led to sagittal malreductions of unstable cadaver syndesmosis injuries. Clamping induced overcompression in all cases.

30. Miller AN, Barei DP, Iaquinto JM, Ledoux WR, Beingessner DM: Iatrogenic syndesmosis malreduction via clamp and screw placement. *J Orthop Trauma* 2013;27(2):100-106.

    Rotational and sagittal malreductions and overcompression were noted with all clamp placements. Certain screw placements also induced malreductions despite clamping.

31. Westermann RW, Rungprai C, Goetz JE, Femino J, Amendola A, Phisitkul P: The effect of suture-button fixation on simulated syndesmotic malreduction: A cadaveric study. *J Bone Joint Surg Am* 2014;96(20):1732-1738.

    Despite purposeful off-axis clamping or malreduction, the suture button facilitated improved reductions compared with screw fixation.

32. Naqvi GA, Cunningham P, Lynch B, Galvin R, Awan N: Fixation of ankle syndesmotic injuries: Comparison of tightrope fixation and syndesmotic screw fixation for accuracy of syndesmotic reduction. *Am J Sports Med* 2012;40(12):2828-2835.

    In this study, 23 patients treated with suture buttons and 23 with screw fixation were compared using postoperative CT. No malreductions were noted in the suture button group, whereas 21.7% of patients in the screw group were found to have malreductions. No functional differences were noted.

33. Sun H, Luo CF, Zhong B, Shi HP, Zhang CQ, Zeng BF: A prospective, randomised trial comparing the use of absorbable and metallic screws in the fixation of distal tibiofibular syndesmosis injuries: Mid-term follow-up. *Bone Joint J* 2014;96-B(4):548-554.

    In this study, 86 patients treated with bioabsorbable screws were compared with 82 patients treated with metallic screws. Function was similar in both groups and the absorbable screws group had increased range of motion.

34. Boyle MJ, Gao R, Frampton CM, Coleman B: Removal of the syndesmotic screw after the surgical treatment of a fracture of the ankle in adult patients does not affect one-year outcomes: A randomised controlled trial. *Bone Joint J* 2014;96-B(12):1699-1705.

    At 1 year, no differences were observed in tibiofibular clear space, functional scores, or range of motion, despite 76% of retained screws showing loosening or breakage.

35. Schepers T, Van Lieshout EM, de Vries MR, Van der Elst M: Complications of syndesmotic screw removal. *Foot Ankle Int* 2011;32(11):1040-1044.

    In this study, 22.4% of patients having screws removed experienced complications, including wound infections and diastasis. Screws were removed quite early in this study, especially in the complication group. Level of evidence: IV.

36. Little MM, Berkes MB, Schottel PC, et al: Anatomic fixation of supination external rotation type IV equivalent ankle fractures. *J Orthop Trauma* 2015;29(5):250-255.

    This study compared transsyndesmotic fixation using screws with soft-tissue repair of the posterior inferior tibiofibular ligament, with and without deltoid repair in the face of syndesmotic instability and increased medial clear space. Radiographic outcomes were similar, but the screw group had higher rates of hardware removal. No differences were found in function, however. Level of evidence: III.

37. Laflamme M, Belzile EL, Bédard L, van den Bekerom MP, Glazebrook M, Pelet S: A prospective randomized multicenter trial comparing clinical outcomes of patients treated surgically with a static or dynamic implant for acute ankle syndesmosis rupture. *J Orthop Trauma* 2015;29(5):216-23.

    This randomized trial compared the fixation device TightRope (Arthrex) to a 3.5-mm screw. Olerud-Molander scores and return to work were better in the TightRope group at 12 months. In the screw group, four ankles had loss of reduction. No correlation was seen between the quality of the reduction and functional scores or return to work. Level of evidence: II.

38. Degroot H, Al-Omari AA, El Ghazaly SA: Outcomes of suture button repair of the distal tibiofibular syndesmosis. *Foot Ankle Int* 2011;32(3):250-256.

    In this study, 24 patients treated with suture button fixation were reviewed. Outcomes were acceptable at 20 months, but 6 patients required device removal. Osteolysis and subsidence commonly were seen.

39. Peterson KS, Chapman WD, Hyer CF, Berlet GC: Maintenance of reduction with suture button fixation devices for ankle syndesmosis repair. *Foot Ankle Int* 2015;36(6):679-684.

    At approximately 6 months, tibiofibular clear space and overlap increased from that seen immediately after surgery. The medial clear space was maintained, and no functional detriments were seen with syndesmosis diastasis. Level of evidence: IV.

40. Smeeing DP, Houwert RM, Briet JP, et al: Weight-bearing and mobilization in the postoperative care of ankle fractures: A systematic review and meta-analysis of randomized controlled trials and cohort studies. *PLoS One* 2015;10(2):e0118320.

    In this meta-analysis of 1,376 patients, no increased incidence of complications was seen with early motion or weight bearing. The authors reported that early motion and walking may shorten the return-to-work time.

41. Lin C-W, Donkers NA, Refshauge KM, Beckenkamp PR, Khera K, Moseley AM: Rehabilitation for ankle fractures in adults. *Cochrane Database Syst Rev* 2012;11:CD005595.

    This meta-analysis of 1,896 patients led the authors to conclude that only limited evidence exists to recommend early weight bearing and motion and that patient compliance was paramount. Specific rehabilitation was not found to impact outcomes.

42. McDonald MR, Bulka CM, Thakore RV, et al: Ankle radiographs in the early postoperative period: Do they matter? *J Orthop Trauma* 2014;28(9):538-541.

    In this study, 7% of patients from whom radiographs were obtained at 7 to 21 days after surgery and 5.9% of those from whom postoperative radiographs were obtained at 22 to 120 days had complications. No differences were noted between fracture types. The authors suggest more critical utilization of routine radiographs. Level of evidence: III.

43. Pelet S, Roger M-E, Belzile EL, Bouchard M: The incidence of thromboembolic events in surgically treated ankle fracture. *J Bone Joint Surg Am* 2012;94(6):502-506.

    Patients with particular risk factors had more venous thromboembolic events; however, no benefit was seen in venous thromboembolic prophylaxis in patients with or without these risk factors. Level of evidence: III.

44. Nåsell H, Ottosson C, Törnqvist H, Lindé J, Ponzer S: The impact of smoking on complications after operatively treated ankle fractures—a follow-up study of 906 patients. *J Orthop Trauma* 2011;25(12):748-755.

    Early complications were seen in 22.3% of ankle fractures. Overall, 30.5% of smokers and 20.3% of nonsmokers had complications. Smoking was a particular risk for deep infection.

45. Miller AG, Margules A, Raikin SM: Risk factors for wound complications after ankle fracture surgery. *J Bone Joint Surg Am* 2012;94(22):2047-2052.

    In this study, 20 of 478 ankles had complications, and 6 required further surgery. Patients requiring additional surgery were older, had complicated diabetes, and were often noncompliant. Level of evidence: I.

46. Wukich DK, Joseph A, Ryan M, Ramirez C, Irrgang JJ: Outcomes of ankle fractures in patients with uncomplicated versus complicated diabetes. *Foot Ankle Int* 2011;32(2):120-130.

    At intermediate follow-up, 50% of patients with advanced diabetes had more complications. Neuropathy and open fractures in particular had higher rates of complications. Level of evidence: III.

47. Ovaska MT, Mäkinen TJ, Madanat R, et al: Risk factors for deep surgical site infection following operative treatment of ankle fractures. *J Bone Joint Surg Am* 2013;95(4):348-353.

    In this study, 6.8% of patients had a deep infection. Multivariate analysis showed that tobacco use and surgical times longer than 90 minutes were independent risk factors. Cast application in the operating room reduced the risk. Level of evidence: III.

48. Donken CC, Verhofstad MH, Edwards MJ, van Laarhoven CJ: Twenty-one-year follow-up of supination-external rotation type II-IV (OTA type B) ankle fractures: A retrospective cohort study. *J Orthop Trauma* 2012;26(8):e108-e114.

    A 21-year review of SER fractures showed overall good results. No worse function was noted with fracture severity. Surgically and nonsurgically treated fractures performed similarly. Level of evidence: IV.

49. Donken CC, Verhofstad MH, Edwards MJ, van Laarhoven CJ: Twenty-two-year follow-up of pronation external rotation type III-IV (OTA type C) ankle fractures: A retrospective cohort study. *J Orthop Trauma* 2012;26(8):e115-e122.

    A 22-year review of PER fractures showed overall good results. No worse function was noted with fracture severity. Surgically and nonsurgically treated fractures performed similarly. Level of evidence: IV.

50. Berkes MB, Little MT, Lazaro LE, et al: Articular congruity is associated with short-term clinical outcomes of operatively treated SER IV ankle fractures. *J Bone Joint Surg Am* 2013;95(19):1769-1775.

    In this study, 108 SER type IV fractures were evaluated with CT and the Foot and Ankle Outcome Score. Of the total, 33% healed with an incongruity greater than 2 mm (most commonly the posterior malleolus), and these patients had more symptoms, pain, and limitations in activity. Level of evidence: IV.

51. Lambers KT, van den Bekerom MP, Doornberg JN, Stufkens SA, van Dijk CN, Kloen P: Long-term outcome of pronation-external rotation ankle fractures treated with syndesmotic screws only. *J Bone Joint Surg Am* 2013;95(17):e1221-e1227.

    In this study, 50 Maisonneuve injuries were fixed with syndesmosis screws alone. Of the total, 49% had PTA at 21 years. Patient pain correlated with function. Depression, limited range of motion, and repeat surgery predicted pain. Level of evidence: IV.

52. Stufkens SA, Knupp M, Horisberger M, Lampert C, Hintermann B: Cartilage lesions and the development of osteoarthritis after internal fixation of ankle fractures: A prospective study. *J Bone Joint Surg Am* 2010;92(2):279-286.

    The authors found that any cartilage damage correlates with poorer clinical and radiographic outcomes. Anterior and lateral talar and medial malleolus lesions deeper than 50% of the cartilage were predictive of worse outcomes. Level of evidence: II.

53. Mayich DJ, Tieszer C, Lawendy A, McCormick W, Sanders D: Role of patient information handouts following operative treatment of ankle fractures: A prospective randomized study. *Foot Ankle Int* 2013;34(1):2-7.

    Patient information handouts for immediate postoperative care and early rehabilitation improved patient satisfaction. Patients had better activity at 6 weeks, but this difference was not noted at 3 months. Level of evidence: I.

54. Shivarathre DG, Chandran P, Platt SR: Operative fixation of unstable ankle fractures in patients aged over 80 years. *Foot Ankle Int* 2011;32(6):599-602.

    In this study, 75 of 87 patients returned to preinjury mobility by 9 months. The superficial wound infection rate was 7% (6 patients), and four deep infections were noted. Level of evidence: IV.

55. Little MT, Berkes MB, Lazaro LE, et al: Comparison of supination external rotation type IV ankle fractures in geriatric versus nongeriatric populations. *Foot Ankle Int* 2013;34(4):512-517.

    In this study, the geriatric population had more incidence of diabetes mellitus and vascular disease but had fewer reports of symptoms and a better return to sports. No difference was seen in the reduction quality or in complications. Level of evidence: III.

56. Assal M, Christofilopoulos P, Lübbeke A, Stern R: Augmented osteosynthesis of OTA 44-B fractures in older patients: A technique allowing early weightbearing. *J Orthop Trauma* 2011;25(12):742-747.

    A construct of an intramedullary wire and cement with overlying plates/screws allowed weight bearing by 13.5 days. All 36 patients healed without displacement.

57. Jonas SC, Young AF, Curwen CH, McCann PA: Functional outcome following tibio-talar-calcaneal nailing for unstable osteoporotic ankle fractures. *Injury* 2013;44(7):994-997.

    The authors report that 21 patients were treated with a TTC nail. Eight of 21 patients did not go on to full union, but none had clinical symptoms of a nonunion.

58. Al-Nammari SS, Dawson-Bowling S, Amin A, Nielsen D: Fragility fractures of the ankle in the frail elderly patient: Treatment with a long calcaneotalotibial nail. *Bone Joint J* 2014;96-B(6):817-822.

This series of 48 patients had good results despite the high mortality rate. The authors chose to use a long nail to avoid the historical 10% risk of periprosthetic fracture.

59. Olsen JR, Hunter J, Baumhauer JF: Osteoporotic ankle fractures. *Orthop Clin North Am* 2013;44(2):225-241.

This article reviews the incidence and treatment considerations for dealing with geriatric ankle fractures. The authors note that outcomes can be obtained but that medical comorbidities correlate with complication rates. The authors also review treatment options including the "comb" technique.

Chapter 46

Distal Tibial Pilon Fractures

Langdon A. Hartsock, MD, FACS Peter H. White, MD

Abstract

A distal tibial pilon fracture is a complex bone and soft-tissue injury occurring after an axial load to the ankle region. Careful evaluation of the bone and soft-tissue injury is recommended before surgical treatment. External fixation is desirable before definitive fixation in the setting of acute swelling. Reduction of the fracture to restore articular congruence and overall alignment is the surgical goal. Timely healing and the avoidance of postoperative complications can be achieved by a variety of methods. Long-term outcomes are related to the severity of the bone and soft-tissue injury and the quality of the reduction. More severe injuries have a poorer outcome.

Keywords: pilon fracture; open reduction; spanning external fixation; bridging external fixation; soft-tissue management

Introduction

Ankle pilon injuries are characterized by an axial load on the ankle that results in a multifragmentary fracture of the articular surface of the distal tibial and metaphyseal area and variable fracture of the fibula. These injuries can vary considerably, depending on the amount of force applied to the ankle at the moment of injury. In addition to the complex fracture of the distal tibia and the fibula, pilon fractures are accompanied by major soft-tissue injury. The severity of the soft-tissue injury can determine the timing and invasiveness of fracture treatment. Along with major swelling, bruising, blisters, and hematoma, open fractures are common with pilon fractures, and the wound can expose the tibia fracture, the fibula fracture, or both.[1]

Ankle pilon fractures are distinctly different from the more common malleolar fractures of the ankle. Malleolar ankle fractures typically result from torsional forces on the ankle joint and result in a predictable and simpler fracture pattern. The results of the treatment of malleolar ankle fractures tend to be predictably good, with the exception of fracture-dislocations.

The mechanism of injury for pilon fractures is direct axial load, occasionally leaving the fibula intact, and the ankle in varus, or a dorsiflexion/valgus injury with lateral comminution of the tibia and fibula. The severity of the fracture makes anatomic reduction and fixation challenging. Unlike malleolar fractures, pilon fractures have a higher rate of postoperative complications including infection, wound breakdown, fixation failure, and loss of reduction. Long-term complications include persistent pain, swelling, stiffness, posttraumatic arthritis, and gait disturbances.

Early reports of anatomic reduction and internal fixation from the AO/ASIF group emphasized four treatment principles for pilon fractures: restoration of the length and alignment of the fibula, anatomic reduction of the tibial plafond, bone graft of any metaphyseal defects, and buttress plating of the medial tibia. Early attempts to replicate the results of the Swiss surgeons in North America often led to poor results, including skin breakdown, deep infection, fixation failure, posttraumatic arthritis, and chronic pain.[1,2]

Over the past 20 years, surgeons have developed treatment strategies to mitigate the risk of poor outcomes related to the surgical treatment of pilon fractures. These strategies include early reduction and splinting of the fracture or bridging external fixation in order to maintain reduction, restore length, correct alignment, and relieve any pressure on the skin from displaced bone fragments.

Dr. Hartsock or an immediate family member serves as a board member, owner, officer, or committee member of the South Carolina Orthopaedic Association, the Southeastern Fracture Symposium, and the Southern Orthopaedic Association. Neither Dr. White nor any immediate family member has received anything of value from or has stock or stock options held in a commercial company or institution related directly or indirectly to the subject of this chapter.

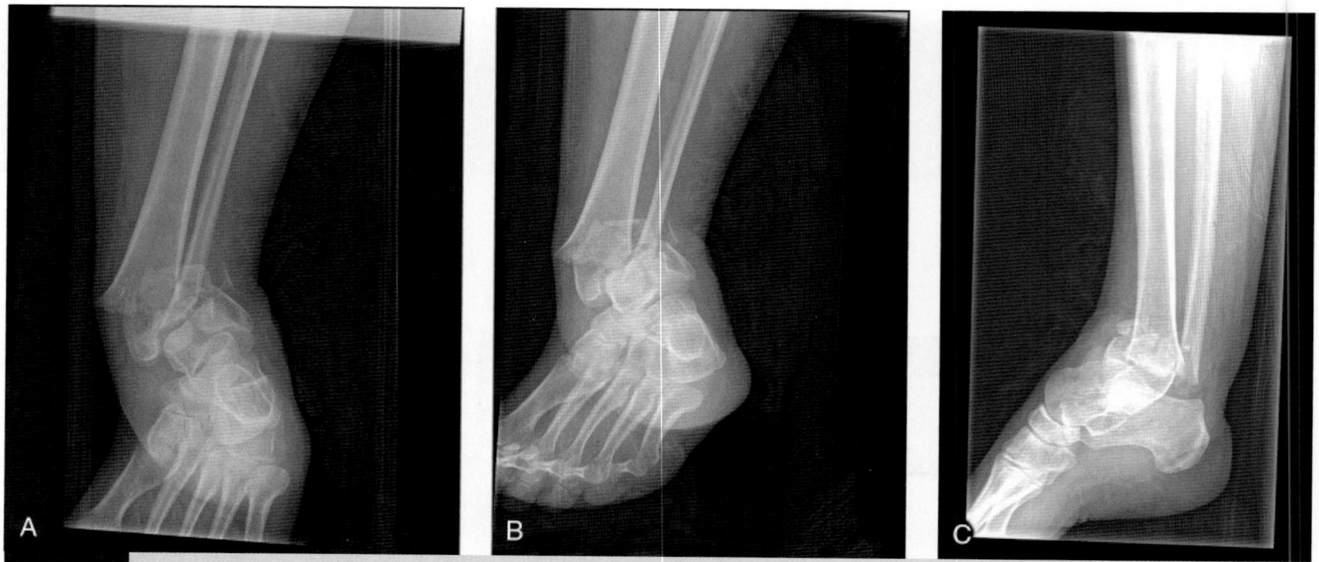

Figure 1 Radiographs show the AP (**A**), oblique (**B**), and lateral (**C**) views of a comminuted pilon fracture dislocation with associated distal fibula fracture.

Open fractures are treated urgently with intravenous antibiotics, excisional débridement and irrigation of the fracture and soft-tissue injury, and application of a bridging external fixator to control the fracture and prevent further damage to the soft tissues.

Definitive treatment, including open reduction and internal fixation (ORIF), is delayed until the soft-tissue injury has improved sufficiently so that surgical incisions can be performed safely. Surgical approaches, reduction methods, and fixation implants have improved, and the principles of treatment have been standardized. The primary determinant of the timing of the procedure is the condition of the soft tissues, not the severity of the fracture. Currently, no objective quantifiable test is available for determining when the soft tissues are amenable to surgery. Generally, the swelling needs to have diminished enough that skin wrinkles are apparent, blisters typically are re-epithelialized, and any wounds or abrasions have healed, with new epidermis covering the old wound. The soft tissues may not be considered ready for surgical intervention for between 2 days and 3 weeks postinjury.

Evaluation

The evaluation of a patient with a pilon fracture begins with a complete history and physical examination. Plain radiographs help identify the fracture and the fracture pattern including whether the fibula is also fractured.[3] Pilon fractures that result from a varus moment tend to create fibula fractures with failure in tension or a combination of tension and rotation. Fractures caused by valgus loading tend to create fibula fractures with comminution at the fracture site from a compressive force. Disruption of the distal tibial syndesmosis can occur with a valgus or varus moment and needs to be addressed during surgery.

Although rare, compartment syndrome in association with pilon fractures has been reported. The treating surgeon should maintain a high index of suspicion for compartment syndrome coupled with close physical examination of these high-energy injuries.[4]

Fracture comminution of the tibial plafond and distal tibial metaphysis is variable, depending on the amount of energy absorbed at the moment of impact. Plain radiographs of a comminuted pilon fracture are shown in **Figure 1**. Complete evaluation of joint surface comminution can be difficult with plain radiography. CT provides useful imaging in the diagnostic workup and should be performed after placement of a spanning external fixator. CT shows the size and shape of the fragment(s) as well as any comminution and impaction of the joint surface. Three-dimensional CT reconstructions are helpful in showing the exterior surface anatomy so that the surgeon has a visual representation of what will be seen during ORIF of the fracture (**Figure 2**).

During a study of a large number of CT scans of pilon fractures, it was determined that a consistent pattern of fracture of the distal tibia occurs. A typical fracture of the tibial plafond consists of a posterolateral fragment, an anterolateral fragment, and a medial fragment. The

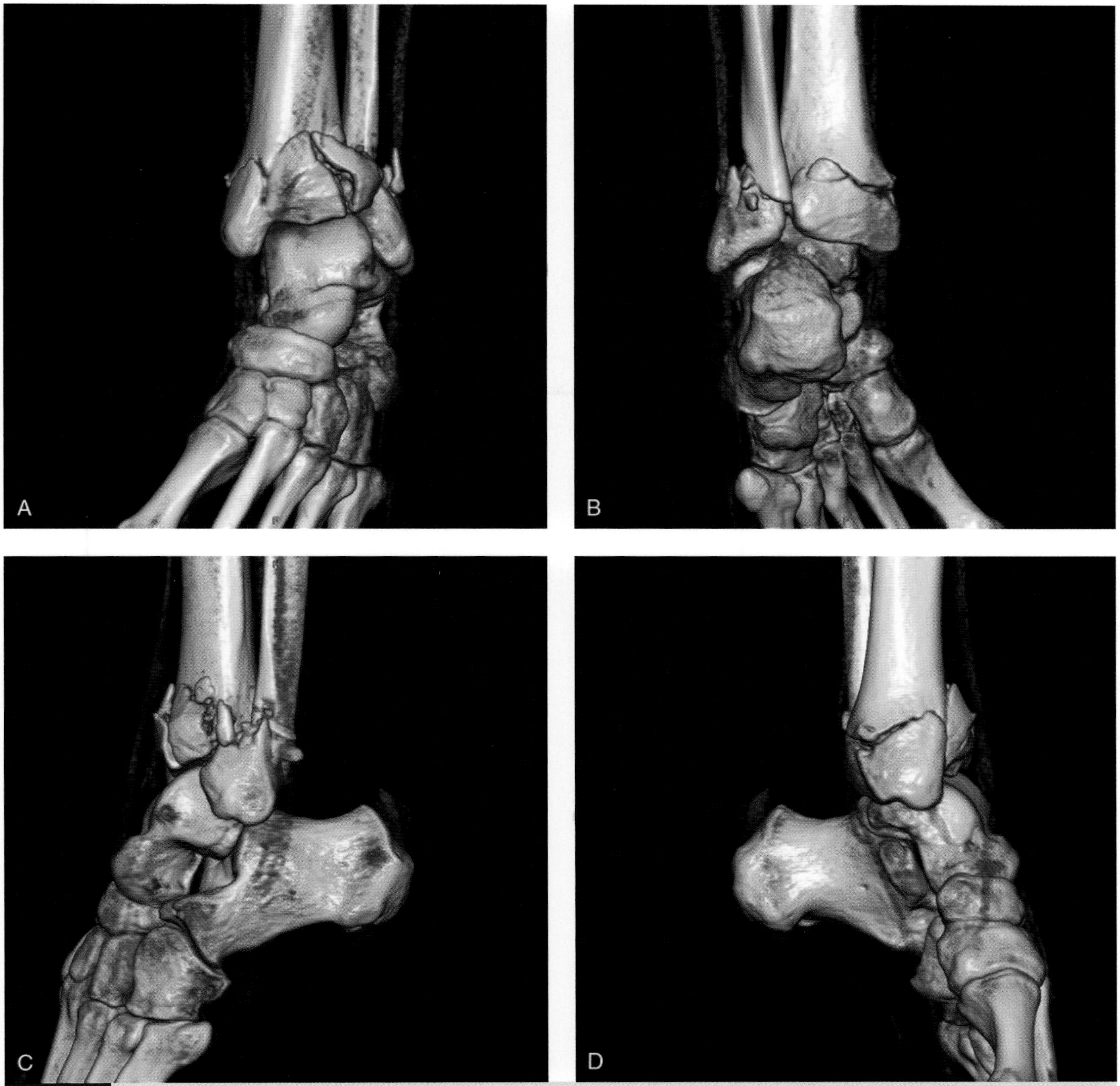

Figure 2 Three-dimensional CT reconstructions demonstrate the anterior (**A**), posterior (**B**), lateral (**C**), and medial (**D**) views of a comminuted pilon fracture dislocation with associated distal fibula fracture.

fragments vary in the size and degree of comminution and in impaction between the major fracture components.[5] The fibula also should be assessed for fracture location and displacement.

Classification schemes have been established including the AO/Orthopaedic Trauma Association (OTA) fracture classification system. The higher grade, more complex fractures tend to have poorer outcomes.

Treatment

The original AO principles remain relevant in the treatment of pilon fractures. The timing of surgical intervention has changed since the early AO reports several decades ago. Initial management is designed to obtain a preliminary reduction to protect the soft tissues from sharp or displaced bone fragments. Preliminary reduction

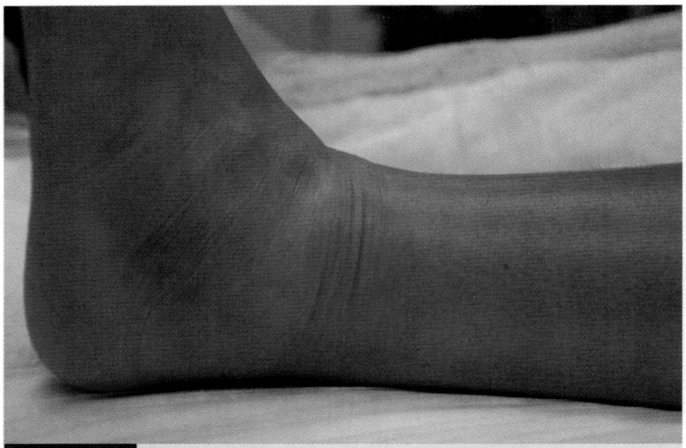

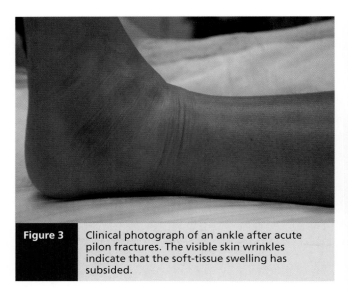

Figure 3 Clinical photograph of an ankle after acute pilon fractures. The visible skin wrinkles indicate that the soft-tissue swelling has subsided.

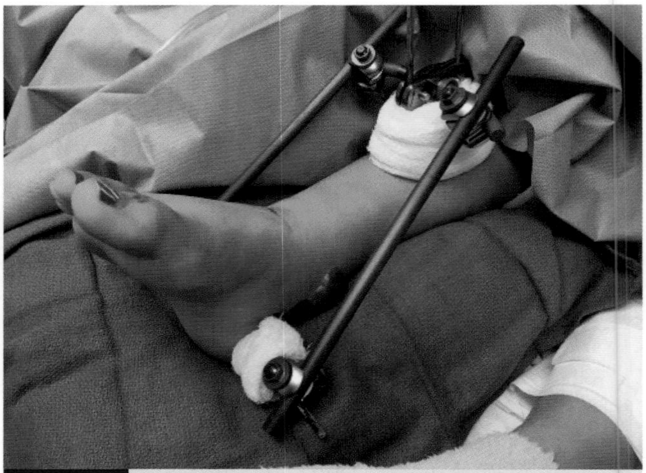

Figure 4 Clinical photograph of a bridging external fixator in place to stabilize an acute pilon fracture.

and stabilization control pain, and the ankle can be elevated to resolve the swelling. It is recommended that CT be performed after the initial reduction and placement of a spanning external fixator because the fracture fragments are better aligned and the anatomy of the fracture fragments can be better appreciated.

Foot pumps may help quickly resolve edema associated with these injuries. A study involving calcaneus fractures that compared elevation and a bulky splint with foot pump, posterior splint application, and elevation in patients with intra-articular calcaneus fractures demonstrated that patients tolerated the foot pump and showed a substantial reduction in foot volume in the first 48 hours after application.[6]

After the soft tissues have improved sufficiently to allow ORIF, the surgeon can choose from several surgical techniques, depending on the fracture pattern and surgeon experience. As shown in **Figure 3**, the appearance of skin wrinkles indicates that the swelling from the initial injury has improved to allow for postoperative skin closure after surgical fixation. The goal of surgery is to obtain an anatomic reduction of the articular surface of the distal tibia and restoration of the normal alignment of the distal tibia as well as the ankle mortise. Fixation methods include plate and screw fixation of the fibula and tibia, fixation of the fibula and limited internal fixation of the tibia with external fixation, or application of a multiplanar external fixator (**Figure 4**). According to a 2015 study, fixation of the fibula is not needed in every case, although it may be helpful in specific cases to aid in tibial reduction or to augment external fixation.[7]

Staged ORIF

A staged repair of pilon fractures, with options including initial application of a bridging external fixator across the ankle joint with or without ORIF of the fibula, is gaining popularity.[8] Whether the fibula should be reduced and fixed acutely is controversial. A malreduced fibula can make anatomic reduction of the distal tibia difficult. When fixation of the fibula and tibia is planned, careful consideration should be given to the placement of the incisions; at least a 5-cm skin bridge should be left between the two approaches.

External fixator pins are placed well above the planned surgical site on the tibia, and a pin is placed in the calcaneal tuberosity and occasionally in the first metatarsal. A first metatarsal pin is useful in controlling equinus. The pins are connected via clamps and connecting bars to control length and alignment. It is important to place the pins away from any planned surgical incision or hardware to reduce the chance of infection. Care should be taken to avoid overlapping definitive plate fixation with the provisional external fixator pin sites. The authors of a 2014 study reviewed 85 pilon fractures and 97 tibial plateau fractures for infection. Internal fixation was performed after provisional external fixation. The authors found that placement of definitive plate fixation overlapping previous external fixator pin sites substantially increased the risk of deep infection in the two-staged treatment of bicondylar tibial plateau and pilon fractures.[9]

After soft-tissue swelling has subsided and fracture blisters have reepithelialized, the fibula is fixed first through a lateral or posterolateral incision. Fixation depends on the fracture pattern. The surgical objective is to restore the length and alignment of the fibula. **Figure 5** shows a distraction technique to regain fibular length with a comminuted fracture pattern. Failure to restore the anatomy of the fibula can make subsequent reduction of the tibia difficult. If there is combined fibular and tibial metaphyseal comminution in an open injury, some surgeons may decide it is preferable to only fix the tibial articular surface and reduce the ankle mortise. Not fixing the fibula and the comminuted distal tibial metaphysis may aid in the closure of transverse medial wounds by allowing the surgeon to shorten the tibia and fibula enough to obtain primary wound closure and avoidance of a free flap.[10]

The reduction of the distal tibia is performed through an anteromedial or anterolateral incision, depending on the fracture pattern (**Figure 6, A and B**). If medial fragments requiring reduction and fixation are present, an anterolateral approach is not recommended. In some instances, the fibula and the tibia can be repaired through a single lateral incision; however, it is difficult to reduce medial fragments through this approach. The tibial reduction usually begins by reducing the posterolateral fragment to the shaft and working progressively to the anteromedial portion of the distal tibia. The fracture is fixed provisionally with Kirschner wires, and the quality of the reduction can be assessed by direct observation and fluoroscopic assessment. Fixation is customized to the fracture pattern and can include a single plate or a combination of plates. Locking plates can assist in maintaining the alignment of the reduced articular fracture fragments to the shaft. A study of the use of locking plates

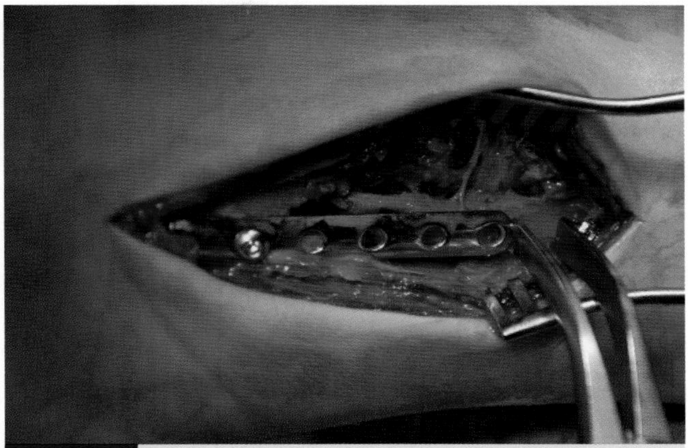

Figure 5 Intraoperative photograph shows a distraction technique to restore fibular length. The plate is fixed to the distal fibular fragment. A screw is placed proximal to the plate on the fibula. The lamina spreader is used as a distraction device between the plate and the screw to restore the length of the fibula.

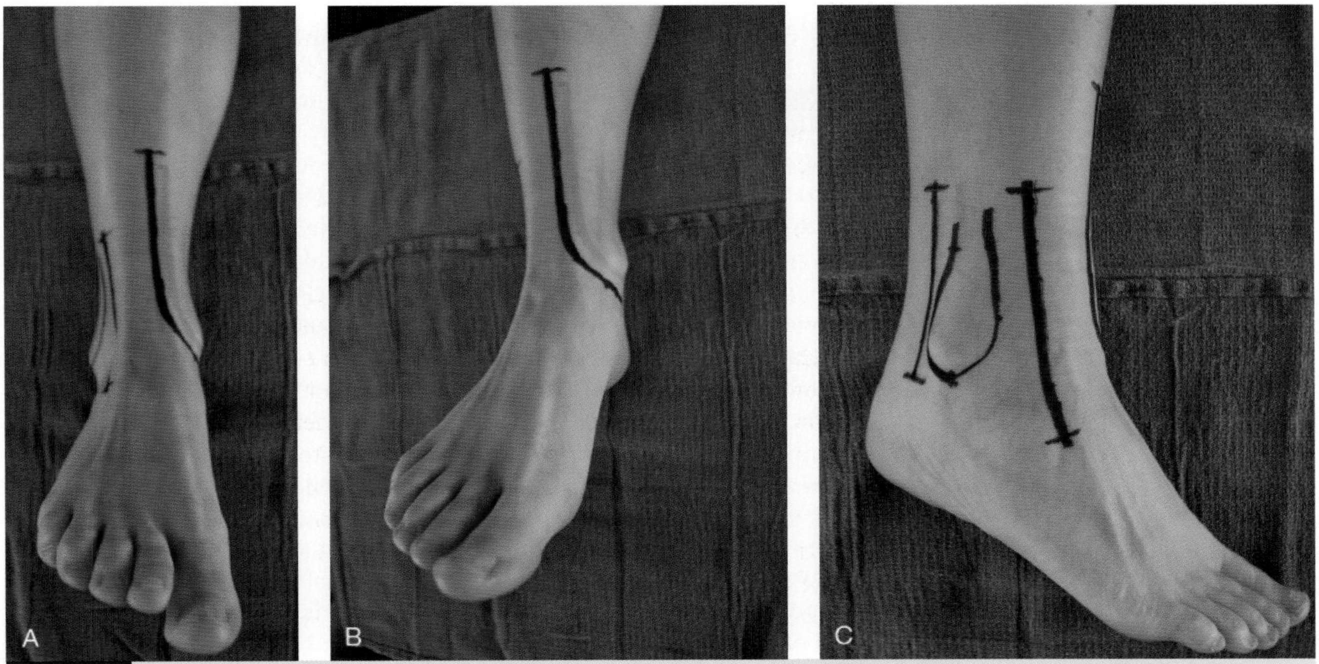

Figure 6 Preoperative photographs show the incisions (marked in black) used in the surgical treatment of distal tibial pilon fractures. The orange line represents the anterior crest of the tibia. **A,** The anteromedial and anterolateral incisions are shown. **B,** The medial view of the anteromedial incision is shown. **C,** The anterolateral and posterolateral incisions are shown.

6: Lower Extremity

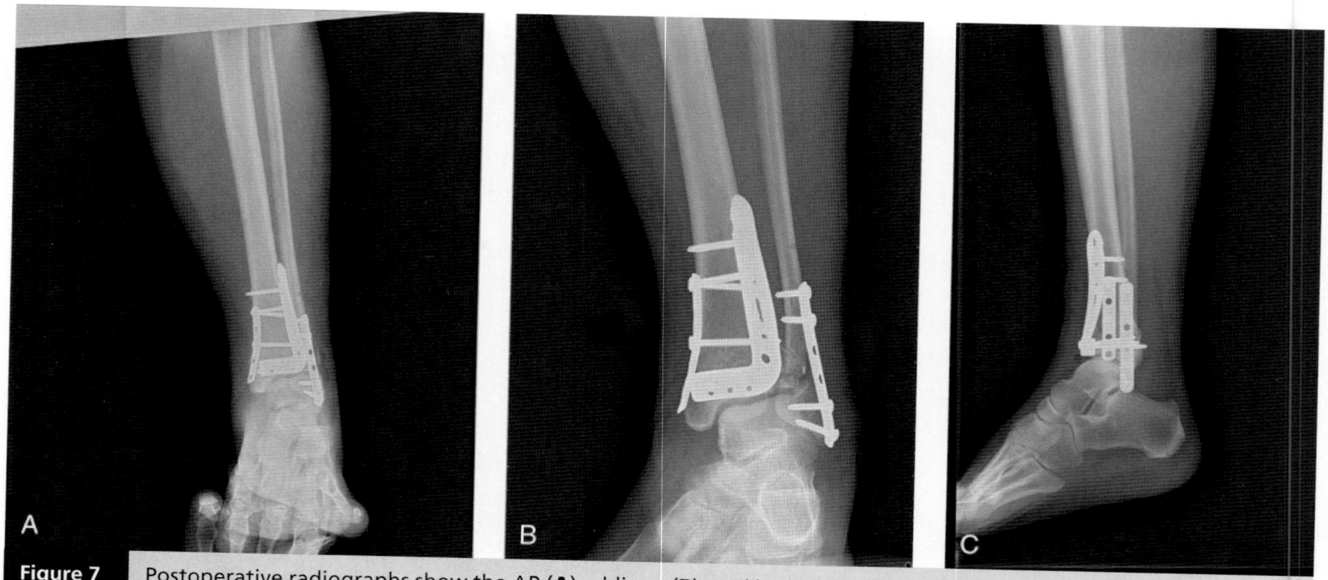

Figure 7 Postoperative radiographs show the AP (**A**), oblique (**B**), and lateral (**C**) views that demonstrate anatomic fixation of the distal fibula fracture with restoration of fibular length, and anatomic reduction of the tibial plafond with both an anterolateral plate and a medial buttress plate.

versus nonlocking plates placed percutaneously for distal tibia fractures demonstrated similar results for both systems, except the locking system was better at maintaining alignment.[11] Fixation and anatomic reduction of the distal fibula and tibial plafond using a standard plate and screw technique is shown in **Figure 7**.

Early ORIF

If the soft tissues allow, early fixation of the fibula and the tibia—within less than 36 hours—can occur at the same time. In most cases, however, it is better to wait until the swelling has subsided and the skin wrinkles have returned. Fixation of the fibula typically is performed through a lateral incision directly overlying the fibula or perhaps slightly posterior to it. The fibula is reduced anatomically and this step often leads to a partial reduction of the tibia through ligamentotaxis. After the fibula has been reduced and fixed, the distal tibia can be approached via the same surgical approaches that would be used in a staged repair. The classic approach is the anteromedial approach (**Figure 6, A**), which uses an extensile incision located just lateral to the tibial crest, gently curving along the lateral border of the tibialis anterior, and curving more medially along the anteromedial border of the ankle joint to the tip of the medial malleolus. The medial and anterior distal tibia can be exposed, and the joint can be visualized. The far lateral aspect of the tibial plafond is difficult to see, but the standard anteromedial approach can provide access to place hardware on the anterolateral tibia. Placement of an anterolateral plate through the anteromedial approach is shown in **Figure 8**.

An alternative procedure is the anterolateral incision (**Figure 6, C**)—a longitudinal incision along the anterior and more lateral aspect of the distal tibia. This incision allows visualization of the anterior and anterolateral aspects of the tibial plafond. It does not allow access to the medial tibia; therefore, a thorough and accurate understanding of the fracture pattern must be obtained before surgery.[12] When planned appropriately, percutaneous fixation of the medial distal tibia also can be performed if needed. If access to the medial tibial plafond is required, the anterolateral incision is not the optimal approach.[13,14]

A 2010 study found that early ORIF performed by experienced orthopaedic trauma surgeons results in a high-quality reduction with a relatively low rate of complications. In the study, 95 patients with OTA type 43C pilon fractures were treated with primary ORIF. Of the total, 70% (66 patients) were treated within 24 hours, and 88% (84 patients) were treated within 48 hours. Reduction was judged to be anatomic in 90% of cases. Six patients were treated for wound dehiscence or deep infection with surgical irrigation and débridement; 4 of these cases involved open fractures.[15]

A similar study published in 2014 found that early ORIF performed within 36 hours resulted in no difference in soft-tissue complications, union rates, and final functional scores at a mean follow-up of 25.8 months compared with definitive fixation delayed 10 days to

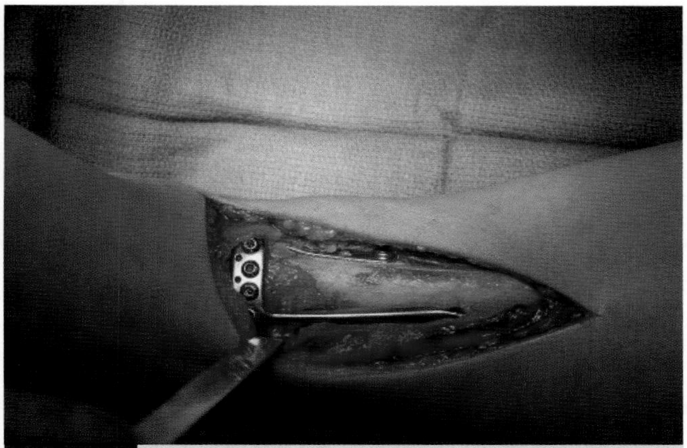

Figure 8 Intraoperative photograph of an anterolateral plate in place.

3 weeks. The study also showed a significantly shorter time to fracture union ($P \leq 0.05$) and a shorter hospital stay ($P \leq 0.01$).[16]

Occasionally, a posterolateral incision (**Figure 6, C**) can be used to repair the posterior part of the tibial plafond. It also can be used in conjunction with an anteromedial or anterolateral approach.[17,18] A posterolateral approach must be planned in advance, based on the size and displacement of the posterior fragment. Additionally, the patient may need to be positioned prone so the surgeon can visualize the reduction and apply fixation. Care must be taken to avoid placing fixation that will hinder reduction and fixation of the remainder of the fracture through another approach.

An alternative to these traditional approaches is the direct anterior approach, which is often used for ankle arthrodesis or total ankle replacement. This approach is gaining popularity because it preserves the possibility of a subsequent salvage procedure in the patient in whom posttraumatic arthritis of the tibiotalar joint develops. If the patient's condition progresses to end-stage ankle arthritis, the traditional anterior approach puts the skin at risk in the presence of prior alternate incisions. This incision is made directly in the midline of the distal tibia, centered over the tibiotalar joint. The distal ankle is approached either between the tibialis anterior and extensor hallucis longus tendons, taking care to protect the anterior neurovascular bundle, or medial to the tibialis anterior tendon, retracting the tendon laterally. If a supplemental posteromedial or posterolateral incision is needed, this anterior incision provides adequate skin bridges to avoid soft-tissue necrosis. If this approach is used in the acute treatment of pilon fractures, additional incisions and the potential for soft-tissue compromise may be avoided in subsequent procedures. **Figures 1** and **7** show the AP, oblique, and mortise views of comminuted pilon fracture dislocation with associated distal fibula fracture.

Intramedullary nailing is another option, and its role was examined in a 2013 study. The authors found that simple AO/OTA type 43C articular fractures of the tibial plafond treated via intramedullary nailing can achieve excellent alignment and union rates with proper patient selection. The additional bone screws or plating options should always be considered to help achieve better anatomic reduction.[19] Intramedullary nails are useful only for specific fracture patterns that have a large block of intact distal tibia in which to seat the nail. Articular fragments require reduction and fixation with interfragmentary lag screws before nail placement. The surgeon must avoid displacement of the prior fixation during insertion of the nail.

External Fixation With Limited Internal Fixation

The fibula can be reduced anatomically, and the tibial plafond can be reduced and fixed with lag screws. Instead of a tibial plate, the external fixator is used to provide control of the tibia. Recent reports demonstrate equivalent outcomes of limited internal fixation with external fixation compared with full ORIF. The external fixator can vary according to surgeon preference. Options include a simple delta frame and hinged external fixator or a multiplanar external fixator.

A 2011 study evaluated 46 patients with OTA type 43C pilon fractures for clinical, radiographic, and functional outcomes. Of the total, 20 patients were treated with a hinged bridging external fixator with supplemental limited internal fixation, and 26 were treated with ORIF. At a mean of 18 and 22 months of follow-up for the external fixation and ORIF groups, respectively, the authors found that both groups appeared to be comparable in treatment of OTA type 43C pilon fractures in the final range of ankle motion, development of arthritis, and hindfoot scores.[20]

Minimally Invasive Plating Techniques

Minimally invasive plating techniques can be useful, especially with simple fracture patterns. The surgeon must be adept at proper plate contouring and using fluoroscopic images to reduce the fracture and secure the fixation. This technique also can be useful in patients with poor skin quality or skin compromise, in whom the traditional open incisions pose a higher risk for wound closure and healing.

Soft-Tissue Management

Management of the soft tissue includes delicate intraoperative handling, careful closure of the skin with a technique that preserves the blood supply, and possibly negative pressure dressings. One study demonstrated that the Allgöwer-Donati suture pattern had the least effect on cutaneous blood flow.[21] A prospective randomized multicenter trial conducted in 2012 showed a decreased incidence of wound dehiscence and total infections after high-risk fractures in patients treated with negative pressure wound therapy applied to the surgical incisions after closure.[22] In addition, a 2013 study showed a trend toward reduction in surgical site infection in patients treated with perioperative supplemental oxygen for 2 hours postoperatively.[23]

A minimum of 5 cm between skin incisions is necessary to prevent soft-tissue compromise. A study of 5-cm or 7-cm skin bridges in pilon fracture repair showed that the complication rate was low with either technique but reinforced that careful planning and meticulous care of the soft tissues was necessary.[24]

Outcomes

Pilon fractures are complex injuries. Outcomes are related to the severity of the fracture, quality of reduction, psychosocial factors, and the occurrence of any complications.[25,26] The experience and skill of the surgeon in obtaining an anatomic reduction and stable fixation are important but are still ill defined. The effect of psychosocial factors on recovery from musculoskeletal trauma has been recognized in general, but the effect on outcomes from pilon fractures is currently unclear. Numerous reports detail the many complications that can occur after surgical intervention for pilon fractures, including wound breakdown, skin loss, fixation failure, bone loss, deep infection, chronic pain, stiffness, swelling, and posttraumatic arthritis.

Outcome studies have tended to show a poor outcome from pilon fractures, particularly when complications have occurred. A 2015 study indicated that Musculoskeletal Functional Assessment scores for patients with pilon fractures improved over 12 months; women experienced greater dysfunction than men at 6, 9, and 12 months after injury; and results in younger patients (ages 18 to 29 years) were better than in older patients.[27] A 2015 retrospective study of 43 patients showed that Medical Outcomes Study 36-Item Short Form scores were significantly worse in patients with pilon fractures than in the general population regardless of surgical technique. Age, education, marital status, fracture pattern, quality of the reduction, and ankle motion all affected results.[28]

Summary

Ankle pilon fractures are complex bone and soft-tissue injuries occurring after an axial load to the ankle region. Careful evaluation of the bone and soft tissue injury is recommended before surgical treatment.

Temporary bridging external fixation across the ankle joint is a useful measure to maintain fracture alignment and gross alignment until acute swelling has subsided enough to perform reduction and fixation of the fracture. Additional radiographs and CT after placement of the external fixator may help the surgeon plan the definitive repair.

Timely healing of the fracture and soft tissues and avoidance of complications can be achieved by a variety of methods depending on the fracture pattern, severity of the soft-tissue injury, and surgeon experience. Surgeons need to be adept at using a variety of methods to treat these challenging injuries. More severe injuries have a worse outcome.

Key Study Points

- Pilon fractures occur from high-energy axial loads.
- The fracture is accompanied by soft-tissue injury, which can be severe.
- The timing of the surgical intervention is important, to avoid soft-tissue complications.
- Surgeons need to be adept at using a variety of surgical approaches to repair the fracture.
- Outcomes are determined by the severity of the injury, psychosocial factors, and the occurrence of any complications.

Annotated References

1. Crist BD, Khazzam M, Murtha YM, Della Rocca GJ: Pilon fractures: Advances in surgical management. *J Am Acad Orthop Surg* 2011;19(10):612-622.

   In individuals with soft-tissue compromise, temporary external fixation and staged management are helpful in reducing further injury and complications. Evidence in support of new surgical approaches and minimally invasive techniques is incomplete. Soft-tissue management, such as negative pressure dressings, may be helpful in preventing complications.

2. Paryavi E, Stall A, Gupta R, et al: Predictive model for surgical site infection risk after surgery for high-energy lower-extremity fractures: Development of the risk of infection in orthopedic trauma surgery score. *J Trauma Acute Care Surg* 2013;74(6):1521-1527.

The authors found that the relative odds of infection among patients with AO type C3 fractures was 5.40 compared with fractures of lower classification. Fractures classified as American Society of Anesthesiologists class 3 or higher and a body mass index less than 30 kg/m^2 also were factors predictive of infection. Level of evidence: II.

3. Graves ML, Kosko J, Barei DP, et al: Lateral ankle radiographs: Do we really understand what we are seeing? *J Orthop Trauma* 2011;25(2):106-109.

   This cadaver study evaluates using the lateral fluoroscopic image to assess the reduction of the tibial plafond articular surface. Even with a perfect lateral fluoroscopic view, displacement still may be present. When small osteochondral fragments are present, direct visualization of the articular surface is necessary.

4. Patillo D, Della Rocca GJ, Murtha YM, Crist BD: Pilon fracture complicated by compartment syndrome: A case report. *J Orthop Trauma* 2010;24(6):e54-e57.

   Pilon fractures associated with compartment syndrome are rare occurrences despite the relatively high-energy mechanisms that cause many of them. The surgeon should maintain a high index of suspicion for compartment syndrome in patients with intractable pain after pilon fracture.

5. Cole PA, Mehrle RK, Bhandari M, Zlowodzki M: The pilon map: Fracture lines and comminution zones in OTA/AO type 43C3 pilon fractures. *J Orthop Trauma* 2013;27(7):e152-e156.

   The authors reviewed axial CT images on OTA type 43C3 fractures. A consistent fracture pattern underlying most of the fractures was observed with three main fragments. The comminution in pilon fractures occurs from secondary fracture lines occurring through the apex of the plafond and in the anterolateral region.

6. Thordarson DB, Greene N, Shepherd L, Perlman M: Facilitating edema resolution with a foot pump after calcaneus fracture. *J Orthop Trauma* 1999;13(1):43-46.

7. Kurylo JC, Datta N, Iskander KN, Tornetta P III: Does the fibula need to be fixed in complex pilon fractures? *J Orthop Trauma* 2015;29(9):424-427.

   Fibular fixation is not a necessary step in the reconstruction of pilon fractures, although it may be helpful in specific cases to aid in tibial plafond reduction or augment external fixation. A higher rate of plate removal was found if the fibula was fixed. Level of evidence: III.

8. Ziran BH, Morrison T, Little J, Hileman B: A new ankle spanning fixator construct for distal tibia fractures: Optimizing visualization, minimizing pin problems, and protecting the heel. *J Orthop Trauma* 2013;27(2):e45-e49.

   The authors describe a novel and simple technique involving placing the calcaneal pins posteriorly and using a U-shaped bar, which creates a construct that reduces or eliminates many disadvantages during the time required for soft-tissue swelling to subside to permit definitive fixation.

9. Shah CM, Babb PE, McAndrew CM, et al: Definitive plates overlapping provisional external fixator pin sites: Is the infection risk increased? *J Orthop Trauma* 2014;28(9):518-522.

   The authors reviewed 85 bicondylar Orthopaedic Trauma Association (OTA) 41C tibial plateau fractures and 97 OTA 43C pilon fractures for deep infection. Placement of definitive plate fixation overlapping previous external fixator pin sites substantially increases the risk of deep infection in the two-stage treatment of bicondylar tibial plateau and pilon fractures. Level of evidence: III.

10. D'Alleyrand JC, Manson TT, Dancy L, et al: Is time to flap coverage of open tibial fractures an independent predictor of flap-related complications? *J Orthop Trauma* 2014;28(5):288-293.

    The authors reviewed 69 patients for flap complications in acute tibia fractures. Even after controlling for known risk factors for complications, including injury severity, the time elapsed until flap coverage was an important predictor of complications.

11. Bastias C, Henriquez H, Pellegrini M, et al: Are locking plates better than non-locking plates for treating distal tibia fractures? *Foot Ankle Surg* 2014;20(2):115-119.

    Both plating systems have similar results for fracture union, complications, and American Orthopaedic Foot and Ankle Society scores. The locking plate may be superior for alignment and implant removal.

12. Eastman JG, Firoozabadi R, Benirschke SK, Barei DP, Dunbar RP: Entrapped posteromedial structures in pilon fractures. *J Orthop Trauma* 2014;28(9):528-533.

    The authors analyzed radiographs and CT of 394 patients with a pilon fracture to identify the incidence of interposed posteromedial soft tissues in the fracture. Failure to recognize an interposed structure could lead to malreduction, impaired tendon function, neurovascular insult, and the need for further surgery. Level of evidence: IV.

13. Hak DJ: Anterolateral approach for tibial pilon fractures. *Orthopedics* 2012;35(2):131-133.

    The anterolateral approach offers improved soft-tissue coverage and the potential for a lower rate of wound-healing complications by avoiding incision placement over the subcutaneous border of the tibia. Additional exposures may be required to address other areas of the fracture, such as the medial malleolus, which cannot be accessed through this approach.

14. Mehta S, Gardner MJ, Barei DP, Benirschke SK, Nork SE: Reduction strategies through the anterolateral exposure for fixation of type B and C pilon fractures. *J Orthop Trauma* 2011;25(2):116-122.

    The authors describe the anterolateral approach in open treatment of pilon fractures and stress the importance of delayed treatment and the meticulous handling of the soft tissues. The anterolateral exposure is not suitable for fractures with medial comminution, medial crush, impaction at the medial shoulder of the joint, segmental medial malleolar injuries, or varus deformity at the time of injury.

15. White TO, Guy P, Cooke CJ, et al: The results of early primary open reduction and internal fixation for treatment of OTA 43.C-type tibial pilon fractures: A cohort study. *J Orthop Trauma* 2010;24(12):757-763.

    Early ORIF performed by experienced orthopaedic trauma surgeons results in a high-quality reduction with a relatively low rate of complications. In the study, 95 patients with OTA type 43C pilon fractures were treated with primary ORIF. Of the total, 70% (66 patients) were treated within 24 hours, and 88% (84 patients) were treated within 48 hours. Reduction was judged to be anatomic in 90% of cases. Six patients were treated for wound dehiscence or deep infection with surgical irrigation and débridement; four of these cases involved open fractures.

16. Tang X, Liu L, Tu CQ, Li J, Li Q, Pei FX: Comparison of early and delayed open reduction and internal fixation for treating closed tibial pilon fractures. *Foot Ankle Int* 2014;35(7):657-664.

    If soft-tissue conditions are acceptable, early ORIF for treating closed type C pilon fractures can be safe and effective, with similar rates of wound complication, fracture union, and final good functional recovery but shorter surgical time, union time, and hospital stay. These results favorably compare with delayed ORIF treatment. Level of evidence: III.

17. Assal M, Ray A, Fasel JH, Stern R: A modified posteromedial approach combined with extensile anterior for the treatment of complex tibial pilon fractures (AO/OTA 43-C). *J Orthop Trauma* 2014;28(6):e138-e145.

    The authors describe a midline posterior approach that could provide better visualization of the posterior column and juxtametaphyseal/diaphyseal parts of the tibia as part of a combined posterior and anterior approach during the same anesthesia for complex tibial AO/OTA 43C pilon fractures in a preliminary study of six patients.

18. Lidder S, Masterson S, Dreu M, Clement H, Grechenig S: The risk of injury to the peroneal artery in the posterolateral approach to the distal tibia: A cadaver study. *J Orthop Trauma* 2014;28(9):534-537.

    In this cadaver study, the authors describe a safe zone of proximal dissection in the posterolateral approach to the distal tibia to avoid injury to the peroneal vessels. Dissection around this region should be performed with care because of the wide variation in vasculature.

19. Marcus MS, Yoon RS, Langford J, et al: Is there a role for intramedullary nails in the treatment of simple pilon fractures? Rationale and preliminary results. *Injury* 2013;44(8):1107-1111.

    The authors reviewed 31 patients who sustained OTA type 43C distal tibial fractures and were treated with intramedullary nailing. Simple AO/OTA type 43C articular fractures of the tibial plafond treated via intramedullary nailing can achieve excellent rates of alignment and union.

20. Davidovitch RI, Elkhechen RJ, Romo S, Walsh M, Egol KA: Open reduction with internal fixation versus limited internal fixation and external fixation for high grade pilon fractures (OTA type 43C). *Foot Ankle Int* 2011;32(10):955-961.

    The authors evaluated 46 patients with pilon fractures for clinical, radiographic, and functional outcomes. Patients were treated with a hinged bridging external fixator with supplemental limited internal fixation or ORIF. Both groups appeared to achieve comparable final range of ankle motion, arthritis, and hindfoot scores. Level of evidence: IV.

21. Sagi HC, Papp S, Dipasquale T: The effect of suture pattern and tension on cutaneous blood flow as assessed by laser Doppler flowmetry in a pig model. *J Orthop Trauma* 2008;22(3):171-175.

22. Stannard JP, Volgas DA, McGwin G III, et al: Incisional negative pressure wound therapy after high-risk lower extremity fractures. *J Orthop Trauma* 2012;26(1):37-42.

    This prospective randomized multicenter trial investigates incisional negative pressure wound therapy. A strong trend also exists for reductions in acute infections after negative pressure wound therapy, which should be considered for high-risk wounds after severe skeletal trauma.

23. Stall A, Paryavi E, Gupta R, Zadnik M, Hui E, O'Toole RV: Perioperative supplemental oxygen to reduce surgical site infection after open fixation of high-risk fractures: A randomized controlled pilot trial. *J Trauma Acute Care Surg* 2013;75(4):657-663.

    This study reports a randomized controlled pilot trial in which the primary outcome measure was surgical site infection. The authors found that using a high concentration of fraction of inspired oxygen (FIO_2) during the perioperative period is safe and shows a trend toward the reduction of surgical site infection. Level of evidence: III.

24. Howard JL, Agel J, Barei DP, Benirschke SK, Nork SE: A prospective study evaluating incision placement and wound healing for tibial plafond fractures. *J Orthop Trauma* 2008;22(5):299-305, discussion 305-306.

25. Korkmaz A, Ciftdemir M, Ozcan M, Copuroğlu C, Sarıdoğan K: The analysis of the variables, affecting outcome in surgically treated tibia pilon fractured patients. *Injury* 2013;44(10):1270-1274.

    The authors reviewed the 1-year follow-up of patients divided into three groups based on the type of treatment: (1) ORIF; (2) mini-open reduction and internal fixation and external fixation; (3) closed reduction and external fixation. The most important factor affecting outcome was the quality of the reduction.

26. Khalsa AS, Toossi N, Tabb LP, Amin NH, Donohue KW, Cerynik DL: Distal tibia fractures: Locked or non-locked

plating? A systematic review of outcomes. *Acta Orthop* 2014;85(3):299-304.

Twenty-seven studies met the inclusion criteria and were included in the final analysis of 764 cases (499 locking, 265 nonlocking). Delayed union was reported in 6% of cases with locked plating and in 4% of cases with nonlocked plating. Nonunion was reported in 2% of cases with locked plating and 3% of cases with nonlocked plating. This study showed that locked plating reduces the odds of reoperation and malalignment after treatment for acute distal tibia fracture.

27. Lundy DW, Agel J, Marsh JL, et al: Musculoskeletal function assessment outcomes scores over time for tibial plafond (OTA/AO 43) and proximal humeral (OTA/AO 11) fractures: A pilot project. *J Orthop Trauma* 2015;29(2):e60-e64.

Patients who sustained isolated proximal humerus or tibial plafond fractures showed gradual improvement over 1 year. Women consistently demonstrated greater dysfunction than men at 6, 9, and 12 months after tibial plafond fracture. Age had an effect on return to function after injury for both fractures. Younger patients (18-29 years) with either type of injury tended to have better scores compared with the older patients. Level of evidence: IV.

28. Cutillas-Ybarra MB, Lizaur-Utrilla A, Lopez-Prats FA: Prognostic factors of health-related quality of life in patients after tibial plafond fracture. A pilot study. *Injury* 2015;46(11):2253-2257.

Tibial plafond fractures have a significant negative effect on general health-related quality of life regardless of the surgical treatment used, which reflects injury severity. In addition, psychosocial characteristics of patients may influence the outcomes.

Chapter 47

Foot Fractures and Dislocations

Anna N. Miller, MD, FACS

Abstract

Foot fractures and dislocations are common traumatic injuries associated with high rates of morbidity and dysfunction. It is important for the orthopaedic surgeon to review calcaneus and talus fracture classifications and indications for nonsurgical and surgical management, along with expected rehabilitation and outcomes for these injuries.

Keywords: calcaneus fracture; Chopart fracture; cuboid fracture; cuneiform fracture; Lisfranc fracture; metatarsal fracture; navicular fracture; talus fracture

Introduction

The wide range of traumatic foot injuries extends from a minimally displaced fracture that can be treated nonsurgically to a mangled limb that must be amputated. In general, anatomic alignment is crucial to allowing the foot structures to resume their normal weight-bearing and mobility functions. Most displaced foot injuries require surgical fixation and a period of non–weight bearing before a return to activity.

Hindfoot Injuries

Talus Fractures and Dislocations

Although talus fractures are rare, accounting for only 2% to 3% of foot fractures, they are associated with decreased functional outcome scores and high rates of posttraumatic subtalar arthritis.[1,2] Almost half of all talus fractures are in the talar neck.[3] The Hawkins classification is used to classify talus fractures[4,5] (**Figure 1**). Osteonecrosis of the talus is correlated with the fracture pattern; it occurs in as many as 64% of Hawkins type III fractures. Osteonecrosis has been attributed to the retrograde blood supply to the talus, although antegrade flow also has been found significant.[2,6] A reevaluation of the Hawkins classification found that subtalar dislocation in Hawkins type II fractures is a predictor of osteonecrosis.[7] The Hawkins sign reliably indicates that the talus has vascularity, but the absence of the Hawkins sign in the talus does not predict osteonecrosis[8] (**Figure 2**).

Urgent reduction of a dislocated talus is mandatory, but the timing of definitive fracture fixation does not determine outcomes, radiographic changes, or functional results.[2,9,10] Although the treatment of a talus fracture is surgical, a nondisplaced fracture can be treated with cast immobilization and non–weight bearing for as long as 12 weeks. Lack of displacement should be confirmed on CT.[11] Nondisplaced talus fractures also can be treated with percutaneous fixation and relatively early mobilization. Posterior-to-anterior constructs were found to provide good biomechanical stability.[12,13]

Two incisions are commonly used for open treatment of a talus fracture.[14] The anterolateral incision is just lateral to the extensor digitorum longus, along the fourth ray. The anteromedial incision is between the anterior and posterior tibial tendons. It is especially important to evaluate comminution, which most commonly is medial. The purpose is to avoid shortening the talus or placing it into varus with fixation, as particularly can occur if the surgeon uses only a lateral incision and relies only on the relatively intact lateral talus fragment for alignment. Plate-and-screw fixation is preferable to compression screw fixation for bridging comminution, although multiple studies found that plate-and-screw constructs have no distinct advantage in strength[12,15,16] (**Figure 3**).

Outcomes after a talus fracture depend on its Hawkins type as well as the presence of an open fracture.[2,9,10] One study found that 100% of displaced fractures led to subtalar arthritis.[9] As many as 50% of patients needed a secondary reconstructive surgery within 10 years of injury.[10] In contrast, patients with an isolated subtalar dislocation without fracture had a good outcome; this finding emphasized that the morbidity is associated with the talus fracture itself.[17] An isolated subtalar dislocation

Dr. Miller or an immediate family member serves as a paid consultant to DePuy Synthes.

6: Lower Extremity

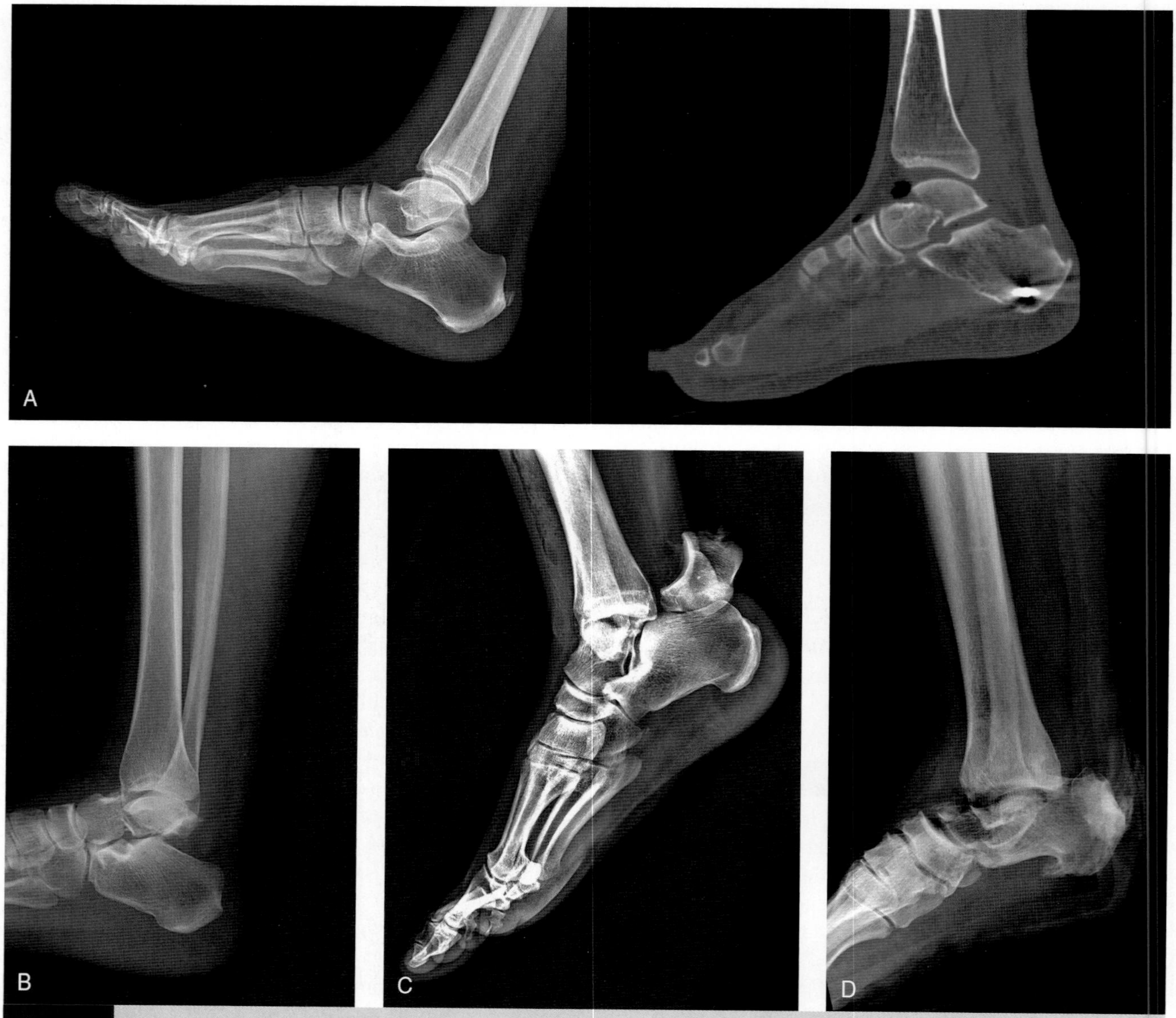

Figure 1 Lateral radiographs showing the Hawkins classification of talar neck fractures. **A**, A nondisplaced fracture (Hawkins type I) (left) with sagittal CT (right) showing the nondisplaced fracture line. **B**, A fracture with subtalar dislocation (Hawkins type II). **C,** A fracture with subtalar and tibiotalar dislocation (Hawkins type III). **D**, A fracture with subtalar, tibiotalar, and talonavicular dislocation (Hawkins type IV).

should be evaluated with CT after reduction to confirm congruency and detect a possible occult fracture or a fragment entrapped in the subtalar joint.

Fractures of the talar body and lateral process are less common than talar neck fractures. A talar body fracture can be treated similar to a talar neck fracture except that a medial malleolus osteotomy may be required for complete visualization of the injury. As with talar body fractures, the presence of other injuries or an open fracture increases the risk of a poor outcome.[18] A lateral process fracture, sometimes called a snowboarder's fracture, may be missed on plain radiographs. Small fragments can be treated nonsurgically, but larger fragments often require fixation to avoid the risk of subtalar arthritis.[19]

Calcaneus Fractures

The calcaneus is the most commonly injured bone of the hindfoot.[20] Most of these injuries have a high-energy mechanism with axial load. Historically, the main fracture line is described as dividing the sustentaculum tali from the main tuber of the calcaneus, leaving the sustentaculum tali as a so-called constant fragment. Displacement was found

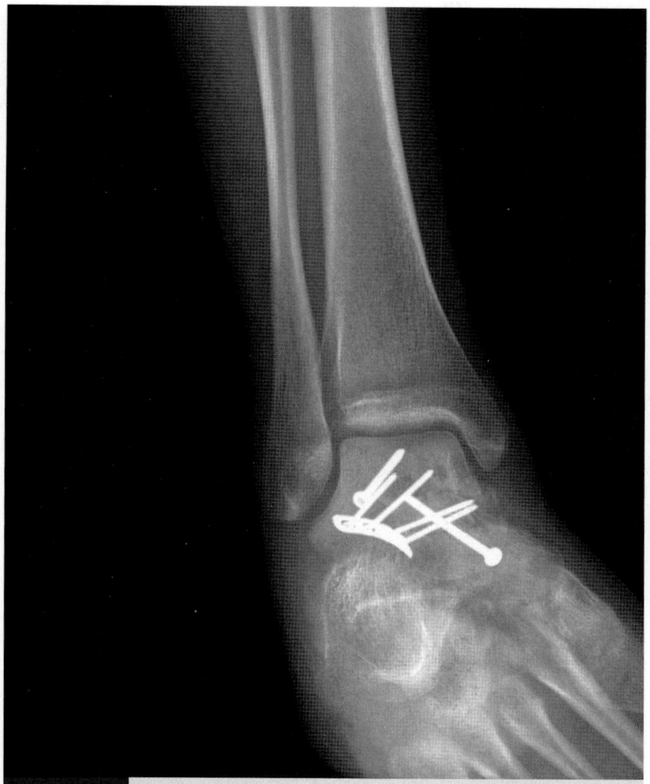

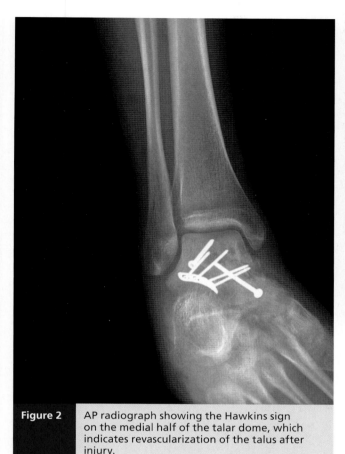

Figure 2 AP radiograph showing the Hawkins sign on the medial half of the talar dome, which indicates revascularization of the talus after injury.

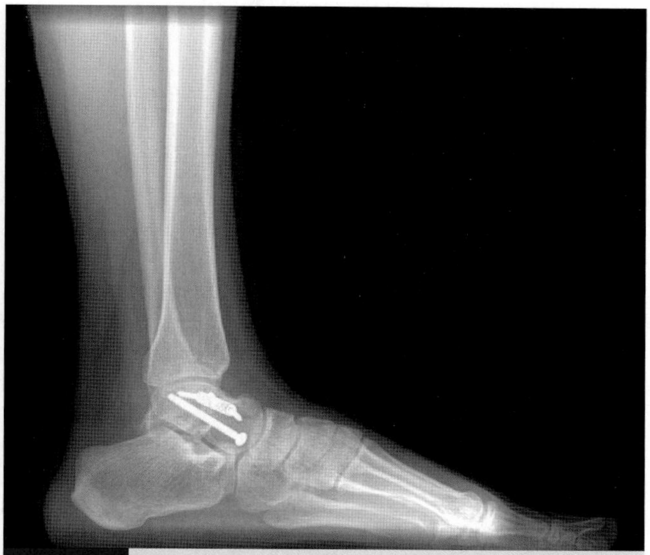

Figure 3 Lateral radiograph showing plate fixation of a comminuted talar neck fracture.

in as many as 40% of fractures, however.[21,22] The primary injury patterns in a calcaneus fracture are height loss, hindfoot varus, heel widening, shortening, and subtalar joint involvement (**Figure 4**). A patient with a calcaneus fracture often has significant soft-tissue damage. Surgery often is delayed until swelling and blistering have resolved and skin wrinkles are visible. In a tongue-type calcaneus fracture, more urgent fixation is required to relieve skin pressure and avoid heel necrosis (**Figure 5**).

The Sanders classification is widely used for joint-depression fractures. This system is CT based and has only fair interobserver reliability.[23,24] Anterior process comminution and the surgeon's overall impression of the fracture were found to be more significantly associated with poor functional outcome than the Sanders classification.[25]

Many patients with a calcaneus fracture are treated nonsurgically because of the high risk of complications in people who have poor skin quality, a long history of smoking, severe diabetes, diabetes-associated vascular disease, immunocompromise, malnutrition, or a chronic disease such as renal failure. A randomized controlled study found that surgical and nonsurgical treatment had equivalent outcomes in these patients.[26] The patient's physiologic condition should be considered; patients older than 50 years were found to have outcomes equivalent to those of younger patients after surgical management of calcaneus fractures.[27] Increased severity of injury (specifically, the size of an open wound and its Gustilo type) was found to be related to the risk for amputation in military personnel.[28] Historically, open calcaneus fractures were believed to have a particularly high rate of poor outcomes, but these rates were found to improve with the use of a standardized treatment protocol, and an open fracture alone should not be considered an indication for avoiding osteosynthesis.[29] Open injury, smoking, and diabetes were cumulative risk factors for the surgical treatment of calcaneus fractures, and the choice of surgical or nonsurgical treatment of a calcaneus fracture should be considered cautiously if the patient has one of these associated conditions.[30] Surgical treatment should be delayed until swelling has subsided and the wrinkle sign returns 2 to 3 weeks after initial injury. Because of the complexity of calcaneus injuries, surgeons and institutions with extensive treatment experience and volume may have the best outcomes.[31]

An extensile lateral surgical approach, which is most commonly used, provides access to the entire extent of the lateral calcaneus and its articulations. The medial side can be reduced only indirectly through this approach. Because the sustentaculum tali is one of the densest areas of calcaneal bone and the sustentaculum fragment often is constant, a screw commonly is placed in this location. Radiographs have shown that this screw is not always

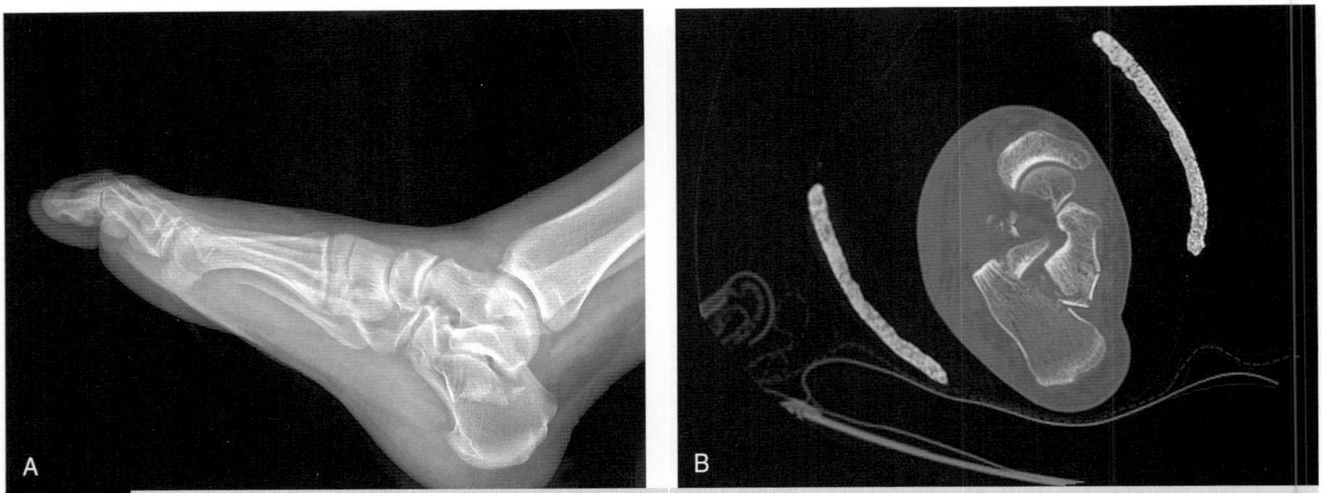

Figure 4 **A,** Lateral radiograph showing a calcaneus fracture with height loss and subtalar joint involvement. **B,** Axial CT showing hindfoot varus and heel widening.

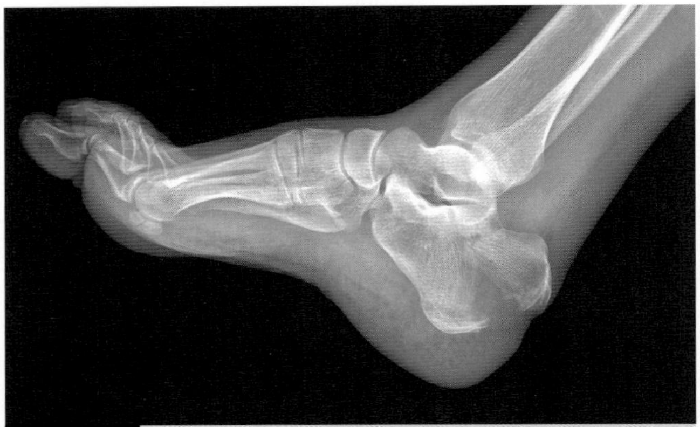

Figure 5 Lateral radiograph showing a tongue-type calcaneus fracture with posterior skin tenting.

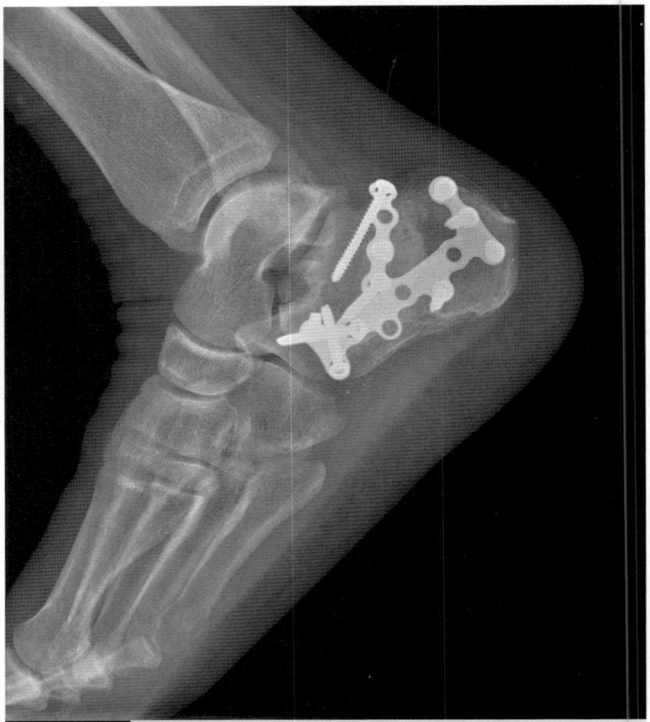

Figure 6 Lateral radiograph showing plate fixation of a calcaneus fracture.

placed accurately, and the placement must be confirmed on multiple views.[32] The use of screws with long tips on the medial side should be avoided to avoid penetration of the neurovascular bundle. Lateral plates also have been used to fix calcaneus fractures. No benefit has been found for the use of a locking construct rather than a nonlocking construct[33] (**Figure 6**). Small percutaneous approaches sometimes can be used with equivalent outcomes and less risk of wound complications or infection compared with a large open approach.[34,35] Long-term studies have not shown a difference in functional outcomes after surgical treatment of calcaneus fractures with or without bone void fillers, although one study found greater height loss after fixation alone compared with fixation and the use of a calcium phosphate filler.[36]

The most common complications of calcaneus fractures are necrosis of the wound-flap edge or the entire wound flap, infection, and posttraumatic arthritis. Wound-flap necrosis can be avoided by meticulous soft-tissue management, including delaying surgery until swelling has subsided, careful intraoperative handling, and avoidance of self-retaining surgical retractors. Meticulous wound closure with absorbable sutures is essential, and the modified Allgöwer-Donati technique for flap closure should be used. The risk of infection is increased in patients who smoke tobacco, have an open fracture, or have diabetes mellitus.[30] Posttraumatic subtalar arthritis is common and affects the outcome in patients with an intra-articular calcaneus fracture.[37]

The outcome after treatment of a calcaneus fracture in general is moderate; most patients are not able to return to employment requiring heavy labor after such an injury.[38] Patients whose initial treatment was surgical were found to have a better outcome than those with initial nonsurgical management, even if subtalar arthritis necessitated further intervention.[37] In patients who had a mangled extremity with severe hindfoot and ankle injury, those treated with a free tissue transfer or ankle arthrodesis had poorer outcomes than those treated with a below-knee amputation.[39]

Midfoot Injuries

The midfoot contains the navicular, the cuboid, and three cuneiforms. The midfoot connects the hindfoot at the Chopart joint with the forefoot at the Lisfranc joint. The midfoot bones are relatively immobile because of their strong plantar ligament attachments, and the midfoot does not contact the ground during weight bearing. The key function of the midfoot is to provide stability to maintain the weight-bearing arch as well as the relationship of the forefoot and hindfoot.[40]

Chopart Dislocations and Fracture-Dislocations

Chopart joint dislocations and fracture-dislocations are quite rare, but they are among the most severe midfoot injuries. These injuries often occur in conjunction with other midfoot injuries, usually during a motor vehicle crash. Combined Chopart and Lisfranc fracture-dislocations are more likely to lead to long-term impairment than any other midfoot injury. [41]Chopart injuries usually require open reduction. Only patients with an isolated pure dislocation have a good outcome after closed reduction.[41] The standard of care is an open anatomic restoration followed by stabilization across the joint. The available methods include external fixation and fixation with 2.0-mm Kirschner wires or 3.5-mm cortical screws. Primary fusion can be considered if severe comminution and/or multiple dislocations are present. Patients with a Chopart injury often need soft-tissue care such as vacuum-assisted wound closure, skin grafting, or fasciectomies for foot compartment syndrome. After surgery, a short leg splint is used, and patients remain non–weight bearing for 6 weeks. A gradual return to full weight bearing extends from 6 to 10 weeks after surgery.

Navicular Fractures

The tarsal navicular has a crucial position in the longitudinal arch and is one of the most important bones in the foot during weight bearing.[42] Because of its key position and the mobility of the talonavicular joint, multiple fracture types are associated with navicular injury. These fractures are relatively rare but more common than cuboid or cuneiform fractures.[43]

Most acute fractures of the navicular are caused by a high-energy axial load, as in a motor vehicle crash. Navicular fractures appear in forms ranging from subtle chronic pain in a stress fracture to an obvious midfoot deformity. If the patient can tolerate standing, weight-bearing radiographs are useful for diagnosing ligamentous instability. CT or a bone scan is especially helpful for evaluating a stress fracture that may not be evident on plain radiographs. Avulsion fractures and simple, nondisplaced tuberosity fractures can be managed with a weight-bearing short leg cast or cast boot for 6 to 8 weeks. All other nondisplaced fractures should be treated in a short leg cast with 6 to 8 weeks of non–weight bearing. The most important goal of surgery for a navicular fracture is to maintain the medial column length and talonavicular articulation, thus restoring stability to the midfoot.

Midbody fractures involve the crucial talonavicular articulation. Displacement of more than 1 to 2 mm should be reduced and fixed. Because of the tenuous central blood supply, it is important to avoid stripping and excessive exposure. The proximal articular surface is the only essential joint. In contrast, the distal and anterior facets have much less motion and can be treated with fusion. With excessive comminution, internal plating or external fixation can be used to maintain medial column length. If less than 60% of the talonavicular joint surface can be reconstructed, an acute talonavicular fusion should be done to maintain the length of the medial column.[44]

Osteonecrosis and late partial collapse of the navicular are common after a body injury, and late medial collapse may necessitate further surgery.

Cuboid Fractures

Cuboid fractures usually occur with another injury such as a talonavicular fracture, Lisfranc injury, or disruption of another midfoot structure. Small medial or dorsal navicular avulsion fractures should be considered as a sign of possible cuboid injury.[45] The cuboid articulates with the lateral cuneiform, navicular, and calcaneus and therefore is involved in almost all midfoot motion. Forced plantar flexion and abduction of the forefoot can cause a so-called nutcracker effect leading to cuboid fracture.[46] Dorsolateral pain and swelling are common with these injuries. The

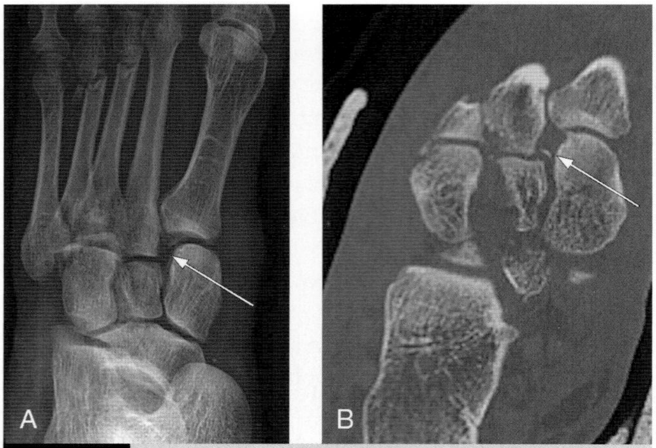

Figure 7 AP radiograph **(A)** and axial CT **(B)** showing a so-called fleck sign indicating tarsometatarsal joint injury (arrows).

presence of another injury to the midfoot bones should raise suspicion for a cuboid fracture.

Nonsurgical management is reserved for an isolated injury with no instability. These fractures are treated with a short leg cast and a period of 6 weeks of non–weight bearing. For a displaced fracture, restoration of length and alignment is the most important goal of surgery. In small studies, anatomic fixation appeared to have better outcomes than aggressive primary calcaneocuboid arthrodesis.[47] In multiple fractures of the midfoot, the cuboid should be fixed first to restore the lateral column before the surgery proceeds medially. Cuboid fractures with relatively little comminution can be directly treated using minifragment plates. For a greatly comminuted fracture, it may be necessary to span the cuboid using spanning plates or external fixation to restore lateral column length. These plates or external fixation pins usually are placed in the fifth metatarsal or calcaneus and must be removed after the fracture has healed. Patients remain non–weight bearing for approximately 6 weeks and slowly progress toward full weight bearing over the next 4 to 6 weeks. Loss of lateral column length and stability are the most worrisome complications after a cuboid fracture. An opening-wedge osteotomy may be necessary if substantial forefoot abduction or loss of midfoot stability develops.

Cuneiform Fractures

Isolated cuneiform fractures are unusual and most commonly are medial. Medial cuneiform injury usually is associated with Lisfranc or other midfoot injuries. Although crush injuries occur, the cuneiforms more commonly are injured as part of a global midfoot injury caused by an indirect axial load. Dorsal dislocation can result from extreme plantar flexion at the time of injury. With intercuneiform ligament disruption, a visible gap may appear as an increase in the size of the first web space, especially during weight bearing.[48] Physical examination findings include tenderness, swelling, and ecchymosis in the dorsomedial midfoot.

Isolated fractures of the medial cuneiform can be treated nonsurgically with 6 weeks of non–weight bearing in a splint. Most cuneiform fractures occur with another injury, such as a Lisfranc fracture, and should be treated as appropriate for the associated injury. The primary goal is to restore proper alignment and stability to the medial side of the foot. Open reduction and internal fixation of adjacent structures should be used as needed to restore stability. Most complications are related to associated injuries of the midfoot. Missed diagnosis of fracture or instability and inaccurate reduction also occur with these injuries.[49]

Tarsometatarsal and Lisfranc Fractures

The annual incidence of tarsometatarsal (TMT) joint injury is approximately 1 in 60,000.[50] Motor vehicle crashes account for almost half of these injuries. TMT injuries can be difficult to diagnose radiographically, and a high index of suspicion is necessary. There is very little mobile articulation at the TMT joints, which form the boundary between the midfoot and forefoot. The lateral column has approximately three times the mobility of the medial column; within the medial column, the first ray is three times more mobile than the second or third rays.[51]

The two main mechanisms of TMT injuries, including ligamentous disruption and bony fracture, are direct dorsal and indirect loads. With a direct dorsal load, as in a crush injury, it is important to pay close attention to soft-tissue damage. Crush injuries have a particularly strong relationship with foot compartment syndrome.[52] An indirect load causes hyper–plantar flexion and dorsal-to-plantar ligament disruption. The bones surrounding the site of injury also may be fractured.[53] The physical examination often reveals pain along the TMT joints in these patients. Plantar ecchymosis in the midfoot also has been described as a sign indicating TMT injury.[54]

The misdiagnosis rate is high for TMT joint injuries, and radiographs are crucial.[55] Weight-bearing views should be obtained, if possible. Any fleck sign of avulsion fracture should lead to suspicion of TMT injury (**Figure 7**). An injury with more than 2 mm of displacement or instability requires surgical treatment. Anatomic reduction and fixation provides the best chance for a good result. Recurrence of instability is most likely to occur with a purely ligamentous injury, and primary fusion may be advisable.[56,57] Most experts recommend using screw fixation across these joints because screws are biomechanically superior to Kirschner wires. The mobile fourth and fifth TMT joints can be fixed with Kirschner wires that are removed relatively quickly to avoid stiffness.[56] Long-term stiffness, pain, and swelling are common after TMT joint injuries, but anatomic realignment improves outcomes.[56] Posttraumatic arthritis is the most common complication that requires reoperation, often with conversion to arthrodesis.

Forefoot Injuries

Appropriate alignment of the metatarsals and phalanges is important for normal foot function and comfort. Multiple metatarsal fractures were found to have worse outcomes than Lisfranc or Chopart joint injuries.[58] Injury to the fifth metatarsal is particularly common, and healing rates vary depending on the fracture location. Along with the tenuous blood supply, the insertion of the peroneus brevis is a factor in the relatively low healing rate of fifth metatarsal base fractures.[59] Many metatarsal and phalangeal fractures can be treated nonsurgically if alignment is maintained. A Jones fracture (at the metadiaphyseal junction of the fifth metatarsal base) often is surgically treated because of high rates of nonunion. A 4.5-mm or larger screw diameter should be used to maximize bony purchase.[60,61] Patients usually are able to return to normal function after these injuries, although they may have occasional pain.[62] The pseudo-Jones fracture is proximal to the fourth-fifth metatarsal articulation and usually heals well without surgical intervention. The dancer's fracture is a spiral fracture of the distal fifth metatarsal shaft that usually can be treated nonsurgically, even in a high-level athlete.[63]

Other types of metatarsal fractures may require surgical fixation, especially with displacement. The overall alignment of the foot can be changed with shortening or flexion-extension of the metatarsal head, neck, or shaft. Malalignment and prominence of the metatarsals can lead to foot ulceration and callus, pain, and shoe wear difficulty. A metatarsal neck or base fracture often can be treated with percutaneous fixation, but a displaced shaft fracture occasionally requires minifragment plating.

Summary

Foot injuries encompass a wide variety of fractures and dislocations. In general, anatomic alignment is crucial to the outcomes of these injuries. Most displaced foot injuries require surgical fixation and a period of non–weight bearing before return to activity. Patient outcomes are moderate to good, depending on the severity of injury. Many of these traumatic injuries later require additional reconstructive or fusion surgery.

Key Study Points

- Talar neck fractures are classified using the Hawkins system. Rates of osteonecrosis correspond to the fracture's Hawkins type and the presence of subtalar dislocation.
- Outcomes after calcaneus fractures are related to the severity of the initial injury. Subtalar fusion may be required for greatly comminuted fractures.
- Midfoot injuries including Lisfranc fracture-dislocations require stable fixation to restore the arch and support the structure of the midfoot.

Annotated References

1. Sanders DW: Fractures and dislocations of the talus, in Court-Brown CM, Heckman JD, McQueen MM, Ricci WM, Tornetta P, eds: *Rockwood and Green's Fractures in Adults*, ed 8. Philadelphia, PA, Lippincott Williams & Wilkins, 2015.

   Chapter overview of talus injuries with reference to surgical and nonoperative treatment.

2. Vallier HA, Nork SE, Barei DP, Benirschke SK, Sangeorzan BJ: Talar neck fractures: Results and outcomes. *J Bone Joint Surg Am* 2004;86(8):1616-1624.

3. Elgafy H, Ebraheim NA, Tile M, Stephen D, Kase J: Fractures of the talus: Experience of two level 1 trauma centers. *Foot Ankle Int* 2000;21(12):1023-1029.

4. Hawkins LG: Fractures of the neck of the talus. *J Bone Joint Surg Am* 1970;52(5):991-1002.

5. Canale ST, Kelly FB Jr: Fractures of the neck of the talus: Long-term evaluation of seventy-one cases. *J Bone Joint Surg Am* 1978;60(2):143-156.

6. Miller AN, Prasarn ML, Dyke JP, Helfet DL, Lorich DG: Quantitative assessment of the vascularity of the talus with gadolinium-enhanced magnetic resonance imaging. *J Bone Joint Surg Am* 2011;93(12):1116-1121.

   A cadaver study of the blood supply to the talus used gadolinium-enhanced contrast MRI and found that the posterior tibial artery contributed almost half of the blood supply. In contrast, earlier studies emphasized the contribution of anterior vascularity.

7. Vallier HA, Reichard SG, Boyd AJ, Moore TA: A new look at the Hawkins classification for talar neck fractures:

Which features of injury and treatment are predictive of osteonecrosis? *J Bone Joint Surg Am* 2014;96(3):192-197.

In talar neck fractures, subtalar dislocation and initial fracture displacement, but not osteonecrosis, were correlated with the timing of reduction.

8. Tezval M, Dumont C, Stürmer KM: Prognostic reliability of the Hawkins sign in fractures of the talus. *J Orthop Trauma* 2007;21(8):538-543.

9. Lindvall E, Haidukewych G, DiPasquale T, Herscovici D Jr, Sanders R: Open reduction and stable fixation of isolated, displaced talar neck and body fractures. *J Bone Joint Surg Am* 2004;86(10):2229-2234.

10. Sanders DW, Busam M, Hattwick E, Edwards JR, McAndrew MP, Johnson KD: Functional outcomes following displaced talar neck fractures. *J Orthop Trauma* 2004;18(5):265-270.

11. Sangeorzan BJ, Wagner UA, Harrington RM, Tencer AF: Contact characteristics of the subtalar joint: The effect of talar neck misalignment. *J Orthop Res* 1992;10(4):544-551.

12. Attiah M, Sanders DW, Valdivia G, et al: Comminuted talar neck fractures: A mechanical comparison of fixation techniques. *J Orthop Trauma* 2007;21(1):47-51.

13. Swanson TV, Bray TJ, Holmes GB Jr: Fractures of the talar neck: A mechanical study of fixation. *J Bone Joint Surg Am* 1992;74(4):544-551.

14. Shakked RJ, Tejwani NC: Surgical treatment of talus fractures. *Orthop Clin North Am* 2013;44(4):521-528.

The pathophysiology, treatment, outcomes, and complications of talus fractures were evaluated.

15. Charlson MD, Parks BG, Weber TG, Guyton GP: Comparison of plate and screw fixation and screw fixation alone in a comminuted talar neck fracture model. *Foot Ankle Int* 2006;27(5):340-343.

16. Fleuriau Chateau PB, Brokaw DS, Jelen BA, Scheid DK, Weber TG: Plate fixation of talar neck fractures: Preliminary review of a new technique in twenty-three patients. *J Orthop Trauma* 2002;16(4):213-219.

17. Jungbluth P, Wild M, Hakimi M, et al: Isolated subtalar dislocation. *J Bone Joint Surg Am* 2010;92(4):890-894.

In 97 patients with isolated subtalar dislocation, intermediate-term results were good. Medial or lateral dislocation direction did not affect outcomes.

18. Vallier HA, Nork SE, Benirschke SK, Sangeorzan BJ: Surgical treatment of talar body fractures. *J Bone Joint Surg Am* 2004;86(Pt 2, Suppl 1):180-192.

19. Valderrabano V, Perren T, Ryf C, Rillmann P, Hintermann B: Snowboarder's talus fracture: Treatment outcome of 20 cases after 3.5 years. *Am J Sports Med* 2005;33(6):871-880.

20. Clare MP, Sanders RW: Calcaneus fractures, in Court-Brown CM, Heckman JD, McQueen MM, Ricci WM, Tornetta P, eds: *Rockwood and Green's Fractures in Adults*, ed 8. Philadelphia, PA, Lippincott Williams & Wilkins, 2015.

Calcaneus injuries with reference to surgical and nonsurgical treatment are discussed.

21. Berberian W, Sood A, Karanfilian B, Najarian R, Lin S, Liporace F: Displacement of the sustentacular fragment in intra-articular calcaneal fractures. *J Bone Joint Surg Am* 2013;95(11):995-1000.

In 100 patients with calcaneus fractures, the sustentacular fragment was displaced in almost half and especially in patients with fractures of more than 50% of the posterior facet.

22. Gitajn IL, Abousayed M, Toussaint RJ, Ting B, Jin J, Kwon JY: Anatomic alignment and integrity of the sustentaculum tali in intra-articular calcaneal fractures: Is the sustentaculum tali truly constant? *J Bone Joint Surg Am* 2014;96(12):1000-1005.

Only 44% of patients with calcaneus fractures had a sustentaculum fracture, and 23% of the sustentaculum fragments were displaced.

23. Sanders R, Fortin P, DiPasquale T, Walling A: Operative treatment in 120 displaced intraarticular calcaneal fractures: Results using a prognostic computed tomography scan classification. *Clin Orthop Relat Res* 1993;290:87-95.

24. Bhattacharya R, Vassan UT, Finn P, Port A: Sanders classification of fractures of the os calcis: An analysis of inter- and intra-observer variability. *J Bone Joint Surg Br* 2005;87(2):205-208.

25. Swords MP, Alton TB, Holt S, Sangeorzan BJ, Shank JR, Benirschke SK: Prognostic value of computed tomography classification systems for intra-articular calcaneus fractures. *Foot Ankle Int* 2014;35(10):975-980.

Three classification systems for calcaneus fractures were compared. The factors most associated with functional outcome were comminution in the anterior process of the calcaneus and the surgeon's impression of fracture severity. These systems were not associated with Musculoskeletal Function Assessment outcome.

26. Griffin D, Parsons N, Shaw E, et al; UK Heel Fracture Trial Investigators: Operative versus non-operative treatment for closed, displaced, intra-articular fractures of the calcaneus: Randomised controlled trial. *BMJ* 2014;349:g4483.

A randomized study of 151 patients with calcaneus fractures found that at a minimum 2-year follow-up patients had the same symptomatic and functional outcomes regardless of assignment to surgical or nonsurgical treatment.

27. Gaskill T, Schweitzer K, Nunley J: Comparison of surgical outcomes of intra-articular calcaneal fractures by age. *J Bone Joint Surg Am* 2010;92(18):2884-2889.

    Patients older or younger than 50 years had similar complication rates a mean 9 years after surgical treatment of a calcaneus fracture. Older patients had better clinical outcomes.

28. Dickens JF, Kilcoyne KG, Kluk MW, Gordon WT, Shawen SB, Potter BK: Risk factors for infection and amputation following open, combat-related calcaneal fractures. *J Bone Joint Surg Am* 2013;95(5):e24.

    In evaluation of 102 combat-related open calcaneus fractures, the factors associated with eventual need for amputation were blast injury mechanism, plantar wound location, large open wound, and severe open fracture classification.

29. Wiersema B, Brokaw D, Weber T, et al: Complications associated with open calcaneus fractures. *Foot Ankle Int* 2011;32(11):1052-1057.

    The overall complication rate after open calcaneus fracture was 23.5% in 112 patients. This rate was lower than previously reported.

30. Folk JW, Starr AJ, Early JS: Early wound complications of operative treatment of calcaneus fractures: Analysis of 190 fractures. *J Orthop Trauma* 1999;13(5):369-372.

31. Poeze M, Verbruggen JP, Brink PR: The relationship between the outcome of operatively treated calcaneal fractures and institutional fracture load: A systematic review of the literature. *J Bone Joint Surg Am* 2008;90(5):1013-1021.

32. Gitajn IL, Toussaint RJ, Kwon JY: Assessing accuracy of sustentaculum screw placement during calcaneal fixation. *Foot Ankle Int* 2013;34(2):282-286.

    A cadaver study evaluated screw fixation into the sustentaculum or misdirected above or below the sustentaculum. Multiple radiographs were needed to correctly identify misplaced screws. In the standard Harris heel view, the screw often appeared to be correctly placed.

33. Blake MH, Owen JR, Sanford TS, Wayne JS, Adelaar RS: Biomechanical evaluation of a locking and nonlocking reconstruction plate in an osteoporotic calcaneal fracture model. *Foot Ankle Int* 2011;32(4):432-436.

    Locking and nonlocking calcaneal plates were compared in a cadaver osteoporotic calcaneus fracture model. Stiffness and cyclic loading displacement were not significantly different for the two constructs.

34. Chen L, Zhang G, Hong J, Lu X, Yuan W: Comparison of percutaneous screw fixation and calcium sulfate cement grafting versus open treatment of displaced intra-articular calcaneal fractures. *Foot Ankle Int* 2011;32(10):979-985.

    In 90 patients randomly assigned to open treatment or percutaneous screw fixation with cement, the quality of reduction was not significantly different, but those with open fixation had greater blood loss, a higher infection rate, decreased range of motion, and decreased function scores.

35. Tomesen T, Biert J, Frölke JP: Treatment of displaced intra-articular calcaneal fractures with closed reduction and percutaneous screw fixation. *J Bone Joint Surg Am* 2011;93(10):920-928.

    At a minimum 2-year follow-up of 37 patients with percutaneous fixation, the mean American Orthopaedic Foot and Ankle Society score was 84, the mean Musculoskeletal Function Score was 86, and the mean Medical Outcomes Study Short Form-36 Health Survey score was 76.

36. Johal HS, Buckley RE, Le IL, Leighton RK: A prospective randomized controlled trial of a bioresorbable calcium phosphate paste (alpha-BSM) in treatment of displaced intra-articular calcaneal fractures. *J Trauma* 2009;67(4):875-882.

37. Radnay CS, Clare MP, Sanders RW: Subtalar fusion after displaced intra-articular calcaneal fractures: Does initial operative treatment matter? *J Bone Joint Surg Am* 2009;91(3):541-546.

38. Potter MQ, Nunley JA: Long-term functional outcomes after operative treatment for intra-articular fractures of the calcaneus. *J Bone Joint Surg Am* 2009;91(8):1854-1860.

39. Ellington JK, Bosse MJ, Castillo RC, MacKenzie EJ;LEAP Study Group: The mangled foot and ankle: Results from a 2-year prospective study. *J Orthop Trauma* 2013;27(1):43-48.

    Patients with severe hindfoot and ankle injury had Sickness Impact Profile scores indicating greater disability than patients with below-knee amputation if they were initially treated with limb salvage and required free tissue transfer or ankle fusion.

40. Benirschke SK, Meinberg EG, Anderson SA, Jones CB, Cole PA: Fractures and dislocations of the midfoot: Lisfranc and Chopart injuries. *Instr Course Lect* 2013;62:79-91.

    The pathophysiology, treatment, outcomes, and complications of midfoot fractures and dislocations were reviewed.

41. Richter M, Thermann H, Huefner T, Schmidt U, Goesling T, Krettek C: Chopart joint fracture-dislocation: Initial open reduction provides better outcome than closed reduction. *Foot Ankle Int* 2004;25(5):340-348.

42. Eichenholtz SN, Levine DB: Fractures of the tarsal navicular bone. *Clin Orthop Relat Res* 1964;34(34):142-157.

43. Miller CM, Winter WG, Bucknell AL, Jonassen EA: Injuries to the midtarsal joint and lesser tarsal bones. *J Am Acad Orthop Surg* 1998;6(4):249-258.

44. Sangeorzan BJ, Benirschke SK, Mosca V, Mayo KA, Hansen ST Jr: Displaced intra-articular fractures of the tarsal navicular. *J Bone Joint Surg Am* 1989;71(10):1504-1510.

45. Sangeorzan BJ, Mayo KA, Hansen ST: Intraarticular fractures of the foot: Talus and lesser tarsals. *Clin Orthop Relat Res* 1993;292:135-141.

46. Hermel MB, Gershon-Cohen J: The nutcracker fracture of the cuboid by indirect violence. *Radiology* 1953;60(6):850-854.

47. Sangeorzan BJ, Swiontkowski MF: Displaced fractures of the cuboid. *J Bone Joint Surg Br* 1990;72(3):376-378.

48. Davies MS, Saxby TS: Intercuneiform instability and the "gap" sign. *Foot Ankle Int* 1999;20(9):606-609.

49. Richter M, Wippermann B, Krettek C, Schratt HE, Hufner T, Therman H: Fractures and fracture dislocations of the midfoot: Occurrence, causes and long-term results. *Foot Ankle Int* 2001;22(5):392-398.

50. Thompson MC, Mormino MA: Injury to the tarsometatarsal joint complex. *J Am Acad Orthop Surg* 2003;11(4):260-267.

51. Ouzounian TJ, Shereff MJ: In vitro determination of midfoot motion. *Foot Ankle* 1989;10(3):140-146.

52. Thakur NA, McDonnell M, Got CJ, Arcand N, Spratt KF, DiGiovanni CW: Injury patterns causing isolated foot compartment syndrome. *J Bone Joint Surg Am* 2012;94(11):1030-1035.

    A review of 364 patients from the National Trauma Data Bank found that the crush mechanism was most strongly associated with isolated foot compartment syndrome, regardless of other injuries.

53. Vuori JP, Aro HT: Lisfranc joint injuries: Trauma mechanisms and associated injuries. *J Trauma* 1993;35(1):40-45.

54. Ross G, Cronin R, Hauzenblas J, Juliano P: Plantar ecchymosis sign: A clinical aid to diagnosis of occult Lisfranc tarsometatarsal injuries. *J Orthop Trauma* 1996;10(2):119-122.

55. Sherief TI, Mucci B, Greiss M: Lisfranc injury: How frequently does it get missed? And how can we improve? *Injury* 2007;38(7):856-860.

56. Kuo RS, Tejwani NC, Digiovanni CW, et al: Outcome after open reduction and internal fixation of Lisfranc joint injuries. *J Bone Joint Surg Am* 2000;82(11):1609-1618.

57. Ly TV, Coetzee JC: Treatment of primarily ligamentous Lisfranc joint injuries: Primary arthrodesis compared with open reduction and internal fixation. A prospective, randomized study. *J Bone Joint Surg Am* 2006;88(3):514-520.

58. Kösters C, Bockholt S, Müller C, et al: Comparing the outcomes between Chopart, Lisfranc and multiple metatarsal shaft fractures. *Arch Orthop Trauma Surg* 2014;134(10):1397-1404.

    In 24 patients with Chopart, Lisfranc, or multiple metatarsal shaft fractures evaluated with pedobarographic analysis and outcomes scores, those with multiple metatarsal fractures had relatively poor results.

59. Morris PM, Francois AG, Marcus RE, Farrow LD: The effect of peroneus brevis tendon anatomy on the stability of fractures at the fifth metatarsal base. *Foot Ankle Int* 2015;36(5):579-584.

    The peroneus brevis tendon insertion effect on two fracture patterns was evaluated in a cadaver study. The Jones fracture had greater widening than the avulsion fracture when force was placed on the peroneus brevis tendon.

60. Ochenjele G, Ho B, Switaj PJ, Fuchs D, Goyal N, Kadakia AR: Radiographic study of the fifth metatarsal for optimal intramedullary screw fixation of Jones fracture. *Foot Ankle Int* 2015;36(3):293-301.

    CT was used to create three-dimensional models of the fifth metatarsal. Screws longer than 68% of the length of the bone increased the likelihood of screw extrusion. Screws should be at least 4.5 mm in diameter.

61. Scott RT, Hyer CF, DeMill SL: Screw fixation diameter for fifth metatarsal jones fracture: A cadaveric study. *J Foot Ankle Surg* 2015;54(2):227-229.

    Transverse section of cadaver fifth metatarsals showed that a 4.5-mm or larger screw should be used to provide sufficient fixation of these fractures.

62. Bigsby E, Halliday R, Middleton RG, Case R, Harries W: Functional outcome of fifth metatarsal fractures. *Injury* 2014;45(12):2009-2012.

    Patients with a fifth metatarsal fracture were evaluated 1 year after injury. As many as 33% continued to have occasional pain but minimal activity limitation.

63. O'Malley MJ, Hamilton WG, Munyak J: Fractures of the distal shaft of the fifth metatarsal: "Dancer's fracture." *Am J Sports Med* 1996;24(2):240-243.

Section 7

Geriatrics

SECTION EDITOR
Kenneth A. Egol, MD

Chapter 48

Perioperative and Postoperative Considerations in the Geriatric Patient

Sanjit R. Konda, MD

Abstract

The incidence of orthopaedic trauma in the elderly is increasing at a rapid pace. Geriatric patients have different perioperative and postoperative issues than young adults. The preoperative evaluation of comorbidities is essential, with particular emphasis placed on the cardiac, pulmonary, and overall functional status of the patient. Anesthesia options for geriatric patients include peripheral nerve blocks, spinal and epidural anesthesia, or general anesthesia; all have different risks and benefits relative to each other. In the postoperative period, geriatric trauma patients are at increased risk of cognitive, pulmonary, cardiac, and gastrointestinal complications, which are associated with considerable morbidity and mortality in this population. Discharge planning to acute inpatient rehabilitation or a skilled nursing facility is the accepted routine in geriatric trauma patients. Increased awareness of the perioperative and postoperative issues facing this cohort of patients will improve overall outcomes.

Keywords: geriatric; perioperative; postoperative; surgery

Introduction

Geriatric (age 65 years or older) trauma currently accounts for 12% of general trauma injuries.[1,2] It is projected that by 2050, geriatric patients will represent 20% of the population and at least 40% of the general trauma patient population.[1,3] Hip fracture is the most well-studied geriatric orthopaedic injury and serves as a good model to explore perioperative and postoperative considerations in the geriatric orthopaedic patient. The incidence of hip fractures is increasing rapidly and is expected to absorb considerable health care resources.[4-6] By 2040, the incidence of hip fractures is expected to reach 650,000 annually, which is more than double the annual incidence of 250,000 observed in 1990.[5,7] To contend with the overall increase in geriatric orthopaedic trauma, it is imperative for orthopaedic surgeons to understand the perioperative and postoperative issues surrounding geriatric orthopaedic care, and take physiologic factors into account.

Neither Dr. Konda nor any immediate family member has received anything of value from or has stock or stock options held in a commercial company or institution related directly or indirectly to the subject of this chapter.

Preoperative Considerations

Evaluation of Comorbidities

The assessment of patient comorbidities is an essential component of the preoperative work-up of any patient. Comorbidities can be classified into chronic-stable, chronic-unstable, and newly diagnosed. Patients with chronic-stable conditions have a known comorbidity such as coronary artery disease (CAD) and typically are followed by their primary care physician, who can help facilitate the medical optimization of the patient before surgical intervention. Patients with chronic-unstable conditions have a known comorbidity with frequent flare-ups (for example, CAD with angina) and may or may not be followed routinely by their primary care physician. An acute exacerbation of the chronic-unstable medical condition may cause the orthopaedic injury (for example, CAD with acute myocardial infarction (MI) leading to a fall with resultant fragility fracture). These patients require an extensive medical evaluation and stabilization of the exacerbated medical condition before any surgical intervention. Patients with a newly diagnosed comorbidity

Table 1

Classification of Comorbidities Based on Chronicity and Disease Stability

Comorbidity Classification	Relationship to Orthopaedic Injury	Intervention Required for Medical Optimization Before Surgery
Chronic-stable	Unrelated	Obtain medical records from primary care physician. Obtain routine preoperative medical evaluation.
Chronic-unstable (acute exacerbation of known preexisting comorbidity)	May have led to injury	Obtain medical records from primary care physician. Obtain medical evaluation to stabilize acute exacerbation of disease. Consider admission to medical service.
Newly diagnosed	May have led to injury	Obtain medical evaluation to determine extent of newly diagnosed comorbidity. Patient may benefit from extensive medical work-up before surgery. Consider admission to medical service.

have not undergone previous evaluation for their disease, which is identified during a routine preoperative work-up incidentally or because the disease led to the orthopaedic injury. These newly diagnosed diseases may be uncontrolled and require more extensive medical evaluation, diagnostic work-up, and management before surgical optimization (**Table 1**).

The treating orthopaedic surgeon should be aware of the many disease processes that contribute to overall surgical risk and perioperative morbidity and mortality. The Charlson Comorbidity Index (CCI) was developed in 1987 as a novel method of classifying prognostic comorbidity for longitudinal studies.[8] It has been validated in numerous studies as a tool that predicts the risk of 1-year, 5-year, and 10-year mortality of patients who may have various conditions. The CCI includes 19 conditions, with each comorbidity assigned a score of 1, 2, 3, or 6, based on the mortality risk associated with each disease. A summary of the scores predicts mortality. Several free online calculators are available to calculate the risk of mortality at 1 year.[9,10] **Table 2** provides a list of common medical comorbidities that should be screened for through a detailed history and/or physical examination, based on the CCI of a geriatric orthopaedic trauma patient.

Table 2

Charlson Comorbidity Index

Comorbidity	Point Value
AIDS	6
Metastatic solid tumor	6
Moderate or severe liver disease	3
Any nonmetastatic solid tumor	2
Malignant lymphoma	2
Leukemia	2
Diabetes with end organ damage	2
Moderate or severe renal disease	2
Hemiplegia	2
Diabetes without end organ damage	1
Mild liver disease	1
Ulcer disease	1
Connective tissue disease	1
Chronic pulmonary disease	1
Dementia	1
Cerebrovascular disease	1
Peripheral vascular disease	1
Congestive heart failure	1
Myocardial infarction	1

Adapted with permission from Charlson ME, Pompei P, Ales KL, Mackenzie CR: A new method of classifying prognostic comorbidity in longitudinal studies: Development and validation. *J Chronic Dis* 1987;40(5):373-383. Online calculator for mortality 1 year after hospital admission available at http://www.pmidcalc.org/?sid=3558716&newtest=Y. Accessed January 12, 2016.

Evaluation of Preoperative Functional Capacity

The metabolic equivalent (MET) is a tool commonly used for cardiac risk stratification and is defined as the resting metabolic rate (the amount of oxygen consumed at rest, such as while sitting quietly in a chair), which normally is 3.5 mL O_2/kg/min or 1.2 kcal/min for a person weighing 70 kg.[11] Therefore, work at 2 METs requires twice the resting metabolic rate (7.0 mL O_2/kg/min), and work at

3 MET requires three times the resting metabolism rate (10.5 mL O_2/kg/min). In individuals able to perform no more than 4 METS, functional status is considered to be poor and additional presurgical cardiac testing may be necessary to identify cardiac risk factors. The ability to perform 1 MET is equivalent to energy expended on basic self-care tasks, whereas 4 METs is equivalent to climbing or walking up a hill, and 10 METs is equivalent to participating in strenuous sports such as swimming or singles tennis (**Figure 1**).

The American Society of Anesthesiologists (ASA) physical status classification is used to determine perioperative risk for anesthesia and is based on the patient's comorbid conditions and functional status. It was developed in 1941 as a tool to standardize communication between anesthesiologists[12] (**Table 3**). The ASA classification subsequently has been shown to correlate directly to an increased risk of inpatient mortality, readmission rates, and overall complication rates.[13] In short, ASA 1 describes a normal healthy patient. ASA 2 describes a patient with mild systemic disease. ASA 3 describes a patient with severe systemic disease, and ASA 4 describes a patient having severe systemic disease that is a constant threat to life. ASA 5 describes a patient who is not expected to survive without the operation, and ASA 6 describes an already declared brain-dead patient whose organs are being removed for donation (**Table 3**).

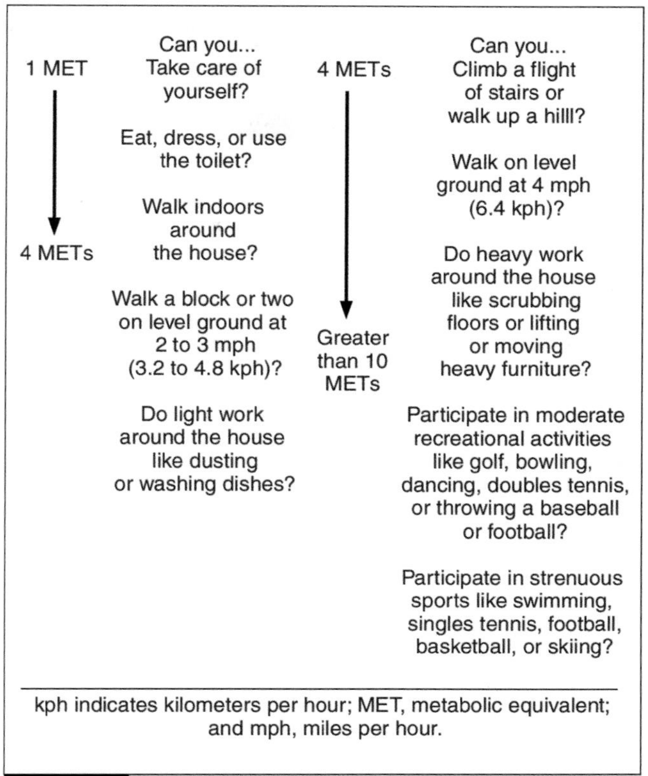

Figure 1 Chart shows the estimated energy requirements in METs for various activities. MET = metabolic equivalent. (Reproduced with permission from Fleisher LA, Beckman JA, Brown KA, et al: ACC/AHA 2007 guidelines on perioperative cardiovascular evaluation and care for noncardiac surgery: A report of the American College of Cardiology/American Heart Association Task Force on Practice Guidelines (Writing Committee to revise the 2002 guidelines on perioperative cardiovascular evaluation for noncardiac surgery): Developed in collaboration with the American Society of Echocardiography, American Society of Nuclear Cardiology, Heart Rhythm Society, Society of Cardiovascular Anesthesiologists, Society for Cardiovascular Angiography and Interventions, Society for Vascular Medicine and Biology, and Society for Vascular Surgery. *Circulation* 2007 Oct 23;116[17]:e418-e499.)

Preoperative Cardiac Risk Assessment

American College of Cardiology and the American Heart Association recommendations provide clear guidelines for preoperative cardiac testing[14] (**Table 4**). In general, additional cardiac testing (echocardiography, stress testing, 24-hour ambulatory monitoring) should be performed only if it would be indicated in the absence of the proposed surgery. Many institutions have policies in place regarding the type of routine preoperative tests necessary before elective and/or emergency surgery can be performed. A baseline preoperative resting 12-lead electrocardiogram (ECG) is standard for the evaluation of baseline cardiac function in the geriatric trauma patient. Additional cardiac testing can be obtained based on the patient's cardiac risk factors, if known, functional capacity tolerance (METS ≤ 4), or abnormalities seen on the baseline ECG. Several studies have documented no improvement in outcome using prophylactic revascularization to prevent ischemia in the setting of preoperative stress testing.[15,16]

Preoperative Pulmonary Risk Assessment

Age has been shown to be an independent predictor of postoperative pulmonary complications, even after adjusting for comorbid conditions.[17] Increasing odds of pulmonary complications have been shown for each decade after the age of 60 years. Although preoperative plain radiographs of the chest are not likely to show abnormalities that change preoperative management, the general consensus is that they should be obtained for all patients older than 50 years as part of the preoperative work-up for medical optimization.[18]

Guidelines established by the American College of Physicians recommend that preoperative spirometry is not indicated to predict the risk of postoperative pulmonary

Table 3

American Society of Anesthesiologists Physical Status Classification

Classification	Definition	Examples
ASA I	A normal healthy patient	Healthy, nonsmoking, no or minimal alcohol use
ASA II	A patient with mild systemic disease	Mild disease only, with no substantive functional limitations; examples include (but are not limited to) current smoker, social alcohol drinker, pregnancy, obesity (BMI between 30 and 40), well controlled DM/HTN, mild lung disease
ASA III	A patient with severe systemic disease	Substantive functional limitations; one or more moderate to severe diseases, examples include but are not limited to poorly controlled DM or HTN, COPD, morbid obesity (BMI ≥40), active hepatitis, alcohol dependence or abuse, implanted pacemaker, moderate reduction of ejection fraction, ESRD undergoing regularly scheduled dialysis, history (>3 months) of MI, CVA, TIA, or CAD/stents
ASA IV	A patient with severe systemic disease that is a constant threat to life	Examples include but are not limited to recent (<3 months) MI, CVA, TIA, or CAD/stents, ongoing cardiac ischemia or severe valve dysfunction, severe reduction of ejection fraction, sepsis, DIC, ARD, or ESRD not undergoing regularly scheduled dialysis
ASA V	A moribund patient who is not expected to survive without the operation	Examples include but are not limited to ruptured abdominal/thoracic aneurysm, massive trauma, intracranial bleed with mass effect, ischemic bowel in the face of substantial cardiac pathology, or multiple organ/system dysfunction
ASA VI	A declared brain-dead patient whose organs are being removed for donor purposes	

ASA = American Society of Anesthesiologists, BMI = basal metabolic index, DM = diabetes mellitus, HTN = hypertension, COPD = chronic obstructive pulmonary disease, ESRD = end-stage renal disease, MI = myocardial infarction, CVA = cerebrovascular accident, TIA = transient ischemic attack, CAD = coronary artery disease, DIC = diffuse intravascular coagulopathy, ARD = acute respiratory distress. Reproduced with permission from ASA Physical Status Classification System by the American Society of Anesthesiologists, 2014. Available at http://www.asahq.org/resources/clinical-information/asa-physical-status-classification-system. Accessed January 12, 2016.

complications.[19] Patients who may benefit from preoperative pulmonary function testing include those with chronic obstructive pulmonary disease (COPD) or asthma whose baseline airflow optimization cannot be determined. Studies have shown that a forced vital capacity (FVC) less than 70% and a forced expiratory volume $(FEV)_1$/FVC ratio less than 65% of the predictive value are predictive of postoperative pulmonary complications.[20] Few studies support using preoperative arterial blood gas analysis to risk-stratify patients for postoperative pulmonary complications; therefore, its routine use is not recommended.

Geriatric Comanagement

Interdisciplinary care by an orthopaedic surgeon and a geriatrician quickly is becoming the gold standard in the United States to improve patient outcomes and provide value-based care, given the potential for complications in geriatric patients with fractures. Interdisciplinary care of geriatric patients with hip fracture was developed in England in the late 1950s.[21] In a 1992 study, the earliest report of interdisciplinary care in the United States, 431 geriatric hip fracture patients were evaluated from 1985 to 1990. The study demonstrated an approximately 50% reduction in postoperative complications, intensive care unit (ICU) transfers, and discharges to nursing homes compared with a control group of hip fracture patients that predated the start of the interdisciplinary care model.[22] More recently, a 2008 study demonstrated that comanagement of the geriatric patient by an orthopaedic surgeon and a geriatrician results in a lower than predicted length of stay, lower readmission rates, a shorter time to surgery, lower complication rates, and lower in-hospital mortality rates.[23] Although most patients are seen by the orthopaedic surgeon in this model, the geriatrician takes ownership of the patient along with the surgeon. The geriatrician takes an active role in managing the preoperative and postoperative medical comorbidities of the patient in addition to making recommendations for medical management. The practice of geriatric comanagement likely will continue to expand as more studies

Table 4

Recommendations for Preoperative Cardiac Testing

The 12-Lead ECG

Preoperative resting 12-lead ECG is reasonable for patients with known coronary heart disease or other substantial structural heat disease, except for low-risk surgery.

Preoperative resting 12-lead ECG may be considered for asymptomatic patients, except for low-risk surgery.

Routine preoperative resting 12-lead ECG is not useful for asymptomatic patients undergoing low-risk surgical procedures.

Assessment of LV Function

It is reasonable for patients with dyspnea of unknown origin to undergo preoperative evaluation of LV function.

It is reasonable for patients with HF with worsening dyspnea or another change in clinical status to undergo preoperative evaluation of LV function.

Reassessment of LV function in clinically stable patients may be considered.

Routine preoperative evaluation of LV function is not recommended.

Exercise Stress Testing for Myocardial Ischemia and Functional Capacity

For patients with elevated risk and excellent functional capacity, it is reasonable to forgo further exercise testing and proceed to surgery.

For patients with elevated risk and unknown functional capacity, it may be reasonable to perform exercise testing to assess functional capacity if doing so will change management.

For patients with elevated risk and moderate to good functional capacity, it may be reasonable to forgo further exercise testing and proceed to surgery.

For patients with elevated risk and poor or unknown functional capacity, it may be reasonable to perform exercise testing with cardiac imaging to assess for myocardial ischemia.

Routine screening with noninvasive stress testing is not useful for low-risk noncardiac surgery.

Cardiopulmonary Exercise Testing

Cardiopulmonary exercise testing may be considered for patients undergoing elevated-risk procedures.

Noninvasive Pharmacologic Stress Testing Before Noncardiac Surgery

It is reasonable for patients at elevated risk for noncardiac surgery with poor functional capacity to undergo DSE or MPI if doing so will change management.

Routine screening with noninvasive stress testing is not useful for low-risk noncardiac surgery.

Preoperative Coronary Angiography

Routine preoperative coronary angiography is not recommended.

ECG = electrocardiogram, DSE= dobutamine stress echocardiogram, HF = heart failure, LV = left ventricular, MPI = myocardial perfusion imaging.
Reproduced with permission from Fleisher LA, Fleischmann KE, Auerbach AD, et al: 2014 ACC/AHA guideline on perioperative cardiovascular evaluation and management of patients undergoing noncardiac surgery: A report of the American College of Cardiology/American Heart Association Task Force on practice guidelines. *J Am Coll Cardiol* 2014 Dec 9;64(22):e77-137.

demonstrate its ability to improve patient outcomes and provide value-based care.

Anesthesia

Spinal and Epidural Anesthesia

The risks and benefits associated with spinal and epidural anesthesia in comparison with general anesthesia are controversial. Regional anesthesia has not been demonstrated conclusively to be superior to general anesthesia. Spinal and epidural anesthesia are associated with greater episodes of intraoperative hypotension, and two large studies using the American College of Surgeons National Surgical Quality Improvement Program (ACS-NSQIP) database have shown conflicting results regarding the increased risk of postoperative complications. A 2015 study evaluated 9,842 patients age 70 years or older who had received spinal or epidural anesthesia rather than general anesthesia for hip fractures and found that general anesthesia was associated with an increased risk of thromboembolic events (odds ratio [OR] 1.90, confidence interval [CI] 1.21–2.89, $P = 0.003$) and any minor adverse events

(OR 1.19, CI 1.24–2.89, $P < 0.001$), as well as a reduced risk of urinary tract infection (OR 0.73, CI 0.62–0.87, $P < 0.001$).[24] A separate 2015 study evaluated 7,764 hip fractures patients from the ACS-NSQIP database who received regional, spinal/epidural, or general anesthesia. The authors found that patients who received spinal or epidural anesthesia had the highest complication rate (19.6%, 1,522 patients) and that spinal or epidural anesthesia was associated with statistically significant greater odds of minor and total complications compared with general anesthesia.[25] Spinal and epidural anesthesia may lead to better oxygenation in the immediate postoperative period.[26] The risks and benefits of spinal and epidural anesthesia should be weighed by the treating surgeon, the anesthesiologist, and the patient.

General Anesthesia

A large 2005 study of more than 800,000 patients demonstrated that age was not an independent risk factor for serious morbidity or mortality in patients undergoing general anesthesia.[27] The induction period is a critical time for general anesthesia. Elderly patients require lower induction doses of propofol because of slower blood-brain circulation, resulting in slower agent onset and a delayed cardiopulmonary depressive effect. In addition, hypotension at induction is more common with general anesthesia because of the less compliant vasculature in the elderly.[28] General anesthesia in patients with an acute exacerbation of pulmonary issues such as COPD, asthma, rib fractures, pneumonia, and pulmonary edema may predispose them to a more prolonged intubation postoperatively, given the greater difficulty in weaning older patients to extubation. Evidence shows that general anesthesia may be associated with a higher incidence of postoperative cognitive dysfunction (POCD) compared with spinal and epidural anesthesia but no increased risk of postoperative delirium (POD).[29]

Peripheral Nerve Blocks

Peripheral nerve blocks have been shown to be effective in providing superior immediate intraoperative and short-term postoperative pain control during many orthopaedic procedures while reducing opioid requirements and minimizing systemic side effects compared with general and spinal anesthesia.[28,30-32] The use of continuously infused peripheral nerve blocks has been shown to reduce the incidence of rebound pain, defined as pain experienced in the immediate postoperative period and before the onset of postoperative pain medication from the wearing off of intraoperative analgesia. Elderly patients have an increased incidence of nerve damage with this technique compared with young adults.[33]

Postoperative Considerations

Postoperative Altered Mental Status

Postoperative patients with an altered mental status can experience one of two types of cognitive dysfunction that carry an increased risk of postoperative mortality: POD or POCD.[34] POD is defined as an acute change in baseline cognitive status associated with the waxing and waning of levels of consciousness. Several etiologies of POD exist, including infection, dehydration, hypoperfusion, medications (most commonly benzodiazepines, histamine blockers, and narcotics), hypoxia, and hypoglycemia. Risk factors for POD include baseline dementia, vision impairment, functional impairment, high comorbidity, and the use of physical restraints.[35] Intervention strategies to minimize POD include the correction of the underlying etiology plus frequent reorientation, the continual use of glasses and hearing aids, the maintenance of a normal sleep-wake cycle, and increased daytime activities.[36] The medical treatment of POD is administration of haloperidol and/or low-dose lorazepam.

Postoperative cognitive dysfunction presents as a nontreatable impairment of memory and concentration during the days to weeks after the index surgery.[37] Up to 10% of elderly patients have been reported to have POCD up 3 months postoperatively. General anesthesia has a slight association with POCD. Patients with POCD may require long-term care unrelated to their orthopaedic injury.

Postoperative Pulmonary Complications

The traditional definitions of postoperative pulmonary complications include atelectasis, bronchospasm, pneumonia, and the exacerbation of chronic lung disease. Geriatric trauma patients, especially those with lower extremity injuries and injuries about the shoulder girdle, are prone to atelectasis and subsequently pneumonia. Shoulder girdle injuries and/or rib fractures may cause pain during deep inspiration and expiration and, therefore, inadequate recruitment of the alveoli may occur during respiration. Lower-extremity injuries predispose the patient to immobility and prolonged recumbency, which can lead to the inadequate recruitment of the alveoli.

Atelectasis usually presents between postoperative days 2 and 5 as the increased work of breathing or hypoxemia. Patients with minimal secretions and atelectasis may benefit from continuous positive airway pressure (CPAP) therapy. In a multicenter trial of 209 patients, those who underwent abdominal surgery were randomized to receive CPAP plus supplemental oxygen or supplemental oxygen alone. Patients who received CPAP had a reduced incidence of intubation (1% versus 10%), pneumonia

7: Geriatrics

(2% versus 10%), infection (3% versus 10%), and sepsis (2% versus 9%).[38] Patients with considerable secretions and atelectasis benefit from suctioning and chest physical therapy.

Bronchospasm can present as dyspnea, wheezing, chest tightness, or tachypnea and may be the result of aspiration, histamine release by opiates or anesthetic agents, exacerbation of a chronic pulmonary condition, or tracheal stimulation from intubation or suctioning. Bronchospasm should be managed in a manner similar to the exacerbation of asthma or COPD. First-line agents include short-acting β-2 agonists (such as albuterol) that are bronchodilators. Ipratropium bromide is an anticholinergic agent that is also a bronchodilator and can be used in conjunction with a β-2 agonist.

Postoperative pneumonia generally presents between postoperative days 0 and 5 and should be suspected in the setting of postoperative fever and new chest infiltrates on radiographs. The diagnosis of pneumonia can be difficult, and chest radiographs are not specific. One study demonstrated that, in a series of 129 consecutive surgical ICU patients, pulmonary infiltrates on chest radiographs were due to pneumonia (30%, 39 patients), pulmonary edema (29%, 37 patients), acute lung injury (15%, 19 patients), and atelectasis (13%, 17 patients).[39] The most common causative bacterial organisms included gram-negative bacteria and *Staphylococcus aureus*. Traumatically injured patients are at increased risk for postoperative pneumonia from *Haemophilus influenzae* or *Streptococcus pneumoniae* infection.[39] Sputum and blood cultures should be obtained, and broad-spectrum antibiotics should be started until definitive speciation and antibiotic sensitivities are noted.

Postoperative Cardiac Complications

Cardiac events are the most common cause of postoperative mortality in the elderly.[40] Specific cardiac events include MI, arrhythmias such as atrial fibrillation, and heart failure. MI is defined as the death of cardiac myocytes caused by ischemia.[41] It is diagnosed by the presence of elevated troponins and at least one of the following factors: symptoms of ischemia, ECG changes consistent with MI (ST segment T wave changes, new left bundle branch block, or pathologic Q waves), echocardiogram evidence of a new regional wall abnormality, or identification of an intracoronary thrombus by angiography. Postoperative screening for MI should be performed by obtaining serial troponin values every 8 hours for the first 24 hours postoperatively. Some authors recommend continuing serial troponins daily on postoperative days 2 and 3 for high-risk patients, defined as patients having in-hospital surgery with one or more risk factors itemized on the Revised Cardiac Risk Index (RCRI, **Table 5**). The RCRI was developed to predict the risk for major noncardiac surgery and has been correlated subsequently to the risk of cardiac arrest.[42,43] Patients with no RCRI predictors have a 0.4% chance of an MI, whereas patients with 3 RCRI predictors or more have a greater than 11% chance of having an MI. In patients older than 85 years, only one-third present with classic chest pain. Therefore, the threshold to obtain serial troponins should be low in the elderly patient with cardiac risk factors.[44]

Table 5

Revised Cardiac Risk Index

Predictors

1. History of ischemic heart disease
2. History of congestive heart failure
3. History of cerebrovascular disease (stroke or transient ischemic attack)
4. History of diabetes requiring preoperative insulin use
5. Chronic kidney disease (creatinine > 2 mg/dL)
6. Undergoing suprainguinal vascular, intraperitoneal, or intrathoracic surgery

Risk for Cardiac Death, Nonfatal Myocardial Infarction, and Nonfatal Cardiac Arrest

0 predictors = 0.4%

1 predictor = 0.9%

2 predictors = 6.6%

≥3 predictors = >11%

Postoperative arrhythmias, including the most common type, atrial fibrillation, can cause changes in mental status and syncope. Patients may be symptomatic with palpitations or asymptomatic. The underlying cause may be postoperative anemia or metabolic derangement. Treatment in the elderly focuses on a rate-control strategy as demonstrated by the Atrial Fibrillation Follow-Up Investigation of Rhythm Management (AFFIRM) and Rate Control Versus Electrical Cardioversion for Persistent Atrial Fibrillation (RACE) trials, which showed equivalent outcomes, with a trend toward a reduction in all-cause mortality with rate control.[45,46] In addition, antiarrhythmic medications are associated with several side effects, including proarrhythmia, which can be devastating in the elderly. Catheter ablation is another rhythm-control strategy that also is associated with complications.

Postoperative heart failure can occur due to anemia, MI, infection, thyroid dysfunction, atrial fibrillation, and dietary-related and medication-related etiologies. Systolic dysfunction presents gradually over time and is associated with decreased ejection fraction and cardiomegaly on echocardiogram. Diastolic dysfunction, in contrast, presents acutely as pulmonary edema and is associated with normal or increased left ventricular ejection fraction and a normal heart size on echocardiogram. Postoperative pulmonary edema should be treated with diuretics to reduce pulmonary congestion and with vasodilator therapy in patients without hypotension. The clinician should maintain a high suspicion for myocardial ischemia or infarction in patients who present with acute postoperative heart failure.

Postoperative Gastrointestinal Complications

Postoperative gastrointestinal (GI) complications can have devastating consequences in the elderly. Complications include but are not limited to GI stress ulcers, GI bleeds, postoperative ileus, and *Clostridium difficile* colitis. The routine GI prophylaxis of elderly orthopaedic trauma patients to prevent stress ulcers of the stomach should not be performed. Several clinical practice guidelines have been published, and all limit the use of GI prophylaxis for stress ulcers to specific patient populations in the ICU setting. The criteria for GI stress ulcer prophylaxis for patients in the ICU setting include mechanical ventilation, coagulopathy, traumatic brain injury, major burn injury, multiple trauma, sepsis, acute renal failure, Injury Severity Score higher than 15, and the requirement of high-dose steroids (more than 250 mg of hydrocortisone or its equivalent per day).[47] First-line treatment choices include histamine 2 receptor antagonists and proton pump inhibitors (PPIs). It should be noted that PPIs lower gastric acidity and can result in reduced calcium absorption. Additionally, PPIs may inhibit bone resorption by osteoclasts directly.[48]

GI bleeds are common in the elderly and have a mortality range of 10% to 25%.[49,50] Bleeds should be investigated as having an upper GI or lower GI source, and adequate resuscitation and treatment should be provided.

Postoperative ileus is defined as obstipation and the intolerance of oral intake following surgery. Risk factors include prolonged pelvic surgery, open surgery, delayed enteral nutrition, nasogastric tube placement, pneumonia, intraoperative and postoperative bleeding and the need for transfusion, perioperative opioid use, and a high body mass index. Patients may present with abdominal distension, diffuse and persistent abdominal pain, nausea and/or vomiting, an inability to pass flatus, and an inability to tolerate a diet taken orally. Plain abdominal radiographs should be obtained and will show dilated loops of bowel. A medical or surgical consultation should be obtained to rule out other sources of mechanical bowel obstruction such as small-bowel obstruction or bowel perforation.

C difficile colitis is an increasingly common cause of morbidity and mortality among the elderly trauma population.[51] In the setting of perioperative antibiotic use for surgical prophylaxis or for the treatment of infection, the normal gut flora is altered, and *C difficile* can colonize the intestinal tract, resulting in a pseudomembranous colitis. If clinical suspicion is high for *C difficile* colitis, then empiric therapy should be started immediately pending definitive results. The initial treatment of nonsevere infection is oral metronidazole, whereas the treatment of severe infection is vancomycin. Concurrently, the inciting antibiotic should be stopped, and infection-control practices should be implemented. These practices include contact precautions and hand hygiene. Soap and water is more effective than alcohol-based sanitizers to eliminate *C difficile* spores. Surgical consultation is warranted if the white blood cell count climbs to greater than 20,000 cells/µL and/or the plasma lactate level ranges between 2.2 and 4.9, because these levels may herald severe disease that is unresponsive to medical therapy.[52] Surgical treatment entails colectomy.

Postoperative Nutrition

More than 70% of hospitalized geriatric patients are malnourished or at increased risk for malnourishment.[53] A standardized definition of adult malnutrition has been provided by the Academy of Nutrition and Dietetics and the American Society for Parenteral and Enteral Nutrition.[54] Identification of two or more of the following six characteristics is recommended for the diagnosis of malnutrition: insufficient energy intake, weight loss, loss of muscle mass, loss of subcutaneous fat, localized or generalized fluid accumulation that may mask weight loss, and diminished functional status as measured by handgrip strength. In the context of acute illness or injury, severe malnutrition is measured most easily by weight loss. Criteria include more than 2% of weight loss from the baseline over 1 week, or more than 5% of weight loss from the baseline over 1 month. Severe malnourishment as a function of energy intake is measured as less than or equal to 50% of the estimated energy requirement for 5 days or more. Malnourishment can contribute to postoperative wound dehiscence, infection, and overall mortality.[55]

The most common reasons for inadequate oral intake are malignancy and depression. Dysphagia is another risk factor. Nutritional supplementation in the form of oral protein and energy supplementation has been shown to reduce morbidity and mortality in malnourished hospitalized patients aged 75 years or older.[56]

Postoperative Deep Vein Thrombosis Prophylaxis

Risk factors for deep vein thrombosis (DVT) include advanced age, previous thromboembolism, malignancy, congestive heart failure, prolonged recumbency, paralysis, obesity, deep venous system disease, and lower-extremity fracture.[57] The rates of DVT after hip fracture surgery range from 30% to 60%.[58] One study showed an overall venous thromboembolism (VTE) event rate of 1.0% in a Danish registry study of 57,619 patients who had undergone fracture surgery distal to the knee.[59] Given this wide discrepancy in VTE rates, DVT prophylaxis for the geriatric orthopaedic trauma patient should be tailored to each patient depending on their injury. Based on the American College of Chest Physicians evidence-based clinical practice guidelines, hip fracture patients should receive low–molecular-weight heparin within 12 hours of surgery preoperatively or postoperatively.[59] Although these guidelines do not comment on pelvic, acetabular, or femur fractures, extrapolation of these guidelines to these specific injuries is prudent. Therapy should continue for 1 month postoperatively because of an increased risk of VTE events in the third postoperative week. In a double-blind multicenter trial of 656 hip fracture patients, low–molecular-weight heparin therapy was extended past the then-current standard of 6 to 8 days postoperatively. The authors showed a reduction in VTE events from 35% to 1.4% at 1 month.[60] For postsurgical patients with fractures distal to the knee, it is reasonable to provide some form of chemical DVT prophylaxis until the patients are fully weight bearing or mobile. Aspirin or low–molecular-weight heparin can be used. It should be noted that, in elderly patients with a history of syncopal episodes or a high risk of falling, anticoagulation medication increases the risk of head bleeding in the event of a fall that results in head trauma. This factor should be taken into consideration when prescribing DVT prophylaxis.

Postoperative Discharge

Many geriatric orthopaedic trauma patients are not discharged home because of ongoing short-term medical and physical therapy needs. Discharge planning is a multidisciplinary effort that includes the orthopaedic surgeon, the medical consultant, the social worker, and the case manager. To qualify for acute inpatient rehabilitation, patients must have the stamina to participate in physical therapy 3 hours a day for 5 days a week, with the expectation that they will make substantial improvements in a reasonable amount of time so that they can be discharged back home or to a similar community setting.[21] These patients may require hospital-level care for medical therapies such as dialysis, wound care, chemotherapy, or radiation therapy. Inpatient rehabilitation units and hospitals must provide 24-hour availability of rehabilitation physicians and nurses 7 days per week.

Patients also may be candidates for discharge to a skilled nursing facility. These facilities differ from acute inpatient rehabilitation units or hospitals in their staffing and other requirements and are less rigorous. At a minimum, the Medicare requirements for a skilled nursing facility include physician visits once every 30 days; however, no requirement is in place for interdisciplinary team conferences, 24-hour registered nurse staffing, or rehabilitation nursing. Additionally, no requirement exists that patients perform 3 hours of physical therapy daily for 5 days, no prosthetic or orthotic service is required, and therapy providers can determine when therapy will end independently of one another.[21]

Summary

Numerous perioperative considerations exist in the geriatric orthopaedic trauma patient. Medical optimization involves determining the baseline functional capacity of the patient as well as the stabilization of newly diagnosed conditions and chronic medical conditions. The choice of anesthesia type can affect postoperative outcome. Finally, postoperative cognitive, cardiac, pulmonary, and GI complications should be evaluated for and treated as they arise. The discharge of severely injured geriatric orthopaedic trauma patients to acute inpatient or skilled nursing facilities may be necessary.

Key Study Points

- Severity of patient comorbidities should be evaluated to determine the preoperative functional capacity of the geriatric trauma patient.
- Preoperative cardiac and pulmonary risk assessment, along with differences in anesthesia in the geriatric trauma patient, affect treatment options.
- Factors affecting outcome include postoperative altered mental status and cardiac, pulmonary, and gastrointestinal complications in the geriatric trauma patient.
- Postoperative nutrition is important to reduce morbidity and mortality in geriatric trauma patients.
- Various discharge options are available for geriatric trauma patients, including acute inpatient rehabilitation and subacute nursing facilities.

Annotated References

1. Koval KJ, Meek R, Schemitsch E, Liporace F, Strauss E, Zuckerman JD: An AOA critical issue. Geriatric trauma: Young ideas. *J Bone Joint Surg Am* 2003;85-A(7):1380-1388.

2. McMahon DJ, Schwab CW, Kauder D: Comorbidity and the elderly trauma patient. *World J Surg* 1996;20(8):1113-1119, discussion 1119-1120.

3. Campbell JW, Degolia PA, Fallon WF, Rader EL: In harm's way: Moving the older trauma patient toward a better outcome. *Geriatrics* 2009;64(1):8-13.

4. Zuckerman JD: Hip fracture. *N Engl J Med* 1996;334(23):1519-1525.

5. Schneider EL, Guralnik JM: The aging of America. Impact on health care costs. *JAMA* 1990;263(17):2335-2340.

6. Morris AH, Zuckerman JD; AAOS Council of Health Policy and Practice, USA. American Academy of Orthopaedic Surgeons: National consensus conference on improving the continuum of care for patients with hip fracture. *J Bone Joint Surg Am* 2002;84-A(4):670-674.

7. Gilbert TB, Hawkes WG, Hebel JR, et al: Spinal anesthesia versus general anesthesia for hip fracture repair: A longitudinal observation of 741 elderly patients during 2-year follow-up. *Am J Orthop (Belle Mead NJ)* 2000;29(1):25-35.

8. Charlson ME, Pompei P, Ales KL, MacKenzie CR: A new method of classifying prognostic comorbidity in longitudinal studies: Development and validation. *J Chronic Dis* 1987;40(5):373-383.

9. Barnett S, Moonesinghe SR: Clinical risk scores to guide perioperative management. *Postgrad Med J* 2011;87(1030):535-541.

   The authors discussed scoring systems that help identify perioperative risk factors.

10. The Charlson Comorbidity Index calculator. Available at http://www.pmidcalc.org/?sid=3558716&newtest=Y. Accessed January 13, 2016.

11. Jetté M, Sidney K, Blümchen G: Metabolic equivalents (METS) in exercise testing, exercise prescription, and evaluation of functional capacity. *Clin Cardiol* 1990;13(8):555-565.

12. American Society of Anesthesiologists Physical Status Classification System. Available at **http://www.asahq.org/resources/clinical-information/asa-physical-status-classification-system.** Accessed January 13, 2016.

13. Radcliff TA, Henderson WG, Stoner TJ, Khuri SF, Dohm M, Hutt E: Patient risk factors, operative care, and outcomes among older community-dwelling male veterans with hip fracture. *J Bone Joint Surg Am* 2008;90(1):34-42.

14. Fleisher LA, Fleischmann KE, Auerbach AD, et al; American College of Cardiology; American Heart Association: 2014 ACC/AHA guideline on perioperative cardiovascular evaluation and management of patients undergoing noncardiac surgery: A report of the American College of Cardiology/American Heart Association Task Force on practice guidelines. *J Am Coll Cardiol* 2014;64(22):e77-e137.

    The authors proposed a series of updated guidelines for the perioperative cardiovascular work-up of patients undergoing noncardiac surgery. In particular, they discussed the current recommendations for 12-lead electrocardiogram (ECG), the assessment of left ventricular function, exercise stress testing for myocardial ischemia and functional capacity, cardiopulmonary exercise testing, noninvasive pharmacologic stress testing, and preoperative coronary angiography.

15. Auerbach A, Goldman L: Assessing and reducing the cardiac risk of noncardiac surgery. *Circulation* 2006;113(10):1361-1376.

16. Young EL, Karthikesalingam A, Huddart S, et al: A systematic review of the role of cardiopulmonary exercise testing in vascular surgery. *Eur J Vasc Endovasc Surg* 2012;44(1):64-71.

    The authors performed a systematic review of cardiopulmonary exercise testing (CPET) in the preoperative evaluation of aortic aneurysm or peripheral vascular disease requiring surgery. They found seven articles that met their inclusion criteria. They concluded that a paucity of data preclude the routine adoption of CPET when risk stratifying patients undergoing major vascular surgery.

17. Smetana GW, Lawrence VA, Cornell JE; American College of Physicians: Preoperative pulmonary risk stratification for noncardiothoracic surgery: Systematic review for the American College of Physicians. *Ann Intern Med* 2006;144(8):581-595.

18. Archer C, Levy AR, McGregor M: Value of routine preoperative chest x-rays: A meta-analysis. *Can J Anaesth* 1993;40(11):1022-1027.

19. Qaseem A, Snow V, Fitterman N, et al; Clinical Efficacy Assessment Subcommittee of the American College of Physicians: Risk assessment for and strategies to reduce perioperative pulmonary complications for patients undergoing noncardiothoracic surgery: A guideline from the American College of Physicians. *Ann Intern Med* 2006;144(8):575-580.

20. Smetana GW: Preoperative pulmonary evaluation. *N Engl J Med* 1999;340(12):937-944.

21. Hempsall VJ, Robertson DR, Campbell MJ, Briggs RS: Orthopaedic geriatric care—is it effective? A prospective population-based comparison of outcome in fractured neck of femur. *J R Coll Physicians Lond* 1990;24(1):47-50.

22. Zuckerman JD, Sakales SR, Fabian DR, Frankel VH: Hip fractures in geriatric patients. Results of an

interdisciplinary hospital care program. *Clin Orthop Relat Res* 1992;274:213-225.

23. Friedman SM, Mendelson DA, Kates SL, McCann RM: Geriatric co-management of proximal femur fractures: Total quality management and protocol-driven care result in better outcomes for a frail patient population. *J Am Geriatr Soc* 2008;56(7):1349-1356.

24. Basques BA, Bohl DD, Golinvaux NS, Samuel AM, Grauer JG: General versus spinal anaesthesia for patients aged 70 years and older with a fracture of the hip. *Bone Joint J* 2015;97-B(5):689-695.

    The authors identified 9,842 patients aged 70 years and older from the American College of Surgeons National Surgical Quality Improvement Program database who underwent spinal or general anesthesia. General anesthesia was associated with a short length of stay but a slightly increased incidence of any adverse event and blood transfusion. Spinal anesthesia was associated with an increased risk of urinary tract infection. The authors observed no clear distinction between the two methods of anesthesia.

25. Whiting PS, Molina CS, Greenberg SE, Thakore RV, Obremskey WT, Sethi MK: Regional anaesthesia for hip fracture surgery is associated with significantly more peri-operative complications compared with general anaesthesia. *Int Orthop* 2015;39(7):1321-1327.

    The authors identified 7,764 hip fractures from the American College of Surgeons National Surgical Quality Improvement Program database and compared patients who underwent general anesthesia with those who underwent spinal anesthesia. Spinal anesthesia was associated with the highest total complication rate (19.6%, 1,522 patients). In a multivariate analysis, spinal anesthesia was associated with greater odds of minor and total complications when compared with general anesthesia.

26. Covert CR, Fox GS: Anaesthesia for hip surgery in the elderly. *Can J Anaesth* 1989;36(3 Pt 1):311-319.

27. Arbous MS, Meursing AE, van Kleef JW, et al: Impact of anesthesia management characteristics on severe morbidity and mortality. *Anesthesiology* 2005;102(2):257-268, quiz 491-492.

28. White PF, White LM, Monk T, et al: Perioperative care for the older outpatient undergoing ambulatory surgery. *Anesth Analg* 2012;114(6):1190-1215.

    The authors summarized the effects of anesthesia on aging patients undergoing ambulatory surgery. The authors believe that ambulatory surgery has several advantages in the elderly; however, importance should be given to the evaluation of comorbid conditions. The authors discussed the different anesthesia techniques that can be used depending on the medical complexity of the elderly patient.

29. Mason SE, Noel-Storr A, Ritchie CW: The impact of general and regional anesthesia on the incidence of post-operative cognitive dysfunction and post-operative delirium: A systematic review with meta-analysis. *J Alzheimers Dis* 2010;22(suppl 3):67-79.

    The authors performed a systematic review of 21 publications, looking at the role of anesthesia in the development of POCD and POD. No anesthesia type had any effect on the development of POD, and general anesthesia was marginally but nonsignificantly related to POCD. The authors concluded that general anesthesia may increase the risk of developing POCD.

30. Aksoy M, Dostbil A, Ince I, et al: Continuous spinal anaesthesia versus ultrasound-guided combined psoas compartment-sciatic nerve block for hip replacement surgery in elderly high-risk patients: A prospective randomised study. *BMC Anesthesiol* 2014;14:99.

    The authors performed a randomized study of 70 high-risk elderly patients undergoing total hip arthroplasty by assigning them to continuous spinal anesthesia (CSA) or a combined psoas compartment-sciatic nerve block (PCSNB). The authors concluded that both CSA and PCSNB provide adequate anesthesia in the elderly, but patients with a PCSNB had less perioperative hemodynamic instability.

31. Goldstein RY, Montero N, Jain SK, Egol KA, Tejwani NC: Efficacy of popliteal block in postoperative pain control after ankle fracture fixation: A prospective randomized study. *J Orthop Trauma* 2012;26(10):557-561.

    The authors evaluated postoperative pain control through a popliteal block in 51 patients with ankle fractures. The authors found that popliteal block provides equivalent postoperative pain control to that of general anesthesia. Patients with a popliteal block experienced a rebound pain phenomenon from 12 to 24 hours postoperatively, however. Early narcotic administration is recommended to minimize this phenomenon. Level of evidence: I.

32. Ding DY, Manoli A III, Galos DK, Jain S, Tejwani NC: Continuous popliteal sciatic nerve block versus single injection nerve block for ankle fracture surgery: A prospective randomized comparative trial. *J Orthop Trauma* 2015;29(9):393-398.

    This study assessed the effectiveness of a continuous popliteal sciatic nerve block compared with that of a single popliteal injection in patients undergoing ankle fracture surgery. The authors found that a continuous popliteal block reduced the rebound pain phenomenon occurring between 12 and 24 hours postoperatively. Level of evidence: I.

33. Auroy Y, Benhamou D, Bargues L, et al: Major complications of regional anesthesia in France: The SOS Regional Anesthesia Hotline Service. *Anesthesiology* 2002;97(5):1274-1280.

34. Steinmetz J, Christensen KB, Lund T, Lohse N, Rasmussen LS; ISPOCD Group: Long-term consequences of postoperative cognitive dysfunction. *Anesthesiology* 2009;110(3):548-555.

35. Inouye SK, Zhang Y, Jones RN, Kiely DK, Yang F, Marcantonio ER: Risk factors for delirium at discharge: Development and validation of a predictive model. *Arch Intern Med* 2007;167(13):1406-1413.

36. Schlitzkus LL, Melin AA, Johanning JM, Schenarts PJ: Perioperative management of elderly patients. *Surg Clin North Am* 2015;95(2):391-415.

    The authors provided a comprehensive review of perioperative management strategies for elderly patients, including the medical work-up, anesthesia requirements, and postoperative hospitalization.

37. Moller JT, Cluitmans P, Rasmussen LS, et al; International Study of Post-Operative Cognitive Dysfunction: Long-term postoperative cognitive dysfunction in the elderly ISPOCD1 study. ISPOCD investigators. *Lancet* 1998;351(9106):857-861.

38. Squadrone V, Coha M, Cerutti E, et al; Piedmont Intensive Care Units Network (PICUN): Continuous positive airway pressure for treatment of postoperative hypoxemia: A randomized controlled trial. *JAMA* 2005;293(5):589-595.

39. Singh N, Falestiny MN, Rogers P, et al: Pulmonary infiltrates in the surgical ICU: Prospective assessment of predictors of etiology and mortality. *Chest* 1998;114(4):1129-1136.

40. Rosenthal RA, Perkal MF: Physiologic considerations in the elderly surgical patient, in Miller TA, ed: *Modern surgical care: physiologic foundations and clinical applications* ,ed 2. New York, Informa, 2006, pp 1129-1148.

41. Thygesen K, Alpert JS, Jaffe AS, et al; Joint ESC/ACCF/AHA/WHF Task Force for the Universal Definition of Myocardial Infarction: Third universal definition of myocardial infarction. *Circulation* 2012;126(16):2020-2035.

    The authors provided an updated definition of myocardial infarction, which is defined as myocardial cell death due to prolonged ischemia.

42. Lee TH, Marcantonio ER, Mangione CM, et al: Derivation and prospective validation of a simple index for prediction of cardiac risk of major noncardiac surgery. *Circulation* 1999;100(10):1043-1049.

43. Devereaux PJ, Goldman L, Cook DJ, Gilbert K, Leslie K, Guyatt GH: Perioperative cardiac events in patients undergoing noncardiac surgery: A review of the magnitude of the problem, the pathophysiology of the events and methods to estimate and communicate risk. *CMAJ* 2005;173(6):627-634.

44. Weaver WD, Litwin PE, Martin JS, et al; The MITI Project Group: Effect of age on use of thrombolytic therapy and mortality in acute myocardial infarction. *J Am Coll Cardiol* 1991;18(3):657-662.

45. Wyse DG, Waldo AL, DiMarco JP, et al: A comparison of rate control and rhythm control in patients with atrial fibrillation. *N Engl J Med* 2002;347(23):1825-1833.

46. Van Gelder IC, Hagens VE, Bosker HA, et al; Rate Control versus Electrical Cardioversion for Persistent Atrial Fibrillation Study Group: A comparison of rate control and rhythm control in patients with recurrent persistent atrial fibrillation. *N Engl J Med* 2002;347(23):1834-1840.

47. Guillamondegui OD, Gunter OL, Bonadies JA, et al: Practice Management Guidelines for Stress Ulcer Prophylaxis: EAST Practice Guidelines Committee. Eastern Association for the Surgery of Trauma, 2008. Available at http://www.east.org/Content/documents/practicemanagementguidelines/stress-ulcer-prophylaxis%20.pdf. Accessed January 13, 2015.

48. Farina C, Gagliardi S: Selective inhibition of osteoclast vacuolar H(+)-ATPase. *Curr Pharm Des* 2002;8(23):2033-2048.

49. Reinus JF, Brandt LJ: Lower intestinal bleeding in the elderly. *Clin Geriatr Med* 1991;7(2):301-319.

50. Rosen AM: Gastrointestinal bleeding in the elderly. *Clin Geriatr Med* 1999;15(3):511-525.

51. Cohen SH, Gerding DN, Johnson S, et al; Society for Healthcare Epidemiology of America; Infectious Diseases Society of America: Clinical practice guidelines for Clostridium difficile infection in adults: 2010 update by the society for healthcare epidemiology of America (SHEA) and the infectious diseases society of America (IDSA). *Infect Control Hosp Epidemiol* 2010;31(5):431-455.

    The authors reported that *Clostridium difficile* remains the most important cause of health–care-associated diarrhea. More virulent strains of *C difficile* are being encountered, and they have a high morbidity and mortality rate. The early recognition and treatment of *C difficile* is important in minimizing complications.

52. Lamontagne F, Labbé AC, Haeck O, et al: Impact of emergency colectomy on survival of patients with fulminant Clostridium difficile colitis during an epidemic caused by a hypervirulent strain. *Ann Surg* 2007;245(2):267-272.

53. Wallace JI, Schwartz RS, LaCroix AZ, Uhlmann RF, Pearlman RA: Involuntary weight loss in older outpatients: Incidence and clinical significance. *J Am Geriatr Soc* 1995;43(4):329-337.

54. White JV, Guenter P, Jensen G, Malone A, Schofield M; Academy of Nutrition and Dietetics Malnutrition Work Group; A.S.P.E.N. Malnutrition Task Force; A.S.P.E.N. Board of Directors: Consensus statement of the Academy of Nutrition and Dietetics/American Society for Parenteral and Enteral Nutrition: Characteristics recommended for the identification and documentation of adult malnutrition (undernutrition). *J Acad Nutr Diet* 2012;112(5):730-738.

    The authors presented a standardized set of diagnostic characteristics that can be used to identify and document adult malnutrition in routine clinical practice.

55. Koval KJ, Maurer SG, Su ET, Aharonoff GB, Zuckerman JD: The effects of nutritional status on outcome after hip fracture. *J Orthop Trauma* 1999;13(3):164-169.

56. Milne AC, Avenell A, Potter J: Meta-analysis: Protein and energy supplementation in older people. *Ann Intern Med* 2006;144(1):37-48.

57. Egol KA, Strauss EJ: Perioperative considerations in geriatric patients with hip fracture: What is the evidence? *J Orthop Trauma* 2009;23(6):386-394.

58. Ennis RS: Postoperative deep vein thrombosis prophylaxis: A retrospective analysis in 1000 consecutive hip fracture patients treated in a community hospital setting. *J South Orthop Assoc* 2003;12(1):10-17.

59. Falck-Ytter Y, Francis CW, Johanson NA, et al; American College of Chest Physicians: Prevention of VTE in orthopedic surgery patients: Antithrombotic therapy and prevention of thrombosis, 9th ed: American College of Chest Physicians Evidence-Based Clinical Practice Guidelines. *Chest* 2012;141(2suppl):e278S-e325S.

    Optimal strategies for prophylaxis to reduce postoperative pulmonary embolism and DVT were discussed.

60. Eriksson BI, Lassen MR; PENTasaccharide in HIp-FRActure Surgery Plus Investigators: Duration of prophylaxis against venous thromboembolism with fondaparinux after hip fracture surgery: A multicenter, randomized, placebo-controlled, double-blind study. *Arch Intern Med* 2003;163(11):1337-1342.

Chapter 49

Femoral Neck Fractures in the Geriatric Population

Anthony V. Florschutz, MD, PhD   Joshua R. Langford, MD   Kenneth J. Koval, MD

Abstract

Femoral neck fracture is a common injury among the elderly (patients at least 65 years old). Unique patient-related and fracture-related aspects must be considered to maximize the long-term function of these patients and minimize the risk of complications. Most femoral neck fractures in these patients require surgical treatment. The appropriate intervention is selected based on individualized patient assessment and planning.

Keywords: femoral neck fracture; elderly; geriatric; arthroplasty; internal fixation

Introduction

Femoral neck fractures represent a substantial cause of morbidity and mortality in the elderly (patients at least 65 years old). The management of these fractures should focus on early postoperative mobilization and a progressive return to preoperative function. To reach these goals, it is important to establish a mechanically stable articulation through internal fixation or arthroplasty.

Epidemiology

More than 250,000 hip fractures occur in the United States every year, and this number is expected to double by 2050.[1,2] Femoral neck and intertrochanteric fractures each account for approximately half of these fractures. Almost all hip fractures (98%) occur in individuals older than 50 years, and the average age at the time of fracture is 72 years.[3] A low-energy fall accounts for 90% of hip fractures, and approximately 75% occur in women.[4] The risk factors for hip fracture include female sex, white racial identity, increasing age, poor general health, tobacco or alcohol use, a history of falls, previous fragility fracture, and low estrogen levels.

Clinical Evaluation

Patients who sustain a femoral neck fracture usually have groin pain and cannot bear weight on the injured extremity. A patient with an impacted fracture or a stress fracture may lack visible deformity and may be able to bear some weight. A patient with a displaced fracture typically has shortening and external rotation of the extremity. It is important to obtain an accurate patient history after a low-energy fracture in an older individual. Loss of consciousness, an earlier episode of syncope, the medical history, chest pain, earlier hip pain related to pathologic fracture, and the preinjury ambulatory status are critical in determining the optimal treatment and postoperative outlook. Patients who sustain a femoral neck fracture as a result of a high-energy injury initially should be treated in accordance with Advanced Trauma Life Support protocols and should undergo a thorough secondary survey to evaluate for the presence of associated injuries.

Dr. Langford or an immediate family member has received royalties from Advanced Orthopaedic Solutions, is a member of a speakers' bureau or has made paid presentations on behalf of Smith & Nephew, serves as a paid consultant to or is an employee of Stryker, and has stock or stock options held in Core Orthopaedic Institute for Better Bone Health, LLC. Dr. Koval or an immediate family member has received royalties from Biomet; is a member of a speakers' bureau or has made paid presentations on behalf of Biomet and Stryker; serves as a paid consultant to or is an employee of Biomet; and serves as a board member, owner, officer, or committee member of the American Academy of Orthopaedic Surgeons and the Orthopaedic Trauma Association. Neither Dr. Florschutz nor any immediate family member has received anything of value from or has stock or stock options held in a commercial company or institution related directly or indirectly to the subject of this chapter.

Radiographic Evaluation

The radiographic evaluation of a suspected hip fracture should include an AP pelvic view and AP and cross-table lateral views of the affected hip. The frog-lateral view should not be used; the positioning for this view may displace an impacted or nondisplaced femoral neck fracture. An internal rotation view of the injured hip, obtained with physician assistance, can be useful for identifying the fracture pattern by bringing the femoral neck into full view. Thin-slice CT is useful for detecting a nondisplaced femoral neck fracture, particularly in a high-energy femoral shaft fracture.[5] MRI is the imaging study of choice for delineating a nondisplaced or occult fracture that is not apparent on plain radiographs. In a patient who has a pacemaker or another contraindication to MRI, a bone scan may show any increased uptake at the fracture site.

Classification

Three classification schemes commonly are used for femoral neck fractures. The Garden classification is based on the extent of displacement of the fracture fragments as seen on an AP radiograph. The four Garden types of femoral neck fractures are as follows: I, incomplete or valgus impacted; II, complete without displacement; III, complete with partial displacement; and IV, complete with total displacement, allowing the femoral head to rotate back to an anatomic position. The Pauwels classification is based on the femoral neck fracture angle deviation from the horizontal. Type I is less than 30°; type II, 30° to 70°; and type III, more than 70°. Greater shear displacement forces correspond to a higher, more vertical fracture angle and greater fracture instability. The AO/Orthopaedic Trauma Association (OTA) classification of femoral neck fractures is used primarily for research purposes. In practice, it is often difficult to precisely classify fracture types using any of these systems, and they have poor intraobserver and interobserver reliability.[6] For prognostic purposes, femoral neck fractures are simply and effectively described as nondisplaced and stable (Garden type I or II) or displaced and unstable (Garden type III or IV).

Management

The treatment of choice for most femoral neck fractures in older patients is surgical. The goals of surgery are to relieve pain, allow early patient mobilization, and facilitate a progressive return to the preoperative functional level. Nonsurgical management should be considered only if the patient is seriously ill and the risk of surgery exceeds the potential benefits. Surgical management is indicated even in patients who were nonambulatory before the fracture, however, to achieve pain relief and facilitate transfers and mobilization.

The choice of a specific surgical procedure should be based on fracture stability and, perhaps more importantly, on patient factors, including age, functional status, and bone quality. In general, surgery should be performed on a semiurgent basis to minimize the risk of perioperative complications, improve patient comfort, and reduce the length of hospitalization.[7,8]

The American Academy of Orthopaedic Surgeons (AAOS) has issued an evidence-based clinical practice guideline on the perioperative and intraoperative management of patients older than 65 years with a hip fracture (http://www.aaos.org/Research/guidelines/HipFxGuideline.pdf).[9] An international multicenter randomized controlled study, Fixation Using Alternative Implants for the Treatment of Hip Fractures (FAITH), is underway to compare using multiple cancellous lag screw (CLS) fixation with sliding hip screw (SHS) devices in femoral neck fractures, with the primary objective of investigating revision rates within 24 months.[10] In addition, the study will analyze the health-related quality of life, functional outcome, state-sponsored health services, fracture healing, mortality, and adverse fracture-related complications in patients with stable and unstable femoral neck fractures.

Stable Femoral Neck Fractures

Active older individuals who sustain a stable valgus-impacted or nondisplaced Garden type I or II femoral neck fracture usually are treated with in situ fixation using multiple CLSs or an SHS device (**Figures 1** and **2**). Surgical treatment of these stable fractures should be geared toward internal fixation to prevent displacement.[11] Compared with SHS fixation, CLS fixation offers a less invasive technique requiring less surgical time and providing sufficient fixation in appropriately selected stable fractures. Typically, three partially threaded cannulated 6.5-, 7.0-, or 7.3-mm CLSs are placed in a parallel, inverted, and triangular pattern in an inferior, posterosuperior, and anterosuperior configuration and are situated adjacent to the inferior (calcar) and posterior cortices (**Figure 1**). The inferior screw resists inferior femoral head displacement, and the posterior screw resists posterior displacement. The starting point for the inferior screw should be at or above the lesser trochanter, because lower entry points generate stress risers in the subtrochanteric region. Screw threads should pass the femoral neck fracture site entirely to ensure a lag effect, and the tip of the screw should be positioned within 5 mm of the subchondral bone in the femoral head.

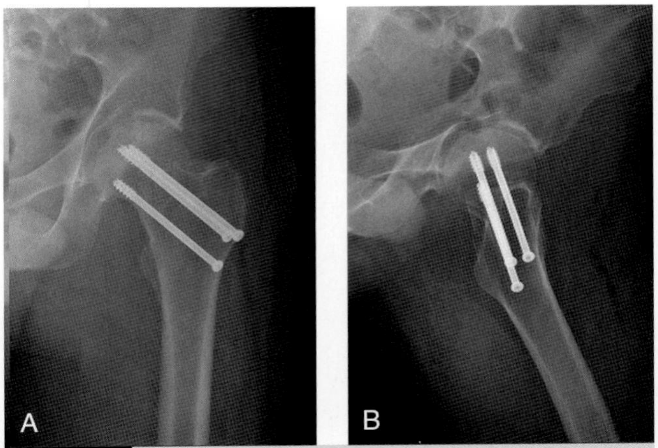

Figure 1 AP (**A**) and lateral (**B**) radiographs show a femoral neck fracture managed with multiple cancellous lag screw fixation in an active 67-year-old patient.

Fracture models comparing different screw configurations and variations in screw number have shown that a parallel inverted triangular CLS pattern achieved the greatest stability for most stable femoral neck fractures.[12,13] A fourth lag screw positioned along the posterior cortex may add stability in the presence of severe posterior comminution.[3,14] The addition of a washer can be useful for avoiding lateral cortex penetration of the screw head in osteoporotic bone and permits greater maximal insertion torque and thread purchase in the femoral head.[15]

CLS fixation for stable femoral neck fractures have an implant survival rate close to 90% at 1-year follow-up.[16] The revision surgery rate was 10% at an average 11-month follow-up in a range of 0 to 5 years. The most common reasons for revision were osteonecrosis, nonunion, loss of fixation, soft-tissue irritation by a prominent screw, and subtrochanteric fracture.[17,18] Advanced age and female sex were cited as the most important risk factors for healing complications.[19] In contrast, the American Society of Anesthesiologists classification, cognitive function, time to surgery, and posterior tilt were not found to be correlated with healing complications.[20]

SHS devices for the internal fixation of stable femoral neck fractures are more preferable than CLS fixation in managing basicervical and higher shear (ie, more vertically oriented) fracture patterns.[21] Although SHS devices exhibit mechanically stronger fixation, comparisons to CLS fixation have shown increased rates of osteonecrosis associated with rotational malalignment resulting from the insertion torque produced during cephalic lag screw advancement. SHS devices also demonstrate longer surgical times and increased blood loss.[22] When using SHS devices, the placement of an antirotation screw or wire helps resist potential rotational displacement[23] (**Figure 2**). Furthermore, a tip-to-apex distance of 25 mm or less should be achieved to prevent cutout of the lag screw.[24]

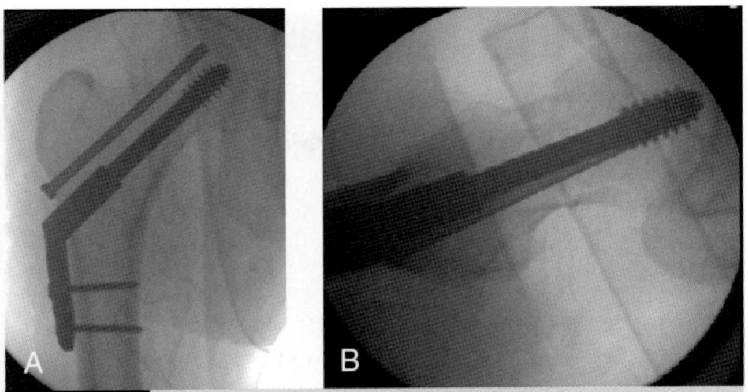

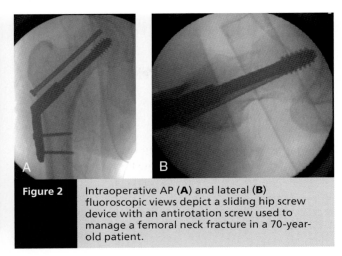

Figure 2 Intraoperative AP (**A**) and lateral (**B**) fluoroscopic views depict a sliding hip screw device with an antirotation screw used to manage a femoral neck fracture in a 70-year-old patient.

An alternative to CLS fixation and SHS devices is currently available in Europe and has shown promising results in managing femoral neck fractures. This new implant is a type of hybrid CLS-SHS fixation with multiple small-diameter sliding cancellous screws that lock into a side plate (**Figure 3**). The design provides rotational stability, controls femoral neck collapse, and eliminates screw toggling. The reported results of this fixation device are comparable functionally to those of CLS fixation and SHS devices, and the design provides decreased shortening of the femoral neck[25] and lower nonunion and revision rates.

Stress Fractures

A distinct type of nondisplaced femoral neck fracture is a stress fracture. These fractures can occur in geriatric patients with impaired bone quality but also can be seen in active individuals of any age. Femoral neck stress fractures result from cyclic mechanically malaligned loading across the femoral neck and diminished bone quality.[26] Early diagnosis is paramount because continued weight-bearing activity may result in displacement and fracture instability. The recognition of fracture morphology on the compression or tension side of the neck is important in dictating management. Compression-side fractures may be treated nonsurgically with protected weight bearing and serial follow-up for 6 to 8 weeks. Tension-side fractures of the femoral neck pose a substantially increased risk for displacement, and surgical fixation is indicated. All insufficiency fractures in the elderly should prompt an endocrine evaluation to manage metabolic bone pathology. Furthermore, education on safe activity techniques

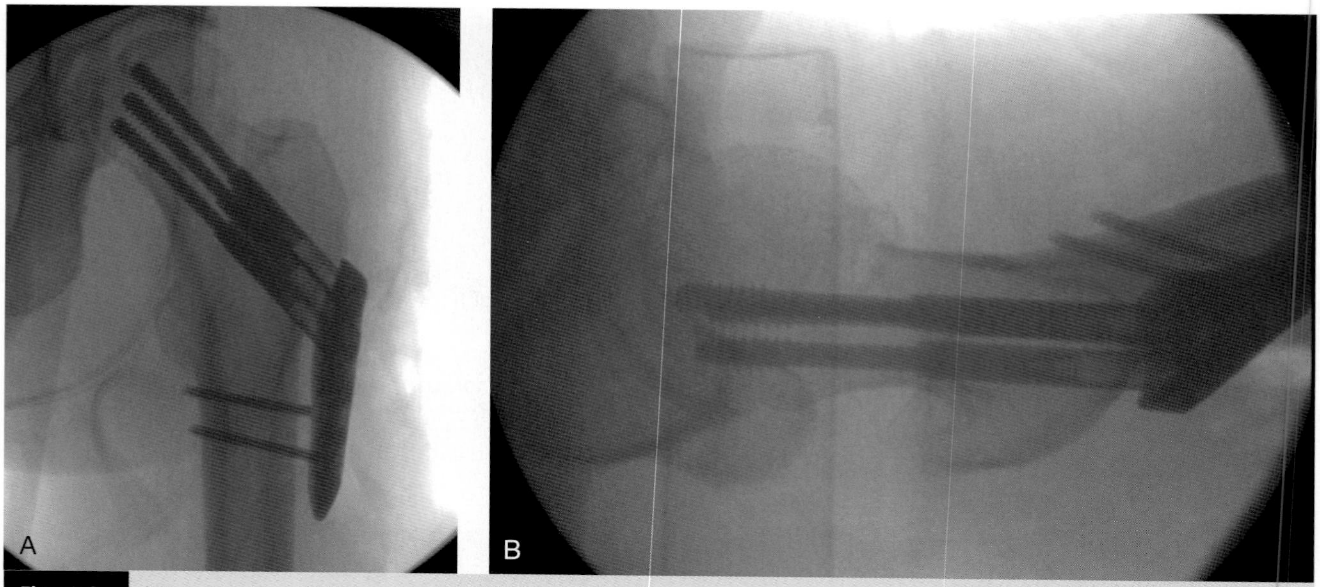

Figure 3 Intraoperative AP (**A**) and lateral (**B**) fluoroscopic views show a hybrid cancellous lag screw-sliding hip screw device used to manage a femoral neck fracture in a 72-year-old patient.

should be a part of fracture management, especially in more active patients.

Unstable Displaced Fractures

Surgical intervention generally is indicated for elderly patients with unstable Garden III and IV femoral neck fractures. Surgical options include closed reduction and internal fixation (CRIF), open reduction and internal fixation (ORIF), hemiarthroplasty (HA), and total hip arthroplasty (THA). The process of selecting a specific surgical option should begin with the evaluation of patient-related factors such as activity, independence, life expectancy, and medical comorbidities. The long-term results of the specific surgical interventions such as reoperation rates and patient function should be considered with respect to individual patient assessment and expectations. The complexity of the decision-making process is highlighted by the heterogeneity of femoral neck fracture management among orthopaedic surgeons. Efforts to establish treatment algorithms and hospital care pathways for patients with femoral neck fractures are ongoing.

Closed or Open Reduction and Internal Fixation

Active elderly patients with unstable femoral neck fractures may be managed effectively with CRIF or ORIF using CLS fixation or an SHS device. CRIF is also a viable fracture stabilization and pain-relieving option in patients who are high-risk surgical candidates, severely infirmed, and nonambulatory and who have a very low functional demand. Although CRIF and ORIF have demonstrated good functional results in appropriately selected patients, studies report that approximately one-third of patients eventually will require subsequent surgical intervention in time.[27]

When performing CRIF or ORIF on active geriatric patients with femoral neck fracture, it is crucial to understand the importance of anatomic reduction and the influence it has on long-term function and complication and reoperation rates. Femoral neck malreduction may be the strongest predictor for bone healing complications, diminished baseline functional recovery, osteonecrosis, loss of reduction, and reoperation.[28] Varus angulation, inferior offset, posterior sag, and retroversion must not be accepted as adequate reductions.[29] The acceptable reduction criteria for femoral neck fractures include a neck-shaft angle between 130° and 150° and neck anteversion between 0° and 15°.[30] Valgus angulation as high as 15° is tolerable and may enhance stability when more severe posterior comminution is present. In many cases, closed reduction maneuvers are successful in gaining acceptable anatomic alignment of a fractured femoral neck; however, if closed techniques fail, an open reduction should be performed through an anterior Smith-Petersen or anterolateral Watson-Jones approach. Studies have noted a higher rate of osteonecrosis of the femoral head with CRIF than with ORIF; this result can be attributed primarily to poorer anatomic reduction.[28] Subsequent fixation then can be performed using CLS fixation or an SHS device, depending on the fracture pattern.

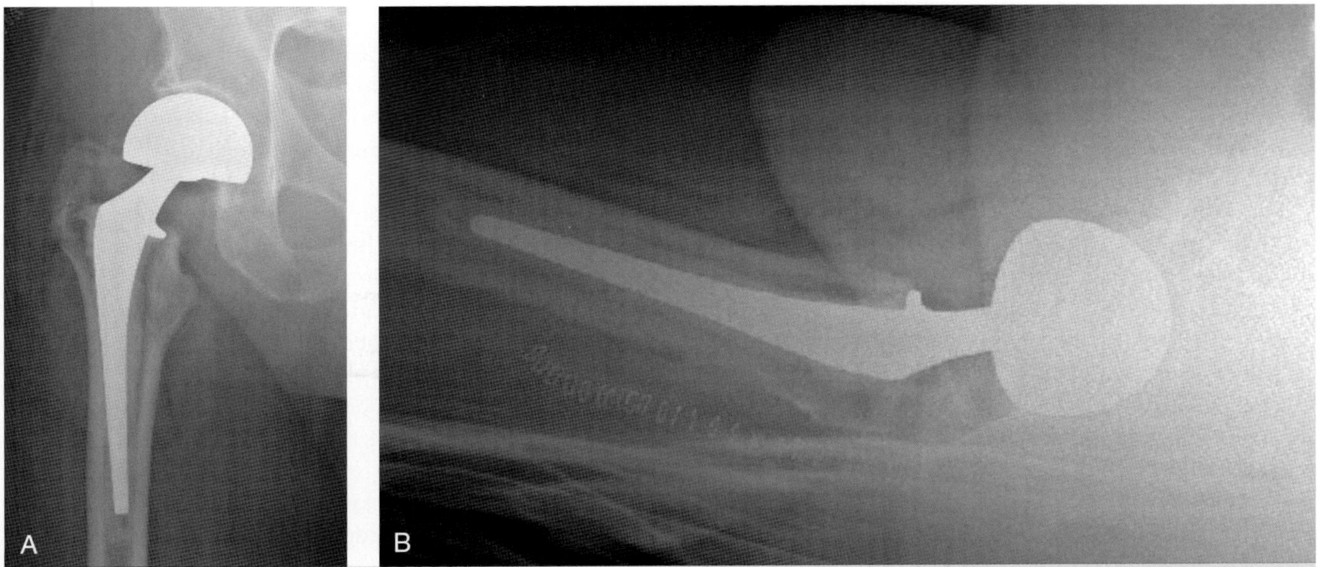

Figure 4 AP (**A**) and lateral (**B**) radiographs show a bipolar hemiarthroplasty with a cemented stem used to manage a femoral neck fracture in an 81-year-old patient.

Even with precise reduction and optimal fixation, collapse of the femoral neck often occurs and may portend to suboptimal patient outcomes. Historically, a shortened but healed femoral neck fracture was considered a satisfactory clinical outcome; however, several studies have reported positive associations between increasing degrees of femoral neck shortening and a lower quality of life as well as higher reoperation rates.[31] Several techniques, including divergent cancellous screws, fully threaded screws, anterior-inferior locked plating of the neck, and fibular strut grafts, have been advocated to prevent or minimize femoral neck shortening.[32,33] Proximal femoral locking plates also were trialed as a solution to prevent femoral neck shortening but demonstrated unacceptably high failure rates and therefore should not be used for managing femoral neck fractures.[34]

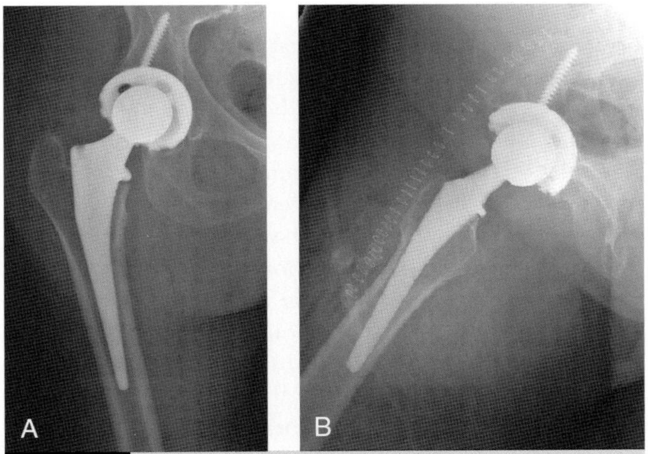

Figure 5 AP (**A**) and lateral (**B**) radiographs depict a total hip arthroplasty used in the management of a femoral neck fracture in an active 78-year-old patient.

Arthroplasty

Arthroplasty is the treatment of choice for most elderly patients with displaced unstable femoral neck fractures. HA (**Figure 4**) and THA (**Figure 5**) both have been employed as feasible long-term options when one of the two implant types has been appropriately selected, depending on patient-specific factors. HA provides excellent pain relief and early mobilization in low-demand patients with femoral neck fracture and, more importantly, delivers good long-term functional recovery. THA is the preferable management choice for healthier active elderly patients and for individuals with a history of symptomatic preinjury osteoarthritis.[35] Acute arthroplasty used for femoral neck fracture management poses increased morbidity risks and a tenfold higher mortality rate than elective arthroplasty.[36] Therefore, selection of the appropriate arthroplasty procedure initially necessitates a thorough inventory of patient factors. Specifically, the patient's general health, medical comorbidities, baseline physical function and activity, cognitive function, social support, and independence are critical parameters to consider in the management decision-making process. Furthermore, the different HA and THA implant options and the surgical approach and technique must be deliberated to optimize individual patient management.

Four main options are available for the surgical approach: the anterior (Smith-Petersen), posterior (Moore), lateral (Hardinge), and anterolateral (Watson-Jones) approaches. The decision to use one approach over another is based on surgeon preference. Although all four of these approaches often are employed, studies suggest higher dislocation rates using the posterior approach.[37] Furthermore, some investigators have found that the direct anterior approach facilitates early mobilization, reduces postoperative pain, and improves overall patient satisfaction.[38] Regardless of the approach, a key difference between HA and THA is that THA requires more extensive exposure and generally has higher blood loss and an increased incidence of perioperative complications.

The implications of the implant design and technique of arthroplasty are important considerations in managing elderly patients with femoral neck fractures. Not uncommonly, suboptimal bone density and considerable comorbidities in the geriatric population increase the complexity of implant selection and technique. The femoral stem component for HA and THA may be cemented or uncemented (press-fit). In patients with osteoporotic bone, cementing the stem provides excellent fixation and mechanically augments weak bone; therefore, it is the standard technique for these patients.[39,40] In the past, intraoperative sudden death secondary to cardiopulmonary insult during cementing was a real concern, but improvements in cementing techniques have reduced the mortality rate from this complication more than threefold.[41] Although press-fit stems preclude the need for cementing and their use is growing in younger patients, fracture around the stem at the time of implantation and postoperatively in elderly patients may affect long-term outcomes considerably.[42-44] Press-fit femoral stems are an option, however, when bone density is determined to be sufficient based on radiographs and intraoperative assessment and in patients who are at high risk for cardiovascular and pulmonary complications. Such stems also have the advantages of a shorter surgical time and reduced intraoperative blood loss while providing complication and reoperation rates similar to those of cemented stems.[45,46]

Another important aspect of the femoral side of arthroplasty implants is the femoral head. HA may be performed with a unipolar or bipolar head component. Most studies have found no measurable difference between these head types, other than the increased cost of bipolar designs.[47-50] In more active geriatric patients, increased rates of acetabular erosion may be observed when using unipolar implants as well as a poorer functional return that may necessitate conversion to THA in certain cases.[51,52] The head component for THA femoral stems may be metal or ceramic, and they articulate with a polyethylene acetabular liner. For aging patients, metal on polyethylene is typically sufficient, although ceramic on polyethylene may be more appropriate for higher functioning active patients.

THA is becoming a more popular option for older patients who are living healthier and more active lives. In the management of femoral neck fractures, THA has shown no difference in 30-day mortality rates and provides better patient-reported function and pain relief as well as lower reoperation rates than HA and ORIF.[53-55] Dislocation rates and respiratory complications are reported to be higher with THA than with HA.[56] Although the immediate cost of acute primary THA is higher than that of HA or internal fixation, analysis has shown a lower long-term economic burden in appropriately selected patients when taking into account the higher reoperation and complication rates of HA and ORIF.[57-59]

Summary

Femoral neck fractures remain a substantial cause of morbidity and mortality in the elderly. A return to preinjury function remains the goal of treatment, which needs to be individualized and should be based on patient and fracture factors. Although an increasing number of higher evidence studies are being conducted to evaluate the prevention and treatment of these devastating injuries, considerable work still needs to be done.

Key Study Points

- The decision-making factors related to the treatment of a femoral neck fracture in an older individual must be understood.
- The risks and benefits of internal fixation and arthroplasty must be weighed when managing femoral neck fracture in the elderly.
- The treatment of femoral neck fractures in the elderly should be individualized and should be based on patient and fracture factors.
- Surgical intervention is indicated for most elderly patients who sustain a femoral neck fracture.
- Older individuals who sustain a valgus-impacted or nondisplaced femoral neck fracture (Garden I or II) usually are treated with in situ fixation using multiple cancellous lag screws or a sliding hip screw device. Arthroplasty is the treatment of choice for most elderly patients who sustain a displaced unstable femoral neck fracture.

Annotated References

1. National Hospital Discharge Survey (NHDS), National Center for Health Statistics: Available at: http://205.207.175.93/hdi/ReportFolders/ReportFolders.aspx?IF_ActivePath=P,18External. Accessed December 31, 2014.

2. Gullberg B, Johnell O, Kanis JA: World-wide projections for hip fracture. *Osteoporos Int* 1997;7(5):407-413.

3. Johnell O, Kanis JA: An estimate of the worldwide prevalence and disability associated with osteoporotic fractures. *Osteoporos Int* 2006;17(12):1726-1733.

4. Jordan KM, Cooper C: Epidemiology of osteoporosis. *Best Pract Res Clin Rheumatol* 2002;16(5):795-806.

5. Tornetta P III, Kain MS, Creevy WR: Diagnosis of femoral neck fractures in patients with a femoral shaft fracture. Improvement with a standard protocol. *J Bone Joint Surg Am* 2007;89(1):39-43.

6. Gašpar D, Crnković T, Durović D, Podsednik D, Slišurić F: AO group, AO subgroup, Garden and Pauwels classification systems of femoral neck fractures: Are they reliable and reproducible? *Med Glas (Zenica)* 2012;9(2):243-247.

   This study assesses the reliability and reproducibility of different femoral neck fracture classification schemes. Results showed that the Garden and AO group classifications were useful for describing displaced and nondisplaced femoral neck fractures.

7. Kim JW, Byun SE, Chang JS: The clinical outcomes of early internal fixation for undisplaced femoral neck fractures and early full weight-bearing in elderly patients. *Arch Orthop Trauma Surg* 2014;134(7):941-946.

   This retrospective study investigated the clinical outcomes of early fixation and early full weight bearing after internal fixation of nondisplaced femoral neck fractures in patients aged 65 years or older. The authors found satisfactory clinical outcomes, noting that 72% of patients returned to their preinjury walking ability, and 7.4% required a secondary procedure.

8. Simunovic N, Devereaux PJ, Sprague S, et al: Effect of early surgery after hip fracture on mortality and complications: Systematic review and meta-analysis. *CMAJ* 2010;182(15):1609-1616.

   This systematic review and meta-analysis assessed the influence of early surgery on the risk of death and postoperative complications in elderly patients undergoing treatment for femoral neck fractures. Earlier surgery was associated with a reduced risk of death and diminished rates of postoperative pneumonia and pressure sores in elderly patients.

9. AAOS Evidence-Based Guidelines for Management of Hip Fractures in the Elderly, Adopted by the American Academy of Orthopaedic Surgeons Board of Directors September 5, 2014. Available at: http://www.aaos.org/Research/guidelines/HipFxGuideline.pdf. Accessed December 31, 2014.

10. FAITH Investigators: Fixation using alternative implants for the treatment of hip fractures (FAITH): Design and rationale for a multi-centre randomized trial comparing sliding hip screws and cancellous screws on revision surgery rates and quality of life in the treatment of femoral neck fractures. *BMC Musculoskelet Disord* 2014;15:219.

    The authors describe the objectives, methods, and design of the Fixation Using Alternative Implants for the Treatment of Hip Fractures (FAITH) study. The trial is registered at ClinicalTrials.gov (Identifier NCT00761813).

11. Bjørgul K, Reikerås O: Outcome of undisplaced and moderately displaced femoral neck fractures. *Acta Orthop* 2007;78(4):498-504.

12. Papanastassiou ID, Mavrogenis AF, Kokkalis ZT, Nikolopoulos K, Skourtas K, Papagelopoulos PJ: Fixation of femoral neck fractures using divergent versus parallel cannulated screws. *J Long Term Eff Med Implants* 2011;21(1):63-69.

    This investigation evaluates a divergent screw technique for the fixation of femoral neck fractures. The results suggest that the parallel placement of screws is not critical for a good clinical outcome and that using the divergent screw technique may offer improved fixation.

13. Selvan VT, Oakley MJ, Rangan A, Al-Lami MK: Optimum configuration of cannulated hip screws for the fixation of intracapsular hip fractures: A biomechanical study. *Injury* 2004;35(2):136-141.

14. Kauffman JI, Simon JA, Kummer FJ, Pearlman CJ, Zuckerman JD, Koval KJ: Internal fixation of femoral neck fractures with posterior comminution: A biomechanical study. *J Orthop Trauma* 1999;13(3):155-159.

15. Bishop JA, Behn AW, Castillo TN: The biomechanical significance of washer use with screw fixation. *J Orthop Trauma* 2014;28(2):114-117.

    Evidence is presented for the use of washers in conjunction with cannulated screw fixation of femoral neck fractures. Synthetic bone models were used to make mechanical measurements.

16. Gjertsen JE, Fevang JM, Matre K, Vinje T, Engesæter LB: Clinical outcome after undisplaced femoral neck fractures. *Acta Orthop* 2011;82(3):268-274.

17. Kain MS, Marcantonio AJ, Iorio R: Revision surgery occurs frequently after percutaneous fixation of stable femoral neck fractures in elderly patients. *Clin Orthop Relat Res* 2014;472(12):4010-4014.

    The purpose of this study is to determine the proportion of hips that required conversion to THA and the proportion of hips that required revision fixation after percutaneous screw fixation of stable femoral neck fractures in patients older than 65 years. The results show that the rate of conversion to THA is 10% at an average of 9 months and that 3.3% required revision fixation for subtrochanteric fracture or removal of symptomatic hardware. Level of evidence: IV.

18. Stiasny J, Dragan S, Kulej M, Martynkiewicz J, Płochowski J, Dragan SŁ: Comparison analysis of the operative treatment results of the femoral neck fractures using side-plate and compression screw and cannulated AO screws. *Ortop Traumatol Rehabil* 2008;10(4):350-361.

19. Parker MJ, Raghavan R, Gurusamy K: Incidence of fracture-healing complications after femoral neck fractures. *Clin Orthop Relat Res* 2007;458:175-179.

20. Lapidus LJ, Charalampidis A, Rundgren J, Enocson A: Internal fixation of garden I and II femoral neck fractures: Posterior tilt did not influence the reoperation rate in 382 consecutive hips followed for a minimum of 5 years. *J Orthop Trauma* 2013;27(7):386-390, discussion 390-391.

    The authors analyze whether preoperative posterior tilt and other factors influence the reoperation rate related to fracture healing complications after internal fixation of stable femoral neck fractures. There was no correlation of reoperation in relation to posterior tilt, patient age, sex, cognitive function, American Society of Anesthesiologists classification, or time to surgery. Level of evidence: II.

21. Aminian A, Gao F, Fedoriw WW, Zhang LQ, Kalainov DM, Merk BR: Vertically oriented femoral neck fractures: Mechanical analysis of four fixation techniques. *J Orthop Trauma* 2007;21(8):544-548.

22. Parker MJ, Stockton G: Internal fixation implants for intracapsular proximal femoral fractures in adults. *Cochrane Database Syst Rev* 2001;4:CD001467.

23. Massoud EI: Fixation of basicervical and related fractures. *Int Orthop* 2010;34(4):577-582.

    This prospective study identifies proximal femoral fractures that may be prone to axial and rotational instability and assesses the results of fixation using a dynamic hip screw and a derotation screw. The authors find that AO types B2.1, A1.1, A2.1, A2.2, and A2.3 fracture patterns have similar instability patterns, and they recommend management using three-plane fixation, in which dynamic hip screw fixation provides two planes and a derotation screw provides a third.

24. Pervez H, Parker MJ, Vowler S: Prediction of fixation failure after sliding hip screw fixation. *Injury* 2004;35(10):994-998.

25. Eschler A, Brandt S, Gierer P, Mittlmeier T, Gradl G: Angular stable multiple screw fixation (Targon FN) versus standard SHS for the fixation of femoral neck fractures. *Injury* 2014;45(suppl 1):S76-S80.

    This comparative analysis of angular stable Targon FN multiple screw fixation (B/Braun) and sliding hip screw device fixation for femoral neck fractures indicates that less head subsidence, a lower conversion to arthroplasty, and a lower incidence of screw cutout has been observed when using the Targon FN device.

26. Egol KA, Koval KJ, Kummer F, Frankel VH: Stress fractures of the femoral neck. *Clin Orthop Relat Res* 1998;348:72-78.

27. Heetveld MJ, Rogmark C, Frihagen F, Keating J: Internal fixation versus arthroplasty for displaced femoral neck fractures: What is the evidence? *J Orthop Trauma* 2009;23(6):395-402.

28. Krischak G, Beck A, Wachter N, Jakob R, Kinzl L, Suger G: Relevance of primary reduction for the clinical outcome of femoral neck fractures treated with cancellous screws. *Arch Orthop Trauma Surg* 2003;123(8):404-409.

29. Weinrobe M, Stankewich CJ, Mueller B, Tencer AF: Predicting the mechanical outcome of femoral neck fractures fixed with cancellous screws: An in vivo study. *J Orthop Trauma* 1998;12(1):27-36, discussion 36-37.

30. Chua D, Jaglal SB, Schatzker J: Predictors of early failure of fixation in the treatment of displaced subcapital hip fractures. *J Orthop Trauma* 1998;12(4):230-234.

31. Zlowodzki M, Brink O, Switzer J, et al: The effect of shortening and varus collapse of the femoral neck on function after fixation of intracapsular fracture of the hip: A multi-centre cohort study. *J Bone Joint Surg Br* 2008;90(11):1487-1494.

32. Boraiah S, Paul O, Hammoud S, Gardner MJ, Helfet DL, Lorich DG: Predictable healing of femoral neck fractures treated with intraoperative compression and length-stable implants. *J Trauma* 2010;69(1):142-147.

    This study reports the outcomes of a treatment algorithm using nonsliding fixation methods aimed at preventing femoral neck shortening after internal fixation of femoral neck fractures.

33. Kunapuli SC, Schramski MJ, et al: Biomechanical analysis of augmented plate fixation for the treatment of vertical shear femoral neck fractures. *J Orthop Trauma* 2015;29(3):144-150.

    This biomechanical analysis compared the strength of augmented and nonaugmented fixation techniques that may be used to manage vertical shear femoral neck fractures. The authors evaluated fixation using 7.3-mm cannulated screws in an inverted triangle configuration and a 135° dynamic hip screw. Augmentation was provided by the placement of a 2.7-mm locking plate placed on the anterior-inferior aspect of the femoral neck. The authors concluded that using the locking plate added substantial strength to the constructs and noted that the cannulated screw construct with augmentation was the strongest.

34. Berkes MB, Little MT, Lazaro LE, Cymerman RM, Helfet DL, Lorich DG: Catastrophic failure after open reduction internal fixation of femoral neck fractures

with a novel locking plate implant. *J Orthop Trauma* 2012;26(10):e170-e176.

This clinical study evaluates a proximal femoral locking plate used in the management of femoral neck fractures. The results demonstrate catastrophic failure of the fixation method.

35. Leighton RK, Schmidt AH, Collier P, Trask K: Advances in the treatment of intracapsular hip fractures in the elderly. *Injury* 2007;38(suppl 3):S24-S34.

36. Parvizi J, Ereth MH, Lewallen DG: Thirty-day mortality following hip arthroplasty for acute fracture. *J Bone Joint Surg Am* 2004;86-A(9):1983-1988.

37. Rogmark C, Fenstad AM, Leonardsson O, et al: Posterior approach and uncemented stems increases the risk of reoperation after hemiarthroplasties in elderly hip fracture patients. *Acta Orthop* 2014;85(1):18-25.

This study identified risk factors for reoperation after hip HAfor femoral neck fractures. A cemented stem and lateral transgluteal approach reduced the risk of reoperation in patients aged 75 years or older. Males and younger patients had a higher risk for reoperation. In the 60- to 74-year-old age group, no significant differences were seen in the risk of reoperation for the variables analyzed.

38. Unger AC, Dirksen B, Renken FG, Wilde E, Willkomm M, Schulz AP: Treatment of femoral neck fracture with a minimal invasive surgical approach for hemiarthroplasty - clinical and radiological results in 180 geriatric patients. *Open Orthop J* 2014;8:225-231.

This investigation shows the clinical and radiographic outcomes in 180 patients managed for femoral neck fractures using the modified direct anterior approach and a bipolar hip HA. High patient satisfaction scores and rapid early mobilization were reported, and major complications were similar to those reported with other approaches.

39. Jameson SS, Jensen CD, Elson DW, et al: Cemented versus cementless hemiarthroplasty for intracapsular neck of femur fracture—a comparison of 60,848 matched patients using national data. *Injury* 2013;44(6):730-734.

This study compares the complications seen in cemented and uncemented hip HA used to manage femoral neck fractures. The study found no significant difference in medical complications or in the return to the operating room. Midterm revision and perioperative chest infections were found to be higher in the noncemented group, however.

40. Viberg B, Overgaard S, Lauritsen J, Ovesen O: Lower reoperation rate for cemented hemiarthroplasty than for uncemented hemiarthroplasty and internal fixation following femoral neck fracture: 12- to 19-year follow-up of patients aged 75 years or more. *Acta Orthop* 2013;84(3):254-259.

This study compares the reoperation rates in patients 75 years or older with displaced femoral neck fractures who were treated with internal fixation, cemented HA, or uncemented HA at 12 to 19 years of follow-up. Cemented HA was found to have a higher long-term survival than internal fixation and uncemented HA.

41. Parvizi J, Holiday AD, Ereth MH, Lewallen DG: The Frank Stinchfield Award. Sudden death during primary hip arthroplasty. *Clin Orthop Relat Res* 1999;369:39-48.

42. Parker MJ, Gurusamy KS, Azegami S: Arthroplasties (with and without bone cement) for proximal femoral fractures in adults. *Cochrane Database Syst Rev* 2010;6:CD001706.

This review of randomized controlled trials compares different arthroplasty types for the management of femoral neck fractures. Evidence shows that cemented prostheses may lead to less postoperative pain and improve mobility. No evidence supports using bipolar implants over unipolar implants, but total hip arthroplasty did trend toward having more improved functional results than HA.

43. Gjertsen JE, Lie SA, Vinje T, et al: More re-operations after uncemented than cemented hemiarthroplasty used in the treatment of displaced fractures of the femoral neck: An observational study of 11,116 hemiarthroplasties from a national register. *J Bone Joint Surg Br* 2012;94(8):1113-1119.

This study compared cemented and uncemented hip HAs for the management of femoral neck fractures. The authors report higher intraoperative complications in the cemented implant group; however, the overall revision rate was higher in the noncemented group.

44. Langslet E, Frihagen F, Opland V, Madsen JE, Nordsletten L, Figved W: Cemented versus uncemented hemiarthroplasty for displaced femoral neck fractures: 5-year followup of a randomized trial. *Clin Orthop Relat Res* 2014;472(4):1291-1299.

This article reports the results of a randomized controlled trial comparing cemented to noncemented fixation for bipolar hip HA used to treat femoral neck fractures. The results demonstrate that both techniques may be used with good midterm results. Harris Hip Scores were higher in the uncemented group, although this advantage was offset by a higher risk for periprosthetic fracture. Level of evidence: I.

45. Luo X, He S, Li Z, Huang D: Systematic review of cemented versus uncemented hemiarthroplasty for displaced femoral neck fractures in older patients. *Arch Orthop Trauma Surg* 2012;132(4):455-463.

This systemic review investigates the effectiveness and safety of cemented versus uncemented hip HA in the management of displaced femoral neck fractures in the elderly population. The authors state that cemented implants do not lead to higher mortality, reoperation, or complication rates; may diminish the risk of lasting pain; and potentially provide improved functional results.

46. Ning GZ, Li YL, Wu Q, Feng SQ, Li Y, Wu QL: Cemented versus uncemented hemiarthroplasty for displaced femoral neck fractures: An updated meta-analysis. *Eur J Orthop Surg Traumatol* 2014;24(1):7-14.

This investigation compares the results of cemented and uncemented hip HA for the management of displaced femoral neck fractures. The study shows no significant difference between the implant types.

47. Ong BC, Maurer SG, Aharonoff GB, Zuckerman JD, Koval KJ: Unipolar versus bipolar hemiarthroplasty: Functional outcome after femoral neck fracture at a minimum of thirty-six months of follow-up. *J Orthop Trauma* 2002;16(5):317-322.

48. Enocson A, Hedbeck CJ, Törnkvist H, Tidermark J, Lapidus LJ: Unipolar versus bipolar Exeter hip hemiarthroplasty: A prospective cohort study on 830 consecutive hips in patients with femoral neck fractures. *Int Orthop* 2012;36(4):711-717.

    In this prospective cohort study analyzing the reoperation and dislocation rates after unipolar and bipolar HA in patients with a displaced femoral neck fracture, the authors observe no difference between the two implant types.

49. Leonardsson O, Kärrholm J, Åkesson K, Garellick G, Rogmark C: Higher risk of reoperation for bipolar and uncemented hemiarthroplasty. *Acta Orthop* 2012;83(5):459-466.

    This prospective observational study focuses on identifying the risk factors for reoperation after femoral neck fracture management using modular hip HA. The study also assesses mortality rates in the same group of patients. The authors recommend using unipolar cemented prostheses and a transgluteal approach.

50. Liu Y, Tao X, Wang P, Zhang Z, Zhang W, Qi Q: Meta-analysis of randomised controlled trials comparing unipolar with bipolar hemiarthroplasty for displaced femoral-neck fractures. *Int Orthop* 2014;38(8):1691-1696.

    This study reviews randomized controlled trials to compare the clinical outcomes of unipolar hip HA with those of bipolar hip HA in the management of displaced femoral neck fractures. The study finds no difference between the implant types.

51. Inngul C, Hedbeck CJ, Blomfeldt R, Lapidus G, Ponzer S, Enocson A: Unipolar hemiarthroplasty versus bipolar hemiarthroplasty in patients with displaced femoral neck fractures: A four-year follow-up of a randomised controlled trial. *Int Orthop* 2013;37(12):2457-2464.

    This randomized controlled trial compares unipolar HA with bipolar HA in patients with displaced femoral neck fractures. The reported results favor bipolar implants, revealing delayed acetabular erosion and higher health-related quality of life.

52. Kanto K, Sihvonen R, Eskelinen A, Laitinen M: Uni- and bipolar hemiarthroplasty with a modern cemented femoral component provides elderly patients with displaced femoral neck fractures with equal functional outcome and survivorship at medium-term follow-up. *Arch Orthop Trauma Surg* 2014;134(9):1251-1259.

    This investigation compares a series of geriatric patients with displaced femoral neck fractures who were managed with a cemented modular unipolar hip HA with another series managed with bipolar hip HA. The study found higher dislocation rates in patients with the unipolar prosthesis, but overall, equivalent function and low revision rates were observed for both prostheses at midterm follow-up.

53. Burgers PT, Van Geene AR, Van den Bekerom MP, et al: Total hip arthroplasty versus hemiarthroplasty for displaced femoral neck fractures in the healthy elderly: A meta-analysis and systematic review of randomized trials. *Int Orthop* 2012;36(8):1549-1560.

    In this meta-analysis and systematic review of a randomized trial comparing THA with HA for the management of femoral neck fractures in fit elderly patients, the authors note improved patient-based outcomes but a higher dislocation rate with THA. They recommend further trials for more definitive evidence.

54. Yu L, Wang Y, Chen J: Total hip arthroplasty versus hemiarthroplasty for displaced femoral neck fractures: Meta-analysis of randomized trials. *Clin Orthop Relat Res* 2012;470(8):2235-2243.

    This meta-analysis of randomized controlled trials assesses whether THA has lower rates of reoperation, mortality, and complications as well as improved functional outcome compared with HA for the treatment of femoral neck fractures. Although a higher dislocation rate was associated with THA, a lower reoperation rate and higher functional scores also were seen.

55. Zi-Sheng A, You-Shui G, Zhi-Zhen J, Ting Y, Chang-Qing Z: Hemiarthroplasty vs primary total hip arthroplasty for displaced fractures of the femoral neck in the elderly: A meta-analysis. *J Arthroplasty* 2012;27(4):583-590.

    This meta-analysis compares the clinical effects of HA with those of primary THA for femoral neck fractures in elderly patients. The authors conclude that THA may provide improved results and pain relief as well as lower reoperation rates in elderly patients, although the dislocation rate is higher.

56. Fisher MA, Matthei JD, Obirieze A, et al: Open reduction internal fixation versus hemiarthroplasty versus total hip arthroplasty in the elderly: A review of the National Surgical Quality Improvement Program database. *J Surg Res* 2013;181(2):193-198.

    The investigators evaluate the 30-day postoperative outcomes of THA, HA, and open reduction and internal fixation for femoral neck fractures in patients older than 65 years. No difference was observed in mortality rates between groups, but a respiratory complication was more likely to develop in patients undergoing THA.

57. Iorio R, Healy WL, Lemos DW, Appleby D, Lucchesi CA, Saleh KJ: Displaced femoral neck fractures in the elderly: Outcomes and cost effectiveness. *Clin Orthop Relat Res* 2001;383:229-242.

58. Aleem IS, Karanicolas PJ, Bhandari M: Arthroplasty versus internal fixation of femoral neck fractures:

A clinical decision analysis. *Ortop Traumatol Rehabil* 2009;11(3):233-241.

59. Hedbeck CJ, Enocson A, Lapidus G, et al: Comparison of bipolar hemiarthroplasty with total hip arthroplasty for displaced femoral neck fractures: A concise four-year follow-up of a randomized trial. *J Bone Joint Surg Am* 2011;93(5):445-450.

This randomized controlled trial compares THA with hip HA for the management of femoral neck fractures. The results show improved function and quality of life after THA in coherent elderly patients with displaced femoral neck fractures.

Chapter 50

Intertrochanteric Hip Fractures in the Geriatric Population

Nirmal C. Tejwani, MD   Vinay Kumar Aggarwal, MD

Abstract

Hip fractures, including intertrochanteric, in elderly patients are among the injuries most commonly encountered by orthopaedic surgeons around the world; therefore, appropriate diagnosis, classification, and treatment of these fractures is paramount to achieve an optimal outcome. The advent of multiple high-profile medical prevention programs has helped decrease the number of hip fractures in the elderly. Nonetheless, the increase in the geriatric population because of the increase in overall life expectancy has led to a higher incidence of hip fractures globally, resulting in substantial economic and societal costs.

Keywords: intertrochanteric fractures; hip fractures; geriatric patients; sliding hip screws; cephalomedullary nailing; outcomes

Introduction

Hip fractures are common injuries in elderly patients.[1] Although the goal of medical prevention programs has been to decrease the incidence of hip fractures in elderly patients, the prevalence of hip fractures has increased in conjunction with increased life expectancy, placing a tremendous economic burden on the healthcare systems in the United States and around the world. Intertrochanteric fractures are equal to femoral neck fractures in incidence.[2]

Epidemiology

The overall incidence of hip fractures in 1990 was between 1.25 and 1.66 million worldwide.[3,4] Although no recently updated large-scale epidemiologic studies regarding hip fracture incidence have been found, prior projection studies indicate that by 2050, this number could increase to between 4.5 and 6.5 million per year around the world.[3,4] In the United States, the total number of hip fractures per year in persons older than 50 years was projected to increase from 238,000 in 1990 to 512,000 by the year 2040.[5] This increase can be attributed to both the increase in the elderly population overall and the rise in the age-specific incidence of hip fractures.[6]

North America and Europe account for about one-half of the hip fractures in elderly people, because of their high at-risk populations of white women. However, large increases in the incidence of hip fractures in Latin America and Asia will play a role in the exponential rise in the coming decades, with the percentage in Asia estimated to increase from 26% of all hip fractures in 1990 to 45% in 2050.[4]

Although there is a 3:1 female-to-male ratio of both femoral neck and intertrochanteric hip fractures, a greater increase in the number of hip fractures in men is expected in the coming years.[7] The exact reason for this trend is unclear, but it is postulated that it is because of the emphasis of treatment and prevention programs aimed specifically at elderly at-risk women during the past decade. Still, the lifetime risk of having a hip fracture is significantly higher in women (14% to 16%) than in men of the same age (6%).[8]

According to data from the Nationwide Inpatient Sample, there were more than 315,000 hospitalizations in the

Dr. Tejwani or an immediate family member is a member of a speakers' bureau or has made paid presentations on behalf of Zimmer and Stryker; serves as a paid consultant to Zimmer and Stryker; and serves as a board member, owner, officer, or committee member of the American Academy of Orthopaedic Surgeons, the Orthopaedic Trauma Association, and the Foundation of Orthopaedic Trauma. Neither Dr. Aggarwal nor any immediate family member has received anything of value from or has stock or stock options held in a commercial company or institution related directly or indirectly to the subject of this chapter.

United States for hip fractures, which accounted for 38% of all injury-related hospital stays in elderly patients—the largest proportion in this age group.[9] The mean cost for a hospital stay after hip fracture was $15,400 per patient, and the average length of stay was 6.3 days. These costs do not account for the long-term rehabilitation costs after hip fracture, which may reach more than $20 billion per year.

Although intertrochanteric fractures are equal to femoral neck fractures in incidence, they may be more costly than femoral neck fractures.[10] Authors of one study noted that patients with intertrochanteric fractures were sicker at baseline, with greater comorbidities, and thus may have higher morbidity and mortality rates.[11]

Medical and Social Issues

Geriatric patients should be assessed before, when, and after a fracture occurs. Primary care physicians and geriatricians now recognize several risk factors for intertrochanteric hip fractures; some are modifiable and others are unavoidable in elderly patients.

The development of osteoporosis and an increased propensity for falls are the top two risk factors for intertrochanteric hip fractures in elderly patients.[12] Ninety percent of these fractures are associated with falls from standing height.[13] Therefore, dedicated fall prevention programs have been established in nursing homes and hospital environments and include avoiding medications such as benzodiazepines, selective serotonin reuptake inhibitors, and anticonvulsants; preventing delirium; supervising patients with dementia; and providing adequate walking aids.

Prevention of bone loss and treatment of established osteoporosis have become commonplace among middle-aged patients in the United States, with widespread bone mineral density (BMD) testing allowing for early identification of patients at risk. Patients with BMD T scores of ≤2.5 SD from normal are candidates for medication therapy to improve their bone mineralization. Depending on specific patient factors, hormonal therapy with estrogens, selective estrogen receptor modulators such as raloxifene, or diphosphonate therapy with alendronate or risedronate may be appropriate choices to prevent osteoporosis and subsequent insufficiency fractures.[14] Nonpharmacologic prevention of osteoporosis also plays a role in the primary care setting; this can include advocating active weight-bearing lifestyles and minimized alcohol consumption and offering smoking cessation programs.

In addition to falls and osteoporosis, there are several medical conditions that studies have identified as independently increasing the danger of sustaining an intertrochanteric hip fracture. These include low body weight; excessive alcohol consumption; cigarette smoking; use of glucocorticoid therapy; vitamin D deficiency; and a variety of chronic medical conditions, including chronic kidney disease, rheumatoid arthritis, diabetes, inflammatory bowel disease, and depression.[15-17] Between 1995 and 2005, the number of hospitalizations for hip fractures in the United States actually decreased, presumably as a result of medical optimization by primary care physicians and of the addressing of some of the aforementioned modifiable risk factors.[18]

When an intertrochanteric hip fracture does occur, a multidisciplinary team should promptly decide on a treatment plan. In addition to the orthopaedic surgeon, this team should include an internist or a geriatrician, an anesthesiologist, a cardiologist, and any other medical specialists, as well as physiatrists, physical and occupational therapists, and social workers or care managers (or both). Several studies have outlined the benefit of such teams with regard to decreased hospital costs, perioperative complications, mortality, time to surgery, and length of hospital stay.[19-21] In a retrospective review, 510 patients older than 65 years who had hip fractures were evaluated. In patients treated after implementation of their multidisciplinary hip fracture team, medical complications decreased from 51% to 36%, the rate of undergoing surgery within 24 hours of admission increased from 35% to 63%, and mean hospital stay decreased from 8.1 to 5.7 days.[20]

An important factor in treating hip fractures is the optimal timing of surgery. An efficient preoperative protocol is beneficial to identify patients who are unfit to undergo surgery or who require medical optimization before surgery. Preoperative cardiac testing may be overused, as one study showed it to be an independent predictor of delay to surgery.[22] Furthermore, it was reported that the cardiac testing in their patient cohort affected neither the orthopaedic nor the medical management of patients with hip fractures, including patients with known cardiac disease.[22]

The typical teaching, which was based on several older landmark studies, was that surgery for hip fractures should be undertaken within 48 to 72 hours of hospital admission to minimize the risk of postoperative mortality.[23] A more recent report, however, suggested that even delaying surgery to hospital day 2 after admission increases the odds of mortality significantly, and that by hospital day 3 or later, the odds ratio of mortality is 1.33.[24] Authors of both of these studies acknowledged that patient comorbidities may be important factors in delays in surgery. In addition to preoperative cardiac testing, other

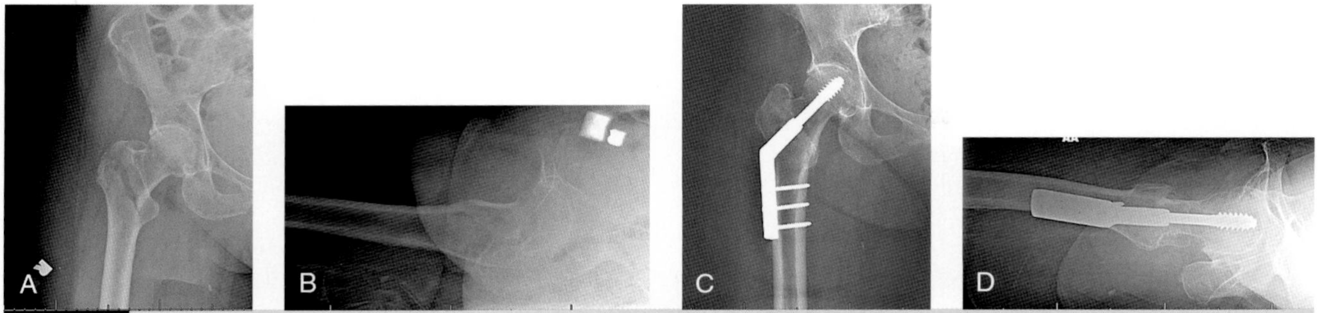

Figure 1 Preoperative AP (**A**) and lateral (**B**) radiographs from an 89-year-old patient with a stable intertrochanteric hip fracture. The lateral wall and the posteromedial cortex are both intact. Postoperative AP (**C**) and lateral (**D**) films show a sliding hip screw implant used for fracture fixation.

factors delaying hip fracture surgery include a higher score on the American Society of Anesthesiologists (ASA) Physical Classification System and the day of the week on which the patient is admitted, with Thursday through Saturday admissions showing greater delays, presumably because of a relative paucity of resources on weekends.[25]

The American Academy of Orthopaedic Surgeons' clinical practice guidelines recommend surgery within 48 hours of admission, with use of a sliding hip screw for stable fractures (**Figure 1**) and cephalomedullary nailing for unstable fractures.[26] Patients should undergo medical evaluation, including nutrition assessment, and surgery should not be delayed in those receiving aspirin or clopidogrel.[26]

Most authorities now agree that medical service management of hip fracture in the perioperative and postoperative periods provides the optimal healthcare result for the patient. This may be a hospitalist service specifically designed for hip fractures, a general medical service, or a geriatrician-driven service now headlined as the "orthogeriatrics model." Each of these co-care models have resulted in shorter lengths of stay, decreased time to surgery, reduction in total costs, and decreased mortality rates postoperatively.[27]

Classification

The diagnosis of hip fracture can be made initially from clinical presentation, as patients will describe a history of a fall from standing height (usually mechanical in nature) and will demonstrate a shortened and externally rotated limb on examination. Plain radiographs of the pelvis and the hip are the next step in diagnosis. The use of a traction-internal rotation view of the affected hip on radiograph may also help elucidate the true fracture pattern[28] (**Figure 2**). In one study, 47 complete sets of hip fracture radiographs were assessed before and after traction internal rotation views. It was concluded that the traction-internal rotation view not only led to better agreement among the involved surgeons in classifying the type of fracture and its stability, but also in some cases led to a change in the choice of the implant used to fix the fracture.[28] In rare instances, when radiographs are nondiagnostic and suspicion is still high, CT scan or, more reliably, MRI may be used to diagnose occult intertrochanteric hip fractures.[29,30]

Intertrochanteric fractures are extracapsular fractures of the proximal femur, as opposed to their femoral neck counterparts, which are intracapsular. This anatomic distinction plays an important role in differentiating the available blood supply to the two proximal fracture regions. Because the blood supply to the intertrochanteric region is so rich and extracapsular fractures offer minimal risk of disrupting blood supply to the femoral head, the rate of healing complications such as nonunion and osteonecrosis is much lower, although not absent, with intertrochanteric fractures.

Several validated classification systems for intertrochanteric fractures are in existence. Most of these—including the Kyle, Boyd and Griffin, and Ender classification systems—are of historical value only.[31] The Evans classification system, which was developed in 1949 and published in 1951, has, in large part, survived the test of time.[32] Fractures were divided into two broad categories: stable and unstable. Type 1 fractures were all true intertrochanteric fractures, with the fracture line extending from the lesser trochanter proximally and laterally along the intertrochanteric line. Within this type, the stable patterns exhibited medial cortex apposition, whereas the unstable patterns did not. Type 2 fractures were reverse obliquity fractures, in which the fracture line extended from the lesser trochanter distally and laterally. Reverse obliquity and intertrochanteric fractures with subtrochanteric extension can be considered

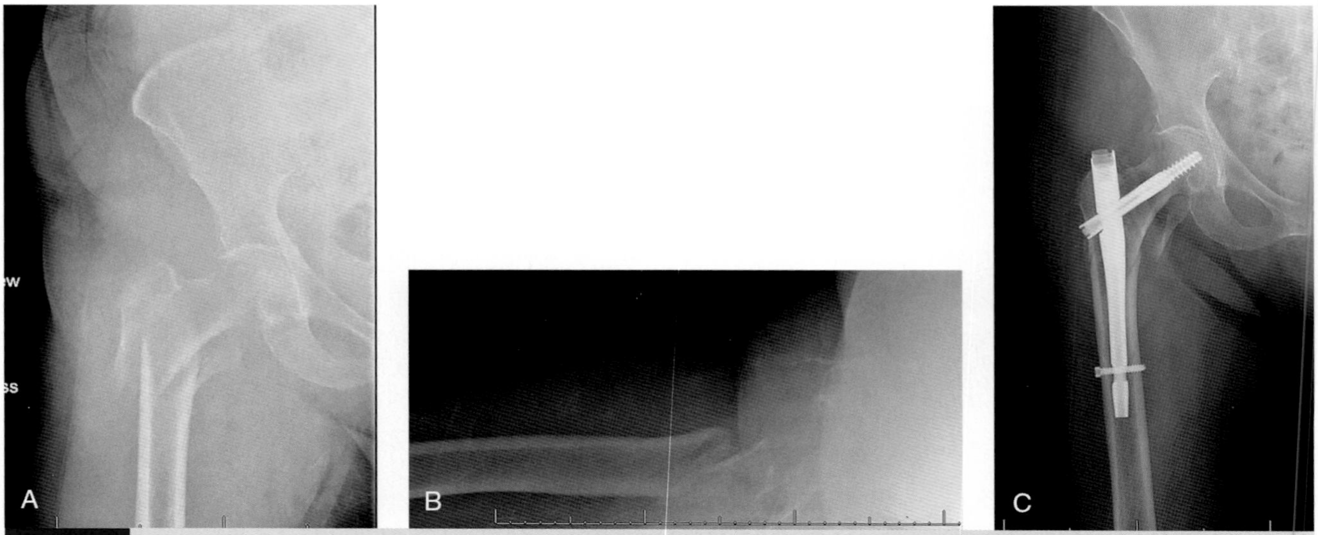

Figure 2 **A** and **B**, Preoperative radiographs from an 87-year-old patient with an unstable intertrochanteric hip fracture. **C**, Postoperative radiograph shows a short cephalomedullary device used for fracture fixation.

a transitional continuum between true intertrochanteric and subtrochanteric fractures and represent an unstable injury (**Figure 3**).

It is becoming well accepted that lateral wall integrity is just as important to the stability of intertrochanteric fractures as is posteromedial cortex apposition. Compromise to the lateral wall can lead to significant revision surgery rates if fixed with sliding hip screws.[33] The AO/Orthopaedic Trauma Association classification of intertrochanteric fractures, types 31-A1 through 31-A3, has been advocated as the most comprehensive and useful classification system to date.[34] It also classifies fractures on the basis of stability and recently was shown to help guide implant choice.[35] For experienced surgeons, the AO/OTA system may even be more reliable, with minimal interobserver variability.[34]

Treatment

Nonsurgical Treatment

Nonsurgical treatment of intertrochanteric fractures is rare and reserved for specific patient populations (nonambulatory patients, patients with dementia, or patients with subacute nondisplaced or impacted fractures who are experiencing minimal pain).[36] Additionally, nonsurgical care may occur in the terminally ill or highly unstable patient with significant uncorrectable comorbidities. Patients treated nonsurgically have shown increased 30-day mortality and loss of independence at 6 months, especially when early mobilization is not possible.[37]

Surgical Treatment

The goal of surgical treatment of intertrochanteric hip fractures is to establish a stable fracture pattern via controlled compression during fracture healing. The main complication to avoid with intertrochanteric fracture treatment is excessive collapse of the fracture fragments. This complication is most commonly related to varus position, penetration of hardware into the hip joint, breakage of the implant itself, or a combination of these factors.

For many decades, extramedullary devices (sliding hip screws with side plate constructs) were used for fixation of intertrochanteric hip fractures. Minimally invasive techniques, as an advancement of the traditional open technique for the dynamic hip screw insertion, have been shown in several comparative studies to be superior with regard to blood loss, hospital length of stay, pain levels, and hip function.[38-40] A minimally invasive percutaneous compression plate has been used in place of the traditional sliding hip screw, and results found to be superior to those of other fixation methods.[41]

In the United States, intramedullary devices have been used often in the treatment of intertrochanteric hip fractures and are the almost exclusive implant of choice for the younger practicing orthopaedic surgeon.[42] The intramedullary nature of the implant allows for buttressing of the fracture against the nail; in the case of lateral wall compromise, fracture stability can be safely achieved with this implant, unlike its extramedullary counterparts, which rely on an intact lateral cortex. An additional advantage of the intramedullary nail devices is the inherent percutaneous nature of insertion, thus ensuring minimal dissection at the fracture site.

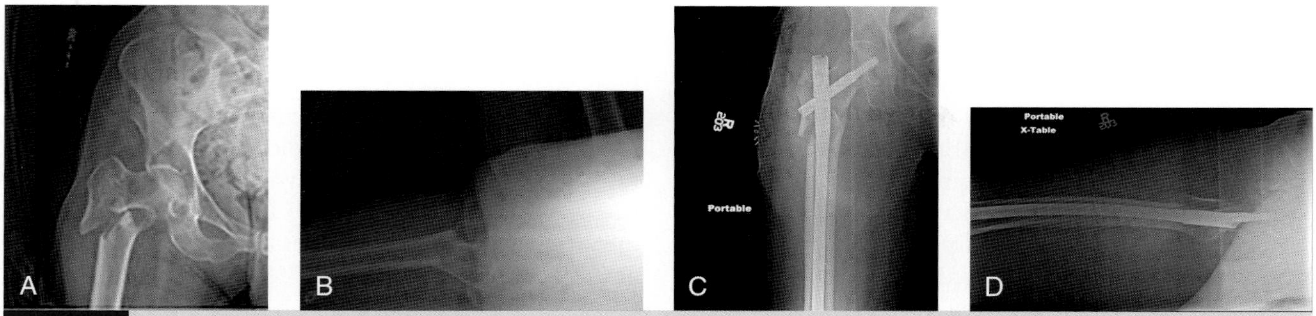

Figure 3 **A** and **B**, Preoperative radiographs from an 80-year-old patient with a reverse obliquity fracture pattern. **C** and **D**, Postoperative radiographs demonstrate fixation using a long cephalomedullary nail.

The short intramedullary nail is less expensive than the long nail and can be used for most intertrochanteric fracture patterns. Authors of a 2014 study reported that in AO/OTA 31-A1 and 31-A2 fractures, shorter nails were associated with significantly shorter surgical times, less blood loss, and lower rates of blood transfusion with no greater rates of complications.[43] The risk of anterior cortex abutment or even penetration, although low, is in theory higher with long cephalomedullary nail devices than with short ones. However, in a 2015 study of failure rates of long versus short nails, the authors found no differences in complication rates with short nails.[43]

Using the American College of Surgeons' National Surgical Quality Improvement Program database, the authors of a 2014 study identified 4,432 patients who underwent sliding hip screw or intramedullary nail procedures for intertrochanteric hip fracture from 2009 to 2012.[44] When examining in-hospital and 30-day outcomes, patients who underwent intramedullary nail procedures had a shorter length of stay by 1.0 day ($P < 0.001$), but no other outcome of adverse events, readmission, or operating room time showed any difference between the two groups.[44]

No matter what implant is used, two basic tenets of trochanteric fracture fixation remain key: the fracture must be adequately reduced before fixation, and hardware must be placed in an accurate position to ensure a positive result. Fracture reduction is especially important before placement of intramedullary devices, and surgeons should realize that the nail will not achieve fracture reduction by itself.

Whether a sliding hip screw or an intramedullary device is used, lag screw placement is important to prevent screw cutout and implant failure, especially in unstable fracture patterns. In one study, a tip-apex distance of less than 25 mm led to a significantly lower rate of screw cutout than did greater distances.[45] Tip-apex distance was described as the sum of the distance from the tip of the lag screw to the apex of the femoral head on an AP radiograph and lateral radiographs. A center-center position of the lag screw in the femoral head was considered ideal on the basis of results from this study. In addition to minimizing tip-to-apex distance, researchers in one study examined additional predictors of screw cutout in sliding hip screw and intramedullary nail implants and determined central-inferior or anterior-inferior positions of the screw were protective against cutout.[46] Recently, the absolute utility of the tip-to-apex distance has come into question. Findings of a biomechanical study in which researchers evaluated lag screw placement in intramedullary nail devices of laboratory-prepared trochanteric fractures suggested that placement of the lag screw in the low-center position was superior to placement in the center-center position even if the tip-to-apex distance exceeded 25 mm.[47]

Newer implant options for both extramedullary and intramedullary devices include sliding hip screws with side plates allowing for locking screws, anatomically contoured proximal femoral locking plates, intramedullary devices with helical blades rather than large lag screws to minimize bone loss, and cephalomedullary nails with dual proximal screw design to control for rotation and prevent migration. In the face of such an expansive array of implant options, some authors emphasize the importance of an algorithmic approach to surgical treatment of intertrochanteric fracture and that such an approach can help optimize implant choice, save significant costs to the practice, and even prevent complications after surgery or readmissions to the hospital.[35]

External fixation has been evaluated in a small number of high-risk elderly patients as a means to minimize surgical morbidity.[48,49] A randomized study in which investigators compared high-risk patients who had trochanteric fractures treated with either dynamic hip screw or external fixation showed the external fixation group to have a significantly shorter surgical time (15 minutes versus 73 minutes, $P < 0.05$), decreased need for blood transfusion (0 patients versus 27 patients, $P < 0.05$), and decreased hospital length of stay (2.2 days versus 8.4 days,

$P < 0.05$) with no compromise in overall long-term outcomes, including Harris Hip Scores and complications such as bedsores.[50] Authors of another study of external fixation in patients 75 years or older with ASA scores of 3 or 4 concluded that external fixators may be used in very high-risk patients with stable fracture patterns but should be used cautiously in elderly patients with unstable fracture patterns owing to prolonged union times, higher rates of varus collapse, and poorer functional outcomes.[51]

Arthroplasty is an uncommonly used option for the treatment of intertrochanteric fractures that is typically reserved for a specific subset of patients who are ambulatory and have associated signs of degenerative arthritis. Reconstruction with hip replacement prosthesis in intertrochanteric fractures can be complex because of the involvement of abductor tendon insertion and incompetent calcar, and therefore should typically be undertaken by surgeons familiar with revision arthroplasty techniques.[52] However, several authors have advocated the use of arthroplasty as a salvage procedure in addressing previously failed fixation of intertrochanteric fracture with good results.[53,54]

Outcomes

The goal of surgical fixation of intertrochanteric hip fractures is pain control, anatomic correction of fracture deformity, return of patients to function in society, and minimizing mortality in elderly patients. Studies have found that patients who sustain an intertrochanteric hip fracture lose some degree of preinjury functional capabilities, including the ability to walk independently, climb stairs, and perform activities of daily living. The most significant predictors of functional recovery after intertrochanteric hip fracture surgery include preinjury functional status (including the ability to walk outdoors) and age.[55] Even in patients who lived independently before injury, it is reported that only 50% to 59% will be able to return to independent living 1 year after surgery.[55]

Patients with unstable intertrochanteric fractures were shown to have worse functional scores at a 2-month follow-up; however, this difference between patients with unstable versus stable fractures had disappeared at 6 months.[56] When comparing specific implant designs and functional outcomes, researchers reporting results of a randomized trial in which proximal femoral nails and dynamic hip screws were compared found no difference at 1 year after surgery in any functional category.[57]

Despite optimization of perioperative medical care, prompt diagnosis, choice of an ideal implant, and swift surgical intervention, mortality after an intertrochanteric hip fracture is a definite risk. Hip fractures in elderly people are a sign of an overall decline in health status and an unavoidable harbinger of an already-deteriorating body system. However, hip fractures in general substantially increase the risk of death in elderly patients. A meta-analysis of prospective studies found relative hazard rates for mortality during the first 3 months after hip fracture to be a relative risk of 5.75 in women and of 7.95 in men.[58] One-year mortality rates have been reported to be as wide ranging as 12% to 37%.[59-61] According to Nationwide Inpatient Sample data from 2005, the in-hospital death rate after hip fracture was 2.8%.[9] Overall, mortality seems to be highest in men, nursing home residents, patients older than 90 years, patients treated nonsurgically, patients with significant cognitive impairment or comorbidities, and patients who are unable to ambulate independently.[62-64]

Summary

Intertrochanteric hip fractures in elderly people are a growing and significant health concern. Appropriate identification of associated medical comorbidities, medical and orthopaedic comanagement, and prompt surgical treatment may minimize the risks of complications, morbidity, and mortality while improving outcomes. The implant choice should be based on fracture pattern, cost, and the surgeon's familiarity, with the goal being to deliver patient appropriate care in a timely fashion.

Key Study Points

- Because of increased life expectancy, the number of elderly individuals alive, and the age-specific incidence of hip fractures, by 2050 there may be more than six million annual hip fractures worldwide.
- The cost for treating patients with hip fractures in the United States is approximately $10 billion per year. The use of multidisciplinary teams, which include primary care providers, geriatricians, internists, social workers, physiatrists, and care managers, can help to lower this cost by decreasing complications and hospital lengths of stay.
- Stable and unstable fracture patterns of intertrochanteric fractures in the Evans classification are differentiated by presence of posteromedial cortex apposition and lateral wall integrity.
- Outcome after intertrochanteric hip fracture depends on the patient's preinjury functional levels and medical comorbidities. One-year mortality rates after fracture are between 10% and 30%.

Annotated References

1. Court-Brown CM, Aitken SA, Forward D, et al: The epidemiology of fractures, in Bucholz RW, Court-Brown CM, Heckman JD, Tornetta P, eds: *Rockwood and Green's Fractures in Adults* ,ed 7. Philadelphia, PA, Lippincott, Williams and Wilkins, 2010, pp 95-113.

   The epidemiology of all fractures in the United States based on large retrospective registry study is described, and information on upper and lower extremity fracture prevalence in the United States is provided. Fractures are categorized by mechanism of injury with regard to high versus low energy, as well as demographics.

2. Fox KM, Magaziner J, Hebel JR, Kenzora JE, Kashner TM: Intertrochanteric versus femoral neck hip fractures: Differential characteristics, treatment, and sequelae. *J Gerontol A Biol Sci Med Sci* 1999;54(12):M635-M640.

3. Cooper C, Campion G, Melton LJ III: Hip fractures in the elderly: A world-wide projection. *Osteoporos Int* 1992;2(6):285-289.

4. Gullberg B, Johnell O, Kanis JA: World-wide projections for hip fracture. *Osteoporos Int* 1997;7(5):407-413.

5. Cummings SR, Rubin SM, Black D: The future of hip fractures in the United States. Numbers, costs, and potential effects of postmenopausal estrogen. *Clin Orthop Relat Res* 1990;252:163-166.

6. Kannus P, Parkkari J, Sievänen H, Heinonen A, Vuori I, Järvinen M: Epidemiology of hip fractures. *Bone* 1996;18(1suppl):57S-63S.

7. Löfman O, Berglund K, Larsson L, Toss G: Changes in hip fracture epidemiology: Redistribution between ages, genders and fracture types. *Osteoporos Int* 2002;13(1):18-25.

8. Lauritzen JB, Schwarz P, Lund B, McNair P, Transbøl I: Changing incidence and residual lifetime risk of common osteoporosis-related fractures. *Osteoporos Int* 1993;3(3):127-132.

9. Russo A, Owens PL, Stocks C: *Agency for Healthcare Research and Quality: Common Injuries That Result in Hospitalization, 2004* .Healthcare Cost and Utilization Project, 2016.

   The report, which features data from 2004, delineates expenditures by the United States healthcare system for hip fractures. It shows that the average length of stay was 6.3 days and the average per-day cost was $15,400.

10. Karagas MR, Lu-Yao GL, Barrett JA, Beach ML, Baron JA: Heterogeneity of hip fracture: Age, race, sex, and geographic patterns of femoral neck and trochanteric fractures among the US elderly. *Am J Epidemiol* 1996;143(7):677-682.

11. Keene GS, Parker MJ, Pryor GA: Mortality and morbidity after hip fractures. *BMJ* 1993;307(6914):1248-1250.

12. Riggs BL, Melton LJ III: The worldwide problem of osteoporosis: Insights afforded by epidemiology. *Bone* 1995;17(5suppl):505S-511S.

13. Leslie MP, Baumgaertner MR: Intertrochanteric hip fractures, in Browner BD, Jupiter JB, Krettek C, Anderson PA, eds: *Skeletal Trauma: Basic Science, Management, and Reconstruction,* ed 5. Philadelphia, PA, Elsevier Saunders, 2015, vol 2, pp 1683-1720.

14. Ettinger B, Black DM, Mitlak BH, et al; Multiple Outcomes of Raloxifene Evaluation (MORE) Investigators: Reduction of vertebral fracture risk in postmenopausal women with osteoporosis treated with raloxifene: Results from a 3-year randomized clinical trial. *JAMA* 1999;282(7):637-645.

15. Berg KM, Kunins HV, Jackson JL, et al: Association between alcohol consumption and both osteoporotic fracture and bone density. *Am J Med* 2008;121(5):406-418.

16. Van Staa TP, Leufkens HG, Abenhaim L, Zhang B, Cooper C: Use of oral corticosteroids and risk of fractures. *J Bone Miner Res* 2000;15(6):993-1000.

17. Kanis JA, Johnell O, Oden A, et al: Smoking and fracture risk: A meta-analysis. *Osteoporos Int* 2005;16(2):155-162.

18. Brauer CA, Coca-Perraillon M, Cutler DM, Rosen AB: Incidence and mortality of hip fractures in the United States. *JAMA* 2009;302(14):1573-1579.

19. Flikweert ER, Izaks GJ, Knobben BA, Stevens M, Wendt K: The development of a comprehensive multidisciplinary care pathway for patients with a hip fracture: Design and results of a clinical trial. *BMC Musculoskelet Disord* 2014;15:188.

   The authors developed a multidiscliplinary care pathway for patients age 60 years or older who had sustained a hip fracture between July 2009 and July 2011. They compared 256 consecutively seen patients in this pathway with 145 patient controls who underwent traditional care between January 2006 and January 2008. The multidisciplinary group demonstrated a considerable decrease in length of stay (7 versus 11 days; $P < 0.001$).

20. Khasraghi FA, Christmas C, Lee EJ, Mears SC, Wenz JF Sr: Effectiveness of a multidisciplinary team approach to hip fracture management. *J Surg Orthop Adv* 2005;14(1):27-31.

21. Swart E, Vasudeva E, Makhni EC, Macaulay W, Bozic KJ: Dedicated perioperative hip fracture comanagement programs are cost-effective in high-volume centers: An economic analysis. *Clin Orthop Relat Res* 2016;474(1):222-233.

   The article described the economic effect of implementing a co-management model of care for geriatric patients with hip fractures at hospitals with moderate volume. Using

7: Geriatrics

decision analysis techniques, the authors concluded that the co-management strategies could expedite preoperative evaluation, improve outcomes, and save money for hospital centers with a moderate to high volume of hip fractures.

22. Ricci WM, Della Rocca GJ, Combs C, Borrelli J: The medical and economic impact of preoperative cardiac testing in elderly patients with hip fractures. *Injury* 2007;38(suppl 3):S49-S52.

23. Zuckerman JD, Skovron ML, Koval KJ, Aharonoff G, Frankel VH: Postoperative complications and mortality associated with operative delay in older patients who have a fracture of the hip. *J Bone Joint Surg Am* 1995;77(10):1551-1556.

24. Ryan DJ, Yoshihara H, Yoneoka D, Egol KA, Zuckerman JD: Delay in hip fracture surgery: An analysis of patient-specific and hospital-specific risk factors. *J Orthop Trauma* 2015;29(8):343-348.

    The authors reviewed more than two million hip fractures by using the National Inpatient Sample database and found that surgery delay of 2 calendar days (odds ratio, 1.13) and 3 days (odds ratio, 1.33) was associated with higher mortality. Same-day or next-day surgery did not increase risk of in-house mortality or morbidity.

25. Ricci WM, Brandt A, McAndrew C, Gardner MJ: Factors affecting delay to surgery and length of stay for patients with hip fracture. *J Orthop Trauma* 2015;29(3):e109-e114.

    The authors identified 635 hip fractures and found that delay in surgery was secondary to day of admission (Thursday to Friday), ASA Physical Classification System score, and need for preoperative cardiac testing (delay, 3.2 days versus 1.7 if no cardiac tests). Length of stay was higher (9.4 versus 7.3 days) if cardiac testing was needed.

26. American Academy of Orthopaedic Surgeons: *Management of Hip Fractures in the Elderly: Evidence-Based Clinical Practice Guideline*. Rosemont, IL, American Academy of Orthopaedic Surgeons, 2014. http://www.aaos.org/research/guidelines/HipFxSummaryofRecommendations.pdf Accessed on Feb. 18, 2016.

    This document presents guidelines from the AAOS regarding management of hip fractures. Moderate recommendations were given to treatment of intertrochanteric hip fractures with either sliding hip screw or intramedullary nail devices. Strong recommendation was also given to use of multimodal analgesia, multidisciplinary teams, and intensive physical therapy programs postoperatively.

27. Boddaert J, Cohen-Bittan J, Khiami F, et al: Postoperative admission to a dedicated geriatric unit decreases mortality in elderly patients with hip fracture. *PLoS One* 2014;9(1):e83795.

    The authors compared hip fractures in patients admitted to a geriatric service versus those admitted to an orthopaedic service. Even after accounting for higher comorbidities, patients on the geriatric service had a lower readmission risk (14% versus 29%) and a lower risk ratio of death (15% versus 24%), with a decrease in number of patients who never walked again (6% versus 22%) over 6 months' follow up.

28. Koval KJ, Oh CK, Egol KA: Does a traction-internal rotation radiograph help to better evaluate fractures of the proximal femur? *Bull NYU Hosp Jt Dis* 2008;66(2):102-106.

29. Gill SK, Smith J, Fox R, Chesser TJ: Investigation of occult hip fractures: The use of CT and MRI. *ScientificWorldJournal* 2013;2013:830319.

    Ninety-two patients included in this study presented to the hospital with clinical suspicion of hip fracture but radiologist review of plain radiographs as negative. Of the 92 patients in the study, 61 were referred for CT scan and 31 for MRI. Of the 34 patients with actual fracture, CT scan picked up fracture in 38% and MRI picked up fracture in 36%. The authors conclude that CT scan may be comparable with MRI in detecting occult hip fractures.

30. Lubovsky O, Liebergall M, Mattan Y, Weil Y, Mosheiff R: Early diagnosis of occult hip fractures MRI versus CT scan (published online ahead of print April 7, 2005). *Injury* 2005;36(6):788-792.

31. Kyle RF, Gustilo RB, Premer RF: Analysis of six hundred and twenty-two intertrochanteric hip fractures. *J Bone Joint Surg Am* 1979;61(2):216-221.

32. Evans EM: Trochanteric fractures; a review of 110 cases treated by nail-plate fixation. *J Bone Joint Surg Br* 1951;33B(2):192-204.

33. Tawari AA, Kempegowda H, Suk M, Horwitz DS: What makes an intertrochanteric fracture unstable in 2015? Does the lateral wall play a role in the decision matrix? *J Orthop Trauma* 2015;29(suppl 4):S4-S9 .

    The authors reviewed the importance of lateral wall integrity in determination of stable versus unstable fracture patterns in intertrochanteric hip fractures. The decision to treat these types of fractures with an intramedullary device is becoming more popular in current orthopaedic literature.

34. Jin W-J, Dai L-Y, Cui Y-M, Zhou Q, Jiang L-S, Lu H: Reliability of classification systems for intertrochanteric fractures of the proximal femur in experienced orthopaedic surgeons. *Injury* 2005;36(7):858-861.

35. Egol KA, Marcano AI, Lewis L, Tejwani NC, McLaurin TM, Davidovitch RI: Can the use of an evidence-based algorithm for the treatment of intertrochanteric fractures of the hip maintain quality at a reduced cost? *Bone Joint J* 2014;96-B(9):1192-1197.

    The study authors implemented a protocol for treating every intertrochanteric fracture with a given fracture pattern by using the exact same implant design. Depending on fracture stability and extent, either a sliding hip screw, a short cephalomedullary nail, or a long cephalomedullary nail was used. The authors found a significant cost savings and trend toward fewer complications by using the new study protocol at their institution.

36. Lyon LJ, Nevins MA: Nontreatment of hip fractures in senile patients. *JAMA* 1977;238(11):1175-1176.

37. Jain R, Basinski A, Kreder HJ: Nonoperative treatment of hip fractures. *Int Orthop* 2003;27(1):11-17.

38. Cheng T, Zhang G, Zhang X: Review: Minimally invasive versus conventional dynamic hip screw fixation in elderly patients with intertrochanteric fractures: a systematic review and meta-analysis. *Surg Innov* 2011;18(2):99-105.

    Several randomized controlled trials or quasirandomized controlled trials were included in an analysis of the ability of a minimally invasive technique to insert dynamic hip screw fixation to minimize complications when compared with traditional dynamic hip screw techniques. The authors concluded the minimally invasive technique resulted in less blood loss, shorter hospital length of stay, decreased pain, faster fracture healing, and better hip function.

39. Wong T-C, Chiu Y, Tsang W-L, Leung W-Y, Yeung S-H: A double-blind, prospective, randomised, controlled clinical trial of minimally invasive dynamic hip screw fixation of intertrochanteric fractures. *Injury* 2009;40(4):422-427.

40. Ho M, Garau G, Walley G, et al: Minimally invasive dynamic hip screw for fixation of hip fractures. *Int Orthop* 2009;33(2):555-560.

41. Cheng T, Zhang G-Y, Liu T, Zhang X-L: A meta-analysis of percutaneous compression plate versus sliding hip screw for the management of intertrochanteric fractures of the hip. *J Trauma Acute Care Surg* 2012;72(5):1435-1443.

    The authors analyzed 14 studies to evaluate the efficacy of the percutaneous compression plate in fixing intertrochanteric fractures and to compare it with that of the sliding hip screw. The meta-analysis shows a decrease in surgical time, blood loss, and transfusion rates. There were no differences found in hospital length of stay, mortality, revision surgery rates, or implant-specific complications. The authors stated that greater evidence is required before widespread use of minimally invasive percutaneous plate options can be advocated.

42. Anglen JO, Weinstein JN; American Board of Orthopaedic Surgery Research Committee: Nail or plate fixation of intertrochanteric hip fractures: Changing pattern of practice. A review of the American Board of Orthopaedic Surgery Database. *J Bone Joint Surg Am* 2008;90(4):700-707.

43. Boone C, Carlberg KN, Koueiter DM, et al: Short versus long intramedullary nails for treatment of intertrochanteric femur fractures (OTA 31-A1 and A2). *J Orthop Trauma* 2014;28(5):e96-e100.

    The authors of this retrospective study evaluated 194 patients with AO/OTA classification 31-A1– or 31-A2–type intertrochanteric hip fractures. They compared patients treated with short and with long intramedullary nails and found significantly shorter surgical times, estimated blood loss, and transfusion rates in the group treated with short nails. One patient in the long-nail group sustained a periprosthetic fracture.

44. Bohl DD, Basques BA, Golinvaux NS, Miller CP, Baumgaertner MR, Grauer JN: Extramedullary compared with intramedullary implants for intertrochanteric hip fractures: Thirty-day outcomes of 4432 procedures from the ACS NSQIP database. *J Bone Joint Surg Am* 2014;96(22):1871-1877.

    Using the American College of Surgeons National Surgical Quality Improvement Program database, the authors reviewed the cases of 4,432 patients who underwent fixation for intertrochanteric hip fractures. The mean postoperative length of stay was shorter (5.4 versus 6.5 days) with intramedullary implants, whereas no difference in surgical times, rates of readmission, or risks of adverse events were identified.

45. Baumgaertner MR, Curtin SL, Lindskog DM, Keggi JM: The value of the tip-apex distance in predicting failure of fixation of peritrochanteric fractures of the hip. *J Bone Joint Surg Am* 1995;77(7):1058-1064.

46. De Bruijn K, den Hartog D, Tuinebreijer W, Roukema G: Reliability of predictors for screw cutout in intertrochanteric hip fractures. *J Bone Joint Surg Am* 2012;94(14):1266-1272.

    A retrospective review of all patients who underwent treatment with either a gamma nail or a sliding hip screw showed that screw cutout was higher with a higher tip-to-apex distance, unstable hip fracture (31-A3 versus 31-A1), and poor fracture reduction. Central-inferior or anterior-inferior positions of the screw were significantly protective against cutout.

47. Kane P, Vopat B, Heard W, et al: Is tip apex distance as important as we think? A biomechanical study examining optimal lag screw placement [published correction appears in Clin Orthop Relat Res 2014;472(8):2499]. *Clin Orthop Relat Res* 2014;472(8):2492-2498.

    In a biomechanical study, the authors found that inferior position of the screw through a cephalomedullary nail was found to be as biomechanically stable as center-center position, even when the tip-to-apex distance was more than 25 mm.

48. Ali AM, Abdelkhalek M, El-Ganiney A: External fixation of intertrochanteric fractures in elderly high-risk patients. *Acta Orthop Belg* 2009;75(6):748-753.

49. Kazakos K, Lyras DN, Verettas D, Galanis V, Psillakis I, Xarchas K: External fixation of intertrochanteric fractures in elderly high-risk patients. *Acta Orthop Belg* 2007;73(1):44-48.

50. Kazemian GH, Manafi AR, Najafi F, Najafi MA: Treatment of intertrochanteric fractures in elderly highrisk patients: Dynamic hip screw vs. external fixation. *Injury* 2014;45(3):568-572.

    A prospective comparison of hip screw and external fixation treatments was done for 60 elderly high-risk patients.

The external fixation group demonstrated shorter surgical time (15 minutes versus 73 minutes), lower risk of blood transfusion (0 versus 27 patients), and significantly shorter length of stay (2.2 versus 8.4 days). The authors thought that the external fixation was well tolerated by their patients, with no difference in quality of reduction, screw cutout, or bed sores. Nine patients in the external fixation group had pin-site infections that were treated with oral antibiotics. The authors recommended this low-cost alternative to sliding hip screw fixation, with its minimal complication rate and no difference in outcomes for high-risk elderly patients.

51. Petsatodis G, Maliogas G, Karikis J, et al: External fixation for stable and unstable intertrochanteric fractures in patients older than 75 years of age: A prospective comparative study. *J Orthop Trauma* 2011;25(4):218-223.

One hundred patients with a mean age of 82.3 years underwent external fixation for treatment of their intertrochanteric hip fractures. Two groups were then compared within this cohort: those with stable fracture patterns and those with unstable fracture patterns according to the AO/OTA classification system. The unstable group saw unfavorable results of prolonged union times, increased incidence of varus position at the fracture site, and inferior functional outcomes.

52. Kim S-Y, Kim Y-G, Hwang J-K: Cementless calcar-replacement hemiarthroplasty compared with intramedullary fixation of unstable intertrochanteric fractures. A prospective, randomized study. *J Bone Joint Surg Am* 2005;87(10):2186-2192.

53. Mortazavi SM, R Greenky M, Bican O, Kane P, Parvizi J, Hozack WJ: Total hip arthroplasty after prior surgical treatment of hip fracture: Is it always challenging? *J Arthroplasty* 2012;27(1):31-36.

When conversion of failed fixation was compared with arthroplasty for hip fractures, there was higher blood loss and longer surgical time for failed intertrochanteric fractures than with femoral neck fractures. Although conversion total hip arthroplasty is a technically challenging procedure, it is safe and yields relatively few orthopaedic complications.

54. D'Arrigo C, Perugia D, Carcangiu A, Monaco E, Speranza A, Ferretti A: Hip arthroplasty for failed treatment of proximal femoral fractures. *Int Orthop* 2010;34(7):939-942.

Of 19 patients treated with hip arthroplasty for failed intertrochanteric fracture, 14 required modular implants with long stems. The authors found a statistically significant improvement when comparing preoperative and postoperative conditions ($P < 0.05$). The authors concluded that total hip arthroplasty is a satisfactory salvage procedure after failed treatment of an intertrochanteric fracture in elderly patients, with few serious orthopaedic complications and acceptable clinical outcomes.

55. Córcoles-Jiménez MP, Villada-Munera A, Del Egido-Fernández MÁ, et al: Recovery of activities of daily living among older people one year after hip fracture. *Clin Nurs Res* 2015;24(6):604-623.

The authors followed a cohort of patients who were fully functional in their activities of daily living (ADLs) and who were without cognitive impairment before hip fracture injury. The authors found a decrease in ADL Barthel Index score, from 90.02 preinjury to 78.09 postinjury. Before injury, 82% walked without assistive devices; after injury, only 65% walked without assistive devices. Older patients and those in nursing homes were at risk of experiencing poorer recovery in ADLs.

56. Cornwall R, Gilbert MS, Koval KJ, Strauss E, Siu AL: Functional outcomes and mortality vary among different types of hip fractures: A function of patient characteristics. *Clin Orthop Relat Res* 2004;425:64-71.

57. Guerra MT, Pasqualin S, Souza MP, Lenz R: Functional recovery of elderly patients with surgically-treated intertrochanteric fractures: Preliminary results of a randomised trial comparing the dynamic hip screw and proximal femoral nail techniques. *Injury* 2014;45(suppl 5):S26-S31.

In a prospective trial in which they compared nailing with plating for stable intertrochanteric hip fractures, the authors found significant loss of function in the first 6 months in the plate group. However, they found no difference in functional scores at 1 year. The mortality rates and complications rates were similar.

58. Haentjens P, Magaziner J, Colón-Emeric CS, et al: Meta-analysis: Excess mortality after hip fracture among older women and men. *Ann Intern Med* 2010;152(6):380-390.

The authors reviewed all articles published from 1957 to 2009 about mortality after hip fracture among older men and women. They identified and selected 37 prospective cohort studies. They found that older adults (older than 50 years) had a fivefold to eightfold increased risk of experiencing all-cause mortality during the first 3 months after hip fracture. Excess annual mortality persisted over time for both women and men, but at any given age, excess annual mortality after hip fracture was higher in men than in women.

59. Wolinsky FD, Fitzgerald JF, Stump TE: The effect of hip fracture on mortality, hospitalization, and functional status: A prospective study. *Am J Public Health* 1997;87(3):398-403.

60. Panula J, Pihlajamäki H, Mattila VM, et al: Mortality and cause of death in hip fracture patients aged 65 or older: A population-based study. *BMC Musculoskelet Disord* 2011;12:105.

This Finnish study of 428 patients with a 3.7-year mean follow-up showed that 1-year postoperative mortality was 27.3% and mortality after hip fracture at the end of the follow-up was 79.0%. During the follow-up, age-adjusted mortality after hip fracture surgery was higher in men than in women. All-cause age- and sex-standardized mortality after hip fracture was threefold higher than that of the general population and included every cause-of-death category.

61. LeBlanc ES, Hillier TA, Pedula KL, et al: Hip fracture and increased short-term but not long-term mortality in healthy older women. *Arch Intern Med* 2011;171(20):1831-1837.

This study aimed to examine the long-term rather than short-term changes in mortality after hip fracture in a cohort of healthy older women. It involved 960 women 80 years or older who were available for follow up for 10 years. After a 1-year period immediately after the fracture in which patients had a twofold increase in mortality compared with healthy age-matched controls, the patients in the older cohort with hip fractures had equal long-term mortality rates.

62. Frost SA, Nguyen ND, Black DA, Eisman JA, Nguyen TV: Risk factors for in-hospital post-hip fracture mortality. *Bone* 2011;49(3):553-558.

The authors evaluated 1,504 patients admitted to the hospital with hip fractures in Australia between 1997 and 2007 for risk factors for hospital mortality. Relative risk ratios were 1.91 for every 10-year increase in age, 2.13 for men compared with women, 3.02 for patients with congestive heart failure, and 4.75 for those with liver disease. The study went on to provide a nomogram model for predicting risk of mortality in patients after hip fracture based on key baseline patient data.

63. Alzahrani K, Gandhi R, Davis A, Mahomed N: In-hospital mortality following hip fracture care in southern Ontario. *Can J Surg* 2010;53(5):294-298.

The authors reviewed the cases of 2,178 patients with hip fracture from 17 hospitals in Canada and found a 5.0% in-hospital mortality rate. An increased risk of death was present in patients transferred to the hospital with hip fracture from a dependent-living facility compared with patients who were previously living unassisted.

64. Mariconda M, Costa GG, Cerbasi S, et al: The determinants of mortality and morbidity during the year following fracture of the hip: A prospective study. *Bone Joint J* 2015;97-B(3):383-390.

The authors analyzed data regarding 568 patients with hip fractures who underwent surgery and found a mortality rate of 18.8% at 1 year; this rate was predicted by both general complications and preoperative morbidities. Surgical delay was the main predictor of length of hospital stay and was directly related to in-hospital and 4-month complication rates.

Chapter 51

Management of Osteoporotic Fractures and Atypical Fractures

David A. Volgas, MD   Shaun Fay Steeby, MD

Abstract

Osteoporosis is a growing problem in the aging population. Conventional methods for fixation of good-quality bone have been associated with high failure rates in osteoporotic bone. Techniques for management of osteoporotic fractures are being developed. Locked plating, bone augmentation, and improved medical management have had good results, but additional techniques and strategic methods are necessary to further improve outcomes in these patients. Atypical fractures, particularly those involving the femoral shaft, are associated with long-term disphosphonate use.

Keywords: osteoporosis; fragility fracture; atypical fracture; locked plating

Introduction

The management of fractures in elderly patients with osteoporosis is much more challenging than a similar fracture in an elderly patient with good bone quality. In addition, medical comorbidities contribute substantially to the mortality and morbidity of elderly patients before and after surgery. Conventional techniques for fixation of fractures in osteoporotic bone have demonstrated high failure rates. Postdischarge orders for physical therapy are frequently omitted from discharge plans, leading to higher complication rates.[1] Complicating matters further, many elderly patients have undergone total joint arthroplasty or prior fracture fixation, which may compromise the treatment of the new fracture.

The treatment of osteoporotic fractures and their sequelae has been the subject of much interest among orthopaedic surgeons during the past 5 years, and there have been several recent advances in the management of these difficult conditions.

Fragility Fracture Center

There has been a general acceptance by orthopaedic surgeons that early surgical stabilization of hip fractures in the elderly along with focused medical comanagement reduces length of hospital stay and mortality in this population.[2,3] The concept of a fragility fracture center that uses a multidisciplinary approach to fracture care in the elderly continues to gain acceptance. More than simple medical comanagement of patients, this multidisciplinary approach involves education and buy-in from the entire team of physicians involved in the care of elderly patients, including anesthesia providers, primary care physicians, and cardiologists. The preoperative workup no longer focuses on all medical comorbidities, but rather on the specific medical problems that might be addressed acutely to favorably influence perioperative outcomes.[4] Routine echocardiography is no longer recommended. Additionally, there is emphasis on education of the patient and family about osteoporosis and communication with the discharge facility about such factors as weight-bearing status and hip precautions. Finally, arranging follow-up not only for the surgical procedure but for the treatment of osteoporosis is important.[5] This team approach does involve additional expense to the hospital, but has been shown to be cost effective.[2,6]

Initiation of medical therapy for osteoporosis in the immediate postoperative period has not been shown to impede bone healing and therefore is becoming more common. The Centers for Medicare and Medicaid Services

Neither of the following authors nor any immediate family member has received anything of value from or has stock or stock options held in a commercial company or institution related directly or indirectly to the subject of this chapter: Dr. Volgas and Dr. Steeby.

has made availability of dual-energy x-ray absorptiometry or initiation of medical therapy one of its menu items for the 2015 Physician Quality Reporting Systems program.[7]

Locked Plating

Locked plating has been a treatment option for more than 15 years. Although initially believed to be primarily useful in the treatment of periarticular fractures, its use in patients with osteoporosis has become widespread. Although failure rates associated with locked plating are lower than with nonlocked plating, multiple studies have demonstrated failure rates that are higher than originally expected.[8-10] Therefore, techniques are being studied to improve fixation with locked plates.

Both biomechanical and clinical studies have been performed to better elucidate optimum screw type, placement, and density. Bone quality was found to be a more reliable predictor of construct failure than working length (the length between the two screws closest to the fracture).[11]

In an osteoporotic synthetic bone model, four screws on each side of the fracture rather than three increased stiffness.[12] When three of these screws were bicortical locking screws, torsional stiffness was also increased by 24%. Locked screws placed between the fracture and nonlocked screws help prevent loosening of the nonlocked screws. Compared with an all-locked plate, hybrid plating (combination of locked and nonlocked screws) offers higher torsional strength.[13]

It is now recognized that fractures that cannot be anatomically reduced must have some, but not too much, strain.[14] An explanation for higher-than-expected failure rates in locked plate constructs is thought to be excessive construct rigidity, which prevents healing of comminuted bone. Far cortical locking constructs attempt to resolve this dilemma by allowing controlled motion at the near cortex, while maintaining rigid fixation in the far cortex. Early biomechanical and animal studies indicate promise for this technology, but it is not yet proven in clinical use.[15,16]

Bone Augmentation

Poor bone quality can contribute to loss of fixation with locked and nonlocked screws. In an attempt to gain better fixation in osteoporotic fractures, many techniques have been used to augment fixation in patients with osteoporosis.

Polymethyl methacrylate (PMMA) has been used for many years to augment fixation in osteoporotic bone. PMMA can be injected through the implant itself or through a bone window. There does not appear to be a significant difference in intraosseous pressure between rapid or slow injection of PMMA into femoral heads.[17] PMMA was noted to have a significantly higher number of load cycles to failure than nonaugmented constructs in a bench study proximal tibial fracture model.[18] Another bench study showed increased stability in a distal femoral model using locked plates.[19] Similarly, in the spine, augmentation with PMMA seems to lessen the incidence of lucency around pedicle screws.[20]

Potential complications can include the thermal effect of the cement causing cellular damage to surrounding tissues including bone and soft tissues such as nerves. Implanting a nonabsorbable material such as cement can impair fracture healing and may lead to difficulty removing the material in the presence of infection.

Augmentation with calcium phosphate products has been studied in femoral neck fractures, tibial plateau fractures, and fractures of the distal radius. A meta-analysis of the use of bone graft substitutes in tibial plateau fractures demonstrated that radiographic subsidence of the reduced joint fragment occurred in 8.6% of patients treated with allograft, demineralized bone matrix, or xenograft, but only 3.7% of patients in the group treated with calcium phosphate.[21]

Injectable calcium phosphate did not reduce the rate of loss of reduction in a randomized study of an osteoporotic hip fracture group treated with cannulated screws.[22] The authors of a 2011 study found that calcium phosphate augmentation of locked volar plating of the distal radius in patients with osteoporosis offered no improvement at any time over locked plating alone.[23]

The use of allograft struts for periprosthetic fractures is a common practice, but there are few level I-II studies examining the optimum construct for these fractures.[24] There is retrospective evidence of the superiority of allograft augmentation of these fractures.[25]

Atypical Femoral Fractures

Although widely used, the diphosphonate class of antiresorptive agents are associated with osteonecrosis of the jaw and atypical fractures. First recognized in 2005, atypical fractures and osteonecrosis of the jaw blunted some of the enthusiasm for diphosphonate use in the second half of the decade. Since 2010, atypical fractures have been more completely characterized by multiple large-database studies. A report summarizing analysis of the FDA Adverse Event Reporting System emphasized the value of diphosphonates in reducing the overall risk of fracture by 100-fold compared to the risk of atypical fractures and noted that diphosphonate use has declined secondary

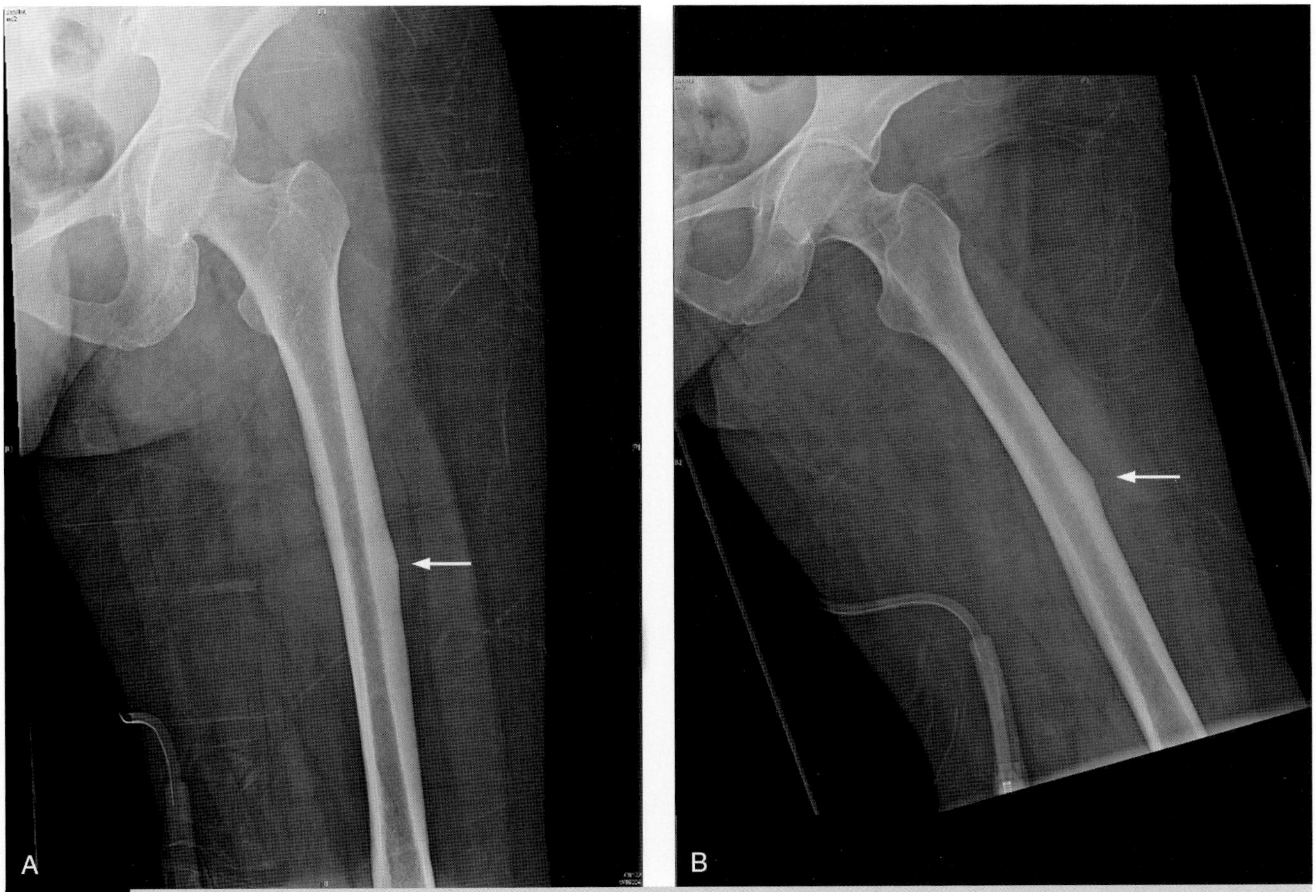

Figure 1 AP (**A**) and lateral (**B**) radiographs of an incomplete atypical femur fracture. Notice the characteristic beaking of the lateral cortex (arrow).

to concerns about atypical fractures.[26] In another large series, the age-adjusted rate of atypical fractures for patients treated for less than 2 years with diphosphonates was 1.7 per 100,000 patients treated, but increased to 113 per 100,000 patients treated for 8 to 10 years.[27] All studies assert that the risk of atypical fracture is orders of magnitude less than the risk of major fracture without the use of diphosphonates.

Atypical femoral fractures usually involve the femoral diaphysis between the lesser trochanter and supracondylar flare and are transverse or with a short, oblique component. They may be complete or incomplete and may be associated with preexisting thigh pain. There is often a thickened lateral cortex or there may be beaking of the lateral femoral cortex (**Figure 1**). The most reliable radiographic signs of an atypical fracture are focal lateral cortical thickening and a transverse fracture pattern.[28]

The population at risk for atypical fracture has also been clearly described. According to a 2014 study, there is an association of atypical fractures in patients with a varus hip.[29] Asian and Hispanic patients have a higher incidence of atypical fractures than other groups. Furthermore, patients with atypical fractures tend to be younger than patients with subtrochanteric femur fractures without diphosphonate use and the incidence of males with atypical fractures is lower than in patients not using diphosphonates long term.[30] There is no clear evidence that teriparatide is associated with atypical fractures.

Nonsurgical management of atypical fractures is generally not recommended because most incomplete fractures will progress to complete fracture.[31] Patients with surgically treated fractures have a longer mean time to union[32] and a higher rate of implant failure than patients who did not undergo diphosphonate therapy.[33]

Current recommendations by the FDA include cessation of therapy with diphosphonates for any patient who has a low-energy femur fracture and consideration of cessation of therapy after 5 years in patients who would be considered low risk for fragility fracture.[34] There is no consensus on how long a drug holiday should be.

Summary

Osteoporosis is prevalent in the aging population, which continues to increase as the baby boomer generation ages. Recent investigations have begun to define better methods to deal with fractures and to define the role of the orthopaedic surgeon in the overall management of patients with fragility fractures.

Key Study Points

- Treatment algorithms continue to evolve for patients with fragility fractures.
- A dedicated fragility fracture comanagement model appears to have substantial benefit for patients with fragility fractures.
- Atypical fractures are associated with prolonged diphosphonate use, and these fractures are associated with a higher rate of complications than fractures not associated with diphosphonate use.

Annotated References

1. Polnaszek B, Mirr J, Roiland R, Gilmore-Bykovskyi A, Hovanes M, Kind A: Omission of physical therapy recommendations for high-risk patients transitioning from the hospital to subacute care facilities. *Arch Phys Med Rehabil* 2015;96(11):1966-72.e3.

   This retrospective cohort study examined the frequency that physical therapy recommendations are included in discharge documentation provided to secondary care facilities, such as skilled nursing facilities. In 54% of patients who had specific therapy precautions, these precautions were omitted from the paperwork they were discharged with. A focus on improved communication between the hospital care team and the accepting facility to limit potential injury is recommended. Level of evidence: III.

2. Kates SL, Blake D, Bingham KW, Kates OS, Mendelson DA, Friedman SM: Comparison of an organized geriatric fracture program to United States government data. *Geriatr Orthop Surg Rehabil* 2010;1(1):15-21.

   This retrospective cohort followed 776 patients over a 50-month period to describe the financial effects of an organized hospital protocol for the care of patients older than 65 years admitted to the hospital with hip fractures. They demonstrated an improvement in both cost and quality of care including an average savings of $18,000 per patient and an average hospital stay 1.5 days shorter than the national average. Level of evidence: III.

3. Schnell S, Friedman SM, Mendelson DA, Bingham KW, Kates SL: The 1-year mortality of patients treated in a hip fracture program for elders. *Geriatr Orthop Surg Rehabil* 2010;1(1):6-14.

   The authors present a retrospective study of 758 patients treated in a comanaged fragility fracture program. One-year mortality was 21%. Age, male sex, Parker mobility score, activities of daily living dependence, and Charlson Comorbidity Index greater than 3 were predictive of worse outcomes. Level of evidence: III.

4. Marsland D, Colvin PL, Mears SC, Kates SL: How to optimize patients for geriatric fracture surgery. *Osteoporos Int* 2010;21(suppl 4):S535-S546.

   This review article discusses the value of a multidisciplinary approach to the geriatric patient. Level of evidence: V.

5. Gardner MJ, Brophy RH, Demetrakopoulos D, et al: Interventions to improve osteoporosis treatment following hip fracture. A prospective, randomized trial. *J Bone Joint Surg Am* 2005;87(1):3-7.

6. Kates SL: Lean business model and implementation of a geriatric fracture center. *Clin Geriatr Med* 2014;30(2):191-205.

   This article outlines a model for the business aspects of care delivery to patients with hip fractures and outlines potential methods for implementing a hip fracture protocol in an effort to assist both surgeons and hospitalists in improving quality of patient care and cost of care. Level of evidence: V.

7. Physician QR: (PQRS): What's new for 2014. April 24 2014. Available at: http://www.cms.gov/Medicare/Quality-Initiatives-Patient-Assessment-Instruments/PQRS. Accessed February 24, 2016.

   This document compiled by the Centers for Medicare and Medicaid Services outlines recommendations for standards of care in patients and what milestones in care physicians are expected to meet.

8. Costa ML, Achten J, Parsons NR, et al; DRAFFT Study Group: Percutaneous fixation with Kirschner wires versus volar locking plate fixation in adults with dorsally displaced fracture of distal radius: Randomized controlled trial. *BMJ* 2014;349:g4807. http://www.ncbi.nlm.nih.gov/pmc/articles/PMC4122170/. Accessed March 22, 2015.

   The authors present a randomized, blinded assessor study of 461 patients treated with closed reduction, percutaneous fixation of distal radius fractures versus open reduction and internal fixation with volar locking plate. This study found no clinically significant difference at 3-, 6-, or 12-month follow-up using the Patient Related Wrist Evaluation. Level of evidence: I.

9. Henderson CE, Lujan TJ, Kuhl LL, Bottlang M, Fitzpatrick DC, Marsh JL: 2010 mid-America Orthopaedic Association Physician in Training Award: Healing complications are common after locked plating for distal femur fractures. *Clin Orthop Relat Res* 2011;469(6):1757-1765.

   A retrospective study of 82 patients treated with locked plating for distal femur fractures is presented. A 20% nonunion rate was associated with the use of stainless steel plates, and almost all of the plate holes near the fracture site were filled, suggesting that too much rigidity inhibits fracture healing. Level of evidence: III.

10. Hou Z, Bowen TR, Irgit K, et al: Locked plating of periprosthetic femur fractures above total knee arthroplasty. *J Orthop Trauma* 2012;26(7):427-432.

    Fifty-two patients were treated with locked plating or retrograde intramedullary nail fixation and studied retrospectively. No clinically significant differences between groups were identified, though both groups had a high complication rate. Level of evidence: III.

11. Pletka JD, Marsland D, Belkoff SM, Mears SC, Kates SL: Biomechanical comparison of 2 different locking plate fixation methods in vancouver b1 periprosthetic femur fractures. *Geriatr Orthop Surg Rehabil* 2011;2(2):51-55.

    A biomechanical study compared a long plate construct with a short plate construct for fixation of a transverse periprosthetic fracture. No difference was identified. Level of evidence: III.

12. Freeman AL, Tornetta P III, Schmidt A, Bechtold J, Ricci W, Fleming M: How much do locked screws add to the fixation of "hybrid" plate constructs in osteoporotic bone? *J Orthop Trauma* 2010;24(3):163-169.

    A biomechanical study compared various configurations of hybrid and nonlocked constructs in an osteoporotic model. At least three bicortical screws on each side of the fracture are required to increase torsional stability. Placing locked screws between the fracture and the nonlocked screws may improve the fatigue life of the construct by protecting the nonlocked screws from loosening. Level of evidence: V.

13. Doornink J, Fitzpatrick DC, Boldhaus S, Madey SM, Bottlang M: Effects of hybrid plating with locked and nonlocked screws on the strength of locked plating constructs in the osteoporotic diaphysis. *J Trauma* 2010;69(2):411-417.

    A biomechanical study compared two constructs, one with three locked screws on both sides of a fracture and the other with two nonlocked and one locked screw on each side of the fracture. The hybrid construct demonstrated higher torsional strength and similar bending strength with slightly lower axial strength. Level of evidence: V.

14. Perren SM: Evolution of the internal fixation of long bone fractures. The scientific basis of biological internal fixation: Choosing a new balance between stability and biology. *J Bone Joint Surg Br* 2002;84(8):1093-1110http://www.ncbi.nlm.nih.gov/pubmed/12463652 Accessed April 29, 2015.

15. Bottlang M, Lesser M, Koerber J, et al: Far cortical locking can improve healing of fractures stabilized with locking plates. *J Bone Joint Surg Am* 2010;92(7):1652-1660.

    This study compares conventional locked plating for an osteotomized tibial defect with far cortical locking using a sheep model. The far cortical locking models were designed to provide lower stiffness permitting parallel gap motion. Far cortical locking specimens had 36% greater callous volume and 54% greater torsional strength than their conventional locked plating counterparts. Level of evidence: V.

16. Bottlang M, Doornink J, Fitzpatrick DC, Madey SM: Far cortical locking can reduce stiffness of locked plating constructs while retaining construct strength. *J Bone Joint Surg Am* 2009;91(8):1985-1994.

    A biomechanical study compared locked plating to far cortical locking in a diaphyseal fracture gap model. Far cortical locking constructs were stronger in torsion and bending, while allowing nearly symmetric closure of the fracture, compared to the locking construct which demonstrated less motion at the near cortex. Level of evidence: V.

17. Blankstein M, Widmer D, Götzen M, et al: Assessment of intraosseous femoral head pressures during cement augmentation of the perforated proximal femur nail antirotation blade. *J Orthop Trauma* 2014;28(7):398-402.

    The effects of cement augmentation technique in osteoporotic bone for pertrochanteric fractures were evaluated in a cadaver study. The difference between rapid or slow injection of PMMA into a cadaver femur in which a basicervical osteotomy had been performed and was then instrumented with the PFNA blade was investigated. Pressures were similar between rapid and slow injection and returned to baseline in both groups within 30 seconds. Level of evidence: V.

18. Goetzen M, Nicolino T, Hofmann-Fliri L, Blauth M, Windolf M: Metaphyseal screw augmentation of the LISS-PLT plate with polymethylmethacrylate improves angular stability in osteoporotic proximal third tibial fractures: A biomechanical study in human cadaveric tibiae. *J Orthop Trauma* 2014;28(5):294-299.

    A cadaver study compared axial load strength of locked screws across an extra-articular proximal tibia fracture with or without cement augmentation of the screws. Cement augmentation with 1 mL PMMA significantly reduced screw migration and varus displacement. Level of evidence: V.

19. Wähnert D, Lange JH, Schulze M, Gehweiler D, Kösters C, Raschke MJ: A laboratory investigation to assess the influence of cement augmentation of screw and plate fixation in a simulation of distal femoral fracture of osteoporotic and non-osteoporotic bone. *Bone Joint J* 2013;95-B(10):1406-1409.

    Cement augmentation of locked screws in osteoporotic versus nonosteoporotic bone was assessed in a cadaver study. The authors found that cement augmentation significantly reduces screw cutout distance in patients with osteoporosis. The same findings were not found to be true in patients with normal bone quality. Level of evidence: V.

20. Sawakami K, Yamazaki A, Ishikawa S, Ito T, Watanabe K, Endo N: Polymethylmethacrylate augmentation of pedicle screws increases the initial fixation in osteoporotic spine patients. *J Spinal Disord Tech* 2012;25(2):E28-E35.

A retrospective study of patients with posterior spinal fusion treated with or without cement augmentation was performed. The augmented group had higher fusion rates and lower rates of loss of deformity correction. In addition, patients experienced some relief of back pain. Level of evidence: III.

21. Goff T, Kanakaris NK, Giannoudis PV: Use of bone graft substitutes in the management of tibial plateau fractures. *Injury* 2013;44(suppl 1):S86-S94.

A literature review was performed of more than 19 studies and 672 patients treated for tibial plateau fractures and the use of several different types of bone graft substitute. There is a lack of sufficient level I evidence for the use of bone graft substitutes, but there is sufficient level II and III evidence to support its use in the treatment of depressed tibial plateau fractures. Level of evidence: III.

22. Mattsson P, Larsson S: Calcium phosphate cement for augmentation did not improve results after internal fixation of displaced femoral neck fractures: A randomized study of 118 patients. *Acta Orthop* 2006;77(2):251-256.

23. Kim JK, Koh YD, Kook SH: Effect of calcium phosphate bone cement augmentation on volar plate fixation of unstable distal radial fractures in the elderly. *J Bone Joint Surg Am* 2011;93(7):609-614.

This randomized controlled trial compared volar locked plating alone with volar locked plating augmented with the injection of calcium phosphate bone cement. There were no significant differences observed between the two groups radiographically immediately postoperatively or 1 year after surgery. Level of evidence: I.

24. Misur PN, Duncan CP, Masri BA: The treatment of periprosthetic femoral fractures after total hip arthroplasty: A critical analysis review. *JBJS Reviews* 2014;2(8):e3.

A review article described the current state of treatment of periprosthetic fractures after total hip arthroplasty. Further high-level studies are needed. Level of evidence: III.

25. Khashan M, Amar E, Drexler M, Chechik O, Cohen Z, Steinberg EL: Superior outcome of strut allograft-augmented plate fixation for the treatment of periprosthetic fractures around a stable femoral stem. *Injury* 2013;44(11):1556-1560.

Twenty-one patients treated with or without a strut graft for periprosthetic fractures around a total hip arthroplasty were studied retrospectively. There was a clinically significant difference in the rate of revision surgery. Five of the 11 patients in the group treated with plating alone required revision. None of the patients in the allograft strut group required revision. Level of evidence: III.

26. Edwards BJ, Bunta AD, Lane J, et al: Bisphosphonates and nonhealing femoral fractures: Analysis of the FDA Adverse Event Reporting System (FAERS) and international safety efforts: A systematic review from the Research on Adverse Drug Events And Reports (RADAR) project. *J Bone Joint Surg Am* 2013;95(4):297-307.

This retrospective study looked at the FDA Adverse Event Reporting System database. An association between the use of diphosphonates and atypical femur fractures was identified. Level of evidence: III.

27. Dell RM, Adams AL, Greene DF, et al: Incidence of atypical nontraumatic diaphyseal fractures of the femur. *J Bone Miner Res* 2012;27(12):2544-2550.

Patients at the Kaiser Healthy Bones Program were studied retrospectively. Of 1,835,116 patients older than 45 years with femur fractures, 142 were identified as being atypical fractures and 128 of those patients had diphosphonate exposure. Of all the patients reviewed, 188,814 had used diphosphonates. The age-adjusted incidence rates for an atypical fracture were 1.78 per 100,000 patients per year in those patients with exposure to diphosphonates ranging from 0.1 to 1.9 years. In those patients whose diphosphonate exposure was from 8 to 9.9 years, the incidence rates increased to 113.1 per 100,000 patients per year. Level of evidence: III.

28. Rosenberg ZS, La Rocca Vieira R, Chan SS, et al: Bisphosphonate-related complete atypical subtrochanteric femoral fractures: Diagnostic utility of radiography. *AJR Am J Roentgenol* 2011;197(4):954-960.

A retrospective radiographic review of two groups of patients with complete subtrochanteric and diaphyseal femur fractures was conducted. One group of patients took diphosphonates and the other group did not. The authors found that atypical femur fractures associated with diphosphonates had reliable radiographic findings including focal cortical thickening and transverse fractures in the subtrochanteric region. Level of evidence: III.

29. Hagen JE, Miller AN, Ott SM, et al: Association of atypical femoral fractures with bisphosphonate use by patients with varus hip geometry. *J Bone Joint Surg Am* 2014;96(22):1905-1909.

This study evaluated the radiographic anatomy of patients receiving chronic diphosphonate therapy who did and did not sustain atypical fractures, looking specifically at the neck-shaft angle of the femoral neck. Radiographic signs such as cortical thickening stress lines and thigh pain in the "fractured" group were included in the assessment. The average neck-shaft angle in the two groups was statistically significant: 129.5° (fractured group) compared with 133.8° (nonfractured group). It can be argued that increased femoral neck varus increases the likelihood of atypical fracture in patients with long-term diphosphonate use. Level of evidence: III.

30. Marcano A, Taormina D, Egol KA, Peck V, Tejwani NC: Are race and sex associated with the occurrence of atypical femoral fractures? *Clin Orthop Relat Res* 2014;472(3):1020-1027.

A prognostic study evaluating if Asian patients and women were more likely to sustain atypical fractures when on long-term diphosphonate use is presented. Conclusions were based on investigation of three different prospective registries that Asian and Hispanic patients were more likely to sustain an atypical fracture when on long-term diphosphonate therapy and should be followed more closely. Level of evidence: III

31. Banffy MB, Vrahas MS, Ready JE, Abraham JA: Nonoperative versus prophylactic treatment of bisphosphonate-associated femoral stress fractures. *Clin Orthop Relat Res* 2011;469(7):2028-2034.

    A retrospective study of patients older than 50 years receiving diphosphonates was performed to evaluate the likelihood of incomplete atypical femoral stress fractures proceeding to completion. The authors found that 5 of the 6 stress fractures treated nonsurgically went on to completion and displacement between 3 to 18 months after the original diagnosis. They also found that patients who underwent prophylactic nailing had a significantly shorter hospital stay than those treated after fracture completion. Level of evidence: III.

32. Egol KA, Park JH, Rosenberg ZS, Peck V, Tejwani NC: Healing delayed but generally reliable after bisphosphonate-associated complete femur fractures treated with IM nails. *Clin Orthop Relat Res* 2014;472(9):2728-2734.

    A retrospective study evaluated the rate of union and return to function of patients treated surgically for complete atypical femur fractures in association with diphosphonates. Sixty-six percent became pain free, 98% went on to radiographic union within 12 months, and 64% reported functional return to baseline within 1 year. Fracture malalignment led to delay in union. Level of evidence: III.

33. Teo BJ, Koh JS, Goh SK, Png MA, Chua DT, Howe TS: Post-operative outcomes of atypical femoral subtrochanteric fracture in patients on bisphosphonate therapy. *Bone Joint J* 2014;96-B(5):658-664.

    The authors retrospectively reviewed 33 consecutive female patients treated surgically for atypical subtrochanteric femur fractures. Mean time to radiographic union was 10 months. Twenty-three patients were treated with an extramedullary device. Implant failure occurred in 7 patients and revision surgery was required in 10 patients. The authors describe this fracture as having a high rate of complications/revisions and a prolonged period of immobilization. Level of evidence: III.

34. FDA Drug Safety Communication: Safety update for osteoporosis drugs, bisphosphonates, and atypical fractures. Page updated January 8, 2016. Available at: http://www.fda.gov/Drugs/DrugSafety/ucm229009.htm Accessed February 24, 2016.

Chapter 52

Periprosthetic Fractures

Richard S. Yoon, MD Frank A. Liporace, MD

Abstract

With an increasing number of elderly individuals undergoing joint arthroplasty, the incidence of periprosthetic fractures is also expected to rise. In the geriatric population, these injuries can have devastating consequences and should be approached with the goals of achieving stable fixation and allowing for immediate mobilization. Prior to surgery, medical optimization and careful preoperative planning is of paramount importance. Surgical management is predicated on the fracture location, the implant stability, and the amount and quality of bone available. Preparation should include options for fixation, revision, or some combination of both. It is helpful to be familiar with the evaluation, management, and technical aspects of periprosthetic fractures in the upper and lower extremities.

Keywords: elbow arthroplasty; periprosthetic fracture; shoulder arthroplasty; total hip arthroplasty; total knee arthroplasty

Introduction

By 2060, it is estimated that approximately 140 million people will be older than 44 years.[1] Advancements in modern medicine have kept patients healthier and living longer, and orthopaedic surgeons have helped improve the quality of life and activity level of patients with musculoskeletal conditions. With the projected increase in the number of older patients, there is also expected to be a concomitant increase in the number of upper and lower extremity joint arthroplasties, along with their subsequent complications.

Although a periprosthetic fracture can develop in any patient with a total joint arthroplasty, these fractures can have a devastating effect on geriatric patients. In geriatric patients that present with this fragility fracture, issues of bone quality and fixation are necessary to address during preoperative planning.

Similar to the care needed for a patient with a hip fracture, preoperative medical optimization is of paramount importance. A thorough patient history, including endocrine, musculoskeletal, and oncologic histories, should be a routine part of the preoperative workup. In addition, identification and review of any previous associated surgeries, including complications, should be done before surgery. Knowledge of the prior surgical approach along with the type of currently implanted hardware improves preoperative planning and allows for a smooth surgical course. An intimate knowledge of the patient's code status, functional activity level, and goals of care are important potential discussion points to consider in the octogenarian population.

In general, fixation of periprosthetic fractures can be approached by applying systematic assessment and methodology. To help facilitate the desired clinical outcomes, it is necessary to consider fracture location, implant stability, the presence of cement mantle and/or infection, bone quality, and expected bone loss. The surgeon also should be prepared to perform fracture fixation, revision, or both.

Typically, the location of the fracture around the implant can help determine the definitive plan. Generally speaking, fractures very proximal or distal in relation to the implant can usually be fixed, whereas treatment options when the fracture lines are located about the stem depend on the stability of the implant. However, it is important to assess overall implant stability regardless of the

Dr. Liporace or an immediate family member has received royalties from Biomet; is a member of a speakers' bureau or has made paid presentations on behalf of Biomet, Stryker, and Synthes; serves as a paid consultant to or is an employee of Biomet, Medtronic, Synthes, and Stryker; and serves as an unpaid consultant to AO. Neither Dr. Yoon nor any immediate family member has received anything of value from or has stock or stock options held in a commercial company or institution related directly or indirectly to the subject of this chapter.

fracture location. An unstable or a loose implant should be revised, whereas a well-fixed implant can usually be left untreated, although recent literature may suggest revision even in stable implants.[2] This strategy must be approached with caution because revision surgery can involve factors such as added surgical time and blood loss.

If cement is present, removal instruments should be available, especially if the implant is being revised. Despite the presence of trauma, it is always prudent to consider concomitant infection, and there should be a low threshold for an associated workup. In addition, an indolent process is common in upper extremity infections. Although *Staphylococcus aureus* is still the most common infecting organism, there is growing concern about infections caused by oral flora such as *Propionibacterium acnes*.[3] These organisms require long-term incubation for speciation and, if untreated, may lead to failure of fracture treatment.[4] Critical assessment of bone quality and the expected amount of bone loss should be completed, and a preoperative list of implants and fixation devices should be determined. Careful planning combined with medical optimization and goals consistent with early mobilization can lead to a consistently reproducible desired clinical outcome.

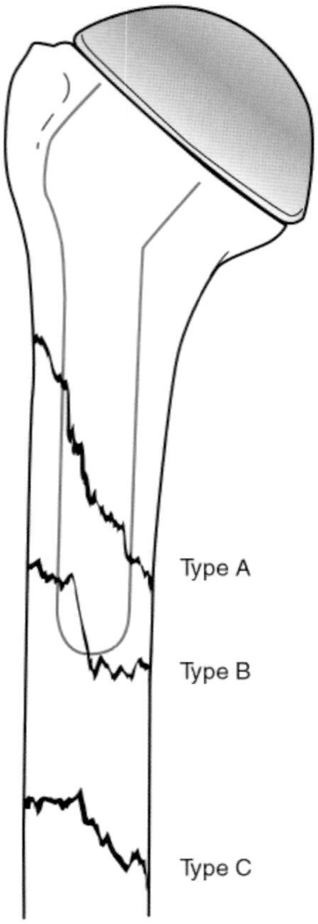

Figure 1 Illustration of the Wright and Cofield classification of periprosthetic humeral fractures associated with shoulder arthroplasty. Type A fractures propagate proximally from the distal stem, type B fractures are centered over the distal stem, and type C fractures are located distal to the tip of the stem.

Upper Extremity Periprosthetic Fractures

Although the number of shoulder and elbow arthroplasties performed each year are substantially fewer than the number of hip and knee arthroplasties, the number of upper extremity procedures continues to increase. Periprosthetic fractures occur in 0.6% to 2.4% of upper extremity arthroplasties, with a concomitant increase expected in the coming decades.[4-6]

Periprosthetic Fractures Associated With Shoulder Arthroplasty

After shoulder arthroplasty, periprosthetic fractures can occur around the glenoid or the humeral stem. Periprosthetic fracture around the glenoid component is rare; when it occurs, it typically occurs intraoperatively. Assessment of the fracture line extension is important; however, a glenoid fracture should be treated with an algorithmic approach similar to that used when preparing for an elective total shoulder arthroplasty with severe glenoid bone loss. In patients with severe bone loss, it may be prudent to use augments or allografts before glenoid component insertion, if warranted.

Most periprosthetic fractures associated with shoulder arthroplasty occur on the humeral side. These fractures can occur both during and after surgery, with women and those with a poor morbidity index score at substantial risk.[6] Treatment, regardless of an intraoperative or a postoperative timing of the fracture, largely depends on the location of the fracture, the stability of the stem, and the quality and amount of bone surrounding the implant. The Wright and Cofield Classification divides these fractures into three categories: type A fractures propagate proximally from the distal stem, type B fractures are centered over the distal stem, and type C fractures are located distal to the tip of the stem[7] (**Figure 1**).

Nonsurgical management is an option for all fracture types and especially for patients with several comorbidities, minimal function, and/or minimal displacement. A 2011 review outlined the specific treatment options for each subtype.[8] Patients with type A fractures with minimal displacement can be treated with a protocol similar to that used for nonsurgical rotator cuff management.

Patients with nondisplaced type B and C fractures also can undergo a trial of nonsurgical management with a fracture brace, but a higher incidence of delayed union and nonunion in these patients has resulted in a recommendation for a low threshold before considering surgical intervention at the 3-month follow-up evaluation.[7-9]

Regardless of the fracture location, careful evaluation of a potentially loose stem is warranted. Even if there is low suspicion of a loose implant, it is prudent to have a long revision component available. For type A, B, and even C fractures with a loose implant, some surgeons have recommended exchange for a longer implant to bypass the fracture by at least two cortical diameters, although this principle may not apply in every instance of a very distal fracture.[10]

Surgical treatment of periprosthetic fractures around a stable humeral implant is amenable to open reduction and internal fixation (ORIF) with several options for fixation.[6,8,11,12] Cerclage cables alone can be used for very proximal type A fractures, especially if the fracture occurs intraoperatively and a simple solution is required. However, in the setting of a postoperative fracture, the surgeon should carefully dissect circumferentially about the humerus to avoid iatrogenic injury to vital neurovascular structures. Although the literature lacks consensus for recommendation of a single, ideal construct, available biomechanical and clinical data support surgical fixation using cables, plates, and/or screws.[4,5,7,9] A plate of an appropriate size and length should not only span the fracture, but it should also provide adequate overlap with the implant to avoid gaps that can be stress risers.[13-16] Especially for type B and C fracture types, implant overlap is a necessary aspect of surgical treatment.[13] Extrapolating from other periprosthetic fracture locations, the effect of lateral plate overlap in a periprosthetic femur model was studied to specifically examine the strain experienced by the hip stem along with overall construct stiffness in the setting of a simulated fall.[13] The results showed that the plate-stem overlap has two main effects. The overlap substantially decreases the amount of strain experienced by the hip stem and simultaneously increases the overall stiffness of the construct.[13] Although adding proximal screws to obtain purchase around the stem increases overall stiffness, this increase is not statistically significant.[13] For type B and C fractures that extend down into the humeral component of an ipsilateral total elbow arthroplasty (TEA), adequate overlap of both stems with a long plate is recommended. Again, if the humeral component is loose with a concomitant fracture in between a distal TEA, exchange to a long-stemmed component with a plate that overlaps both stems (to avoid stress risers) should be performed.[13]

There is a paucity of literature regarding outcomes after either surgical fixation or revision for periprosthetic shoulder fractures.[11,12] A large 2013 series summarized outcomes for 36 patients; 17 were treated with ORIF alone, and 19 were treated with ORIF and revision.[11] Overall, a 97% union rate was reported, with acceptable outcome scores at follow-up; however, a 39% complication rate also was reported. The revision rate was nearly 19%, with most revisions needed because of failed hardware (stem breakage, loosening, subsequent periprosthetic fracture, or dislocation). Only one infection and one nonunion occurred. Larger studies are needed to analyze and improve on reported techniques to decrease the complication rate.

Periprosthetic Fractures Associated With TEA

Fractures about a TEA occur either on the humeral or ulnar side. The O'Driscoll and Morrey classification of TEA fractures delineates fracture type based on location[17] (**Figure 2**). Type A fractures occur in the periarticular region (distal humerus, proximal ulna). Type B fractures occur in the midportion to the tip of either the humeral or ulnar stem. Type C fractures occur either proximal to the humeral stem or distal to the ulnar stem. There is little published literature regarding the treatment algorithm for periprosthetic TEA fractures; however, many of the general principles previously discussed can be applied to each situation about the elbow.[8,18,19]

Type A fractures typically are minimally displaced and often can be managed nonsurgically. However, with substantial displacement of either the medial or lateral epicondyles or the proximal olecranon, surgical fixation may be recommended to avoid pain or maintain muscular attachments. For displacement of the condyles about the distal humerus, periarticular plates can offer stout fixation for larger, reconstructible fragments; however, condylar excision may be appropriate in the setting of severe comminution.

For type B fractures, treatment is determined based on implant stability. Loose implants on either the humeral or ulnar side should be revised to longer stems that bypass the fracture site.[18,19] Because bypassing the fracture with a longer stem alone will not provide enough stability, including plate-and-screw fixation to add further stability is recommended. On the humeral side, if stems are stable and well fixed, cables can be used to re-create the tube and maintain reduction and, if needed, additional fixation with overlapping plates and screws can be used.[20,21] Again, adequate plate-implant overlap and a minimum span of at least two cortical diameters in either the proximal (humerus) or distal (ulnar) direction is recommended.

For type C fractures, a loose implant should warrant

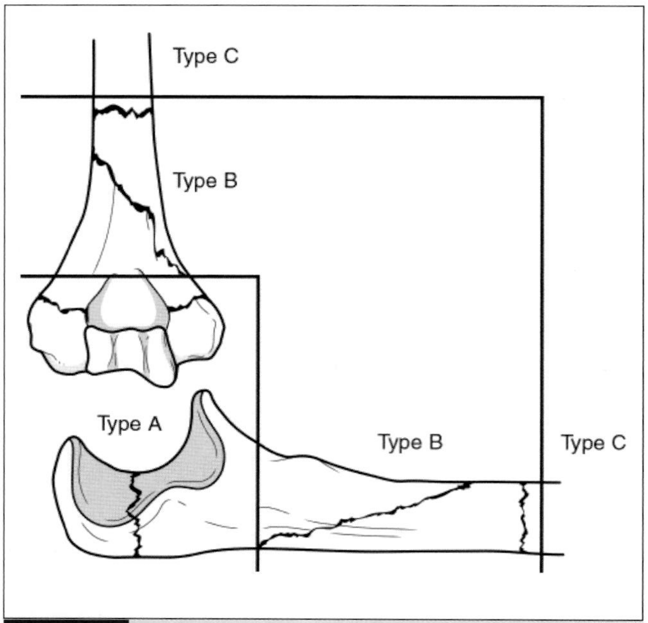

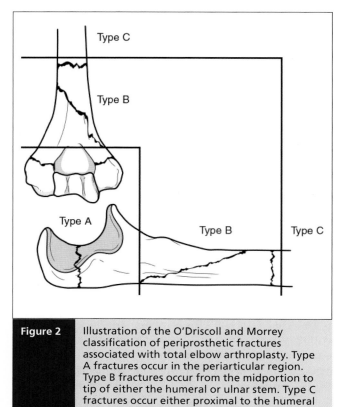

Figure 2 Illustration of the O'Driscoll and Morrey classification of periprosthetic fractures associated with total elbow arthroplasty. Type A fractures occur in the periarticular region. Type B fractures occur from the midportion to tip of either the humeral or ulnar stem. Type C fractures occur either proximal to the humeral stem or distal to the ulnar stem.

a revision to a longer stem with plate-and-screw fixation added when necessary for re-establishment of the "tube's integrity." For type C fractures with a well-fixed implant, standard plate osteosynthesis should be performed. Appropriate plate-implant overlap is necessary to decrease the strain on the humeral stem while maximizing overall construct stiffness.[13]

Lower Extremity Periprosthetic Fractures

Because of excellent clinical outcomes, reliable implant survivorship, improved engineering, and an increasing number of more active and healthier elderly individuals, the number of hip and knee arthroplasties continues to rise. A concomitant increasing incidence of associated periprosthetic fractures is also expected. Because of the greater volume of lower limb arthroplasties compared with upper limb arthroplasties, periprosthetic fracture in the lower limb is much more studied and reported on in the literature.[22]

Hip Arthroplasty

Periprosthetic fractures can occur about an associated total hip arthroplasty (THA), hemiarthroplasty, or resurfaced hip. This chapter will focus on fractures about a THA on both the acetabular and femoral sides. Periprosthetic fractures about a hemiarthroplasty can be treated based on the femoral-side recommendations for a THA. Typically, fractures about a resurfaced hip occur about the femoral neck and require revision to THA.

Fractures on the Acetabular Side

Addressing periprosthetic acetabular fractures depends mainly on implant stability, which is determined by fracture displacement and available bone stock. The Paprosky classification for periprosthetic fractures about the acetabulum summarizes recommendations based on these characteristics[23] (**Table 1**). In general, for both intraoperative and postoperative fractures about the acetabular cup, assessment of fracture displacement and available bone stock can help determine treatment. Stable, minimally displaced fractures can usually be managed nonsurgically, whereas unstable components with displaced fractures with or without adequate bone stock require surgical intervention.[23]

For unstable, intraoperative acetabular fractures, upsizing to a larger cup may provide a stable construct; however, if cup stability is questionable (even with screw fixation), an additional posterior column buttress should be provided. This can be achieved via further proximal dissection and contouring and placing a reconstruction plate along the posterior column for additional buttressing.

For periprosthetic fractures with an obviously loose cup, a thorough CT assessment should be performed to determine the amount of associated bone loss as well as the location of fracture lines to help in surgical planning. An anterior approach (for example, an ilioinguinal or a modified Stoppa approach) to the inner table is rarely required for the surgical treatment of these fractures. However, depending on the fracture pattern, access to the quadrilateral plate may be necessary to achieve adequate fixation, especially if gross acute discontinuity is noted between the anterior and posterior columns. Depending on the amount of bone loss, the surgeon should have a low threshold for revision to a jumbo cup and for the use of a cage construct to help re-create a stable acetabular side.

Fractures on the Femoral Side

Treatment of periprosthetic fractures that occur around the femoral implant can often be reasonably guided by the Vancouver classification system (**Table 2**). The Vancouver system, which is similar to others, separates the fracture patterns by location. For fractures about the stem, the classification is further stratified by implant stability and available bone stock, which are classification

Table 1

Paprosky Classification of Periprosthetic Acetabular Fractures

Type and Subtype	Location and Characteristics
Intraoperative (during implant insertion)	
A	Recognized, stable, nondisplaced fracture
B	Recognized, unstable, displaced fracture
C	Unrecognized fracture
Intraoperative (during implant removal)	
A	Less than 50% bone stock
B	Greater than 50% bone stock
Traumatic	
A	Stable component
B	Unstable component
Spontaneous	
A	Less than 50% bone stock
B	Greater than 50% bone stock
Pelvic Discontinuity	
A	Less than 50% bone stock
B	Greater than 50% bone stock
C	Associated with pelvic radiation

Table 2

Vancouver Classification of Periprosthetic Femoral Fractures

Type and Subtype	Location and Characteristics
Type A	
A_G	Greater trochanter
A_L	Lesser trochanter
Type B	
B_1	Around stem/tip, well-fixed
B_2	Around stem/tip, loose stem
B_3	Around stem/tip, loose stem, poor bone stock
Type C	Distal to stem

principles that apply throughout this chapter and help dictate treatment. In addition, preoperative assessment of the acetabular component also should be performed, and the surgeon should have a low threshold for cup revision to obtain longevity of the hip.

Vancouver type A fracture subtypes depend on location; either about the greater or lesser trochanters. Intraoperative fractures that occur about the trochanters can typically be addressed with cerclage wiring. However, it is imperative to assess the integrity of the calcar. If the calcar is fractured or unstable, subsidence and subsequent instability may result and lead to dislocation or potential implant instability. To avoid such complications, the surgeon should have a low threshold for changing the femoral stem to a calcar-replacing diaphyseal fitting or a modular diaphyseal fitting stem. When occurring postoperatively, many fractures about the trochanters are often minimally displaced and can be managed nonsurgically with motion restriction. However, with substantial displacement, nonunion can occur, and surgical fixation with a trochanteric grip plate (with or without cerclage wires) is recommended. It is imperative to assess implant stability intraoperatively; if there is any possibility that the stem is loose, revision is recommended.

Of note, if there is a greater trochanteric fracture with concomitant lesser trochanteric involvement, there should be high suspicion for potential implant loosening because the fracture line may be continuous and hidden by the implant on plain radiographs. CT evaluation may be helpful; however, image artifact caused by the femoral implant can make a full evaluation difficult to achieve.

Vancouver type B fractures generally require surgical treatment. Definitive classification of stem stability is usually made intraoperatively; therefore, provisions should be made for fixation and implant revision. Type B fractures, by definition, occur about the distal tip of the stem, and each subclassification depends on the stability of the implant and the surrounding bone stock. Type B_1 fractures occur about well-fixed implants with good bone stock and are most often amenable to surgical fixation after intraoperative assessment of the stem. An extensile, lateral approach to the femur without devascularizing the muscle is a powerful approach that allows full visualization of the fracture. Fixation strategies typically recommend the application of an "appropriate" amount of plate-implant overlap, with the amount of overlap a subject of debate. With increased distance of fixation past the overlap between the plate and the stem, the potential of a stress riser at the tip of the stem becomes negligible.[10] However, the ideal plate length is still unknown and controversial because of the lack of high-level evidence.[13-16] In proximal fractures, biomechanical studies have failed

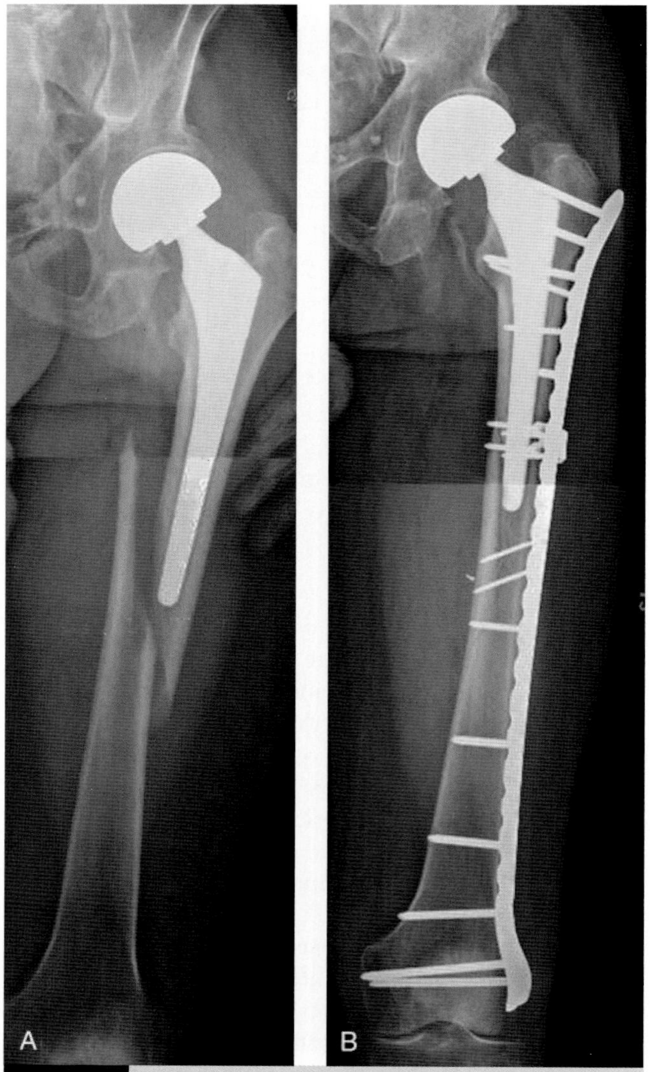

Figure 3 **A,** Preoperative radiograph of the femur of 78-year-old man who sustained a Vancouver B_1 fracture in a fall. Intraoperatively, the implant was deemed stable, and the patient underwent open reduction and internal fixation using an extensile lateral approach. **B,** Postoperative radiograph shows placement of a locking plate that spans the entire femur.

to find substantial differences between plates that reach the greater trochanter and those that stop short of the trochanter. Some authors have recommended maximizing the distance from the overlap based on the availability of the intact bone, thus maximizing the working length of the fixation.[13-15,20,24] In distal fractures, there is emerging literature that spanning the entire femur from the femoral condyles may further decrease nonunion rates and allow for prophylactic fixation to avoid future injury[14,15,25,26] (**Figure 3**).

The ideal fixation strategy also remains controversial. Although biomechanically superior to conventional plating, locked plating has not consistently decreased nonunion rates in all case series.[24-26] The authors of a 2014 study did not report significant complication rates with locked plating but recommended the use of a combination of cables and locked screws in the proximal femur.[26] The authors did note a substantially higher rate of failure and infection with concomitant allograft use and recommended against such use.[26]

Recent level IV studies have attempted to compare the results between ORIF and revision arthroplasty to determine if one modality was superior to the other.[2,27] A comparison of the two treatment methods found a twofold higher rate of complications in the ORIF cohort.[27] Other authors reported a substantially higher mortality rate in the ORIF group compared with those who underwent revision arthroplasty.[2] It has been suggested that revision with or without supplementary fixation may prove beneficial to geriatric patients by allowing for earlier mobilization and at least immediate partial weight bearing.[2,27] However, both of these studies were severely underpowered subgroup comparisons with inherent selection biases that likely represent statistical error. Larger prospective studies are needed to offer a definitive comparison.

The treatment of type B_2 periprosthetic femoral fractures is often more extensive in complexity and exposure. Implant removal can be facilitated by approaching the fracture in a manner analogous to that used for an extended trochanteric osteotomy.[28] By booking open the fracture site, implant removal can be facilitated. In this setting, revision procedures often use diaphyseal-fitting stems, many of which are modular. The proximal hip approach can be continued into an extensile lateral femoral approach and is the preferred method to accomplish surgical goals.

To protect against fracture propagation when prepping the intact femur for the distal aspect of a revision femoral stem, a prophylactic cable can be placed distal to the fracture site before reaming. At this point, it may be beneficial to ream and pot the distal end of the implant before reducing the fracture fragments around the stem. Potting the diaphysis of a modular implant not only allows confirmation of a good fit, but it also allows temporary building of the trial proximal body while the greater trochanter is used as a reference for overall sizing before trialing stability.

Type B_3 fractures are characterized by poor proximal bone stock and a loose stem. Depending on the amount of proximal bone stock available, options for revision include full-coated stems, fluted tapered stems, prosthesis-strut

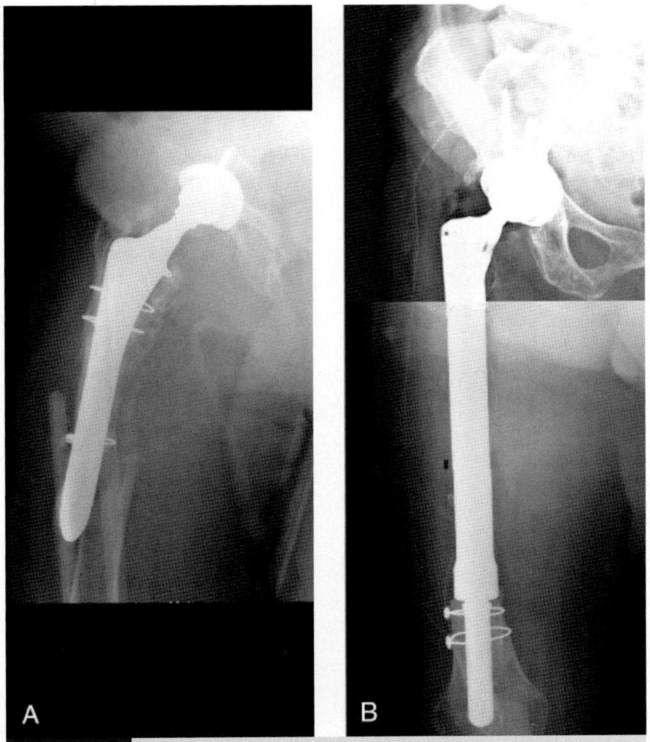

Figure 4 Imaging studies from an 84-year-old woman with a history of total hip arthroplasty complicated by two previous periprosthetic fractures who experienced another fall. **A,** AP radiograph shows a fracture about the stem. Because the patient had very little available bone stock, the decision was made to proceed with proximal femoral replacement. Intraoperatively, the cup was also found to be in poor position, and was revised. **B,** AP radiograph shows the proximal femoral implant and the revised cup.

allograft composite constructs, and proximal femoral replacement.[29-34] Although often used in the past, prosthesis-strut allografts are becoming less common because of the prolonged time to incorporation, infection risks, and modern improvements in fixation and revision implants. Implant removal strategies are similar to those previously described in this chapter. Encouraging short and midterm implant survivorship and function have been reported with modular fluted tapered stems, even in the setting of poor proximal bone stock.[32-34]

In type B_3 fractures, however, definitive assessment of available bone stock typically does not occur until after the incision is made. Some surgeons have recommended having a proximal femoral replacement available. A low threshold for proceeding with proximal femoral replacement has been advocated to minimize surgical time and blood loss and allow for immediate weight bearing; this is especially important in elderly, low-demand patients[35]

Table 3

Lewis and Rorabeck Classification of Periprosthetic Supracondylar Fractures

Type	Characteristics
I	Nondisplaced, stable prosthesis
II	Displaced, stable prosthesis
IIIA	Displaced, loose prosthesis
IIIB	Nondisplaced, loose prosthesis

(**Figure 4**). As in any revision setting, the integrity of the abductors should be considered along with an assessment of cup position and stability. Following the assessment, there should be a low threshold for addressing the acetabular side with revision or the use of a dual-mobility cup or a constrained liner to minimize the dislocation risk.

Type C fractures, which occur distal to the stem, are often treated as distal femoral fractures, with many surgeons using distal femoral plates. Similar to the controversy concerning type B_1 fractures, adequate overlap of the femoral stem and the plate (with a combination of cables and screws) is also recommended to provide the best biomechanical construct. However, there is no general consensus on the ideal length and type of construct.[13]

Periprosthetic Fractures Associated With Knee Arthroplasty

Although there are some classification systems for periprosthetic fractures about total knee arthroplasties (TKAs), treatment is guided by fracture location (above or below the implant), bone quality, and implant stability.[28]

Fractures on the Femoral Side

The treatment of fractures occurring on the femoral side of a TKA depends on the stability of the implant (**Table 3**). The Lewis and Rorabeck system classifies periprosthetic TKA fractures into three types: type 1 is nondisplaced with a stable implant; type II is a displaced fracture with a stable implant; and type III fractures are displaced (IIIA) or nondisplaced (IIIB) fractures with unstable or loose implants.[36]

Type I fractures can sometimes be treated nonsurgically, especially in patients with severe comorbidities. However, even in the most minimally displaced fracture, fixation may provide a more stable construct to promote earlier mobilization and avoid progressive deformity. Type I and II fractures are treated similarly, with options including either the use of a lateral plate or a retrograde nail. There is a paucity of definitive level I or II evidence to support one method over the other. Both

7: Geriatrics

fixation methods are well accepted and depend on surgeon preference.[37-39] Several key pearls dictate the choice of implant. First and foremost, the presence of an implant in the proximal femur, whether it is a femoral stem or a short intramedullary nail, should dictate the use of a construct that spans the entire femur. If a lateral plate is used, it should extend proximally enough to overlap with the femoral implant.[13] If a retrograde intramedullary nail is used and stopped short of the femoral implant, a plate can be placed to overlap both implants and avoid the creation of a stress riser. Recently, evidence reporting the biomechanical benefits of linking these implants together has been published.[21]

Revision is recommended for grossly loose implants with concomitant fractures. If the bone stock is good and the femoral implant can be easily removed, fixing the fracture and placing another primary component is possible but rare. Typically, the femur is revised with a stemmed component with or without augments for areas with defects, and flexion and extension gaps are matched. Although some manufacturers have revision components that can be mated to primary components, revision of the femur typically will require revision of the tibial component to achieve a mated system (**Figure 5**). For very low fractures with questionably stable implants with or without poor bone stock, a distal femoral replacement can offer a faster, lower morbidity procedure that also allows immediate weight bearing and mobilization in elderly patients.[40,41]

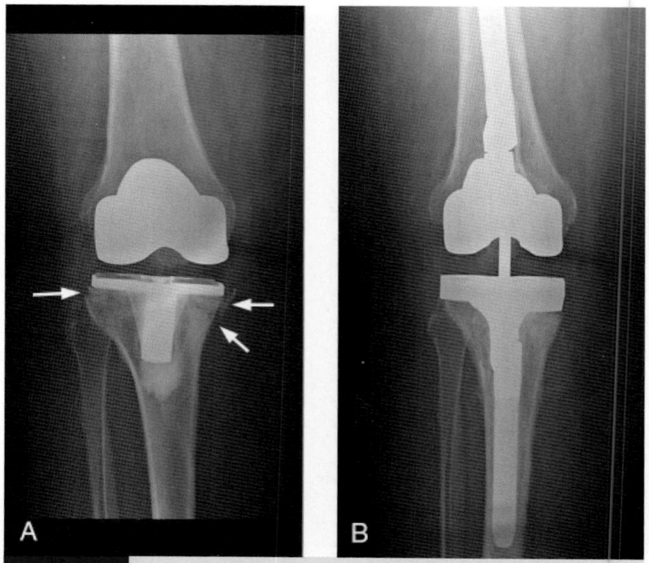

Figure 5 **A,** AP radiograph of the tibia of 76-year-old woman after a fall shows subtle fracture lines (arrows) about an already loose tibial component of a 10-year-old total knee arthroplasty (TKA). **B,** AP radiograph after revision of the TKA to stemmed components because of poor bone stock. The height of the joint line was maintained with a medial augment.

Fractures on the Tibial Side

There is little published literature about periprosthetic fractures on the tibial side of a TKA; however, treatment principles remain the same as for other periprosthetic fractures. Nondisplaced fractures around stable implants can often be treated nonsurgically with either a cast or brace and protected weight bearing. However, many surgeons prefer surgical fixation to allow immediate mobilization and prevent joint contracture. Minimally invasive fixation techniques can achieve stability with low morbidity. A stable implant with a displaced fracture typically can be fixed with plate-and-screw constructs. It is imperative to assess the anatomic axis and restore the appropriate parameters about the joint line. When plating around the tibial component, variable-angle locked screws can be helpful in obtaining good purchase while avoiding the stem. Nonanatomic reduction may lead to increased wear and failure of the TKA. A loose implant warrants revision with long-stemmed components, with or without augments. Although some manufacturers have components that allow for mixed mating of primary and revision components, revision on one side typically requires revision on the other side to create a mated system (**Figure 5**).

Midshaft and distal tibial fractures occur rarely in association with TKA and typically occur independent of the implant. However, the implant and the mechanical and anatomic axes should be assessed and the surgeon should have a low threshold for fracture fixation (**Figure 6, A**). Plate-and-screw constructs can provide excellent fixation with minimal soft-tissue disruption, especially in patients with poor bone quality. The surgeon may choose to span the entire length of the bone to avoid stress risers and future fracture (**Figure 6, B**).

Summary

Periprosthetic fractures are common and the incidence is increasing. Treatment of upper and lower extremity periprosthetic fractures is achieved using a systematic approach, including identifying the location of the fracture relative to the prosthesis, assessing the inherent implant stability, and considering the surrounding bone quality and available bone stock. The surgeon should consider and be prepared for revision arthroplasty. Methods that promote early mobilization and avoid postoperative complications are preferred. For proximal and distal femur fractures with substantial bone loss, there should be a

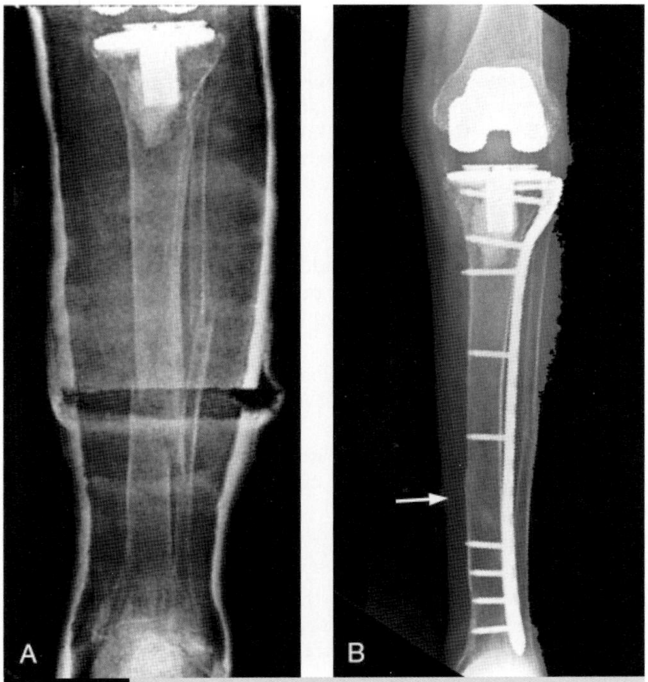

Figure 6 **A,** Preoperative AP radiograph shows a diaphyseal fracture distal to a stable tibial component. **B,** AP radiograph shows anatomic reduction (arrow) and placement of a locking plate to span osteoporotic bone and avoid stress risers and future fracture. (Reproduced from Liporace FA, Donegan DJ, Langford JR, Haidukewych GJ: Contemporary internal fixation techniques for periprosthetic fractures of the hip and knee. *Instr Course Lect* 2013;62:317-332.)

low threshold for revision to a proximal or distal femoral replacement. When performing internal fixation, extensile approaches should be used and spanning the entire long bone should be considered to increase stability and avoid the creation of stress risers.

Key Study Points

- Treatment of periprosthetic fractures is determined by fracture location, implant stability, available bone stock, and bone quality.
- The surgeon should always be prepared for revision and, in certain situations, should use end-segment replacing prostheses.
- Elderly patients with periprosthetic fracture should be treated in a manner similar to those with geriatric hip fractures—medical optimization and mobilization are key principles to maximize outcomes.

Annotated References

1. Colby SL, Ortman JM: Projections of the Size and Composition of the U.S. Population: 2014 to 2060: Population Estimates and Projections. Census Bureau, U.S. Department of Commerce. Available at: https://www.census.gov/content/dam/Census/library/publications/2015/demo/p25-1143.pdf. Accessed February 15, 2016.

   The latest summarized report by the US Census Bureau indicates that there will be a projected 140 million people older than 44 years by 2060. More than 80 million people will be older than 65 years. Level of evidence: II.

2. Bhattacharyya T, Chang D, Meigs JB, Estok DM II, Malchau H: Mortality after periprosthetic fracture of the femur. *J Bone Joint Surg Am* 2007;89(12):2658-2662.

3. Hudek R, Sommer F, Kerwat M, Abdelkawi AF, Loos F, Gohlke F: Propionibacterium acnes in shoulder surgery: True infection, contamination, or commensal of the deep tissue? *J Shoulder Elbow Surg* 2014;23(12):1763-1771.

   In this study of 118 patients undergoing first-time shoulder surgery, the authors analyzed specimens from several different layers from superficial to deep. Infection with *P acnes* was reported in 36% of cases. Notable risk factors were male sex and an anterolateral approach. Most of the infections occurred within the deep tissue layer. Level of evidence: III.

4. Athwal GS, Sperling JW, Rispoli DM, Cofield RH: Periprosthetic humeral fractures during shoulder arthroplasty. *J Bone Joint Surg Am* 2009;91(3):594-603.

5. Kumar S, Sperling JW, Haidukewych GH, Cofield RH: Periprosthetic humeral fractures after shoulder arthroplasty. *J Bone Joint Surg Am* 2004;86(4):680-689.

6. Singh JA, Sperling J, Schleck C, Harmsen W, Cofield R: Periprosthetic fractures associated with primary total shoulder arthroplasty and primary humeral head replacement: A thirty-three-year study. *J Bone Joint Surg Am* 2012;94(19):1777-1785.

   This prospective registry analysis conducted at the Mayo Clinic evaluated more than 2,000 shoulder arthroplasties over a 30-year-period. Logistic regression analysis determined that significant risk factors for intraoperative fracture were female sex and an underlying diagnosis of posttraumatic arthritis. Postoperatively, a higher Deyo-Charlson index was associated with an increased risk of periprosthetic fracture. Level of evidence: II.

7. Wright TW, Cofield RH: Humeral fractures after shoulder arthroplasty. *J Bone Joint Surg Am* 1995;77(9):1340-1346.

8. Dehghan N, Chehade M, McKee MD: Current perspectives in the treatment of periprosthetic upper extremity fractures. *J Orthop Trauma* 2011;25(suppl 2):S71-S76.

   This literature review provides a concise update on the prevalence, incidence, evaluation, and treatment strategies available for periprosthetic fractures that occur in the upper extremity. Recommendations and general guidelines of management are reviewed. Level of evidence: V.

9. Cameron B, Iannotti JP: Periprosthetic fractures of the humerus and scapula: Management and prevention. *Orthop Clin North Am* 1999;30(2):305-318.

10. Dennis DA, Dingman CA, Meglan DA, O'Leary JF, Mallory TH, Berme N: Femoral cement removal in revision total hip arthroplasty. A biomechanical analysis. *Clin Orthop Relat Res* 1987;220:142-147.

11. Andersen JR, Williams CD, Cain R, Mighell M, Frankle M: Surgically treated humeral shaft fractures following shoulder arthroplasty. *J Bone Joint Surg Am* 2013;95(1):9-18.

    In this single surgeon, retrospective comparative series, the authors report on the outcomes of ORIF versus revision arthroplasty after periprosthetic fracture about the shoulder. A total of 36 patients were included; 17 patients were treated with ORIF and 19 with revision arthroplasty. All stable, well-fixed stems were fixed, whereas loose implants were revised. The authors reported acceptable outcomes and function in each cohort; however, the overall complication rate was nearly 40%. There were no differences in complication rates in the cohorts, and most complications in both groups involved implant failure. Level of evidence: IV.

12. Mineo GV, Accetta R, Franceschini M, Pedrotti Dell'Acqua G, Calori GM, Meersseman A: Management of shoulder periprosthetic fractures: Our institutional experience and review of the literature. *Injury* 2013;44(suppl 1):S82-S85.

    The authors present a retrospective analysis of 36 periprosthetic fractures in 35 patients treated either with ORIF or revision arthroplasty. A 97% union was reported; however, there was a 19% reoperation rate and an overall 39% complication rate. Level of evidence: IV.

13. Kubiak EN, Haller JM, Kemper DD, Presson AP, Higgins TF, Horwitz DS: Does the lateral plate need to overlap the stem to mitigate stress concentration when treating Vancouver C periprosthetic supracondylar femur fracture? *J Arthroplasty* 2015;30(1):104-108.

    A biomechanical study was performed to determine the necessity of plate and stem overlap in the treatment of Vancouver type C fractures. A simulated fall model as well as cyclic loading were used in the study. The authors determined that the hip stem alone decreased the strength of the native femur. They recommended proximal overlap with plates and cable to decrease strain on the implant and provide the most rigidity.

14. Bryant GK, Morshed S, Agel J, et al: Isolated locked compression plating for Vancouver Type B1 periprosthetic femoral fractures. *Injury* 2009;40(11):1180-1186.

15. Moloney GB, Westrick ER, Siska PA, Tarkin IS: Treatment of periprosthetic femur fractures around a well-fixed hip arthroplasty implant: Span the whole bone. *Arch Orthop Trauma Surg* 2014;134(1):9-14.

    This retrospective cohort comparison reviewed results of two groups of patients treated with ORIF for Vancouver type B_1 fractures. The authors noted a high rate of failure when the plate did not span the entire femur and recommended routine plating down to the femoral condyles. Level of evidence: III.

16. Zdero R, Walker R, Waddell JP, Schemitsch EH: Biomechanical evaluation of periprosthetic femoral fracture fixation. *J Bone Joint Surg Am* 2008;90(5):1068-1077.

17. O'Driscoll SW, Morrey BF: Periprosthetic fractures about the elbow. *Orthop Clin North Am* 1999;30(2):319-325.

18. Liporace FA, Kaplan D, Stickney W, Yoon RS: Use of a hinged antibiotic-loaded cement spacer for an infected periprosthetic fracture in a total elbow arthroplasty: A novel construct utilizing Ilizarov rods. A case report. *JBJS Case Connect* 2014;4:e122.

    This case report reviews the management of a chronic, infected nonunion after fracture about the humeral stem of a TEA. Level of evidence: V.

19. Kawano Y, Okazaki M, Ikegami H, Sato K, Nakamura T, Toyama Y: The "docking" method for periprosthetic humeral fracture after total elbow arthroplasty: A case report. *J Bone Joint Surg Am* 2010;92(10):1988-1991.

    The authors describe the use of a "sleeve" to place over the humeral component to "dock" the component within the proximal length of the intramedullary canal and adequately bypass the fracture site. Level of evidence: V.

20. Demos HA, Briones MS, White PH, Hogan KA, Barfield WR: A biomechanical comparison of periprosthetic femoral fracture fixation in normal and osteoporotic cadaveric bone. *J Arthroplasty* 2012;27(5):783-788.

    This biomechanical study compared fixation strategies in both normal and osteoporotic bone. Results showed that the stiffest, most reliable construct was a combination of screws (locked or nonlocked) with cables, providing a well-balanced construct for Vancouver type B_1 fractures.

21. Dubov A, Kim SY, Shah S, Schemitsch EH, Zdero R, Bougherara H: The biomechanics of plate repair of periprosthetic femur fractures near the tip of a total hip implant: The effect of cable-screw position. *Proc Inst Mech Eng H* 2011;225(9):857-865.

    This biomechanical analysis tested the proximal screw-cable combinations for the repair of periprosthetic femoral fractures. The authors noted that the stiffest constructs used screw-cable constructs, with a specific location near the fracture site providing the best stability.

22. Della Rocca GJ, Leung KS, Pape HC: Periprosthetic fractures: Epidemiology and future projections. *J Orthop Trauma* 2011;25(suppl 2):S66-S70.

This literature review provides a concise overall look at the current and future states of periprosthetic fractures and the potential effects on the US healthcare system. Level of evidence: V.

23. Della Valle CJ, Momberger NG, Paprosky WG: Periprosthetic fractures of the acetabulum associated with a total hip arthroplasty. *Instr Course Lect* 2003;52:281-290.

24. Froberg L, Troelsen A, Brix M: Periprosthetic Vancouver type B1 and C fractures treated by locking-plate osteosynthesis: Fracture union and reoperations in 60 consecutive fractures. *Acta Orthop* 2012;83(6):648-652.

    In this retrospective analysis of 60 consecutive patients undergoing ORIF for type B_1 and C Vancouver fractures, the authors specifically evaluated failure rates and potential causes. Overall, 8 of 60 fractures required revision surgery. Three patients sustained subsequent falls and failure of fixation, which the authors hypothesized was caused by the less than 50% overlap with the implant. This study was limited by its retrospective nature and the high rate of loss to follow-up (28 patients unavailable at a mean follow-up of 24 months). Level of evidence: IV.

25. Dehghan N, McKee MD, Nauth A, Ristevski B, Schemitsch EH: Surgical fixation of Vancouver type B1 periprosthetic femur fractures: A systematic review. *J Orthop Trauma* 2014;28(12):721-727.

    In this systematic review conducted via a search of Cochrane, PubMed, and MEDLINE, the authors analyzed outcomes of surgical fixation of Vancouver type B_1 periprosthetic femoral fractures and compared ORIF with cortical strut grafts alone, ORIF with cable plate/compression plates alone, ORIF with both, and ORIF with locking plates alone. A total of 333 patients were included in the analysis. The overall complication rates were low, and union rates were high; however, the authors noted a significantly higher rate of nonunion as well as a higher rate of hardware failure in the group treated with locking plates. Level of evidence: III.

26. Moore RE, Baldwin K, Austin MS, Mehta S: A systematic review of open reduction and internal fixation of periprosthetic femur fractures with or without allograft strut, cerclage, and locked plates. *J Arthroplasty* 2014;29(5):872-876.

    This study searched MEDLINE over a 10-year period and included 682 patients from 37 papers. Comparisons between the use of allograft struts, plates (locking and nonlocking), and cerclage showed that the results for all methods were reproducibly reliable and achieved good union and complication rates. However, the authors cautioned against the routine use of allograft struts in type B_1 fractures because of the higher rate of infection and nonunion in this subset. Level of evidence: III.

27. Laurer HL, Wutzler S, Possner S, et al: Outcome after operative treatment of Vancouver type B1 and C periprosthetic femoral fractures: Open reduction and internal fixation versus revision arthroplasty. *Arch Orthop Trauma Surg* 2011;131(7):983-989.

    In this retrospective cohort study, the authors compared ORIF versus revision arthroplasty for type B_1 and C Vancouver fractures. With 16 patients in each group, functional outcomes using the Timed Up and Go test were comparable in each cohort. However, the ORIF group had a substantially higher complication rate, with most complications related to implant failure. Although this was an underpowered comparison, the authors hypothesized the high failure rates resulted from unrecognized loose stems (in type B_2 fractures) and advocated for a true assessment of implant stability intraoperatively. Level of evidence: III.

28. Liporace FA, Donegan DJ, Langford JR, Haidukewych GJ: Contemporary internal fixation techniques for periprosthetic fractures of the hip and knee. *Instr Course Lect* 2013;62:317-332.

    This case-based instructional lecture reviews the technical aspects and tips for treating periprosthetic fractures with the most contemporary implants and techniques. Special attention is given to more complex cases with severe bone loss. Level of evidence: V.

29. Berry DJ: Periprosthetic fractures associated with osteolysis: A problem on the rise. *J Arthroplasty* 2003;18(3suppl 1):107-111.

30. Macdonald SJ, Paprosky WG, Jablonsky WS, Magnus RG: Periprosthetic femoral fractures treated with a long-stem cementless component. *J Arthroplasty* 2001;16(3):379-383.

31. Wong P, Gross AE: The use of structural allografts for treating periprosthetic fractures about the hip and knee. *Orthop Clin North Am* 1999;30(2):259-264.

32. Abdel MP, Lewallen DG, Berry DJ: Periprosthetic femur fractures treated with modular fluted, tapered stems. *Clin Orthop Relat Res* 2014;472(2):599-603.

    In this study, 44 type B_2 and B_3 fractures were treated with modular fluted tapered stems. Good results were reported. The mean Harris hip score at a minimum follow-up of 2 years was 83, and there were five revisions for instability. The authors recommended having a low threshold for using a larger diameter femoral head to decrease the risk of further dislocation. Level of evidence: IV.

33. Amenabar T, Rahman WA, Avhad VV, Vera R, Gross AE, Kuzyk PR: Vancouver type B2 and B3 periprosthetic fractures treated with revision total hip arthroplasty. *Int Orthop* 2015;39(10):1927-1932.

    This retrospective review included outcomes and survivorship for 76 elderly patients who had undergone revision arthroplasty for Vancouver type B_2 and B_3 fractures. Midterm follow-up of approximately 6 years showed implant survivorship at 89.6%. The authors reported high patient mortality of 77.9% during the same interval. Level of evidence: IV.

34. Munro JT, Masri BA, Garbuz DS, Duncan CP: Tapered fluted modular titanium stems in the management of Vancouver B2 and B3 peri-prosthetic fractures. *Bone Joint J* 2013;95-B(11suppl A):17-20.

This study reported midterm implant survivorship in 55 patients. Kaplan-Meier analysis reported 96% modular, fluted stem survival at 54 months' follow-up in patients with type B_2 and B_3 Vancouver fractures. Level of evidence: IV.

35. Klein GR, Parvizi J, Rapuri V, et al: Proximal femoral replacement for the treatment of periprosthetic fractures. *J Bone Joint Surg Am* 2005;87(8):1777-1781.

36. Rorabeck CH, Angliss RD, Lewis PL: Fractures of the femur, tibia, and patella after total knee arthroplasty: Decision making and principles of management. *Instr Course Lect* 1998;47:449-458.

37. Aldrian S, Schuster R, Haas N, et al: Fixation of supracondylar femoral fractures following total knee arthroplasty: Is there any difference comparing angular stable plate fixation versus rigid interlocking nail fixation? *Arch Orthop Trauma Surg* 2013;133(7):921-927.

    This retrospective, cohort study compared ORIF and intramedullary nailing for periprosthetic supracondylar fractures. Eighty-six patients were evaluated (48 in the ORIF group and 38 in the intramedullary nailing group). Union rates and return to function were similar; however, those treated with intramedullary nailing exhibited slightly higher functional outcomes and satisfaction, although the outcomes were not statistically significant. Level of evidence: IV.

38. Gliatis J, Megas P, Panagiotopoulos E, Lambiris E: Midterm results of treatment with a retrograde nail for supracondylar periprosthetic fractures of the femur following total knee arthroplasty. *J Orthop Trauma* 2005;19(3):164-170.

39. Horneff JG III, Scolaro JA, Jafari SM, Mirza A, Parvizi J, Mehta S: Intramedullary nailing versus locked plate for treating supracondylar periprosthetic femur fractures. *Orthopedics* 2013;36(5):e561-e566.

    In this retrospective multicenter cohort study, the authors compared the union rates and outcomes for patients with supracondylar periprosthetic femoral fractures after ORIF with locked-plate fixation (n = 28) or intramedullary nailing (n = 35). The authors reported a significantly higher rate of union at 36 weeks for the group treated with locked-plate fixation and an overall lower rate of revision surgery. The authors recommended the use of a lateral locked plate. Level of evidence: IV.

40. Jassim SS, McNamara I, Hopgood P: Distal femoral replacement in periprosthetic fracture around total knee arthroplasty. *Injury* 2014;45(3):550-553.

    This retrospective case series reports the early 33-month results after distal femoral replacement in low-demand, ill patients with supracondylar femoral fractures. The authors used distal femoral replacement as a salvage procedure. No revision surgeries and an overall low complication rate were reported. Level of evidence: IV.

41. Saidi K, Ben-Lulu O, Tsuji M, Safir O, Gross AE, Backstein D: Supracondylar periprosthetic fractures of the knee in the elderly patients: A comparison of treatment using allograft-implant composites, standard revision components, distal femoral replacement prosthesis. *J Arthroplasty* 2014;29(1):110-114.

    This retrospective study compared outcomes between three groups: those with periprosthetic supracondylar knee fractures fixed with an allograft prosthesis composite (n = 7), those treated with complete revision (n = 9), and those treated with a distal femoral replacement endoprosthesis (n = 7). Although the study was underpowered, notable results were the shortest length of hospital stay and earliest mobilization in the group treated with a distal femoral replacement prosthesis. There was also less blood loss in the distal femoral prosthesis group than in the allograft composite group. Level of evidence: IV.

Section 8

Pediatrics

SECTION EDITOR

John M. Flynn, MD

Chapter 53

Fractures of the Upper Extremity in Children

Robert L. Wimberly, MD   Anthony I. Riccio, MD

Abstract

Upper extremity injuries are common in children and traditionally are treated without surgery; however, the literature continues to evolve. Most injuries quickly achieve union and rapid return of function is expected. Increased surgical management of clavicle fractures has been studied due to recent literature demonstrating better results after surgery in adults. Radial neck fractures continue to frustrate the surgeon, both in management and diagnosis. There is an abundance of literature on the most common fracture of the pediatric elbow, the supracondylar humerus fracture, but the treatment of the pink and pulseless elbow remains unresolved. Medial epicondyle fractures of the humerus and lateral humeral condyle fractures have good expected outcomes, but defining the original displacement is challenging. The treatment of forearm fractures is widely guided by the assumed skeletal maturity of the patient. Adolescent injuries are a focus of attention in the upper extremity, especially when remodeling is more limited.

Keywords: pediatric trauma; upper extremity trauma

Introduction

The traditional management of pediatric musculoskeletal injuries is largely nonsurgical given the remodeling potential of the growing skeleton. It is well understood that injuries adjacent to the physis in a skeletally immature patient will remodel well, especially when the deformity is in the plane of motion of the joint and the child has substantial growth remaining. The thick periosteum of the growing skeleton can aid in reduction and improve outcomes. Most injuries heal readily and children rapidly return to preinjury activities.

Dr. Wimberly or an immediate family member serves as a board member, owner, officer, or committee member of the Pediatric Orthopaedic Society of North America. Dr. Riccio or an immediate family member has received research or institutional support from Synthes and serves as a board member, owner, officer, or committee member of the Pediatric Orthopaedic Society of North America.

Clavicle Fractures

The treatment of clavicle fractures in children usually is nonsurgical, but findings from several studies have expanded the use of surgical treatment in adolescents. A 2007 multicenter randomized study compared the clinical outcomes of adults with a clavicle fracture after surgical or nonsurgical treatment. Patients who underwent surgery had better Constant Shoulder and Disabilities of the Arm, Shoulder and Hand scores as well as better malunion and nonunion rates and more rapid radiographic union than those treated nonsurgically.[1] According to a 2011 survey, most members of the Pediatric Orthopaedic Society of North America preferred nonsurgical management of clavicle fractures, regardless of the pattern.[2] However, there was an increase in the surgical treatment of adolescent patients near skeletal maturity with a displaced injury, especially if the injury was treated by a relatively young surgeon.

Before surgical treatment of a pediatric clavicle fracture is considered, it is important to examine the possibility of a complication or a poor outcome associated with nonsurgical management. The most common complications of nonsurgical management of a displaced fracture are nonunion, malunion, and impaired function. However, children usually do not have loss of function from a foreshortened malunion or pain from a nonunion. If a symptomatic malunion or nonunion does occur, later surgical correction has a good outcome.[3,4]

If necessary, plate fixation of a clavicle fracture can be done safely and predictably, with minimal morbidity. Union can be expected. The risk of malunion is potentially less than after nonsurgical treatment and the risk of loss of function is decreased. It is common for the patient to request removal of the implant because of its prominence, and many patients have peri-incision numbness.[2,5]

The indications for surgical treatment of displaced clavicle fracture are likely to continue to expand, especially for adolescent patients. Until a large prospective study defines the risks and benefits of fixation of clavicle fractures in patients who are skeletally immature, surgeons must continue to be guided by experience and small outcome studies. There is little current support for surgical treatment of closed, displaced clavicle fractures in pediatric patients.

Radial Neck Fractures

Radial neck fractures account for 5% to 10% of pediatric elbow injuries, and 30% to 50% of radial neck fractures are associated with another elbow injury.[6] Most pediatric proximal radial fractures are classified as a Salter-Harris type I or II injury. These fractures rarely involve the articular surface. Anatomic alignment is not required because remodeling is expected with growth. Most surgeons agree that angulation of less than 30° and translation of less than 2 mm is reasonable at any age, but that angulation of more than 60° is poorly tolerated at any age.[6] With 30° to 60° of angulation, there is less agreement on the treatment strategy. The maximum angulation may not be adequately represented on routine radiographic views of the elbow, and therefore the fracture should be examined under fluoroscopy. This study can be done in the emergency department, usually without anesthesia, while the extremity is gently manipulated to bring the maximum angulation into view. With translation, the radial head may tend to subluxate out of the capitellum with a cam type of displacement, and the potential for remodeling is decreased in this type of fracture.[6]

The most commonly reported complications after treatment of a radial neck fracture include loss of range of motion, radial head osteonecrosis, malunion, nonunion, heterotopic ossification, and proximal radioulnar synostosis. Acute compartment syndrome has been described after an isolated radial neck fracture.[7]

If the radial neck fracture is acceptably aligned or an acceptable alignment can be achieved with closed or percutaneous reduction, the typical treatment involves 3 to 4 weeks of immobilization in a long arm cast. Many methods of achieving a closed reduction have been described, including the use of an Esmarch bandage, to reduce the radial head and neck and the use of manual pressure over the radial head to reduce it back onto the proximal radial diaphysis. Percutaneous methods typically involve the insertion of a wire into the fracture to correct the angular deformity, after which the fragment is manipulated medially to correct translation (**Figure 1**). Regardless of the method, it is important to ensure that an acceptable, stable reduction has been achieved.[6]

Multiple surgical techniques are available for treating an unacceptably aligned radial neck fracture. Some radial neck fractures require an aggressive open approach to achieve acceptable alignment. A fracture that has early callus formation or is rotated 180°, is 90° to the radial shaft, or is medially displaced often requires an open reduction.

Retrograde intramedullary fixation and reduction is a popular surgical option.[8] In a partial modification of the original Métaizeau technique, the radial neck fracture is partially reduced percutaneously and the final translation or angular correction is achieved by passage of the retrograde intramedullary implant that crosses into the radial epiphysis. The reduction is achieved by rotation of the implant. The implant often is left external to the skin at the distal radius and is removed in the clinic 3 to 4 weeks later. The reported final outcomes of intramedullary management of radial neck fractures generally are good, but not always excellent, because of loss of motion, radial head overgrowth, or persistent malunion.[9-11]

Despite surgical improvement of alignment, many patients lose range of motion after healing. The most common factors contributing to poor final motion are patient age older than 10 years at the time of injury, the need for an open reduction to achieve alignment, and the presence of a severe injury pattern.[12] At final evaluation, patients treated with a noninvasive method generally have better motion than those treated surgically.[13]

The management of radial neck fractures remains imperfect. Acceptable alignment is necessary for achieving a satisfactory outcome, but the techniques used to reduce these fractures, as well as the injury itself, may lead to a less than ideal outcome.

Supracondylar Humerus Fractures

The Gartland classification is the most commonly used system to describe extension-type supracondylar humerus fractures. Type I fractures are nondisplaced. Type II fracture are displaced with an intact posterior hinge and type III fractures are displaced with no cortical continuity. Nondisplaced supracondylar humerus fractures can be safely and effectively treated using 3 to 4 weeks of cast immobilization. The preferred treatment of most displaced fractures is with closed reduction and percutaneous Kirschner wire fixation.[14] The management of type II supracondylar humerus fractures and supracondylar humerus fractures with an associated vascular abnormality or neurologic injury is controversial.

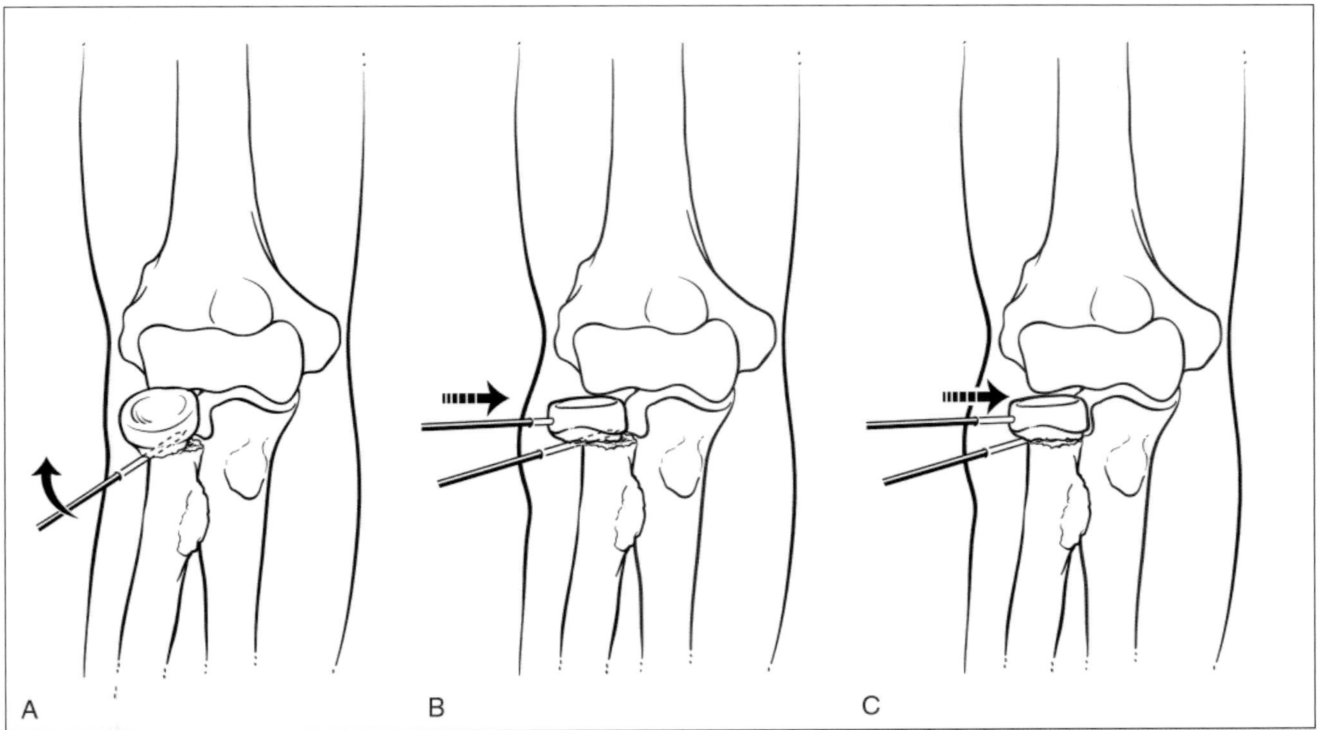

Figure 1 Schematic drawings showing percutaneous reduction of a displaced radial neck fracture. A 2.0 Kirschner wire is inserted into the fracture and used to lever the radial head into position **(A)**. If further translation of the fragment is needed, a second wire can be used **(B** and **C)**. (Courtesy of Stuart Almond, Dallas, TX.)

Certain type II supracondylar humerus fractures can successfully be managed nonsurgically in the absence of rotation, coronal plane angulation, or severe extension.[15] Delaying surgery more than 24 hours after a type II fracture occurs does not increase the risk of complications or an inferior clinical outcome.[16] Although nonsurgical management without reduction is rare, most children treated without surgery for a type II fracture have a good functional outcome despite possible cosmetic cubitus varus and elbow hyperextension.[17]

The management of patients with a well-perfused but pulseless hand in the presence of a supracondylar humerus fracture remains controversial. An emergency reduction should be done in an attempt to restore a palpable pulse. If the reduction fails to improve the vascular examination, the options include immediate vascular exploration or prolonged inpatient observation to monitor for diminishing perfusion or ischemia. Good evidence supports observational management, and one high-quality study reported universal recovery of a palpable radial pulse and a good functional outcome at final follow-up in all patients, despite documented occlusion of the brachial artery.[18]

Intraoperative and postoperative Doppler examination can be helpful in the absence of a palpable pulse. Clinical observation without vascular exploration in patients who have a nonpalpable, dopplerable pulse and good perfusion of the hand has led to low rates of vascular decline and near-universal return of a palpable pulse before hospital discharge or the initial follow-up visit.[19]

Approximately 11% of patients with a supracondylar humerus fracture have an associated neurapraxia. Injury to the anterior interosseous nerve is the most commonly encountered neurapraxia in an extension-type fracture.[20] Anterior interosseous nerve injury without sensory changes was once believed to require urgent treatment, but treatment as late as 24 hours after injury has not led to an increase in the time to recovery of neurologic function or an increased incidence of complications.[21] Urgent treatment may be needed if there is concomitant nerve injury, a vascular deficit, severe soft-tissue swelling, sensory deficits, or an ipsilateral forearm fracture. A twofold increase in associated neurologic injury was found in patients with an ipsilateral forearm fracture requiring manipulative reduction.[22]

Pin constructs and pin diameters used in the surgical fixation of supracondylar humerus fractures have been extensively studied.[23,24] Biomechanical studies found that stability of the fixation construct does vary with both pin pattern and the use of a large-diameter wire, but no study found a difference in clinical outcomes based

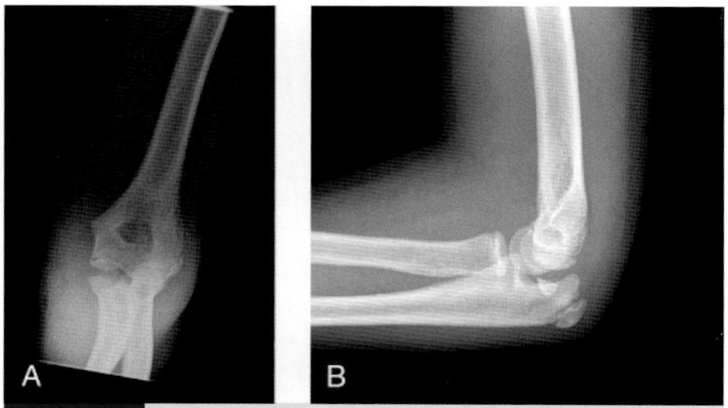

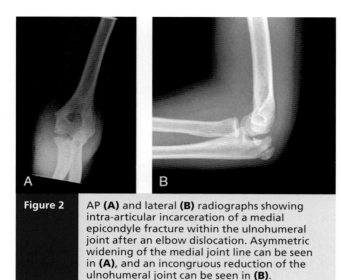

Figure 2 AP **(A)** and lateral **(B)** radiographs showing intra-articular incarceration of a medial epicondyle fracture within the ulnohumeral joint after an elbow dislocation. Asymmetric widening of the medial joint line can be seen in **(A)**, and an incongruous reduction of the ulnohumeral joint can be seen in **(B)**.

on the choice of pin construct or diameter. Regardless of the fixation technique, the surgeon should assess the reduction for stability after fixation.

Medial Epicondyle Fractures of the Humerus

No classification system of medial epicondyle humerus fractures is widely accepted for guiding treatment. In addition, no evidence is available to support the choice of surgical or nonsurgical treatment of these fractures based on displacement, nor is there consensus on the best means of measuring fracture displacement. Plain radiography alone may be insufficient to accurately determine displacement, and CT may be required.[25]

A fracture that is nondisplaced or minimally displaced (less than 5 to 10 mm) often is managed with a brief period of immobilization. The recommended treatment involves a 3-week period of immobilization in a long arm cast, followed by active range-of-motion exercises and limited activity until full range of motion is restored and the fracture is radiographically or clinically healed.

Surgical treatment is absolutely indicated for an open fracture or a fracture with incarceration of the medial epicondyle fragment in the ulnohumeral joint. Approximately 50% of all medial epicondyle fractures are associated with an elbow dislocation, and intra-articular incarceration is not rare.[26] An entrapped bony fragment is detected as joint incongruity on lateral or AP radiographs (**Figure 2**). Surgical treatment is relatively indicated if the patient has gross elbow instability or ulnar nerve dysfunction or is an athlete requiring use of the upper extremity. Patient satisfaction and functional outcomes do not vary significantly based on whether the treatment is surgical or nonsurgical.[27]

In a medial humeral epicondyle fracture, the flexor-pronator mass of the forearm displaces the medial epicondyle fragment distally and anteriorly. Relaxation of the deforming musculature can be achieved with the patient in a prone position and the elbow flexed 90° to facilitate reduction and fixation. Although the ulnar nerve is in proximity to the fracture bed, it does not require routine mobilization. Fixation is achieved with a single, partially threaded cannulated screw placed over a threaded guidewire, often with a washer to distribute compressive forces and minimize comminution during final tightening. The use of a second guidewire is recommended for provisional fixation, and the use of a derotation device is recommended during screw placement. The provisional or derotational guidewire may inhibit compression and should be removed prior to final screw tightening. Kirschner wire fixation may be preferable if the epicondyle is too small to accommodate a screw. Because stiffness has been reported after fixation, active range-of-motion exercises should begin within 3 to 4 weeks.

Lateral Condyle Fractures of the Humerus

Nondisplaced lateral condyle fractures and those with less than 2 mm of intra-articular displacement often are managed with 4 weeks of long arm cast immobilization. Weekly radiography can be helpful to ensure maintenance of reduction. The follow-up radiographs are best obtained without the cast and should include an internal oblique view, which often reveals articular displacement that cannot be seen on an AP view.

Classification systems have attempted to differentiate stable and unstable lateral condyle fracture patterns based on the extent of the fracture line and amount of displacement.[28] A stable fracture that hinges through an intact articular surface is treated with closed reduction and percutaneous Kirschner wire fixation. An unstable fracture or a fracture displaced more than 2 mm is best managed with open reduction and wire fixation to ensure anatomic alignment of the articular surface, although closed reduction and pin fixation has also proved successful.[28,29] Two- or three-pin fixation with maximal pin divergence at the fracture site usually provides sufficient stability.[30] Leaving the pins exposed rather than burying them in a subcutaneous position is safe and cost-effective, and this technique avoids the need for pin removal under anesthesia.[31]

Forearm Fractures

The management of forearm fractures usually is nonsurgical in children and many adolescents. The expectation of remodeling with growth permits acceptance of significant displacement in many injuries, especially if the fracture is adjacent to the physis or is displaced in the plane of motion of the adjacent joint. The use of a short arm cast molded only to reduce angular deformity was reported for treatment of overriding distal radius fractures in children age 3 to 10 years.[32] Near-complete remodeling was achieved at 1-year follow-up. Analgesia or sedation was not used in the treatment. The expense of treatment was five to six times greater if general anesthesia was used during injury reduction and as much as nine times greater if percutaneous pin fixation was used.

For nonsurgical treatment of a forearm fracture, immobilization in a long arm cast often is chosen to limit pronation and supination and reduce the risk of redisplacement. Although a well-molded, well-fitting cast undoubtedly is critical to the maintenance of reduction, the choice of a long arm or short arm cast is under scrutiny. In the treatment of displaced distal-third forearm fractures, some evidence supports the use of a well-fitted short arm cast. The benefits of short arm casting include greater ease in activities of daily living and a decrease in the number of missed school days.[33,34] Recent studies assessed the risk factors for redisplacement of forearm fractures. Relatively great initial displacement, nonanatomic initial reduction, poor casting technique, patient age older than 10 years, and a proximal-third fracture were associated with a greater likelihood of loss of reduction.[35-37]

Open forearm fractures and fractures that cannot be adequately maintained in a cast often require surgical treatment. Intramedullary fixation of the radius and/or ulna through closed or open reduction often is done in a skeletally immature patient, although some surgeons prefer open reduction and plating. There has been an increase in the number of forearm fractures managed with surgical fixation. Studies have found approximately 90% good to excellent outcomes after surgical fixation of forearm fractures using an intramedullary device or plating.[38-41] If intramedullary fixation is chosen, the fracture site may need to be opened to allow safe passage of the implant. An opened fracture site, whether in an open fracture or for nail passage, is associated with a well-established increase in the rate of delayed union, especially in patients older than 10 years.[38-41] This issue has led physicians to attempt single-bone fixation for certain forearm injuries, which can lead to good clinical results but may increase the rate of radius malunion, especially in an open fracture. Both-bone fixation may be beneficial in older patients to avoid loss of motion from a radius malunion.[42]

The traditional management of open forearm fractures involves the use of antibiotics, formal irrigation and débridement of the open wound site in the operating room, and often internal stabilization to achieve soft-tissue rest. The possibility of managing these fractures with short-term use of antibiotics as well as irrigation and débridement in the emergency department continues to be investigated. Small studies found no increase in the risk of infection in comparison with traditional surgical débridement.[43,44] Until better-powered studies are completed, the recommendation is to continue to treat an open fracture with immediately administered antibiotics followed by surgical irrigation and débridement, with or without implant stabilization.

Summary

As patients approach skeletal maturity, the remodeling potential of injuries is reduced and the need for an anatomic reduction becomes more important. In pediatric upper extremity fractures, the surgeon must not only understand the injury and possible sequelae of treatment, but also consider the risks and benefits of surgery when compared to nonsurgical management. Rapid healing of the fracture and return to normal activity can be expected in most pediatric injuries. The literature continues to evolve and will improve surgeons' ability to manage upper extremity pediatric orthopaedic injuries.

Key Study Points

- Nonsurgical management is the mainstay of treatment for most pediatric orthopaedic upper extremity injuries in skeletally immature patients.
- Skeletally mature adolescent patients with significantly displaced clavicle fractures may benefit from surgical fixation.
- There is not a consensus in the management of the pink, pulseless supracondylar humerus fracture. In the presence of a supracondylar humerus fracture with ischemia, urgent reduction should be performed in an attempt to re-establish perfusion.
- The pediatric orthopaedic surgeon must be confident in identifying and assessing the displacement of medial humeral epicondyle and lateral humeral condyle fractures in skeletally immature patients.
- With good technique, almost all skeletally immature forearm fractures can be managed without surgery.

Annotated References

1. Canadian Orthopaedic Trauma Society: Nonoperative treatment compared with plate fixation of displaced midshaft clavicular fractures: A multicenter, randomized clinical trial. *J Bone Joint Surg Am* 2007;89(1):1-10.

2. Vander Have KL, Perdue AM, Caird MS, Farley FA: Operative versus nonoperative treatment of midshaft clavicle fractures in adolescents. *J Pediatr Orthop* 2010;30(4):307-312.

   In a study of consecutive adolescent patients with a clavicle fracture, the 17 patients treated with plate fixation had a more rapid time to union than the 25 patients treated nonsurgically. Four patients treated without surgery went on to corrective osteotomy for symptomatic nonunion.

3. Schulz J, Moor M, Roocroft J, Bastrom TP, Pennock AT: Functional and radiographic outcomes of nonoperative treatment of displaced adolescent clavicle fractures. *J Bone Joint Surg Am* 2013;95(13):1159-1165.

   In a retrospective study of 16 adolescent patients treated without surgery for a midshaft clavicle fracture, little or no difference in pain, strength, shoulder range of motion, or subjective outcome scores was found, regardless of patient age, sports participation, or final clavicle shortening.

4. Bae DS, Shah AS, Kalish LA, Kwon JY, Waters PM: Shoulder motion, strength, and functional outcomes in children with established malunion of the clavicle. *J Pediatr Orthop* 2013;33(5):544-550.

   Sixteen skeletally immature patients with malunion of the clavicle had excellent functional outcomes after nonsurgical management. Routine fixation of a displaced clavicle fracture in a skeletally immature patient is unwarranted if based solely on concern about loss of future shoulder function or strength.

5. Namdari S, Ganley TJ, Baldwin K, et al: Fixation of displaced midshaft clavicle fractures in skeletally immature patients. *J Pediatr Orthop* 2011;31(5):507-511.

   A review of 14 skeletally immature patients with plate fixation of a clavicle fracture found that the procedure was reproducible and safe at a minimum 24-month follow-up. Peri-incision numbness was reported by 8 patients (57%), and 4 had elective removal of symptomatic implants after union.

6. Pring ME: Pediatric radial neck fractures: When and how to fix. *J Pediatr Orthop* 2012;32(Suppl 1):S14-S21.

   Current recommendations on the treatment of radial neck fractures were summarized based on reports presented to an expert panel of surgeons at the 2010 annual meeting of the Pediatric Orthopaedic Society of North America.

7. Peters CL, Scott SM: Compartment syndrome in the forearm following fractures of the radial head or neck in children. *J Bone Joint Surg Am* 1995;77(7):1070-1074.

8. Metaizeau JP, Lascombes P, Lemelle JL, Finlayson D, Prevot, J: Reduction and fixation of displaced radial neck fractures by closed intramedullary nailing. *J Pediatr Orthop* 1993;13(3):355-60.

9. Tarallo L, Mugnai R, Fiacchi F, Capra F, Catani F: Management of displaced radial neck fractures in children: Percutaneous pinning vs. elastic stable intramedullary nailing. *J Orthop Traumatol* 2013;14(4):291-297.

   At an average 42 months after surgery, approximately 70% of patients with percutaneous pinning or intramedullary fixation of a radial neck fracture had an excellent Mayo Elbow score.

10. Wang J, Chen W, Guo M, Su Y, Zhang Y: Percutaneous reduction and intramedullary fixation technique for displaced pediatric radial neck fractures. *J Pediatr Orthop B* 2013;22(2):127-132.

    At an average 37-month follow-up of 21 patients after treatment of a radial neck fracture with percutaneous reduction and intramedullary fixation, 15 patients had an excellent outcome, 6 had a good outcome, and 3 had a malunion.

11. Luo J, Halanski MA, Noonan KJ: The Métaizeau technique for pediatric radial neck fracture with elbow dislocation: Intraoperative pitfalls and associated forearm compartment syndrome. *Am J Orthop (Belle Mead NJ)* 2014;43(3):137-140.

    Two radial neck fractures associated with elbow dislocation were treated using the Métaizeau intramedullary technique.

12. Zimmerman RM, Kalish LA, Hresko MT, Waters PM, Bae DS: Surgical management of pediatric radial neck fractures. *J Bone Joint Surg Am* 2013;95(20):1825-1832.

    A retrospective analysis of 151 children with a radial neck fracture assessed posttreatment range of motion and outcome. Patients older than 10 years, those with a severe fracture, and those with an open reduction were most likely to have a poor outcome.

13. Basmajian HG, Choi PD, Huh K, Sankar WN, Wells L, Arkader A: Radial neck fractures in children: Experience from two level-1 trauma centers. *J Pediatr Orthop B* 2014;23(4):369-374.

    Radial neck fracture treatment at two centers over 17 years were retrospectively reviewed and compared. The surgical treatment required to achieve an acceptable fracture reduction was a surrogate for injury severity. A poor outcome was most likely to occur after aggressive treatment.

14. Mulpuri K, Wilkins K: The treatment of displaced supracondylar humerus fractures: Evidence-based guideline. *J Pediatr Orthop* 2012;32(Suppl 2):S143-S152.

    A review of 44 scientific articles included evidence-based recommendations on the treatment of displaced supracondylar humerus fractures, selection of fixation constructs, and complications of open reduction of irreducible fractures.

15. Spencer HT, Dorey FJ, Zionts LE, Dichter DH, Wong MA, Moazzaz P, Silva M: Type II supracondylar humerus fractures: Can some be treated nonoperatively? *J Pediatr Orthop* 2012;32(7):675-681.

    In a comparison study of outcomes after type II supracondylar humerus fractures were treated surgically or nonsurgically, 21% of fractures treated nonsurgically lost alignment and required surgery. Fractures without rotational deformity, coronal angulation, or significant extension were most likely to be successfully treated without surgery.

16. Larson AN, Garg S, Weller A, Fletcher ND, Schiller JR, Kwon M, Browne R, et al: Operative treatment of type II supracondylar humerus fractures: Does time to surgery affect complications? *J Pediatr Orthop* 2014;34(4):382-387.

    In 399 type II supracondylar fractures, no differences were identified in the rate of major or minor complications based on whether patients were treated within 24 hours of injury or later.

17. Moraleda L, Valencia M, Barco R, González-Moran G: Natural history of unreduced Gartland type-II supracondylar fractures of the humerus in children: A two to thirteen-year follow-up study. *J Bone Joint Surg Am* 2013;95(1):28-34.

    At long-term follow-up, 46 children with an unreduced type II supracondylar humerus fracture had a small but significant increase in elbow extension and cubitus varus compared with the contralateral elbow. Validated outcome measures found low disability and good function in most patients.

18. Scannell BP, Jackson JB III, Bray C, Roush TS, Brighton BK, Frick SL: The perfused, pulseless supracondylar humeral fracture: Intermediate-term follow-up of vascular status and function. *J Bone Joint Surg Am* 2013;95(21):1913-1919.

    Twenty patients with a pulseless, well-perfused supracondylar humerus fracture treated with closed reduction, pinning, and observation had a palpable radial pulse at 20-month follow-up and good to excellent outcomes scores, although five patients had a brachial artery occlusion on duplex ultrasound.

19. Weller A, Garg S, Larson AN, et al: Management of the pediatric pulseless supracondylar humeral fracture: Is vascular exploration necessary? *J Bone Joint Surg Am* 2013;95(21):1906-1912.

    In a review of 54 supracondylar humerus fractures without a palpable pulse, absence of a radial pulse after reduction and fixation was found not to be an absolute indication for vascular exploration as long as the hand was perfused and the patient received careful postoperative inpatient monitoring.

20. Babal JC, Mehlman CT, Klein G: Nerve injuries associated with pediatric supracondylar humeral fractures: A meta-analysis. *J Pediatr Orthop* 2010;30(3):253-263.

    In a meta-analysis of 5,154 displaced supracondylar humerus fractures, the incidence of nerve injury was 11.3%. In extension-type fractures, 34% of neurapraxias involved the anterior interosseous nerve. In flexion-type injuries, 91% of neurapraxias involved the ulnar nerve.

21. Barrett KK, Skaggs DL, Sawyer JR, Andras L, Moisan A, Goodbody C, Flynn JM: Supracondylar humeral fractures with isolated anterior interosseous nerve injuries: Is urgent treatment necessary? *J Bone Joint Surg Am* 2014;96(21):1793-1797.

    A review of 35 patients with a supracondylar humerus fracture and isolated anterior interosseous nerve palsy without sensory deficits found that a delay in surgery up to 24 hours was not associated with an increased rate of complications or an increased time to recovery of nerve function.

22. Muchow RD, Riccio AI, Garg S, Ho CA, Wimberly RL: Neurological and vascular injury associated with supracondylar humerus fractures and ipsilateral forearm fractures in children. *J Pediatr Orthop* 2015;35(2):121-125.

    Patients with a surgically-treated supracondylar humerus fracture and an ipsilateral forearm fracture had twice the rate of neurologic injury as patients with an isolated, surgically-treated supracondylar fracture (14.8% versus 7.8%).

23. Gottschalk HP, Sagoo D, Glaser D, Doan J, Edmonds EW, Schlechter J: Biomechanical analysis of pin placement for pediatric supracondylar humerus fractures: Does starting point, pin size, and number matter? *J Pediatr Orthop* 2012;32(5):445-451.

    In this biomechanical study using a synthetic supracondylar humerus model, 2.0-mm pins provided greater rotational stability than 1.6-mm pins. A capitellar starting point provided greater rotational stability than a lateral starting point.

24. Srikumaran U, Tan EW, Belkoff SM, et al: Enhanced biomechanical stiffness with large pins in the operative treatment of pediatric supracondylar humerus fractures. *J Pediatr Orthop* 2012;32(2):201-205.

    In a biomechanical study using a synthetic supracondylar humerus model, two 2.8-mmpins placed in either a crossed medial and lateral configuration or a divergent lateral configuration conferred greater sagittal plane stability than two 1.6-mmpins placed in a divergent lateral configuration. Crossed 1.6-mm wires provided greater construct stiffness than lateral divergent 1.6-mm wires.

25. Edmonds EW: How displaced are "nondisplaced" fractures of the medial humeral epicondyle in children? Results of a three-dimensional computed tomography analysis. *J Bone Joint Surg Am* 2010;92(17):2785-2791.

    Displacement of 11 medial epicondyle fractures was assessed with plain radiography and CT. CT identified significantly greater anterior displacement and significantly less medial displacement than plain radiographs.

26. Patel NM, Ganley TJ: Medial epicondyle fractures of the humerus: How to evaluate and when to operate. *J Pediatr Orthop* 2012;32(Suppl 1):S10-S13.

A review article explored current controversies and treatment recommendations for medial epicondyle fractures of the humerus.

27. Lawrence JT, Patel NM, Macknin J, Flynn JM, Cameron D, Wolfgruber HC, Ganley TJ: Return to competitive sports after medial epicondyle fractures in adolescent athletes: Results of operative and nonoperative treatment. *Am J Sports Med* 2013;41(5):1152-1157.

In a comparison of functional outcomes after surgical or nonsurgical treatment of medial epicondyle fractures in young athletes, all patients, regardless of treatment, reported high levels of satisfaction, had excellent Disabilities of the Arm, Shoulder and Hand scores, and were able to return to overhead throwing activities.

28. Song KS, Kang CH, Min BW, Bae KC, Cho CH, Lee JH: Closed reduction and internal fixation of displaced unstable lateral condylar fractures of the humerus in children. *J Bone Joint Surg Am* 2008;90(12):2673-2681.

29. Song KS, Shin YW, Oh CW, Bae KC, Cho CH: Closed reduction and internal fixation of completely displaced and rotated lateral condyle fractures of the humerus in children. *J Orthop Trauma* 2010;24(7):434-438.

The feasibility of closed reduction and fixation of displaced rotated lateral condyle fractures was evaluated. Twelve of 24 displaced rotated lateral condyle fractures were successfully reduced to less than 2 mm of displacement, without complications, using a closed reduction technique.

30. Bloom T, Chen LY, Sabharwal S: Biomechanical analysis of lateral humeral condyle fracture pinning. *J Pediatr Orthop* 2011;31(2):130-137.

In two-pin constructs, increased pin divergence provided greater stability in torsional and valgus loading in a lateral condyle fracture model. The use of a third pin conferred greater torsional stability and stability in valgus and varus loading than the use of two pins.

31. Das De S, Bae DS, Waters PM: Displaced humeral lateral condyle fractures in children: Should we bury the pins? *J Pediatr Orthop* 2012;32(6):573-578.

Patients with a displaced lateral condyle fracture who were treated with pin fixation using buried wires had higher rates of skin and implant complications without a decrease in the rate of nonunion, compared with those in whom the wires were left exposed.

32. Crawford SN, Lee LS, Izuka BH: Closed treatment of overriding distal radial fractures without reduction in children. *J Bone Joint Surg Am* 2012;94(3):246-252.

Fifty-one children with an overriding distal radius fracture were managed with simple alignment of the coronal and sagittal deformity and application of a short arm cast without anesthesia. Parental satisfaction was high, alignment was excellent, and the treatment was cost-effective.

33. Webb GR, Galpin RD, Armstrong DG: Comparison of short and long arm plaster casts for displaced fractures in the distal third of the forearm in children. *J Bone Joint Surg Am* 2006;88(1):9-17.

34. Bohm ER, Bubbar V, Yong Hing K, Dzus A: Above and below-the-elbow plaster casts for distal forearm fractures in children. A randomized controlled trial. *J Bone Joint Surg Am* 2006;88(1):1-8.

35. Bowman EN, Mehlman CT, Lindsell CJ, Tamai J: Nonoperative treatment of both-bone forearm shaft fractures in children: Predictors of early radiographic failure. *J Pediatr Orthop* 2011;31(1):23-32.

Patients older than 10 years, those with a proximal-third radius fracture, and those with ulnar angulation greater than 15° had the greatest risk for unsuccessful nonsurgical management of a forearm fracture.

36. Kamat AS, Pierse N, Devane P, Mutimer J, Horne G: Redefining the cast index: The optimum technique to reduce redisplacement in pediatric distal forearm fractures. *J Pediatr Orthop* 2012;32(8):787-791.

A review of more than 1,000 patients with a distal forearm fracture treated with reduction and casting found that fractures with a cast index higher than 0.81 were most likely to lose alignment.

37. McQuinn AG, Jaarsma RL: Risk factors for redisplacement of pediatric distal forearm and distal radius fractures. *J Pediatr Orthop* 2012;32(7):687-692.

Twenty-one percent of patients had a loss of reduction in a distal forearm fracture. In comparison with other patients, those at highest risk had greater initial displacement, a nonanatomic initial reduction, and a less well-molded cast upon cast index review.

38. Flynn JM, Jones KJ, Garner MR, Goebel J: Eleven years experience in the operative management of pediatric forearm fractures. *J Pediatr Orthop* 2010;30(4):313-319.

An increasing frequency of surgical management of diaphyseal forearm fractures was found over an 11-year period. Intramedullary nailing had a 14.6% complication rate, and delayed union was found when fracture sites were opened. In 29% of surgical procedures for intramedullary nailing, the fracture site had to be opened to allow nail passage.

39. Baldwin K, Morrison MJ III, Tomlinson LA, Ramirez R, Flynn JM: Both bone forearm fractures in children and adolescents: Which fixation strategy is superior - plates or nails? A systematic review and meta-analysis of observational studies. *J Orthop Trauma* 2014;28(1):e8-e14.

A meta-analysis found that orthopaedic research supports both intramedullary fixation and plate fixation for the surgical treatment of forearm fractures in children.

40. Martus JE, Preston RK, Schoenecker JG, Lovejoy SA, Green NE, Mencio GA: Complications and outcomes of diaphyseal forearm fracture intramedullary nailing:

8: Pediatrics

A comparison of pediatric and adolescent age groups. *J Pediatr Orthop* 2013;33(6):598-607.

Intramedullary nailing leads to a good to excellent outcome in 90% of patients. The reported complication rate was 17%. Patients older than 10 years were twice as likely as younger patients to have delayed union or another complication.

41. Lobo-Escolar A, Roche A, Bregante J, Gil-Alvaroba J, Sola A, Herrera A: Delayed union in pediatric forearm fractures. *J Pediatr Orthop* 2012;32(1):54-57.

    In a case-control study, patients with a forearm fracture were most likely to have a delay in union after treatment with an open reduction.

42. Dietz JF, Bae DS, Reiff E, Zurakowski D, Waters PM: Single bone intramedullary fixation of the ulna in pediatric both bone forearm fractures: Analysis of short-term clinical and radiographic results. *J Pediatr Orthop* 2010;30(5):420-424.

    Thirty-four percent of patients treated with single-bone intramedullary fixation of the ulna had more than 10° of radial angulation at final follow-up. Loss of alignment of the radius was most common in open fractures. Both-bone fixation should be considered in older children.

43. Iobst CA, Spurdle C, Baitner AC, King WF, Tidwell M, Swirsky S: A protocol for the management of pediatric type I open fractures. *J Child Orthop* 2014;8(1):71-76.

    Forty-five consecutive patients with a type I open forearm fracture were treated with a protocol of intravenous antibiotics as well as emergency department irrigation and débridement with reduction and casting. No infections were reported.

44. Bazzi AA, Brooks JT, Jain A, Ain MC, Tis JE, Sponseller PD: Is nonoperative treatment of pediatric type I open fractures safe and effective? *J Child Orthop* 2014;8(6):467-471.

    Forty patients with a type I open forearm or tibia fracture were treated in the emergency department with irrigation and débridement and closed reduction and casting. There were no reported infections. A retained foreign body was surgically removed after 4 weeks in one patient.

8: Pediatrics

Chapter 54

Pediatric Spine Trauma

Daniel Hedequist, MD

Abstract

Traumatic spinal injury is rare in children; the age of the patient and mechanism of injury are factors related to the injury. Management begins with transport from the field as well as appropriate initial physical examination. Radiographic studies include plain films followed by CT and MRI when needed. Analysis of plain radiographs must take into account normal anatomic variations in children. Younger children are predisposed to injuries of the upper cervical spine secondary to a relatively large head-to-body ratio, whereas adolescents sustain injuries more commonly seen in adulthood. Pediatric injuries such as odontoid fractures through the synchondrosis, spinal cord injury without radiographic abnormality, and Chance fractures resulting from inappropriately applied lap belts are unique to children. Management of fractures ranges from closed treatment with an orthosis to surgical treatment of unstable fractures or fractures associated with a neurologic deficit.

Keywords: pediatric; spine trauma; vertebral fractures

Introduction

Spine fractures represent about 1% of all fractures seen in children in level 1 trauma centers. The actual incidence is difficult to ascertain given the variation in reporting. The pattern and cause of spinal injury are age related. The anatomic differences in children vary. Younger children, who have a large head-to-body ratio, account for more upper cervical spine injuries, whereas adolescents sustain mostly lumbar injuries. Motor vehicle accidents (MVAs) are the leading cause of fracture in all age groups. Falls are the second most common injury mechanism in younger children, whereas sports injuries are the second most common injury mechanism in older children. According to a 2014 review article, spinal injuries in toddlers younger than 3 years are associated with nonaccidental trauma in up to 19% of cases and have a 25% mortality rate.[1] A retrospective 20-year review of spinal trauma has shown that noncontiguous spinal injuries also become associated with nonspinal injuries as the patient's Injury Severity Score increases.[2]

Dr. Hedequist or an immediate family member serves as a board member, owner, officer, or committee member of the American Academy of Orthopaedic Surgeons and the Pediatric Orthopaedic Society of North America.

Anatomy

The anatomic differences between children and adolescents predispose each age group to differing injury patterns. Children younger than 8 years have more horizontally aligned cervical facets, greater ligamentous laxity, and a larger head-to-body ratio, all of which predispose them to upper cervical spine injuries at occiput-C1 and C1-C2. Younger children also have open cartilaginous growth centers known as synchondroses, and the largest of these is located at the dens, which makes odontoid fractures much more common in younger children. The dentocentral synchondrosis fuses at around 6 years of age. Before that age, younger children are at risk of sustaining an injury at the dens through this growth center. Subaxial spine fractures, thoracic burst/compression fractures, and lumbar injuries become more common as children develop more adult-like anatomy after 10 years of age.

Initial Evaluation

The initial evaluation of a child with suspected spinal trauma begins on the field. Children pose unique transport challenges because of their small size and anatomic differences. On the field, children must be placed in cervical collars, and increased stability must be obtained by taping their heads to sandbags or intravenous bags placed on either side of the head to further minimize cervical motion. The larger head size in children predisposes them to inadvertent flexion because of the occipital prominence;

this flexion must be counteracted by placing the child on a backboard with an occipital recess or by elevating the body with blankets. The initial physical examination should focus on Advanced Trauma Life Support surveys, followed by a thorough secondary survey of the child that includes a detailed neurologic examination. The evaluation of a child with suspected thoracolumbar spine trauma should begin after a thorough primary survey, given the association of spinal trauma with other injuries. The clinical evaluation of the back is performed via standard inspection and palpation of the entire area, with care taken to logroll the patient using spine precautions. A detailed neurologic examination needs to be performed and documented, given the potential association with spinal cord injury (SCI). Because of the risk of lap belt injuries in children, inspection and palpation of the anterior abdominal wall and pelvic region are critical in younger children involved in MVAs.

Radiographic Studies

In the acute trauma setting, standard radiographs remain the initial imaging modality of choice for pediatric patients. At minimum, the required radiographs should include a cross-table lateral view with an anterior posterior view of the cervical spine. Plain radiographs of the thoracic and lumbar spine should be obtained in cases of suspected injury, based on physical examination findings, associated injuries, or the history. The analysis of pediatric radiographs is challenging, especially before 8 years of age, because normal anatomic variations exist that may be mistaken for fractures or ligamentous injury.[3] Ossification centers—most commonly the dens before age 5 years—can be mistaken for a fracture line. Vertebral height differences and differences in morphology exist that may be mistaken for compression fractures. These differences need to be considered in the context of the physical examination findings. Cervical pseudosubluxation due to ligamentous laxity (most commonly C2 on C3), the loss of normal cervical lordosis, and increased apparent anterior soft-tissue swelling from crying all are examples of normal variants that could be encountered in the pediatric cervical spine. Subtle wedging of the thoracic and lumbar vertebra and apparent disk irregularities such as Schmorl nodes all must be considered in the context of the history and physical examination. Further imaging should be based on a complete evaluation.

CT is used when evaluating a suspected bony or ligamentous injury. The use of CT in cervical screening has become more commonplace, especially in more severely injured children. According to a 2013 study, CT has been shown to be as efficacious as MRI in clearing the cervical spine of severely injured children, avoiding the need for cervical collars and spine precautions in obtunded patients.[4] In pediatric patients who are obtunded and require clearance, MRI remains the gold standard. Routine use of CT as a screening tool for cervical injuries is not appropriate, however, because of the high radiation dosing and the ability to diagnose most suspected injuries using plain radiographs and the physical examination. The use of CT for thoracic and lumbar spine injuries should be limited to the study of documented fractures. Before ordering these studies, discussion with the trauma team regarding any potential need for thoracic or abdominal CT for associated injuries is warranted. In patients who have already undergone abdominal or chest CT as part of their trauma work-up, additional dedicated spine CT is not needed, because the trauma CT can yield information regarding fractures. CT angiography should be considered in patients with cervical facet fractures or fractures through the foramen, given the potential for vertebral artery injury with these associated patterns.[5]

In spinal trauma, MRI may be obtained for clearance and for the documentation of known injuries. The authors of a 2013 study reported that in children with multiple injuries or those who are obtunded, MRI remains an excellent cervical screening tool, yielding high sensitivity and specificity within the first 48 hours of injury.[6] MRI remains a critical study in the evaluation of suspected ligamentous injuries, disk injuries, and SCIs. Any patient with a neurologic deficit should have undergo MRI to determine the extent of neurologic injury and/or compression, because the information it produces may aid in treatment decisions. Patients who require the surgical treatment of spinal trauma also should undergo MRI of the associated area as well as CT, to clearly identify the extent of bony, ligamentous, and neural injuries.

Types of Injuries

Spinal Cord Injury Without Radiologic Abnormality

SCI without radiologic abnormality is a traumatic entity seen in children who present with neurologic dysfunction of varying degree with no evidence of injury on radiologic or CT studies. It is seen most frequently with cervical injuries, although it may be observed in other areas of the spine. It is thought to result from the elasticity of the younger child's spine and a stretch phenomenon to the spinal column during injury. This stretch returns the bony and ligamentous structures back to the preinjury level, thus making radiographic determination of injury difficult, but the spinal cord, which inherently does not tolerate stretch, becomes injured, resulting in neurologic injury. The neurologic dysfunction ranges from mild to complete SCI. MRI has become very useful in documenting the injury to the spinal cord and the surrounding structures when other studies reveal no injury. Management is based on the determination of any occult bony or ligamentous injury, which requires treatment to prevent further deterioration. Neurologic outcomes depend on the degree of injury to the spinal cord and the initial physical examination of the neurologic system. The more severe the neurologic findings on initial examination, the greater the potential for permanent neurologic injury. The prognosis for less severe injuries is improved.

Atlanto-occipital Dissociation

Injuries to the cranial-vertebral junction include ligament injuries, fractures, and combined injuries. Occipital condyle fractures are more common in the adolescent population than in younger children and necessitate further evaluation of the supporting ligamentous structures to rule out more substantial injury. Injuries to the atlanto-occipital region are high-energy injuries caused by a sudden deceleration while the head is moving forward on the cervical spine. These injuries can be subtle and difficult to diagnose, or they may be highly unstable injuries such as atlanto-occipital dissociations. Usually they are fatal injuries; however, improvement in modern emergency medical systems that provide rapid stabilization and transport have allowed survival in some children. Modern imaging techniques and a high degree of suspicion by the clinician also account for improved diagnostic capabilities for these injuries. They often can be difficult to ascertain, given the challenges in assessing the craniovertebral junction with plain radiographs. Correlation of MRI findings with the degree of injury can be difficult; however, any distraction is highly suggestive of an unstable injury. Patients present with neck pain and associated injuries and may have a lateral gaze palsy due to cranial nerve injury. In patients with true atlanto-occipital dissociations, an instrumented occiput-to-cervical fusion is required. The authors of a 2013 retrospective review found that halo immobilization is insufficient for these ligamentous injuries.[7]

Jefferson Fractures

Fractures of the ring of C1 in children may occur through the synchondroses of C1 (**Figure 1**). Frequently, these fractures result from an MVA and are not associated with neurologic dysfunction because of the ample space available for the spinal cord at C1. These fractures are difficult to diagnose on plain radiographs and may be seen better with CT or MRI in a child who is suspected to have such a fracture based on physical examination findings or the mechanism of injury. Jefferson fractures are managed with an orthosis or a halo vest. The stability of the fracture is determined by any lateral overhang of the lateral mass of C1 on C2, which can be appreciated best with the reformatted coronal CT images. A substantial overhang greater than 5 mm on either side is indicative of a transverse atlantal ligament (TAL) injury, which may be studied best with MRI. The injuries having greater severity ultimately require proof of ligamentous stability on flexion-extension radiographs after a period of treatment in a halo vest. Early stabilization and fusion are recommended only if substantial displacement and evidence of complete ligamentous disruption are present.

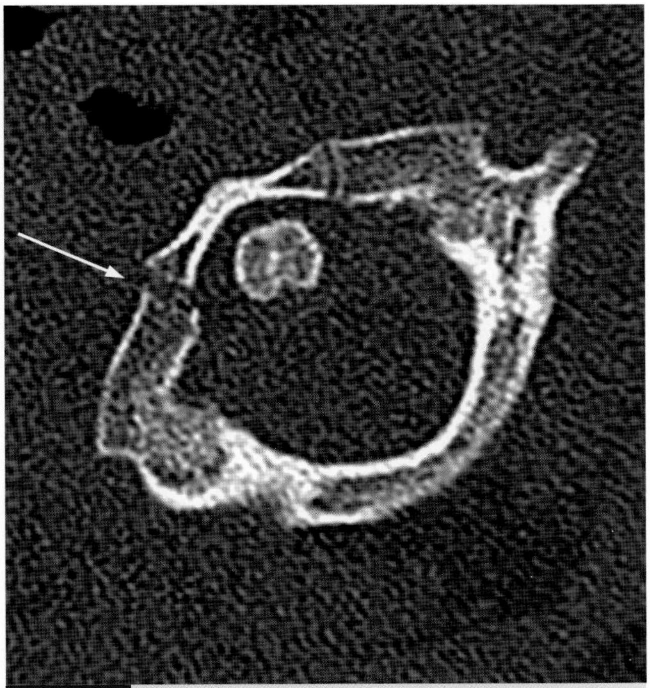

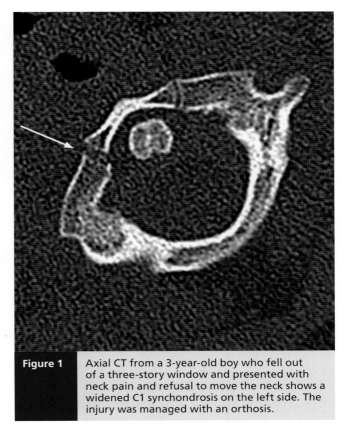

Figure 1 Axial CT from a 3-year-old boy who fell out of a three-story window and presented with neck pain and refusal to move the neck shows a widened C1 synchondrosis on the left side. The injury was managed with an orthosis.

Odontoid Fractures

Odontoid fractures are the most common pediatric cervical spine fracture and usually are seen in younger children. The fracture occurs through the dentocentral synchondrosis in children (**Figure 2**). Sudden deceleration with hyperflexion of the head, usually occurring during an MVA, is the mechanism of injury seen most commonly in these patients. Presentation usually reveals considerable apprehension and cervical pain, and radiographs demonstrate the anterior and flexed position of the dens through the dentocentral synchondrosis. CT is usually sufficient to clarify the injury, although MRI also may be used. Neurologic function is usually intact because

8: Pediatrics

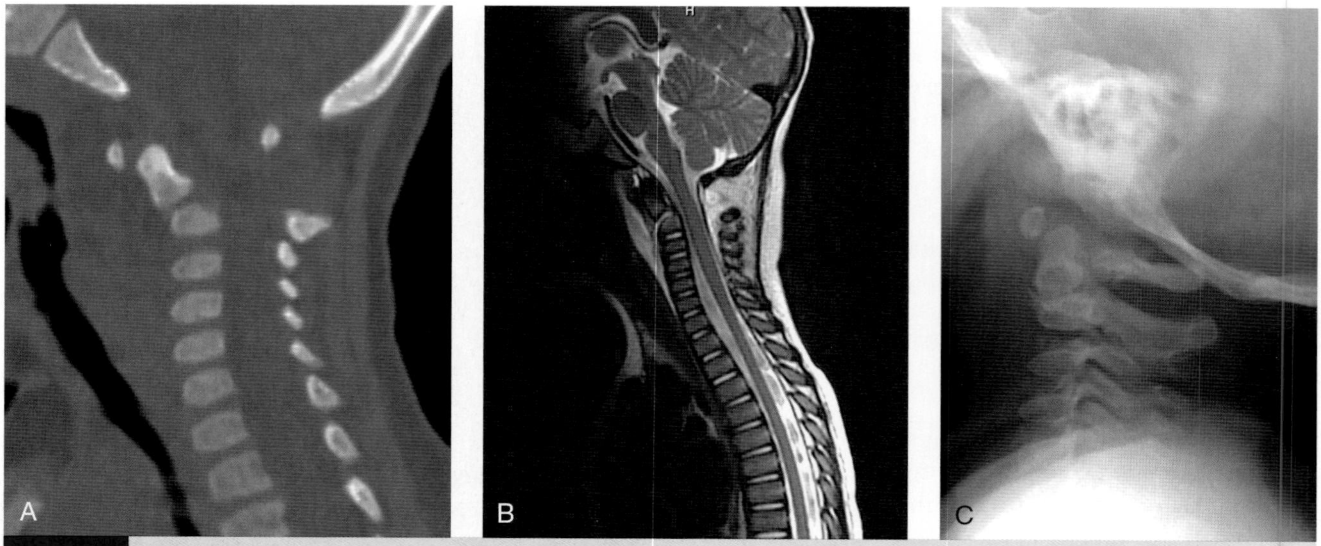

Figure 2 Images demonstrate fracture occurring through the dentocentral synchondrosis. **A**, Sagittal CT scan from a 2-year-old child who sustained an odontoid fracture through the dentocentral synchondrosis shows the flexed position at the fracture. **B**, T2-weighted MRI from the same patient shows the fracture through the synchondrosis. **C**, Lateral radiograph demonstrates the healed fracture and good alignment 3 months after the injury, which was managed with closed reduction and a halo vest for 8 weeks.

of the ample space available for the cord at that level. MRI is required to assess the spinal cord in the presence of a neurologic deficit. Management involves reduction under anesthesia, with translation and hyperextension under fluoroscopy and immobilization in a halo vest for 6 to 8 weeks.

Atlantoaxial Rotatory Subluxation or Traumatic Torticollis

C1-C2 fixed subluxation may result from infection, head positioning at surgery, such as turning the head for access to one side of the head and neck, or trauma. Patients present with neck pain and spasm, hold the head rotated to one side, and keep the chin tilted. Attempts at movement are resisted by the patient secondary to pain. Confirmation of the subluxated C1-C2 complex is obtained with CT. The Fielding and Hawkins classification is used to categorize these injuries and is related to the severity of displacement; however, treatment usually is mandated, depending on the presentation and the length of the symptoms. High-speed mechanisms such as those resulting from an MVA, with acute torticollis, deserve further work-up with MRI to rule out a traumatic C1-C2 ligamentous injury. Low-speed mechanisms need no further imaging and can be managed with a soft collar, NSAIDs, and antispasmodic agents for the first week. Patients who have no initial response after 1 week may need to be admitted and placed in halter traction or halo traction. Reduction usually is seen, with an improvement in pain and a return to a normal clinical appearance. Failure of traction to reduce the subluxation requires reduction by positioning the head in a neutral position under anesthesia with halo vest placement or surgical fusion via an instrumented C1-C2 fusion. Traumatic torticollis with ligamentous injury seen on MRI frequently requires a C1-C2 fusion. Patients may be trialed with a halo vest but ultimately need documented stability on flexion-extension radiographs.

Subaxial Cervical Injuries

Subaxial cervical spine injuries are more common in children older than 10 years and usually occur following an MVA or during sports. These injury patterns tend to resemble those in adults. Such injuries include spinous process avulsion fractures and ligamentous injuries, including facet subluxations/dislocations, facet fractures, compression fractures, and burst fractures with multicolumn involvement. Treatment depends on the injury pattern, the potential for stability, and the neurologic deficit/cord compression. Facet alignment, focal kyphosis, translation, and posterior spinous process distraction all are factors in determining injury stability. CT and MRI are paramount in the decision making. Stable injury patterns may be treated with cervical collars, whereas unstable injuries require stabilization and fusion with segmental rigid instrumentation. Ultimately, cervical stability is determined by flexion-extension radiographs in the nonacute setting.

Thoracic Compression Fractures

Compression fractures are commonly seen in children and usually are observed in the thoracic spine over two or three contiguous levels. Frequently, these fractures are related to a fall or to athletic injuries and have a shock-wave effect through the spine, hence the multilevel nature of the injury. Radiographs reveal a subtle loss of height over a few different levels, which should correspond to the region of back pain. Frequently, children have normal morphologic variations that resemble compression fractures, making it difficult to determine whether the injuries are in fact real. In patients with associated tenderness, the radiographs should be interpreted as suggestive of fracture. These injuries are self-limiting, and a thoracic hyperextension type of brace may be placed for symptoms but is not required for stability.

Burst Fractures

Burst fractures are high-energy injuries seen in older children and adolescents. The mechanisms of injury usually include vehicular trauma or high-velocity sports such as skiing or all-terrain vehicle motocross.[8] Although most patients remain neurologically intact, some present with partial or incomplete SCIs. The risk of SCI is higher in patients with thoracic burst fractures who have associated injuries to the posterior ligamentous complex, and recovery is related directly to the severity of the neurologic injury.[9] Neurologic compression also can be seen readily on the MRI. Treatment ranges from bracing with a thoracolumbosacral orthosis to surgical stabilization and is based on a variety of factors such as canal compromise, loss of vertebral height, the location of the fracture, and the neurologic status of the patient. Most surgeons believe that the absolute indications for surgery are a burst fracture in the setting of incomplete or complete neurologic injury. Focal kyphosis with a loss of height in the setting of an insufficient posterior longitudinal ligament is suggestive of the need for surgical stabilization. Nonsurgical treatment in neurologically intact patients is associated with good functional outcomes; however, care must be taken to monitor patients for worsening focal kyphosis, especially at the level of the thoracolumbar junction, where loss of alignment adversely affects the overall sagittal alignment.

Chance Fractures

Correct placement of a lap belt is dependent on the size of the child. Positioning the belt so that it is in contact with the pelvis is inherent to safety. This positioning is facilitated by placing younger children in a booster seat. Chance fractures in children result from the sudden deceleration of a vehicle, causing the momentum of the child to move forward and flex over an incorrectly applied lap belt placed at the abdominal/umbilical level. This sudden deceleration results in a flexion injury to the anterior column and a resulting distraction of the posterior column. The resulting Chance fracture may be ligamentous, bony, or mixed. Frequently, a delay in diagnosis occurs, because the association of this fracture with intra-abdominal injuries requiring laparotomy is high. Intra-abdominal injuries need to be ruled out by the trauma team in any patient with a Chance fracture. These injuries frequently occur in children younger than 10 years. The authors of a 2011 multicenter review reporteed that most cases occur in the upper lumbar spine and are associated with neurologic deficit in more than 40% of cases.[10] Chance fractures may be treated nonsurgically with hyperextension casting or bracing if the injury is purely bony in nature with no substantial kyphosis and no neurologic injury. The tendency for kyphosis to develop persuades most surgeons that surgery is needed. Patients with ligamentous injuries and those with neurologic deficits are treated best with reduction and rigid posterior instrumentation and fusion (**Figure 3**).

Ring Apophysis Injuries

In growing children, the disk attachment to the end plate is an apophysis, which may become avulsed during trauma. Frequently, this injury is observed in adolescents with a trauma sustained during athletic events. Usually, evidence of a previous apophysitis is present. Injuries usually are located at the thoracolumbar junction, and the patient may present with neurologic deficit if retropulsion into the canal has occurred. Lumbar ring apophyseal injuries frequently present as a radiculopathy. Treatment usually entails bracing if no neurologic deficit is present, followed by physical therapy. The presence of a motor deficit usually requires surgical treatment, comprising diskectomy and fusion.

Pars Fracture

Orthopaedists frequently are called on to evaluate athletic injuries to the lumbar spine in athletes. Many of these injuries are acute exacerbations of chronic repetitive injury to the pars interarticularis. Pars fractures are usually subacute and present as back pain in the lumbar spine. Most patients with spondylolysis have pain related to hyperextension mechanisms, and the diagnosis may be made via plain radiographs or MRI. A continuum of stress fractures is present, including those characterized by signal changes in the pedicle on MRI without a definitive fracture line to chronic united fractures with sclerosis and nonunion. Most pars injuries require bracing, the avoidance of hyperextension, and eventual physical

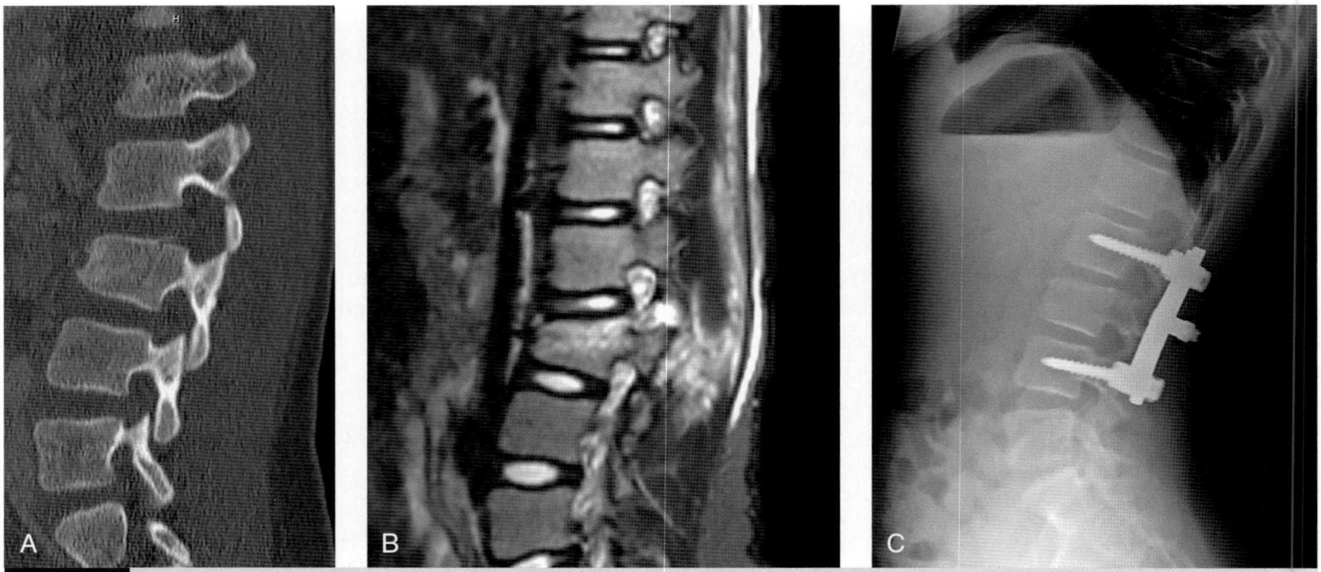

Figure 3 Images depict radiographic evidence of a Chance fracture. **A**, Sagittal CT scan from a 9-year-old patient who sustained a Chance fracture with a small bowel injury requiring emergent laparotomy demonstrates fracture through the vertebral body and the subluxated posterior facet, indicative of a highly unstable injury. **B**, T2-weighted MRI depicts the posterior ligamentous injury as revealed by the signal changes and facet disruption. **C**, Lateral radiograph obtained 4 months after reduction and posterior instrumented fusion shows the restoration of alignment.

therapy because of the association of pars fractures with tight hamstrings. In a small subset of patients, pars repair is desirable if the disk looks healthy. In the case of a chronic fracture with a desiccated disk, fusion is warranted. Treatment of a pars fracture with bracing may help the fracture heal in cases of acute bony injuries; however, with chronic injuries bracing is done for symptomatic relief only and not for fracture healing.

Summary

Successful management of pediatric spine trauma begins with recognition of potential injuries in the field and appropriate transport methods. Radiographic imaging should be done after initial physical examination and if injuries are documented, then imaging modalities such as CT and MRI are warranted. Treatment of injuries ranges from simple immobilization with an orthosis to surgical treatment of unstable fractures or fractures with neurologic deficit.

Key Study Points

- Children have unique anatomic differences from adults that predispose them to spinal injuries based on age.
- In children younger than 8 years, upper cervical spine trauma is the most common area of injury.
- Age-related anatomic variants, which are seen radiographically, exist in children and need to be understood in order to avoid misdiagnosis.

Annotated References

1. Knox JB, Schneider JE, Cage JM, Wimberly RL, Riccio AI: Spine trauma in very young children: A retrospective study of 206 patients presenting to a level 1 pediatric trauma center. *J Pediatr Orthop* 2014;34(7):698-702.

   This article is a review of 206 patients younger than 10 years with spinal fractures. Upper cervical spine injuries were more frequent in the younger children. The older children sustained more thoracic compression fractures. Nonaccidental trauma was the cause of 19% of all injuries. Level of evidence: IV.

2. Hofbauer M, Jaindl M, Höchtl LL, Ostermann RC, Kdolsky R, Aldrian S: Spine injuries in polytraumatized pediatric patients: Characteristics and experience from a Level I trauma center over two decades. *J Trauma Acute Care Surg* 2012;73(1):156-161.

This retrospective 20-year review of spinal trauma in polytraumatized children with stratification by age showed that cervical injuries occur in younger children more commonly, whereas lumbar injuries were seen only in adolescents. Level of evidence: IV.

3. Lustrin ES, Karakas SP, Ortiz AO, et al: Pediatric cervical spine: Normal anatomy, variants, and trauma. *Radiographics* 2003;23(3):539-560.

4. Gargas J, Yaszay B, Kruk P, Bastrom T, Shellington D, Khanna S: An analysis of cervical spine magnetic resonance imaging findings after normal computed tomographic imaging findings in pediatric trauma patients: Ten-year experience of a level I pediatric trauma center. *J Trauma Acute Care Surg* 2013;74(4):1102-1107.

This study looked at the use of high-resolution CT as a screening entity for pediatric cervical spine clearance. The authors suggest high-resolution CT for clearance when MRI is not readily available. Level of evidence: III.

5. Tolhurst SR, Vanderhave KL, Caird MS, et al: Cervical arterial injury after blunt trauma in children: Characterization and advanced imaging. *J Pediatr Orthop* 2013;33(1):37-42.

This retrospective study looked at the incidence of cervical vascular injuries (CVIs) associated with spinal trauma in children. Foraminal fractures, fracture-dislocations, and C1-C3 injuries are high risk for CVI. Level of evidence: IV.

6. Henry M, Scarlata K, Riesenburger RI, et al: Utility of STIR MRI in pediatric cervical spine clearance after trauma. *J Neurosurg Pediatr* 2013;12(1):30-36.

This article described a level I trauma center's experience using Short TI Inversion Recovery (STIR) MRI for cervical spine clearance in children. STIR MRI was associated with a high specificity and sensitivity for clearance in trauma patients. Level of evidence: III.

7. Astur N, Klimo P Jr, Sawyer JR, Kelly DM, Muhlbauer MS, Warner WC Jr: Traumatic atlanto-occipital dislocation in children: Evaluation, treatment, and outcomes. *J Bone Joint Surg Am* 2013;95(24):e194,(1-8).

A retrospective review of 14 pediatric patients with atlanto-occipital dislocation, this article reported that the preferred management in this series was occiput-to-cervical fusion. Level of evidence: IV.

8. Sawyer JR, Beebe M, Creek AT, Yantis M, Kelly DM, Warner WC Jr: Age-related patterns of spine injury in children involved in all-terrain vehicle accidents. *J Pediatr Orthop* 2012;32(5):435-439.

This retrospective database review of children who sustained spinal injuries using all-terrain vehicles showed that these injuries are associated with nonspine injuries and noncontiguous spine injuries. Level of evidence: IV.

9. Vander Have KL, Caird MS, Gross S, et al: Burst fractures of the thoracic and lumbar spine in children and adolescents. *J Pediatr Orthop* 2009;29(7):713-719.

The authors present a retrospective review of patients treated for burst fractures at two institutions. Thoracic burst fractures had a higher degree of neurologic injury and prognosis was related to the severity of initial neurologic injury. Level of evidence: IV.

10. Arkader A, Warner WC Jr, Tolo VT, Sponseller PD, Skaggs DL: Pediatric Chance fractures: A multicenter perspective. *J Pediatr Orthop* 2011;31(7):741-744.

This article is a multicenter review of 35 patients younger than 18 years with a Chance fracture. These fractures tend to be in the lumbar spine, frequently have associated neurologic deficit, and commonly require surgery. Level of evidence: IV.

Chapter 55

Fractures of the Lower Extremity in Children

Kevin Latz, MD

Abstract

Lower extremity fractures in children and adolescents are common, and continue to be a substantial portion of a pediatric orthopedic trauma surgeon's surgical practice. Pelvic fractures are often stable and can often be treated conservatively; however, open pelvic fractures can be associated with visceral and vascular injuries and should be managed in conjunction with a general surgeon. Femoral neck fractures are fraught with complications and require anatomic reduction and internal fixation. Femur fractures are best managed with internal fixation in all but the youngest patients. Periarticular and intra-articular fractures of the knee require management that allows early motion to avoid the development of arthrofibrosis. Most tibia fractures can be managed nonsurgically; however, fractures that occur in adolescents and open fractures may best be managed with internal or external fixation. Triplane and Tillaux fractures, termed transitional fractures, require anatomic intra-articular reduction.

Keywords: pelvic fractures femoral neck fractures; tibial spine; fractures; tibial tuberosity fractures; triplane fractures; Tillaux fractures; femur fracture; medial malleolus; tibia fractures

Introduction

Pediatric lower-extremity fractures are common injuries. Many of these fractures occur as a result of the unique properties of the growth plates of the lower extremity. These fractures can lead to major complications even when managed appropriately. Knowledge of the unique anatomy of the child and adolescent combined with awareness of the potential complications of these fractures can improve the chance of their successful treatment.

Pelvic Fractures

Pelvic fractures are relatively rare injuries in children. No single classification system is used to describe such injuries, but the Torode and Zeig classification provides a concise description of these injuries.[1] Type I pelvis fractures are avulsion fractures. Type II represent iliac wing fractures. Type III are simple ring fractures, and Type IV fractures produce an unstable segment. An even more simplified classification divides these injuries into those that involve a mature or immature pelvis or a stable or unstable injury. Standard radiographs and CT are generally sufficient for stable and unstable pelvic fractures. MRI may be useful for posterior wall acetabular fractures, which often are associated with posterior hip dislocations, as ossification of the posterior acetabulum does not occur until adolescence.[2]

Avulsion fractures can originate from the anterior superior (sartorius) or the anterior-inferior (rectus) iliac spines, the ischial tuberosity (hamstrings), or the lesser trochanter (psoas). Most of these injuries can be treated with activity modification, crutch use for a limited period of time, and a supervised return to activity. Surgical management of displaced anterior superior iliac apophyseal fractures has been advocated to return patients to sports more quickly.[3]

Fractures of the iliac wing and stable pelvic ring fractures can similarly be treated with activity modification and protected weight bearing until the patient is pain free. Unstable pelvic ring fractures can be associated with injuries to the vascular structures, the abdominal viscera, the genitourinary system, and the spine. Such fractures should be managed concomitantly with the trauma

Dr. Latz or an immediate family member serves as a board member, owner, officer, or committee member of the Pediatric Orthopaedic Society of North America.

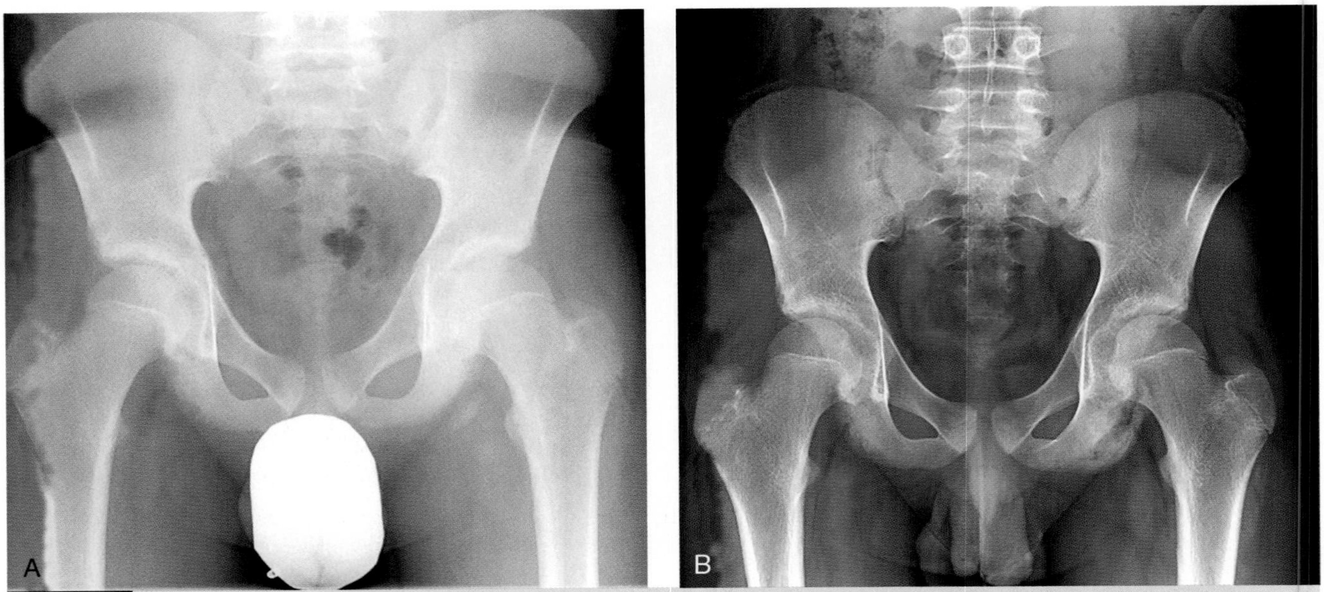

Figure 1 AP pelvis radiographs show an ischial tuberosity fracture. **A**, Fracture at presentation. **B**, Healed fracture.

surgery service and with a high degree of suspicion for additional injuries (**Figure 1**).

Proximal Femur Fractures

Femoral neck and intertrochanteric fractures are usually the result of high-energy trauma and are associated with a high incidence of complications. These injuries have been classified by Delbet. Type I fractures are transphyseal, type II are transcervical, type III are cervicotrochanteric, and type IV are intertrochanteric. Type I and II fractures are intracapsular, and type III may be intracapsular.[4] The treatment principles for displaced fractures include prompt reduction and anatomic reduction, usually with internal fixation. The risks associated with types I and II fractures include osteonecrosis, coxa vara, premature physeal arrest, and delayed union or nonunion. Osteonecrosis may be associated with the degree of the initial displacement of the fractures. Osteonecrosis is most common in Delbert type I fractures and in those fractures for which treatment is delayed longer than 24 hours. The utility of capsule decompression for the prevention of osteonecrosis is controversial. Nonunion, coxa vara, and premature physeal arrest are the most common complications associated with type I fractures.[5] For type II and III fractures, improved fracture reduction and better results, as determined by the Ratliff criteria, can be anticipated with open rather than closed reduction.[6] Fixation should cross the proximal femoral physis as necessary for stabilization of the fracture. Femoral neck stress fractures should be considered in the differential diagnosis of a pediatric patient presenting with hip pain.[7] Slipped capital femoral epiphysis is a rare complication associated with the nonunion of a femoral neck fracture[8] (**Figure 2**).

Femoral Shaft Fractures

Femoral shaft fractures are relatively common injuries in children. These fractures are often the result of considerable trauma, but can be the result of rather innocuous injuries in younger children. Nonaccidental trauma should be considered for any femur fracture that occurs in a child who is not yet ambulatory. Pathologic fractures should be considered, particularly in an older child whose injury occurred as a result of a relatively low-velocity injury.

Treatment decisions generally are based on the age of the child, the location of the fracture, the stability of the fracture, and surgeon experience or preference. Treatment options typically include closed reduction and spica cast placement, flexible or rigid intramedullary (IM) nailing, or plating. External fixation still has a limited role in femur fracture management, particularly in open fractures.

Spica casts continue to be used effectively in the management of femur fractures, particularly in younger children. Spica casts can be placed in the emergency department or in the operating room. Casts placed in the emergency department have been associated with a reduced length of hospital stay, reduced cost of the cast application, and a shorter interval between the time of presentation to the hospital and cast placement. The

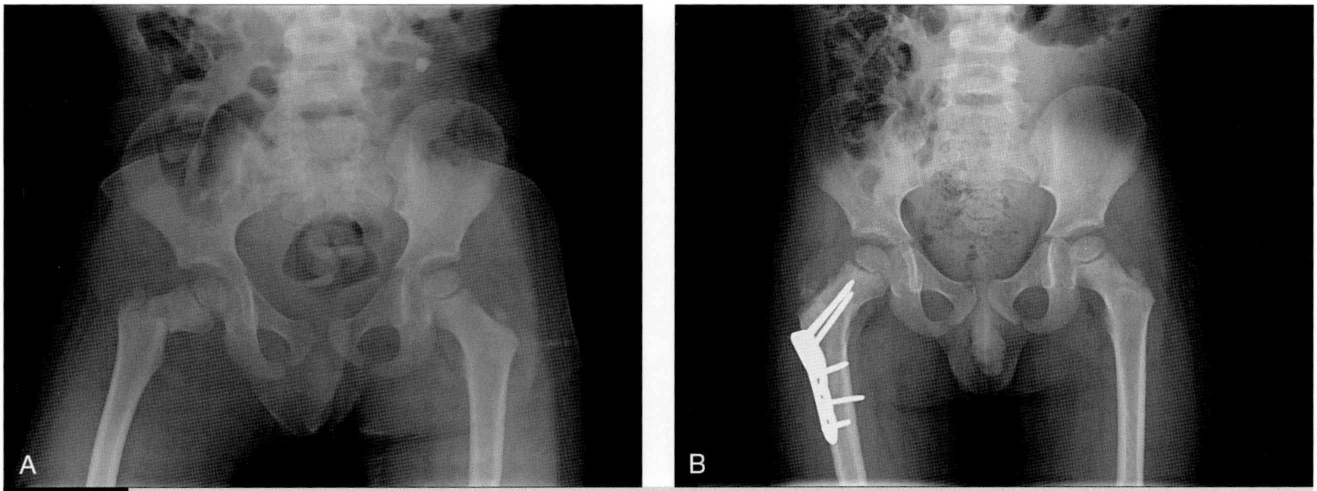

Figure 2 Preoperative (**A**) and postoperative (**B**) AP pelvis radiographs depict a Delbet type III fracture, which was managed with open reduction and internal fixation.

quality of outcomes between the two groups are similar, despite the fact that casts placed in the emergency department typically are applied by residents.[9] Spica casts have been compared with titanium IM nails for use in children younger than 6 years with an isolated femur fracture. Improved sagittal, rotational, and coronal alignment and less shortening have been noted in those fractures managed with flexible nails. The length of the hospital stay and the rate of fracture union are similar for each treatment option. A second surgery to remove the implants may be necessary for fractures treated with IM fixation.[10]

Flexible IM fixation is often used for the management of femur fractures in school-age children aged 6 to 12 years. Sagittal plane deformity is not unusual in patients treated with titanium flexible IM nails. Malunion is most common in older and heavier patients. Sagittal plane deformity (procurvatum) can be avoided by pointing at least one proximal nail tip anterior.[11] Flexible IM nails should be used with caution for a femur fracture in older heavier patients, because malalignment in this patient population is not unusual.[12] Results have been reported to be similar when using flexible titanium nails or rigid locked nails in heavier patients weighing more than 47 kg for stable femur fracture patterns.[13,14] Stainless steel and titanium flexible IM nails have been used for stable diaphyseal femur fractures with similar results, but because of the reduced cost of stainless steel nails, some advantage may be obtained in using these implants, particularly in under-resourced settings.[15] Flexible nails can be modified by adding end caps or interlocking screws. The use of locked Ender nails has been associated with less fracture shortening and fewer prominent nails when compared with unlocked Ender nails in the management of length-unstable femur fractures.[16] Similarly, flexible IM nails with end caps have been associated with increased stiffness in torsion and axial bending in an unstable distal femur fracture model when compared with flexible nails without end caps in this fracture pattern.[17] Prebending of the titanium nail to 45° or greater has a deleterious effect on the sagittal stiffness of the nail construct in a synthetic bone model with a transverse or stable femur fracture.[18]

Plates are valuable tools in the management of femur fractures, particularly in proximal, distal, or unstable femur fractures. Similar outcomes have been noted with open and submuscular plates, with the exception of increased blood loss during surgery when using open plating and increased rotational asymmetry when using submuscular plating.[19] Precontoured plates may be useful.[20] Implantation and the removal of a sliding plate that spans the distal femoral physis have been used to stabilize an unstable distal femur fracture.[21] Submuscular plates and rigid IM nails have been used to stabilize adolescent diaphyseal femur fractures, with similar outcomes. Diminished surgical time, reduced fluoroscopy use, and a rapid return to weight bearing have been noted with rigid IM implants.[22] One risk associated with using rigid IM implants in children and adolescents is the development of osteonecrosis of the femoral head. An increased incidence of osteonecrosis has been associated with the use of the piriformis fossa and to a lesser degree the tip of the greater trochanter as entry sites compared with rigid nails placed through a lateral trochanter entry site.[23]

Physeal Fractures of the Distal Femur

Physeal fractures of the distal femur can lead to considerable morbidity from partial or complete physeal arrest, which may lead to shortening of the limb, angular deformity, or both. Knee stiffness also can occur with these fractures. Salter-Harris type II fractures are the most common fractures of the distal femur. Plain radiographs may underestimate the degree of displacement with Salter-Harris type III and IV fractures; thus, these fractures may be evaluated best with CT or MRI in addition to standard radiographs. An arthrotomy and internal fixation to confirm the reduction and provide stability of these fractures may be helpful.[24] Fractures with a higher Salter-Harris classification and injuries that result from high-energy mechanisms are more likely to develop a physeal arrest. Antegrade or retrograde smooth Kirschner wires (K-wires) often are used to stabilize Salter-Harris type I or II distal femur fractures. Placing smooth, smaller 1.8-mm to 3.2-mm K-wires across the physis and removing them at 6 weeks does not appear to contribute to physeal arrest.[25] Cannulated screws in the metaphyseal fragment can be used to augment K-wire fixation of Salter-Harris type II fractures. Intraepiphyseal cannulated screws generally are used for the fixation of Salter-Harris type III and IV fractures.

Most femur fractures in children younger than 4 years occur as a result of a fall. In children aged 4 to 12 years, most fractures occur during sports, and in children older than 12 years, most occur during traffic accidents. Specific injury-prevention strategies should be targeted to each age group based on their unique fracture mechanism.[26]

As noted previously, physeal fractures of the distal femur can lead to partial or complete physeal arrest. Close clinical follow-up is prudent, including the consideration of standing radiographs at regular intervals. Alerting families that deformity can occur and enlisting them to watch for deformity may be of benefit. Physeal bar excision, epiphysiodesis, or limb lengthening may be necessary if physeal arrest results from these injuries.

Tibial Spine Eminence Fractures

These fractures are relatively uncommon injuries that occur at the base of the tibial spine. Although these injuries can occur in adults, they are more common in children and adolescents. Tibial spine fractures have been classified by Meyers and McKeever as type I, type II, and type III.[27] This classification system has been modified to include type IV.[28] Type I fractures are nondisplaced or minimally displaced. Type II fractures are displaced anteriorly with an intact posterior hinge, and type III fractures are completely displaced. Type IV fractures are comminuted. The traditional mechanism of injury for these fractures is a hyperextension injury often incurred during a bicycle accident. These injuries also can occur during sports.

Plain radiographs help determine the degree of fracture displacement. MRI can be useful in identifying meniscus tears, chondral injuries, and entrapment of the meniscus or intermeniscal ligament. MRI may be particularly useful to identify underrecognized meniscal or chondral injuries.[29] Additionally, MRI may be more accurate than open surgery in identifying injury to the meniscus.

The treatment of these fractures generally is based on the degree of displacement and the presence of any concomitant injury. Treatment can be administered closed or nonsurgically, through bracing or casting, or surgically, using open or arthroscopic techniques. The goals of surgery include obtaining reduction of the fracture while maintaining range of motion. Common complications of these fractures include arthrofibrosis and instability. Arthrofibrosis can be defined as a loss of 10° of extension, compared with the opposite knee, and/or less than 90° of knee flexion. This complication can occur in fractures treated arthroscopically or with open surgery, but it is unlikely to occur in fractures treated in a closed manner. Manipulation under anesthesia to treat arthrofibrosis without accompanying arthroscopy and lysis of the adhesions can lead to distal femur physeal fractures.[30]

Nondisplaced or minimally displaced fractures of less than 5 mm usually can be managed successfully closed. Displaced fractures usually require surgical intervention. Similar results can be achieved with open or arthroscopic techniques, as well as with screw or suture fixation of displaced fractures. As expected, a greater loss of motion and greater laxity are more likely to occur with type III and IV fractures.[31] Nonunions are more likely to occur with type III fractures treated nonsurgically.[32] Closed management of type III fractures has been associated with decreased success of reduction of the fracture and an increased rate of delayed surgery, particularly in fractures displaced more than 5 mm at presentation.[32] For suture fixation of these fractures, a similar strength of repair was obtained with absorbable No. 5 Vicryl suture (Ethicon) and nonabsorbable No. 5 FiberWire (Arthrex) suture in a cadaver model.[33]

Tibial Tubercle Fractures

Tibial tubercle fractures are relatively rare injuries that can be associated with substantial complications. These injuries occur as the result of a forceful concentric or eccentric contraction of the quadriceps and often occur

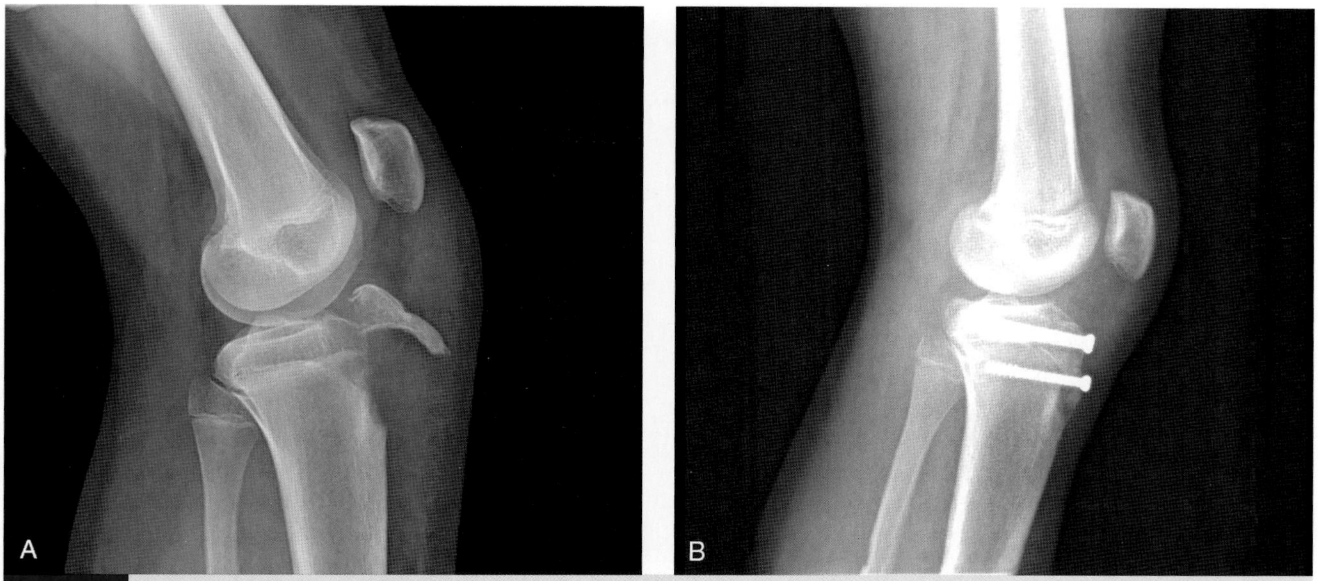

Figure 3 Preoperative (**A**) and postoperative (**B**) lateral radiographs show an Ogden type III fracture, which was managed with open reduction and epiphyseal and metaphyseal fixation.

during sports activities such as jumping in basketball or kicking in soccer. Traditionally, these injuries have been classified as Ogden types I, II, and III.[34] Type I fractures occur through the tubercle apophysis. Type II fractures occur at the apophysis-physis junction, and type III fractures extend into the joint through the epiphysis of the proximal tibia. Type IV injuries have been described as extending posteriorly through the proximal posterior tibial metaphysis and potentially extending intra-articularly.[35,36]

The proximal tibial physis generally closes at age 13 to 14 years in girls and at age 15 to 16 years in boys. The physis is uniquely vulnerable during this time of pending physeal closure. In a manner similar to the distal tibia, the proximal tibial physis closes in stages from posterior to anterior and from medial to lateral. The apophysis closes from proximal to distal. As noted previously, these fractures are major injuries and are associated with the possible development of compartment syndrome, vascular injuries, growth arrest, and loss of knee motion.

Plain radiographs traditionally have been used to identify these fractures, but CT and/or MRI may be useful in identifying the full extent of these injuries. Based on CT findings, a new classification system has been proposed that categorizes these fractures as type A, tubercle youth; type B physeal; type C intra-articular; and type D, tubercle teen.[37]

Nondisplaced or minimally displaced fractures can be treated closed. Displaced fractures require open reduction and internal fixation. Ogden type II fractures often can be managed with unicortical metaphyseal fixation. Ogden type III fractures require additional epiphyseal fixation. Type IV fractures may require bicortical screws to secure the posterior cortex.[36] Intra-articular fractures may be managed best with preoperative MRI or intraoperative arthrotomy or arthroscopy to better delineate the degree of intra-articular injury[37] (**Figure 3**).

Tibial Shaft Fractures

Tibial shaft fractures are common injuries in children. These fractures can occur as a result of minimal trauma in younger children, but are often associated with substantial trauma in older children. These fractures can be classified by their location, fracture pattern, and associated soft-tissue injury. Most low-energy injuries can be treated effectively with cast immobilization. Injuries that result from higher-energy trauma and open fractures can be treated with cast immobilization, flexible IM nails, external fixators, and plating. Older adolescents with higher-energy unstable fractures can be treated with rigid IM fixation. Surgical stabilization has been recommended for open fractures and for patients with polytrauma, specifically floating knee. Surgical stabilization should be considered for comminuted fractures, tibial fractures with an intact fibula, and fractures in adolescents.[38] For open or closed fractures that cannot be stabilized effectively with casting, surgical stabilization is often beneficial with flexible or rigid nails. As expected, open fractures take longer to heal and are associated with an increased number of surgeries for an individual fracture.[39] A Taylor Spatial Frame (Smith & Nephew) can be used for the management of unstable or open tibial fractures in children. This fixator has been found to be particularly useful in open fractures, very proximal or very distal fractures, and fractures with comminution. This frame is useful because of the ability to adjust the fixator, and thus the fracture, after external fixator placement without the need for anesthesia.[40,41]

Ankle Fractures

Ankle fractures are relatively common injuries in children. Physeal fractures of the ankle are fairly common and generally are categorized using the Salter-Harris classification. Juvenile Tillaux and triplane fractures, termed transitional fractures, are unique fractures that occur in adolescents reaching skeletal maturity.

Juvenile Tillaux fractures occur because the distal tibia physis closes in a predictable manner, first centrally, then medially, and finally, laterally. These fractures are Salter-Harris type III fractures involving the anterior lateral distal tibial epiphysis, which occur at the insertion of the anterior tibiofibular ligament. Nondisplaced or minimally displaced fractures can be managed closed and can be reduced as necessary with internal rotation of the ankle. That same rotation maneuver can be used when performing an open reduction. Fixation, when necessary, usually can be accomplished with a single screw that can cross the physis as necessary, given the near skeletal maturity of most of these patients.

Triplane fractures are tibia fractures that appear to be Salter-Harris type III fractures on the AP radiograph and Salter-Harris type II fractures on the lateral radiograph. They can be two-part, three-part, or four-part fractures. Treatment generally is based on the degree of displacement of the intra-articular portion of the fracture. As in Tillaux fractures, fixation can cross the physis as necessary to obtain reduction. Using CT in addition to plain radiographs for these transitional fractures does not always lead to a change in the measurement of fracture displacement but may increase the likelihood of surgery.[42]

Medial malleolus fractures are Salter-Harris type III or IV fractures, which have a tendency to result in physeal arrest. Displacement greater than 2 mm generally requires surgical intervention using closed or open techniques with internal fixation. Factors that may predispose these fractures to physeal arrest include an initial displacement greater than 6 mm, a lack of anatomic reduction, and a delay in treatment longer than 24 hours.[43]

Physeal fractures of the fibula are thought to be common injuries and have been considered the pediatric version of an ankle sprain. MRI studies of patients who present with an inversion injury of the ankle and who have pain at the site of the distal fibula physis have determined that few of these injuries are physeal fractures.[44]

Summary

Although many lower extremity fractures can be managed nonsurgically, restoration of function is often maximized with surgical management. Physeal fractures of the lower extremity can result in angular deformity or length inequality despite conscientious care. A thorough understanding of anatomy and awareness of the complications that can result from these fractures and their surgical management is essential to successful care of these fractures.

Key Study Points

- Many pelvic fractures are stable injuries and can be managed nonsurgically. A high index of suspicion is required for open pelvic fractures.
- A number of techniques are available for the successful management of femur fractures. Most femur fractures in all but the youngest children are best managed with internal fixation.
- Displaced tibial tubercle fractures and tibial spine fractures are effectively managed with stable internal fixation to allow early motion.
- Tibial tubercle fractures are complex injuries and benefit from axial imaging.
- Many tibial diaphyseal fractures can be effectively managed with closed reduction and casting. Open fractures and fractures in adolescents may be best managed with internal or external fixation.

Annotated References

1. Torode I, Zieg D: Pelvic fractures in children. *J Pediatr Orthop* 1985;5(1):76-84.

2. Hearty T, Swaroop VT, Gourineni P, Robinson L: Standard radiographs and computed tomographic scan underestimating pediatric acetabular fracture after traumatic hip dislocation: Report of 2 cases. *J Orthop Trauma* 2011;25(7):e68-e73.

8: Pediatrics

Posterior acetabular fractures associated with hip dislocations may be under appreciated on CT and radiographs because portions of the acetabulum are cartilaginous in pediatric patients.

3. Li X, Xu S, Lin X, Wang Q, Pan J: Results of operative treatment of avulsion fractures of the iliac crest apophysis in adolescents. *Injury* 2014;45(4):721-724.

   In a case series of surgically treated pelvic avulsion fractures in adolescents, the patients experienced a rapid return to sport.

4. Colonna PC: Fracture of the neck of the femur in children. *Am J Surg* 1929;6(6):793-797.

5. Yeranosian M, Horneff JG, Baldwin K, Hosalkar HS: Factors affecting the outcome of fractures of the femoral neck in children and adolescents: A systematic review. *Bone Joint J* 2013;95-B(1):135-142.

   This systematic review of the literature noted a higher risk of complications with Delbet type I fractures. It also observed no change in rates of osteonecrosis with capsule decompression.

6. Song KS: Displaced fracture of the femoral neck in children: Open versus closed reduction. *J Bone Joint Surg Br* 2010;92(8):1148-1151.

   This retrospective review compared outcomes from Delbet type II and III fractures with closed and open reduction. Better reduction and more good results were achieved with open reduction.

7. Er MS, Eroglu M, Altinel L: Femoral neck stress fracture in children: A case report, up-to-date review, and diagnostic algorithm. *J Pediatr Orthop B* 2014;23(2):117-121.

   There should be a high level of suspicion for femoral neck stress fractures in children with hip and groin pain.

8. Gopinathan NR, Chouhan D, Akkina N, Behera P: Case report: Bilateral femoral neck fractures in a child and a rare complication of slipped capital epiphysis after internal fixation. *Clin Orthop Relat Res* 2012;470(10):2941-2945.

   SCFE is an uncommon complication of nonunion of a femoral neck fracture.

9. Mansour AA III, Wilmoth JC, Mansour AS, Lovejoy SA, Mencio GA, Martus JE: Immediate spica casting of pediatric femoral fractures in the operating room versus the emergency department: Comparison of reduction, complications, and hospital charges. *J Pediatr Orthop* 2010;30(8):813-817.

   In this retrospective review of casts placed in the emergency department compared with casts placed in the operating room, similar quality outcomes were seen in each group. Level of evidence: III.

10. Assaghir Y: The safety of titanium elastic nailing in preschool femur fractures: A retrospective comparative study with spica cast. *J Pediatr Orthop B* 2013;22(4):289-295.

    This retrospective review of 104 femur fractures in children younger than 6 years reported improved radiographic outcomes with flexible titanium nails.

11. Sagan ML, Datta JC, Olney BW, Lansford TJ, McIff TE: Residual deformity after treatment of pediatric femur fractures with flexible titanium nails. *J Pediatr Orthop* 2010;30(7):638-643.

    This article described a retrospective review of 70 fractures treated with flexible titanium nails and a femoral fracture model treated with flexible titanium nails. Procurvatum is a common sagittal plane deformity that can be avoided by using a specific pin tip position. Level of evidence: III.

12. Baldwin K, Hsu JE, Wenger DR, Hosalkar HS: Treatment of femur fractures in school-aged children using elastic stable intramedullary nailing: A systematic review. *J Pediatr Orthop B* 2011;20(5):303-308.

    A systematic review of the use of flexible nails for management of femur fractures in children 6 to 12 years old is presented. Caution should be exercised when using flexible nails in older and heavier patients.

13. Garner MR, Bhat SB, Khujanazarov I, Flynn JM, Spiegel D: Fixation of length-stable femoral shaft fractures in heavier children: Flexible nails vs rigid locked nails. *J Pediatr Orthop* 2011;31(1):11-16.

    This retrospective review of stable femur fractures in heavier children compared rigid and flexible nails. Similar rates of malunion were observed with each implant. A shorter surgical time and less blood loss were noted with flexible nails.

14. Ramseier LE, Janicki JA, Weir S, Narayanan UG: Femoral fractures in adolescents: A comparison of four methods of fixation. *J Bone Joint Surg Am* 2010;92(5):1122-1129.

    This retrospective cohort study examined four methods of fixation for adolescents with femur fractures. Similar outcomes were observed with rigid and flexible nails and plate fixation. External fixation had the highest rate of complication. Level of evidence: III.

15. Goyal N, Aggarwal AN, Mishra P, Jain A: Randomized controlled trial comparing stabilization of fresh close femoral shaft fractures in children with titanium elastic nail system versus stainless steel elastic nail system. *Acta Orthop Belg* 2014;80(1):69-75.

    The stabilization of stainless steel and titanium nails for management of femur fractures was compared in children 6 to 12 years with similar outcomes and complications.

16. Ellis HB, Ho CA, Podeszwa DA, Wilson PL: A comparison of locked versus nonlocked Enders rods for length unstable pediatric femoral shaft fractures. *J Pediatr Orthop* 2011;31(8):825-833.

    Locked versus unlocked nails for management of length for unstable femur fractures were compared in a retrospective study of pediatric patients. Shortening of the fracture and prominence of the implant were more common in unlocked Enders nail cases.

17. Volpon JB, Perina MM, Okubo R, Maranho DA: Biomechanical performance of flexible intramedullary nails with end caps tested in distal segmental defects of pediatric femur models. *J Pediatr Orthop* 2012;32(5):461-466.

    Elastic nails with and without end caps for management of a femur fracture with bone loss were compared in a model. End caps provided increased stiffness of nails in axial loading and torsion.

18. Doser A, Helwig P, Konstantinidis L, Kuminack KF, Südkamp NP, Strohm PC: Does the extent of prebending affect the stability of femoral shaft fractures stabilized by titanium elastic nails? A biomechanical investigation on an adolescent femur model. *J Pediatr Orthop* 2011;31(8):834-838.

    This study was performed on synthetic bones with femur fractures to determine the biomechanical effects of prebending titanium flexible nails. A statistically significant decrease in sagittal plane stiffness occurred with a prebending of 60°.

19. Abbott MD, Loder RT, Anglen JO: Comparison of submuscular and open plating of pediatric femur fractures: A retrospective review. *J Pediatr Orthop* 2013;33(5):519-523.

    Open versus submuscular plating for management of pediatric femur fractures was compared. Open plating was associated with greater blood loss. Submuscular plating had an increase in asymptomatic rotational asymmetry. Level of evidence: III.

20. Eidelman M, Ghrayeb N, Katzman A, Keren Y: Submuscular plating of femoral fractures in children: The importance of anatomic plate precontouring. *J Pediatr Orthop B* 2010;19(5):424-427.

    The results of precontoured plates for management of pediatric femur fractures were good in 11 patients.

21. Lin D, Lian K, Hong J, Ding Z, Zhai W: Pediatric physeal slide-traction plate fixation for comminuted distal femur fractures in children. *J Pediatr Orthop* 2012;32(7):682-686.

    This case series outlined the use of a slide traction plate for comminuted distal femur fractures in children with good outcomes. Level of evidence: IV.

22. Park KC, Oh CW, Byun YS, et al: Intramedullary nailing versus submuscular plating in adolescent femoral fracture. *Injury* 2012;43(6):870-875.

    This prospective study compared the results of adolescent diaphyseal femur fractures treated with submuscular plates with those of fractures treated with rigid IM nails. Similar radiographic results were observed in each group, but less surgical time, fluoroscopy time, and time to weight bearing were seen in the IM group.

23. MacNeil JA, Francis A, El-Hawary R: A systematic review of rigid, locked, intramedullary nail insertion sites and avascular necrosis of the femoral head in the skeletally immature. *J Pediatr Orthop* 2011;31(4):377-380.

    This review of the literature compared the piriform fossa, the tip of the trochanter, and the lateral aspect of the trochanter as entry sites for rigid IM nails in the management of femur fractures. No reports of osteonecrosis were reported after using the lateral trochanter entry site. The highest rates of osteonecrosis were associated with the piriform fossa entry site. Level of evidence: III.

24. Lippert WC, Owens RF, Wall EJ: Salter-Harris type III fractures of the distal femur: Plain radiographs can be deceptive. *J Pediatr Orthop* 2010;30(6):598-605.

    Salter-Harris type III distal femur fractures at one hospital were studied with both plain radiographs and MRI or CT scan. Open reduction and internal fixation of these fracture types was recommended. Plain radiographs underestimated the degree of fracture displacement. Level of evidence: IV.

25. Garrett BR, Hoffman EB, Carrara H: The effect of percutaneous pin fixation in the treatment of distal femoral physeal fractures. *J Bone Joint Surg Br* 2011;93(5):689-694.

    This retrospective review of distal femoral physeal fractures focused on the development of physeal arrest. An increased risk of physeal arrest was observed in higher-energy injuries and in injuries having a higher Salter-Harris class. Placing smooth pins across the physis was not linked to the development of physeal arrest.

26. Heideken Jv, Svensson T, Blomqvist P, Haglund-Åkerlind Y, Janarv PM: Incidence and trends in femur shaft fractures in Swedish children between 1987 and 2005. *J Pediatr Orthop* 2011;31(5):512-519.

    This registry review revealed that femoral fractures results from falls, sports participation, and traffic accidents in children younger than 4 years, age 4 to 12 years, and older than 13 years, respectively. Level of evidence III.

27. Meyers MH, McKEEVER FM: Fracture of the intercondylar eminence of the tibia. *J Bone Joint Surg Am* 1959;41-A(2):209-220, discussion 220-222.

28. Zaricznyj B: Avulsion fracture of the tibial eminence: Treatment by open reduction and pinning. *J Bone Joint Surg Am* 1977;59(8):1111-1114.

29. Mitchell JJ, Sjostrom R, Mansour AA, et al: Incidence of meniscal injury and chondral pathology in anterior tibial spine fractures of children. *J Pediatr Orthop* 2015;35(2):130-135.

    In this retrospective review of 58 patients with tibial spine fractures, 29% of type II injuries had meniscal entrapment and 33% had meniscus tears. Of all type III injuries, 48% had meniscal entrapment. MRI or arthroscopy was recommended for type II and III injuries. Level of evidence: IV.

30. Vander Have KL, Ganley TJ, Kocher MS, Price CT, Herrera-Soto JA: Arthrofibrosis after surgical fixation of tibial eminence fractures in children and adolescents. *Am J Sports Med* 2010;38(2):298-301.

In this retrospective review of 32 patients with arthrofibrosis after tibial spine fractures, manipulation of the knee without arthroscopy and lysis of adhesions resulted in three femoral physeal fractures. Level of evidence: IV.

31. Gans I, Baldwin KD, Ganley TJ: Treatment and management outcomes of tibial eminence fractures in pediatric patients: A systematic review. *Am J Sports Med* 2014;42(7):1743-1750.

In this systematic review of the literature for tibial spine fractures, no difference in outcomes was observed between open and arthroscopic management or between screw and suture fixation. Greater laxity and loss of motion were seen with type III and IV fractures. Level of evidence: IV.

32. Edmonds EW, Fornari ED, Dashe J, Roocroft JH, King MM, Pennock AT: Results of displaced pediatric tibial spine fractures: A comparison between open, arthroscopic, and closed management. *J Pediatr Orthop* 2015;35(7):651-656.

This article described a retrospective review of 76 children treated with displaced tibial spine fractures. A greater risk of subsequent surgery was observed when closed management was chosen for fractures with an initial displacement greater than 6.7 mm. A similar quality of reduction was achieved using open and arthroscopic techniques. Level of evidence: III.

33. Schneppendahl J, Thelen S, Twehues S, et al: The use of biodegradable sutures for the fixation of tibial eminence fractures in children: A comparison using PDS II, Vicryl and FiberWire. *J Pediatr Orthop* 2013;33(4):409-414.

Three suture types for fixation of a tibial eminence fracture were compared in a cadaver study. Vicryl and FiberWire resulted in similar clinical results. Polydioxanone II use was not recommended.

34. Ogden JA, Tross RB, Murphy MJ: Fractures of the tibial tuberosity in adolescents. *J Bone Joint Surg Am* 1980;62(2):205-215.

35. Vyas S, Ebramzadeh E, Behrend C, Silva M, Zionts LE: Flexion-type fractures of the proximal tibial physis: A report of five cases and review of the literature. *J Pediatr Orthop B* 2010;19(6):492-496.

Five patients who sustained a flexion type fracture of the proximal tibial physis were retrospectively reviewed. This study describes the characteristics of this unusual fracture pattern, and it was determined that this fracture type can safely and effectively be managed with closed reduction.

36. Pace JL, McCulloch PC, Momoh EO, Nasreddine AY, Kocher MS: Operatively treated type IV tibial tubercle apophyseal fractures. *J Pediatr Orthop* 2013;33(8):791-796.

Twenty-four type IV or flexion type tibial tubercle fractures were retrospectively reviewed. All patients eventually were treated with open reduction and internal fixation. Three patients who underwent initial closed treatment eventually required open reduction and internal fixation. Level of evidence: IV.

37. Pandya NK, Edmonds EW, Roocroft JH, Mubarak SJ: Tibial tubercle fractures: Complications, classification, and the need for intra-articular assessment. *J Pediatr Orthop* 2012;32(8):749-759.

In this retrospective review of 41 tubercle fractures, the use of standard radiographs and Ogden classification was compared with a new classification system developed with CT or MRI. The authors found that plain radiographs underestimate the degree of injury. Open or arthroscopic evaluation is required for intra-articular fractures. Level of evidence: III.

38. Gordon JE, O'Donnell JC: Tibia fractures: What should be fixed? *J Pediatr Orthop* 2012;32(suppl 1):S52-S61.

The literature was reviewed to identify which tibia fractures benefit from surgical stabilization. Open fractures, fractures associated with ipsilateral femur fractures, comminuted fractures, fractures associated with an intact fibula and tibia fractures that occur in adolescents benefit from surgical stabilization.

39. Economedes DM, Abzug JM, Paryavi E, Herman MJ; Economedes Dm Fau: Outcomes using titanium elastic nails for open and closed pediatric tibia fractures. *Orthopedics* 2014;37(7):e619-e624.

Thirty-eight pediatric patients with open and closed tibia fractures treated with titanium elastic nails were retrospectively reviewed. Open fractures take longer to heal and are associated with more surgeries when compared with closed tibia fractures.

40. Zenios M: The use of the taylor spatial frame for the treatment of unstable tibial fractures in children. *J Orthop Trauma* 2013;27(10):563-568.

Twelve skeletally immature patients with unstable tibia fractures treated with the Taylor Spatial Frame were retrospectively reviewed. The Taylor Spatial Frame was particularly useful for very proximal or distal fractures or fractures with bone loss or comminution. Level of evidence: IV.

41. Monsell FP, Howells NR, Lawniczak D, Jeffcote B, Mitchell SR: High-energy open tibial fractures in children: Treatment with a programmable circular external fixator. *J Bone Joint Surg Br* 2012;94(7):989-993.

Ten pediatric patients with open, high-energy tibia fractures treated with a programmable circular external fixator were retrospectively reviewed. All patients achieved bony union and satisfactory wound healing.

42. Liporace FA, Yoon RS, Kubiak EN, et al: Does adding computed tomography change the diagnosis and treatment of Tillaux and triplane pediatric ankle fractures? *Orthopedics* 2012;35(2):e208-e212.

The use of CT versus plain radiographs for evaluation of Tillaux or triplane fractures was studied by six blinded orthopaedic surgeons. CT did not substantially change the interpretation of degree of displacement, but the surgeons were more likely to recommend surgical management.

43. Petratos DV, Kokkinakis M, Ballas EG, Anastasopoulos JN: Prognostic factors for premature growth plate arrest as a complication of the surgical treatment of fractures of the medial malleolus in children. *Bone Joint J* 2013;95-B(3):419-423.

This article is a retrospective review of 20 children with Salter-Harris type III or IV medial malleolar fractures who underwent open reduction and internal fixation of their fractures. An increased rate of physeal bar formation was associated with substantially displaced fractures at presentation, a delay in surgery, and a less-than-anatomic reduction of the fracture.

44. Boutis K, Narayanan UG, Dong FF, et al: Magnetic resonance imaging of clinically suspected Salter-Harris I fracture of the distal fibula. *Injury* 2010;41(8):852-856.

In a prospective cohort study involving 18 patients with suspected distal fibula physeal fractures based on clinical examination who underwent MRI of the ankle, no patient had MRI findings consistent with a physeal fracture.

Index

Page numbers with *f* indicate figures
Page numbers with *t* indicate tables

A

B

C

D

E

F

G

H

I

J

P

Q

R

U

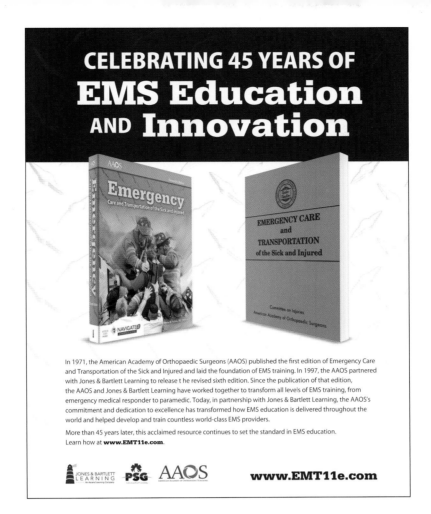

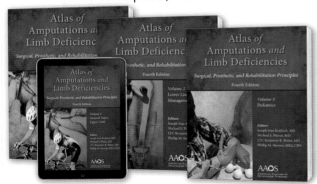

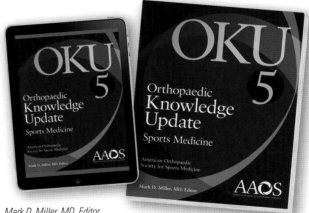